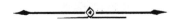

ISBN 978-0-428-95430-7
PIBN 10647148

THE

MEDICAL NEWS.

𝔄 Weekly Medical Journal.

EDITED BY

HOBART AMORY HARE, M.D.

VOLUME LVII.

JULY–DECEMBER, 1890.

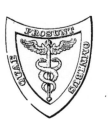

PHILADELPHIA:
LEA BROTHERS & CO.
1890.

PHILADELPHIA:
DORNAN, PRINTER,
No. 100 N. Seventh Street.

CONTRIBUTORS

TO

VOLUME FIFTY-SEVEN.

HARRISON ALLEN, M.D., of Philadelphia.
OSCAR H. ALLIS, M.D., of Philadelphia.
A. C. AMES, M.D., of Reynolds, Nebraska.
JOHN AULDE, M.D., of Philadelphia.
JOHN H. AYRES, M.D., of Accomack C. H., Va.
J. A. BACH, M.D., of Milwaukee, Wis.
J. F. BALDWIN, M.D., of Columbus, Ohio.
J. M. BALDY, M.D., of Philadelphia.
A. L. BARR, M.D., of Calamine, Ark.
SIMON BARUCH, M.D., of New York.
W. A. BATCHELOR, M.D., of Milwaukee, Wis.
WILLIAM T. BELFIELD, M.D., of Chicago.
CHARLES D. BENNETT, M.D., of Newark, N. J.
WILLIAM H. BENNETT, M.D., of Philadelphia.
JOHN S. BILLINGS, M.D., LL.D., of Washington, D. C.
J. T. BINKLEY, M.D., of Tacoma, Washington.
SETH S. BISHOP, M.D., of Chicago.
CARL E. BLACK, M.D., of Jacksonville, Ills.
R. H. BOLLING, M.D., of Philadelphia.
L. DUNCAN BULKLEY, A.M., M.D., of New York.
WILLIAM T. BULL, M.D., of New York.
CHARLES H. BURNETT, M.D., of Philadelphia.
SWAN M. BURNETT, M.D., of Washington, D. C.
HENRY T. BYFORD, M.D., of Chicago.
W. C. CAHALL, M.D., of Philadelphia.
J. M. G. CARTER, M.D., Sc.D., Ph.D., of Waukegan, Ills.
S. C. CHEW, M.D., of Baltimore.
J. E. COVEY, M.D., of Lexington, Ills.
WARRICK M. COWGILL, Ph.B., M.D., of Paducah, Ky.
B. FARQUHAR CURTIS, M.D., of New York.
CHARLES L. DANA, M.D., of New York.
J. L. DAWSON, JR., M.D., of Charleston, S. C.
H. A. DEEKENS, M.D., of Philadelphia.
LESLIE DEWEES, M.D., of Shelbyville, Mo.
THEODORE DILLER, M.D., of St. Louis.
ARCH DIXON, M.D., of Hendersonville, Ky.
GEORGE DOCK, M.D., of Galveston, Texas.
LOUIS A. DUHRING, M.D., of Philadelphia.

WILLIAM A. EDWARDS, M.D., of San Diego, Cal.
JOSEPH EICHBERG, M.D., of Cincinnati.
HUGO ENGEL, A.M., M.D., of Philadelphia.
GEORGE J. ENGELMANN, A.M., M.D., of St. Louis.
J. T. ESKRIDGE, M.D., of Denver, Colorado.
JOHN FERGUSON, M.A., M.D., L.R.C.P., of Toronto, Canada.
HENRY M. FISHER, M.D., of Philadelphia.
LAWRENCE F. FLICK, M.D., of Philadelphia.
ROBERT T. FRENCH, M.D., of Rochester, N. Y.
A. H. GARNETT, M.D., of Colorado Springs.
HENEAGE GIBBES, M.D., of Ann Arbor, Mich.
PAUL GIBIER, M.D., of New York.
VIRGIL P. GIBNEY, M.D., of New York.
WILLIAM GOODELL, M.D., of Philadelphia.
GEORGE M. GOULD, M.D., of Philadelphia.
JOHN W. S. GOULEY, M.D., of New York.
J. E. GRAHAM, M.D., of Toronto, Canada.
SCHUYLER C. GRAVES, M.D., of Grand Rapids, Michigan.
J. P. CROZER GRIFFITH, M.D., of Philadelphia.
ALLAN MCLANE HAMILTON, M.D., of New York.
SAMUEL L. HANNON, M.D., of Washington, D. C.
HOWARD FORDE HANSELL, M.D., of Philadelphia.
H. A. HARE, M.D., of Philadelphia.
T. A. HARRIS, M.D., of Parkersburg, W. Va.
C. M. HAY, M.D., of Morris Plains, N. J.
GERSHOM H. HILL, M.D., of Independence, Iowa.
BARTON COOKE HIRST, M.D., of Philadelphia.
K. HOEGH, M.D., of Minneapolis.
ORVILLE HORWITZ, B.S., M.D., of Philadelphia.
L. HUBER, M.D., of Rocky Ford, Colorado.
GEORGE F. HULBERT, M.D., of St. Louis.
EDWARD JACKSON, M.D., of Philadelphia.
W. W. JAGGARD, M.D., of Chicago.
W. W. KEEN, M.D., of Philadelphia.
JOHN H. KELLOGG, M.D., of Battle Creek, Mich.
HOWARD A. KELLY, M.D., of Baltimore.
CHARLES B. KELSEY, M.D., of New York.
FRANCIS P. KINNICUTT, M.D., of New York.
PROFESSOR ROBERT KOCH, of Berlin, Germany.

GEORGE M. KREIDER, A.B., M.D., of Springfield, Ills.
ERNEST LAPLACE, M.D., of Philadelphia.
A. H. LEVINGS, M.D., of Appleton, Wis.
J. A. LIPPINCOTT, M.D., of Pittsburgh, Pa.
SIR JOSEPH LISTER, M.D., of London, England.
JAMES HENDRIE LLOYD, M.D., of Philadelphia.
RICHARD LEA MACDONELL, B.A., M.D., of Montreal, Canada.
J. A. MACK, M.D., of Madison, Wis.
WILLIAM MACKIE, M.A., M.D., of Milwaukee, Wis.
DONALD MACLEAN, M.D., of Detroit, Mich.
THOMAS MANLEY, M.D., of New York.
EDWARD MARTIN, M.D., of Philadelphia.
WILLIAM MARTIN, M.D., of Bristol, Pa.
THOMAS E. MCARDLE, A.M., M.D., of Washington, D. C.
CHARLES MCBURNEY, M.D., of New York.
A. MCPHEDRAN, M.B., of Toronto, Canada.
ARTHUR V. MEIGS, M.D., of Philadelphia.
MIDDLETON MICHEL, M.D., of Charleston, S. C.
A. B. MILES, M.D., of New Orleans, La.
B. L. MILLIKEN, M.D., of Cleveland, Ohio.
F. H. MILLIKEN, M.D., of Philadelphia.
C. V. MOORE, M.D., of Fairmount, Ind.
E. R. MORAS, M.D., of Cedarburg, Wis.
THOMAS G. MORTON, M.D., of Philadelphia.
HAROLD N. MOYER, M.D., of Chicago.
CHARLES P. NOBLE, M.D., of Philadelphia.
FREDERICK G. NOVY, Sc.D., M.D., of Ann Arbor.
CHARLES A. OLIVER, M.D., of Philadelphia.
WILLIAM OSLER, M.D., of Baltimore.
E. R. PALMER, M.D , of Louisville, Ky.
EDWARD F. PARKER, M.D., of Charleston, S. C.
CHARLES B. PENROSE, M.D., Ph.D , of Philadelphia.
WILLIAM PEPPER, M.D., LL.D., of Philadelphia.
MILES F. PORTER, A.M., M.D., of Fort Wayne, Ind.
CHARLES A. POWERS, M D., of New York.
D. W. PRENTISS, M.D., of Washington, D. C.
JOSEPH PRICE, M.D , of Philadelphia.
B. ALEX. RANDALL, A.M., M.D., of Philadelphia.
JOSEPH RANSOHOFF, M.D., F.R.C.S., of Cincinnati, Ohio.

J. C. REEVE, M.D., of Dayton, Ohio.
ROBERT REYBURN, M.D., of Washington, D. C.
JOHN B. ROBERTS, M.D., of Philadelphia.
W. L. ROBINSON, M.D., of Danville, Va.
KARL VON RUCK, B.S., M.D., of Asheville, N. C.
L. SCHOOLER, M.D., of Des Moines, Iowa.
E. A. v. SCHWEINITZ, Ph.D., of Washington, D. C.
HENRY SEWALL, M.D., of Denver, Col.
EDWARD O. SHAKESPEARE, A.M., M.D., Ph.D., of Philadelphia.
E. L. SHURLY, M,D., of Detroit, Mich.
MANNING SIMONS, M.D., of Charleston, S. C.
WHARTON SINKLER, M.D., of Philadelphia.
A. A. SMITH, M.D., of New York.
STEPHEN SMITH, M.D., of New York.
D. A. K. STEELE, M.D., of Chicago.
ALFRED STENGEL, M.D., of Pittsburgh, Pa.
GEORGE M. STERNBERG, M.D., U. S. Army.
C. W. STROBELL, M.D., of Middletown Springs, Vermont.
E. STUVER, M.S., M.D., of Rawlins, Wyoming.
GEORGE B. TAYLOR, M.D., of Barclay, Pa.
ROBERT W. TAYLOR, M.D., of New York.
FRANK W. THOMAS, M D., of Germantown, Pa.
EDWARD PAYSON THWING, M.D., Ph.D., of Canton, China.
LOUIS MCLANE TIFFANY, M.D., of Baltimore.
ROBERT TILLEY, M.D., of Chicago.
F. TISCHER, M.D., of San Francisco, Cal.
LAWRENCE TURNBULL, M.D., Ph.G., of Philadelphia.
AP MORGAN VANCE, M.D., of Louisville, Ky.
A. VANDER VEER, M.D., of Albany, N. Y.
VICTOR C. VAUGHAN, M.D., of Ann Arbor, Mich.
MARIE B. WERNER, M.D., of Philadelphia.
H. R. WHARTON, M.D., of Philadelphia.
J. WILLIAM WHITE, M.D., of Philadelphia.
CUNNINGHAM WILSON, M.D., of Birmingham, Alabama.
JAMES C. WILSON, M.D., of Philadelphia.
U. B. O. WINGATE, M. D., of Milwaukee, Wis.
H. C. WOOD, M.D., LL.D., of Philadelphia.
HAL C WYMAN, M.S., M.D., of Detroit Mich.

THE MEDICAL NEWS.

A WEEKLY JOURNAL OF MEDICAL SCIENCE.

VOL. LVII.   SATURDAY, JULY 5, 1890.   No. 1.

ORIGINAL LECTURES.

REMARKS ON THE FREQUENCY AND CHARACTER OF THE PNEUMONIAS OF 1890.

An Address
delivered before the New York Academy of Medicine,
April 17, 1890.

BY WILLIAM PEPPER, M.D., LL.D.,
OF PHILADELPHIA.

IN attempting to give, in the few minutes at my disposal, a statement of the prevalence and peculiarities of pneumonia as it has presented itself in Philadelphia during the epidemic of influenza, I have tried to secure some reliable statistics by addressing nearly three thousand circulars to the physicians living in Philadelphia. To these I have had 272 replies, each more or less full. Dr. Benjamin Lee, the Secretary of the State Board of Health of Pennsylvania, has kindly given me the following returns, extending up to April 5th, as made to that Board, of the pandemic of influenza :

Total number of physicians giving returns	. .	187
" " adults affected	. .	19,868
" " children "	. .	8,258
Total	. . . .	28,126
Total number of nervous (as per returns)	. .	5,275
" " catarrhal "	. .	13,249
" " inflammatory "	. .	4,976
" " deaths, directly caused	.	36
" " " indirectly "	.	147
Total	. . . .	183
Immediate cause of death, bronchitis	. .	4
" " pneumonia	. .	86
" " phthisis	. .	24
" " nervous symptoms	. .	12

Through the kindness of my correspondents, to whom I desire to return my sincere thanks for their coöperation in this inquiry, I am able to submit statistics of 35,413 cases reported as above stated by 272 practitioners. From my personal knowledge of the profession in Philadelphia, I am disposed to believe that these figures do not represent a fair average, but that I have secured returns from an undue proportion of those who treated a considerable number of cases; I believe, however, that, so universally prevalent was the disease, not less than two out of every three, or, possibly, three out of every four of the eleven hundred thousand population of Philadelphia suffered from the disease in a greater or less severity. The figures which I have secured are probably sufficiently large to warrant some deductions as to the mortality of the disease, directly or indirectly, and as to the number of cases in which pneumonia appeared as a complication. The number of deaths in the 35,413 cases is given as 257, or 0.72 per cent. Of these 257, 84 are reported as directly due to influenza without pneumonia. Out of the total number

of cases of influenza, pneumonia occurred in 1485, with a mortality of 173, or 11.65 per cent. There were also reported as occurring independently of influenza, 2471 cases of pneumonia, with a mortality of 324, or 13.11 per cent. Of these, 1046 are given as croupous, with a mortality of 151, or 14.43 per cent., and 1749 as catarrhal, with a mortality of 173, or 9.89 per cent.

It will be observed that of the 28,126 cases reported to the State Board of Health by 187 physicians in various parts of Pennsylvania, there were only 86 deaths from pneumonia. No mention is made of the total number of cases of pneumonia occurring, although it is probable that under the heading "Inflammatory cases," a considerable number of pneumonias were included. The individual experience of physicians has, however, varied greatly in this respect; thus, one of the most reliable of my respondents reports 1000 cases, with only three cases of pneumonia, each case of pneumonia terminating fatally. There were 10 other fatal cases, and it may be suspected that in some of these a concealed pneumonia was the cause of death, or at least was coexistent. Another respondent, of the highest distinction as a clinical observer, reported 850 cases of influenza with but 5 pneumonias and not a single death in the entire series. It is needless to say that the experience of those largely engaged in consulting practice is wholly without value from a statistical standpoint, and the same remark must be held applicable to the returns from hospitals.

A more complete notion of the great prevalence of pneumonia during the past season may be obtained from a chart, kindly prepared for me by Dr. Frederick A. Packard from the weekly returns of the Board of Health of Philadelphia. It is seen that during the period embraced between September 7th and December 28th there were, in 1888, 428 deaths from pneumonia, and during the same period of 1889 there were 453, or about an equal number of deaths from this disease; while during the period from December 28th to March 8th the deaths from pneumonia were, in 1889, 459; and, in 1890, 810. There was also a notable, but not equal, difference in the returns of deaths from bronchitis, and it cannot be doubted that the cases of death from pneumonia in 1890 would be further increased by the fact that some such cases are included under the head of bronchitis. In addition to this, the total number of deaths returned as from influenza, without specific mention of pneumonia, is 138, and unquestionably a large proportion of pneumonias are therein concealed. Finally, it will be noticed that during the five weeks from December 28th to February 1st, the number of deaths from pneumonia were, respectively, 71, 145, 182, 131, 82, a total of 611; while during the same weeks of the previous year the figures were, respectively, 44, 50, 38, 34, 55, a total of 221. The maximum number of deaths from pneumonia in one week in the winter 1888–9 was 64—in the week ending March 8th.

In attempting to estimate the relative proportion of the croupous and catarrhal varieties, the returns made to me (and which I must regard as more reliable than the aggregate returns to the city health office) would indicate that the catarrhal were almost twice as frequent as the croupous. It is no argument against this conclusion, as would be expected, when I say that Dr. Da Costa and myself saw at least as many cases of croupous as of catarrhal, in consultation, since this might be explained by the fact that the former were the more severe and dangerous (giving a mortality of 14.43 per cent. as against 9.89 per cent.).

In passing from this merely statistical return to the peculiarities of the pneumonias of the past season, I would first note the large preponderance of cases affecting the right lung. I should be inclined to say that this side was affected at least twice as often as the left. There was also an unusual proportion of cases of apex pneumonia where the entire upper lobe was completely consolidated without implication of any other part. As usual in such cases, there seemed to be a special predominance of cerebral symptoms.

It would appear that the association with pleurisy was even more constant and marked than usual. The side pain was often intense and sudden. The pleurisies were usually plastic; in one case, coming on with pneumonia immediately after exposure during convalescence, aspiration secured a pint and a half of pus on the third day and a few ounces of sero-pus from the pericardium on the following day.

I would offer merely as a suggestion resulting from personal observation that there has been an unusual prevalence of pericarditis, both plastic and purulent, in all probability, in some cases at least, associated with and preceding influenza. Corresponding prevalence of endocarditis has not been noted.

Jaundice has been observed in Philadelphia in a considerable proportion of cases, especially in those accompanied with pneumonia of the right lung. The evidence as to the cause of jaundice is not conclusive. In the cases where careful examinations were made bile pigment was detected. In the following case (Case I.), which may be quoted in full as typical, there were hæmin crystals found in the first examination of the urine, which was made prior to the development of the jaundice, and subsequently bile pigment was detected. In the only cases where autopsies were made the bile-ducts seemed pervious, although, as is well known, a preceding catarrhal swelling may have subsided just before or after death. Jaundice was certainly a symptom of highly unfavorable omen in pneumonic cases; when it occurred merely in the catarrhal form in influenza not complicated with pneumonia it was not necessarily grave.

CASE I.—N. C., aged twenty-five, unusually vigorous and athletic, was in excellent condition when attacked by a very slight form of influenza. He was not confined to bed at all and took no medicine and did not consult a physician. He stayed in the house but went to his meals, and in four or five days announced that he felt so well that he would go out after dinner to visit a friend a few blocks distant. The night was damp and raw. After sitting and conversing about an hour he was suddenly seized with a violent pain in the right side, which grew so intense that he fell upon the floor and vomited a quantity of blackish matter. It was not said, but it is not improbable that there was blood mixed with it. The vomiting was perhaps induced by brandy and ginger which was given to him. He was taken home in a carriage and I saw him within an hour from the time of the attack, and found him with temperature over 105° and with the evidences of the congestive stage of pneumonia of the right lower lobe. He had a hypodermic of morphine to allay pain, took aconite at short intervals during the night with antipyrine and salicylate of sodium, each 5 grains. During the night pain was intense, the respirations were short and gasping and the face wore an anxious expression. The hypodermic of morphine and atropine had to be repeated. The following morning the temperature had fallen to 103° and at no time subseqently did it reach 105° till just before the fatal ending. Complete consolidation of the right lower lobe developed at the end of forty-eight hours; the cough was painful with rusty sputa; until the fourth day the temperature averaged from 102° to 103° and the pulse between 90 and 100. The stomach was irritable and retained only very small quantities of liquid. The tongue was heavily coated; the bowels were quiet. The urine was scanty, dark, and contained albumin and granular casts. He was treated with large doses of quinine by suppositories, and repeated half-grain doses of calomel until 10 grains had been taken. At the close of this time, about the fifth day, there were several loose stools of light color. The patient seemed to be doing extremely well and frequently expressed himself as improving. By this time the rapid extension of disease began and soon led to consolidation of nearly all of the upper lobe on the right side while the middle lobe remained free. On the sixth day sudden and violent pleuritic pain developed on the left side, low down, followed by rapid consolidation of the lower lobe, extending upward and producing complete consolidation of the entire lung. Deep jaundice developed on the sixth day and the urine showed the following changes:

January 12, 1890. Acid, 1031. No albumin, sugar, or casts. *Evening*—Acid, 1027. No albumin, sugar or casts. Many triple phosphate crystals.

15th. Acid, reddish color, 1024. Distinct amount of albumin. No sugar. No casts. No red blood-corpuscles. Teichmann's crystals.

16th. No hæmin crystals. Bile pigment detected by Gmelin's test.

17th. Acid. Trace of albumin. Bile pigment. No sugar. No casts. A few bile-stained leucocytes.

There were no cerebral symptoms, but a most singular persistence of a feeling of comfort, of strength and of improvement within a few hours before death; with a perfectly clear mind and a natural tone of voice he asserted that he felt well enough to sit up and walk across the room. The temperature rose progressively to 105°, the respirations steadily grew more rapid up to 50 to 60, and the pulse lost strength and grew very rapid. There was increased cyanosis. He died of heart-failure on the beginning of the eighth day. No microscopical examination of the sputa was made. The autopsy showed typical croupous consolidation of the entire left lung and, on the right side, of the entire lower lobe and of scattered patches in the apex. The middle lobe remained entirely free but was not fully expanded. The bronchial tubes were not obstructed; on both sides there were layers of plastic lymph; there was no pericarditis; no ante-mortem clots or valvular lesions. The liver was stained yellow, its tissue presented no marked change to the naked eye and the bile-ducts seemed pervious. No lesions of the gastro-intestinal canal. The blood seemed somewhat more liquid than normal.

Albumin in the urine was, I think, found in nearly all cases of pneumonia where it was carefully looked for, though not rarely there were no casts. Both hyaline and epithelial casts were found in some cases as early as the second day. It is clear that infectious nephritis was a frequent complication of influenza and especially in cases with pneumonia.

Many cases of pneumonia were associated with an unusual degree of gastro-intestinal irritability. Vomiting frequently occurred spontaneously at the onset and was readily caused by food or medicines during the course of the disease. Diarrhœa was also often easily caused. Both of these symptoms were highly unfavorable. Hæmorrhage from the bowels occurred in one case which came under my observation where there had been marked abdominal distress and fulness. A case is quoted here in full not only on this account but as illustrating peculiar physical signs and nervous symptoms.

CASE II.—Mr. X., aged forty-six, of excellent health, but probably somewhat overtaxed and depressed in vitality, having recently suffered from a very severe carbuncle, had a sharp attack of influenza. His whole family suffered at the same time. He went out and attended to business while still relaxed and with a hard, dry cough. He exposed himself on the evening of January 8th, going out in a damp, raw air and was attacked about midnight with chills, violent pains on the right side of chest, cough, and rapid development of fever. On physical examination there was found an extraordinary weakness of respiratory murmur over the right lung, especially over the two lower lobes. It was scarcely possible to hear the vesicular murmur, and crepitant râle was developed only after cough. Even on the left side there was no compensatory exaggeration of the respiratory murmur. The case developed into typical lobar pneumonia, involving the entire posterior part of the right lung and the anterior part of its lower lobe. There were a few râles at the base of the left lung, but no pneumonia developed there. The temperature never became very high (103°, maximum). The tongue was heavily coated and the stomach was very sensitive, but he was doing apparently well when there occurred sudden collapse with marked heart-failure and abdominal distress, which was explained soon after by several bloody discharges from the bowels. There had been a great deal of hebetude and mind-wandering before this, and this increased greatly after the pain extended, so that he was desperately ill until the twelfth day, after which improvement began and increased steadily until recovery. The urine showed:

January 10, 1890. Acid, 1018. Marked amount of albumin. No sugar. No casts.

11th. Acid, 1021. Marked amount of albumin. No sugar. No casts.

13th. Acid, 1018. Marked amount of albumin. No sugar. One hyaline and one epithelial cast in three slides. '

15th. Acid, 1017. Marked amount of albumin. No sugar. No casts.

The pyrexia deserved more critical study than could be given, owing to the excessive pressure of work. I would observe, in the first place, that there seemed to be a highly pyrogenic state of the system widely prevalent throughout the community during the season. I am sure that such observations as the following must be familiar to all: One of my own children, aged five, seemed somewhat dull late in the afternoon, but did not appear at all unwell otherwise. I found his temperature 104°. In the case of a child, aged twelve, whose mother is a trained clinical observer, but who merely remarked that the child seemed feverish and dull, but did not need any attention, I found the temperature 105°. The pyrexia subsided in thirty-six hours with a development of no local lesion or the evidence of a specific influenza. Naturally, therefore, hyperpyrexia would be expected in complicated cases of influenza, and very many records have been furnished supporting this view. A striking phenomenon was a very rapid rise of the temperature at the commencement of the disease; and not rarely, this initial rise continuing for the first eighteen or twenty-four hours, was followed by a distinct drop with no subsequent rise equal to the initial temperature. Temperatures of 105° and 106°, and in two cases of 107°, have been reported, the latter occurring toward the fatal close of the cases, one of whom was quite clear in his mind and the other fairly rational. On the other hand, in a few cases strikingly low temperatures were noted throughout the course of croupous pneumonia. In a case involving all of the left lung except the tip of the apex, and terminating in abscess, the initial temperature reached 102° for a brief period, but at no subsequent time was it above 101⅔° until hectic fever set in. It is proper here to call attention strongly to the fact that the vast majority of pneumonias occurred as a sequel, rather than a complication, and that they were clearly traceable to exposure to damp and raw weather while the patient had a relaxed system and while slight pyrexia persisted after the subsidence of the more marked symptoms of his influenza. Experience furnishes many instances of this fact. Both the cases above quoted are striking examples. It was not even necessary that the patient should leave the house to meet with this fate. In a marked case which I saw, a man aged thirty-five, heavily taxed with important professional work and depressed by the loss of a favorite child of three with apex pneumonia of a cerebral type, had an ordinary influenza, from which he improved so greatly by the fourth day that, in opposition to his physician's orders, he rose, dressed, and went to his library at some distance from his bed chamber. He soon had a chill, followed by temperatures of 105° and 106°, with right-sided pneumonia, rapidly developing delirium and deepening stupor, and with rapid and furious convulsions before death, which occurred on the fourth day. The practical lesson taught to all of us by this case must be embodied impressively in the records of this epidemic, and in all future cases of influenza must serve as a most important guide in the management of this disease, especially in this state of convalescence.

Allusion has already been made to the nervous and cerebral symptoms attending the influenza pneumonia of this past season. I am not aware that the cases of pneumonia which occurred unassociated with influenza presented any marked peculiarities in this respect, but, as should naturally be expected, the pneumonias which occurred during or after influenza proved otherwise. In the first place they were often associated with exceptionally severe pain about the chest and with pains in different parts of the body. There is much evidence to show that these pains might be considered partly due to general neuritis or perineuritis of varying degrees of intensity. It is not now the time to discuss the question whether this affection of nerve-trunks was of purely infectious origin or was due to atmospheric influences acting upon systems relaxed and sensitive to an almost unprecedented degree. It would seem, however, that the view of its infectious origin is strongly supported by many facts. The existence of such neural trouble has been made clear in a number of cases by muscular and sensory sequelæ. I refer to it partly in this connection because it has seemed probable to others besides myself that such a condition of the intercostal and respiratory nerves, and possibly of the pneumogastrics themselves, may be invoked to explain not only the chest pains, but the extraordinary weakness of the respiratory murmur noted in so many of our pneumonia cases. Another explanation of this striking phenomenon that has been advanced is the hypothetical enlargement of the bronchial glands. I do not know anything in direct evidence in support of this view, but merely mention as of interest in connection with the matter that Dr. John Todd, of Pottstown, Pa., reports to me that in the cases of influenza occurring in that town there was diffuse enlargement of the lymphatics, even advancing to suppuration. We had no such reports from Philadelphia.

The cerebral symptom which attended the pneumonias here were dulness, at times amounting to deep hebetude, or, in the latter stages of fatal cases, coma. In the following case (Case III.) this type of stupor was strongly marked for two days prior to the clear development of physical signs of consolidation. I am doubtful whether the case was one of influenza at all. It is more probable that it was a typical example of the ordinary infectious type of pneumonia, where, as is well known, the constitutional symptoms may precede by hours or even several days the development of the local lesions.

CASE III.—H., aged twenty-two years, an athlete in splendid condition, though overworked and exposed in a malarial district. He had felt unwell for several days but continued at business. On Friday, December 6th, he felt very tired in the evening, but put on evening clothes and went to the theatre with only a light overcoat. He had fever during the night and slept badly, but rose the following morning and went three miles to work, walking one and one-half miles. He had to go home, however, had a hard chill, and when seen that evening had a temperature of $104\frac{3}{8}°$ with evident congestion of the upper lobe of the right lung. He was stupid and heavy, but had scarcely any cough and made no complaint of pain, other than a slight soreness about the right nipple. Consolidation of the right upper lobe was not evident until December 9th. The temperature

reached 105° on the second day and for five days remained between 103° and 104°. It began to fall toward the close of the seventh day and by the morning of the eighth day had reached normal. He continued in a state of deep hebetude until the sixth day, but without delirium. Throughout the whole course of the case there were only two slight coughing spells, and only on the fifth day did he raise any sputa and then but two small portions of viscid, rusty-colored exudation. A careful microscopical examination of the blood showed no plasmodium. The entire upper lobe of the right lung and part of the back of the middle lobe were solid. When the temperature fell there was rapid resolution, with complete absorption without any expectoration. There was abundant herpes at both corners of the mouth. He took 10 grains of quinine the first day and on the second day he took 20 grains in one dose in the morning. The stomach then became irritable and he was treated with carbonate of ammonium, 5 grains every three hours, and antipyrine and sodium salicylate, 4 grains each about three times daily. On the seventh day he took five doses of 5 grains of quinine each. The rapid fall in temperature which followed on the next day was probably in large part a coincidence. Quinine was continued in decreasing doses. He made a complete and rapid recovery. The urine contained albumin but no casts. Chlorides were present on every examination.

Delirium was frequently met with and varied much in type and degree. In many cases there was continual mind wandering and delirium, and such cases were not rarely followed by emotional sensibility and weakness. Another type was of wild and maniacal delirium. This came on in some cases at an early stage, even as an initial symptom; it was sometimes persistent, and in not a few cases there was subsequent temporary dementia. Lastly, in other cases, especially in neurasthenic females or in anæmic and exhausted males, there was an excited delirium with garrulousness and even with hysteroidal phenomena. In other cases there was evident irritation, meningeal or cerebral, with wild excitement, passing into stupor with convulsions; or spinal, with stiffness and retraction of the head, muscle-soreness and hyperæsthesia.

Finally, in regard to thoracic symptoms. Cough was at times almost or entirely absent (of course, generally in cases where cerebral symptoms were present). In some instances it was almost suppressed, with no adequate cerebral symptoms to explain it. Ordinarily it was a marked symptom and often severe, paroxysmal, and painful in both croupous and catarrhal forms. I regret to say that there seem to have been in Philadelphia very few careful microscopic or culture studies of the sputa; in the cases where search was made, the pneumococcus is reported to have been found. I am unable to report any new facts in regard to the pneumonic lesions. Certainly in such cases as the first, above reported, the lesions present were to all appearance the typical ones of croupous pneumonia, and the same statement is made of other cases with and without microscopic examination.

There is nothing especial about the sputum except that in cases with little or no cough even extensive consolidation terminated in rapid absorption without expectoration (as in Case III.).

The physical signs were deeply interesting and in many cases were difficult to understand. To such an extent was this the case that I doubt not that in many examinations the diagnosis as to the extent and nature of pneumonia, or even as to the existence of pneumonia at all, was erroneous. The most evident cause of this difficulty was the excessive weakness of the respiratory murmur as above mentioned, and the poor development of all auscultatory phenomena. Further, the co-existence of bronchial catarrh, even in croupous cases, often complicated the physical signs, and not only were the breath-sounds weak in the early stages of congestion, but with complete consolidation the bronchial breathing was at times imperfectly developed.

A careful observer reports that he deliberately punctured a case of croupous pneumonia to establish a differential diagnosis because the bronchial murmur was so feeble as to justify the suspicion that there might be a considerable amount of fluid. Although in many cases of the croupous type there was typical crepitus, it was often developed only on the deep breathing following coughing. In most cases, also, the râles were coarser and heard somewhat in expiration, though chiefly in inspiration, and in cases which were clearly croupous. After the exudation was absorbed, the affected area continued in some cases for a considerable time to give impaired resonance, weak breath-sounds, and fine expansion crepitus.

CASE IV.—Mrs. W. was seen in consultation with Dr. James Collins. She was a woman in good general health when she was attacked with a slight chill, followed by fever and coughing, which soon became associated with some pain, especially in the right side. There were also pains throughout the body evidently due to influenza. The fever was of the regular type, with a maximum of $104\frac{3}{8}°$ and with daily variations of from 2° to $3\frac{1}{2}°$. At the close of the fourteenth day the temperature reached 100°, but did not remain down long as symptoms of increased pulmonary trouble in the form of catarrhal pneumonia developed, and for the next five days the fever ranged between 100° and 103°, dropping again on the seventeenth day to $99\frac{3}{8}°$. The next two days presented an even greater range of remission from $104\frac{3}{8}°$ to $99\frac{3}{8}°$, and the following day rose from 100° to $104\frac{3}{8}°$; from the eighteenth day to the twenty-eighth day the fever ranged from 103° to 105°, reaching $105\frac{1}{2}°$ once. It then gradually fell and reached 99° on the thirtieth day, and during convalescence did not again rise above 100°. From the thirteenth day to the thirtieth day the patient was so ill that her life was despaired of. Both lungs were extensively involved, but at no point was there any considerable area of dulness. The respiratory murmur was extremely feeble and in many places almost inaudible. At other points it was feebly blowing, with prolonged expiration. Percussion resonance on very light percussion gave very irregular results at different points of the pulmonary area. The cough was feeble and there was very little expectoration. It was not rusty-colored at any time. The pulse was extremely feeble and ranged from 96 to 136. The râles heard were irregularly distributed and at certain points, both anteriorly and posteriorly, there were quantities of small subcrepitant râles. The respirations were not very rapid in comparison with the temperature, the average being from 24 to 26 in a minute. The treatment consisted of nutritious enemata, small doses of morphine with quinine by suppositories, and by the mouth strychnine in large doses with aromatic spirits of ammonia. The patient made a complete recovery.

It is not designed to make any remarks in reference to treatment. The general type of the disease forbade the use of depletives or of depressing remedies. The general course of treatment which seems most useful may be inferred from the cases above reported.

ORIGINAL ARTICLES.

ON THE RADICAL CURE OF HERNIA, WITH RESULTS OF ONE HUNDRED AND THIRTY-FOUR OPERATIONS.[1]

BY WILLIAM T. BULL, M.D.,
SURGEON TO THE NEW YORK HOSPITAL; PROFESSOR OF SURGERY IN
THE COLLEGE OF PHYSICIANS AND SURGEONS, NEW YORK.

AT the meeting of last year this Association had the benefit of a thorough critical paper on the various methods of radical cure of hernia, from Dr. Mastin, who used these words in closing the discussion: "But at this date the operation which is best calculated to offer general satisfaction remains a mooted question, and until more accurate experience decides it, the selection of the special operation must still remain *sub judice*." It goes without saying, that in the solution of this problem, "accurate experience" is not the only desideratum. Observations which cover a number of years are equally important. The tendency of hernia to relapse after apparent cure was a well-established fact when mechanical treatment was the general rule of practice, and, except in the case of children, patients were encouraged after the hernia ceased to appear, to continue the use of trusses as a safeguard against relapse. In illustration of this fact Segond,[2] in his thesis on "Radical Cure," presents a table of 39 cases, collected by Berger, in which, after apparent cure by the truss, relapse was noted at periods varying from five to sixty years.

But in the commendable zeal to perfect some method of cure for this disabling conditions, operators seemed to have overlooked this tendency to relapse, and have been ready to propose one modification after another, with a confidence justified by only months of observation. Even since the experience of surgeons has shown that the majority of relapses occur within a year after radical operation,[3] there have been plenty of new methods, or justifications of older ones after a brief period of waiting.

As an illustration of this undue haste in forming conclusions, I may refer to a paper read before a

---

[1] A paper read at the meeting of the American Surgical Association, at Washington, May 14, 1890.

[2] Cure Radicale des Hernia, p. 356. Paris, G. Masson, 1883.

[3] Anderegg: Deutsche Zeitschrift für Chirurgie, 24, 207.

society in New York, during the past winter, in which the writer reported, as cured, some cases operated on within a year, by the "open method," approved by McBurney, with some personal modifications. In less than three months later, three of the patients were reported to the surgeon from the Hospital for Ruptured and Crippled, as having applied for trusses for the relapsed herniæ. I was, myself, an example of this short-sightedness when, in 1882, I reported to the Surgical Society of New York, 5 cures in 21 cases of reducible hernia, by Heaton's method of injection, the oldest having been observed for one year and nine months only. Within the next year all these cases relapsed.

The difficulty of tracing patients after their discharge from hospital or private treatment has undoubtedly much to do with the incompleteness of the evidence offered in support of different procedures. A patient, who at the end of a few months is known to have no relapse, is counted as cured; if he then disappears the record is completed, and he stands as a "cure," of equal significance with one which has been examined after a much longer period of observation. The number of such cures, the continuance of which varies greatly, is a prominent factor in estimating the value of any method. This is not the accurate and continued observation which is needed.

It will be of decided advantage in comparing methods in the future, if we discard altogether the word "cure," and estimate their relative merits by a statement, first, of the total number of operations with result as to recovery, wound-complications and healing, then by an enumeration of the cases which have been examined at later periods with the proportion of relapses.

It is in accordance with these considerations that I present the results of my own work during the past seven years. In many respects the data are not so complete as they ought to be; but this shortcoming seems unavoidable in work done, as this has been, in four different hospitals, with a constantly changing staff of internes. After the injection treatment (Heaton) proved so unsatisfactory, I took up in 1883, shortly after the publication of Leisrink's statistics,[1] the more modern methods. An examination of the methods on which Leisrink reported, satisfied me that the most essential feature of any effective procedure was that proposed by Riesel, viz., the ligature of the sac at its highest point. This has since been generally adopted. But there was some doubt in my mind as to the relative advantage of the closure of the pillars of the external ring with sutures, proposed by Czerny, or the plan adopted by Socin, of merely leaving the canal to

granulate over the sutured integuments. In the first series of cases, 40 in number, I followed this plan. After exposure of the neck of the sac, by dividing the integuments and anterior wall of the inguinal canal, the sac was isolated and ligated at its neck with catgut; the portion below was dissected out when it was small; when large, or containing the testicle, it was merely drained through the bottom of the scrotum. The wound was sutured over a drain in the inguinal canal, which was left for three or four days. This method, which may for brevity be termed the method of "ligature and excision of the sac," has been adhered to and favorably reported on by Socin,[1] of Bâle.

In a second series of cases, 39 in number, the method has been the same with the addition of catgut sutures to the pillars of the external ring and the divided aponeurosis. This may be denominated the method of "Ligature, excision, and suture." It is Czerny's method with the addition of the high ligature of the sac, as Riesel proposed, and has been extensively employed by Banks, of Liverpool,[2] who, however, used silver wire for suture.

I compared these two methods in a paper before the New York State Medical Association, in September, 1889, and found that, estimating the "cures" and relapses in accord with the plan adopted by others, the results were almost identical. Twenty patients in each series had been followed for periods varying from six months to four years; forty per cent. had relapsed, and sixty per cent. were "cured" when heard from. All of these patients had been operated on more than one year previously, but some of them could not be found at a later period than a few months after operation. I have subjected these patients to a fresh scrutiny,[3] in the past three months, with the help of Dr. Albert H. Leyton, and, as will be seen later, more time having elapsed, the percentage of so-called "cures" has suffered no diminution.

The third series embraces 39 cases, all operated on in 1889; in these the sac had been treated as before, but the anterior wall of the canal has been more respected and only divided when it was impossible to reach the neck by drawing down the sac. But the canal has been sutured with two layers of silk or catgut sutures, the deeper ones uniting the muscular fibres, the more superficial ones the aponeurosis and the pillars of the external ring. I would call this the method of "Ligature, excision and suture of canal."

The fourth series consists of sixteen operations

1 Die moderne radical-operation des unterleibsbruches. Hamburgh. Leopold Foss, 1883.

1 Revue de Chirurgie, April 10, 1888, 264.
2 British Medical journal, December 10, 1887.
3 In rearranging these cases, one case has been lost from the second series, making the number now 39 instead of 40, as before reported.

on children, between the ages of four and four-teen. Here no one method has been adhered to because the condition of the herniæ varied greatly. All operations have been performed within the past six months, but enough relapses have been noted within that time to warrant some conclusions.

The total number of cases may be advantageously considered with reference to indications, mortality, complications, and wound results. As to indications, of the 134 cases, 77 were reducible, 42 irreducible, and 15 strangulated. In nearly one-half, then, the radical cure was added to the operation for the relief of irreducibility or strangulation. This is in accordance with the general belief, I think, that it should be done in such cases with few exceptions. In irreducible herniæ I would except only scrotal enteroceles of long standing and voluminous contents, where the adhesions between loops of intestine are firm, and the return of the long-protruded mass is sure to be a matter of difficulty. It necessitates a prolonged operation with much bleeding and many raw surfaces, and the aperture is sure to be large and little likely to be closed long by any method of suture. In general, I believe that irreducible cases are best treated by operation ; they do not bear the pressure of any truss with comfort, and are constantly liable to have fresh contents descend into the sac. It must be remembered, however, that many small irreducible ruptures, both inguinal and femoral, of a few days' duration, will undergo spontaneous reduction by rest in bed, or even while on the feet, with the pressure of a spica bandage.

In strangulated hernia, when the gut is not returned, the radical cure must naturally be omitted. When patients are too feeble to warrant any prolongation of the operation, it is undesirable.

Of the reducible cases, the majority have presented difficulties in the management of a truss, or, in a few instances, have been anxious to try the radical cure as a means of dispensing with it, or of being able to wear one with lighter pressure. There have been more of these cases in the third series, as shown by the following table :

Series.	Reducible.		Irreducible and Strangulated.
I. contains	11	and	29
II. "	21	"	18
III. "	29	"	92

All the cases in Table IV. have been reducible.

At the outset of my experience, I was disposed to operate without regard to age. The first series shows in regard to age :

2 patients under 20
6 patients from 20 to 30
10 "   "   30 " 40
8 "   "   40 " 50
9 "   "   50 " 60
5 "   over 60

Of these 40 patients, the earliest operated on, 14 were over 50. In the second series there were but 5 over 50, as I had begun to think it undesirable to attempt the radical cure at this age, unless in connection with irreducible or strangulated cases. The ages in Series II. are :

2 patients under 20.
12 patients from 20 to 30.
7   "   "   30 " 40.
11 "   "   40 " 50.
4   "   "   50 " 60.
1 patient over 60.
2 patients not given.

In the third series of cases, the ages are about the same as in the second. The fourth series of patients were all between the ages of 4 and 14. The indication for operation was either difficulty of retaining the rupture with a truss, or absence of any improvement in its condition as the child continued under observation. In one or two instances, inability of the parents to adjust the truss, or inattention or irregular attendance constituted impediments to the mechanical treatment. In one instance, an adherent appendix, in another a thin slip of adherent omentum, in a third a testicle arrested in the canal explained the difficulty of retention.

There are three deaths in the entire number of 134 cases, two in the first series and one in the second. The third and fourth lists represent 55 cases in succession with no fatal result. The first death was (Case 5, Table I.) a man of eighty, in apparently good health, who was subjected at the same time to the radical operation for hydrocele (Volkmann's) on the opposite side. The hernia was a large, scrotal entero-epiplocele, and a portion of omentum was excised after ligating. Death resulted in twenty-four hours from the shock of slight hæmorrhage into the peritoneal cavity from an atheromatous artery in the omentum, which had been cut by the ligature. The second fatal result was in a healthy patient (Case 26, Table II.), twenty-six years of age, whom I advised to undergo the radical operation for an irreducible epiplocele ; a large bunch of omentum was removed after ligating with great care, the attention of those present being called to the advantage of using heavy silk for this purpose. Bleeding occurred after the stump was replaced in the cavity ; a large incision was necessary in order to withdraw the omentum and re-ligate the vessels. The ligature had slipped. The cavity was cleansed of blood and no further oozing took place, but death resulted from septic peritonitis in twenty-four hours. The third death (Case 15, Table II.) was from shock in a large, scrotal strangulated case of twenty-four hours' duration.

These fatal results are worthy of notice in so far as they serve to emphasize my conviction that old and feeble subjects should not be subjected to operation in reducible cases, and that too much attention cannot be given to management of the omentum. In cases of strangulated hernia the radical measures should be omitted, if patients are not in condition to endure safely prolongation of the operation.

The complications existing at the time of operation were a large uterine fibroid in one case, hydrocele of the tunica vaginalis in three cases. The latter condition was managed simultaneously by simple drainage with good results.

In the course of the operation there was bleeding from a faulty ligature in one case (ending fatally, as just mentioned), wound of the intestine in four instances, and division of the vas deferens in one case. The intestinal wounds were all made in separating adhesions; all were promptly sutured and no accident resulted. In one case there were five tears made in separating intestine from the wall of a suppurating sac (an irreducible case, 34, Table I.). The wounded vas deferens was not sutured; suppurative orchitis followed, with burrowing of pus in the abdominal wall. The patient was a healthy farmer, forty-seven years of age, and was eighty-five days under treatment. There were no accidents or complications among the children.

Following the operation, the general complications to be noted are acute mania in a woman sixty-eight years of age, who could not be traced after removal from hospital (Case 4, Table I.), and erysipelas in one case, which developed from a slowly healing sinus. Septic fever has been so exceptional as to be hardly worth noting, though the wounds have healed primarily in only about one-half the cases, as the following table shows:

Series.	Prim. union.	Suppur.	Died.	Not stated.
I.	16	21	2	1
II.	21	16	1	1
III.	12	14	0	13
	49	51		

IV. All wounds healed primarily but one; this was in an unruly boy of defective intellect who tore off his dressings.

By primary union is meant the occurrence of prompt healing of the wound which, with the exception of the drainage-tube opening, has closed within a few days with but a few drops of pus. Many of the cases noted as healing by suppuration were simply slow-healing drainage openings. Profuse suppuration has been rarely noted. Of the adult cases the duration of treatment on the average was 26½ days, the shortest being 10, and the longest 85 days. Bichloride irrigation and moist dressings have been uniformly employed; drains were of rubber (a few of glass); catgut was prepared according to Kocher's formula with oil of juniper.

My practice has been to make the first dressing at the end of two or three days for the purpose of re-

moving the tubes, and to permit the second dressings to lie in place a week, if no complication occurred. Silk was used for buried sutures in about a dozen cases, boiled in five per cent. carbolic acid solution immediately before and sometimes during the operation; yet in spite of these precautions, all the cases heard from had small abscesses after leaving hospital and discharged one or more sutures.

Of the varieties of hernia, there were 116 inguinal, 15 femoral, and 3 ventral. In the different series there are reported as follows:

		Series I.	Series II.	Series III.	Series IV.
Inguinal.	26	9 reducible. / 13 irred. / 4 strang.	36 { 22 reducible. / 11 irred. / 3 strang.	38 { 28 reducible. / 6 irred. / 4 strang.	16 reducible.
Femoral.	12	1 red. / 7 irred. / 4 strang.	2 irred.		
Ventral.		2 reducible.	1 irreducible.		

The subsequent observation of these patients gives the following results as to relapse:

Of the 40 cases operated on in the first series, by the method of ligature and excision of the sac, only 22 have been traced:

	Total Number.	No Relapse.	Relapse.
Cases under obs over 5 years	1	1	0
" " " from 4 to 5 years	3	3	0
" " " 3 " 4 "	2	1	1
" " " " 2 " 3 "	0	0	0
" " " " 1 " 2 "	9	8	1
" " " less than 1 year	7	1	6
	22	14.	8

Of the 39 cases operated on by the method of ligature, excision and suture of the external ring, but 20 have been traced, with this result:

		No Relapse.	Relapse.
Under obs. from 3 to 4 years	1	0	1
" " " 2 " 3 "	4	3	1
" " " 1 " 2 "	10	8	2
" " less than 1 year	5	1	4
	20	12	8

Of the 39 cases operated on by the method of ligature, excision and suture of the canal and external ring, 20 have been followed for less than one year with the result that 11 have recurred.

Of the 16 children, all operated on within a year, 5 have already presented relapses—at the end of one month in 2 cases, two months in 1 case, three months in 1 case, and four months in 1 case. In 6 patients, the sac was cut across just below its neck, the remainder drained and the canal sutured. But 1 of these herniæ has reappeared as yet. In the 10 others, all small, the sac was not found, and the pillars of the external ring were sutured; 4 of these have relapsed.

In comparing these methods, without reference to the time of observation, we find that:

By method I., ligature and exision of sac, there are 36.36 per cent. of relapses in 22 cases.

TABLE I.—CASES OPERATED ON BY LIGATURE AND EXCISION OF THE SAC (SOCIN).

No.	Sex.	Age.	Variety and duration.	Date. Complication.	Result.	Duration of treatment.	Last observation.
1	M.	30	Inguinal.	April 8, 1883; omentum removed.	Recovered	30 days.	
2	M.	32	Strangulated inguinal, few hours. Hernia 12 years.	August 13.	Recovered	10 days; primary union.	July, 1889. No relapse. Truss.
3	F.	55	Irreducible inguinal, 3 years.	March 3, 1884; omentum removed.	Recovered	53 days.	
4	F.	58	Strangulated inguinal, 2 days. Hernia 30 years.	May 25; insanity developed.	Recovered	12 days; primary union.	
5	M.	80	Double inguinal, right, 25 years; left, 3 years. Left hydrocele radical cure at same time.	July 7; omentum removed. Hæmorrhage into peritoneal cavity.	Died		
6	M.	40	Inguinal. Small.	September 11.	Recovered	15 days; primary union.	
7	M.	5	Irreducible inguinal, 4 mos. Small.	October 27; omentum and appendix removed.	Recovered	12 days; primary union.	February, 1886. Died. No relapse at time of death.
8	M.	46	Inguinal, 14 years. Herniotomy 4 years previous. Hernia returned in 2 days. Large.	November 6; omentum removed.	Recovered	18 days; primary union.	May, 1889. Relapsed three and a half years later.
9	F.	48	Irreducible femoral, 3 years. Small.	December 9; omentum removed.	Recovered	37 days.	July, 1886. No relapse. No truss.
10	F.	11	Irreducible femoral, 8 months.	December 10; omentum removed.	Recovered	42 days.	
11	M.	55	Inguinal, 8 years. Large.	January 21, 1885.	Recovered	57 days.	
12	M.	61	Strangulated femoral, 8 days. Hernia 10 years.	January 23.	Recovered	31 days.	August, 1886. Relapsed. Truss.
13	F.	38	Strangulated femoral. Hernia 3 years.	January 29.	Recovered	21 days.	July, 1886. Relapsed soon afterward. Truss.
14	M.	93	Strangulated inguinal, 12 hrs. Hernia 5 years. Radical cure 1 year ago. No relapse until 12 hours previously.	February 15.	Recovered	46 days.	January, 1886. No relapse. No truss.
15	M.	35	Irreducible inguinal, 15 years.	March 9; omentum removed.	Recovered	20 days; primary union.	
16	F.	43	Irreducible femoral, 5 years.	June 29; omentum removed.	Recovered	32 days.	July, 1886. No relapse. Truss for nine months.
17	M.	18	Irreducible inguinal, life time Small.	June 30; omentum removed.	Recovered	34 days.	
18	F.	49	Irreducible inguinal, 6 years. Small. Fibroid of uterus.	July 27.	Recovered	39 days.	
19	M.	31	Irreducible inguinal, 5 years. Very large.	August 4; omentum removed.	Recovered	55 days.	January, 1890. No relapse. Truss.
20	M.	39	Irreducible inguinal, 15 years. Large. Strangulation reduced by taxis.	August 13.	Recovered	39 days.	
21	M.	28	Inguinal, 3 years.	August 25; omentum removed.	Recovered	13 days; primary union.	January, 1890. No relapse. Truss for two years.
22	F.	29	Femoral, 2 months. Small.	September 18.	Recovered	12 days; primary union.	January, 1890. No relapse. No truss.
23	M.	23	Inguinal. Small.	November 17; omentum removed.	Recovered		
24	F.	61	Irreducible femoral.	January 16, 1886; omentum removed.	Recovered	Primary union.	
25	F.	60	Strangulated femoral, 3 days. Hernia 3 years.	June 16; omentum removed.	Recovered	12 days; primary union.	
26	M.	36	Irreducible inguinal, 5 years.	August 3; omentum removed. Hæmorrhage from stump into peritoneal cavity. Stump drawn out; vessel tied.	Died	....	Autopsy. Septic peritonitis.
27	M.	71	Strangulated inguinal, 12 hrs. Hernia 12 years.	September 5; omentum removed.	Recovered	31 days.	January, 1890. No relapse. No truss.
28	M.	29	Irreducible ventral, 5 years. Small.	March 16, 1887; omentum removed.	Recovered	16 days; primary union.	
29	M.	20	Inguinal, 8 months. Small.	May 11; omentum removed.	Recovered	42 days; primary union	
30	M.	46	Ventral, 12 years. Small.	July 14; omentum removed.	Recovered	38 days.	January, 1889. No relapse.
31	M.	59	Irreducible inguinal, 20 years	September 2.	Recovered	25 days; primary union.	Relapsed in one month.
32	M.	35	Inguinal, 16 years.	May 15, 1888, omentum removed.	Recovered	51 days.	January, 1890. No relapse. No truss.
33	M.	20	Irreducible inguinal, 5 years.	May 19; omentum removed.	Recovered	24 days.	January, 1890. No relapse. Truss. Hernia on opposite side.
34	M.	47	Irreducible inguinal, 4 years. Hydrocele.	June 5; abscess of omentum and sac; intestines wounded. Drainage of abdominal cavity.	Recovered	38 days.	October, 1888. Relapsed. No truss.
35	F.	37	Strangulated femoral, 24 hrs. Hernia 6 years.	July 14; omentum removed.	Recovered	13 days; primary union.	January, 1890. No relapse. Truss.
36	M.	55	Irreducible inguinal, 4 years. Small	July 18; omentum removed	Recovered	85 days.	January, 1890. Relapse.
37	F.	76	Irreducible femoral, 13 years. Small.	July 26.	Recovered	18 days.	January, 1889. Relapsed. No truss.
38	M.	51	Irreducible inguinal, 35 years.	September 3; omentum and appendix removed.	Recovered	28 days.	August, 1889. Relapsed.
39	F.	60	Irreducible femoral, 4 years.	September 15; omentum removed.	Recovered	17 days; primary union.	
40	F.	49	Irreducible femoral, 6 months. Small.	December 7; omentum removed.	Recovered	11 days; primary union.	January, 1890. No relapse.

TABLE II.—CASES OPERATED ON BY LIGATURE AND EXCISION OF SAC, WITH SUTURE OF EXTERNAL RING (BANKS).

No.	Sex.	Age.	Variety and duration.	Date. Complications.	Result.	Duration of treatment.	Last observation.
1	M.	14	Inguinal. Small.	June 1, 1885; omentum removed.	Recovered	19 days; primary union.	July, 1886, Relapsed. Truss.
2	M.	45	Inguinal, 3 years. Small.	July 9.	Recovered	15 days.	
3	M.	...	Inguinal, 1 year. Small.	July 24.	Recovered		
4	F.	40	Irreducible femoral, 2 years. Small.	November 23; omentum removed, and stump sutured in ring.	Recovered	39 days.	
5	.	36	Inguinal, 8 years.	December 23.	Recovered		
6	.	46	Inguinal, 3 years. Small.	February 25, 1886.	Recovered	27 days; primary union.	August, 1889. Relapsed.
7	.	63	Irreducible inguinal, 10 years.	March 11; omentum removed.	Recovered	42 days; primary union.	February, 1888. No relapse.
8	.	43	Irreducible inguinal, 11 years.	July 31.	Recovered	36 days.	
9	.	45	Inguinal, 34 years.	August 6.	Recovered	25 days.	
10	.	31	Incarcerated inguinal, 3 yrs.	August 17.	Recovered	34 days.	
11	.	23	Inguinal.	September 17; no sac found.	Recovered	36 days.	October, 1887. Relapsed.
12	.	...	Inguinal, 25 years.	September 25; omentum removed.	Recovered	49 days; primary union.	July, 1889. Relapsed.
13	.	...	Inguinal, 2 months. Small.	February 26, 1887.	Recovered	16 days; primary union.	
14	.	25	Irreducible inguinal. Small.	June 11.	Recovered	21 days.	July, 1889. No relapse. No truss.
15	M.	59	Strangulated inguinal, 1 day. Hernia 2 years. Large hydrocele.	July 17: gut congested.	Died.	....	Death from shock
16	M.	25	Strangulated inguinal, 2 days.	July 26.	Recovered	14 days; primary union.	February, 1889. Relapse 8 months later.
17	.	50	Inguinal, 26 years.	August 1.	Recovered	25 days; primary union.	
18	M.	22	Strangulated inguinal, 3 days. Hernia 14 years. Small.	August 2; omentum removed.	Recovered	32 days.	January, 1889. No relapse. No truss.
19	.	41	Irreducible inguinal, 15 years. Small.	September 5; omentum removed.	Recovered	19 days; primary union.	January, 1890. No relapse. Truss.
20	.	22	Inguinal, 4 years Small.	October 4.	Recovered	37 days.	
21	.	48	Inguinal, 17 years. Small.	October 4.	Recovered	11 days; primary union	December, 1888. Relapsed in six months.
22	M.	35	Inguinal, 20 years. Operation two years previously. Relapse in two days.	December 15; omentum removed.	Recovered	39 days.	July, 1888. Relapse. See Table III., No. 17.
23	M.	25	Inguinal, 19 years. Small.	January 12, 1888.	Recovered	22 days; primary union.	January, 1890. No relapse. Truss.
24	M.	43	Inguinal, 6 weeks.	January 12.	Recovered	36 days.	August, 1889. No relapse.
25	M.	28	Inguinal, 7 years.	May 3.	Recovered	27 days; primary union.	
26	M.	19	Irreducible inguinal, 18 mos.	June 19; omentum removed	Recovered	18 days; primary union.	January, 1890. No relapse. Truss.
27	M.	26	Irreducible inguinal, 2½ yrs.	June 23; omentum removed.	Recovered	18 days; primary union.	January, 1890. No relapse. No truss.
28	M.	45	Inguinal, 10 years. Large.	June 25.	Recovered	24 days; primary union.	
29	M.	24	Irreducible inguinal, 2 years.	July 16; omentum removed	Recovered	28 days.	
30	M.	23	Irreducible inguinal, 8 years.	August 4; omentum removed.	Recovered	16 days; primary union.	January, 1890. No relapse. No truss.
31	M.	55	Irreducible Ventral, 4 years. Small.	August 27; omentum removed.	Recovered	10 days; primary union.	January, 1889. Relapsed.
32	M.	38	Inguinal, 7½ years. Large.	September 1.	Recovered	41 days.	January, 1889. No relapse. Truss.
33	F.	20	Inguinal, 18 months. Small.	December 13.	Recovered	10 days; primary union.	
34	M.	36	Inguinal (left), 10 years.	December 20.	Recovered	25 days.	
35	.	...	Inguinal (right), 1 year.	December 20.	Recovered	25 days; primary union.	
36	M.	46	Inguinal (right), 6 months.	December 20.	Recovered	12 days.	January, 1890. No relapse.
37	M.	30	Irreducible inguinal, 2 years. Hydrocele.	December 24.	Recovered	15 days.	
38	M.	59	Irreducible inguinal, 39 years.	December 27.	Recovered	30 days.	
39	F.	31	Irreducible femoral, 8 years.	January 2, 1889.	Recovered	15 days; primary union.	January, 1890. No relapse. No truss.

By method II., ligature and excision of sac, and suture of external ring, there are 40 per cent. of relapses in 20 cases.

This is a very trifling difference, and seems to my mind to prove that there is little choice between the two procedures. The first method has been the longer on trial by two years. It is simpler and more rapidly executed.

But the results of the first two methods are about the same, when the period of observation is taken into account. Of the cases under observation for less than a year, six out of seven relapsed in the first,

TABLE III.—CASES OPERATED ON BY LIGATURE, EXCISION, AND SUTURE OF CANAL (SILK OR CATGUT).

No.	Sex.	Age.	Variety and duration.	Date. Complication.	Result.	Duration of treatment.	Last observation.	Truss.
1	M.	21	Inguinal, 17 years.	January 3, 1889.	Recovered	35 days.		
2	M.	46	Inguinal, 1 year.	January 19.	Recovered	20 days.		
3	M.	15	Irreducible inguinal, 5 months. Small hydrocele	Omentum removed.	Recovered	14 days.		
4	M.	26	Inguinal, 6 months.	February 12.	Recovered	10 days ; primary union.		
5	M.	37	Inguinal, 2 years.	February 12.	Recovered	20 days ; primary union.		
6	M.	35	Inguinal (right), 19 years.	February 15.	Recovered	10 days ; primary union.	January, 1890.	No relapse. Truss.
7	...	...	Inguinal (left), 2 years.	February 15.	Recovered	Primary union.		
8	M.	18	Inguinal (left), 15 years. Cured by truss in 7 months.	February 23.	Recovered	16 days.		
9	...	...	Inguinal (right), 3 months.	February 23.	Recovered	Primary union.		
10	M.	55	Inguinal, 18 months.	March 6.	Recovered	14 days ; primary union.	January, 1890.	No relapse.
11	M.	25	Inguinal, 4 weeks.	March 16.	Recovered	12 days ; primary union.		
12	F.	34	Irreducible inguinal, 7 years.	March 16.	Recovered	14 days ; primary union.	January, 1890.	Relapsed in one month.
13	M.	35	Inguinal, 5 years.	March 23.	Recovered	14 days.		
14	M.	21	Inguinal, 3 years.	April 6.	Recovered	20 days.	January, 1890.	Relapsed.
15	M.	18	Inguinal, 4 years.	April 15.	Recovered	12 days ; primary union.	January, 1890.	Relapsed.
16	M.	35	Inguinal, 21 years.	March 9.	Recovered	11 days.	January, 1890. Relapsed. See Table II., No. 22.	
17	M.	42	Inguinal, 11 years.	March 1.	Recovered	34 days.		
18	M.	18	Inguinal, 3 years.	April 11.	Recovered	25 days.		
19	M.	40	Inguinal.	April 11.	Recovered	28 days.		
20	M.	29	Strangulated Inguinal.	April 22.	Recovered	57 days.	January, 1890.	Relapsed.
21	M.	57	Inguinal, 8 years.	May 10.	Recovered	40 days.	January, 1890.	No relapse.
22	M	37	Irreducible inguinal, 10½ yrs.	May 15.	Recovered	42 days.	January, 1890.	No relapse. Truss.
23	M.	28	Strangulated inguinal. Hernia 23 years.	May 29. (Gut nicked.)	Recovered	28 days ; primary union.		
24	M.	19	Inguinal, lifetime.	June 1.	Recovered	41 days.	January, 1890.	No relapse. Truss.
25	M.	43	Strangulated inguinal. Hernia 4 years.	May 30. (Gut nicked twice.)	Recovered	30 days ; primary union.		
26	M.	25	Inguinal, 5 years.	May 4. Wound of vas deferens ; erysipelas.	Recovered	138 days ; suppuration ; abscess of testicle ; cellulitis of abdomen.	January 1890. No relapse. No truss.	
27	M.	26	Inguinal, 6 years.	August 31.	Recovered	13 days ; primary union.	January, 1890. No relapse. Truss.	
28	F.	17	Inguinal, 2 years.	August 31.	Recovered	21 days ; primary union.	February, 1890. No relapse. Truss.	
29	M.	31	Inguinal, 1½ years.	September 11.	Recovered	15 days ; primary union.	January, 1890. No relapse. Truss.	
30	F.	40	Incarcerated inguinal, 5 yrs.	September 11. Gut wounded four times.	Recovered	20 days ; primary union.	January, 1890. Relapsed. Truss.	
31	M.	35	Irreducible inguinal, 2 years.	September 9. Double hydrocele.	Recovered	29 days.		
32	M.	33	Inguinal. Operation for strangulation July 11, 1888. Relapsed Sept. 12, 1889.	September 14.	Recovered	29 days.		
33	M.	33	Inguinal, 9 years.	September 14.	Recovered	23 days ; primary union.		
34	M.	19	Inguinal, 3 months.	September 18.	Recovered	13 days ; primary union.	January, 1890. Relapsed in canal. Truss.	
35	M.	65	Strangulated inguinal, 2 days. Hernia 20 years.	September 17.	Recovered	29 days ; primary union.	January, 1890. Relapsed. Truss.	
36	M.	42	Irreducible inguinal, 5 days. Hernia 12 years.	October 15 ; omentum removed.	Recovered	81 days.		
37	M.	47	Femoral, 8 weeks.	November 9.	Recovered	20 days ; primary union.	January, 1890. No relapse. Truss.	
38	M.	74	Inguinal, 8 months.	November 25.	Recovered	15 days ; primary union.	January, 1890. No relapse. Truss.	
39	M.	21	Inguinal, 18 months.	December 28.	Recovered	10 days ; primary union.		

TABLE IV.—CASES OF HERNIA IN CHILDREN OPERATED ON AT THE HOSPITAL FOR RUPTURED AND CRIPPLED 1889–90.

The duration stated by parents is of doubtful value: all the cases where sac was found were anatomically congenital, except one.

No.	Sex.	Age.	Variety and duration.	Date. Complication.	Result.	Duration of treatment.	Last observation.
1	M.	6	Congenital, inguinal, scrotal; difficult.	December 3, 1889. Suture of ring. Sac not found. Wound closed; no drain.	Recovered	Primary union.	Relapsed in scrotum at end of one month. Truss.
2	M.	8	Incomplete inguinal, 6 mos. ?	January 4, 1890. Suture of ring. Wound closed; no drain.	Recovered	Primary union.	Relapsed in 2 months.
3	M.	12	Inguinal, 5 years ?	January 7. Removal of sac. Suture of ring; scrotal drain.	Recovered	Primary union.	Relapsed in three mos.
4	M.	7	Inguinal, 2 months ?	October 30, 1889. Removal of sac. Suture of ring and canal; scrotal drain.	Recovered	Primary union.	
5	M.	12	Inguinal, 5 years ?	January 28, 1890. Suture of ring.	Recovered	Primary union.	
6	F.	13	Inguinal, small, 5 years ?	November 12, 1889. Suture of ring.	Recovered	Primary union.	March 8. 1890. Relapsed. Truss.
7	F.	12	Inguinal, 3 years ?	October 22. Suture of canal and ring.	Recovered	Primary union.	
8	M.	6	Inguinal, 6 years ? Treated twice before ; wearing plaster for Pott's disease.	November 19. Excision, ligature, and suture.	Recovered	Primary union.	February 27, 1890.
9	M.	9	Congenital, inguinal.	October 30. No sac found. Suture of ring.	Recovered	Primary union.	November 25, 1890. Relapsed.
10	M.	13	Inguinal ? Small.	November 19. No sac found. Suture of ring.	Recovered	Primary union.	
11	M.	14	Inguinal ?	November 12. No sac found. Suture of ring.	Recovered	Primary union.	March 6, 1890. No relapse. Truss in daytime.
12	M.	8	Inguinal, 1 year ? Unable to hold.	May 8. Excision and suture; scrotal drain.	Recovered	Primary union.	
13	M.	4½	Inguinal, 4 years ?	February 14, 1890. Suture of ring.	Recovered		
14	M.	5½	Inguinal, 1 year ?	February 21. Suture of ring.	Recovered		
15	M.	10	Inguinal, double, 8½ years.	February 1. Left ligature and suture.	Recovered		
16	M.	13¾	Inguinal, 9 years.	February 21. Excision of sac. Suture of canal. Small hydrocele of cord incised.	Recovered	April 3, suppuration.	

and four out of five in the second. In the second year the proportion of failures is about the same, but it is much less in each. Thus of nine cases operated on by the first method only one, and of ten by the second method only two recurred. In both, the tendency to relapse during the first year is markedly shown, and the inspection of cases traced after two or three years shows a much larger proportion of cases that have not reappeared.

A comparison between these two and the third method, ligature, excision and suture of the canal, can be made only roughly by noting the proportion of cases recurring during the first year. This should be compared, however, with the number of cases by the other methods that have been longer under observation. If we do this we find that:

In the first series of 22 cases, 6, or 27.27 per cent., relapsed within one year.

In the second series of 20 cases, 8, or 40 per cent., relapsed within one year.

In the third series of 19 cases, 8, or 42 per cent., relapsed within one year.

If this third method has no better showing in the first year it is not likely that it will after longer observation, and it is not, therefore, entitled to greater confidence.

Of the cases in children it may be said that they

prove or disprove nothing ; but the prompt recurrence in cases where the sac was not found shows the importance of obliterating it in any method of cure, as well as the uncertainty of simple closure of the pillars of the external ring with sutures.

Of the effect of the use of trusses after the radical operation I can form no positive conclusion. Of the cases which relapsed where this fact was inquired into, six used trusses, three did not. Of those which did not relapse, eighteen wore trusses, eleven used none. I have usually directed patients to wear a very light support, and shall continue to do so. It seems to me important that no strong pressure should be made upon the recently healed parts ; but that, on the other hand, they should be supported against the weight of the abdominal contents.

There is no advantage shown by the comparison of these methods in the femoral and inguinal varieties of hernia. If suture of the inguinal canal or the external ring leads to no better result than that of leaving the wound to heal after a drainage-tube, we cannot hope to close the femoral-canal opening any more securely.

In eight femoral herniæ, the method of ligature and excision has given me three relapses, and five apparent cures ; while in inguinal hernia there are thirteen cases, eight without and five with relapse.

Of two ventral herniæ, situated between the sternum and umbilicus in the median line, one has recurred, the other has not. Another similar hernia, treated by the same method, the aponeurosis being sutured, has recurred.

Of the ages in reference to relapse, I can merely say that the majority of relapsed cases are over forty.

In reflecting on the experience of these cases I am obliged to conclude that in these methods, which I have faithfully tried, there is no prospect of attaining a radical cure of any form of hernia, and that the majority of cases will be found to relapse, if followed for a sufficient time. I am convinced, however, that the attempt to cure is desirable, since the majority of patients are in better condition than before. This is certainly true of irreducible cases, and of all reducible ones which are subjected to operation because mechanical treatment is difficult or painful. The patient who wears his truss with comfort and safety is only bettered by the operation so long as the rupture remains out of sight. The attempt to cure is furthermore desirable, since it can be made witht rifling risk to life, except in feeble, old, or unhealthy patients, and with little chance of complications or accidents. My own results as to relapse being no better by the complicated method of suture of the ring alone, or of the ring and canal, than by the simpler method of excision of the sac after ligature, I shall confine myself to that method of operation till other procedures, which have stood the test of years, make a more promising showing.

This method has the further advantage of being applicable to all forms of herniæ.

Of the newer operations, of which there are a multitude, I have not been unmindful in framing these conclusions. Each one has its earnest advocate ; with a large number of theoretical advantages, or any brief period of observation, I doubt if any, subjected to the same continued scrutiny that my methods have been, will show better results. I am becoming confirmed in that judgment day by day in witnessing the relapsed cases that apply for trusses to the Hospital for Ruptured and Crippled. Between January and October, 1889, there were forty-five such cases, and in the past nine months there have been fully as many more. I am trying to trace the history of all these patients, about 100 in number, in order to obtain accurate knowledge of the methods employed. It will be of interest to know that thus far, of the forty-five patients above mentioned, twenty-two have been thus investigated. Of these, eleven had been operated on by McBurney's method, the shortest period of relapse being one month, the longest eleven months. Two had been subjected to treatment by injection, according to Heaton, with relapse at two months and eighteen

months. In four operated on by ligature and excision, recurrence occurred on the average at the end of one year. One, by Macewen's method, recurred in seven months. One relapse took place four years after ligation and excision of the sac with suture of the external ring. Another, five years after treatment, by purse-string suture and inversion of the sac. Two patients, in whom the sac was sutured at its neck, had relapses in four and five months, respectively. These observations will, without doubt, be duplicated in the cases yet to be traced, and go to strengthen the conviction that all methods of radical cure will be found unsatisfactory.

THE ETIOLOGY OF PLEURITIS, ESPECIALLY IN ITS RELATION TO TUBERCULOSIS.[1]

BY A. A. SMITH, M.D.,

PROFESSOR OF MATERIA MEDICA AND THERAPEUTICS IN THE BELLEVUE HOSPITAL MEDICAL COLLEGE, NEW YORK.

THE frequent occurrence of pleuritis, its apparent harmlessness in some cases, its very serious character in others, and the great variety of conditions under which it may arise must make it always a subject of interest. Since the discoveries of Koch, and the interest in the whole subject of tuberculosis excited by those discoveries, the study of the etiology of pleuritis and the significance of its relation to tuberculosis have received a new stimulus. Many careful observations have been made and very different conclusions have been reached by observers.

If one follows the discussions of the past few years on the subject of the relation of pleuritis to tuberculosis, he must have been thoroughly impressed with the difficulties of arriving at a satisfactory conclusion. If, as is claimed by many excellent observers, almost all cases of pleuritis not traceable to the ordinarily recognized causes are of tubercular origin, then not only must much more care be given to the diagnosis and probable etiology, but to the prognosis and treatment. If a case of pleuritis, sooner or later, goes on to the development of pulmonary tuberculosis, it is easy to accept the view that the pleuritis was of tubercular origin. The most earnest advocates of the tubercular origin of pleuritis admit that it is very difficult to prove in any given case, unless there is evidence of tubercular lesions elsewhere.

Ehrlich is of the opinion that tubercle bacilli can be demonstrated in all exudations of tubercular nature except the sero-fibrinous.

Fränkel believes it very difficult to discover the bacillus of tuberculosis in the fluids effused into the thoracic cavity, and yet he is of the opinion that

---

[1] Read before the Association of American Physicians, May, 1890.

the large majority of these cases are of tubercular origin.

Von Ziemssen says that even if it is not possible to show in most sero-fibrinous pleuro-exudates the microörganisms, this is no proof of their non-existence, as they may be lost in the perforation made in the pleura by the exploring-needle, or they may only occur in the form of spores.

From October 1, 1889, to April 1, 1890, I had under special observation, with a view to careful investigation and examination of the pleural exudates and sputa, 9 cases of pleuritis in Bellevue Hospital; 5 of sero-fibrinous exudations and 4 of purulent. The fluids were repeatedly examined, and were taken from the lowest portion of the pleural sac as the situation most likely to contain the cell constituents, if any were present. In not a single instance were any tubercle bacilli found. Likewise the sputa were carefully and repeatedly examined, and in only one instance were tubercle bacilli found and that was in a case in which the exudate was purulent. This was the only evidence of tuberculosis in the case; careful physical examination failed to reveal evidences of pulmonary tuberculosis. In one case of sero-fibrinous exudation the patient was aspirated twice in October. After the second aspiration the patient's condition improved very materially until early in March, when she developed an acute febrile attack with evidences of peritonitis, and died in three weeks. The autopsy was interesting in that it showed evidences of tubercular peritonitis, a tubercular lesion in the left Fallopian tube and a few miliary tubercles on the left pleural surface of the diaphragm. No tubercular lesions were found in the lungs. It was the *right* pleural sac from which the fluid had been drawn in October. These cases are mentioned to show the difficulties in the way of determining the origin of pleural exudates. They are not given as instances of tubercular or of non-tubercular pleurisies.

The study of the results of inoculation of the pleural exudates has been unsatisfactory, at least in so far as the production of tuberculosis is concerned. The most recent observations in this direction have been made by von Ziemssen, who concludes that although fresh pleural exudates injected into the serous cavities of dogs, and into their subcutaneous cellular tissue, has not produced true tuberculosis, they have acted injuriously, "but the infecting potentiality could not be isolated."

It is well known that tuberculous sputa and tuberculous material from the lungs can be injected into the tissues of animals and produce tuberculosis. On the other hand the material from so-called tuberculous joints has only, to a very moderate extent, the power of producing tuberculosis in animals. The potentiality seems to be limited to certain tissues. A number of observers confirm these conclusions of von Ziemssen.

From a clinical standpoint some recent observations are of great interest. At a meeting of the Leeds and West Riding Medico-Chirurgical Society, January 10, 1890, Dr. Barrs read a paper on an investigation of 74 cases of pleuritis under treatment from 1880–1884 inclusive, and which had apparently recovered from pleuritis, but showing at the present time a death-rate of 57 per cent. Excluding the empyema of children, he thinks the majority of cases of pleuritic effusion are of tubercular origin. Such a series of cases lends strength to the theory of the tubercular origin of pleuritis.

Coriveaud, on the other hand, reports a series of twenty-seven cases followed for from twenty-five years to eight years, and found that none of them became tubercular after attacks of sero-fibrinous pleuritis. Such a series certainly confirms the view, held by probably the vast majority of observers, of the primary and non-tubercular origin of many cases of pleurisy with effusion.

In a paper read before the American Climatological Association, Dr. Vincent Y. Bowditch gives results of an investigation of the subsequent histories of ninety cases of pleuritis occurring in his father's practice, in thirty years, and the conclusions he arrives at, are: that a large percentage of the patients who were afflicted with pleuritis, often in apparently chronic forms, recovered their health, and have not had a recurrence of the trouble, nor developed subsequent pulmonary or other tubercular trouble.

In the last twelve years, of eleven cases of pleuritis with effusion seen in private practice, of which I have records, and the subsequent histories to date, seven were purulent and four sero-fibrinous.

Of the seven purulent, six have apparently recovered, and only one has developed tuberculosis. Five of the seven followed pneumonia. Of the four sero-fibrinous, two have apparently recovered and two developed tuberculosis. It must be admitted, however, that sufficient time has not yet elapsed to give these cases much value. The advocates of the tubercular origin of pleuritis contend that many years may elapse before the pulmonary tuberculosis manifests itself—twenty-four years is the longest period I have found reported. It is very difficult to believe that there is any connection between the pleuritis and the subsequent pulmonary tuberculosis after so long a period, but it is not difficult to find observers who can believe much more improbable associations than this. Baumgarten believes that a child may be born with tubercle bacilli in some of its tissues, and that they may remain inactive for years, or even throughout life. Verneuil goes still farther. He believes that the tubercle bacillus can exist throughout life in a parasitic form, and then manifest itself in a succeeding generation.

It will be noticed that six of my seven cases of empyema have apparently recovered. I have made no reference to a large number of hospital and dispensary cases observed, as it is impossible to get satisfactory subsequent histories, and the cases would have no value in connection with the subject of this paper. The favorable progress of purulent pleural exudate is in accordance with the experience of von Ziemssen. He reports eighteen cases of empyema. Fifteen of these were treated, of which thirteen recovered. It should be stated that all of these cases of von Ziemssen's followed pneumonia. Many other observers have had a similar experience.

In sixteen cases of dry pleuritis more or less extensive, of which I have kept records, five have thus far developed pulmonary tuberculosis. These were cases occurring in private practice; hospital and dispensary cases are not included for the same reason that such cases were not included in my series of pleurisies with effusions namely, unsatisfactory subsequent histories. Nor were cases included in which at the time there were unmistakable evidences of pulmonary disease. The observations extend over a period of fourteen years and it may be objected that this is not a sufficiently long time to determine the question of a possible development of pulmonary tuberculosis later. Still, up to date, eleven are in such a condition as to justify the opinion that they have recovered.

During the past two years I have had observations made in 140 autopsies in which there were evidences of old or recent changes in the pleura, all cases being included in which such changes were found. These autopsies were performed on subjects from Bellevue and Charity Hospitals, the hospitals of the workhouse and almshouse of the city of New York, and a few were cases of sudden death (coroner's cases) occurring outside of hospitals. There were changes in the pleura, more or less extensive, in nearly 80 per cent. of another series of autopsies, numbering 120, in which this was looked for, not including those cases where only a few fibrous threads connected the surfaces of the pleura. These changes consisted for the most part either in old adhesions, tubercular pleuritis, or recent acute pleuritis secondary to some other disease. These 120 cases were taken at random from autopsies made by Dr. Hermann M. Biggs at different hospitals in New York.

In the 140 cases 47, or 33.5 per cent., died from pulmonary tuberculosis, or else showed quite extensive pulmonary disease; of these, 9 presented unmistakable evidences of tubercular pleuritis. In 50, or a little over 35 per cent. of the remaining cases, cheesy or calcareous nodules were found in the lungs, making in all 97 cases, or 68.5 per cent. in

which the lungs showed evidences of recent or old tuberculosis. Taking these two series as a whole, it is found that a little over 60 per cent. of the autopsies showed evidences of old or recent pulmonary tuberculosis, and of these less than one-half died of tuberculosis.

In 27 of the series of 140 cases the pleuritis was recent (in ten of them there were also rather extensive old adhesions), and in 5 instances it was double and associated with pericarditis. In 5 there was anthracosis with fibrous new formations in the lungs, without tuberculosis, but associated with adhesions, as a rule, rather extensive. In 16 other cases there were changes in the pleura, in which the tubercular lesions were found. Of these, 5 were cases of tertiary syphilis, 2 were associated with new growths in the lungs, 5 others showed quite marked renal disease. In one rheumatic case there was acute pleuritis, pericarditis and endocarditis; in one, chronic bronchitis and bronchiectasis; in one, an aneurism of the aortic arch, and one was a case of scleroderma with advanced heart disease.

In speaking of an old process, reference is made to the cheesy or calcareous nodules so frequently found in the lungs, and surrounded by fibrous tissue capsules. Recent investigations have clearly shown that in the vast majority of cases these nodules have resulted from a local tuberculosis; and that the cheesy masses generally, and the calcareous masses frequently, still contain the tubercular virus and will, when inoculated, produce tuberculosis in animals. It should also be distinctly understood, that the nodules found in some of the cases were very small, not more than 3 mm. in diameter, and that in some instances not more than one nodule was found in the lungs. These have been included on the ground that they are exactly the same in nature as the larger masses, and if they are tubercular the question of size does not come into consideration. Fibrous cicatrices without cheesy nodules were not taken into consideration, although many of these unquestionably result from tuberculosis.

As regards the extent and distribution of adhesions, it was found that there was no constant relation between the degree of lung involvement and the extent of the adhesions. In some cases of very advanced disease the pleura showed only a few adhesions. This was especially the case where the process did not involve to any great extent the pleural surface. On the other hand, small nodules in one lung were not infrequently associated with extensive adhesions on both sides, and often the adhesions were more marked in the lung that contained no cheesy nodules.

The observations in these cases do not confirm the assumption that the adhesions are primary, and that they predispose to the development of a tubercular process in the lungs. The cheesy and calcareous nodules were generally found in the upper lobes, and near the apices, and were not infrequently found in other parts of the lungs also, especially in the upper portion of the lower lobes. When these nodules were found in the lungs, the bronchial glands usually showed similar changes macroscopically.

In the series of 140 cases only 9 showed unmistakable evidences of tubercular pleuritis, although 97 showed evidences of either recent or old tuberculosis in the lungs, and 47 of these showed very extensive involvement.

Post-mortem researches seem to show that tubercular pleuritis is, a rare disease, even though the lungs in many cases may be extensively diseased. Undoubtedly many cases of tuberculosis have their first manifestation in a pleuritis, and many cases of pleuritis are secondary to pulmonary tuberculosis. *Possibly* a pleuritis may favor the development of pulmonary tuberculosis by depressing vitality, by lessening the proper lung expansion or by interfering with the nutrition of the adjacent lung ; but more probably the same underlying cause produces both.

In the absence of evidences of tuberculosis in other situations there is no sufficiently precise clinical history to warrant an absolute diagnosis of tubercular pleuritis. If it is an effusion, the appearance of the fluid is not characteristic. Unless tubercle bacilli are found one cannot positively affirm its nature, and as has been shown the bacilli are very rarely found.

From my own researches and a study of the researches of others, I offer the following conclusions:

First. If it be true that the very large majority of cases of pleuritis, not traceable to ordinarily recognized causes, are tubercular, we have no clinical method by which the fact can be proven, and the assumption that they are tubercular can only be by inference.

Second. If such a large majority of pleurisies, as many seem to believe, are of tubercular origin, recovery from tuberculosis of the pleura is much more frequent than from pulmonary tuberculosis.

Third. The prognosis in purulent pleural exudate is more favorable as to the subsequent development of tuberculosis than in sero-fibrinous exudate.

Fourth. That even though at an autopsy, evidences of pleuritis recent or old may be found, it does not necessarily follow that the pleuritis is tubercular, because there are tubercular lesions in the lung.

Fifth. It is fair to assume from the frequent association, post-mortem, of recent and old changes in the pleura with pulmonary tuberculosis, that many of these changes are tubercular in origin, although at the time of death tubercles are not found in the pleura.

Sixth. In cases of pleuritis, although evidences of tuberculosis exist in the lungs, as shown by physical signs, and by the presence of tubercle bacilli in the sputa, it does not necessarily follow that such cases of pleuritis are tubercular in origin, although they probably are.

Seventh. In cases in which pulmonary tuberculosis develops subsequent to a pleuritis, there is probably the same underlying cause for each.[1]

ACUTE PERITONITIS FROM GONORRHŒA.

BY CHARLES B. PENROSE. M.D., PH.D.,
SURGEON TO GYNECEAN HOSPITAL AND TO OUT-PATIENT DEPARTMENT
OF PENNSYLVANIA HOSPITAL, PHILADELPHIA.

PERITONITIS in women is generally the result of disease of the Fallopian tubes. The sequence of events is, in most cases, slow—salpingitis, closure of the fimbrinated end of the tube by peritoneal adhesions, and distention of the tube with pus or other material more or less septic. The resulting peritonitis, if acute and general, is caused by sudden rupture and escape of the tube-contents into the peritoneum ; or, if chronic, by gradual leakage from a small rupture, or by direct extension of inflammation through the tubal or abscess wall.

In this way gonorrhœa in women often produces peritonitis and death. But the causative attack of gonorrhœa generally occurs several months or years before the final fatal peritonitis, the peritonitis being a remote sequel of the gonorrhœa, and the infecting virus being of a mixed character. The case which I am about to describe followed a very much more unusual course. The inflammatory process travelled directly from the vagina, through the previously healthy uterus, and along the Fallopian tubes, and thence throughout the general visceral and parietal peritoneum. The action was too rapid to permit the formation of preservative adhesions and occlusion of the fimbriated ends of the tubes.

Similar rapid peritonitis from a septic focus in the vagina or uterus occurs in the puerperal state, after criminal abortion, and after surgical traumatism to the uterus, as in cases reported by Coe (*N. Y. Med. Journ.*, May 15, 1886), when death followed the operation of hystero-trachelorrhaphy, and the autopsy showed septic inflammation, traceable directly from the wounded cervix, along the endometrium and tubes, and thence throughout the general peritoneum. It is, however, probable that in many cases of so-called puerperal peritonitis the rupture during labor of a previously diseased tube, or pelvic tumor of any kind, is the cause of the peritonitis, rather than septic infection from the uterus

[1] I desire to acknowledge my indebtedness for much valuable assistance in the preparation of this paper to Dr. Hermann M. Biggs, one of the Curators of Bellevue Hospital and a director of the Carnegie Laboratory.

or vagina. And it is also very probable that the same cause which was active in the case here reported — that is, gonorrhœa acquired immediately after labor—may be present, though unrecognized, in other cases of peritonitis following childbirth :

In October, 1889, a young colored man came to the Surgical Clinic of the Pennsylvania Hospital with a violent inflammatory attack of gonorrhœa, of several days' duration. He had great dysuria, a very profuse purulent discharge, inflammatory swelling of the whole penis, and œdema of the prepuce. He stated that this was his first attack of gonorrhœa, and that he had acquired the disease by being unfaithful to his wife during her convalescence from childbirth. Seven days after his first visit he had a violent attack of epididymitis on the left side, which obliged him to take to bed.

On October 29th he came at night to my office, walking with crutches, and suffering intense pain. He asked me to see his wife, who was very sick. On visiting the house I found a large colored woman, over 200 pounds in weight, presenting all the symptoms of general peritonitis. The pulse was 130. Temperature 100°. The abdomen was distended and very tender. There was a profuse purulent vaginal and urethral discharge, and redness and inflammatory swelling of the external genitals. Vaginal examination caused great pain, and revealed nothing more definite than fulness on each side of, and posterior to, the uterus. She had free diarrhœa, which had appeared a few hours after the onset of general abdominal pain, and which had greatly relieved the pain.

She and her husband gave me separately the following history. She had always been perfectly healthy, and had had two children, the last on September 24, 1889, one month before the present sickness. The child was healthy in every respect, and the mother convalesced without trouble of any kind, leaving bed on the eleventh day. She had connection with her husband, for the first time after delivery, on October 23d. This was six days before my visit to her, and, as I have said, at this time I was treating the husband for a violent attack of gonorrhœa. Coitus was followed in two days by burning micturition, swelling and inflammation of the vulva, and profuse purulent discharge. Three days later she began to have pelvic pain, greatest on the right side, and free bleeding from the vagina. This was speedily followed by general abdominal pain, tenderness, and distention. Diarrhœa appeared shortly after the general abdominal pain. The bleeding from the vagina lasted four days. As her surroundings were of the worst kind. I sent her to the Gynecean Hospital, and performed abdominal section the next day.

The parietal peritoneum was hypertrophied, being about one-eighth inch in thickness. It did not present the usual smooth surface, but was red and granular, and bled easily. The intestinal loops were adherent to the parietes and to each other in the region of the incision, throughout the pelvis, and in the right iliac and hypogastric regions. All the loops of intestine which were visible were distended, and presented the same red, granular appearance, and bled very easily, even on contact with soft sponges.

There was no lymph, pus, or fluid of any kind in the peritoneum. There were no organized adhesions, all adhesions being very recent and easily separated. The Fallopian tubes were six inches long, and as thick as the index-finger. They were bound by recent adhesions to the surrounding intestines. There was no sign of old tubal disease. The walls of the tubes were thickened, hard, and rigid. The distal ends were not closed. The fimbriæ stood out turgid and stiff. The whole organ was hypertrophied and rigid from recent inflammatory exudation throughout all the structures. A very small quantity of thin, puriform fluid was in the tubes. The tubes and ovaries were removed close to the cornua. The abdomen was freely flushed with hot distilled water, and a large glass drain was introduced. A small quantity of sanguinolent serum was discharged from the drainage-tube, which was removed on the third day. The convalesence was uneventful. She continued to suffer from urethritis and vaginitis for five weeks after the operation, but is at present well in every respect.

The unusual course followed by the gonorrhœal disease in this case was due to two causes: the virulence of the infecting pus, which was shown by the intensity of the inflammation in the husband, and the patulous condition of the uterus and tubes incident to parturition. Both causes prevented the chronic course of the disease—the gradual formation of peritoneal adhesions and occlusion of the tubes. This would have happened if the patient had survived without operation. The operation accomplished the same result by shutting off the uterus from above, rendering the peritoneum a closed sac, safe from further infection.

I subjoin the report of the microscopic examination of the Fallopian tubes, which was made by Dr. L. Coplin, of the Jefferson Medical College Laboratory of Pathology :

"The tubes show well-marked inflammation, masked by thickening and young cell-deposit through their entire structure. Cocci are present in both tubes, the right more than the left, and in this the processes of inflammation are most developed. The cocci are not gonococci; as they are not diplococci, as not all of them within the perinuclear protoplasm, and do not stain by gonococci stain. They are larger, and are found both inter- and intra- cellular. They are rarely found singly, but as zooglœic masses, the size of which vary from $\frac{1}{2500}$ to $\frac{1}{1500}$ of an inch, and in these masses may be counted from 25 to 75 or more cocci. They have very much the appearance of some of the staphylococci of suppuration. None of them are streptococci. They are not in the epithelium of the tube, but in the younger connective tissue corpuscles of the margin of the tube. The epithelium is for the most part normal."

University of Halle.—After many erroneous announcements regarding the successor of Volkmann at Halle, the fact is that Professor Bramann is there and has begun his clinics.

CLINICAL MEMORANDA.

MEDICAL.

Case of Slow Pulse.[1]—This patient has continued in much the same condition during the past year. In November, 1889, he had a relapse of which the following is the record:

Nov. 24, 1889. Pulse 11. Frequent attacks of unconsciousness. During the attacks his pulse ceases to beat for ten, fifteen, and twenty seconds.

25th. Pulse 36. Quinine and iron prescribed.

Dec. 1. Pulse 32. Twenty attacks daily.

7th. Pulse 12. Pulse irregular for three or four beats, and then a long interval. Fainting attacks are very frequent.

13th. Pulse 34. Ammonium bromide and belladonna given.

21st. Pulse 12. Fifteen to twenty spells per day.

24th. Pulse 36. Spells not so frequent.

31st. Pulse 13. Very severe attack of syncope.

Jan. 14, 1890. Pulse 26. Very severe attack of syncope.

15th. Pulse 18. For a time thought to be dead.

17th. Pulse 18. Better. Temperature 99.6°.

Feb. 6. Pulse 23.

8th. Pulse 13. Slight attacks.

TRACING I.

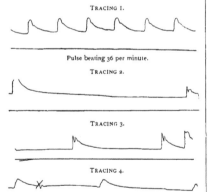

Pulse beating 36 per minute.

TRACING 2.

TRACING 3.

TRACING 4.

Tracings 2, 3 and 4 taken when pulse was beating 12 per minute. They show the long diastole—5 seconds.

(Tracings were taken by Dr. R. T. Edes.)

9th. Pulse 48. At 8.20 A. M., fell on floor unconscious ; black in face ; no motion for one hour ; choking sound in throat. At 9.15 A. M. constant rolling of the head, then jerking, kicking, and bellowing constantly as though in greatest distress. Takes no notice of surroundings, but put out tongue when told to sharply. Nitrite of amyl and hypodermic injection of morphine and atropine.

10th. Pulse 32. Recovered from attack of yesterday.

15th. Pulse 24.

21st. Pulse 28. Better and sitting up.

27th. Pulse 28. Swelling of face.

April 8. Pulse 28.

On May 14th, when the patient was brought before the Association, his pulse was 24. He was apparently comfortable and was able to be about, though he still had occasional attacks of syncope.

D. W. PRENTISS, M.D.

WASHINGTON, D. C.

MEDICO-LEGAL.

Collapse of the Lung from Hanging.—Collapse of the lungs in hanging is of such rare occurrence that this case may be of some importance in legal medicine. This condition of the lungs is mentioned once in Taylor's *Medical Jurisprudence ;* and I am informed by Dr. John J. Reese, Professor of Medical Jurisprudence in the University of Pennsylvania, that this is the only case recorded.

The case is as follows : B. E., colored, aged twenty-two years, was hung in this city, April 18, 1890, and was given a fall of six feet. Heart-action ceased in twelve minutes after the drop fell. Post-mortem examination held one hour afterward. Temperature in axilla at this time was 98⅞°. Body well nourished, but not very muscular.

Opening the chest, the lungs were found completely collapsed, otherwise normal.

The pleural cavities were entirely free from fluid and were without pleuritic adhesions. The right heart was distended with dark blood. The stomach contained a small amount of blood but no food, and there was marked capillary engorgement. Bowels were empty. The vessels of the liver and kidneys were engorged. Spleen normal.

Bloodvessels of brain distended.

Careful dissection of the neck showed that the articulations of the vertebræ were intact.

CUNNINGHAM WILSON, M.D.

BIRMINGHAM, ALABAMA.

MEDICAL PROGRESS.

Experimental Studies in Tuberculosis.—At the Heidelberg congress of German naturalists and physicians Schottelius stated that some years ago he instituted a series of experiments with tuberculous lungs interred in a wooden box at a depth of five feet, the usual mode of sepulture of bodies. After two years and a half he removed from the surrounding earth a quantity of tubercle bacilli, for the most part spore-producing. From these he obtained pure cultures which furnished positive results in 80 per cent. of his experiments in inoculation. He is now engaged in investigations with the object of ascertaining whether the virulence resides in the bacilli taken from the soil or in their spores. Soyka expresses the opinion that the greater number of the bacilli perish, but that

---

[1] Patient was brought before the meeting of the Association of American Physicians, May 14, 1890. The patient was also shown to the Association in 1889. For more full account of the case see Proceedings of The Association of American Physicians for 1889.

some possess durability and may recover their virulence under favorable conditions. Gärtner has observed bacilli in a cemetery abandoned for twenty-five years.

As a practical outcome of his investigations, Schottelius advises the disinfection of bodies of persons dead from infectious diseases.

Gebhardt has experimented with the sputum of consumptives, his object being to test the virulence of the sputum in different grades of dilution, and to ascertain whether the potentiality of the tubercular virus is essentially modified by the organ first infected—that is to say, by the manner of infection. With this object he practised hypodermic and intraperitoneal inoculation and experiments in inhalation and alimentation, and ascertained that in the subcutaneous connective tissue, the peritoneum, and the lungs the tuberculous virus multiplies in about an equal degree, while the digestive apparatus offers resistance. Hence tubercular virus may, especially in small quantities, pass through certain organs without provoking local alterations. As the point of ingress is not always the seat of the disease, pulmonary tuberculosis is not to be invariably attributed to infection by inhalation.

Sputum which contains bacilli is exceedingly infectious, retaining its virulence even in dilution of 1 : 100,000, apparently without regard to the manner of infection. The virulence of the sputum being in proportion to the quantity of bacilli present, Gebhardt employed pure cultures of the bacilli of tuberculosis, on the hypothesis that equal quantities of the same culture contain quantities of bacilli. With a subcutaneous inoculation of 1 c. c. of a dilution in the proportion of 1 : 400,000 and an inhalation of 0.5 c. c. of the same dilution in a culture of agar-agar he obtained positive results. Hence the pure cultures retain their virulence when enormously diluted.

Malassez and Vignal desiccated the sputum of tuberculosis, moistened it with water, again desiccated and pulverized it, and this repeatedly, endeavoring to realize, as far as possible, the conditions to which the sputum daily ejected in our streets is subjected. After successive desiccation and moistening the bacillus of the sputum retained all its virulence.

With regard to the penetration of tubercle bacilli into the organism, Dobroklonski states, as the result of his experiments in the Cornil laboratory at Paris, that tuberculosis may attack the organism by way of the digestive apparatus. For this to occur, no lesion of the intestinal wall, epithelial desquamation, local modification, nor previous inflammation is necessary. The tuberculous virus (bacilli and spores) may easily traverse the completely normal epithelial lining of the intestine, but it does not determine inflammation unless it remains for a length of time in contact with the intestinal wall. Dobroklonski asserts that the spores and bacilli do not penetrate the organism by any fixed means, but that they are carried by the current of the lymphatic system, and, being arrested by the tissues, determine in them the formation of tubercles.

As a natural inference from Hirschberger's experiments demonstrating that tubercular cows, or cows infected with tubercular phthisis, produce, in 55 per cent. of cases, infectious milk, it was supposed that milk from large dairies would contract virulent properties from the infectious milk of one tuberculous cow. A series of ex-

periments, conducted by Gebhardt, under the direction of Bollinger, in the Pathological Institute of Monaca, show that tuberculous milk loses its virulence at a certain dilution. The mixing of milk practised in large dairies diminishes the danger, and in most cases renders the milk innocuous. Milk served by large dairies is always to be preferred to the continued use of milk from one cow.

Studies in the transmission of tuberculosis from animals to men by means of tuberculous milk, directed the attention of hygienists to the derivatives of milk, the most important of these being butter. Gasparini inoculated guinea-pigs with butter containing the bacillus of Koch, and by microscopic observation verified tubercular lesions in almost all cases.

Referring to his studies of the infectious property in the flesh of tuberculous animals, Kastner stated that the object of his experiments was to ascertain if such flesh contained virus, and to what extent the consumption of such flesh as meat was dangerous to man. From the results of his experiments he concludes that the danger is slight, unless the nodules of tuberculosis are formed in the meat, which is rarely the case.— *Weekly Abstract of Sanitary Reports, U. S. Marine Hospital Service,* June 13, 1890.

Effects of Caffeine.—In an able article on the study of caffeine Dr. Edward T. Reichert reached the following conclusions:

1. The pulse-rate may be diminished during the first and last stages of the poisoning, but is generally decidedly increased. During the first stage the diminution is due to stimulation of the cardio-inhibitory centres in the medulla oblongata and heart, and during the last stage to a direct depression of the heart. The increase in the pulse-rate is due to a depression or paralysis of the above-mentioned cardio-inhibitory centres.

2. Arterial pressure during the first stages of poisoning is generally either unaffected or diminished, but occasionally a trifling increase is noted ; during subsequent stages it is diminished. The increase is due to a direct stimulant action upon the bloodvessel walls increasing vascular tension. The diminution is due chiefly to a direct depression of the heart, and to some extent, doubtless, to a secondary paralysant action on the vessel walls.

3. The acceleration of the heart-beats may be accompanied by no appreciable alteration in blood-pressure, but generally by a more or less decided diminution, which is dependent upon cardiac depression.

4. Caffeine diminishes the heart's efficiency for work, arrests it in diastole, sometimes induces sudden paralysis, and is, therefore, a cardiac depressant.

5. The asserted stimulant action upon the circulation is, doubtless, subjective, and dependent upon an excitation of the cerebral centres.

The Effect of Opiates on Gastric Secretion.—According to the *Lancet,* Dr. Abutkoff has examined the effects of opium and two of its alkaloids on the digestive functions of healthy people. He found that the three substances experimented with—viz., opium, morphine, and codeine—all exert a retarding action on gastric digestion by diminishing the general acidity of the gastric juice. Neither the quantity of pepsin nor the absorbent power of the stomach appeared to be affected by any of the three substances. As to their relative effects in such doses as can be given medicinally, opium had decidedly the most marked influence, and codeine the least. Dr. Abutkoff suggests that in the case of patients with weak digestion, due to deficiency of acid in the gastric juice, opiates should be given some hours after a meal, but that where the hydrochloric acid is excessive, they may be given with meals.

Surgical Treatment of Tubercular Peritonitis.—CZERNY, of Heidelberg, has recently published his views upon surgical interference in cases of tubercular peritonitis. It is pointed out that though the records of operations seem to show that the disease is amenable to such treatment, it should be remembered that tubercular inflammation of a serous membrane usually indicates that tuberculosis has reached an advanced stage and has become diffused. Czerny grants that surgical treatment of tubercular lesions may, under certain circumstances, bring about an improvement in the nutritive processes, and thus aid in eliminating the virus, and, in cases of restricted localization, lead to a definite cure. It is different, however, when there are many infecting foci.

It is held that the prospects offered by surgical interference will depend upon a distinction being made between the variety of this affection characterized by the presence of a fluid exudate with miliary tubercles, and the dry form in which large tubercular nodules are found; operation in the latter variety being very unpromising. In the former variety the author regards incision and removal of the fluid much preferable to any other plan of treatment, but he also holds that the ultimate results of such treatment are not very encouraging.—*London Medical Recorder*, March 20, 1890.

Intubation of the Larynx.—DR. G. HUNTER MACKENZIE describes the following cases illustrative of the complications which may arise during intubation of the larynx (*British Medical Journal*, May 24, 1890).

CASE I.—A child of twenty-one months intubated for membranous croup (laryngeal diphtheria?). The insertion of the tube was immediately followed by great relief, and all went well until six hours later, when profuse bleeding from the mouth and nose began, and the child very quickly died. Post-mortem examination showed a blood-clot firmly plugging the tube, and an erosion of the inferior laryngeal artery and vein. The erosion was evidently not caused by the tube.

CASE II.—A child of three and a half years suffering from "croup" (no mention of false membrane is made). The immediate results of the operation were excellent, the child breathing easily for seventy-two hours. At the end of this time he suddenly died, and on removal the tube was found blocked by a firm dry purulent mass.

CASE III.—In this case the insertion of the tube was difficult and, as Dr. Mackenzie doubted that the tube was in the larynx he did not remove the silk cord, but fixed it externally by means of adhesive plaster. A few hours before death the child gnawed through the cord, and at the *post-mortem* the tube was found in the lower part of the œsophagus. The difficulty in introduction was due to supra-glottic narrowing and distortion of the larynx.

Dr. Mackenzie has in a few instances seen the tube expelled by coughing, but writes that this need not cause alarm as there is usually sufficient time for reinsertion.

Since his experience with the second case above reported he has made it a rule to remove and examine the tube within forty-eight hours after its insertion. If dyspnœa then returns, which is the exception, the tube is replaced. The difficulty in swallowing is another reason why the tube should not be left in position longer than absolutely necessary.

Dr. William Hales in the same number of the *British Medical Journal* reports one hundred cases of intubation with 38 per cent. of recoveries and with seven consecutive successful cases.

Nitrite of Amyl in After-pains.—WINTERBURN employs nitrite of amyl for the relief of severe after-pains. His method of using it is as follows: A small piece of tissue-paper is saturated with five or six drops of the nitrite, then placed in a two-drachm vial, which is tightly corked.

The patient is directed to take out the cork and inhale from the bottle when the pains are severe.—*Archives of Gynecology*, June, 1890.

Powder for Fœtid Perspiration.—

R.—Powdered rice   .   .   2   ounces.
    Bismuth subnitrate   .   . 7   drachms.
    Potassium permanganate   3   "
    Powdered talc   .   .   . 1½   "   —M.

To be dusted upon the perspiring parts.—*College and Clinical Record.*

Prescription for Removal of Comedones.—McCASKEY uses the following application in the treatment of comedones:

R.—Sulphuric ether   .   .   . 8 drachms.
    Ammonium carbonate   .   .   1 drachm.
    Boric acid   .   .   .   . 20 grains.
    Water, sufficient to make   2 ounces.—M.

To be applied locally twice daily.—*Peoria Medical Monthly.*

Ferruginous Tonic Pills.—The following formula is quoted in the *Archives of Gynecology:*

R.—Powdered digitalis ⎫
    Ext. of nux vomica ⎬ of each   8 grains.
    Carbonate of iron   ⎭
    Sulphate of quinine   .   . 1 drachm.
    Ext. of gentian, sufficient quantity.

Mix and divide in thirty pills, of which one should be taken three times daily.

Prescription for Cases of Pin-worms.—The *Pittsburgh Medical Review* quotes the following formula, to be used in cases of pin-worms:

R.—Tincture of rhubarb   .   . 30 minims.
    Magnesium carbonate   .   3 grains.
    Tincture of ginger   .   .   1 minim.
    Water   .   .   .   . 1½ drachm.—M.

Three or four such doses should be given in twenty-four hours.

THE MEDICAL NEWS.

A WEEKLY JOURNAL
OF MEDICAL SCIENCE.

COMMUNICATIONS are invited from all parts of the world. Original articles contributed exclusively to THE MEDICAL NEWS will be liberally paid for upon publication. When necessary to elucidate the text, illustrations will be furnished without cost to the author.

Address the Editor: H. A. HARE, M.D.,
·   1004 WALNUT STREET,
                                    PHILADELPHIA.

Subscription Price, including Postage.
PER ANNUM, IN ADVANCE . . . . $4.00.
SINGLE COPIES . . . . 10 CENTS.
Subscriptions may begin at any date. The safest mode of remittance is by bank check or postal money order, drawn to the order of the undersigned. When neither is accessible, remittances may be made, at the risk of the publishers, by forwarding in *registered* letters.

Address,   LEA BROTHERS & CO.,
              NOS. 706 & 708 SANSOM STREET,
                                    PHILADELPHIA.

SATURDAY, JULY 5, 1890.

GONORRHŒA IN WOMEN.

THE serious complications which may result from gonorrhœa in women have only been fully recognized within very recent years. Noeggerath's statement that over one-half of the women of New York have some disease the result of gonorrhœa, seemed very much exaggerated when it was first made ; but the results of abdominal surgery have strengthened this opinion.

Gonorrhœa in women is not only a cause of salpingitis, and resulting sterility and invalidism, but it is not infrequently the cause of death. The mortality of untreated cases of pyosalpinx is difficult to determine ; we have seen it variously estimated at from ten to twenty-five per cent. In a consecutive series of fifty cases of pyosalpinx which were operated upon, we have found general peritonitis present in six cases. These six women were in a dying condition, and they alone, if not subjected to operation, would have given a mortality of twelve per cent. for this series of cases—a mortality certainly much too small when we consider the dangers to which the remaining forty-four women were constantly exposed. It is often difficult to estimate the part played by gonorrhœa in the production of salpingitis. The great majority of women who have pyosalpinx have been exposed to gonorrhœal contagion ; but they have also been exposed to other

causes of pyosalpinx, a very frequent one of which is criminal abortion. The presence of the gonococcus in the Fallopian tube is pathognomonic ; but we believe that there are many cases of salpingitis caused primarily by gonorrhœa, in which careful search fails to reveal the specific diplococcus. This opinion is based on the examination of many specimens of tubal disease, with an undoubted clinical history of gonorrhœa, in which no gonococci were discoverable.

A case recently reported by DR. E. CAPPI (*Gaz. Hebd. des Sciences Méd. de Montpellier*, May 24, 1890) is of interest in this connection. A woman was operated upon for encysted peritonitis, and the gonococcus was found not only in the pus from the abdomen, but also in the discharge from the os uteri. Though the operation failed to show the primary cause of the abdominal abscess, yet it most probably originated from the rupture of a pyosalpinx of gonorrhœal origin. This case followed the usual course ; the sequence of events being : vaginitis, endometritis, salpingitis, and closure of the Fallopian tubes ; and finally, encysted peritonitis with the formation of a pelvic or an abdominal abscess, or general diffuse peritonitis following rupture of the tubal abscess. The case of peritonitis from gonorrhœa reported by DR. PENROSE in this number of THE MEDICAL NEWS followed a very unusual course. The progress of the disease was not delayed by local peritoneal adhesions resulting in closure of the Fallopian tubes. We know of no case with a similar history ; and though the gonococcus was not discovered, yet the clinical history points so definitely to the cause that we must conclude that the disease was of gonorrhœal origin.

This case exemplifies in a forcible way the dangers of gonorrhœa in women. The physician should always remember that neglected gonorrhœa is dangerous not only on account of the consequences to the male, such as urethral stricture, cystitis, and epididymitis, but also on account of the much more frequent and more serious sequelæ which may occur in the female.

TRICHLORACETIC ACID IN INTRA-NASAL DISEASES.

THOUGH the galvano-cautery has to a great extent supplanted chemical agents in the treatment of hypertrophic rhinitis, in many cases the cicatrix produced by the application of pure chromic acid is sufficient to cause contraction of the turbinated bodies, and possesses the advantages of not alarming the patient and of requiring comparatively little manipulative skill. Its disadvantages are that unless considerable care is exercised the acid spreads, causes an unnecesarily large slough and an undesirable amount of inflammatory reaction.

Trichloracetic acid, recently introduced in Germany as a cauterant, apparently has all the advantages and none of the disadvantages of chromic acid. Von Stein and Stanislaw, of Moscow (*Journal of Laryngology and Rhinology*, June, 1890), recommend it not only in the treatment of hypertrophy but in that of acute nasal catarrh (coryza), ozæna, adenoid vegetations, and of various laryngeal diseases. Making due allowances for the enthusiasm of the experimentalists, their assertions are are still so positive that the drug should certainly be given a fair trial, although we believe its field will eventually be restricted to the cauterization of hypertrophies and possibly as a stimulant in the treatment of ozæna.

As a cauterant a crystal of the pure acid should be applied by means of a probe, precisely as chromic acid is ordinarily used, and, of course, during cocaine anæsthesia.

In ozæna a weak solution (five-tenths of one per cent.) should be rapidly brushed over the diseased mucous membrane. It is stated that this treatment, if repeated daily, corrects fœtor, softens the crusts and prevents their formation.

CORRESPONDENCE.

"DETACHMENT AND EXPULSION OF THE VAGINAL PORTION OF THE CERVIX DURING LABOR."

To the Editor of The Medical News,

Sir : Under the above title, in the last issue of your journal, Dr. Hirst reports a case which is of considerable interest. The treatment of the case, however, strikes one as somewhat peculiar. Is it considered orthodox practice in Philadelphia to allow a multiparous woman to remain in labor attended by " vigorous uterine contractions," supplemented by " energetic abdominal action," for *twelve* hours, or, in fact, until the " vaginal portion of the cervix " is extruded from the vulva, without extending to her a helping hand? Could not the os uteri have been dilated artificially? And, if other means failed, could not the tissues surrounding the os (even though they had undergone " cicatricial infiltration ") have been subjected to multiple incision (*débridement multiple*), and then the delivery have been carefully effected with forceps under chloroform? Dr. Hirst says: " the absence of serious symptoms after an injury of this gravity is remarkable." It is still more remark-

able, in view of the practice adopted, that the body of the uterus did not rupture before the cervical portion gave way under the influence of the *vis a tergo*. Dr. Hirst seems to think that the recovery of the patient, without " serious symptoms," speaks well for the *asepsis* of the Maternity Hospital. We think that it speaks well for the *vis medicatrix naturæ*, and are inclined to attribute the recovery of the patient more to good luck than good management.   A Reader of The News.

June 16, 1890.

Before printing this note the Editor of The Medical News submitted it to Dr. Hirst for reply, which is appended:

To the Editor of The Medical News,

·Sir : As I did not see the case reported by me in the last number of The News until after the cervix had been detached and expelled, the rather harsh criticism of "A Reader of The News " applies to the conduct of the resident physician in charge. Her action did not appear so heinous to me as to this critic. Would he, in a first stage of labor, which had only lasted twelve hours, uncomplicated by rise of the contraction-ring, by elevation of temperature, by marked disturbance of pulse, by anything, in fact, but delayed dilatation of a rigid cervical canal—would he, I ask, resort to the forced dilatation of the cervix, or to its incision? If so, he would find his " meddlesome midwifery " more dangerous than the conservative course pursued by the young graduate of not a year's standing, who was in charge of the case.

Barton Cooke Hirst, M.D.

PTOMAINES AND BACTERIA.

To the Editor of The Medical News,

Sir : My attention has just been called to a short article on ptomaines by Professor Ernst, of Harvard, in Volume V. of the *Annual of the Universal Medical Sciences*, 1889, and while the entire article might justify some comment, I am certainly at a loss to understand what authority Professor Ernst has for saying that Mr. Novy and myself in our little volume on *Ptomaines and Leucomaines* make "the suggestion that bacteria may be the *products* of these alkaloids." Will Professor Ernst be kind enough to inform me on what page of the volume I will find the suggestion? As the author of that portion of the volume in which a ptomaine is defined and its nature discussed, I had never heard of the " suggestion " until I had the pleasure of reading the article by Professor Ernst. Respectfully,
V. C. Vaughan, M.D.

The above having been submitted to Professor Ernst, he replied as follows:

To the Editor of The Medical News,

Sir : The statement to which I referred and to which Dr. Vaughan wishes to be directed will be found in *Ptomaines and Leucomaines, or the Putrefactive and Physiological Alkaloids*, by Victor C. Vaughan, M.D., and Frederick G. Novy, page 86, sixth line from the bottom, reading " we are justified in saying that the microörganism may be an accompaniment or a consequence of the disease."

My attention was first called to the statement by a review of the book in the *American Journal of the Medical Sciences*, October, 1888, page 394.

Respectfully,
HAROLD C. ERNST, M.D.

TYPHOID FEVER IN CHATTANOOGA.

To the Editor of THE MEDICAL NEWS,

SIR : In an interesting paper by Dr. James E. Reeves, of Chattanooga, Tennessee, on "Some Points in the Natural History of Enteric or Typhoid Fever," read before the Association of American Physicians, in May last, and published in THE MEDICAL NEWS of June 7th, the author claims for Chattanooga a remarkable and almost entire immunity from typhoid fever, and quotes several well-known physicians of that city to prove that typhoid fever is a disease of extremely rare occurrence—one physician, in active practice for more than thirty years, having seen only three or four cases within that period.

The official records of the Chattanooga Board of Health, as favorable as they are, scarcely justify these extraordinary claims. The reports of the board charge 107 deaths to typhoid fever during the last four years. This mortality probably represents over 1000 cases of the disease. At all events, there appears a marked discrepancy between Dr. Reeves's conclusions and the official figures of the Health Department.

I observe, furthermore, that the Board of Health calculates the rate of mortality upon an estimated population of 40,000 instead of 60,000, the estimate adopted by the writer of the paper.

In studying the natural history of any disease as influenced by local conditions and environment, the official figures adopted by competent persons charged with the responsibility of collecting and publishing statistical data are entitled to serious consideration, and should outweigh, it seems to me, the random estimates of individuals, however capable and honest they may be.

The line between facts and mere opinions should be sharply drawn, and the opinions, to be trustworthy, should be supported by the facts ; otherwise confusion may ensue, innocent persons may be misled, and evil may come when only good was intended.

Respectfully,
JAMES B. BAIRD, M.D.
ATLANTA, GEORGIA.

IODOFORM AND IODOL IN DIABETES MELLITUS.

To the Editor of THE MEDICAL NEWS,

SIR : I have just read a very interesting inaugural thesis by Dr. Fructuoso V. Valdés, presented last year to the National School of Medicine of Mexico. The subject of Dr. Valdés' essay is "Iodol," and in it he reports the excellent results obtained, by the local use of the drug, in the treatment of ulcers in general. The observations were made in the different hospitals of the Mexican capital, under the supervision of the ablest clinical professors. Among other cases, he reports, through the kindness of Dr. José Olvera, of the City of Mexico, in whose private practice they occurred, two of diabetes mellitus, in one of which the most flattering

success followed the use of iodoform, in the other from the use of iodol.

I will translate the details of both cases, as they are extremely interesting, one of them corroborating the results obtained in a case recently reported by me.[1]

Dr. Olvera writes as follows : "Last year I attended a lady about fifty years of age, who was then suffering from glycosuria accompanied with polyuria (about 2½ litres of urine daily), general debility, intense thirst, and a very disagreeable dryness of the mouth and fauces. The first time that the urine was analyzed by Professor Morales it gave 33 grammes of glucose and 30 grammes of urea per thousand of the liquid. The patient, four years previously, had suffered for six months from nephritis with albuminuria. She recovered completely, but afterward had a rheumatic facial paralysis of the right side. It was impossible for me to ascertain, at the time of consultation, the length of time since she began to have the diabetic affection, nor the cause of the disease. She was submitted to a rigorous diet, excluding all sugary and amylaceous food, but was allowed to use bran bread. I prescribed a daily dose of 0.005 milligramme of strychnine, and at the end of the second month the 33 grammes of glucose determined by the first analysis had only been reduced by 2 grammes. I then administered a combination of iodoform and strychnine. The third time the urine was analyzed, the reduction was very noticeable, as the liquid gave only 18 grammes of glucose, which encouraged me to continue the treatment. At the end of three months the sugar had *entirely* disappeared from the urine. I deemed it prudent to continue the same diet and medicines for a month and a half longer, after which she was allowed to use gradually amylaceous and sugary articles of food. Notwithstanding the free ingestion of these in the course of time, no glucose could be detected by later analyses, a fact which greatly strengthens my belief that it was, undoubtedly, a case of perfect cure.

"Mrs. R. L. presenting an emphysematous condition and symptoms of a slow, progressive medullary sclerosis, began to notice last December an increase in the secretion of urine, especially at evening, which was the cause of sleepless nights. At first she attached no importance to this circumstance and attributed the disturbance to cold ; but the continuous and gradually increasing dryness of the mouth and fauces decided her to consult me at the end of January last. The urine was analyzed by Professor Morales, who found 29 grammes of sugar per thousand of the liquid. The amount of urine passed in twenty-four hours was calculated to be 1200 grammes. Remembering the good results obtained from the combined use of iodoform and strychnine in the previous case, I immediately proceeded to treat the present one with the same agents. These were administered during one week only and then, according to the suggestion of Dr. Valdés, I decided to substitute the iodoform with *iodol*, but continuing to give strychnine. The analysis of March 3d gave only *three grammes* of glucose per thousand of urine. The total amount of urine passed in the twenty-four hours has also diminished considerably. It is, perhaps, needless for me to say that the patient's diet has been properly regulated.

"From what has been here stated I think we ought to

[1] THE MEDICAL NEWS, vol. lvi., March 8. 1890.

congratulate ourselves on the happy results obtained in the latter case. In the first case it may be that, while the diminution of the glucose was slower under the use of iodoform and strychnine than that of the second case under iodol and strychnine, the more rapid disappearance of the sugar was due not to the action of the drugs, but to the constitution of the patient, the nature of the cause or causes of the disease, idiosyncrasies and what not; however, setting these considerations aside, we have sufficient reason to continue our experimentation in this matter, and further experience will, in the future, decide the usefulness or worthlessness of the drug in question."

I can only add that there is, undoubtedly, sufficient clinical evidence to show that iodol deserves further and continuous trials at the hands of the profession, and not simply as a substitute for iodoform but as a drug possessing its own and highly valuable therapeutical properties.

I am about to make an experimental physiological study of iodol, which will form the substance for a future article.   DAVID CERNA, M.D.

Laboratory of Experimental Therapeutics,
University of Pennsylvania.

NEWS ITEMS.

A New Hospital at Zanzibar.—The Emperor of Germany has subscribed 20,000 marks to help in the establishment of a new German hospital at the capital of Zanzibar, in East Africa.

University of Berlin.—*The Lancet* announces that the chair of mental pathology at the University of Berlin, made vacant by the death of Professor Westphal, has been accepted by Dr. Grashey, of Munich.

· Protection of the Insane against Fire.—In view of the frightful loss of life from the burning of asylums at Montreal, Canada, and Utica, N. Y., the Committee of Charities of the Massachusetts Assembly have framed a bill requiring iron fire-escapes to be constructed on the outside of all asylums for the insane throughout the State. Suitable apparatus for the distribution of water-hose within the buildings will be required, and the trustees are directed to cause a regular monthly inspection to be made of these life-saving appliances.

The Death-rate of England.—The death-rate in England in 1889 was 17.9 per 1000; in 1888, 17.8 per 1000. For each of the nine years, 1881–1889, the rate was lower than in any year prior to 1881, and the average annual rate for that period was only 18.9 per 1000. For the ten years, 1871–1880, the average annual rate was 21.4 per 1000. This shows a saving of 2.5 in every 1000 of the population, comparing the last two decades with each other. The Registrar General of England estimates that not less than 600,000 people in England and Wales at present survive by reason of the declining mortality rate—that is, if the rate 21.4 per 1000 had persisted in the past nine years instead of falling to 18.9, there would have been 600,000 more deaths.

This improvement is no doubt largely referable to the improved sanitary condition of the United Kingdom, more especially in the great cities. One proof of this is seen in the decreasing mortality from zymotic diseases, such as smallpox, scarlet fever, and typhoid fever. Infant mortality, also, has shown a marked decline, and is another index of the life-saving results of an improved sanitation.

OFFICIAL LIST OF CHANGES IN THE STATIONS AND DUTIES OF OFFICERS SERVING IN THE MEDICAL DEPARTMENT, U. S. ARMY, FROM JUNE 24 TO JUNE 30, 1890.

By direction of the Secretary of War, leave of absence for two months, to take effect August 6, 1890, is granted to WILLIAM N. SUTER, *First Lieutenant and Assistant Surgeon.*—Par. 3, *S. O. 140, A. G. O.,* June 26. 1890.

By direction of the Secretary of War, leave of absence for three months and fifteen days, to take effect as soon as his services can be spared, is granted WILLIAM C. BORDEN. *Captain and Assistant Surgeon*—Par. 11, *S. O. 46, A. G. O.,* June 23, 1890.

Captain HOWARD CULBERTSON (Retired) died June 18, 1890, at Zanesville, Ohio.

Appointments in the Medical Department. U. S. Army, to be Assistant Surgeons, with the rank of First Lieutenant. June 6, 1890:

KEEFER, FRANK R., of Pennsylvania, vice Woodruff, promoted.

RAYMOND, THOMAS U , of Indiana, vice Newton, resigned.

SNYDER, HENRY D., of Pennsylvania, vice Wilson, resigned.

SMITH, ALLEN M., of New York, vice Matthews, promoted.

HEYL, ASHTON B., of Pennsylvania, vice Hall, promoted.

CLARKE, JOSEPH T., of New York, vice Porter, resigned.

By direction of the Secretary of War, CHARLES R. GREENLEAF, *Major and Surgeon,* will attend the encampment of the Pennsylvania National Guard at Mount Gretna, Pennsylvania, from the 18th to the 26th of July, 1890, for the purpose of accompanying the Surgeon General of Pennsylvania in his inspection of the camp.—Par. 11, *S. O. 144, A. G. O.,* June 20, 1890.

OFFICIAL LIST OF CHANGES IN THE STATIONS AND DUTIES OF THE MEDICAL CORPS OF THE U. S. NAVY, FOR THE TWO WEEKS ENDING JUNE 28, 1890.

PAGE, JOHN E., of Berryville, Va.—Commissioned Assistant Surgeon in the Navy.

KENNEDY, ROBERT M., of Pottsville, Pa.—Commissioned Assistant Surgeon in the Navy.

WHITFIELD, JAMES M., of Richmond, Va.—Commissioned Assistant Surgeon in the Navy.

STONE, LEWIS H., of Litchfield, Conn.— Commissioned Assistant Surgeon in the Navy.

ATLEE, LOUIS W., *Assistant Surgeon.*—Detached from the U. S. S. " Marion, and granted three months' leave.

OFFICIAL LIST OF CHANGES OF STATIONS AND DUTIES OF MEDICAL OFFICERS OF THE U. S. MARINE-HOSPITAL SERVICE, FROM MAY 31 TO JUNE 21, 1890.

GASSAWAY, J. M., *Surgeon.*—When relieved at Cairo, Ill.. to proceed to New Orleans, La., and assume command of the Service at that station, June 4, 1890.

STONER, G. W., *Surgeon.*—Granted leave of absence for three days, June 18, 1890.

WASDIN, EUGENE, *Passed Assistant Surgeon.*—Granted leave of absence for fourteen days, June 5 and 10, 1890.

WHITE, J. H., *Passed Assistant Surgeon.*—To proceed to Savannah, Ga., on special duty, June 9. 1890.

HEATH. F. C., *Assistant Surgeon.*—Granted leave of absence for fifty-eight days. June 10, 1890.

MAGRUDER, G. M., *Assistant Surgeon.*—Granted leave of absence for twenty days, June 2, 1890. Ordered to examination for promotion, June 5, 1890.

WOODWARD, R. M., *Assistant Surgeon.*—Relieved from duty at Chicago, Ill., to assume command of Service at Cairo, Ill., June 4, 1890.

CONDICT, A. W., *Assistant Surgeon.*—Upon expiration of leave of absence, to report to Medical Officer in command at Chicago, Ill., for duty, June 4, 1890.

RESIGNATION.

HEATH, F. C., *Assistant Surgeon.*—Resignation , to take effect August 31, 1890, accepted by the President. June 10, 1890.

THE MEDICAL NEWS.

A WEEKLY JOURNAL OF MEDICAL SCIENCE.

VOL. LVII.   SATURDAY, JULY 12, 1890.   No. 2.

ORIGINAL ARTICLES.

THE PATHOLOGY AND TREATMENT OF CLUB-FOOT, ESPECIALLY VARUS AND EQUINO-VARUS.

With Brief Reports of Fifteen Excisions of the Astragalus for Correction of the Deformity.[1]

BY THOMAS G. MORTON, M.D.,

SURGEON TO THE PENNSYLVANIA HOSPITAL, PHILADELPHIA.

CLUB-FOOT is not a product of modern civilization; it existed as far back as our records extend; and it presented the same problems to the early physicians that it does to the surgeon of to-day. It is only our ideas as to its pathology and methods of treatment which have been changed. If, at the present time, we can make a more correct diagnosis and have more successful results, we can justly ascribe our advances to the genius and practical skill of Stromeyer, and preëminently to Lister, under whose teachings operations have become possible the results of which may be justly claimed as among the triumphs of modern surgery.

If we consider the history of the operative treatment of club-foot, we find that it naturally divides into three periods, or stages of development. In ancient medicine such poor results followed cutting operations that they were practically abandoned. During this first period little advance was made, and for over two thousand years the teachings of Hippocrates upon the subject had full sway in the medical world. All operative interference was condemned, and the treatment of the deformity consisted in the use of manipulation and bandages, or fixed apparatus, and hygienic measures. With the simpler forms of club-foot this sufficed, as it still does in many cases to-day; but during this period the graver forms of deformity were regarded as hopeless malformations beyond relief, and were the opprobrium of surgery. Even so recently as 1839, we find Dr. Little stating in the preface to his classical treatise on Club-foot, that "until within three years such cases had been to a considerable extent confined to the care of the instrument-maker."

The second period began about 1834, when Stromeyer published an account of his new method of tenotomy, and directed attention anew to the treatment of club-foot. Although it was left for

Stromeyer to make this operation a practicable one by subcutaneous tenotomy, division of the tendo-Achillis had been previously successfully performed by Lorenz, in 1784, and by Petit, of England, in 1779. It had also been successfully performed in 1816, by Delpech, to whom the credit is due of having first indicated the principle, which he was unable to carry out, of keeping the wound secure from contact with the air, in order to obtain satisfactory results.

The third and present period began with the introduction of antiseptic wound treatment, first scientifically formulated by Sir Joseph Lister, less than a score of years ago.

With thorough antisepsis the dangers of inflammation and suppuration may be said to exist no longer. The operator may now safely explore the ankle-joint, divide tendons or fascia by open incision; remove a wedge from the tarsus; extirpate the astragalus, cuboid, or any other portion of the joint; in short, do whatever may be deemed necessary to secure proper redressment of the foot, without fear of the consequences, or causing more reaction, as the rule, than that from a simple incision.

Pathology and Morbid Anatomy.—The pathology of congenital club-foot, in some points, is perhaps still unsettled. In the acquired non-traumatic form it is generally admitted that the majority of cases have their origin in infantile paralysis, although other influences and lesions may likewise cause the deformity.

Regarding the intimate nature or the cause of congenital club-foot, there are good reasons for believing that in most cases, if not in all, the affection in its pathology resembles very closely the infantile form of spinal paralysis, if, indeed, it be not identical with it. In any given case of congenital club-foot, however, we will find in one or more of the muscles or groups of muscles of the leg and foot more or less paresis or actual paralysis, and in other opposing or correlated muscles tonic spasm, or contraction. In consequence of the nerve lesion, the supply of nerve force to the limb is defective, disturbances of nutrition naturally follow, and more or less atrophy results, which even under the most favorable circumstances is never more than partially recovered from.

This may be easily understood when we recall the fact that not only is the growth of muscle and bone impaired, but as Cruveilhier pointed out, even the

---

[1] Read before the American Surgical Association, May, 1890.

nerves and bloodvessels are imperfectly developed, and are smaller than in the normal limb. Where there is double club-foot, we can say positively that there never will be even fairly well-formed extremities; the legs are much more spindle shaped than in the single form, because the central lesion has been more severe. That cell-life and cell-growth are seriously affected by the original lesion is manifested by the general atrophy, involving all the structures of the foot, leg, and thigh; the circulation is defective, as is demonstrated by the blueness of the skin and the comparative coldness of the extremity. The leg and thigh bones are shorter and of smaller size than on the sound side, and this want of symmetry of the limbs becomes more and more evident as the patient advances to adult age.

It seems only reasonable to assume in explanation of the difference between the various grades of congenital club-foot, that the amount of deformity is dependent upon the extent of the lesion, and also upon the period of intra-uterine life during which the nerve lesion or palsy occurred. If the palsy occurred at an early stage of fœtal development, it is likely to give rise to the more marked forms of tarsal distortion, because the tarsus when cartilaginous is more readily affected by the force exerted by abnormal muscular action. On the contrary, should the paralysis occur toward the close of gestation, the tarsus being already formed, there is less likelihood of malformation or displacement of the bones, and the distortion is mainly in the soft structures.

It is perhaps not possible to determine positively when the intra-uterine paralysis occurs, which results in the formation of any case of club-foot. In some cases we find one or more of the tarsal bones involved in the deformity, in others only the soft structures; and when the bones are displaced and misshapen it seems probable that there must have been long-continued paralysis of some muscles and contraction or spasm of others. If the palsy occurred very early in fœtal life an entire change in the bony joint may result, the principal variation in such a case being likely to involve the position of the astragalus. When the palsy has occurred at a later period of intra-uterine life, the anterior tarsus may become somewhat displaced, and later on, when the os calcis and the astragalus are fairly well ossified (or subsequent to the seventh month), the distortion will probably be found almost entirely in the soft parts. Later on in life we find severe, aggravated, or so-called inveterate forms of varus, or equino-varus, due either to ineffectual or improper treatment, to neglect after operation, or to the entire want of treatment.

The most important features in the pathology of club-foot, therefore, may be said practically to consist in:

1. The period of life at which it occurs.
2. Whether the foot has been used in walking.
3. Whether there has been any previous treatment or unsuccessful operations.

A consideration of these points will naturally indicate the general outline of treatment.

Varieties of Club-foot.—In every case of club-foot we find interference with the function of the ankle and foot, with limitation of the normal range of mobility, usually accompanied with more or less deformity or distortion. When this limitation exists in the antero-posterior plane we have either inversion or eversion of the sole of the foot (talipes varus or valgus); or we may have combinations of both forms (talipes equino-varus or valgus, talipes calcaneo-varus or valgus).

At birth there is one form of club-foot which is of such constant occurrence that it may be regarded as the typical congenital variety; it is varus or equinovarus. In comparison with this all other forms of club-foot are very infrequent.

Treatment.—The more modern treatment of talipes, by the aid of which we are enabled to accomplish so much for its relief, is the direct result of our present methods of wound treatment. I repeat, that it would not have been possible to perform the operations now practised, nor to have improved so generally upon the old methods of treating these deformities, without the aid of antiseptics. We can now, without danger, and in a very short time, accomplish more than could ever have been gained by the former measures, even after months or years of treatment. Therefore, it may safely be asserted that the introduction of the modern wound dressing has completely revolutionized the treatment of the severer forms of talipes, and thus the way has been opened for early and absolute correction of all malpositions, whether congenital or acquired, by operations peculiar to modern surgery.

There still exists a very decided diversity of opinion among surgeons in regard to the treatment of talipes. It is maintained by some, that, with proper management from birth all cases of club-foot, without exception, can be cured, and that even tenotomy is seldom, if ever required. Some advise tenotomy soon after birth, while others condemn tendon-section as totally unjustifiable and premature, until the child is ready to walk and exercise the foot. Even in the more inveterate forms of talipes of young persons or adults, where there has been no treatment, or improper treatment, or neglect after operation, we may state that the operation as yet has not been established. It is most unfortunate that such widely different views should still exist, and it would seem that by this time some well-defined rule for guidance should have been formulated. We have but to observe the diverse opinions, the array of surgical methods recommended, the great variety of apparatus devised, and the unsatisfactory results, to demonstrate that the question of treatment of club-foot is yet practically unsettled.

From what has been stated regarding the pathology of the deformity, it can readily be understood why there can be no successful plan of routine treatment for club-foot. Each case must be studied by and for itself, the object being to restore the deformed foot to the normal or as near to it as can be done, to retain it in this position, and to restore its function as soon as possible. Excluding all varieties of foot deformity which include valgus and calcaneus, and which give rise to little, if any, difficulty in their treatment, I shall confine myself strictly in this discussion to the two really important varieties of congenital club-foot, namely *varus* and *equino-varus*.

The other varieties of congenital talipes, which include the different forms of valgus and calcaneus, are rarely met with at birth. These deformities always present more serious nerve-lesions than are found in varus and equino-varus. The acquired forms of valgus and calcaneus are also the result of a more marked paresis or general paralytic muscular condition.

Recently, in a case of acquired calcaneus in a boy four years of age, in whom the paralysis occurred at the age of two years, I found the normal limb one inch longer than the deformed one, while the calf and thigh measurements showed a variation of two inches in circumference; the deformed foot was one inch short.

In the treatment of calcaneus and valgus the application of an apparatus, and perhaps tenotomy, is generally sufficient, and rarely will any severe operation upon the tarsus be required.

Confining our remarks, therefore, to the consideration of varus and equino-varus, we may group these deformities in two classes, as follows:
:   1. The simple, or uncomplicated.
    2. The complicated.

1. *Simple, or uncomplicated.* In this division are those cases which, if seen at, or shortly after birth, can be rectified by traction, stretching, massage, electricity, and the use of proper apparatus. In such cases there is little or no change in the shape, or articulation, of the bones of the tarsus. Flexion and extension are nearly normal, the deformity being entirely in the soft parts. Such cases are so amenable to treatment that by the time the child is able to stand, or ready to walk, the sole of the foot can usually without much, if any effort, be placed upon the ground. Although the varus in these cases can always be corrected without operation, there may develop during this period (or it may

have existed from birth) a disposition to equinus, so that when the child is ready to walk, if equinus exists, even to a moderate extent, the tendo-Achillis should be divided, but tenotomy should never be performed until this time. Afterward the child should be encouraged to walk, so as to keep the foot well stretched, the ankle motion free, and the ends of the divided tendon well apart. An appropriate, light apparatus, should be worn from early age, and subsequently until all tendency to contraction has disappeared. With careful watching, the result in such cases will usually be a perfect cure.

2. *Complicated.* But again we meet at birth with a form of talipes which I have designated as the "complicated" variety. Cases of this kind will not yield to treatment suited to the mild or uncomplicated form. In such cases we likewise find varus and equinus, and although we can usually overcome the varus, the equinus cannot be corrected; the foot cannot be brought into the right-angle position with the leg. In such it will be found that the normal depression on the dorsum of the foot, just in front of the fibula, is filled with a prominent irregular mass of bone which can be readily outlined, especially if the foot be placed in a position of extreme varus. This projecting bone, arch-shaped, is the astragalus which has been forced out of its normal position of articulation with the os calcis. The tibia and fibula are found more posterior than in the normal condition; in other words, from long tendo-Achillis contraction, exerted probably from an early period of fœtal life, a partial or complete backward dislocation of the tibia and fibula has occurred, while the astragalus, at the same time, is pushed forward from its natural position and is rotated. In this manner the equinus is produced and maintained.

In the deformity just described the leg-bones rest in part or absolutely upon the calcis, forming a new joint, while the displaced astragalus represents a sort of a wedge in front of the ankle which interferes with the joint motion, and effectually prevents flexion of the foot to a right angle.

In these cases the astragalus will be found to be the source of obstruction, and it is principally to this pathological condition that our attention must be directed.

It is beyond question, I am quite confident, that a large proportion of the unsuccessful results from operations in talipes, and the subsequent occurrence of the inveterate or severe forms of foot-deformity, are due to this condition not having been recognized or thoroughly appreciated. I am also inclined to believe that tarsotomy, tarsectomy, and the "open incision," so-called, will, if this view be correct, rarely, if ever, be required in the congenital form of equino-varus which I have described. I have on a number of occasions in times past operated on such by tarsectomy and open incision, and although improvement has followed, yet the operation has failed to overcome completely the equinus; and subsequently I have been compelled to remove the astragalus in order to correct the deformity, to bring the foot properly on the ground, and to secure proper flexion of the joint. In all of the cases of the congenital equinus in which I have excised the astragalus, the removed bone was so altered from the normal as to be unrecognizable.

I recently sent two of these bones to Professor Leidy for examination, with a note asking him to identify them, to which he replied as follows:

" The two specimens of bone, submitted to my examination a few days since, are so altered from the normal form that I utterly failed to recognize them as being the astragalus."

Under these circumstances, it is not possible to force the astragalus between the malleoli because of its altered shape and fixed position. In other words, the altered or abnormal condition has become the normal one, and it is not possible to reconstruct the articulation. When the condition just described is present, nothing will relieve the deformity except the removal of the astragalus. This displacement of the astragalus forward, and of the tibia and fibula backward, appears to be the result of traction of the gastrocnemius, with relative weakness of the anterior muscles, having had its origin at an early period of fœtal development before the tarsal bones were ossified and their articular surfaces or facets fully formed.

The removal of the astragalus in no wise shortens the limb, because the tibia and fibula in these cases do not articulate with this bone, but with the os calcis.

We may now consider those cases of aggravated or so-called inveterate deformities, whether congenital or acquired, which have resulted from improper treatment, or from neglect after operation, or which have not had any treatment at all.

Inveterate Club-foot.—Cases of congenital or acquired equinus and equino-varus which have never been treated readily become aggravated by walking, partly by the action of the stronger muscles which are constantly twisting the foot inward, but more particularly on account of the weight of the body. The tarsus becomes more and more misshapen, the inversion increases, the sole of the foot is upturned, and soon the patient walks on the cuboid, or even on the dorsal region, where a dense bursa forms. Gradually the tarsus becomes more and more solid and unyielding, while the foot and ankle are deprived of flexion and extension.

Whether the deformity is congenital or acquired, the object will be to rectify effectually the malposi-

tion. The correction should be so complete that no disposition to contraction can be observed at the time of the operation, and I would lay down the rule that all interfering structures, soft parts or bone, whether the tarsus is considered as a whole or as individual bones, should be sectioned or excised. It will probably be found, as I have shown, that the astragalus is very commonly the obstruction to rectification in the congenital form.

When tarsectomy is proposed, it should be clearly demonstrated that the distortion is due to the anterior tarsus alone, and not to dislocation of the astragalus. If there is equinus with varus, and it is found impossible to flex the foot to a right angle, or if the ankle motion is greatly restricted, and if, at the same time, the region anterior to the fibula is occupied by the mass of bone already referred to, it is certain that the astragalus is prominently concerned in the deformity. In such cases, if the astragalus is removed the tarsus will unfold by moderate manual force, and the foot can be brought into good position ; for it will be found that the space gained by removal of the astragalus will permit, to a very remarkable degree, a replacement of the anterior tarsus. It is true that occasionally there is so great fore-shortening of the skin and deep soft structures on the inner side of the foot as to interfere with the unfolding of the foot and its being brought into normal shape ; and if this condition be found, it may be necessary to also divide very freely the tissues on the inner side. It should be remembered, however, that this open wound may be of considerable size, and must contract in its final healing, and so dispose to the re-formation of the varus. To obviate this, I have suggested and successfully made a plastic operation, by turning upon the wound a flap of integument from the dorsum of the foot.

The treatment of talipes varus and of equino-varus, congenital or acquired, simple, complicated, or inveterate, we may briefly sum up as follows :

1. *Simple or uncomplicated* congenital varus and equino-varus can be cured without operation other than an occasional tenotomy of the tendo-Achillis.

2. *Complicated* congenital equino-varus which is associated with dislocation or displacement forward of the astragalus, requires excision of this bone and tenotomy of the tendo-Achillis.

3. *Mild, severe, or inveterate* talipes, whether congenital or acquired, which has never been treated, or has been neglected after treatment, or improperly operated upon, may require, according to the deformity, tenotomy, excision of the astragalus or cuboid, tarsectomy or open incision, or combinations of these operations.

Operation for Excision of the Astragalus.—The operation presents no special difficulty. The

Esmarch bandage should be used. The astragalus being, in this case, merely subcutaneous, it is readily exposed by an incision, which should include the most prominent part of the bone, extending from the end of the external malleolus in a straight or slightly curved line to the base of the metatarsal bone of the middle toe. The knife is then carried around the circumference of the bone and the attachments severed, when the bone may be grasped and ·lifted with bone-forceps; the sub-astragaloid ligament and other tissues can be divided either with the knife, curved scissors, or blunt-hook knife devised by Lund. The tendo-Achillis should always be divided. The wound is brought together with interrupted gut-suture, and a few strands of the same are carried to the bottom of the wound to insure drainage. Before, during, and after the operation rigid antiseptic measures should be used. Immediately after the operation the foot should be capable of being placed in an easy, natural position without any tension. If there should be the slightest disposition in the foot to reassume an abnormal position, search should be made for all contracted tissues, and such should be sectioned. The line of sutures is covered with protective, over which is applied the bichloride-gauze dressing, or the mercury and zinc moist gauze; this is held in position by a wet sublimate-gauze bandage, leaving the extreme ends of the toes exposed. Antiseptic cotton, another wet, and then a dry bandage completes the dressing.

A posterior, well-padded, right-angle, flat, tin splint is then applied. Care should be taken to have the heel well down and the deformity *slightly* over-corrected. If there is no soiling of the dressings they need not be disturbed for several weeks. Usually at the end of a month the wound is firmly closed, and shortly after this, or so soon as the child makes any effort, he should be encouraged to walk, when the tin splint must make way for the ordinary talipes walking-shoe.

Tarsectomy.—That no less than eleven different forms of tarsectomy have been described for the cure of club-foot would seem to show that surgeons have not found any one of these operations giving perfectly satisfactory results. The very fact that relapses have occurred after the most carefully conducted tarsectomies, shows that probably the pathology of the deformity has not been properly understood. A year ago a boy four years of age was brought to me with double equino-varus, a typical congenital case to which no treatment had ever been directed. I performed tarsectomy, made the open incision, divided the anterior and posterior tibial tendons, the plantar fascia and the tendo-Achillis in each foot. Although a fairly satisfactory result was obtained, yet the feet could not be planted squarely on the ground when the child stood up-

right, nor could they be brought to a right angle with the leg. I observed that flexion was from the first markedly restricted, but hoped that in time this would be overcome.

The boy was again brought to me a year later (in March last) with marked equino-varus of both feet with great contraction on the inner side where the open incision was made. There was total inability to flex the feet to a right angle, and the obstruction to ankle motion was found upon examination to be due to a displaced astragalus. At the time of the first operation the pathological conditions which I now believe prevail in all cases of congenital equino-varus of the complicated form were not so fully recognized, and I can understand why the tarsectomies were of but little, if any, benefit. Finding that another operation would be necessary, I removed the astragalus in each foot with entirely satisfactory results.

· I am, therefore, quite prepared, after considerable experience, to believe that tarsectomy and the open incision, except possibly in the inveterate deformities of more mature years or in adults, will seldom if ever be required.

To illustrate the foregoing principles, I submit the following notes of cases in which the treatment by excision of the astragalus gave results that could be attained by no other method with which I am acquainted.

CASE I. *Congenital equino-varus; unsuccessful operations in early life; excision of the astragalus; cure.*—Thomas C., aged fourteen, was admitted to the Orthopædic Hospital June 12, 1889. He had been operated upon for club-foot when nine months

FIG. 1.

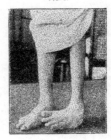

Case I. Congenital equino-varus. Unsuccessful operation in early life.

old by general tenotomy, and had worn braces for several years without benefit. His condition was as follows: Left foot, congenital equino-varus with great outward displacement and rotation of astragalus, its fibular articular process presenting subcntaneously in the central plane of the leg. . Considerable atrophy. Right foot normal, three-fourths of an inch longer than the left. (Fig. 1.)

July 16, the astragalus was excised through a curvilinear incision extending from half an inch above the external malleolus to the base of the metatarsal bone of the ring toe. The bone had to be split with cutting pliers before the sub-astragaloid ligament could be divided; otherwise the operation was easy. Tendo-Achillis divided. Catgut drain, permanent antiseptic dressing, and right-angle tin splint were used.

August 11, twenty-six days after the operation, dressed for the first time; foot in excellent position and condition; wound healed, save a very superficial ulcer.

13th. Wound entirely cicatrized.

28th. Brace applied, and he was able to walk; the foot presented no tenderness.

FIG. 2.

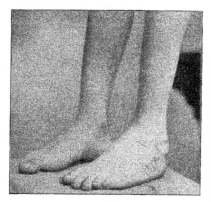

Case I. Condition, May, 1890.

April, 1890. Good ankle-motion; excellent use of foot and limb; position normal. (Fig. 2.)

CASE II. *Congenital equino-varus (double); unsuccessful operation in infancy; excision of left astragalus; cured.*—George H., aged three years, was admitted to the Orthopædic Hospital, August 21, 1889.

Right foot: congenital equino-varus, operated upon in infancy and tendons divided, but foot greatly deformed at present.

Left foot: also operated on previously, but in much worse condition, the astragalus being rotated through nearly half a circle with its tibial articulating surface subcutaneous.

August 22. Left astragalus removed entire, without difficulty, through an incision extending in a curvilinear direction from just above the external malleolus to the base of the metatarsal bone of the

ring toe. Catgut drain, permanent dressing, and right-angle tin splint.

Right foot: Open incision with extensive division of tendons.

September 3. Feet dressed. Right foot: wound closed. Left foot: slight superficial wound.

October 5. Walks well; good motion; position of foot a right angle.

May, 1890. Left foot in excellent position. Right foot, some disposition to recurrence of varus; excision of astragalus advised, and will soon be performed.

CASE III. *Congenital equino-varus; excision of astragalus; cured.*—Alex. G., aged two and a half years, was admitted to the Orthopædic Hospital on September 26, 1889, with severe left equino-varus, the astragalus markedly rotated, and its tibial articulating surface subcutaneous.

September 27. The usual incision was made from the external malleolus forward, and the astragalus removed. The wound was dressed in the usual manner with catgut drain, permanent dressing, and a right-angle tin splint.

November 3. Dressed; perfect cure.

April, 1890. Present condition: position excellent; walks without lameness.

CASE IV. *Congenital equino-varus (double); unsuccessfully treated by manipulation and stretching; excision of astragalus from each foot; cured.*—Phœbe A. N., from Milton, Penna., came under care, February, 1889, when five months old. The deformity was very marked, and the tarsus rigid. Under ether the feet were thoroughly stretched—neither foot, however, could be brought to a right angle with the leg—tin splints were applied, removed each day, and massage and traction used.

April 10. Stretched under ether, and applied apparatus.

October 1, 1889. No special benefit from previous treatment; upon examination astragalus of each foot found displaced forward and rotated. Operation at once performed; the bones were excised through the usual incision. Two dressings. Three weeks subsequently the child was able to stand; and in ten weeks subsequent to operation was walking without difficulty.

April, 1890. Position of feet good; result excellent; walks with freedom.

CASE V. *Congenital equino-varus (double); unsuccessful treatment by tenotomy; subsequently excision of astragalus from each foot; cured.*—Leon H., aged two months, from Woodstown, N. J., was brought to the Orthopædic Hospital October 20, 1887, with marked equino-varus; both feet involved to about the same extent. Ordered manipulation, massage, and apparatus.

March 1, 1888. Condition about the same; marked equinus; tenotomy of tendo-Achillis and stretching; apparatus to be continued.

October 24, 1889. Deformity has increased; astragaloid equinus very marked; flexion of feet greatly hindered by the displaced astragalus. Operation performed this day, and the astragalus excised from each foot, with perfect rectification of position and motion.

March, 1890. In every respect the result has been most satisfactory ; flexion and extension, and position of the feet excellent.

CASE VI. *Congenital talipes equino-varus ; unsuccessfully treated by massage and apparatus for three years ; excurvation of the knee ; astragaloid equinus ; excision of astragalus ; cured.*—Alvin W., aged four years, no family history of deformity, was brought to the Orthopædic Hospital in February, 1886. He was then but a few months old ; there was marked equino-varus of the right foot ; a weak ankle and slight valgus of left foot. Traction, massage, and an apparatus were ordered.

February 20, 1890. Returned to hospital with marked equino-varus, and unable to flex the foot ; astragalus displaced ; tendo-Achillis rigid. The child, finding it impossible to place the sole of the foot on the ground, had gradually developed excurvation of the knee, which allowed the heel to come down.

22d. Astragalus was removed by the usual incision ; tendo-Achillis divided ; gut ligature and drainage. Dressed on the fifth and again on the twenty-third day, when the union was firm, with perfect position and good motion.

April, 1890. Result most satisfactory, both as regards position and good motion.

CASE VII. *Congenital equino-varus (double) ; stretching ; excision of astragalus from each foot.*— Raymond J. P., aged fifteen months ; has been able to walk for several weeks. No treatment has ever been attempted except daily stretching. Came under my care March 22, 1890.

Present condition : right foot, varus and equinus marked. Impossible to flex either foot to right angle. Astragalus displaced and subcutaneous. Left foot, more severe equino-varus ; otherwise, condition the same as in other foot.

March 22. Excision of astragalus and division of tendo-Achillis in each foot. Feet brought to perfect position and placed upon right-angle tin splints.

Present condition most satisfactory.

CASE VIII. *Congenital talipes equino-varus (double) ; tarsectomy and open incision ; failure. Second operation one year later ; astragalus excised from each foot ; cured.*

Wolf S., aged five years, was admitted into the Orthopædic Hospital in February, 1889, with a very marked deformity of both feet. (Fig. 3.)

March 10. Tarsectomy and open incision, division of tendo-Achillis, of anterior and posterior tibial tendons and plantar fascia.

May 1. Discharged in apparently fair condition of improvement ; directed to wear braces and to continue stretching.

March 20, 1890. Re-admitted with aggravated equino-varus. Tarsus rigid ; astragalus evidently the cause of the deformity ; very limited amount of joint-flexion ; unable to stand alone.

22d. Excision of the astragalus from each foot. The bones were found quite anterior to the tibia, and rotated. The usual incision, crossing the most prominent subcutaneous part of the astragalus, was made ; gut drain ; right-angle tin splints. After the excision the feet could, without the least difficulty, be placed at a right angle with the leg.

FIG. 3.

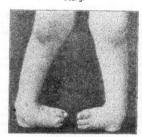

Case VIII. Double congenital equino-varus. March 1, 1889. No previous treatment.

April 26. Position of the feet perfect ; ankle-motion good ; cure perfect. (Fig. 4.)

May 10. Walking without apparatus and with ordinary shoes ; limbs straight ; feet turn out.

FIG. 4.

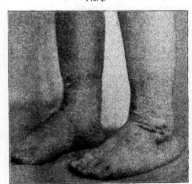

Case VIII. Condition after excision of each astragalus. Feet at right-angle to legs.

CASE IX. *Congenital talipes equino-varus : manipulation, stretching, and apparatus : no improvement ; excision of astragalus ; cure.*

Harry W., aged sixteen years, was admitted to the Orthopædic Hospital, April 14, 1890. The right limb normal. Left, severe equino-varus and marked atrophy of entire limb ; for many years has been walking without any apparatus. Ankle very rigid ; general atrophy of the limb. The right thigh measures in circumference fifteen and one-half inches ; calf, eleven and one-half inches.

The left thigh measures ten inches; calf, eight and one-half inches. The left foot is much shorter than the right.

April 19. Astragalus excised through usual incision; tendo-Achillis divided; foot placed without tension in normal position; usual dressing; catgut drain; right-angle tin splint.

May 10. Dressed; position excellent; superficial ulcer.

CASE X. *Congenital equino-varus (double); unsuccessful operations in infancy; deformity excessive; excision of astragalus, cuboid, cuneiform, and part of the scaphoid.*

Dorothea R., aged seven, from Towanda, Pa., was admitted to the Orthopædic Hospital, April 22, 1890. General health good; no family history of deformity; weight, forty-six pounds.' When five months old was operated upon by general tenotomy, stretching, and fixed dressings. The feet became inflamed and ulcerated; all treatment was abandoned; contractions increased; subsequently apparatus was applied and worn for some months. During the past three years has had no treatment.

Condition on admission.—The thighs, legs, and feet markedly atrophied and spindle-shaped; thigh-and leg-bones small; feet more solid and deformed than I have ever known at such an age. Patient walks on the cuboid bones; great contraction of all the soft parts, including the sole and inner side; ankle-joints apparently ankylosed.

April 26. Right foot; the usual incision made for astragalus excision. The tarsus was found so dense and distorted and the bones so firmly wedged that it was with the greatest difficulty that the articulations could be identified.

The astragalus, cuboid, external cuneiform, and a portion of the scaphoid required removal, in order to bring the foot to a right angle with the leg. The tendo-Achillis was divided; likewise the plantar fascia and the flexor tendons of all the toes. The wasting and contraction of the soft parts on the inner side and the sole of the foot presented great impediment to rectification. The left foot required exactly the same treatment. The wound was closed by interrupted gut-sutures, drained by a few strands of same material, and dressed in the usual manner. The feet were placed upon right-angle, well-padded tin splints.

May 12. Doing well; has not been dressed since the operation; feet in excellent position.

Résumé.—The records of these cases present fifteen excisions of the astragalus for congenital equino-varus upon ten patients, all males with the exception of one. Five had been unsuccessfully treated in infancy or early life by tenotomy, tarsectomy, or otherwise; in four cases both feet were operated upon at the same time. Four of the patients were under two years; the others were, respectively, three, four, six, seven, fourteen, and sixteen years old. The line of incision in the operations extended from half an inch or so above the external malleolus to near the base of the metatarsal bone of the fourth or ring toe, crossing the most prominent part of the astragalus; the tendo-Achillis was always sectioned. No vessel required ligation. The peronei tendons were not involved in the operation. A few strands of catgut were inserted in the wound to secure drainage. Strict antiseptic precautions were observed before, during, and after the operation. The limb was placed upon a right-angle tin splint and kept elevated for a day or two. Immediate union followed; the primary dressings were not disturbed before the end of the third, generally in the fourth, week.

Although, perhaps, sufficient time has not elapsed to give a positive opinion as to all of these cases, yet, so far, the results have been much more satisfactory than in any former operations for similar deformities in my experience.

I believe that we have more reason to expect permanent correction of the deformity after the operation of excision of the astragalus, from the fact that the cause of the obstruction is removed, so that the foot can be brought to a right angle and the whole of the sole of the foot can be normally placed upon the ground when the patient stands. The motion of the joint is also increased by the removal of the bony wedge which so seriously interferes with flexion. There has not been in any case a tendency to ankylosis nor any tenderness or want of strength in the ankle as a result of the operation. If I have correctly appreciated the pathology of these cases, I think that we are warranted in claiming that, by the means proposed, better and more permanent results will be obtained than by any other method which has been devised for the relief of these complicated forms of club-foot.

It is well, however, to bear in mind that no matter what form of operation is performed for the correction of talipes, nor how perfect may be the immediate result, a disposition to recurrence of the deformity may continue for a long time from the persistent unequal muscular action, which demands watchful care to insure a permanent successful result.

THE RELATION OF PERIPHERAL IRRITATION TO DISEASE; CONSIDERED FROM A THERAPEUTIC STANDPOINT.[1]

BY SIMON BARUCH, M.D.,

PHYSICIAN TO MANHATTAN GENERAL HOSPITAL, AND TO THE NEW YORK JUVENILE ASYLUM, ETC.

THE most important element in the discussion of this question is the influence of its decision upon our therapeutic procedures.

Whether peripheral irritations be etiological factors by reason of sympathetic effect, as was formerly

---

[1] Discussion at Stated meeting of New York Academy of Medicine, May 1, 1890.

taught, or, as a more refined pathology and more scientific inquiry into pathological processes claim to have ascertained, it be due to reflex agencies acting through the spinal cord, the chief aim of our therapeutic endeavors must be at the point of irritation. The removal of the source of peripheral irritation becomes imperative. If, on the other hand, as Dr. M. Allen Starr has correctly pointed out and as the general practitioner but too often has occasion to observe after much bootless attacking of peripheral disturbing causes by specialists, many so-called neuroses are really but the manifestations of a slight or serious defect of control by the higher centres due to their impaired nutrition and consequent impaired activity, the course of the medical attendant must be clear.

Who shall decide these different problems which now more than ever press for solution?

The method of arranging a symposium on the great medical questions of the day must be of advantage. It brings out prominently the elements of each question as viewed from different standpoints, if the essayists are selected for the diversity as well as the honesty of their respective views.

It was a wise suggestion, too, of Dr. Jacobi to afford the general practitioner a hearing on the subject offered for discussion, for he stands, as it were, upon neutral ground, watching eagerly the friendly contests of his colleagues and co-laborers, the specialists, and appropriating the wheat as they sift it from the abundant chaff by the threshing of contending views.

Therapeutic questions have ever possessed a fascination for me. In the course of the past thirty years it has not infrequently been my privilege to observe the budding forth of plausible theories, to watch them as they developed into lusty plants, only to see them blighted when the clear light of strict clinical test beat upon them.

When the lamented Hack called the attention of the profession to the attractive theory of reflex neuroses traceable to the nose, I was, although he offered us such positive clinical illustrations, somewhat reluctant in recognizing the validity of his claim. Some of the arguments which were brought against the idea of sensitive areas in the nose as the cause of reflex troubles of diverse and utterly incompatible characters confirmed the therapeutic scepticism which is the natural outgrowth of advancing years, and the doubts thus aroused were somewhat strengthened by the enthusiasm of the author. But a case presented itself shortly after reading Hack's original pamphlet which enlisted my interest. A man aged twenty-four years was brought to me by Dr. L. Peiser, with the following history :

He had been complaining for one year of a "sticking pain on the right side of the neck"

about the apex of the carotid triangle. This pain was so severe at times that it deprived him of sleep. He also suffered from a dry cough and, what annoyed him more, violent attacks of sneezing ten or twelve times in succession, recurring four or five times a day. His acquaintances twitted him because he "sneezed like a cat." His appearance was worn and dull. The right lower turbinated covering was cavernous and doughy, and touching the septum which presented numerous sensitive spots. The lower turbinated on the left side also touched the septum and was sensitive but not doughy. The uvula was elongated. Posterior rhinoscopy revealed spongy hypertrophies on the lower turbinated. The right anterior turbinated swelling was thoroughly cauterized with the galvano-caustic point, under cocaine. Ten days later he claimed an improvement ; two sensitive spots on the septum were now cauterized. Six days later pains in the neck had disappeared. Cough continuing, a portion of the elongated uvula was cut off and the left lower turbinated was cauterized. After two more cauterizations of sensitive spots on the septum, his nasal fossæ were clear and free. Sneezing, cough, and pain subsided.

The attacks of sneezing in this case were probably due to mechanical irritation, for, as Hack has shown, and as I have frequently observed, the "erectile" turbinated coverings are subject to enlargement and to diminution by mental and physical causes. The cough, too, was probably due to the elongated uvula. But the pain in the neck was probably reflex.

It is just as important to adopt local treatment, whether the peripheral irritation produces symptoms through mechanical or through reflex channels. But it is well to differentiate these conditions for the sake of scientific accuracy, as was done in this case. The first positive case which removed my scepticism on the reflex influence of nasal irritation is a cure of true epilepsy, the only one which has ever occurred under my observation :

A. K., aged sixteen years, a robust boy, had been suffering from distinct attacks of *grand mal* since the summer of 1884.

The free use of bromide, by my friend, the late Dr. Wm. Frothingham, diminished the number of attacks and finally gave immunity for one year. But they returned with greater frequency, and continued despite increased quantities of bromide. Dr. Frothingham having referred the case to me on April 1, 1886, it occurred to me that an enchondroma on the left side of the anterior portion of the septum, which filled the entire fossa in front, forcing the ala far beyond its normal line, might be a peripheral irritant bearing etiological relations to the epilepsy. After failure with the galvano-cautery, as advised by Woakes, I removed the entire growth with a Bosworth saw. The bromides were continued until September, 1889. He had an attack a week after the operation, but since then he has been entirely exempt, although during the past seven months he has taken no bromides.

An immunity from attacks for four years may probably be regarded as a recovery from the disease. Similar cases are on record in recent literature, the most recent addition being six cases of epilepsy reported by Schneider.[1] These cases cured, after the failure of active bromide treatment, by removal of pathological conditions in the nose, furnish interesting reading to those who are sceptical regarding the influence of peripheral irritation in disease.

A disease like epilepsy, in the presence of which we stand almost helpless, demands the utmost scrutiny of search for possible etiological factors.

There are a sufficient number of cases recorded by reliable observers to warrant us in adding the nose to the field of possible points of reflex irritation. Empirical though such treatment may be and probably inexplicable upon strictly scientific principles, it behooves us to remove all pronounced abnormal conditions existing in the nose, *as an auxiliary therapeutic measure.*

With regard to asthma, migraine, trigeminal neuralgia, and minor nervous affections, the conditions are different.

The nose presents a field for thorough study of the question at issue, and it should be utilized to the fullest extent. Unlike the ovaries and urethra or other internal organs, we may subject it to tests which are impossible in these organs. It is not difficult to ascertain the presence of sensitive areas in the nose, even if the patient's attention has not been directed to them by actual symptoms. If irritation by the probe produces the paroxysm of migraine, asthma, or neuralgia, we have evidence that can be obtained from no other organ. And if in addition to this, we succeed in removing the attack, either artificially or spontaneously produced, by complete cocaine anæsthesia of the sensitive areas, the etiological connection is demonstrated beyond a doubt, and the treatment is clear. In a recent paper on asthma, Professor Dielafoy of Paris, recommended a cocaine application to the nose as the first step in the treatment. This is a wise suggestion, for if, as our *confrères*, the rhinologists, claim with some show of reason, nasal irritation may be the starting-point of an asthmatic paroxysm, the latter must surely be abated by inhibiting the sensitiveness of these spots. But here an error may creep in. It will not suffice simply to brush the nose with a two-per-cent. solution of cocaine. A bulb-pointed syringe or atomizer with numerous fine openings introduced just within the nostrils, would distribute half a drachm of a four-per-cent. solution of cocaine over the accessible portion of the nasal fossa. If

[1] Berliner klin. Wochenschrift, October 28, 1889.

the patient will press the bulb or piston of the syringe during expiration, hold his head downward and avoid swallowing the fluid, no possible harm can ensue, while complete anæsthesia of the entire nasal tract would be attained. If an attack of asthma or neuralgia be averted by such anæsthesia the proof is clear. How many of our enthusiastic friends apply such a test or any other test in these cases? Except the *post hoc ergo propter hoc,* than which none is at times more misleading, we have in these tests a perfectly available method, which I trust will be more frequently resorted to, of discovering the actual connection between peripheral irritation and disease at a distance.

I am of the opinion that the so-called peripheral irritations should only be treated as etiological factors, if they manifest themselves to the patient.

This holds good, however, of all organs except the nose. The latter is, as the epithelium covering its lining mucous membrane indicates, a respiratory as well as an olfactory organ. As an olfactory organ its function may be greatly disturbed or entirely lost without actual damage to the economy. Even as a respiratory organ its functions may be interfered with, without much embarrassment, because the mouth furnishes a vicarious channel for the entrance of air; hence only when very positive stenosis exists does the system rebel and call the patient's attention to its presence, by embarrassment of the respiration or other symptoms. Sensitive areas, swollen and cavernous turbinated coverings, polypi, etc., may exist within the nose, as the cases I have cited witness, without being sufficiently recognized by the patient to call the physician's attention to them. It therefore becomes our duty to search for these abnormal conditions in all those functional nervous disturbances which have been reported as possibly connected with nasal irritation. The tests I have referred to are then readily applied, and the treatment is rendered more effective and less difficult than in many other disturbances. A word of warning may, however, be not inopportune at this point. Operations on the nose are not so free from danger as they have often been represented by some enthusiastic specialists. I am personally cognizant of two cases, in which deviations of the septum were removed by the saw; one with serious, the other with fatal results. The first, operated on while apparently in good health, by one of the most noted rhinologists of the present time, suffered from hæmorrhages and septic fever, which seemed to be the starting-point of a state of cachexia lasting over a year, during which a malignant and fatal disease of the stomach developed. The second case, also in good health when operated on by one of our most active septum-sawers, whose skill cannot be impugned, awoke the night succeeding the operation with vomiting of blood and with epistaxis. He fell ill, and was attended for three weeks by no less than eleven physicians and surgeons. When I took charge of him, the gentleman who had operated gave an obscure history in the patient of feeble heart, loss of appetite, and great apprehension of a fatal issue. I found the urine had been reduced below 20 ounces daily, without microscopic or other evidence of renal disease. An unfavorable prognosis was given. Dr. A. Jacobi, who had previously seen the patient, was called in consultation. The patient died thirty-six hours after I first saw him, simply from exhaustion due to loss of blood and subsequent inanition. A post-mortem discovered no trace of organic disease. There is no doubt in my mind that this death was directly due to the operation for deviated septum, which had been properly and skilfully done, *for relief of embarrassment to respiration.*

When you are told, by our friends, the rhinologists, that the operation for deviated septum, if skilfully performed, is free from danger, bear in mind this testimony of a general practitioner, and let it not be done except for good cause.

In other organs the difficulty of discovering points of irritation is not so marked as in the nose, because interference with their functions becomes more or less burthensome, and in a large proportion of cases calls for remedy.

The eye, for instance, does not brook infringement upon its normal condition without protest—a protest which may or may not be heeded, according to the intelligence of the patient and his capacity for resisting encroachments upon normal functions. Here it is important to inquire cautiously for symptoms, lest by leading questions we be led astray. But here too the connections, if such exist, between peripheral irritation and the existing functional nervous disturbance may be traced, and it should be clearly traced ere the diagnosis is regarded as exact.

Surely nothing is easier for the general practitioner than the inquiry for eye-strain in connection with or independent of the attacks whose causative relations he is endeavoring to fathom. And, if he is in doubt, nothing is easier than to refer such a case to his friend the ophthalmologist. This has been my constant practice since it first suggested itself in my own case, which may be of interest in this connection. Up to within nine years ago I was a martyr to migraine, suffering one or more attacks weekly, which disabled me from work. Although I was conscious of a difference in the refraction of my eyes, I was assured by two eminent oculists that the difficulty was a simple myopia affecting the right eye, with which it was not advisable to meddle. On coming to New York and taking a course of instruction on the eye and ear, I discovered a double astigmatism. Dr. R. H. Derby was kind enough to make a thorough examination of the refraction under homatropine, by which he discovered a high degree of myopic astigmatism in the right and a minor degree in the left eye. The correction of the error of refraction not only endowed me with perfect vision, but the agreeable discovery that the migraine was removed was an additional and unexpected result. Not a single attack has occurred since the glasses were adjusted.

If we do not succeed in relieving the patient of the functional nervous disease for which the ophthalmic examination was advised, we may at least be content that no damage has been inflicted by the correction of any error of refraction that may have caused distress from eye-strain.

This is quite a different matter, however, from the mutilations which have been recently recommended by some of our *confrères.* The mournful record of these mutilated eyes and disappointed patients is indeed, as has been remarked by another, a sad chapter in the history of this subject. The fact that the novel view that "asthenopia," from which nervous diseases of all kinds are now said to result, "is chiefly dependent upon muscular insufficiencies, and is generally to be relieved by operations upon these muscles," is entertained and urged by only a very small number of men who stand alone in this country, and that this idea has not received the slightest recognition in Europe, where the opportunities for testing its correctness are so abundant, appeals to the general practitioner as a cogent reason against its acceptance. The Neurological Society of this city has fairly weighed the arguments advanced by these innovators, and now Dr. Roosa has added one of those valuable practical observations, of which he is so admirable an adept, which must remove the question from the arena of discussion. He has shown us that, among over one hundred healthy persons, 84 per cent. presented a want of muscular equilibrium, so-called heterophoria, and that, moreover, a great deal depends, as has been well-known since Graefe's time, upon uncorrected astigmatism. I was somewhat surprised that Dr. Roosa deemed the refutation of this novel and unsubstantiated theory a cause worthy of his steel. But he has offered us a clinching argument which must lay this all too lively ghost to everlasting rest.

From a therapeutic standpoint the eye as a source of peripheral irritation demands as careful and painstaking investigation as the nose. I am convinced that both promise satisfactory therapeutic results. But our efforts must not be indiscriminate. *Nil nocuisse* should be our motto so long as uncertainty haunts our course. Fortunately we have in these organs means for ascertaining positively the existence of points of peripheral irritation and of remedying them harmlessly. I plead for the more general adoption of these tests before active treatment is adopted.

The sexual organs as sources of peripheral irritation have been ably discussed from the gynecological standpoint.

From a therapeutic standpoint I desire simply to plead for the same principles that I have enunciated regarding the eye and nose. Here, however, we meet greater difficulties. The male genital organs are more accessible to investigation and treatment than those of the opposite sex. Alexander Peyer, our own Otis, and many others have studied this subject from the specialist's point of view. They have offered us clinical data which cannot be controverted. But let us proceed cautiously, and always bear in mind the motto, "*Nil nocuisse.*" Mutilation of these important organs must be avoided, unless the existence of a point of peripheral irritation is clearly established. We have no tests here as we have in the nose and eye, so every other means must be exhausted before local surgical treatment is resorted to. Another point of therapeutic importance is to be remembered, viz., the danger of directing the patient's attention to the sexual organs as a possible cause of his functional troubles. Such a course is almost certain to increase the latter.

The existence of peripheral irritation in the utero-ovarian system has long been a vexed question. While I am convinced that a lacerated cervix is frequently an etiological factor of pronounced type, and while I regard the removal of the local pathological conditions connected with the latter as a *sine qua non* to the improvement of the health of many suffering women, I am also convinced that these lesions rarely if ever give rise to the reflex functional nervous troubles that have been attributed to them. The latter may almost invariably be traced to conditions of general ill health and anæmia, resulting from the local processes which give rise to muco-purulent discharges, to infection from raw surfaces on the cervix, and to interference by pain with comfortable locomotion, rather than to the pressure of cicatricial plugs, etc. These views I have fully set forth in a paper on the therapeutic significance of the cervical follicles,[1] and I must now be content with this simple reference to a subject which has given rise to more acrimonious and bootless discussion than even the insufficiencies of the ocular muscles.

The idea of the connection of ovarian irritation with functional nervous diseases is coeval with the history of medicine. Since gynecology has become a full-fledged offspring of medicine this question has persistently clamored for solution. There has been so wide a schism in the ranks of the special worker in this branch, a schism which is happily narrowing to a more conservative point in recent years, that a general practitioner may well be excused from expressing his views, except to urge respectfully the warning, "*Nil nocuisse.*" I have searched the literature of this subject industriously for the clinical proof that the removal of the uterine appendages has been instrumental in removing pronounced functional nervous diseases. While I am convinced that the ablation of *diseased* ovaries and tubes must and does contribute to the improvement of health in some women by removing foci of infection, distress, and pain, and by removing a barrier to exercise and to the pursuit of the duties of life, I cannot bring myself to the belief that the removal of ovaries or tubes not presenting palpable and well-defined pathological changes is ever called for ; and I deem such a procedure an outrageous violation of the highest aims of our calling, which demands the condemnation of every decent physician.

There are many other points of peripheral irritation whose relation to disease demands discussion. As one speaker has referred somewhat contemptuously to peripheral irritation as productive of nervous diseases, it may be well to mention that we have the authority of Professor Thomsen, of Berlin, for the statement that even serious psychoses may be traced to peripheral irritation. In the *Charité Annalen* for 1888 he gives the histories of five cases of reflex psychoses resulting from wounds of the head, with concentric narrowing of the field of vision and unilateral hallucinations ; and two other cases in which scars in the periphery produced epileptic attacks, and later also psychoses, which were cured by excision of the scars. All these patients suffered anæsthesia or hyperæsthesia, and in all the extent of the field of vision was an index to the amount of the psychical disturbance.

The relation of peripheral irritations existing in the gastro-intestinal tract to diseases elsewhere, has been recognized from the earliest time of medicine as an empirical observation, by which the harmful practice of indiscriminate purging has been upheld. Our literature abounds in well-defined clinical evidence upon this subject. Among the most recent and interesting observations I find one which in this day of over-zealous specialism may serve as an illustration of scientific conservatism. Professor Gussenbauer has published[1] twenty-eight cases of intermittent trigeminal neuralgia, which were referred to him for surgical treatment, and among which he found only four that required surgical interference. The remaining twenty-four yielded to careful attention to existing intestinal torpor. Some of our enthusiastic specialists would do well

---

[1] New York Medical Journal, June and July, 1885.

[1] Prager medicinische Wochenschrift, No. 3. 1886.

to emulate the example of this conservative surgeon and ponder well and long ere they inflict lasting deformities upon the patients committed to their care.

Nothnagel has clearly shown in his *Klinik für Darmkrankheiten* that intestinal activity depends upon the functionating capacity of the intestinal glands, and that many cases of constipation may be traced to the diminution of automatic action in the nervous apparatus of the intestines. That pathological changes in the ganglia of the intestinal muscles, producing constipation, may convey nervous impulses through the sympathetic to the cerebro-spinal system, and then produce abnormal sensations, has been often practically demonstrated.

Nothnagel believes that hemicrania from constipation is due to a venous stasis in the intestines, which impairs the functions of the latter by reason of an insufficient supply of oxygen, so that intestinal irritability or automatic activity is diminished. The latter produces abnormal excitation of the cerebro-spinal system, resulting in an irritation or paresis of the vaso-constrictor fibres of the cervical sympathetic, which in turn produces the vaso-motor phenomena of hemicrania.

Sciatica, formerly supposed to be due to pressure from fæcal masses in the sigmoid flexure, may be similarly explained. This brief reference is made in order to illustrate that many functional nervous conditions may be removed by the old-fashioned and rationally explicable treatment of constipation, and to emphasize thereby the lesson that careful and industrious search for foci of peripheral irritation should be made *in every direction* before the eyes and nose, the urethra, or worst of all the uterus and ovaries are attacked and mutilated.

In conclusion, permit a general practitioner who has endeavored by many years' service in the eye, ear, throat and gynecological departments of our city dispensaries, and by industrious attendance upon the clinics of our metropolitan hospitals, to keep himself abreast of the advances of special departments in medicine, to sum up his views on the therapeutic significance of peripheral irritations, as follows:

1. The existence of peripheral irritation as an etiological factor is well established.

2. There need be no conjecture in the search for such causes of functional nervous diseases in many cases, because we have means, in at least the more recently discovered sources of peripheral irritation, the eye and nose, of detecting and testing their existence.

3. All harmless methods of treatment should be exhausted before mutilating procedures are adopted.

4. Whenever there is a doubt the local condition should receive the benefit of that doubt and treat-ment should be directed to the improvement of the general health, the re-establishment of defective secretions and to the removal of the patient from unfavorable environment.

47 EAST SIXTIETH STREET.

AN OVARIAN CYST, COMPLICATING PREGNANCY; OBSTRUCTING LABOR AND BECOMING GANGRENOUS IN THE PUERPERAL STATE.

BY BARTON COOKE HIRST, M.D.,
PROFESSOR OF OBSTETRICS IN THE UNIVERSITY OF PENNSYLVANIA

MRS. S., married for thirteen years, had one child twelve years ago, when she was delivered by forceps. The lying-in period was complicated and since that time the patient has been in bad health. She was told by one physician that there was backward displacement of the womb with fixation, and that she could never again be impregnated. Another said there was a pelvic tumor. A gynecologist of New York believed the tumor to be a fibroid and prescribed fluid extract of ergot in teaspoonful doses; this was taken three times a day for two months, and afterward in daily doses of a teaspoonful for two years until last July, when the medicine was discontinued on account of the nausea and general distress which it produced. After this time the menses failed to appear, and there soon developed all the presumptive signs of pregnancy; there occurred at this time several sharp attacks of abdominal inflammation. A physician who was then consulted took such a gloomy view of the case that the patient became thoroughly alarmed, and, having heard of Dr. S. Weir Mitchell as a famous physician, travelled to Philadelphia to consult him in regard to her condition. She was bitterly disappointed when Dr. Mitchell refused the case and kindly referred it to me. On examination I found an abdominal tumor corresponding in size to the uterus at the seventh month of gestation. Palpation detected the outline of a fœtal body and intermittent contractions of the tumor walls. Fœtal heart-sounds were plainly heard. On vaginal examination the cervix was discovered, with some difficulty, high up and far forward, directly over the symphysis pubis. Back of it the posterior vaginal vault projected downward with an even dome-like shape to within an inch of the vulva—too soft for a fibroid, too firm for a cyst. On balancing the fœtal head between the fingers placed above the symphysis externally and those within the vagina, the impact upon the latter was so distinct and the head entered the pelvic inlet so readily that the idea of sacculated uterus occurred to me. The diagnosis rested between this condition and some form of tumor blocking up the pelvis, with the stronger inclination on my part to the former opinion. Arrangements were made to induce labor two weeks before term by dilating the cervical canal and then to proceed according to the indications. When the dilatation was sufficient to insert a finger in the uterus the nature of the trouble was discovered to be, not sacculation of the uterus, but a tumor in the pelvis which gave an indistinct sensation of fluctuation.

On the chance of the tumor containing fluid an aspirating-needle was plunged through the vaginal vault and eight ounces of a thick, grayish sebaceous-like liquid slowly flowed into the aspirator bottle. This reduced the tumor in size sufficiently to permit combined version and the extraction of an infant, alive but so deeply asphyxiated that it could not be revived.

The mother did perfectly well for four days, when the temperature began to rise. The fever at first was slight, but gradually increased until on the tenth day it was evident that there was serious trouble. Being obliged to leave town on that day, I requested a colleague to operate for me. Returning a week later, I found the operation not yet performed and the patient in a desperate condition. She had high fever, was reduced to the last degree, and had a rapid, fluttering, almost imperceptible pulse. She certainly had not more than twenty-four hours to live. A laparotomy was immediately done, under partial anæsthesia. A large tumor with dark-colored walls was seen to the right of and behind the uterus, immovably fixed by dense adhesions. It was punctured and discharged several pints of horribly fœtid fluid mixed with putrefying solid particles. Enucleation of the tumor was out of the question. The empty sac was stitched to the abdominal walls and drained, the peritoneal cavity was well washed out, the lower part of the omentum, congested, œdematous, and thickened to about one and a half inches, was amputated, and the abdominal wound closed without drainage. As there was a constant discharge of fœtid pus from the sac, the abdominal wound was simply dusted with iodoform and covered with a piece of absorbent cotton which was changed every half hour, as no occlusive dressing could have been kept clean. The wound healed by first intention. The day following the operation the woman's temperature was normal. There have been a few rises of temperature during convalescence, due to imperfect drainage of the cyst. This has been overcome by a counter-opening made into it through the vault of the vagina. The case at present (eight weeks after the operation) bids fair to end in a speedy and complete recovery.
248 SOUTH SEVENTEENTH STREET.

CLINICAL MEMORANDA.

THERAPEUTICAL.

Is Aconitine "Always Unsafe Internally"?—The above question, which I shall endeavor to answer in the negative, was suggested to my mind by noticing in the table of doses in the *National Medical Dictionary* the statement that aconitine is "always unsafe internally," and also that the dose is from "$\frac{1}{400}$ to $\frac{1}{500}$ of a grain."

From actual experience I am convinced that aconitine is far from being an unsafe internal remedy, but that, on the contrary, it is one of the most valuable and safe therapeutical agents, if given in proper doses, and with the judgment that is always necessary in administering the alkaloids. Like all drugs of its class, it is very powerful; but this makes it the more useful, as the dose

is consequently small, and its physiological and therapeutical effects are rapidly obtained. For nearly thirty years I have used aconitine in place of all other preparations of aconite, and in no instance have I observed any dangerous symptoms follow. I have given it, both by the mouth and hypodermically, in doses ranging from $\frac{1}{500}$ to $\frac{1}{100}$ of a grain, and I would have no hesitation in giving $\frac{1}{100}$ of a grain in proper cases. The latter dose would correspond to about one grain of aconite root.

To employ therapeutic agents to the best advantage, the physician must be able to prescribe the exact dose required. This is impossible with drugs of variable strength. That a crude vegetable drug will vary greatly in this respect is a fact that all must admit, and, consequently, drugs in this form are now comparatively little used. They have given place to solid and fluid extracts which are more uniform in strength. These, ere long, must give place to remedies whose strength has been definitely fixed by assay. It is unreasonable to suppose that the active principle of any drug is an unsafe remedy, for it is to this principle that all drugs owe their virtue. True, the active principles are a great deal more powerful for good or harm; and, consequently, it is necessary to handle them with more care and judgment. By using aconitine we obtain a more rapid and decided effect than we can with aconite, and one that is preferable in many respects.

In concluding this note, I wish to say that I believe, if any intelligent physician will give the active principles an unprejudiced trial for one year, at the expiration of that time he will agree with me that they are far more desirable than any other form of medication, and that, if handled with care, they are far less dangerous.
                                                    A. L. BARR, M.D.
CALAMINE, ARK.

HOSPITAL NOTES.

EXCISION OF A BRANCHIOGENIC CYST. RADICAL CURE OF INGUINAL AND VENTRAL HERNIA. OPEN OPERATION FOR VARICOCELE.

Abstract of a Clinical Lecture delivered at the Roosevelt Hospital, New York.

By CHARLES McBURNEY, M.D.,
ATTENDING SURGEON.

A man thirty-five years old with a large cystic tumor on the front of the neck was the first subject for operation. This tumor was perfectly round and smooth and projected just beneath the symphysis and body of the jaw, with a deep attachment on the left side beneath the edge of the sterno-cleido-mastoid muscle. It was about four inches in diameter. The tumor had been first noticed when the patient was six years of age, but had caused no disturbance of function and no great discomfort, but had grown very much during the last four years. Dr. McBurney said that it was a branchial cyst, produced from the remnant of a fœtal branchial cleft, one of the four openings between the branchial arches, which are seen at the end of the first or the beginning of the second month of fœtal life. Owing to defective closure of these clefts embryonic structure becomes included in the tissues of the neck, and this is capable of producing large and very serious cysts. Although their origin is so remote, it by no means follows that the development of the tumor is noticed at birth or even soon after, for they may not make their existence known for many years. They are lined with epithelium, sometimes ciliated, but usually of the tessellated variety. This epithelium is the element which has made it so difficult to obtain a complete cure; for, so long as a portion of this epithelium-lined cyst remains, unless there is sufficient active inflammation after the operation to destroy the lining there will most probably be a recurrence.

There was a difference in the situation of this cyst from that of a cyst of the thyroid gland; for the thyroid gland was below the site of the tumor, which did not participate in the movements of deglutition. There was no pulsation to be felt in the tumor.

Dr. McBurney said that in the treatment of this condition all such methods as the seton, which have for their object the establishment of inflammatory action within the sac for the purpose of obliterating it, should be discarded. Evacuation of the contents of the sac and the injection of tincture of iodine are inefficient and unscientific procedures; for the cysts often have prolongations running deep into the tissues of the neck which cannot be reached by such means. Treatment by simple incision and drainage has so often failed that it holds out no special inducements. If the wound were packed with gauze the obliteration might be only superficial, and a second operation is much more difficult on account of the inflammatory thickening of the tissues. Some cases of excision of the cyst are very simple, the tumor shelling out with comparative ease; while others are so difficult as to force the boldest operators to abandon the operation. One difficulty frequently met with is the close attachment of the cyst to the jugular vein. This vein is readily displaced, and is often emptied of blood by the tension made by the tumor, so that a safe dissection of this region is extremely difficult. The plan proposed in this case, which was apparently an easy one, was to dissect down to the tumor and then decide upon the propriety of performing a complete excision. If this were found to be too dangerous, the exposed portion would be cut off, and the wound allowed to granulate in the hope of securing obliteration of the remainder.

A thick reddish-brown fluid, which was first removed by hypodermic puncture, under the microscope showed epithelial cells, fat and cholesterin. An incision was made in the median line over the whole extent of the tumor, the overlying tissue being found very vascular. There was not a single and easily dissected capsule, but rather a number of capsules, each one of which partly surrounded the mass. There was no attachment to the jugular vein, although this vein lay immediately under the left edge of the tumor, which was removed entire without any special difficulty. The wound was irrigated with bichloride solution (1 : 2500), and a few small vessels tied. A rubber drainage-tube was inserted at each side through separate openings and the wound was closed with a continuous silk suture. A final irrigation and the application of antiseptic dressings completed the operation.

CASE II.—The next patient was a young and healthy woman with a tumor in the right groin. The tumor was reducible, and had never been strangulated or inflamed, but had been very painful. It proved to be an indirect inguinal hernia coming well down into the labium. Dr. McBurney said that the radical cure of hernia was especially desirable in women, and he did not acknowledge any contra-indication to the performance of his operation for radical cure, except alcoholism or some advanced chronic ailment like Bright's disease, which would make one hesitate to do any important operation. The mortality from the operation had been extremely low, he having lost only two patients out of a large number, and both of these developed acute alcoholism very soon after the operation. His cases had never had peritonitis, hæmorrhage, or general septic infection, although some of the herniæ had been large and the intestines had been handled pretty freely. He does not consider some other methods of radical cure equally safe; for, in his operation there is no tissue deprived of vitality included under the skin or sutures, and no opportunity for concealed sepsis. Brilliant as had been the results of Macewen's method, he could only regard it as founded on unsound surgical principles. The return to a concealed position beneath the abdominal wall of a tissue like the sac which had been dissected out and deprived of its vitality he could not endorse.

The incision was begun just beyond the situation of the internal ring following the line of the canal as far as the pubes, and the dissection was continued at the upper part until the external oblique aponeurosis was exposed. Then the remainder of the incision external to the sac could be completed in safety. This exposed the pillars of the ring and the hernial sac. The sac appeared to be empty. The canal was then opened, exposing the lower border of the conjoined tendons, and the sac dissected out. If the sac should be cut off at the level of the external ring and left in the canal or sewed up at any point below the internal ring, the remnant would invite a recurrence of the hernia. If twisting the sac were resorted to a portion of intestine might be injured. It was imperative that the sac should be opened, for there might be some omentum or intestine adherent within it. There was an additional advantage in being able to push the finger in and being sure that nothing but the sac was included in the ligature, which could then be applied just above the level of the internal ring. Some claim that if the conjoined tendon be brought against Poupart's ligament and sewed there it will unite with that ligament; but it cannot do so with any strength, for tissues so unlike in their structure can be made to unite only by first freshening their surfaces or by forcing them to granulate. Dr. McBurney does not allow the granulation tissue to form loosely in too wide a wound; for it is not intended that the cicatricial tissue itself shall support the abdominal pressure, but only that it shall firmly bind together the walls of the wound. To accomplish this the wound was harrowed by the use of tension sutures.

CASE III.—The next case was a woman with a ventral hernia, the result of the yielding of the cicatrix left after some abdominal operation. The incision had been quite extensive, and the cicatrix was said to be three or four years old. The patient said that about three months ago, while making some unusual exertion, the swelling first appeared. The hernia was easily reducible, and as it was covered with thin cicatricial tissue it threatened to enlarge rapidly. This case permitted entirely different treatment from the preceding; for these tissues could be incised and homologous structures brought together and made to heal by first intention. He thought it safer to cut down at either side of the hernia to avoid possible injury to adherent intestine. After some dissection the finger was introduced into the subperitoneal tissue. The operator said that it would be desirable to obliterate this loose pouch of peritoneum which had been in the sac, but as the intestine was evidently adherent such a procedure might involve injury to the gut. The tissues were united by a continuous catgut suture, layer by layer, the skin wound being brought together with silk. No drainage was needed. Healing by first intention and strong union should be obtained in three weeks.

CASE IV.—Dr. McBurney next exhibited a young man who had had a swelling in the left scrotum for eleven years. He stated that it had appeared suddenly after making some unusual exertion, and that it caused more or less discomfort. It became much larger a short time ago, after a sudden effort, but it had never been acutely inflamed. It had a peculiar feeling, not unlike that of a lipoma. There was the usual impulse on coughing noticed in varicoceles. The case resembled the kind of varicoceles sometimes seen in connection with abdominal tumors, but the patient had not been examined under ether with reference to this point. No abdominal tumor could now be found.

The subcutaneous method is excellent for small varicoceles; but for large ones Dr. McBurney prefers the open method. An incision was made from the external ring down into the scrotum. The case proved to be one of ordinary varicocele with much condensed areolar tissue which could not be dissected, as usual, by tearing, but required cutting with scissors. Apparently there had been considerable inflammation. The veins were separated from the cord and ligated at the external ring and again a short distance above the testis, and the portion included between these two ligatures excised. There were always enough healthy veins remaining to carry on the circulation. The two stumps were then stitched together with catgut, which brought the testis near the external ring, a position which would be permanent. The skin wound was closed with a continuous silk suture, and a drainage-tube inserted. An antiseptic dressing with rubber tissue and a spica bandage completed the operation.

MEDICAL PROGRESS.

A Successful Case of Inguinal Colotomy for Absence of Rectum in a Child Five Days Old.—DR. T. A. HELME, in the *British Medical Journal,* june 7. 1890, reports a case of this kind. He says: Complete obstruction of the bowels in the newborn child is not a very rare occurrence, and is dependent on one or other of a variety of pathological conditions. Most commonly the cause is found in the imperfect development of the lower bowel. It is a matter of importance, whenever the bowels of a newborn child do not move naturally, to make a careful examination for any gross lesion of the anus or rectum before proceding with purgative treatment; otherwise

the only result may be aggravation of the child's suffering and hastening the commonly fatal issue. The history of the case related suggests the necessity of this precaution, and at the same time the successful result of the operative treatment adopted shows what may be hoped for from timely interference.

A male child, aged five days, came under observation on the evening of April 18, 1890, with the following history : The child was born on the evening of April 13th, when it presented every outward appearance of full and healthy development; the mother was a strong and healthy woman of twenty-six, and this was her first child. Two days later, April 15th, as the bowels had not yet moved, castor oil was administered. The desired effect not being brought about, the castor oil was repeated several times on the three succeeding days, and on the evening of April 18th, as the bowels still remained obdurate, the nurse was ordered to give the child a soap-water enema. As this could not be satisfactorily done, the child, presenting a most pitiable appearance, was brought to Dr. Helme. Its face was pinched and emaciated, its arms and body in constant movement, its legs repeatedly drawn up in a piteous manner on the abdomen, while it moaned continuously ; evidently the child was in extreme pain. On examination, the abdomen was found to be greatly distended, the walls so thinned that the intestinal coils could be seen and their movements watched.

The perineal region presented a normal appearance, but on introducing the little finger into the anus the canal was found blocked by a membranous septum about half an inch from the skin surface. No bulging could be felt during the child's straining, from which it was evident that the lower end of the rectum was not in contact with the septum. Nevertheless, it was decided to puncture the membrane. No escape of intestinal contents following, Dr. Helme therefore carefully dilated the opening already made and introduced his finger into the peritoneal cavity. This examination confirmed his opinion ; the rectum was altogether wanting, the blind bulging extremity of the sigmoid flexure being felt at the pelvic brim. Inguinal colotomy was, therefore, decided upon.

The operation, after washing the anal depression with weak sublimate solution, and introducing a strip of iodoform gauze, was done in the usual way on the left side. The abdominal wall was incised down to the peritoneum, the incision being about one inch and a half in length, parallel to the outer part of Poupart's ligament, and commencing externally a little above the anterior superior spine of the ilium. After compressing one or two bleeding points the peritoneal sac was carefully opened, when the bowel immediately presented in the wound. Two silk sutures were passed through the skin and parietal peritoneum of the one side of the incision (the muscular tissue being avoided), then through the bowel, the peritoneum and the skin of the other side. The bowel was then incised longitudinally for half an inch, the silk sutures were hooked up in a loop, divided, and tied on their respective sides; additional sutures were put in, completely closing the peritoneal sac. An immense quantity of material escaped from the bowel.

For several days after the operation there was considerable redness encircling the wound, and some sloughing of cellular tissue around the adherent peritoneal surfaces. Gradually, however, this healed, the child, fed on peptonized milk, was discharged in an excellent state of health on the seventeenth day after operation. The mucous membrane had retracted within the bowel and the wound had healed perfectly. The sound introduced through the false anus passed in a downward direction for little more than half an inch, striking there the blind extremity of the colon.

This condition, complete development of the anus with absence of the rectum, is rare, and is likely to mislead the practitioner unless a very careful examination is made. Even on careful inspection the child appears to be perfectly developed, and unless the finger is passed into the anus the cause of the obstruction cannot be ascertained.

The history of this case of obstruction in the newborn child serves to emphasize the necessity of a careful digital examination of the bowel before resorting to any medicinal treatment. After the condition has been recognized the choice of operation seems to me a simple one. There are two alternatives, viz., inguinal or lumbar colotomy. But the three facts, namely (1) the small amount of space available; (2) the frequency with which one finds a long mesocolon in the infant, and the consequent displacement of the colon; (3) the relatively large size of the kidney and the consequent risk of injuring it, turn the balance in favor of opening the bowel in the groin.

On the Treatment of Metrorrhagia.—DR. A. W. EDIS, in the *Brit. Med. Journ.*, June 7, 1890, writes that in metrorrhagia a correct diagnosis being the first and most important element of treatment, it follows as a matter of course that having ascertained the presumed cause we know then what our plan of action should be. Still there are some practical hints which may be found to be of value to some. Where the hæmorrhage results from constitutional or general conditions it is not always wise to attempt to check the flow at once, unless it is producing such an effect upon the system as to suggest the expediency of arresting it at all hazards. In certain cases of heart disease uterine hæmorrhage, in place of aggravating, seems to relieve the cardiac symptoms, and should not, therefore, be hastily repressed. Strophanthus, digitalis, and aconite here prove most useful. Where the action of the liver seems to be at fault, attention to diet, abstention from alcohol, and the administration of a few grains of calomel, blue mass, or euonymin, followed by a brisk saline aperient, will probably be indicated. If albuminuria be present, or if the kidneys seem to be at fault, encourage vicarious action of skin and bowels by means of diaphoretics and purgatives, and follow out any other indications suggested. In cases of menorrhagic chlorosis, bromide of potassium in half-drachm doses has proved of service, iron with strychnine being given between the periods and attention being also given to ordinary hygienic details, to avoidance of tight lacing and of physical overwork. It is well to remember that hæmophilia, scurvy, malaria from residence in damp or marshy districts, lead-poisoning, and other unusual conditions will occasionally explain the presence of metrorrhagia. The mere recognition of the cause will be at once a suggestion as to the proper course of treatment.

Where uterine hæmorrhage persists, notwithstanding the employment of constitutional measures, and there is no apparent local cause to account for it, we should without further delay dilate the cervix uteri and explore the interior of the uterus. Numerous instances have been recorded of patients dying from uncontrollable hæmorrhage, where a *post-mortem* examination revealed the existence of some intra-uterine growth, such as a polypus or submucous fibroid, retained product of conception, or fungoid condition of the endometrium, which could readily have been removed or dealt with had appropriate measures been adopted in time.

The insertion of a sponge tent into the cervix uteri arrests the hæmorrhage for the time being, and facilitates subsequent exploration of the uterine cavity. As to any risk of reflux through the Fallopian tube, as sometimes spoken of, it is a mere visionary objection, and need not deter us from employing dilatation in suitable cases. Plugging the vagina is a very unscientific procedure, as well as being unsatisfactory and inefficient. It should seldom, if ever, be resorted to.

It would clearly be impossible in these brief remarks to indicate in detail the methods of local treatment, such as curetting for villous endometritis, removing polypi, operating for cancer, the use of electricity in cases of myoma, the best method of dealing with cases of incomplete abortion, or replacing an inverted uterus. If we have once clearly made out the indications for treatment the remainder is merely a matter of detail. But now and again instances occur where no assignable cause, either constitutional or local, can be made out, and where remedies fail to restrain the hæmorrhage In such cases the hot vaginal douche may prove of service, or even washing out the uterine cavity with hot water through a double-current catheter, provided the cervix be patulous enough to admit it. Should this fail it may be considered requisite to wash out the interior of the uterus with a strong solution of iodine or of iron. As a *dernier ressort*, the insertion of a sponge tent into the cervix uteri may be effected.

The reliable remedies at our disposal for checking or arresting uterine hæmorrhage are really very few. Ergot is unquestionably one of the most potent; Hydrastis Canadensis is a valuable agent and far too little generally known. In cases of myoma it often proves of service when ergot has failed. Hamamelis, which forms the basis of the American nostrum hazeline, is sometimes useful. Quinine and strychnine, alone or in combination, often succeed in checking or arresting hæmorrhage in those cases where the system is much depressed from repeated or prolonged losses. Bromide of potassium in cases of ovarian irritation, and even in hæmatocele, possesses the power of checking hæmorrhage and is equal, if not superior, to any remedy we possess. Chlorate of potassium in combination with ergot has lately been strongly recommended. Opium is beneficial in cases where the loss has already been severe. Sulphuric acid and opium formerly were, and still are, with some practitioners, favorite remedies; also, acetate of lead and opium in the form of pill.

The ordinary astringents, such as gallic and sulphuric acids, have really very little influence in restraining hæmorrhage, and are far too often relied upon. Iron is often of much benefit in those cases where the loss has been very profuse, as in myomata, and where the blood has become so attenuated as to pass readily through the capillaries. Digitalis, in combination with iron, proves most valuable in cardiac complications.

In place, however, of attempting to deal empirically with the effect, we should always endeavor to arrive at a definite opinion as to the cause of the hæmorrhage, and, if we can deal with this satisfactorily, the treatment is very simple.

Prescription for Impetigo Contagiosa.—SAALFELD recommends the following somewhat elaborate ointment in the treatment of impetigo contagiosa (*Medicinische-chirurgische Rundschau*):

R.—Potassium carbonate . . . I part.
Olive oil . . . . . 10 parts.
Zinc oxide ⎱ of each . . . 15 "
Starch ⎰
Salol . . . . . . 5 "
Sulphur . . . . . 6 "
Lanolin . . . . 100 " —M.

Local Application for Diphtheria.—This formula, to be used as a local application in the treatment of diphtheria, is quoted in the *Medicinische-chirurgische Rundschau:*

R.—Carbolic acid . . 1¼ to 2½ drachms.
Camphor . . 5 to 7½ "
Tartaric acid . . 4 to 10 grains.
Olive oil . . 9 to 12 drachms.
Alcohol . . 2½ "

To be applied with a soft brush.

Tiersch's Method of Skin-grafting.—In a thoroughly practical paper upon skin-grafting, MR. W. WATSON CHEYNE gives the following advice upon the methods to be employed (*Practitioner,* june, 1890):

1. The proper time for grafting is when cicatrization is distinctly advancing at the borders of the wound. If we wait much longer than this an unnecessary amount of granulation tissue will form, and the contraction of the scar will be excessive.

2. Before attempting to graft, the surface of the ulcer should be aseptic ; if it is not, suppuration between the granulations and the graft will prevent union. Asepsis of the sore is best secured by washing the surrounding skin with carbolic and sublimate solutions, mopping the ulcer with zinc chloride solution (40 grains to the ounce), then dusting it with iodoform, and dressing with borated lint which has been dipped in a 1-to-2000 sublimate solution. Excepting the zinc chloride, this treatment should be repeated for several days before applying the grafts.

3. just before grafting, the superficial layer of the ulcer should be shaved or scraped off, checking hæmorrhage by the pressure of a sponge under which is a piece of protective.

4. While the bleeding is being arrested the grafts should be taken, preferably from the thin skin of the flexor surface of the forearm. The skin which is to be used should be shaved and disinfected by scrubbing with a 1-to-500 sublimate solution, then with a 1-to-20

carbolic solution. A strip of skin about one inch wide and as long as desired is then dissected off, avoiding the subcutaneous tissue. The strip is cut into pieces about half an inch long, and planted on the prepared surface. The grafts should be numerous and nearly touching one another. It must be remembered that they shrink considerably.

5. When the operation is completed, the surface is covered with protective, and gentle pressure is made to squeeze out any blood that may be between the grafts and the surface of the ulcer. The remainder of the dressing is boric lint, salicylated cotton, and a bandage. The dressing may be renewed on the third day.

The Preparation of Beef Juice.—According to the *Dietetic Gazette*, the following is the proper method of extracting the juice from beef: Broil half a pound of beef for a moment over a hot fire, then score it thoroughly, and with a lemon-squeezer press out the juice. Add a pinch of salt, and warm before administering.

Formula for the Hypodermic Administration of Ergotinin.—BARONI uses the following formula for the hypodermic administration of ergotinin:

R.—Ergotinin ⎱ of each . . 3 grains.
Lactic acid ⎰
Cherry-laurel water . . 5 drachms.
Distilled water . . . 3 ounces.—M.

The dose of this is from fourteen to eighteen drops.—*Gazette de Gynécologie,* june 1, 1890.

An Antiseptic for Midwives.—The Paris correspondent of the *Pharmaceutical Era* writes that the Academy of Medicine has formulated the following antiseptic powder to be dispensed to midwives, upon their order in writing:

Corrosive sublimate, . . . 3.8 grs.
Tartaric acid, ... 15.4 "
Five per cent. solution of indigo-carmine, 1 drop.
Mix and dry.

Each powder to be dissolved in one quart of water, must bear the regulation orange-red label, with the words " Corrosive Sublimate. Poison."

Iodine in the Treatment of Retinal Detachments.—In the Berlin Medical Society, on May 7th, SCHOELER made a further report on the use of intra-ocular injections of iodine in the treatment of retinal detachment. A total of twenty-eight cases had been so treated, and details were given as to the five successful and the remaining more or less successful cases—three of the latter being really nearly complete successes. A number of the cases had been desperate, and hardly suitable, from their long duration, the presence of cataract, etc. Serious hæmorrhage ruined the result in three eyes ; minor extravasations lessened it in two cases ; and in five a brilliant success proved but transient. Based upon a series of studies upon animals, and already attended with some success, the method seems worthy of fuller study, especially by laboratory experiments ; and while an expectant treatment by rest, etc., should always be tried first, there is great likelihood that the method can be used in otherwise hopeless cases with moderate safety and considerable hope of cure.

THE MEDICAL NEWS.

A WEEKLY JOURNAL
OF MEDICAL SCIENCE.

COMMUNICATIONS are invited from all parts of the world. Original articles contributed exclusively to THE MEDICAL NEWS will be liberally paid for upon publication. When necessary to elucidate the text, illustrations will be furnished without cost to the author.

Address the Editor: H. A. HARE, M.D.,
1004 WALNUT STREET.
PHILADELPHIA.

Subscription Price, including Postage.

PER ANNUM, IN ADVANCE . . . . $4.00.
SINGLE COPIES . . . . 10 CENTS.

Subscriptions may begin at any date. The safest mode of remittance is by bank check or postal money order, drawn to the order of the undersigned. When neither is accessible, remittances may be made, at the risk of the publishers, by forwarding in *registered* letters.

Address.   LEA BROTHERS & CO.,
NOS. 706 & 708 SANSOM STREET,
PHILADELPHIA.

SATURDAY, JULY 12, 1890.

THE TREATMENT OF TUBERCULOSIS IN SANITARIA.

GERMAIN-SÉE, with the collaboration of M. JOURMON, discusses in *La Médecine Moderne* (May 15, 1890, No. 21) the utility of special hospitals for the treatment of phthisical patients of moderate means. This is a subject of very great importance, and the attitude of the profession is constantly becoming more and more favorable to the method.

There are many reasons why this should be so. In the first place, it is much more generally recognized that pulmonary phthisis is an affection in the treatment of which mere drug-giving is utterly useless; and measures designed to promote nutrition, as well as special therapeutic means directed against various incidents of the disease, must be faithfully, assiduously, persistently, and hopefully applied in order to be effective.

The average practitioner has not the familiarity with these measures, the hopefulness or the facilities necessary to carry them out in the proper manner. Hence, institutions, with their corps of trained physicians, experienced nurses, specially instructed cooks, their inhalatoriums, baths, sun-parlors, parks, and other desiderata, occupy a vantage-ground in the struggle against this disease immeasurably superior to that which can ordinarily be gained in the homes of any but the most wealthy patients; while some of the advantages of certain institutions cannot be obtained even by the greatest wealth.

Sée and Jourmon advance the following arguments:

In the first place, they claim that the treatment of tuberculosis may be reduced to two terms: first, the hygienic management of the patient; and second, prophylaxis.

They admit that all endeavors to find a parasiticide which would destroy the bacillus tuberculosis and allow the patient to live, have proved futile. Creasote is the only medicament which has retained the slightest credit in this direction, and it is extremely doubtful whether even this has any direct influence whatever upon the life of the microbe. When it has a good effect, this is to be attributed to the favorable influence which it exercises upon the character of the secretions. The problem, therefore, is reduced to the best means of rendering the tissues invulnerable; in other words, to bring about a "normal sterilization." The experience of the most competent observers in all countries shows that measures directed toward conserving and improving the nutrition of the patient, and varying with the idiosyncrasies of the individual, are the only means of accomplishing this. For the vast majority of patients these means are not attainable except in hospitals.

In the second place, the recognition of the specific nature of the disease, especially when one takes into consideration the great number of persons affected, makes it evidently injudicious to place them in general hospitals; even were it practicable there to devote to them the special attention which the peculiar nature of the treatment demands.

A further advantage in the establishment of special institutions is the fact that their location can be selected with due regard to climatic influences: and that all the details of internal arrangement and of surroundings, can be so managed as to reduce to a minimum the disadvantages of civilization, while retaining its comforts.

If typhoid fever alone can be excluded, and there is no reason why it should not be, from among the dangers to which the person of phthisical tendencies is exposed, there will be a great gain. The authors admit that it is vexatious and unnecesary to insist on the sequestration of phthisical patients as a measure of public health, on the ground of the supposed contagiousness of the disease. With proper precautions all danger of its spread from person to person can be obviated.

In discussing this subject all honor and credit must be paid to the late Dr. Hermann Brehmer, who, in 1855, established his sanitarium at Goerbersdorf, in the face of much opposition, winning a success which has led to the multiplication of similar institutions in Germany and elsewhere. The institution at Goerbersdorf, with its accretions of thirty-five years, remains the model to which we must still turn for instruction as to the best means of securing the objects in view. It is now conducted by the assistants of Brehmer and by his widow.

A beginning has been made in this country, and the sympathy and interest of the profession should be sufficiently aroused to induce them to lend every encouragement to make the attempt successful.

It is not of charitable institutions that we are now speaking, it must be remembered, but of resorts for persons of moderate means, who can afford to pay for their board and care, but who cannot afford to pay for the skilled nursing and therapeutical appliances necessary to successful treatment, when the entire cost of these must be defrayed from individual resources. In special institutions, this expense being divided among many does not bear too hardly upon any one. We hope that some practical philanthropist will be induced to found such a sanitarium in the neighborhood of Philadelphia. If it merely accustoms the profession in this vicinity to a hopeful view of the resources of intelligent therapeutics, it will do much to save the lives even of patients beyond its walls.

THE RADICAL CURE OF CANCER OF THE CERVIX UTERI.

ON this important and interesting topic two opinions stand in opposition at the present day. Some operators regard vaginal extirpation of the uterus as offering an excellent prospect for recovery. Others limit their operations to ablation of the cervix with cauterization of infiltrated tissues, regarding the disease as incurable, and seeking in this way to prolong the patient's life and to relieve her sufferings. In his studies upon the catheterization of the ureters, PAWLIK (*Archives de Tocologie*, May, 1890) observed that cancer of the cervix usually spreads laterally before involving the body of the uterus. He also found that the ureters were rarely involved in this infiltration, and that it would be possible to extirpate the pelvic tissue with the uterus without injuring the ureters. Accordingly, in four cases of cancer of the cervix, he inserted a catheter into the ureters and extirpated the connective tissue of the pelvis with the affected organ. His results justified the inference which he drew from his observations. So far as a recurrence is concerned—only one of his patients could not be heard from subsequently—two of the women were in good health without recurrence over a year after operation; the fourth had cystitis with uretero-vaginal fistula. An operation to close this was refused, but the patient's general health continued good.

While the number of cases is too small to base a definite conclusion upon, yet it seems rational to follow Pawlik's suggestion. The catheterization of the ureters, however, while not exceedingly difficult, requires constant practice. We remember very well the skill with which Professor Pawlik illustrates and performs this little manipulation, and under his eye we have successfully followed his example; but when we remember that he embraces every opportunity to practise the exploration of the ureters, and that he finds constant practice requisite to maintain his remarkable dexterity, it is evident that the average operator may have difficulty in following his example. Without a guide in the ureter, it would certainly be unsafe to attempt the extirpation of the peri-uterine connective tissue, and also it would be impossible to tell whether malignant infiltration had not attacked these important channels. In the hands of an operator as skilful as Pawlik the method should certainly receive fair trial, but those less experienced and skilful should attempt it with caution. It is applicable to cases in which the pelvic connective tissue is only partially affected, in which the uterus is movable, and in which the fundus remains intact.

REVIEWS.

PRACTICAL ELECTRICITY IN MEDICINE AND SURGERY. By G. A. LIEBIG, JR., Ph.D., and GEORGE H. ROHÉ, M.D. Philadelphia and London: F. A. Davis, 1890.

THIS book having the stamp of johns Hopkins University upon its title-page at once excites the expectations of the reader. The first part is devoted to a careful consideration of the various forms of the electrical and magnetic apparatus commonly used in medicine, together with the theory of the chemical actions taking place in the storage cell, a description of the electric motor, and the telephone and the phonograph. Though in this part of the book one is somewhat appalled by weird spiral figures, and pages of algebraic formulæ, it must be admitted that a student who has already acquired a thorough knowledge of mathematics and is well grounded in physics will have little difficulty in catching the drift of the subject-matter. To those not so thoroughly prepared an omission of this portion of the work will be found, perhaps, as useful as a careful. perusal, and will, moreover, be less confusing.

Part second is devoted to electro-physiology, electro-diagnosis, and electro-medical apparatus. Into this subject the authors have dipped with great thoroughness, and though their descriptions are not always clear, they are invariably comprehensive. The sins of omission are few. In the chapter upon special electro-therapeutics specific directions are given for the electrical treatment of each disease. Thus, insomnia is treated by galvanization of the brain and medulla, general faradization, subaural and spinal galvanization, and static electricity. These concise yet comprehensive suggestions will, we think, be found of great service to the general country practitioner. Enlargement of the spleen, ascites, diabetes mellitus, and many other conditions are, it is claimed, benefited or cured by the electrical treatment.

We would say, in general, that this book suggests a compilation rather than the result of ripe experience, and that, like all other works constructed on this plan, it has not given the profession exactly what is needed.

PRACTICAL PHOTO-MICROGRAPHY, BY THE LATEST METHODS. By ANDREW PRINGLE, F.R.M.S. New York: The Scovill & Adams Co., 1890.

NOTWITHSTANDING that the book before us, as we are told by the author, was "written deliberately and confessedly for the natural and medical sciences rather than for those who use the microscope as a pastime," American workers in these fields will feel that their needs have been but partially appreciated. What the investigator wants is the simplest possible method of arriving at thoroughly satisfactory results.

Illumination—that matter of the greatest importance for successful photo-micrography—is very inadequately discussed. While admitting that sunlight is, perhaps, the best of all illuminating agents, the author confesses that he has had but little experience with this illuminant, and, therefore, allows the unfortunate condition of British skies to so warp his judgment, that he gives utterance to the regret that those older notably successful cultivators of photo-micrography—Woodward among others—had not the advantages of " equable radiants and very sensitive plates." Does the author imagine that Dr. Woodward continued to use sunlight because the capabilities of the electric, magnesium, or lime-light were unknown to him ? While Woodward's experiments showed that these were useful and fairly satisfactory substitutes for sunlight, he, as well as every experienced worker who has made comparison since, clearly recognized the great superiority of sunlight over all other sources of illumination. Let every one who seriously desires to produce the highest class of work, determine, from the start, to use sunlight, regarding the proper management of which, however, he will find little in the present volume.

Having expressed our dissent from what we are convinced is mistaken advice, it is a pleasure to endorse heartily the author's high estimate of the value of color.

screens and of the apochromatic objectives. The examples of work serving as illustrations are very creditable, especially so when it is remembered that all were taken by artificial light—this, with one exception, being the lime-light. The confusion arising from printing the figures of Plate IV. over the descriptions of Plate V., and vice versâ, possibly extends to only a small part of the edition. Debarring the opinions already discussed, and a few slight inaccuracies, there is an abundance of hints valuable to all interested in photo-micrography.

CORRESPONDENCE.

NEPHRITIS FOLLOWING INFLUENZA.

To the Editor of THE MEDICAL NEWS,

SIR : In *The Lancet* of May 10th, Dr. E. Mansel Sympson describes a case of acute nephritis following influenza, and I have a similar case to report, as well as four cases to mention, in which disease of the kidneys became prominent after attacks of " La Grippe."

CASE I.—Patrick D., private of Marines, aged twenty-five years, a native of Ireland, was admitted to the United States Naval Hospital, Washington, on February 25, 1890, with catarrhal fever, which began on the day before with severe muscular pains, nausea, anorexia, a temperature of 103° F., and a pulse of 90 per minute. About this time the epidemic of influenza was nearing its end here. The patient had also been treated for gonorrhœa from February 11, 1890.

On his arrival at the hospital he was very restless, complained of frontal headache, and of pain in the muscles of his back and in the calves of his legs ; his eyes were red and watery ; nausea, bilious vomiting, and looseness of the bowels were present, with a temperature of 101° at 2 P.M., rising to 101.4° at 6 P.M., and a pulse of 100. Lungs and heart normal ; no cough or expectoration. Quinine was given, but otherwise the treatment was expectant.

26th. No better ; temperature 102.6° ; nausea and vomiting continue.

27th. Much worse ; pulse 96, temperature 102° ; is very restless ; complains of almost constant nausea and uneasiness in the stomach. At 5 P.M., pulse 100, temperature 99.4° ; somewhat better.

28th. Rested well last night after a dose of chloral and potassium bromide ; temperature 99.2° in the morning. and 101.2° at 5 P.M.

March 1. Temperature 98.4° at 8 A.M., rising to 100.6° at the evening examination. Improving ; discontinued medicines.

2d. Temperature normal.

5th. Is up and about the ward. Ordered the following injection for his gonorrhœal discharge: Sulphate of zinc and acetate of lead, of each 4 grains ; distilled water 2 ounces.

9th. Discharge from the penis has almost stopped ; at 8 P.M. he went to bed with a chill, which was followed by a rise in temperature.

10th. Is better ; the urethral injection continued.

11th. Much worse ; had a chill during the night, followed by a temperature of 103.2°.

12th. Somewhat better ; temperature 101.2° in the morning, and 101.6° at 4 P.M. ; complained of uneasy sensations in his stomach and pain in the back; discharge from the urethra had ceased.

13th. Temperature normal in the morning, but rose to 102° in the evening; discharge from the urethra returned.

14th. Temperature normal in the morning, rising to 100.4° in the evening; complained of nausea and uneasiness in the stomach, and of great pain in the right lumbar region; tongue much coated.

15th. Not so well; temperature 100°, rising to 104° in the evening.

16th. Temperature 100°, rising to 103° in the evening.

17th. Urine this morning contained blood, pus, and some *casts;* it is also highly *albuminous;* temperature 101°, rising to 103° in the evening; complained of pain over the right kidney.

18th. Better; temperature normal in the morning, but rose to 100° in the afternoon.

20th. Much better; temperature normal.

24th. Urine still cloudy, contains blood and pus-corpuscles, but the patient is improving.

31st. Urine clearing up; still of low specific gravity and pale.

April 3. Urine pale, specific gravity 1011; contains a little blood and mucus, but no casts.

13th. Urine clearing up; specific gravity 1016; patient much better.

22d. Patient restored to health, and discharged to duty.

As with Dr. Sympson's case, a complication exists in mine. His patient had ancestors who suffered from renal calculus and gravel; and the doctor suspects "hereditary weakness or predisposition" to renal disease. My patient had gonorrhœa, which was treated with copaiba before he came to the hospital, and with a fairly strong urethral injection here.

These two cases resemble many others in which "la grippe" seems to have found a nidus for its redundant germs to work mischief in organs already enfeebled by other causes.

For a time I was in doubt about the cause of nephritis in the case I have reported, attributing it to an extension of the gonorrhœal inflammation to the right kidney, which had been the seat of acute pain; but Dr. Sympson's case, together with some others which I will mention, leads me to believe that influenza was at least one of the chief exciting causes of the nephritis.

CASE II.—A patient died with uræmia at this hospital on January 24, 1890. He had suffered with influenza on January 5th, and was sent here for acute pleuritis on the 9th of the month. Autopsy revealed recent adhesions on both sides, but more on the left side. He had a urinary fistula at the root of his penis, resulting from a urethral stricture; his urine had only dribbled away for several years. There was hydronephrosis on each side. The left kidney weighed four ounces, its cortical portion having almost entirely disappeared; its pelvis and calyces were dilated. The right kidney weighed seven and a quarter ounces, its cortical portion having undergone some degeneration also from the existing hydronephrosis. The Malpighian bodies were small and indistinct; pelvis and ureter very much dilated, and discharging a dirty, brownish-looking liquid when cut open.

CASE III.—On February 28, 1890, a lieutenant in the U. S. Navy was admitted to this hospital with albuminuria; the hospital ticket stated as follows: "Albumin first noticed in urine following an attack of epidemic influenza in the latter part of December, 1889, and the beginning of January, 1890, at U. S. Naval Training Station at Newport, Rhode Island.' A very few hyaline casts were found, and albumin to the extent of about ¼ of one per cent. persisting, with symptoms of lung irritation, cough, cold extremities, etc."

The patient has the lithæmic diathesis, and is subject to rheumatoid pains, and a slight swelling of the feet.

On March 16th the examination of his urine showed a very faint trace of albumin, very few hyaline and granular casts, a specific gravity of 1016, and an acid reaction. He felt stronger, and on going out into the city he came back less fatigued than on other days recently.

On May 2d he was detached from this hospital and placed on sick-leave, his urine still showing albumin and casts.

On May 17th I had a letter from him dated two days earlier, in which he stated that he had not kept up the modified milk-diet on which I had placed him, that he did not feel so well, and had more albumin in his urine than he had while here.

CASE IV.—On March 5, 1890, a patient was admitted to this hospital with pneumonia of the right lung. His hospital ticket described him as having been ailing for ten days before he was received here. His case resembled the numerous cases of pneumonia that followed "la grippe" in this vicinity about the same period. As he came from a tender that had no medical officer on board, he was not examined until pneumonia had set in, and this fact renders it probable that his preceding ailment was due to the then prevailing epidemic of influenza. His sputum was very much tinged with bile, he was intensely jaundiced, and for weeks after his convalescence from pneumonia his urine looked like brown-stout.

The most interesting point in this case is that, about the beginning of May, 1890, his urine was found to have a very low specific gravity, though albumin has never been found in it. On May 6th the record reads: "Urine clear, but of low specific gravity (1005)." In other respects he was quite comfortable, and on May 22d he was discharged to do duty as a servant. His conjunctivæ were still a little yellow; his skin did not reveal anything, as he is a negro; and his urine was normal in appearance. Could the influenza germs have irritated both liver and kidneys, as well as the right lung, in this case?

For the notes relating to the foregoing cases, and for the examinations of the urine, and the necropsy in the fatal case, I am indebted to Dr. D. O. Lewis, U. S. Navy, the resident medical officer of this hospital.

CASE V.—Another case bearing upon this subject has come to my knowledge. A friend and fellow medical officer recently died of pneumonia following an attack of influenza, during the height of the epidemic at Mare Island, California; he had suppression of urine before death, and at the necropsy he was found to have the "large white kidneys of Bright," in fact they were said to have been double the normal size.

While the five cases reported by me do not prove that

the germ of "la grippe" alone caused the renal complications, yet I believe they do show that an attack of influenza often brings to the patient's notice the existence of serious or even fatal kidney disease previously unsuspected. A. A. HOEHLING, M.D.,

WASHINGTON, D. C. Medical Inspector, U. S. N., in charge.

NEW YORK.

To the Editor of THE MEDICAL NEWS,

SIR: The busy round of society meetings, lectures and clinics has given place to the usual lethargy of the heated term, and medical men are more interested just now in planning for a short season of recreation than in medical matters. Those less fortunate ones, who are compelled to remain in the city all summer, are either dazed at the prospect, or, making the best of their lot, have begun their annual struggle with the problem of summer diarrhœa, and are endeavoring to determine the best methods of infant feeding.

New York has not had to wait this year until the "dog days" to record a case of hydrophobia; for a genuine case of this much dreaded disease was brought to Bellevue Hospital the other day. The patient was a middle-aged man, bitten by a dog several weeks previously. He was brought to this city for the purpose of receiving the Pasteur treatment; but he arrived too late for this to be of any avail. Dr. Paul Gibier, who has treated at his institute here about thirty-five cases since last February, says that inoculations made after the appearance of the symptoms of hydrophobia are useless; although he has successfully treated one patient who had already begun to complain of tingling at the seat of the bite, which had been received about six weeks before. I understand that a sufficient donation has been offered Dr. Gibier to enable him to erect a properly equipped Pasteur Institute. The most recent statistics of this mode of treatment lead him to believe that the mortality may be reduced to absolutely nothing.

The ex-internes of our hospitals seem to have suddenly awakened to the advantages of forming themselves into associations, and this spring has witnessed the organization of two such—*i. e.*, the Alumni Association of Charity Hospital and that of the Mount Sinai Hospital. It is to be hoped that they will strive to equal the admirable record already made by the Bellevue Alumni. At a recent meeting of the latter Society, Professor A. L. Loomis discussed the relations of digitalis to cardiac disease. He believes digitalis to be the most reliable of all the so-called heart tonics; but that it requires exceptional skill and judgment to administer it efficiently. It should never be given so long as the compensatory hypertrophy is sufficient to maintain a good general circulation; but when the first signs of irregularity and failing strength are discernible, after careful and repeated examination, the drug should not be longer withheld. It is, he thinks, a mistake to give it in large doses, except in emergencies; and when the case seems to demand doses of more than five or ten drops of the tincture, he makes it a rule to insist upon the patient remaining in the recumbent position. A neglect of this precaution not infrequently leads to sudden and fatal syncope. His guide in the administration of digitalis is the quantity of urine excreted. If the quantity increases while the patient is taking the digitalis, the remedy is doing good; but if the quantity remains small or diminished it is an indication that the drug is not accomplishing the desired object. Where he wishes a tonic effect, he prescribes the tincture; but where large doses are required in cases of advanced cardiac insufficiency, or where it is desirable to produce diuresis, he prefers the infusion. Several of the members spoke of the large doses of digitalis that are sometimes tolerated, and Dr. Van Santvoord said that he knew of a case of pneumonia under the care of a homœopathic practitioner, where the tincture of digitalis had been administered in teaspoonful doses, the patient experiencing no disagreeable effects. Such a case as this is interesting, both on account of the tolerance exhibited by the patient and the disregard of the doctrine of infinitesimals displayed by this disciple of Hahnemann. Certainly, if this practitioner is a worthy representative of his clan, the homœopaths of this degenerate age need have no fears concerning the effect of the tariff reform upon the price of milk-sugar.

At the last meeting of the New York Academy of Medicine, Dr. George M. Sternberg briefly described some of his bacteriological researches in yellow fever, and exhibited a series of lantern slides showing photographic representations of many of the organisms which he has studied in connection with the subject. He said that when one considers the mode of distribution of the disease, and the great success which has attended the treatment of it simply by sanitary measures, it is difficult to resist the conclusion that yellow fever is due to a particular germ, which probably finds a favorable nidus in the fæces. Notwithstanding the fact that he undertook his researches with the full expectation of finding such a germ, no characteristic organism has been as yet discovered. It is interesting to note that throughout his investigations he has never met with anything resembling the cholera bacillus.

At the close of Dr. Sternberg's remarks, the President, Dr. Loomis, reminded the Fellows of the Academy that this was the last meeting to be held in the old building, which has been the home of the Academy for nearly twenty years. During this time its membership has nearly doubled, and these years represent an important epoch in its history; for it was during this time that the sections had come into life. It has been estimated that the collective work of the Academy is greater than the total of all the other medical societies in the State. It is true, he said, that the present building has been the scene of some pretty active skirmishes, both scientific and ethical, but he hoped that all petty jealousies would be left behind in the old building, and that the Fellows would enter their new home with the determination to do better scientific work, and to promote that sociability among the members which is the best prophylactic for those bickerings and petty squabbles, which too often interfere with the proper unity of the profession.

NEWS ITEMS.

The Pasteurian Institute in New York.—The work of Dr. Paul Gibier, in the prevention of hydrophobia, is constantly increasing, and he inoculates about twenty persons daily. The quarters in which his work was begun about four months ago have been outgrown, and a removal to a larger permanent building must be made very soon. Already there have been offers of valuable property made to Dr. Gibier by citizens interested in promoting his work. One offer, that of a large dwelling surrounded by spacious grounds, and not far from Central Park, has many suitable features, and will probably become the future home of the Institute. It is stated that during the current summer Dr. Gibier will visit Europe, and that his place will be temporarily filled by one of Pasteur's principal assistants who will come to this country for the purpose.

The Italian Sanitary Council and the Sale of Nostrums.— The *British Medical Journal*, May 24, refers to the consequences in Italy of certain new laws for the suppression of the sale of patent medicines and other "specialties." The article says " the golden age of nostrums in Italy is past and the iron age has begun. No proprietary nostrums may now be offered for sale in that country unless they are favorably passed upon by the Superior Sanitary Council. Over 200 such articles have .been rejected, and at a meeting on May 13th every article then before the Council was disallowed, and the grounds of this action were made public, namely, that all these rejected 'specialties' contained remedies which cannot be used with safety except under the direction of a medical man ; that many of the articles were actually dangerous, and that many others possessed none of the virtues attributed to them."

The Origin of Hospitals.—In the *Lancet*, May 31, is an archæological summary of the most recent discoveries and researches regarding primitive institutions for the care and cure of the sick and wounded. Hospitals existed in India as early as the fifth century, B. C. In Ceylon, according to the English Orientalist, Turnour, King Pandukabhayo, established a hospital in his palace, and one of his successors, King Dutthagamini, in the second century before Christ, established eighteen such institutions in as many different localities, with a medical staff for each, and the remedial agents of those days. The Buddhist King, Asoka, as shown by Dr. Bühler, had, about the year 250 B. C., hospitals both for man and animals. There were doubtless many other founders of hospitals whose names are lost, but the *Lancet* thinks that their work was less important than that of the hospitals which developed from temporary relief as the result of the spread of Christianity.

· **Beaumont Hospital Medical College.**—According to the *St. Louis Courier of Medicine*, the corner-stone of the Beaumont Hospital Medical College, laid on May 31st, contained a copy of Lawson Tait's *Diseases of Women and Abdominal Surgery*, presented for the purpose by the author.

A Relief Fund for Dr. J. H. Douglas.—Dr. T. Gaillard Thomas has written to the *New York Medical Journal* a letter in which a plea is made on behalf of a physician who is ill and in want, Dr. J. H. Douglas, best known as the physician of General Grant, in his last illness. Dr. Douglas is now an inmate of the Presbyterian Hospital, of New York. Dr. Willard Parker may be addressed by those desiring to co-operate in the raising of a fund for the relief of their afflicted *confrère*.

American Otological Society.—The twenty-third annual meeting of the American Otological Society will be held on Tuesday, July 15th, at the Hotel Kaaterskill, Catskill Mountains. Papers will be read by Drs. C. H. Burnett, A. H. Buck, B. Alexander Randall, F. M. Wilson, Huntington Richards, S. Theobald, Charles A. Todd, O. D. Pomeroy and Lucien Howe.

OFFICIAL LIST OF CHANGES IN THE STATIONS AND DUTIES OF OFFICERS SERVING IN THE MEDICAL DEPARTMENT, U. S. ARMY, FROM JULY 1 TO JULY 7, 1890.

GARDINER, JOHN DE B. W., *Captain and Assistant Surgeon.* —Having been found incapacitated for active service by an Army Retiring Board, and having complied with Par. 12, S. O. 135, June 10, 1890, from this office, is, by direction of the Acting Secretary of War, granted leave of absence until further orders, on account of disability.—Par. 3, *S. O. 153, A. G. O., Washington, D. C.,* July 2, 1890.

ROBINSON, SAMUEL Q., *Captain and Assistant Surgeon.*—Is relieved from temporary duty at the U. S. Military Academy, West Point, New York, to take effect upon the arrival there of W. Fitzhugh Carter, Captain and Assistant Surgeon, and will report in person to the commanding officer, Fort Du Chesne, Utah Territory, for duty, relieving Curtis E. Price, Captain and Assistant Surgeon. Captain Price, on being relieved by Captain Robinson, will proceed to Fort Wadsworth, New York Harbor, and report in person to the commanding officer of that post for duty, relieving Robert B. Benham, Captain and Assistant Surgeon. Captain Benham, on being thus relieved from temporary duty at Fort Wadsworth, will report in person, without delay, to the commanding officer Fort Hamilton, New York Harbor, for duty.— —Par. 12, *S. O. 153, A. G. O., Washington, D. C.,* July 2, 1890.

By direction of the Acting Secretary of War, leave of absence for four months is granted JAMES P. KIMBALL, *Major and Surgeon,* to take effect when an officer of the Medical Department is assigned to his department commander to relieve him.—Par. 6, *S. O. 152, A. G. O., Washington, D. C.,* July 1, 1890.

By direction of the Secretary of War, the following named Assistant Surgeons (recently appointed, with the rank of First Lieutenant) will report in person to the commanding officers of the posts designated opposite their respective names:

KEEFER, FRANK R., Fort Leavenworth. Kansas.
RAYMOND, THOMAS U, Fort Sherman, Idaho.
SNYDER, HENRY D., Fort Reno, Indian Territory.
SMITH, ALLEN M., Fort Snelling, Minnesota.
HEYL, ASHTON B., Fort Niobrara, Nebraska Territory.
CLARKE, JOSEPH T., Fort Riley, Kansas.—Par. 6, *S. O. 151, A. G. O., Washington, D. C.,* June 28, 1890.

CORBUSIER, WILLIAM H., *Captain and Assistant Surgeon.*— Is relieved from duty at Fort Lewis, Colorado, and will report in person to the commanding officer Fort Wayne, Michigan, for duty.—Par. 7, *S. O. 151, A. G. O., Washington, D. C.,* June 28. 1890.

BALL, ROBERT R., *First Lieutenant and Assistant Surgeon.*— Is relieved from duty at Fort Riley, Kansas, and will report in person to the commanding officer Fort Spokane, Wash., for duty. —Par. 7, *S. O. 151, A. G. O., Washington, D. C.,* June 28, 1890.

OFFICIAL LIST OF CHANGES IN THE STATIONS AND DUTIES OF THE MEDICAL CORPS OF THE U. S. NAVY FOR THE TWO WEEKS ENDING JULY 5, 1890.

PAGE, JOHN E., *Assistant Surgeon.*—Ordered to Hospital, Mare Island, California.
KENNEDY, ROBERT M., *Assistant Surgeon.*—Ordered to the League Island Navy Yard, Pennsylvania.

THE MEDICAL NEWS *will be pleased to receive early intelligence of local events of general medical interest, or of matters which it is desirable to bring to the notice of the profession.*

Local papers containing reports or news items should be marked.

Letters, whether written for publication or private information, must be authenticated by the names and addresses of their writers— of course not necessarily for publication.

All communications relating to the editorial department of the NEWS *should be addressed to No. 1004 Walnut Street, Philadelphia.*

THE MEDICAL NEWS.
A WEEKLY JOURNAL OF MEDICAL SCIENCE.

VOL. LVII.   SATURDAY, JULY 19, 1890.   No. 3.

ORIGINAL ARTICLES.

LEUKÆMIA AND PREGNANCY.[1]

With Report of a Case.

BY W. W. JAGGARD, M.D.,

PROFESSOR OF OBSTETRICS IN THE CHICAGO MEDICAL COLLEGE, AND OBSTETRICIAN TO MERCY HOSPITAL, CHICAGO.

THE purpose of this communication is to place on record an example of fatal lienal leukæmia, that seems to have sustained some necessary relation to pregnancy, or to prolonged lactation during pregnancy, or to both these factors.

The notion of some necessary relation between the female generative organs and leukæmia has long been accepted. Thus Virchow,[2] the discoverer of leukæmia, writes on the etiology of the disease:

" The only thing that can be asserted with any degree of certainty is the connection with the sexual functions in woman."

And Mosler[3] says:

" Disturbances of the sexual functions in woman have an influence in the origin of leukæmia that is numistakable. There exists a certain connection between the female genital organs and spleen. An acute splenic tumor with slight increase of the white blood-corpuscles often arises in consequence of anomalies of menstruation."

Within a recent period, however, the nature of the evidence upon which this notion rests has been called in question by Sänger,[4] in an excellent critical review of the literature of the subject. This testimony, he writes, is not the language of modern gynecology.[5]

" The question, up to the present surrendered entirely to internal medicine, must be investigated anew by gynecologists, who hitherto have interested themselves in leukæmia and splenic tumors only in their relation to differential diagnosis for the purpose of laparotomy."

It is a fact that leukæmia occurs twice in men to once in women. Among 91 cases Ehrlich found 60 males and 31 females, while among 201 cases Birch-Hirschfeld found 135 males and 66 females. This unequal occurrence exists in spite of, or perhaps on account of, the greater demands on the blood-glandular system of women. Now, if men-

[1] Read before the Chicago Medical Society, June 16, 1890.
[2] Gesammelte Abhandlungen, Frankfurt, 1856, p. 209.
[3] Die Pathologie und Therapie der Leukämie, Berlin, 1872, p. 113.
[4] Ueber Leukämie bei Schwangeren, etc.
[5] Archiv für Gyn., Bd. xxxiii. H. 2.

strual disturbance, so commonly observed, were always of primary, causal moment, the world would swarm with leukæmics. On the other hand, does it not seem probable that the more active blood-metabolism is the factor that tends to shield the female sex from leukæmia?

On the reciprocal relations of leukæmia and menstruation it can be said that in most cases the menstrual blood-flow is lessened in the course of the disease even to the degree of complete amenorrhœa. Oligomenorrhœa and amenorrhœa, however, are secondary. They arise in consequence of the leukæmic blood-dyscrasia, just as they occur in chloro-anæmia, in the anæmia of obesity, in pulmonary tuberculosis and after severe hæmorrhages. With reference to sudden suppression of the menses, whose causal importance is insisted upon by Mosler, it is more probable that the same pernicious influence that effected the suppression at the same time produced the leukæmia.

It is alleged that among women the climacteric period has the greatest number of cases, and Mosler goes so far as to attach causal significance to the senile retrograde changes in the genitalia. But it is irrational to suppose, as he does, in a single case that the numerous severe labors and abortions with considerable loss of blood should first avenge themselves at the menopause instead of immediately upon the reception of the injury. And, in general, it may be remarked that the recorded cases furnish no evidence that can incriminate the change of life.

No evidence whatever has been presented to prove a connection between primary affections of the ovaries and secondary leukæmia. It has been shown, however, that in the course of leukæmia these organs, or their analogues, are sometimes involved. Hérard demonstrated the formation of lymphomata in the ovaries in one case; Robin, in the testicles; Gillot, in the mammary glands.

The coincidence of pregnancy and leukæmia is rare. Still, in the cases of Cameron, Greene and Sänger conception occurred. The conclusion is justified that leukæmia, as such, does not inhibit capability to conceive, but, at the most, limits the function, though even limitation is not probable, since repeated conceptions have been observed in leukæmia.

From these considerations the opinion seems justified that disturbances of menstruation, of ovulation and of conception in leukæmia have either a secondary significance or are entirely independent of the disease.

Turning now to the connection between pregnancy and leukæmia, it seems to me that the evidence in hand does not warrant Sänger's absolute denial of all causal relation.

The history of my case is briefly as follows :

Mrs. F. G., thirty-four years old ; born in Boston of German parents; wife of a mechanic ; VI.-para. When in health a large, fine-looking woman, five feet four inches in height, 150 pounds in weight. Menstruation, established in sixteenth year, was regular every four weeks, painless and of three days' duration.

No serious illness during girlhood with the exception of an attack of "inflammation of the bowels" that lasted six weeks during her fourteenth year. No history of syphilis, alcoholism, injury nor of rheumatism. Patient has lived in Boston, Mass. ; Milwaukee and Menasha, Wis., and in Chicago, and never suffered from malarial infection.

Married Jan. 12, 1875, while in her twentieth year.

First child, male, born February 1, 1876, died of cholera infantum when eight months old (Dr. Root's certificate).

Second child, male, born September 7, 1877, nursed sixteen months; living and in health.

Third child, female, born November 12, 1879, nursed sixteen months; living and in health.

Fourth child, male, born May 4, 1882, nursed eighteen months; living and in health.

Fifth child, female, born December 12, 1886, nursed during her sixth pregnancy up to and on the morning of her confinement, July 8, 1888; child is now living and in health.

Sixth child, female, born July 8, 1888, small (premature). This child she was not able to suckle. At the end of the first week the child was artificially fed and died in convulsions at the end of the third week.

All her labors were easy and rapid. She was attended exclusively by a midwife. No miscarriages. With the exception of the sixth all the children large and vigorous. The four survivors, seen and examined June 1, 1890, present every appearance of health.

The course of the sixth pregnancy was normal. Three weeks before the sixth labor patient was a large and apparently healthy woman, with well-developed bust, and weighed 158 pounds. At this time she had a photograph taken, because, to use her own words, "she never looked so well."

Sixth puerperium, with the exception of the failure of lactation, was apparently normal. At the end of tèn days she was up and at work as usual. At this time she first noticed stinging paroxysmal pains in the region of the left hypochondrium, although no tumor was perceptible. About six weeks after labor, August 22, 1888, menstruation was reëstablished, but was very scanty.

Menstruation for the second and last time, January 2, 1889; scanty.

Pains of a lancinating character in the region of the spleen became more severe, the loss of weight was progressive and weariness and general malaise became marked. About eight weeks after this labor she first noticed, and called to her husband's attention, a painful lump in the region of the left hypochondrium, which seemed to grow in size from week to week. Finally she consulted her physician, Dr. Glenn M. Hammon, of Chicago, who made an examination, January 21, 1889. He writes: "I found a large, densely hard nodular mass extending downward from the spleen and filling nearly the whole of the left half of the abdominal cavity. It was easily outlined because of the emaciation. There were no other glandular enlargements. There was considerable pain of a lancinating character." The case came under my observation January 31, 1889, and remained under my control for four weeks. Patient greatly emaciated, pulse 116, temperature 100.3° F. Heart, lungs, and liver negative. Urine free from sugar and albumin. Palpation of the abdominal tumor, rendered easy by the disappearance of the panniculus adiposus and by the marked diastasis of the recti, revealed an enormously enlarged spleen that filled out the left half of the abdominal cavity and below the navel extended obliquely to a point near the right iliac fossa. The hilum and the free notched anterior margin were easily outlined. The organ, symmetrically enlarged and immobile, was painful spontaneously and on pressure. There were some ascites and slight œdema of the legs and feet.

Pelvic genitalia absolutely normal.

Lymphatic glands and long bones negative.

A drop of blood, notably viscid, showed an enormous increase of the white corpuscles. The white corpuscles apparently equalled in number the red disks.

Diagnosis.—Leukæmia lienalis.

February 4, 1889, Dr. Frank Billings saw the case with me, and together we made a careful examination of the blood.

Blood-count (Hayem's hématimèter).—Red disks, per c.mm., 3,255,000 ; white corpuscles, per c.mm., 1,178,000; ratio of white to red as 1 : 2.7+.

On account of the viscosity of the fluid, due to the increase of white corpuscles, we encountered difficulty in the estimation of the hæmoglobin by Gowers's instrument. After many trials, however, we were successful, and fixed the quantity at 50 per centum. At this time we went over the history of the case and made a thorough physical examination, but discovered nothing new. We detected no enlargement of lymphatic glands, no change in the bones.

Retina not examined.

Family history good. Both parents aged, but in health. Blood of father and only sister (II.-para) upon examination, normal.

Prognosis.—Absolutely unfavorable.

Treatment.—Nutritious food, arsenic, iron, anodynes.

Subsequent course of disease. — February 11. Paroxysms of terrible pain ; vomiting large quantities of blood. Diarrhœa ; dejecta streaked with blood. Rapid progressive emaciation. Pain always referred to the splenic tumor. Dr. J. M. Hutchinson, of Chicago, who saw the case later, kindly informs me that the paroxysms of terrible pain, always accompanied with violent vomiting, continued, the tumor increased in size, considerable ascites and œdema of the feet and legs developed; and that cachexia and emaciation progressed.

A few days before death patient weighed less than 100 pounds.

She remained conscious to within three hours of death, which occurred June 27, 1889. Autopsy could not be obtained.

This case presents several points of interest:

1. The certificate, returned to the city Board of Health, I am informed, assigns cancer of the spleen as the cause of the death of this woman. Now, as an ingenious figure of speech, it may be permissible to speak of leukæmia as carcinoma of the blood (Bard), or as sarcoma of the blood (Sänger), but it is a gross error to call a leukæmic spleen a cancer. Under adequate microscopical examination of the blood is it not possible that some of the examples of splenic cancer and of ague-cake reported here and elsewhere might be resolved into instances of leukæmia?

2. Exploratory laparotomy was actually proposed and very seriously considered in this case. But in view of the professional insanity that has attended the evolution of the "abdominal instinct," this proposal cannot be regarded as phenomenal. Splenotomy, according to Collier, has been performed in 29 cases. Out of these, 18 were in cases of leukæmia —all patients died immediately after the operation. Of the rest, 61 per cent., recovered. The operation of extirpation of the leukæmic spleen is justly looked upon as an art error.

3. The family history of the patient is good. As before remarked, the father and mother, though aged, are in excellent health. The only sister is the healthy mother of a robust child. The patient's four living children are sound and active.

4. The history of the case seems to point to some necessary relation between pregnancy or between prolonged lactation during pregnancy, or both these factors, and the leukæmia. The evidence, indeed, is only probable, but it is sufficient to create a presumption. As pertinent to the discussion, I beg to submit the following sentence, taken from the Introduction of Butler's *Analogy:*

" In questions of difficulty, or such as are thought so, where more satisfactory evidence cannot be had or is not seen, if the result of examination be that there appears upon the whole the lowest presumption on any one side and none on the other, or a greater presumption on one side, though in the lowest degree greater, this determines the question even in matters of speculation, and in matters of practice will lay us under an absolute and formal obligation, in point of prudence and of interest, to act upon that presumption or low probability,

though it be so low as to leave the mind in very great doubt which is the truth."

This view of the nature of the case receives some support from its antecedent probability. During gestation the organs of the blood-glandular system, notably the spleen, the thyroid and lymphatic glands, increase in size and their functional activity is augmented. According to Birch-Hirschfeld,[1] the normal average weight of the spleen in the non-gravid woman is 140 grammes, while at term it is 180 grammes. Virchow says that the number of white corpuscles is normally increased during pregnancy. Sänger, indeed, questions the evidence upon which this assertion rests, but he does not prove that the physiological leucocytosis does not occur. Clinical experience teaches that physiological processes are liable to undergo pathological exaggeration during pregnancy. Restricting attention to the blood we have examples of the truth of this statement in the chlorosis, hydræmia, and pernicious anæmia of the gravid woman. It is conceivable that under certain conditions the physiological leucocytosis of pregnancy and the normal splenic hypertrophy may undergo pathological exaggeration and terminate in leukæmia. This notion is not forced nor strange, but is altogether in harmony with what we know of the constitution and the course of nature.

As to the exact effects of lactation during the usual period, upon the blood-glandular system but little is known, and our ignorance is still greater when we come to lactation during pregnancy. From carefully conducted examinations of the mammary glands of guinea-pigs, during and after pregnancy, Rauber concludes that:

" Milk owes its origin to the entrance of countless leucocytes into the lumen of the gland-vesicles. The emigrated lymphoid elements penetrate the alveolar walls, passing through the single layer of epithelial cells which lines them. Arrived in the interior of an ultimate acinus, the leucocytes undergo fatty metamorphosis and thus furnish the most essential and characteristic ingredient of milk, viz., the milk-globule."

Satterthwaite says:[2]

" Thus the primitive opinion advanced by Empedocles, describing milk as white pus, is in a measure revived, and milk is held to be directly derived from the white corpuscles of the blood."

But, as at present informed, Rauber's ingenious hypothesis has never been definitely corroborated, and it is not positively asserted that in this case the excessive demand by the lacteal secretion upon the white corpuscles was the cause of the splenic tumor.

The probable time of the commencement of the leukæmia in this case coincides with the latter days of the sixth pregnancy. This is the period

---

[1] Berliner klin. Wochenschrift, 1878, p. 324.
[2] Manual of Histology, 1881.

when the blood-glandular organs are most severely taxed by pregnancy itself. Add to this the additional strain of suckling a vigorous babe, and it seems that there is presented a cause adequate to the phenomenon.

This proposition rests chiefly upon the history of the case, obviously a precarious basis. Still, three weeks before labor the woman was the picture of health, as shown by her photograph, and by her weight, 158 pounds. Soon after labor and after the failure of the milk the pains were felt in the side, and the splenic tumor, small then, appeared. All these facts fix with tolerable accuracy this time as the date of the commencement of the disease. This impression is confirmed by the duration and by the character of the course of the disease. The patient died eleven months and nineteen days after her sixth confinement, and the course of the disease was steadily progressive.

Out of the 63 cases tabulated by Gowers, the duration of the disease was under a year in the 13 examples whose symptoms more or less closely resemble the clinical picture of this case, and in general the average duration of the malady may be reckoned as between one and two years (Eichhorst).

The history of the case offers no other explanation of the leukæmia. Trauma, syphilis, alcoholism, can be absolutely excluded. The patient never resided in a malarial region, and to the best of her knowledge never suffered from malarial infection.

A few cases have been published that seem to point to a causal relation between some phase of the puerperal state and leukæmia. Sänger, indeed, insists that this connection has never been established. On the one hand, he thinks that pregnancy does not affect the origin or course of leukæmia; on the other hand, he seeks to prove that leukæmia affects pregnancy in the determination of premature labor only indirectly by the greatly increased intra-abdominal tension, on account of the presence of the splenic tumor, ascites, meteorism of the intestines and the like. "The leukæmic quality of the blood, as such," he writes, "does not need to be invoked in explanation." But, as before remarked, the weight of evidence, as it seems to me, is in favor of the older view, of some necessary reciprocal relation between pregnancy and leukæmia. For my purpose, it is sufficient to mention merely one old and three new cases.

Leube[1] and Fleischer describe a case of a myelogenic leukæmia. A woman, strong and healthy up to the time of examination, developed four months after a normal labor, signs of a somewhat rapidly increasing leukæmia, without demonstrable cause.

There were impairment of nutrition and strength, syncope, headache, anorexia, and also painfulness and swelling, which finally in part disappeared, of the left lower extremity. Five weeks later, there were signs of a high degree of anæmia, blowing murmur over the heart and a small compressible pulse. No enlargement of spleen, liver, or lymphatics. The number of red corpuscles was significantly decreased and there were both relative and absolute increase of the white corpuscles. The left tibia and left tarsus were painful on pressure. On account of rapidly increasing gangrene of the skin, amputation of the left foot was performed and was followed by death, six days later. Section revealed extreme anæmia of all internal organs, advanced degeneration of the cardiac muscle and chronic ulcer of the stomach, but no change in the liver, spleen or lymphatics. The bone-marrow was red and hyperplastic, with numerous nucleated red blood-corpuscles (transition forms, and numerous marrow cells).

According to Osler's[1] interpretation:

"This was no doubt a case of post-partum anæmia aggravated by the presence of ulcer of the stomach, and the great interest of the case lies in the transition of the anæmia into leukæmia."

In Cameron's[2] case, there were presented among others, the following points of interest:

"1. Splenic tumor was first noticed by her at the beginning of her sixth pregnancy."

"2. Spleen and liver always enlarge during pregnancy and become tender."

"3. The progressively enormous increase of white cells and decrease of red cells, as pregnancy advances."

"4. The rapid subsidence of œdema and dyspnœa after the termination of labor, together with the rapid increase of red and decrease of white cells."

Of the later course of this case, Dr. Cameron, under date of June 3, 1890, writes me:

"My patient is still living and has been confined twice since the Washington meeting. The first time she made an excellent recovery and regained her health so much that she was able to do all her own housework. The child was premature and died very shortly after birth, but was quite free from all trace of leukæmia. During her last pregnancy her health was poor. She became very anæmic and suffered so much from dyspnœa, palpitation, and threatenings of heart-failure that I was obliged to induce labor about the seventh month. The fœtus had perished some days previously. She barely escaped with her life, and is slowly going down-hill. The splenic tumor and her blood-count remain about the same."

James L. Greene's[3] report of two cases, of leukæmia, so sharply criticised by Sänger, while defective, is still of a certain value. His first case, during a first pregnancy, was an example of acute lienal leukæmia that was fatal within six months of the apparent outset. Although malarial infection cannot be

[1] Ein Beitrag zur Lehre von der Leukæmie, Virchow's Archiv, lxxxiii. p. 1124.

[1] Pepper's System of Medicine, vol. iii. p. 920.
[2] Transactions of the International Medical Congress, Ninth Session, Washington, 1887. Vol. ii. p. 330.
[3] New York Medical Journal, February 11, 1888. p. 144.

absolutely excluded in this case, the course of the disease creates the presumption that malaria, if present, must have played a minor *rôle*. It is to be hoped that the history of Greene's second case will be filled out in the near future, since, as at present described, the diagnosis of leukæmia, to say nothing of the variety, is not established. The case is that of a young primipara, the sister of the patient of the first example, who suffered from symptoms pointing to leukæmia. Upon the artificial induction of abortion, the patient promptly recovered. Of this case, Dr. Greene, under the date of May 30, 1890, writes me :

"The second case mentioned by me, Mrs. C., has conceived since the report was published, and with this condition returned all of the symptoms of leukæmia. An abortion was produced and she regained her health as before."

On account of the antecedent probability of the view, on account of the coincidence of the apparent onset of the disease with the later days of pregnancy, on account of the absence of any other demonstrable adequate cause, and finally, on account of the evidence accumulated from the cases cited, it seems to me to be highly probable, that in this case, the leukæmia sustained some necessary relation to pregnancy, or to prolonged lactation during pregnancy, or to both these factors.

2330 INDIANA AVENUE.

RECENT OBSERVATIONS IN THE ETIOLOGY AND TREATMENT OF MIGRAINE.[1]

BY WHARTON SINKLER. M.D.,
PHYSICIAN TO THE PHILADELPHIA HOSPITAL AND TO THE INFIRMARY FOR NERVOUS DISEASES, ETC.

IT has seemed to me well to gather together some of the experience of the past few years in the treatment of migraine, and to cull from the journals and elsewhere what is of value in regard to conditions which may cause it.

This form of headache is of unending interest to the medical profession, for its cure or the alleviation of the paroxysms is a constant problem. Moreover, as Gowers remarks, " The disease is often associated with high intellectual ability and many distinguished men have suffered from it and have supplied more careful observations of the subjective symptoms than we possess of any other malady." We may almost say of it, as Sydenham said of gout, that "More rich men than poor men and more wise men than fools, are victims of the affection." Among the prominent men who have had migraine are DuBois-Reymond, Dr. Fothergill, Dr. Lauder Brunton, Dr. Anstie, Sir John Herschell, Sir George Airy and his son, Dr. Hubert Airy, and we all have

among our own medical friends many who suffer from attacks. It is by no means, however, confined to the more prosperous classes, for we meet with it in all conditions of men and at all ages.

The attacks of migraine from uterine disorders have been known to the profession for years, and there is a large amount of literature on the subject. Recently much has been written on headaches from eye-strain and many of these are of the hemicranic type. Numerous cases have been reported which have been relieved by correcting refraction errors of the eye. The connection between migraine and disorders of vision has been pointed out by several authorities, amongst others, Mr. John Tweedy, Dr. Savage,[1] Mr. Carter, Dr. William Thomson, Dr. S. Weir Mitchell,[2] and quite lately, by Dr. George F. Stevens,[3] whose writings on the relief of various disorders of the nervous system by tenotomy of the ocular muscles have attracted much attention. This author thinks that ocular defects play a conspicuous *rôle* as causative conditions in migraine. He refers to a few cases of "blind headache" in which the fundus of the eye was examined during the period of visual disturbance preceding an attack. The retina has been found pale and brilliant, the optic nerve unusually white, and the main arteries somewhat irregularly contracted in their course. In these cases the field of vision was found to be contracted in a striking manner, in some cases, one-half of the field being lost, and in others the central field was gone and imperfect sight remaining in the periphery. He finds that, unlike ordinary forms of headache, hemicrania does not easily yield to the simple measure of adapting glasses to correct refraction errors. It is often caused by a complication of refraction trouble and muscular insufficiency. This requires tenotomy and suitable glasses. Mr. Bendelack Hewetson[4] has removed migraine by paralyzing the power of accommodation by atropine. Henry S. Oppenheimer[5] considers eye-strain to be a frequent cause of headache and believes that it is often overlooked. He relates a case of headache and severe tinnitus aurium cured by the proper application of prisms combined with convex cylinders.

He recommends in the treatment of headaches from eye-strain, first, that all hygienic and medical indications be carefully carried out ; secondly, a most careful correction of the refraction and accom-

---

[1] Read before the Association of American Physicians. May 14. 1890.

[1] Medical and Surgical Reporter. July 29, 1882.
[2] Ibid., July 25. and Aug. 1. 1874.
[3] Functional Nervous Diseases, by George T. Stevens. M.D. New York, 1887.
[4] The Relation between Sick Headache and Defective Sight. Leeds. 1885.
[5] Headaches and other Nervous Symptoms caused by Functional Anomalies of the Eye. Gaillard's Medical Journal, New York. January. 1880.

modation; thirdly, correction of muscular insufficiencies by prisms, beginning with a low degree and, when necessary, increasing in power; and should this prove insufficient, tenotomy.

T. Lauder Brunton[1] speaks of migraine from caries of the teeth. He says:

"The most common causes of headache, indeed, are decayed teeth and irregularities of vision. When the teeth are decayed rinsing out the mouth with a lotion of bicarbonate of sodium, or applying a little cocaine to the exposed pulp will relieve the headache."

He refers to his own case in which, during the attack, the pain was limited to a spot in the left temple. On one occasion he accidentally discovered, under the angle of the jaw, a small gland, which was hard and painful to the touch. This led him to examine his teeth, and these he tested by percussing with a steel instrument until he discovered a tender spot on the last lower molar on the left side. He went to a dentist who found that caries had begun at that spot but had, as yet, caused no cavity. He also describes the case of a clergyman who began to suffer from headaches so intense as completely to incapacitate him. He took various medicines in vain and went for a continental tour, but came back little benefited. Dr. Brunton saw him shortly after his return and examined his teeth, all of which looked healthy. He then took a steel bodkin and probed and percussed each tooth in succession until he came to one which was tender. The dentist found that this tooth was carious. It was properly filled, and the headaches disappeared. He further says:

"In cases of headache depending upon a decayed tooth when no toothache is felt, it is not improbable that the irritation in the tooth does not give rise directly to the sensation of pain in the head, but does so by acting through the sympathetic system on the vessels, so as to cause the spasm which leads to the sensation of pain."

J. S. Dixon[2] reports several cases in which the removal of carious teeth stopped attacks of hemicrania.

Dr. Louis Starr[3] speaks of headaches being frequent in children during the period of second dentition. He says:

"Headache is common. The pain is usually temporal or unilateral. It may be seated, however, in the occipital region or in different parts of the face, and sometimes shifts suddenly from the occiput to the temporal region. One or more painful points can often be detected and generally there is a hard, tender, markedly enlarged lymphatic gland in the sub-maxillary or cervical region."

He suggests that the method of production of the headache is one of direct nervous connection, the sub-maxillary ganglion acting, in the case of the lower teeth and the spheno-palatine in the case of the upper, as mediums of transfer of irritation to the vaso-motor nerves.

The nose and ear are now recognized as means by which external irritation may operate in producing headaches. Dr. Brunton[1] finds that in his experience headache depending on disease of the nose is at the top of the head just behind the commencement of the scalp, and headache here should always lead to an examination of the nose.

Dr. Hack, of Freiburg, (quoted by Brunton), has observed several cases, both of migraine and of frontal headache, depending upon congestion of the mucous membrane covering the anterior turbinated bones, and has been able to effect a radical cure in several cases by the application of the galvano-cautery to the inflamed and swollen mucous membrane.

Thomas E. McBride[2] relates four cases of migraine which were cured by relieving the post-nasal catarrh which had existed in each case.

Harrison Allen, in a paper read before the Philadelphia Neurological Society,[3] refers to a patient in whom merely touching the right middle turbinated bone with a probe instantly caused intense vertex pain. He reports a second case in which there were attacks of general headache and clavus over the right parietal eminence. In this patient he found disease confined to the middle turbinated bone on the right side. He also mentions the case of a lady in whom there were frequent attacks of "sick headache" which were dependent upon deep-seated infiltration of the pharynx. The headaches were removed by curing the pharyngeal disease.

John O. Roe[4] has contributed a paper on "The Frequent Dependence of Persistent and So-called Congestive Headaches upon Abnormal Conditions of the Nasal Passages."

Most of his cases had constant, dull, general headache, but in two or three the attacks were migraine, and were accompanied with nausea and vomiting. In all some obstructive disease was found in the nose and removal of the obstruction was followed by relief from the headaches.

Migraine has been known as a disorder of childhood for many years and I have elsewhere pointed out its frequency in very young children.[5] I have seen at least one case in which a child of two years had periodical attacks, with every characteristic of mi-

1 Disorders of Digestion. London, 1888.
2 Atlanta Medical and Surgical Journal, December, 1856, vol. II. p. 201.
3 A Study of the Relationship between the Eruption of the Permanent Teeth and the Ailments of late Childhood, Therapeutic Gazette, April 15, 1890, p. 228.

1 Loc. cit., p. 107.
2 THE MEDICAL NEWS, January 30, 1886, p. 136.
3 On the Headaches which are Associated Clinically with Chronic Nasal Catarrh. THE MEDICAL NEWS, March 13, 1886, p. 289.
4 New York Medical Record. August 25, 1888, p. 200.
5 Transactions Philadelphia County Medical Society. 1887.

graine. A medical friend has described to me the case of one of his own children whom he believes to have had attacks of hemicrania from the age of two years. Gowers[1] says one-third of the cases begin between five and ten years of age.

Russell Sturgis[2] has described a form of recurrent headache in children, which he considers to be similar to the migraine of adults, with the difference that the pain is more likely to be across the forehead, and is less often confined to either side of the head than that of migraine. He describes these. attacks as occurring in children of a nervous temperament, who sleep poorly, with bad dreams and night terrors, and who are fretful and often chilly and have a heavy expression about the eyes. There were in many of his cases optical illusions of sparks or spots, and bands of color. The treatment which he has used successfully in some twenty cases, consists in the administration of ten minim doses of the fluid extract of ergot, more being added if there is coëxisting anæmia. The ergot should be continued for several weeks after the cessation of the headaches.

Migraine sometimes begins late in life. A patient, whose case I shall report later, never had an attack until his thirty-eighth year, and Gowers speaks of a man in whom the attacks began at sixty years.

The visual phenomena of an attack of migraine have been discussed for many years. Lately some interesting cases of transient hemianopsia and unusual forms of scotomata have been reported. Dr. de Schweinitz has kindly given me an account of two cases in which the form of scotoma was unusual. In one it was described as being like the wavy appearance of heat rising from a chimney. The cases are as follows :

"A man, aged thirty-two, whose family physician reports general health good, and who, as far as my own examination is concerned, has no organic disease. For a number of years this patient has had attacks of typical migraine ; the invariable prodrome is an appearance as if heat were rising in the air, which is followed by numbness of one hand, or else numbness of the tongue and, although of this I am not absolutely sure, aphasia. This condition lasts from fifteen to twenty minutes, sometimes as long as an hour, and is succeeded by a terrific explosion of hemicrania. His attacks average one a month, but they have occasionally come as often as once in two weeks. He has a moderately high degree of compound hypermetropic astigmatism, together with insufficiency of the internal recti of eight degrees in accommodation. There are no other muscular anomalies. He is at present under treatment for the eyes.

"The other case is one of a man aged forty-seven, typically neurasthenic, and of bilious temperament, who, for many years, has had severe migraine, the

attacks averaging one every two weeks. He has no definite or always present prodrome, but in a certain number of instances this has consisted of a large, dark, circular object, composed from within outward of a dense black rim, a broader grayish-black circle, a central nucleus of yellow color, and a nucleolus of dense black. It is needless to remark that I, not he, have used these technical terms to describe it, but you observe that this curious appearance which he drew for me, contains the components of a compound cell, the dark outer rim corresponding to the capsule, the gray portion to the cell contents, the yellow spot to the nucleus, and the dark spot to the nucleolus. This patient has a high mixed astigmatism, with insufficiency of the external recti of four degrees."

- Dr. Charles A. Oliver kindly referred to me a case of migraine in whom there existed that rather unusual condition of contraction and dilatation of the pupil known as hippus, in connection with the attacks of migraine, and in whom there were other interesting visual phenomena accompanying the attack. The following notes were made by Dr. Oliver :

"*January 8, 1886*. L. L., aged twenty-five years, unmarried.

"For two weeks past she has had a spasmodic action of the right iris, causing the pupil to dilate and contract irregularly ; this spasmodic action being felt by the patient as a twitching or a series of movements. During the past eleven months she has had a number of severe attacks of migraine, blindness appearing simultaneously before the right side of each field of vision and quickly moving across to the left side, lasting for fifteen minutes and followed by clearing up of the visual fields in the same sequence ; that is, commencing at the right periphery of each field and ending on the extreme left side. The attacks terminate with the usual signs of headache, nausea, etc. She has had the headaches, which have been worse at the time of menstruation, for several years. She complains of asthenopic symptoms and she has never worn glasses. She had four brothers and one sister, she being the third child. A younger brother had a 'cast' in his eye and the mother has worn glasses for years. The patient was overworked, neurasthenic, and her menses were scanty and irregular. Ocular symptoms show :

$$\propto \text{O. D. V.} = \frac{5}{7}, \frac{1}{2}? \quad \text{Sn. } 1\frac{1}{2} \ 6''\text{-}26''.$$

$$\propto \text{O. S. V.} = \frac{5}{7}, \frac{1}{2}. \quad \text{Sn. } 1\frac{1}{2} \ 6''\text{-}26''.$$

"Eyes are slightly *in* under hand-cover.

"The ophthalmoscope showed gray disks with a tortuous condition of somewhat undersized retinal veins, with the characteristic changes of disturbed ametropia. Patient was advised an estimation and correction of refraction error, but she refused to have glasses. thinking that rest from work would relieve the necessity for wearing them.

---

[1] Diseases of the Nervous System, 1888, p. 1172.
[2] Archives of Pædiatrics, 1889, vol. vi. p. 293.

"*November 5, 1886.* The last attack began as a large, central scotoma,' which she says was about the size of a silver half-dollar, associated with fronto-temporal pain on both sides and lasting about twenty minutes, followed by numbness of the left upper extremity, commencing in the ring and little finger.

" Patient failed to report for over two years, when she stated that she had been free from attacks until the day when she was seen. This attack appeared as a central, blind area which was not surrounded by any brilliant lines or zigzags. This lasted for about fifteen minutes, and was followed by giddiness but no numbness. The right-sided hippus was again complained of, and upon careful study was found just as pronounced as at the previous examination. The iris excursions which were quite extensive were found to be fifteen times in each half minute upon monocular exposure, and but six times in the same length of time upon binocular exposure.

" The patient was next seen April 29, 1890. No attack until three weeks before, when one unexpectedly appeared four days before menstruation. Patient was then highly neurasthenic and nervous."

In June, 1887, Dr. S. Weir Mitchell read at the College of Physicians[1] a paper on some remarkable visual hallucinations, which took the place of the ordinary balls of light and zigzag lines which are so commonly met with as a precursor of an attack of headache. He relates four cases, the first of which is of so much interest that I will repeat it in full :

"Miss W., aged thirty, was in good general health, and able to bear great fatigue, and to use her mind and body incessantly as a teacher. About once a week for many years she had attacks of migraine of great severity. When nineteen years old she began, just before the headaches, to see a bright, gold-tinted cloud, and with it an appearance of parti-colored rain. There was most clouding of vision when the sequent pain was over the right eye, and these visual phenomena were not constant. When twenty-eight years old, and still subject to prolonged headaches, the attacks changed their type. After a few weeks of freedom, one day when going up-stairs she was abruptly aware of being accompanied on her left by a large, black, and very hairy dog. In some alarm she ran into a room and sat down, but still found the dog beside her. Being a woman of courage, she put out her hand to touch it,· but could feel nothing, although her ghostly companion was still visible. At this moment severe pain began over the left eye, and the dog was gone. The attacks recurred at intervals, as well as the now ordinary brow-pain, without the dog vision, but the ' dog-headaches,' as she called them, were always the most severe. The visual phenomena left her after some years, but as she went to live abroad I lost sight of her. I should add as a curious detail that nearly always, but not invariably, the dog appeared as she was going up-stairs.

" In the second case the apparition consisted in the appearance of a sister who had long been dead.

" The first time it appeared the patient, who was in the fourth month of lactation, was dressing in front of a mirror when she was suddenly aware of the dead sister standing beside her. The vision was followed by a severe pain in the left eye, lasting for many hours, which ended with an attack of nausea and a great flow of pale urine.

" In the third case, the form of a near relative appeared just before the attack of headache, and faded as the pain increased, but she was left for some days with a strong desire to kill the person whose image she had seen. The patient came of a highly neurotic family. Two brothers died of epilepsy, and two sisters had been insane. The patient afterward had attacks of melancholia, but ultimately made a complete recovery after removal of both ovaries.

" In the fourth case a man of thirty saw a variety of visions, complex figures of brilliant pink or red, multiple red circles in rapid rotation, which apparently came from the distance. Once there appeared a crescent of silver on the wall, suspended from which were numerous heads in profile. Some were strange to him, and some the revival of faces which had long been forgotten. In one attack a red spider appeared which merged into a series of rectangles, revolving in swift motion."

De Schweinitz[1] reports six additional cases of migraine hallucinations of vision which preceded or accompanied the attacks. In one of these patients a large green snake was seen just before the attack. In another, marked visions of animals, always either mice or dogs, were associated with headache. Once in the morning the vision took the form of the water-pitcher in the room, through the handle of which a constant stream of running mice playfully chased each other. Once in church the vision was that of a small black dog, that curled himself at her feet.

The hallucinations of vision in connection with epileptic attacks have been observed by many authors to resemble markedly those described by Mitchell and de Schweinitz. I have recently seen a patient who had some interesting visual phenomena connected with epilepsy :

Mrs. A., aged forty, has three children, and has had three miscarriages. There is no neurotic family history, and she has never been subject to headaches. From the age of nine or ten years she has had attacks in which everything seems far off, or, as she expresses it, "like looking through the large end of an opera-·glass." There always appeared in these attacks a face with unpleasant expression, which was very distinct for a time, but gradually faded away. She was not unconscious during the attack, but felt powerless to move or exert herself, and would call to any one in the room to shake her so that she might regain self-control. The attacks continued with greater or less frequency until November, 1889, when she

---

[1] Neuralgic Headache with Apparitions of Unusual Character. Transactions of the College of Physicians of Philadelphia, vol. ix. p. 175.

[1] University Medical Magazine, May, 1889, p. 450.

had an attack of epilepsy (*grand mal*) in her sleep. Again, in April, she had another attack while driving in her carriage. These are the only attacks of *grand mal* which she knows of having had, and both were preceded by the vision of the unpleasant face.

P. Blocq thinks that ophthalmic migraine should be separated from the other migraines. This variety has pain in the head and visual troubles in the simple form, to which are added at times aphasia and sensory or motor troubles. He reminds us that Charcot has already called attention to the fact that ophthalmic migraine may be prodromic to general paralysis. Therefore, its liability to this serious ending must be borne in mind. Blocq relates three cases of migraine associated with general paralysis, the first of which is a typical one of ophthalmic migraine, reported by Charcot, the second reported by Parinaud, and the third case by himself. In all the cases heretofore described the attacks of migraine had preceded the general paralysis, but in the case reported by Blocq the attacks of migraine accompanied the paresis.

Suckling[1] has reported a case of migraine in a youth of eighteen years, in which the attacks were followed by paralysis of the upper eyelid on the left side, which lasted forty-eight hours. The patient had been subject to attacks of sick-headaches since infancy, and the temporary paralysis of the third nerve had occurred since that time. The paroxysms lasted two days, during which time the patient was confined to bed, and was unable to eat. There was a nasty taste in the mouth, and a copious flow of saliva.

The periodicity of the attacks of migraine has been known for many years. It is spoken of by Liveing,[2] but I can find only one writer besides myself[3] who has observed that the attacks may recur on a certain day of the week. Tissot[4] says that Salins relates the case of an Italian monk who, for three years and seven months, had an attack of violent hemicrania every Monday, the attacks lasting from twenty-eight to thirty hours.

Liveing, who refers to Tissot's case, thinks that an exact periodicity like this is probably due to the diet or engagements of the day preceding the attack. This is undoubtedly the case in many instances, but in some of the cases which I have seen there was nothing done on the day previous to the attack different from that done on any other day of the week. I will relate some examples of cases of this kind which I have seen.

CASE I.—Miss C. J. H., aged thirty years, teacher. Menstruation regular, painless. From twelve until twenty-two years of age she had attacks of "regular sick-headache." For the past eight years the attacks have been confined to the left side of the head, chiefly in the left brow. The attacks recurred with great regularity and came always either on Monday or Tuesday. The attacks were often brought on by fatigue or by a draught of cold air.

Cannabis indica was given in increasing doses and the patient was greatly relieved. The periodicity of the attacks was broken up and the intervals became from eight to ten weeks.

CASE II.—Mr. A. H. W., aged thirty years, temperate, uses tobacco in moderation. He has a sister who frequently suffers from attacks of headache which come almost always on Sunday.

Mr. W. had sick-headaches in childhood, and when about sixteen years of age began to have attacks in which the pain was confined to one side of the head. They occurred almost every Sunday morning for several years. He usually got up with a dull headache and soon after breakfast had scotomata (red and yellow spots), floating at the upper and external angle of the eye. This was followed by violent pain in one brow or in the occiput. The attack would last eight or ten hours, terminating in vomiting or in a sharp attack of diarrhœa, after which he felt entirely relieved. Occasionally the crisis was accompanied by an exceedingly copious flow of urine. The patient usually rose at about 6.30 A. M., but on Sunday lay in bed until 9. This, and the culmination of a hard week's work, probably induced the headache. For the past two or three years his work has not been so hard and his life has been more regular; he now but seldom has a severe headache (not more than three or four in the course of the year), and his general health has become excellent.

CASE III.—Mr. J. D. F., aged forty-one. Married. A grain merchant.

He had had headaches since he was eight or nine years of age. The attacks were not periodical until five or six years ago when he became actively engaged in business. He then began to have attacks with regularity every Sunday. They usually came on about midday without ocular or other prodromes. The pain was always located in the occipital region and lasted with great severity for five or six hours when vomiting occurred, after which he was relieved of pain.

I gave him cannabis indica and regulated his diet and the attacks were very much relieved in frequency and severity. The Sunday attacks recurred for about nine months. He ascribed the attacks to the result of a week's hard work. As he expressed it himself, on Saturday night he would "unbuckle," feeling that his work was done until Monday. Instead of rising at six, as was his habit, he did not get up until nine on Sunday morning. He now very rarely has attacks and they are not so severe as formerly.

CASE IV.—Mr. J. M. H., aged fifty. Bookkeeper and has close desk-work. Of a nervous tem-

---

[1] Brain, vol. x. p. 241.

[2] On Megrim or Sick Headache, p. 36. London, 1873.

[3] Pepper's System of Medicine, vol. v. p. 407. Philadelphia, 1886.

[4] Traité des Nerfs, vol. viii. p. 102. Lausanne, 1788.

perament. His habits have always been good as to stimulants and he never uses tobacco. He had no headaches in childhood. Twelve years ago, at the age of thirty-eight, after a plain, wholesome dinner, he noticed waves and floating spots before his eyes. These were followed by a severe pain in the head. Since that time he has averaged five attacks in a year. The attacks are very much alike. They are always preceded by scotomata and occasionally there is partial hemianopsia. This is followed by pain over the entire head, which lasts for from twelve to fifteen hours. There is nausea, but no vomiting or crisis of any kind. The attacks almost always occur on Sunday. He rises later on Sunday than on other days, takes a bath about midday, and it is after his bath that he usually has the attack of headache. For some years he has had a permanent scotoma before the eyes. He does not notice it when he is at work, but when he is in a bright light or out of doors the spots are very bright, sometimes irregular in shape with a double outline and always seem to be falling.

CASE V.—A. W., aged thirty-three years. Single. Seamstress. She has suffered from headaches since she was seventeen years of age. For some years her attacks have occurred about once a week and almost always on Sunday.

The attack is usually hemicrania, but the pain is occasionally over both eyes. Sometimes there are intervals of three weeks between the attacks, but on each of the last three Sundays she has had her usual form of headache. When at the seashore or in more robust health she has had less frequent attacks of headache.

CASE VI.—M. C., aged thirty-five. Lady's maid. Both parents are dead. Father died of pneumonia, the mother in confinement. She has one brother and one sister. The brother is healthy. The sister is thirty-eight years of age and has always had violent headaches. For many years the sister had the attack on Sunday. Her occupation and mode of life on that day or the day preceding seemed to have nothing to do with the attacks.

The patient's headaches began with the catamenial period, and have always preceded the menses. About nine years ago she began to have headaches on almost every Sunday. There was no change in her manner of life at this time and for three or four years the attacks came with regularity on this day. Then she began to have them on Saturdays, sometimes for two or three months at a time. At present she does not have the attacks so often. She has been free from headache for as long a time as two or three weeks, but she always has an attack before the menstrual period, and does not remember to have ever gone longer than two months without an attack. She has been abroad two or three times, and then she escaped the attacks of migraine for a long period. Sometimes she wakes with pain in the head. At other times the attack begins later in the day. The pain is always confined to one side of the head, and generally the left side. She has no ocular symptoms except wavy spots like smoke. Occasionally there is vomiting, but not generally. The face and lips are pale during the attack. Her general health is good. Her catamenia are regular and she has no amenorrhœa. Her sleep is excellent and she is not overworked.

Treatment.—The drugs which have attracted the most attention of late are, undoubtedly, antipyrine, phenacetin, and the host of antipyretic and analgesic coal-tar derivatives, which have been introduced in the past few years. White[1] claims to have first used antipyrine in headache. At all events, it has been very universally employed in every variety of head-pain since its analgesic properties became known. T. S. Robertson[2] has used it in 88 cases of migraine; in 54 the action was satifactory in the course of from thirty minutes to two hours, and in 15 cases the administration of other drugs was rendered more effective by the use of the antipyrine. A negative result was obained in the remaining 8 cases. He recommends that 22 grains be taken at the onset, and in case the headache continues an additional dose of the same size. Bokenham[3] has used the remedy in 26 cases with entire success, but instead of using the large doses usually recommended, he gives only 3 or 4 grains, repeating the dose in an hour, if necessary.

Müller[4] has given phenacetin in migraine and various other forms of headache, but has found that large doses, as much as from 2 to 3 drachms, have been needed to produce good results.

Pesce has used[5] antifebrin with advantage in migraine. P. Guttman[6] uses phenacetin in small doses and gets as good results as from the use of antipyrine. The great advantage that phenacetin has over antipyrine is that it is much safer, as it does not depress the heart. During the recent epidemic of "grip" phenacetin proved efficacious in relieving the violent headache associated with that disease.

Rabuske[7] after trying quinine, arsenic, caffeine, antipyrine, electricity, change of climate, etc., was successful in the treatment of a very bad case of long-standing hemicrania by the administration of 8 grains of phenacetin night and morning. The cure was effected after the sixth dose.

Antifebrin has been used quite largely of late. Faust[8] has found this remedy, in doses of ½ to 1 drachm, of great use, the headache being relieved.

A. L. Clark[9] has found that 8 to 10 grains of antifebrin will relieve pain in the head in twenty to thirty minutes. S. Merkel,[10] from an experience of

[1] Annual of the Universal Medical Sciences. 1888, vol. iv. p. 444.
[2] Medical Record, May 7, 1887.
[3] London Practitioner, February, 1888.
[4] Therapeutische Monatschrifte, August, 1888.
[5] Le Bulletin Médical, May 30, 1888.
[6] Deutsche medizinal Zeitung, July 12, 1888.
[7] Ibid., Sept. 13, 1888.
[8] Ibid., June 30, 1887, p. 575.
[9] Chicago Medical Times, Sept. 1888. p. 401.
[10] Munchener med. Wochenschrift, June 12, 1888.

49 cases of migraine and headaches of like nature, considers this a valuable drug. James Little[1] recommends, in the treatment of migraine, that during the intervals between the attacks the follow-pill be given twice a day:

R.—Arseniate of sodium . . $\frac{1}{12}$ grain.
  Extract of cannabis indica . $\frac{1}{8}$ "
  Extract of belladonna . . $\frac{1}{3}$ " —M.

He gives in addition to this 2 grains of valerianate of zinc twice daily. To cut short a paroxysm he gives 20 grains of the salicylate of sodium in a wineglassful of water made effervescent by the addition of a dessertspoonful of the granular citrate of caffeine, a second or third dose to be taken after an interval of two hours.

Nitrate of cytisine (a poisonous alkaloid extracted from the seeds of the cytisus laburnum) has been given by Kräpelin in the angio-paretic form with excellent results in two cases.[2] He gives it hypodermically and was led to use it on account of its power of causing contraction of the bloodvessels. In two cases of the spastic form of migraine in which he used it the symptoms were aggravated.

De Schweinitz and Lewis[3] had a certain amount of success in the treatment of hemicrania with the oil of eucalyptus, and I myself had two or three patients in whom this drug was of marked utility. These authors have lately told me that further investigation has proved that its value is by no means general, although certain cases are relieved by its use. In cases where migraine is associated with the gouty diathesis, treatment of the latter is attended with success as far as relief of the headache is concerned. Haig[4] states that he has relieved many attacks in this form of the disease by giving 20 to 30 drops of dilute nitro-muriatic acid in water, repeated once or twice at intervals of a half hour.

Cannabis indica, which has been given in migraine for many years, still holds a prominent place among the medicinal agents used in its treatment. For myself, I may say that I consider it of more value in the majority of cases of migrainous headache than in any other headache. It must be given for some length of time and the dose should be increased until slight toxic symptoms are felt. We must remember the great variability in the strength of the drug, and be careful to begin with a minimum dose. I have but recently seen a patient who had marked toxic effects from $\frac{1}{8}$ of a grain of the extract. Seguin[5]

several years ago pointed out the benefit of cannabis indica in this form of headache and insisted on its long-continued use.

Dr. Richard Green, who first recommended Indian hemp in migraine,[1] has continued to use it with success. He maintains that its effect is not simply palliative, but curative, and that in nearly all cases it gives permanent relief.[2] E. J. Overend[3] believes caffeine to be as complete a specific in migraine as quinine is in malarial fevers. He is himself a victim to the affection. He advises the administration of citrate of caffeine in doses of from 3 to 5 grains as soon as the first indication of an attack is felt, and its hourly repetition until relief is experienced. Electricity is of more or less value and many cases have been greatly helped by galvanism. I have found this means of marked benefit, but have not depended upon it alone in any case. Labbé[4] has cured a severe case of eight years' standing by thirty-four applications of static electricity. A number of other new remedies have been used to a limited extent in this affection. Among them is exalgine, which I found of use in shortening an attack. Ringer has successfully used tincture of nux vomica in drop doses repeated every half hour.

Amongst the latest remedial agents proposed for the cure of migrainous attacks is hypnotism. In a work on the subject by Albert Moll[5] he expresses his belief that either post-hypnotic or auto-hypnotic suggestion may be used to cure this disease.

Most authors now agree as to the prime importance of hygienic measures in connection with any remedy used for the relief of this disease. Removal from care and work, with fresh air, good food, and change of climate will do more to relieve the frequency of the attacks than any drug. In connection with this the rest-treatment of S. Weir Mitchell is of the greatest value, and I have seen many cases of chronic migraine relieved by this means.

STUDIES IN THE ETIOLOGY OF MALARIAL INFECTION AND OF THE HÆMATOZOA OF LAVERAN.[6]

BY GEORGE DOCK, M.D.,
OF GALVESTON, TEXAS.

THE present condition of the search for the *contagium vivum* of malaria is such as to make expedient the collection and recording of even isolated experiences. Proof in regard to the causal relation

[1] Note on the Relief of Migranous Headache. Transactions of the Royal Academy of Medicine in Ireland, Dublin, 1888, vol. vi. p. 55.
[2] Neurolog. Centralblatt, Jan. 1, 1888.
[3] THE MEDICAL NEWS, July 20, 1889.
[4] British Medical Journal, Jan. 12, 1888.
[5] Paper read before Section on Medicine, New York Academy of Medicine, Nov. 20, 1877.

[1] The Practitioner, Nov. 1872.
[2] Ibid., July, 1888.
[3] Pacific Medical Journal, Jan. 1889.
[4] Journal de Médecine de Paris, Nov. 11, 1889.
[5] Der Hypnotismus. Second edition. Berlin, 1890.
[6] Read before the Section of Practice of Medicine, Materia Medica and Physiology of the American Medical Association, May 20, 1890.

of the organisms first described by Laveran is so strong as to be all but convincing, yet there are still certain links to be added to the chain of evidence. In bringing forward some observations of my own I shall omit a detailed account of the investigations of others, presuming that from the works of Councilman, Osler, Sternberg, and James, they are already known to the reader.

The observations to which I wish particularly to call attention are those which deal with the flagellate organisms ; but partly to preserve a better order, partly as an additional contribution to the subject, I will give my general experience with the malarial parasites.

The observations here reported were made in Galveston, Texas, and after I had become practically familiar with the parasites while acting as Dr. Osler's laboratory assistant. Malaria is uncommon in Galveston. Only three cases which could have originated on the island have come under observation. The other cases, thirty in all, came from various points of the interior of Texas, whose river "bottoms" have a well-deserved reputation as malaria breeding-places. These cases, with few exceptions, were seen in the hospital. In all of them some of every form of the parasite heretofore described by authors have been found. Most of the cases were seen but once, so that detailed studies could not be made. In 12 cases, however, I was able to make more extensive observations, amounting in all to over 50, in which the blood was examined in one or several preparations for from one-half to four hours.

To supplement this I must add another series of more than thirty cases of fevers of various kinds, including enteric fever, pneumonia, phthisis, septic conditions, etc. Some were suspected cases of malaria, and in them quinine had been used. In none of these were organisms found, nor anything (with an exception to be noted later) resembling them. I have also examined the blood of a large number of persons from the interior, some of whom had had chills, but at the time of examination were well ; others of whom, though exposed, had never had ague—and in none did I find organisms, nor did ague occur in them as long as they remained under observation.

It is almost needless to say that in many cases the blood-examination led to important changes in the therapeusis. One of the most striking examples is the following : On February 13, 1890, I examined the blood of a foreign sailor just arrived from a South American port, who had had no chills, and on account of muscular pains was thought to have "grippe." Finding a number of nearly "ripe" plasmodia I diagnosed malaria and predicted a chill, which followed in seven hours. Quinine was given and the patient rapidly recovered without another chill.

In all cases I examined the blood from the finger-tip, at the ordinary temperature. In some cases in addition dried preparations were made and stained, but I had no opportunity of making extensive investigations of that kind. Necessary as such studies are in determining some facts regarding the organisms, fresh preparations are for many reasons more valuable. In all the observations I used a Zeiss one-twelfth homogeneous immersion, ocular iv.

This seems the proper place to explain the above statement regarding the bodies resembling the plasmodia, but found in non-malarial blood. The exception alluded to concerns the unpigmented hyaline forms, which are sometimes simulated by certain appearances in the red blood-corpuscles. Some of these appearances are the so-called vacuoles ; others, and more deceptive, are reflections caused by bosses on the surfaces of the corpuscles ; still others, often seen in patients with hyperpyrexia, are caused by an increase in the biconcavity of the disks. All of these can be distinguished, with care and experience, from the true plasmodium.

For purposes of description the various forms may be classified into endoglobular bodies,[1] including the rosettes ; free bodies, including flagellates and crescents. I shall follow this order as well as circumstances allow me.

With the bodies in the first class my experience has been similar to that of others. That is, I have found them in all cases of acute intermittent fever (not cinchonized) and in many protracted cases, and therefore look on them, on the whole, as the most important from a clinical standpoint. I have made several attempts to follow up Golgi's theory of the cyclical development of the plasmodium, the general truth of which is accepted by many observers. My own studies seem to prove the truth of Golgi's law, the practical importance of which is seen in the case cited ; but most of my cases have been of mixed type and could not be left to their natural course long enough to establish the relations. I have not yet seen a case of quartan fever, and as all the many rosettes I have observed correspond with those Golgi has described as peculiar to tertian fever, this may be looked on as additional confirmation of his views.

In addition to those forms which perform the cyclical development, terminating in the segmentation of the rosettes, there are other endoglobular bodies which have a different series of phases. Many of these forms have been seen and described by various authors. Celli and Guarnieri looked on them as irregularly segmenting forms, and possibly

---

[1] Plasmodium malaria of Marchiafava and Celli.

as degenerations. Golgi described a very common form as a modification of division, but was uncertain whether it really was so. I have had very favorable opportunities for studying these bodies, and can confirm the observations of the authors named, as well as carry them further in some respects.

For convenience I shall speak of them as atypical plasmodia. They differ so much in minute details, that it is difficult to classify them, and indeed it would probably not be profitable to do so, since the differences can hardly be important. I have studied these bodies carefully in six cases, and have seen them in several others. Four were cases of acute vernal intermittent. In the two other cases there had been no chills for one month, but the temperature rose from one to three degrees at irregular periods. ("Dumbague," "bone-fever," of common parlance.) In the former cases there were typical forms, in the latter none.

These atypical bodies develop from small hyaline forms which cannot be distinguished from the typical plasmodia. The process of development is rather rapid, and is apparently unconnected with the course of the fever. They seem to have a special tendency to escape from the blood-corpuscles at early periods (Fig. 1). A little later than the

FIG. 1.

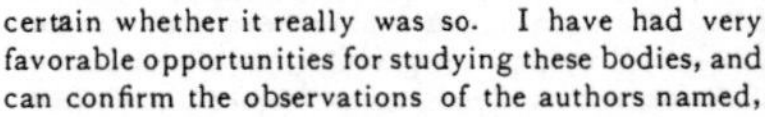

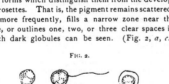

Changes of form in a small, free, hyaline body. Observation lasting five minutes.

stage shown in the figure, but where the corpuscle is not entirely destroyed, they form, on escaping, small spherical bodies, single or in rows connected by fine filaments, which have a fibrinous appearance. When the bodies reach a size almost equal to that of the corpuscle, they begin to assume the characteristic forms which distinguish them from the developing rosettes. That is, the pigment remains scattered, or, more frequently, fills a narrow zone near the edge, or outlines one, two, or three clear spaces in which dark globules can be seen. (Fig. 2, *a*, *c*.)

FIG. 2.

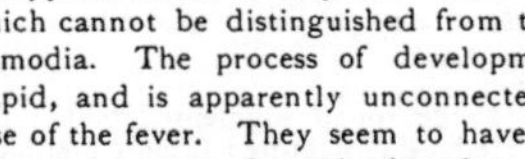

Developing atypical plasmodia. Nuclear bodies not shown.

The later stages of this process are not often seen in blood from the finger, which fact makes me think that part of the development of these bodies is in internal organs. This opinion is supported by the analogous development of the rosettes in the brain-

capillaries in pernicious malarial fever; and I have seen the stage often enough to know that the substance of the corpuscle is gradually destroyed, a shell-like, colorless rim being left for some time, but ultimately disappearing. (Fig. 2, *b*.) Even before the final disappearance of the corpuscle a filament may form on the plasmodium (Fig. 2, *c*.), as I have seen in one observation. We thus have the free pigmented bodies, which, though varying in details, correspond in general to the later forms of the atypical endoglobular forms.

As my observations show a relation between these and the flagellate organisms, I shall consider other of their characteristics in connection with the latter.

Regarding the nature and origin of the flagellate bodies there still exist the greatest differences of opinion among authors. Laveran, in his earliest as in his latest communication, described them as the most characteristic and most important forms of the parasite of malaria, but admitted that they are comparatively seldom seen (in 92 out of 432 cases), as they appear only in a certain stage of development. Councilman came to similar conclusions, and found the bodies in 15 out of 20 cases in which splenic blood was examined. On the whole, the mass of testimony is against these views. Space does not permit a review of all that has been written on the subject recently, and I shall submit my own observations with only occasional reference to the contradictory or confirmatory studies of others.

In regard to the occurrence of the flagellate bodies I can say from my own earlier experience that they were often overlooked because the bodies on which they form were mistaken for pigmented leucocytes. It is remarkable how cautious in this respect were the older observers of malarial blood (Virchow, Frerichs, and J. F. Meigs), and how near some of them came to anticipating Laveran's discovery (Kelsch and Joseph Jones).

The occurrence of flagellate bodies in three successive cases of acute intermittent seen this spring led me to look over my notes, and I was surprised to find how frequent flagellate bodies had been observed in my experience. Of the 12 cases carefully observed, in 7 acute cases they were found six times, and in 5 chronic cases twice or probably three times. The description of the bodies which follows is based on observations made in 4 cases of vernal intermittent, of from three days to one week's duration.

Corresponding to the stage at which they escape from the corpuscles (or are formed by budding, as described below), the free bodies vary in diameter from one-fourth of to quite that of a red blood-corpuscle. A large majority are slightly smaller than the latter. At rest, and when fresh, they are round, with positive but faint outlines, and always contain black or reddish-brown pigment, in short rods. The pigment is usually gathered in a zone near the margin, the centre being clear and very bright and containing a dark globular body (nucleus?), as seen in Fig. 3. In some the nucleus is divided, or in dumb-

FIG. 3.

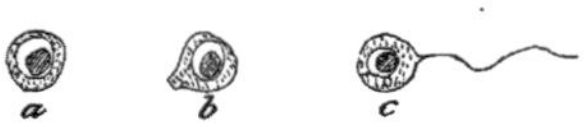

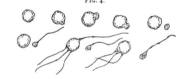

a   *b*   *c*

Flagellate body. The changes shown were observed within a period of ten minutes.

bell shape, or there are two or three clear spaces with pigment around them, as in the endoglobular forms (Fig. 2). In others the pigment is scattered over the optical surface, and in such it may be seen by focussing that the body is spherical, or spheroidal. In most of the bodies the pigment exhibits, at once, or soon after the preparation of a specimen, a peenliar motion. This was accurately described by Laveran, and quoted by Sternberg, but not mentioned, so far as I know, by other observers, who speak of the motion ·as "Brownian." Celli and Guarnieri have described a similar motion in bodies derived from crescentic forms.[1] Laveran's words are very vivid: "*Les grains pigmentés . . . . sont animés de mouvements très vifs, comparables à ceux des particules solides qui se trouveraient dans un liquide en ébullition.*" That the motion is not Brownian may be seen by comparing the melanin granules in the bodies with others free in the plasma. It seems to depend on currents or contractions in the protoplasm of the bodies. The outlines of the bodies appear almost structureless, but at times the edges show an active undulation, when a membrane is apparently present. The undulation of the margin seems to be connected in some way with the formation of the filaments, and I have often been struck by the aptness of the comparison Richard drew between the process observed and the struggles of an animal. The edge waves violently, small projections are formed, pigment grains are ejected, and finally, in the words of Laveran, the filament shoots out. It may be apparently retracted again, but at last rhythmically oscillates or lashes to a length of twenty to thirty micromillimetres. Not all the filaments make so much commotion on their first appearance. Sometimes they appear on a side where there was little motion. It is usually said that filaments are never seen until from fifteen to twenty minutes after the preparation of a slide, but some observers have seen them earlier without a warm stage, and I have "focussed down" on a body with active filaments, with a surrounding temperature of 80°.Fahr. Frequently I have seen the whole process end within fifteen minutes. The

[1] Canalis mentions it in a recent work received after this paper was finished. Fortschritte der Med., 1890, No. 8.

delicate structure of the filaments ·cannot easily be portrayed. They taper off rather abruptly from the bodies. Terminal knobs I have never seen, except those caused by pigment granules, but dilatations on the filaments have been rather frequent, and were always caused by movable pigment. In some cases the filaments appear to be tubular, as described by Laveran. I have often seen, as have others, the filaments, with or without pigment grains in them, tearing loose from the bodies, when they can be seen moving in a not very active manner, but often making wide excursions.

The production of filaments is not the only capability of the free bodies. Frequently a process of budding may be seen, the daughter-cells·so formed having also a filament and dancing pigment.[1] I could trace no connection between the budding and the nuclear globules described.

In order to make clearer the characteristics of the bodies under consideration I reproduce sketches and notes made on a single one, in an observation lasting half an hour:

Fig. 4. Large round pigmented body; pigment marginal; edges undulating; intense motion of pig-

FIG. 4.

ment on side opposite eccentric nucleus (not shown in sketch); formation of a bud, in which pigment is intensely aggregated and dancing. The portion of the bud on the wall varies as much as 40 degrees; bud gradually constricted off; a filament four times as long as a red corpuscle formed on daughter-cell; mother continues undulating and pigment motion (the melanin rods) having an excursion of 20 degrees to 40 degrees around the periphery. Three filaments appear on mother-cell; opposite them a very long filament appears, strongly agitating adjacent blood corpuscles; daughter-cell approaches and indents a red corpuscle repeatedly, but does not enter it. Daughter-cell is larger, pear-shaped, pigment running up and down in filament.

When preparations containing free (flagellate) bodies are kept for some hours—though a half-hour may suffice—their dissolution may be seen. The edges become more vague, the body flattens out and

[1] Celli and Guarnieri (loc. cit. p. 528) describe the formation of flagellate daughter-cells from atypical segmenting bodies, but do not mention the formation of filaments on the mother-cell. I have recently seen both, in bodies which correspond in other respects with those described by the authors.

finally remains as a shapeless, hyaline mass, with motionless pigment-granules scattered over it.

As already intimated, what I have said of the flagellate bodies is based on observations in the early stage of intermittent fever. Bodies similar in every respect, and accompanied with typical endoglobular forms and crescents, have been seen in protracted cases of severe intermittent; also in cases in which malarial infection could not easily be recognized without the microscope. In the latter they were the only forms, as in the following case :

M. R., laborer, living in the western part of Galveston, a swampy region. Admitted April 14, 1890, for diarrhœa. Had three chills six weeks ago, with intervals of one day. Took "Chill-cure." No more chills, but is peevish at times ; spleen enlarged. In the blood numerous large, endoglobular, atypical bodies are found, together with many free bodies and flagellates. Kept on spirit of Mindererus for four days. The temperature rose to 99.8° F. from 2 to 4 o'clock P. M. daily. Patient expressed himself as feeling well. The bodies persisted as before ; there were no typical forms. The diarrhœa having ceased spontaneously the patient left the hospital.

In a case of two months' duration seen last fall, which began as tertian but became quotidian, I found numerous free and flagellate bodies and crescents, but no endoglobular forms. The patient had been cinchonized for some time. Tonic treatment, with small doses of quinine, was carried out. There were no more chills. Flagellate bodies, and later the crescents, ceased to appear.

Other histories could be cited, but I think enough has been said to show not only the number, but the variety of cases in which the flagellate bodies occur, confirming in the latter respect what Councilman has said of the bodies.

As regards numbers, the flagellate bodies and free pigmented bodies seem to vary more in different cases than in the same case at different times (except under treatment). In some cases one only may be seen in a preparation. In one case every field had at least one, sometimes two or three. At times one can see a medium-size pair together. Not all of these free bodies had filaments, but some filaments could always be found, and no doubt many were overlooked in the brief time of the examination.

As to the origin of the bodies, my observations show beyond doubt that they are derived from certain endoglobular forms. From their occurrence in recent cases it would seem that they are simply varieties of the forms which carry on the typical process in malaria. But on the other hand, cases like the two described make it probable that they have an independent existence. To make this supposition stronger we must discover the unknown parts of the cycle of development—*i. e.*, the origin of the atypical endoglobular forms from the free bodies — as has been done for the typical bodies. In the first case here described I saw the nucleus of a free body break up into a number of oval globules, smaller than those of the tertian cyclical forms, but could not see their ultimate liberation. The most inviting solution of the question may possibly be found in the theory of Celli and Guarnieri[1] that the plasmodia can go into the reproductive phase at any stage of their development. It has occurred to me that perhaps the atypical and flagellate bodies are the results of such processes, and that they represent resting states of the organism, capable of existing independently, perhaps even of reproducing themselves, but also able, under favorable circumstances, of reproducing the typical growth of the parasite. Biology supports such a theory as much, I believe, as it does the theories which make them simply degenerative or post-mortem phenomena. In endeavoring to get some light on this question I thought of the action of drugs as perhaps giving some assistance. The effect of quinine on the parasites has long been known ; *i. e.*, that it stops the development of the plasmodium, but has no effect on the crescentic bodies. In all the reports I have access to, large doses of quinine have been used. I endeavored to make the process less abrupt in the following case :

J. H. Acute quotidian intermittent ; second chill. In the blood, developing plasmodia (rosettes) and flagellate bodies were found. He was given tincture of gentian for two days, the chills and condition of the blood continuing. Five grains of quinine given in solution three hours before the next expected chill prevented the paroxysm, but the blood contained bodies as before. That is, there were large, "ripe" plasmodia and free bodies with very active filaments. No rosettes. On the next day, after thirty-five grains of quinine had been given, the endoglobular forms were fewer, but the flagellates numerous and active. On the following day, with twenty grains of quinine, endoglobular bodies were not to be found, and of the few free bodies all were motionless, as was their pigment, and they developed no flagella. The patient was discharged at his own request and has not since reported.

In another case I tried a remedy which may prove a valuable addition to our list, viz.: nitrate of potassium, recommended by Dr. J. D. Hunter.[2] After my friend Dr. Hadra had told me of his success with this remedy in ague, I tried it, but, in order to observe the blood-changes more readily, gave it, not as advised by Hunter, in

---

[1] Loc. cit., p. 527.
[2] Virginia Medical Monthly, February, 1890.

large doses before and during the paroxysm, but in smaller doses, fifteen grains every three hours. The case was one of quotidian (double tertian) intermittent, of one week's duration, and had been treated by whiskey alone. I may add that the effect of saltpetre on a *potator's* stomach was much better than that of quinine. After beginning treatment there were no more chills, but the temperature rose on two successive days to 101.2° and 101.8° F. respectively. The manner of disappearance of the parasites was precisely similar to that in the other case ; but as the patient was kept under observation ten days after the last chill the final and complete disappearance of the flagellate bodies could be followed.

In a third case quinine and saltpetre were used together, as follows : At the beginning of a chill (the second of a tertian) the patient took ten grains of quinine in capsules. The temperature rose to 100° F. Examined in the defervescence the blood showed organisms, endoglobular, free and flagellate. Saltpetre was given in the dose of thirty grains every three hours and the parasites disappeared in the same order as in the preceding cases.

These observations show a greater resistance to specific or antiperiodic remedies on the part of the flagellate bodies, and support the view I have advanced as to their nature—*i. e.*, as resting forms. A temporary cessation of intermittent fever prevents me from carrying these observations further, so that for confirmation as well as for learning additional details regarding the atypical bodies we must await future investigations. It is in the hope that others may take up the matter that I bring forward these few observations.

My observations on the crescentic bodies, though rather numerous, are all imperfect from the fact that I could not observe my cases in their natural condition for a long enough period. Observers are unanimous in considering these bodies the constant parasites of the chronic irregular forms of malaria, and of malarial cachexia, but as to their origin and development and relation to the other forms there is still great difference of opinion. Most recent investigators ascribe to these bodies an endoglobular development, but the accounts of various authors differ radically. Golgi, who looks on the endoglobular development as undemonstrated thinks they represent a later stage in the development of the flagellate bodies. I have not yet seen his latest contribution on the subject.

I have never seen a crescent in a red blood-corpuscle, although in some of my cases crescents were so numerous that six or seven could be seen in a single field. Still, I am inclined to believe in the endoglobular development of these forms, on account of the numbers in which they occur, the destruction of blood corpuscles in those cases, and the

difficulty of accounting in any other way for the melanin they contain. The most interesting explanation of the origin of the crescents is that suggested by Grassi and Feletti (p. 434), viz., that it takes place in the bone-marrow. This explains why undeveloped crescents are so seldom found in blood from the finger, and receives support from observations of Danilewsky on certain parasites of reptiles, probably belonging to the same class as those of malaria.

Crescentic bodies are seldom found in recent cases. The following history shows the most rapid development I have yet seen.

October, 1889, a man who had never before had malaria lived for four weeks in one of the most noted ague localities in Texas. A week after his arrival a quotidian intermittent became manifest and soon the paroxysms were doubled, one in the day and one at night. Quinine was taken to cinchonization during the first week ; after that not at all. Examined three weeks after the first chill. His blood then showed many crescents, but no endoglobular or flagellate forms. The blood corpuscles numbered 2,335,000 per c.mm.

Under the energetic use of quinine, arsenic, strychnine and iron there was steady improvement and there were no more chills. Crescents gradually disappeared.

The changes the crescents undergo have often been described and need not be repeated here. That they are cadaveric I have no doubt. The production of filaments on them, however, I have never seen, although I have looked for it long and frequently. In all cases where filamentous bodies were found with crescents, the flagella could be seen to develop only on the bodies already described.

A word in regard to an important subject, namely phagocytosis. I have endeavored to study this in malarial blood, but the results were disappointing. I have often seen the atypical bodies enclosed, while still active, in leucocytes (large polynuclear and eosinophile), and have followed their gradual disintegration. But considering the number of free bodies and leucocytes encountered, the process, on the whole, is infrequent, and "pigmented leucocytes" do not figure so largely in our notes on malarial blood as before the parasites were known (James, p. 270).

As said at the outset, it is not the object of this paper to consider the whole aspect of the pathology of malaria, and I have purposely avoided discussing the biological and etiological relations of the malarial parasite.

As to the former I can add nothing to the latest conclusions of those who have given most thought to the subject. The lowest classes of animal organisms, to which the hæmatozoa malariæ are evidently related, are so imperfectly understood that at present we learn but little from them. The investigation of malarial blood by biologists with special training must throw a great deal of light on that subject. Though culture methods and ordinary inoculations are not available much can be done, with no danger and but slight discomfort, by inoculations in man.

As regards etiology, while the strict methods of bacteriology cannot be applied to malaria, proof as to the causal relation is stronger, it may be remarked, than it is for some parasites whose pathogenic nature is not questioned, *e. g.*, the trichina spiralis. Inoculations by many observers have shown that the virus of malaria exists in and is transmissible by the blood. In the latter we find the organisms, whose cyclical, combined with irregular, polymorphous development furnishes so perfectly what clinical pathology requires of the germ of malaria. Added to this we have the action of quinine, which, specific as it is for some forms of the disease, is so probably only by virtue of its power over amœboid organisms in general.

The value of the organisms in diagnosis has been emphasized by all who have tested the matter. The use of the microscope in clearing up the nature of a host of vague complaints, called by both profession and laity "malarial," and in limiting the application of that term to the proper class of diseases, should be general.

Not only in diagnosis is the microscope of practical value in malarial diseases, for with its assistance specific remedies can be used more rationally than heretofore, and with a certainty not otherwise possible.

Works referred to.

Councilman : Transactions of Assoc. of American Physicians, 1886; THE MEDICAL NEWS, vol. i., 1887, No. 3; Medical and Surgical Reporter (abstract), vol. lviii., 1888, No. 4.

Osler : Transactions of Phila. Pathological Society, vol. xiii., 1887; Medical Record, vol. xxxv., 1889, p. 393; Johns Hopkins Hospital Bulletins, vol. i. No. 1.

Sternberg : Medical Record, vol. xxix., 1886, Nos. 18, 19.

James : Medical Record, vol. xxxiii., 1888, 269.

Golgi : Fortschritte der Med., Bd. 7, 1889, No. 3.

Celli and *Guarnieri :* Ibid. Bd., 7, 1889, Nos. 14, 15.

Laveran : Compt. rend., No. 17, 1882; Archiv de Med. Exp. etc., 1889, p. 798, and 1890, p. 1; reference in Fortschritte der Med., Bd. 8, 1890, p. 231.

Grassi and *Feletti :* Centralblatt f. Bakt. u. Parasitn., Bd. vii. 1890, 13, 14.

CLINICAL MEMORANDA.

SURGICAL.

Mucous Polypi of the Bladder in a Child. Suprapubic Operation. Death on the 23d Day.—The following case is reported somewhat in detail: first. because cases of vesical tumor are by no means common; and, second, that it may add to the data available in forming a prognosis in such cases, although some doubt as to the exact cause of death makes the case one of uncertain value in determining the prognosis of future operations.

The case is as follows: March 11, 1890, I saw for the first time R. B., aged four and a half years. The boy was considerably emaciated, but there was no satisfactory evidence of any disease other than that of the bladder. The symptoms dated back eight months, and had been gradually increasing in severity. At the date above mentioned, there was frequent micturition, with much vesical tenesmus and pain; some dribbling of urine (urine was never bloody); prepuce elongated from frequent handling. Micturition was distinctly easier when the body was in a horizontal position. Microscopical examination of urine revealed nothing more than evidences of cystitis. There were the ordinary symptoms of stone, but with more than the ordinary amount of pain and tenesmus. The boy was accordingly examined for stone on two different days and under chloroform : the instruments used were a small, ordinary urethral sound, and a small, flexible, metallic olive-tipped urethral bougie. The results of these examinations were not satisfactory. With a finger in the rectum, the bladder felt thick and boggy even after the urine had been drawn off by a catheter. The sound could be felt through the base of the bladder, and once upon entering there was a faint suspicion of a "click." At another place there was a suspicion of a grating sensation that was also suggestive of a calculus. These suspicions, however, did not warrant a cutting operation—certainly not cutting for *stone.* The only fact that might have been suggestive of the true condition of affairs was that the amount of urine that could be drawn off with a catheter did not correspond with the suprapubic percussion dulness, which persisted in a considerable degree after withdrawal of the urine. Another fact already mentioned, and particularly noticed by but one of several authorities consulted upon the subject, was the *inordinate* vesical tenesmus. Although no blood appeared during or after the two examinations referred to, the pain and tenesmus were increased thereby, and an operation was decided upon as the best means of curing the cystitis and relieving the bladder.

A suprapubic cystotomy was therefore made under some disadvantages. Owing to circumstances beyond the control of the operator, the child could not be moved to a hospital; the house was small and the surroundings decidedly unattractive from a surgeon's point of view. No rectal distention was used, the bladder being moderately distended and irrigated at the same time by a stream of warm, boiled water from a fountain syringe at an elevation of three feet above the bladder. A median incision two inches long and just above the symphysis gave access to the bladder-wall, which was incised between two supporting tenacula. The peritoneum was not seen. The incision was made large enough to admit a finger, and the bladder was found completely filled with pedunculated mucous polypi varying in size from one-eighth to one inch in diameter and variously attached to the base of the bladder, but grouped more closely about the vesical neck. These were carefully removed with the finger-nail and forceps, and when removed half filled a one-ounce quinine bottle. The hæmorrhage was unimportant. The bladder-wall was not sutured. Two or three deep sutures closed the abdominal wound about a Trendelenburg drainage-tube—no perineal drainage, or catheter in the urethra. The pain and tenesmus were entirely relieved by the operation, and the child's general condition seemed much improved. The wound was dressed daily, and the drainage-tube removed on the sixth day. The temperature was normal until the seventeenth day, when there was slight fever and some looseness of the bowels. The wound looked healthy, and the cause of the disturbance evidently was one or two recent errors in the management of his diet. On the eighteenth day there were two general convulsions, with loss of consciousness, lasting two or three minutes; looseness of the bowels continued, with pronounced though not excessive tympanites. On the two following days there was some general improvement. There were no more convulsions and no higher temperature, but on the twenty-third day the patient died with no more marked symptoms than those above described.

W. A. BATCHELOR, M.D.

MILWAUKEE, WIS

OBSTETRICAL.

A Case of Placenta Prævia ; Death.—The following case is that of an Italian woman aged thirty-four, who had had three children, all of which are living. The labors were easy. To this case my friend Dr. Cheston, of Chestnut Hill, called me in. The woman, according to our informant, had been bleeding so profusely for fifteen hours that the bedclothes and surroundings were soaked. On arrival we found a very pale, though fairly well-nourished woman. Her pulse was weak, and respiration hurried. She was not bleeding at this time. We were informed that she was in the seventh month of pregnancy. On vaginal examination the os was found the size of a half-dollar, and on introducing the examining finger, all antiseptic precautions being carefully observed, the placenta was found firmly adherent around and across the os, and bleeding when touched. The woman being very weak from the excessive loss of blood, and not bleeding at this time, version and delivery were delayed. As she had some bearing-down pains, one drachm of ergot every two hours was ordered, and the vagina was tamponed.

The foot of the bed was raised. Hot black coffee, and half an ounce of whiskey with tincture of digitalis were given also, every two hours.

In the evening, about eight hours later, we found her bleeding, but in a somewhat better condition. Having been allowed to get up out of bed to bear down, she had forced out the tampon. She had vomited her ergot and stimulants.

We decided to perform version and delivery by the breech. External version was done, the os still about the size of a half-dollar, and the feet were brought down. The woman was given her coffee and milk, and hypodermic stimulation was resorted to, but the pulse was failing. The breech being delivered, the arms were extracted, but great difficulty was experienced in delivering the head, and after some effort the forceps were applied. After the child was delivered the uterus commenced to contract under the action of external abdominal stimulation.

The placenta was apparently normal. The child, rather large, was born dead. The mother never reacted from the profound collapse, and died an hour after labor.

R. H. BOLLING, M.D.,
Resident Physician, Germantown Hospital.

MEDICAL PROGRESS.

Treatment of Granular Lids with Strong Solutions of Bichloride of Mercury.—In the *University Medical Magazine* for July, 1890, is the following report from the hospital service of DR. G. E. DE SCHWEINITZ:

The favorable reports which from time to time have appeared in regard to the value of strong solutions of bichloride of mercury in the treatment of granular lids have led to an extensive trial of this remedy in the eye wards of the Philadelphia Hospital. The method adopted is as follows: Every alternate day the everted lids are carefully touched with a solution of bichloride of mercury, 1 : 300 or 1 : 120, according to the size of the granulations, while three times a day the conjunctival cul-de-sac is irrigated with a warm solution of the same drug, 1 : 7000. No other medicine is employed. The results have been almost uniformly favorable. In no single instance has the disease been aggravated ; in a few it has apparently undergone no modification, while in the vast majority, after four or five applications of the character described, there has been increased comfort, lessening in the size of the granulations, dissipation of the discharge, and not infrequently amelioration of pannus, if this was present. Perhaps the strongest testimony in favor of this application is that given by most of the patients themselves, all of the chronic cases having, either in this institution or elsewhere, had all manner of local astringents applied to their everted lids. Their testimony is practically unanimous that this has given the greatest comfort. It is a painful application, and in sensitive patients, as has been recommended, the eyes may be cocainized. In most of the instances, however, this precaution has not been deemed necessary. These observations are based upon the experience of about thirty cases.

The Pathogenesis of Yellow Fever.—DRS. FINLAY and DELGADO (*Lancet*, June 21, 1890), who have for some time been engaged in investigating the bacteriology and pathology of yellow fever in Cuba, recently read a paper on the subject before the Havana Academy of Sciences, in which they detailed their experiments and discussed their significance, with special reference to the researches of Dr. Sternberg. They say that Sternberg's micrococcus Finlayensis has been found by Dr. Kinyoun on the skin of patients suffering from malarial fever in localities where yellow fever does not occur, and that it is, therefore, impossible that this microörganism can bear any relation whatever to the causation of yellow fever. The micrococcus tetragenus versatilis has been found in the serous fluid of blisters on yellow fever patients in spite of the most careful disinfection of the skin, in one-half ot the cases examined, and in three-eighths of the specimens on which observations were made. This micrococcus was found in the blister serum of persons resident in Havana and acclimatized, in two out of seven cases examined, and in three-thirteenths of the specimens taken, but only in cases where the disinfection of the skin had been omitted, or in which it had been but imperfectly performed. Nothing of the sort was found in any of the eight specimens taken from four persons whose skin had been as thoroughly disinfected as that of the cases of yellow fever.

The Dangers of Tonsillotomy.—Removal of the tonsils by the bistoury or guillotine is a popular operation in England and America. The French are less partial to it, and MM. Quénu and Lucas-Championnière have recently dwelt on its dangers at the Paris Société de Chirurgie. The latter surgeon referred to two cases in Broca's practice where profuse hæmorrhage followed removal of the tonsils. In one of these instances the patient, a medical student, died almost immediately after one tonsil was cut, so violent and uncontrollable was the bleeding. In a case in M. Lucas-Championnière's own experience the patient, a middle-aged man, had enlarged tonsils, quite free from inflammation, and he was not suffering from any morbid condition likely to prevent the natural arrest of hæmorrhage. On removal of one tonsil hæmorrhage took place, and could not be checked until after two hours of digital pressure with a tampon soaked in ergotine. M. Quénu always uses the galvano-cautery three or four times, at intervals of a fortnight, and atrophy of the tonsil always follows. MM. Marc Sée and Chauvel do not dread the knife. There can be no doubt that hypertrophy of the tonsils require active treatment, especially in youth; and the evil consequences of neglect are well known. In the majority of cases the risk of dangerous hæmorrhage is very slight; but the possibility of its occurrence should always be borne in mind, and the use of ice or of a styptic gargle should be enforced as a measure or precaution immediately after the operation. —*British Medical Journal*, June 21, 1890.

Prescription for Exophthalmic Goitre.—According to the *Weekly Medical Review*, DR. A. F. WATKINS recommends the following prescription in the treatment of exophthalmic goitre :

> R.—Picrotoxin   .   .   .   . $\frac{1}{30}$ grain.
> Aqueous extract of ergot   .   2½ grains.

Make into a pill. One pill should be taken three times daily.

Aseptic Wound Treatment.—BLOCH, of Norway, deprecates the use of corrosive sublimate as an antiseptic in surgical practice, and believes that with proper precautions as good results can be obtained without this agent as with it. The author's usual method of procedure is as follows : The region to be operated on is cleansed with soap and water, ether, and carbolized water (3 per cent.); the instruments are sterilized by exposure to steam, and then laid in carbolic solution (3 per cent.). At the end of the operation the wound is irrigated with carbolic solution of the same strength (sometimes it is first swabbed with chloride of zinc, 10 per cent.); all ligatures and sutures are of catgut, prepared by steeping first for forty-eight hours in 5 per cent. watery, then in 5 per cent. alcoholic, solution of carbolic acid. The author has discarded Schede's sublimated catgut, culture experi-

ments having shown it to be not invariably sterile. Drainage-tubes (red rubber) are kept in 3 per cent. carbolic solution. Two layers of sterilized gauze are interposed between the absorbent dressing and the wound to keep the cotton-wool from sticking to the stitches. The drainage-tubes are removed on the third, fourth, or fifth day, and the dressing then applied remains on for two or three weeks.

After summing up the results of twenty-nine cases managed in this manner, the author is able to say that wounds treated with sterilized cotton-wool heal in an ideal manner. Nevertheless, on examining the secretions of the wounds, as was done in every case, there were found microbes even in the "aseptic" clots from the drainage-tubes withdrawn on the third, fourth, and fifth days. None the less he is able to record perfect union, by first intention, without any suppuration whatever.

The microbes found were monococci, diplococci, and staphylococci. Cultures usually showed these to be staphylococcus albus; rarely staphylococcus pyogenes aureus or bacilli were found.

Cases treated with a layer of iodoform gauze next the wound give equally good results. Here, too, there were microbes in the clots; from one case, which healed ideally, there was obtained the staphylococcus pyogenes aureus.

With carbolized gauze next the wound the results were the same: the wounds healed in perfect manner, but microbes were present. In only two out of seventeen cases could they not be found. They probably lodge in the epidermis, and are practically ineradicable from it; and it must be supposed that their development is inhibited by the antiseptics applied to the wound during and after the operation.

Conclusions.—1. Large operation wounds may heal as perfectly, in a clinical sense, when dressed with sterilized materials not containing any antiseptic agents as when treated with antiseptic dressings.

2. Large aseptic operation wounds, dressed simply with sterilized cotton-wool, heal generally by first intention.

3. The secretions of wounds, healing without any suppuration whatever, contain microbes, as a rule, whether the dressing contains bactericide agents, or consists simply of sterilized materials.

4. Wounds containing microbes (abscesses, etc.), dressed simply with sterilized cotton-wool, may pursue a course identical with that which they would have pursued had they been treated with antiseptic dressings.

The logical issue of the investigation would be the recommendation of sterilized cotton-wool as the best form of dressing. For private operations, where two intelligent persons can divide the work between them, it is available with full security. But in large hospitals, where the carrying out of details is divided among a number of persons, a certain security is gained by the addition of an antiseptic agent.

For this reason the author recommends the treatment of wounds by carbolic acid, with the modification that the outer layer of the dressing shall be not of macintosh, but of sterilized non-absorbent cotton-wool.—*Glasgow Medical Journal*, June, 1890.

The Dangers of Constipation in Children.—In a lecture recently delivered before the Paris Hospital for Sick

Children, DR. JULES SIMON (*Journal de Médecine et de Chirurgie*, May, 1890) called attention to the fact that while diarrhœa occurring in children is the object of the most extreme solicitude both on the part of parents and of physicians, constipation, which possesses almost as great danger, is almost entirely neglected. He called attention to the case of a girl, fifteen years of age, who was brought into the hospital suffering from extreme abdominal pain, caused by a fall upon the abdomen, and followed by an abscess in the abdominal walls. The symptoms, however, rapidly increased in intensity, and were followed by vomiting and diarrhœa, and the patient died at the end of a few days. At the autopsy there was noted general peritonitis, with a perforation of the cæcum, surrounded by an old purulent deposit in this region. There was thus typhlitis, followed by perforation, which led to the formation of an encysted abscess in the pelvis, and only as the result of injury was general peritonitis produced. Dr. Simon believes, from the nature of the lesion observed, that the inflammation and the perforation were the consequences of marked constipation, leading to a rapidly fatal termination by traumatism. He believes that cases similar to the one reported are much more common than is ordinarily supposed, and he thinks that in many cases faulty development and numerous digestive disturbances are attributable to more or less obstinate constipation. Indeed, even in some cases death itself may follow either through the production of typhlitis and the perforation of the cæcum, as in the present case, or from intestinal obstruction. Dr. Simon stated that in another case he had seen death produced by a fæcal tumor the size of a child's head. In such cases the author has frequently obtained satisfactory results from electricity, but when the obstruction has been overcome by this means, it must be recognized that the patients are constantly exposed to a return of a similar state of affairs ; for the intestinal tube, after such great distention, becomes the seat of structural modifications, and is almost incapable of resuming its normal condition. There is thus a practical point to be observed, whose neglect may be followed by the most serious complications, and in examination for the cause of obscure infantile troubles the occurrence of constipation as a possible factor should never be overlooked, especially as constipation may be actually obscured by an apparent diarrhœa.—*Therapeutic Gazette*, June, 1890.

Condensed Milk as an Infant-food.

—DR. LOUIS STARR considers condensed milk a good food for infants while travelling, or under circumstances in which good cow's milk cannot be procured. If possible, he gives it in the following mixture :

Cream	. . .	1 tablespoonful.
Condensed milk	. .	2 tablespoonfuls.
Water	. . .	11 "
Mellin's food	. . .	1 tablespoonful.

In preparing this, the water should be heated to the boiling point, adding first the Mellin's food, then the condensed milk, stirring constantly until the solution is complete. After the mixture has slightly cooled, the cream is added. This amount is sufficient for one meal for a child of eight months.—*Annals of Gynæcology and Pædiatry*, June, 1890.

Ointment for Chapped Hands.

—According to the *Journal of Cutaneous and Genito-urinary Diseases*, the following is an excellent application for chapped hands: Dissolve one part of boric acid in twenty-four parts of glycerin ; add to this solution five parts of anhydrous lanolin and seventy parts of vaseline. The mixture may be colored and perfumed.

A Plaster-of-Paris Splint for the Treatment of Fractures of the Leg.

—DR. A. G. R. FOULERTON describes the following method of applying plaster dressings to fractures of the leg (*Lancet*, June 28, 1890) :

In the case of a fracture, say, at the junction of the middle and lowest thirds of the leg, three measurements are taken: (1) The length of the limb from a point an inch and a half above the knee to the sole of the foot ; (2) the circumference of the thigh at the level of about an inch and a half above the knee ; (3) the length of the foot from the heel to the ball of the big toe. An oblong piece of shrunken flannel or old blanket is then cut to such dimensions that it is in one direction an inch and a quarter longer than measurement 1, in the other an inch and a half less than twice the measurement 2. The limb is laid on the flannel, which is then held up by its edges, supporting the leg as in a sling. Next, the flannel is tacked together with needle and thread close to the limb, down the front of the leg, along the sole, and then along the dorsum of the foot. It is better to sew the flannel in the order given, along the sole first and along the dorsum afterward, because by doing so the foot will be held by the flannel in the position in which it should be—at a right angle with the axis of the limb. The leg is thus closely encased in flannel, while along the front of the leg and the dorsum and sole of the foot a double free edge of flannel is left beyond the seam. These free edges along the dorsum of the foot, as high as the ankle, and along the sole, are trimmed off close to the seam. There now remain two considerable wings of flannel extending down the front of the leg as far as the ankle. Each wing, when turned back from the middle line in front, will reach to within about half an inch of the middle line behind. These wings are then trimmed from below upward, so as to shape them to the form of the leg. Two side splints with rectangular foot-pieces are then cut out of flannel, so that each piece, when applied to the limb, shall reach to within about a quarter of an inch of the middle lines in front and behind. Care must be taken that the anterior edge of each side-piece is quite straight ; the posterior edge may be shaped so as to allow for the swelling of the calf muscles. Traction is then applied to the limb, and these side-pieces, having been thoroughly saturated with plaster-of-Paris mixture, are placed over the flannel casing, one on each side of the leg. The wings of flannel are then quickly folded back, each over its respective side-piece, and smoothed down. Plaster-of-Paris is then rubbed well into the outer surface of the two flannel wings, avoiding, however, a border about a quarter of an inch wide down the front of the leg on either side of the seam. The perfect adaptation of the splint to the limb may then be secured by applying a thin muslin roller-bandage over the whole from the toes upward. After ten minutes the muslin bandage is unrolled, and the splint is then finished. The plaster will probably be quite dry in the course of an hour.

ically THE MEDICAL NEWS.

A WEEKLY JOURNAL
OF MEDICAL SCIENCE.

COMMUNICATIONS are invited from all parts of the world. Original articles contributed exclusively to THE MEDICAL NEWS will be liberally paid for upon publication. When necessary to elucidate the text, illustrations will be furnished without cost to the author.

Address the Editor: H. A. HARE, M.D.,
1004 WALNUT STREET,
PHILADELPHIA.

Subscription Price, including Postage.

PER ANNUM, IN ADVANCE . . . . $4.00.
SINGLE COPIES . . . . 10 CENTS.

Subscriptions may begin at any date. The safest mode of remittance is by bank check or postal money order, drawn to the order of the undersigned. When neither is accessible, remittances may be made, at the risk of the publishers, by forwarding in *registered* letters.

Address,   LEA BROTHERS & CO.,
Nos. 706 & 708 SANSOM STREET,
PHILADELPHIA.

SATURDAY, JULY 19, 1890.

THE RELATION OF THE HOSPITAL PHYSICIAN TO THE HOSPITAL SURGEON.

THE existing unwritten, yet inflexible, laws governing the actions of the members of a hospital staff in regard to one another are becoming, at the present time, so unsuited to the demands made by the rapid progress and subdivisions of medical science as to require serious innovations if the benefit of patients is to be considered as a more important matter than the preservation of professional ethics. Our attention is called to this growing evil by the generally acknowledged fact that the various branches of medical science are each becoming so vast in their scope and minute in their individual technique that no one is capable of carrying out successfully all of the operations or therapeutical measures which patients of every class may present. We fear that some surgeons and physicians still believe themselves able to treat all the ills to which man is subject, without calling in the aid of any of their brethren, and that there are others who, from pecuniary motives alone, neglect to send a patient to a more experienced friend because they will lose the case. This lack of humanity and abuse of professional confidence are not, however, the evils at which this editorial is aimed. What we complain of is the lack of recognition on the part of the boards of managers of hospitals of the fact that the staff should consist of a body of men not all general surgeons or physicians, but some of them specialists in the important parts of medicine and surgery. Either this fact must be recognized, or the individual members should be allowed to call into their wards, in consultation or for operation, friends who in their opinion are qualified to assist or take entire charge of a given case. At present this is considered a professional impossibility, yet every one who has occupied a position on a hospital staff must have experienced the difficulties of referring a patient to the care of his colleague, knowing when he did so that while his friend was an accomplished physician or surgeon, he was in reality utterly without adequate training for that particular emergency.

As an instance of this we may cite a case which was recently brought to our notice, in which a woman suffering from peritonitis of a frequently recurring type came under the care of a physician who had charge of a ward in a large hospital. The history of gonorrhœa and the entire atmosphere of the case showed it to be one demanding operative interference of a most skilled and experienced character, an experience confessedly lacking in the eminent surgeon on service at the same institution during the course of the case. Under these circumstances this surgeon would have been bound to operate if called on, since he could not refuse to perform an act so plainly indicated, nor could he confess his inability to do so through ignorance. There was, therefore, but one path left for the physician in charge; namely, to wait until the inflammation remitted in its violence, and then hurriedly to discharge the patient with a recommendation to call on a surgeon qualified to relieve her without exposing her life to unnecessary risk. In the case before us the surgeon attached to the hospital had enough conceit to believe himself capable of operating on anything, but the subsequent history of the case proved that only the most dexterous and experienced of men could have possibly saved the woman's life, because of the extensive abdominal lesions produced by her disease.

If the physician had referred his case to his colleague with his knowledge of his colleague's inability to treat it, the one would have been but an accomplice to a professional murder. and the other a man who, by the force of existing laws and his conceit, must forever have the awful responsibility of the loss of a human life resting upon his shoulders. In this instance the remittance of the disease permitted the physician to do the best he could for his case, and he practically advised her to flee from the hands of his colleague; but had no remittance in the disease taken place, he would have had to be content with letting her die on his hands, or of sending her to her death in the surgical wards. We cannot clearly see our way toward remedying this evil, but the evil exists, and as such should be remedied, and if any of the readers of THE MEDICAL NEWS can recommend a plan we shall be glad to hear from them. The mere appointment of specialists does not entirely avert the danger, since the individual so appointed may not entirely command the professional confidence of his colleagues in every case which appears. No practitioner sends all his private cases to one surgeon or physician, but selects for each case the professional brother best qualified to take care of the diseased process suffered from.

CORRESPONDENCE.

MILK INSPECTION IN CINCINNATI.

To the Editor of THE MEDICAL NEWS,

SIR: In THE MEDICAL NEWS of June 21st your Cincinnati correspondent indulges in some statements in regard to the dairies and milk-supply of this city, which are not only sensational and untruthful, but reflect very unfavorably upon all who have heretofore held the position of Health Officer. No such state of affairs as is depicted by your correspondent has existed for years, if ever, in this city. All of Dr. Prendergast's predecessors have paid much attention to the dairies and milk-supply, and very few cities in the country have had better milk than this has had.

For the last four years the office of milk inspector has been filled by an honest physician, who was very attentive to his duties, and was well versed in chemical analysis, and who had as assistants competent and trustworthy inspectors of dairies; and their weekly reports to the Health Office showed that their duties were not neglected.

If your journal were read only by Cincinnati subscribers no reply to your correspondent would be necessary; but to those who do not know the absurdity of his letter, I desire to say that his statements that "the dairies were in an appalling condition," that "in some, the cows stood up to the knees in filth," and that "many of them had not been liberated from their stalls for more than a year," are utterly devoid of truth, and that his letter is but an attempt to write into notoriety a set of newly appointed men who were absolutely ignorant of the duties they were expected to perform.

Yours respectfully,

BYRON STANTON, M.D.,

Ex-Health Officer of Cincinnati.

To the above letter our Cincinnati correspondent replies as follows:

To the Editor of THE MEDICAL NEWS,

SIR: In the letter which I had the honor of contributing to THE MEDICAL NEWS of June 21st, it was my aim to give you the opinions of the local medical profession, and not my own ideas; and I was particularly careful to consult the best available authorities with reference to the truth of every statement before its publication. When, therefore, Dr. Stanton takes exception to my letter, he flatly denies, not merely the veracity of a newsmonger, but the official action of the Cincinnati Academy of Medicine, of which he is a member, the verdicts of the daily press, compiled at great length and with many illustrations, not from the reports of the Health Office, but from personal investigation by reporters, and, I might add, from the confessions of dairymen who made no denials but pleaded inability to obey the law profitably. What there was, therefore, of the "sensational" in my letter was of the character which is inherent in the description of a dire calamity of large proportions, though it be the slaughter of innocent babes through the ignorance and carelessness of milk-producers. Through personal regard for Dr. Stanton and the esteemed physician who was associated with him as milk-inspector during his term of office, as well as at the request of the present Health Officer when interviewed, I not only refrained from criticism or censure of previous officers, but distinctly stated in the letter referred to, that "In the revelations which have been made there has been no attempt to reflect unfavorably on the official career of previous health officers, and no such reflection should be made. The fault lies not with those who have occupied the office . . . but with the city government." I heartily agree with Dr. Stanton as to the official honesty and professional ability of himself and associates in office, and have still no desire to criticise them.

But, when the ex-health officer selects from my letter the statements that the "dairies were in an appalling condition," that "in some the cows stood up to the knees in filth," and that "many of them had not been liberated from their stalls for more than a year," and asserts that they are utterly devoid of truth, I most respectfully but emphatically deny and refute his statement. On the evening of May 12th, the Cincinnati Academy of Medicine unanimously adopted a resolution of which the following is a part:

"*Resolved*, That we have witnessed with much surprise and alarm the exposures recently made by the Health Department of our city under the direction of Health Officer Prendergast, of the appallingly unsanitary condition of a large number of the dairies which supply us with milk, but we fully endorse the efforts of the Department to correct the existing evils . . . that we tender to the Health Officer our earnest support, and urge him to continue his efforts to increase the efficiency of the Department in the same energetic and fearless manner as he has begun."

"Filth to the knees" was the condition described in the daily press, and I am informed that it is correct. It might have been an inch or two less deep, if the Jersey cow was taken as the standard of measurement, but the fact remains that the filth was there, and that the cows stood in it. Even worse, an eye-witness informs me that in at least one instance the cow's udder was so besmeared that this same filth dropped from the fingers of the milker into the pail, and remained there until the milk was strained.

The *Cincinnati Lancet-Clinic*, May 17, 1890, says editorially:

"From time out of mind Cincinnati has been greatly cursed with a stock of dairies that have had a place and habitation within the city precincts, where the cows were almost wholly fed on distillery slops and starch grains. As if this were not bad enough, the poor unfortunate animals are, month after month, confined within the stables, and often standing in their own filth; while, to make the condition as bad as possible, the frame sides of the sheds are, in the fall, as hermetically sealed as possible with the dung of the cattle."

Now, whom are we to believe? If the letter of June 21st was so "utterly devoid of truth," what of these other statements? and if these were false why did not the injured ex-health officer immediately cry aloud and at home? Why did he select for refutation (?) a letter in which his official career was vindicated in preference to those in which he had been less kindly dealt with? His statement, that no reply would be necessary if read only by Cincinnati subscribers, is as aqueous as any of our milk.

If the letter of June 21st was "intended to write into notoriety a set of newly appointed men," it came too late, when prompt and energetic devotion to duty had already made them "notorious." And if these neophytes were "utterly ignorant of the duties they were expected to perform" (can he refer to obligations to the dairymen?), then may we thank the kind Providence that sent us men thus ignorant, Democrats though they be!

MODIFIED CHEYNE-STOKES RESPIRATION.

To the Editor of THE MEDICAL NEWS:

SIR: The article in THE MEDICAL NEWS of May 31, 1890, by Dr. Norton Downes, on "Cheyne-Stokes Respiration," brings to mind a case that I met with last autumn.

A boy, between three and four years of age, had had a severe attack of diphtheria, but had recovered from its immediate effects. The membrane had disappeared from his throat and nostrils, and his physician thought that there would be no further obstacle to recovery. The child, however, continued debilitated, and seemed unable to regain his strength. Some days later I was called in. The parents had become alarmed at a peculiarity of the breathing that had developed. This peculiarity was like that of the cases referred to by Dr. Downes as having been reported by Dr. William O'Neil, viz., deep inspirations, with long intervals of rest. This was particularly noticeable when the child was sleeping, either in the night or day. Sometimes there was very little noticeable in his respiration except an occasional long breath, but when he fell asleep the peculiar respiration would occur, sometimes to such an extent as to alarm the parents and friends. At no time was there the quick shallow respiration, followed by the period of apnœa, so marked in well-developed cases of Cheyne-Stokes respiration. Examination showed that his heart was weak but regular in action, the pulsations ranging from 110 to 120 per minute. Throughout the case there was

no cyanosis or rise of temperature. On testing the urine, which was diminished in quantity, I found abundance of albumin, but at no time was there any dropsy, other than slight puffiness about the eyelids and lips. Constipation was present, and the complexion was of that clayey, unhealthy appearance, not uncommon after diphtheria, and always present in anæmic and dropsical patients. Some days after my first visit, paralysis of the palate began, and continued until it was almost complete. In spite of the fact that the condition of the kidneys improved, as shown by urinary tests, and by the improvement in the respiration, the child continued to grow weaker, and while there was no actual paralysis of the lower limbs, the patient was unable to walk. After careful treatment for about six weeks, I regarded him as convalescent, and he finally completely recovered.

The points of peculiar interest in this case are, that the difficulty in respiration increased during sleep, yet at no time was it sufficient to keep him awake; and that there was no cyanosis. My explanations of these peculiarities is that the case was one of uræmic poisoning, and the centres of respiration were benumbed by the poison circulating in the blood, yet not sufficiently so to prevent the child's recognizing the want of air when awake.

Now, during sleep the centres failed to act, except when the *non-aërated* blood roused them to action, and when the need of oxygen was felt. By the expression "*non-aërated* blood," I mean blood deprived of a certain amount of oxygen, and carrying enough carbonic acid or uræmic poison, or both, to overcome that state of inactivity, and to cause the respiratory centres to respond. In thinking over the matter of cyanosis, I have concluded that the deep, full inspirations at intervals, really furnished almost as much air in a given time as is normally furnished, and that while the respiratory centres were so influenced as to cause irregular breathing, yet they were sufficiently active to respond before the lack of air was so great as to cause cyanosis.

W. R. CUSHING, M.D.

DUBLIN, VA.

ABSORPTION OF BONE-SPLINTERS.

To the Editor of THE MEDICAL NEWS,

SIR: The question as to the extent to which splinters of bone detached from the periosteum may be absorbed is an interesting one. It has seemed to me that the possibility of absorption might be greatly increased by appropriate measures. The cases that have come under my observation in which this condition was supposed to exist were not verified by post-mortem examination, and it is on this account that I take the liberty of suggesting the following points as perhaps worthy of the attention of those who may have greater opportunities for their verification.

It is evident that even slight irritation due to motion of the fragments of the delicate granulation tissue surrounding splintered bone tends to produce swelling and stasis, which prevent absorption. If in the effort to prevent such motion bandages are drawn too tightly, absorption is interfered with. I have seen two instances, at least, in which, so far as could be judged from the symptoms, a long bone had been splintered so as apparently to separate fragments from the source of their periosteal blood-supply. In both, however, absorption seemed to have taken place and to have become complete without suppuration, at the end of several months. It was thought that this result was due, in part at least, to the treatment adopted, which consisted in the prolonged application of the ideal elastic pressure secured by means of splints which had been upholstered with curled hair. By means of such splints it is possible to hold the parts immovable with comparatively gentle pressure and without any tendency to strangulation and consequent pain and swelling. Moreover, they are light, cool, and comfortable. Certainly, in the difficult and tedious cases mentioned, they contributed to the favorable result, whatever may have been the precise pathological condition.

M. A. VEEDER.

LYONS, NEW YORK.

NEWS ITEMS.

A Successful Cæsarean Section by Candle-light.—D. F. Albert Mouillot, in the *British Medical Journal*, June 28, 1890, reports a successful case of Cæsarean section in a woman four feet eleven inches in height. The distance between the anterior superior spinous processes was only eight inches. The operation was done by candle-light in a peasant's house, and with no other instruments than those of a pocket-case. Dr. Mouillot attributes the recovery to the fact that the woman was not exhausted before the operation, and that strong uterine contractions followed.

A Fatal Epidemic of Whooping-cough.—The *British Medical Journal* states that the mortality from the epidemic of whooping-cough now prevailing in Aberdeen, Scotland, is exceptionally high. During the month of May one case in every eight proved fatal.

Increase of Insanity in England and Germany.—It is computed that there is an annual increase of 300 to 400 lunatics in London. A new asylum for the accommodation of 2000 patients has been begun, and will be finished in about two years. At the present rate of increase of lunacy in that city a new asylum will be required every five years. The population of the city is stated to increase about 80,000 per annum, so that a large lunacy increase is explicable.

It is stated that in the German Empire during the past five years there has been an increase of 25 per cent. in the number of cases of insanity, against an increase of 3.5 per cent. in the population.

Artesian Water-supply at Memphis.—The new artesian water-supply of Memphis, Tenn., is probably as perfect as that of any city in this country. According to the *Bulletin of the Tennessee State Board of Health*, the supply is practically inexhaustible, such is the capacity of the water-bearing sand, and it is estimated that, however great the amount of water used, no impression can be made on the subterranean river of supply. It is assured that clear water, free from admixture with river water or surface drainage, can always be obtained. This is rendered probable by the fact that there is an upward

pressure from the wells to a point that is higher than the high-water mark of the Mississippi River. The water, as delivered from the wells, is sparkling and transparent, and is unaffected by rains or by turbidity of superficial streams. Its fountain-head must be at a distance of many miles. The system for gathering, storing, and distributing, has been constructed in an unique and admirable manner, and, from a hygienic point of view, its introduction is a blessing to all concerned, and the system will be a model to other cities in the valley of the Mississippi.

The Code of Ethics of Oregon.—In a bill before the Oregon legislature, for the regulation of medical practice, there is a singular clause providing that licences to practise may be revoked for "unprofessional conduct," which is defined in the bill as: (1) Participation in criminal abortion; (2) employing "drummers or steerers;" (3) promising to cure an incurable disease, and taking a fee therefor; (4) betrayal of a professional confidence; (5) advertising in a false or exaggerated manner; (6) advertising to regulate the menses of women; (7) conviction under some charge implying "moral turpitude;" (8) habitual intemperance. Like many other newly settled communities, Oregon has greatly suffered from quacks and advertising adventurers.

THERE is a movement on foot at Paris to establish a polyclinic, conducted similarly to those of Vienna and Berlin.

OFFICIAL LIST OF CHANGES IN THE STATIONS AND DUTIES OF THE MEDICAL CORPS OF THE U. S. NAVY FOR THE TWO WEEKS ENDING JULY 12, 1890.

P. H. RIXEY, *Surgeon.*—Leave of absence granted for fifteen days.
F. M. OGDEN, *Assistant Surgeon.*—Promoted to be a Passed Assistant Surgeon.
S. STUART WHITE, *Assistant Surgeon.*—Promoted to be a Passed Assistant Surgeon.
L. W. ATLEE, *Assistant Surgeon.*—Granted three months' leave of absence
T. WOLVERTON, *Medical Inspector.*—Awaiting orders to the U. S. S. "Philadelphia."
P. A. LOVERING, *Passed Assistant Surgeon.*—Awaiting orders to the U. S. S. "Philadelphia."
D. MCMURTRIE, *Medical Inspector.*—Granted leave of absence for thirty days.

OFFICIAL LIST OF CHANGES IN THE STATIONS AND DUTIES OF OFFICERS SERVING IN THE MEDICAL DEPARTMENT, U. S. ARMY, FROM JULY 8 TO JULY 14, 1890.

By direction of the Secretary of War, the leave of absence on surgeon's certificate granted MARCUS E. TAYLOR, *Captain and Assistant Surgeon,* in S. O. 45, June 13, 1890, Division of the Pacific, is extended five months on surgeon's certificate of disability, with permission to go beyond sea.—Par. 6, *S. O. 159, A. G. O.,* July 10, 1890.

THE MEDICAL NEWS *will be pleased to receive early intelligence of local events of general medical interest, or of matters which it is desirable to bring to the notice of the profession.*

Local papers containing reports or news items should be marked.

Letters, whether written for publication or private information, must be authenticated by the names and addresses of their writers—of course not necessarily for publication.

All communications relating to the editorial department of the NEWS *should be addressed to No. 1004 Walnut Street, Philadelphia.*

THE MEDICAL NEWS.

A WEEKLY JOURNAL OF MEDICAL SCIENCE.

VOL. LVII.   SATURDAY, JULY 26, 1890.   No. 4.

ORIGINAL LECTURES.

AMPUTATION OF THE NECK OF THE CERVIX UTERI. DYSMENORRHŒA FROM CERVICAL STENOSIS.

A Clinical Lecture
delivered at the Hospital of the University of Pennsylvania.

BY WILLIAM GOODELL, M.D.,
PROFESSOR OF GYNECOLOGY IN THE UNIVERSITY OF PENNSYLVANIA.

[Reported by LEWIS H. ADLER, Jr., M.D.,
RESIDENT PHYSICIAN EPISCOPAL HOSPITAL; LATE RESIDENT PHYSICIAN
UNIVERSITY HOSPITAL.]

GENTLEMEN: My first case to-day is one upon which I operate under a sort of protest, because I am not certain that it will be followed by success. Yet, taking all the circumstances together, I feel that it is the safest and best thing that can be done.

The history of the patient is briefly as follows: The woman is thirty-three years old, married, but sterile and very anxious to become a mother. A few years ago she began to lose much blood at her menstrual periods. This menorrhagia has now become a serious matter. The cause of this excessive hæmorrhage is a multiple fibroid tumor of the womb: more than this, she labors under the physical defect of having the surgical neck of the womb elongated to the length of one and a half inches, and this mechanically interferes with coition to the extent of preventing any semen from entering the uterus. I operate to-day, first, on account of the tumor, and, in the second place, on account of the sterility. On account of this tumor the woman is losing each month a serious quantity of blood ; now, if through an amputation of the cervix she be enabled to become pregnant, two very important objects are gained—in addition to the sterilty being cured, the pregnancy will stop her menstruation, and thus for the time prevent the loss of blood, and probably, also during her lactation. By the blood-currents being directed into other channels during these two periods—of pregnancy and of lactation—and by the positive influence that the act of involution will exert to divert the blood from the uterus, there will be a strong tendency and even a great probability that the fibroids in the walls of the womb will become actually smaller.

I have in two instances delivered women with uterine fibroids, in whom the tumors afterward became smaller, although for a time there was excessive hæmorrhage ; because, in both cases the tumors, being intra-mural, acted as splints to the walls of the uterus, and prevented the womb from contracting. I know of another case in which a doctor delivered a woman who had a fibroid tumor weighing thirty pounds. In that case the labor came on and ended without difficulty, the hæmorrhage being very slight, because the tumor was subperitoneal. The final result was not so successful, as the woman died in two days from septicæmia, which disease was caused, as the post-mortem examination revealed, by broken-down uterine tissues, which in many places had become necrotic and had further degenerated into pus.

There are, in general, three ways in which fibroids of the uterus prevent conception :

The first of these ways is by menorrhagia. The excessive flow of blood washes away the ovum before it is impregnated, or, at any rate, prevents its becoming moored to the side of the womb, to undergo there its complete development. For this reason the fibroid that causes the greatest hæmorrhage will be the most apt to prevent conception. So that pregnancy is more common with subperitoneal fibroids than with the other two varieties.

The second way that a fibroid prevents conception is by causing the Fallopian tubes to become tortuous, which condition, by narrowing the calibre of their canals, delays or prevents the passage of the ovum to the uterus.

Lastly, in the vast majority of cases of fibroid tumors the ovaries and tubes are themselves the seat of disease ; in some instances being affected with inflammatory changes ; in others, with cystic degeneration.

Now, in the case before us, the woman is anxious to have a child, and I would feel warranted in removing the tumor, provided I was certain that she would then become pregnant ; but really, with the elongated condition of her cervix uteri, I think that, if all other obstacles were removed, she would still be mechanically incapacitated from conceiving. For, as I press down the womb from above, and, at the same time, dilate the vaginal canal, you can see in this instance a redundancy in both lips of the cervix, which condition has been compared to a shark's mouth or to a tapir's nose, and as you know the latter resemblance has given rise to the expression of the "tapiroid cervix." The measurement of the normal uterus gives minus five inches, while from the beginning of the present cervix, I get a measurement of plus five inches. Therefore what I propose doing to-day is to amputate about one inch and a half of this redundant cervix with the hope that she will then become pregnant and that thereby the menorrhagia may be stopped and the fibroid tumor grow smaller.

In this case, the operation of amputating the cervix is complicated by the presence of the fibroid tumor, which has for a long time been inviting a large quantity of blood to the uterus, so that from this excessive nutrition of the endometrium there is upon it an outgrowth of vegetations. These will have to be scraped off, and in order to do this the cervical canal must be made large enough to allow the curette to pass through. Therefore, the operation to-day would naturally divide itself into three stages :

1. Dilating the cervical canal ;
2. Scraping the cavity of the womb ; and,
3. Amputating the redundant part of the cervix.

But, I find that in this instance I cannot follow these stages of the operation in the order given; because the cervix is so long that when I attempt to dilate it the shoulder of my dilator will not allow the instrument to pass far enough in, so that I find myself obliged to begin with the amputation.

The first step is to disinfect thoroughly the instruments. For this purpose I prefer to use a 1-to-2000 solution of the bichloride of mercury. I am fast giving up the use of carbolic acid as a disinfectant, not only on account of its odor, but also because it does not compare with the solution of the bichloride of mercury as a germicide. The drawbacks to the use of the latter are that it is a very poisonous drug to handle, and that it is injurious to instruments, especially dulling the edges of sharp tools.

The vagina may be thoroughly washed out with a 1-to-1000 or 1-to-1500 solution of the bichloride solution.

The patient, now being fully under the influence of the anæsthetic, is placed upon the table in the lithotomy position, on the left side, and a Sims's speculum is introduced and given to my assistant to hold. I now bring the womb fully into view and introduce into the bladder a well-curved sound in order to determine its situation in relation to the uterus ; next, the cervix uteri is transfixed with a long, straight skewer just above the point at which I propose to amputate, and another one is placed at right angles to it. Behind these an elastic noose of rubber tubing is tied to control the hæmorrhage, after which the redundant portion of the cervix is removed in a cone-shaped piece.

One danger in this operation is the possibility of accidentally getting into Douglas's pouch. I am certain that during my professional career I have opened this pouch once and possibly oftener, but with very little bad effects.

The little hæmorrhage which you notice is no more than will be controlled by the stitches. When it is excessive Paquelin's cautery is the quickest and surest means of stopping it. Having now removed the redundant part of the cervix, which, as it is now bloodless, appears much smaller than it did a minute ago, I prepare to unite the mucosa of the os uteri with the mucosa of the vagina by means of silver-wire stitches, which, in their radiating arrangement, resemble that of the spokes of a wheel. I say, I prepare to unite, because I shall not complete that part of the operation, but when I have finished the remaining two stages of the operation Dr. William L. Taylor will kindly take her outside and unite the sutures.

I next proceed to dilate the cervix to one and one-sixteenth of an inch, which, in this woman, is rendered more difficult than usual on account of the long, narrow cervical canal. This being done, I now prepare to use the curette, which instrument I grasp gently, both that I may not inflict any injury on my patient and that I may the better appreciate the character of the surface over which it moves. Upon inserting the instrument I feel as I pass it around within the cavity of the uterus projections here and there, also a ridge of fibroid tissue over which the curette passes.

I should have told you that the instrument which I use for this purpose is always the sharp curette, which makes great care necessary.

Before beginning this curetting I had washed my in-

struments in a strong bichloride of mercury solution and also had the vagina syringed out with a 1-to-1000 solution of the same material. Now that it is over I wish to disinfect the parts once again with this 1-to-1000 solution. I therefore syringe out the vagina, and, as I want some of the solution to go into the cavity of the scraped womb, I gently swab out the endometrium. It would be highly dangerous to syringe the uterine cavity in this condition, because if the organ were to contract and the os not remain patulous so that the solution could readily pass out, the imprisoned liquid might be forced through the Fallopian tubes into the cavity of the peritoneum. Therefore, the rule is never to syringe into the uterine cavity unless you have a perfect avenue of escape.

[The patient was now removed.]

This condition of cervical elongation upon which I have just operated was a congenital defect. There is, however, a hypertrophic elongation of the cervix, following laceration, and due to the parts being rendered more plastic than normal by their increased blood supply. The operation on the laceration in these cases does not, in my experience, cure the elongation. There happens just now to be in my private hospital a case of this kind that has been operated on by another physician for laceration of the cervix and yet the organ protrudes from her person.

After these operations there will be around the os uteri a raw surface that will heal by granulation ; this fact, together with the irritation set up by from fifteen to twenty sutures, may cause so great a degree of retrograde metamorphosis that a womb that gave a measurement of from four to five inches may be made to shrink to only two inches. The weight of the organ is correspondingly diminished, and as the uterus rises in the pelvis the cervix will then seem shorter than it really is. Paquelin's cautery may also cause cicatricial contraction.

There are two accidents to avoid in this operation. They are, getting into the bladder and as before stated getting into Douglas's pouch. The first of these is guarded against by passing a catheter into the bladder or by passing the finger through the dilated urethra, that it may serve as a guide. I have never yet met with this accident, though I fear I shall some day, for it has happened already to a good many of my brother practitioners. If such an accident were to happen to me, I would at once close the wound with sutures. The other accident, as I said before, has happened to me at least once, but without fatal result. In Die Allgemeine Krankenhaus of Vienna there are no special precautions taken by the operators to avoid opening Douglas's pouch, and they show most excellent results in their operations. The great secret is to have everything antiseptically clean, and then there is comparatively little danger even if we enter either place.

DYSMENORRHŒA FROM CERVICAL STENOSIS.

This woman is married and has had no children, although she has wished for them. She seems to be, physiologically, a perfect woman, and her husband also presents all the qualities of being a perfect physiological man. In the vast majority of virgins and barren wives you will find an anteflexion of the womb, and, while I have not yet examined this woman and so cannot be positive, I think it most probable that I shall find here a case of exaggerated anteflexion and that it is this condition that makes the cervical canal narrower at the os uteri. I often compare this condition to a bent rubber hose, in which the angle causes a lessening in its calibre; and just as the normal calibre of the hose can be restored either by means of straightening or by dilating it at that point, so the diameter of the cervical canal may be made normal either by overcoming the anteflexion or by forcible dilatation.

The first of these objects is attained by means of the pessary. All kinds of these instruments, especially the intra-uterine stem pessary, have been used with more or less benefit. But they are all fast going out of fashion and are much less popular than they were ten years ago. As a rule, I do not advocate their use; but I do like and can most heartily recommend the use of forcible dilatation. By this latter means the result desired is attained without the discomfiture of carrying a pessary; the woman becomes pregnant, and the birth of the child straightens out any angles that may exist in the canal. I have performed this operation about three hundred and fifty times and have never had cause to regret it, and neither will you, provided you are careful to use the one great precaution which may be embraced under the expression "thorough antisepsis." The steps of this operation are as follows: First I introduce into the rectum a suppository of the aqueous extract of opium. This is done before I begin to dilate, so that its effects will be manifest by the time the operation is completed. Next, before introducing the speculum, I disinfect the vaginal canal by thoroughly swabbing it with a 1-to-1000 solution of the bichloride of mercury. I now put in the speculum, not greased, but rendered antiseptic with this same solution. This being done, I again disinfect the vagina and then feel that at least the avenues are antiseptically clean. The passage of the sound caused the discharge of about half a teaspoonful of mucus, which is always a good sign. I now introduce my smallest dilator; upon it I have no rachet, for I consider it both unnecessary and dangerous to the operator, as the rachet is liable to slip and cut the hands. After using this instrument until I have made the canal large enough for my larger dilator, I withdraw the smaller one and insert the larger size, with which I enlarge the canal to the extent of one and a quarter inches in diameter.

There is here a little bleeding, as is often the case, and it would be of no consequence except that it interferes with the means of antisepsis. However it quickly stops. If it were to bleed too much, I would use injections of alum or of vinegar; and then, if it were to continue, I would tampon the vagina with antiseptic lint. But in this case all such measures are unnecessary. I again syringe out the vagina with a strong solution of the bichloride of mercury and then, after drying it with an antiseptic swab, I introduce a ten-grain suppository of iodoform, and the operation is done.

When she comes from under the influence of the ether, she will have another opium suppository: two hours later, if she be suffering much, she will have a third, which will be repeated in a couple more hours, if it be necessary. This is generally all that is needed. To-morrow the nurse will syringe out the vagina, both morning and evening, with a 1-to-4000 bichloride of mercury solution, and will repeat this as often as neces-

sary. I formerly used a 1-to-2000 solution, but I collected thirty or forty cases in which I think that it proved injunous, so that I have ceased to use it so strong. This patient will stay in bed until all soreness is over, and I shall continue to use every antiseptic precaution until all danger is past.

ORIGINAL ARTICLES.

WHAT CAN AND SHOULD BE DONE TO LIMIT THE PREVALENCE OF TUBERCULOSIS IN MAN?[1]

By EDWARD O. SHAKESPEARE, A. M., M.D., PH. D.,
OF PHILADELPHIA.

UNDOUBTEDLY the great majority of advanced thinkers of our profession in Europe and America, to-day admit that Villemin (whatever may have been the reception first accorded his publications) announced a most important truth in 1865 when he declared, from the standpoint of experimentation, that tuberculosis is a specific infectious disease; and unquestionably the same men now acknowledge that Koch in 1882 not only signally confirmed this truth of Villemin, but greatly increased its practical importance by proving that the tubercle bacillus constitutes the sole specific infection of this disease.

It is not my purpose, and, in my opinion, it would waste valuable time to review even cursorily the evidence which now unshakably supports the claims of these two distinguished investigators. Nor can I hope to present anything new.

I think I may safely advance the assertion that there is no fact within the whole range of medical knowledge for the demonstration of which a greater mass of the most exact, positive, convincing proof can be marshalled, than that the bacillus tuberculosis is the sole active exciting cause of tuberculosis, and that without the agency of this micro-vegetable parasite there can be no genuine tuberculosis, no matter how susceptible the individual or how favorable the so-called predisposing causes may be.

Is tuberculosis essentially *infectious* and at the same time essentially *hereditary*? Although we have some examples of infectious diseases which are also at times hereditary, and at least one striking instance where a highly infectious disease—namely, syphilis—which is perhaps as frequently transmitted directly to the offspring *in utero* as it is acquired after birth by direct infection, there is strong reason for holding that, as a rule, diseases which are essentially infectious are also essentially non-hereditary.

What relation has this rule to tuberculosis? Of the analysis of clinical experience upon this question the best that can be said in favor of heredity is that the latter utterly fails to account for the origin of

[1] Read before the Association of American Physicians, May, 1890.

from 66 to 80 per cent. of the cases of this disease. On the other hand, autopsy records show that tuberculosis *in utero* is the rarest of all affections, in spite of the fact that death from tuberculosis is far more frequent in man after birth than is death from any other disease. In truth, all the fairly authentic observations of tuberculosis in the human newborn can be counted on the fingers of one hand, and I am cognizant of but two of these where the lesions have been shown to be genuine, and not pseudo-tubercles, by the presence of the bacillus tuberculosis or by the test of inoculation. In the bovine species, notwithstanding the great prevalence of tuberculosis among them, such observations are also exceedingly rare.

It seems therefore that we have ample ground for the belief that while tuberculosis is essentially infectious it is *essentially non-hereditary;* at least the burden of proof now rests upon those who hold the contrary opinion; and the character of the proof they would offer must be unimpeachable and convincing, affording no opportunity for dubious conclusions. Until such proof to the contrary shall be forthcoming, there seems to be sufficient warrant for regarding the non-hereditary nature of tuberculosis in man as not only highly probable but as well enough established to constitute a very important factor in determining upon a series of judicious, practical, and comprehensive measures of prevention.

To express thus positively acceptance of the conclusion that tuberculosis in man is essentially infectious and essentially non-hereditary, is by no means to affirm that the influence of heredity has nothing to do in any case with the existence of this disease. That the tubercle bacillus is the sole active infectious agent in the causation of tuberculosis is no more certain than that the influence of predisposition or susceptibility of the invaded organism greatly favors the pathogenic action of that parasite after it has found a lodgement in the tissues of the body, and that it oftentimes alone makes the development of the implanted seed possible, where otherwise a comparatively barren soil or other unfavorable conditions might prevent fructification. Marked predisposition or susceptibility to the development of tuberculosis upon *post-natal* infection may undoubtedly be an inheritance transmitted from a tuberculous parent to a child—a transmitted vulnerability which, let us hope, may be within the power of the family physician, through wise counsels respecting hygienic surroundings, wholesome nutritious food, and judicious physical culture, to do much ultimately to remove.

In recent discussions concerning tuberculosis and the practical value of the lately acquired knowledge of the pathogenic and biological characters of the bacillus tuberculosis, we hear much, especially from those chiefly interested in clinical medicine, of the complaint that this great discovery has not yet contributed, and probably never will contribute, anything toward the cure of the disease.

What if the great Koch and his co-laborers in that new field of etiological research have utterly failed to strengthen our hands by placing therein an efficient means of curing tuberculosis! Cannot a very similar reproach be applied with equal justice to Pasteur and his discoveries concerning the cause of morbid fermentations in beer and wine; concerning the cause of *cholera des poules,* of charbon, of *rouget du porc,* and of rabies? Yet what reasonable man would question the fundamental importance and immense practical value for prophylaxis of Pasteur's discoveries because he has not also shown how beer and wine once ruined by the products of morbid fermentation can be restored; or how a chicken seized with cholera, a sheep attacked with anthrax, a hog suffering with rouget, a human being already in the frightful convulsions of hydrophobia, can be cured? Who would demand of him who should come to us with a new and far more effective means than we now possess of arresting or markedly impeding the spread of an epidemic of scarlet fever, diphtheria, yellow fever, or cholera, that he shall first add something to the treatment of these diseases before his proposed measures of prophylaxis, which might be freely acknowledged to be broadly based upon entirely adequate experimental tests and supported by the strongest theoretical deductions, shall have a practical and thorough trial?

In dismissing this point, permit me to suggest that untenable as such a position would be, it is nevertheless very similar ground upon which those stand, in this country and elsewhere, to-day who, acknowledging the infectious nature of tuberculosis and the tubercle bacillus as the sole active cause of the disease, attempt to excuse or justify inaction upon the valuable knowledge we already possess concerning etiology and prophylaxis by lamenting that Koch and all other bacteriologists have failed to suggest, with their prophylactic measures, an effective mode of treatment.

In view of the admitted inefficiency of all present modes of treatment of actual cases of tuberculosis, I hold that effective prophylactic measures are infinitely more important to the general public, and should also be to the physician, than the most skilful therapeutic treatment of the disease can possibly be at the present time.

If ever there were reason for quoting the time-worn saying, "an ounce of prevention is worth a pound of cure," there certainly is when discussing the relative importance of treatment and prophylaxis of tuberculosis—a malady which more than decimates the human race, and against the ravages of which even the most skilful physician has ever been powerless.

" What can and should be done to limit the prevalence of tuberculosis in man?" This, in my opinion, is one of the most important questions with which we as physicians can deal. It is for this reason and also because it seems to interest the clinician but little at present, in comparison with the therapeutics of the disease, that I selected this subject for presentation before a society formed mainly of clinicians, with the hope of provoking a discussion and thereby hastening the time when the clinician shall earnestly unite with the hygienist in an active incessant warfare for the extermination of that terrible scourge of man, the deadly tubercle bacillus.

While, on the one hand, the discovery of the bacillus tuberculosis has, as far as we now can see, little advanced the clinical management and cure of tuberculosis except by furnishing a reliable and ready means of early diagnosis; on the other hand, it has revealed most important principles upon which to base efficient means of preventing, or, at least greatly limiting the extension of the disease—an end which may be rightly regarded as of far greater moment.

Ernst rightly declares that "Proper methods of management of tuberculosis, both in human beings and animals, involve more important interests—pecuniary as well as vital—than any other subject that engages the attention of medical men."

What are the general principles which underlie a comprehensive and effective system of prophylaxis of tuberculosis?

I hold them to be essentially these :

1. Destruction of the vitality of the tubercle bacillus wherever it may be found outside of the human body.

2. Avoidance by the unaffected of unnecessary risk of introduction within the organism of the living bacillus tuberculosis.

3. Improvement of the vitality of the individual, his personal hygiene and that of his dwelling in order that conditions unfavorable to the presence, vitality, and development of the tubercle bacillus shall prevail as widely as possible.

I have named these three fundamental principles in what appears to me their order of relative importance, well aware that many distinguished clinicians look upon the last named as that which alone should receive their hearty sanction and support. I have rated the last as least important for three reasons, each of which I regard as sufficient:

(a) Because analysis of the fullest records we have, bearing upon the relation of family history to the causation of tuberculosis, can possibly account, through the influence of hereditary predisposition or

4*

vulnerability, for little more than one-fourth of the actual cases of tuberculosis.

(b) Because, in the first place, the percentage of the so-called predisposed who could be induced to coöperate intelligently with the physician would be small; and, in the second place, it is highly probable that by no means all of even that small percentage could be so built up permanently that every vestige of inherited vulnerability would be removed.

(c) Because, even when this inherited susceptibility may be successfully removed by such efforts, we have to deal with an infectious poison which, if not destroyed, is virulent enough to produce the disease not alone in the comparatively few who may be born with an hereditary predisposition, but even to cause tuberculosis in the great majority who succumb notwithstanding the absence of an hereditary weakness.

I have not thus estimated the value of this means of combating the prevalence of tuberculosis for the purpose of indicating that it should be wholly discarded. On the contrary, I hold that it is incumbent upon us to wage an incessant and relentless warfare against the cause of this disease, "with all the means which God and nature have placed in our hands." But, let us not indulge the delusive hope that only by the selection and even skilful use of the weakest and shortest-ranged weapons we can "successfully cope with so formidable an adversary;" and let us not imagine that when we have done so we have performed our whole duty as physicians.

It is the seed of the disease, without the implantation of which there can be no harvest of death, that we are now most able to reach and destroy, and I hold that, both as clinician and hygienist—interested as well in the prevention as in the cure of disease—the true physician should do his utmost to eradicate the seeds of this malady.

It is, therefore, in my estimation, the first two general principles which should form a basis for development of details of the means which can and should be adopted at the present time for the limitation of tuberculosis.

But it has not been my purpose here to suggest in detail the prophylactic measures which should be widely adopted and enforced against the spread of tuberculosis. Excellent regulations—the general observance of which would certainly accomplish much toward the ultimate extermination of this disease, at least in its present pandemic form—have been presented by numerous physicians and health authorities.

My sole object has been to lay this important matter before the Association of American Physicians in such a manner as to elicit some action, or, at least, expression of opinion, relative to the urgent necessity of doing something—as a representative body of leaders and advanced thinkers in our profession—which shall aim at the limitation of this disease by effective prophylaxis.

Do we admit that tuberculosis is an infectious disease? Then let us so declare. Do we believe that this disease rarely, if ever, has a truly hereditary origin? Then let us not hesitate to publish that belief. Do we acknowledge that the tuberculous, especially in the active stages of the affection, throw off in the sputa or in other discharges the infectious principle of the disease, and thereby jeopardize, whether little or much, the safety of the healthy? Then let us boldly publish our knowledge, for the benefit of the public who are not in possession of it. Are we convinced that the meat and milk of tuberculous animals often contain the infectious poison and produce the disease in the healthy consumer? Then let us, without further delay, strenuously and unitedly demand the vigorous inspection of the meat and milk supply and the prompt destruction of the affected animals. Do we agree that habitations become infected with virulent sputum from the consumptive and constitute a danger to the other inmates? Then let us insist upon thorough disinfection and immediate destruction of that dangerous matter. Is it probable that an injured condition of the lungs or of other exposed organs increases the risk of development of tuberculosis after exposure to the infection? Then let us prevent many a case of consumption by insisting upon the removal of phthisical patients from the general medical wards of hospitals. Are we convinced that the unfortunate subject of tuberculosis constitutes a migrating centre of possible infection? Then let us warmly advocate the establishment of special consumption hospitals.

Now, brother clinicians, I hold that all these things can and should be done to limit the prevalence of tuberculosis in man. But they can be done only through your influence in forming public sentiment by spreading broadcast the knowledge which we possess concerning these vital matters, and thus limiting to no inconsiderable extent public dissemination of tubercle bacilli.

AMPUTATIONS WITH REFERENCE TO THE ADAPTATION OF ARTIFICIAL LIMBS.[1]

BY A. H. GARNETT, M.D.,
OF COLORADO SPRINGS.

I AM not of those who believe that, "An amputation is an opprobrium to the art of curative surgery," nor am I ready to subscribe wholly to the faith, "that in the present rapid advance in the science, and the greater perfection in the art, the time is not far removed, when amputations for cause other than gangrene, will be rare." That in the thorough observ-

[1] Read before the National Association of Railway Surgeons. May, 1890.

ance of the practice of asepsis, founded upon the bacterial origin of disease, the saving of life and limb under conditions seemingly hopeless, is now made possible, I am free to admit; but so long as there are incurable diseases, so long as there are unavoidable accidents, just so long will the necessity for amputation exist. Mechanical skill and ingenuity find a rich and varied field in the domain of surgery, for the exercise of inventive genius, and with a perseverance worthy of so good a cause, the laborer here, by the application of principles based upon the study of physiological anatomy and mechanical philosophy, has in this country brought the art of prothesis to a degree of perfection that has exerted and must continue to exert a potent influence upon amputations with reference to the successful adaptation of artificial limbs.

Statistics compiled from authentic sources show that nearly 33⅓ per cent. of the limbs lost are traceable directly to railroad accidents. Add this fact to the philanthropic spirit which prompts in many instances the generous hand of corporations to furnish appliances to the unfortunates thus crippled in their employ, and to those of us engaged in the medical service of a railroad, and we have a subjcet at once of personal interest.

Singularly enough, and unfortunately, the textbooks, including Ashhurst's *Encyclopædia*, are content to pass this subject by with scarcely a reference, with the single exception, so far as I have been able to find, of Dr. S. D. Gross, who with a just appreciation of its growing importance, and with that intuitive grasp of the practical in his chosen profession, for which he was so notably and eminently endowed, after paying a graceful tribute to the manufacturer's worth, aptly says:

"Great improvements have of late years been effected in the construction and adaptation of artificial limbs, and there is reason to believe that the inconvenience and suffering occasioned by their use are more frequently attributable to the misconduct of the surgeon than to the want of skill on the part of the manufacturer of the substitute."

Here then we have the key-note as it were from the "Nestor of American Surgery" upon the subject under consideration, who in a single terse sentence makes the relation of operator and manufacturer one of mutual dependence and profitable study.

In the absence of any literature upon the subject at my command, and without that individual experience which carries with it the force of authority, I have been obliged to consult by letter some of the leading makers of artificial limbs, whose daily observations in the construction and adjustment of these substitutes and of every variety of method practised by various operators entitle their opinions and suggestions to a respectful hearing, and to them for their kind responses I owe my thanks.

There is a unanimity of opinion among the makers that the surgeon should have some knowledge of the mechanism, construction, points of bearing, etc., of artificial limbs. I opine that from this position none of us are prepared to dissent, since the ignorance of the average medical man in this particular direction is admitted, at least among ourselves.

A few hours devoted to the perusal of the descriptive pamphlets issued by the more prominent and larger dealers will be all that is needful to acquire this knowledge.

In considering the subject proper, let us begin with amputations between the articulations, or, more definitely speaking, through the shafts of the long bones. The method generally adopted is either that of anterior and posterior, or of lateral flaps, and, as usually performed, the flaps are of the same length, or very nearly so. The stump at the extremity is frequently in consequence but poorly protected, the tissues are more or less adherent, the bone is protruding, and the cicatrix is immediately over the projecting surface; the weight is necessarily taken upon the sides, and upon the enlarging part of the stump. In the thigh, for example, the weight is taken above the end and about the ischium. This necessitates to some extent traction upon the cicatricial tissues covering the end, and this tissue from its non-elasticity and hardness exerts a certain amount of pressure upon unyielding parts; nerve filaments are caught and compressed in the opposing surfaces and as results we have painful sensations and disturbances of nutrition and circulation. To obviate this in a measure we are asked to carry the flap well to the posterior, having taken the precaution to protect the bone with periosteal covering. The cicatrix, by observing this rule, will be distant from the end of the bone, and removed from pressure. A good cushion without cicatricial tissue will form the covering of the extremity, and although it is not intended that the apparatus shall press principally on this point, if it should do so to a slight degree no harm will result. The nerve conditions resulting from adhesions, cicatricial pressure, etc., will be in a measure avoided and the liability to these altogether too frequent complications will be greatly lessened.

The above rule applies with equal force to amputation between the knee and the ankle. Teale's method here as in the thigh seems to fulfil the indications admirably and is well and favorably spoken of. When a choice is possible between the knee-joint and a position immediately above or below, preference is given to disarticulation.

The practice with some operators of trimming the condyles, is condemned upon the grounds of removing the natural cushions, rendering the end incapable of bearing weight, which, contrary to the teachings of some authors, is taken preferably at the

extremity, particularly if the patella can be made to fit into the condyloid space without the probability of becoming displaced. The flap here too should be long and anterior so that the cicatrix will not be pressed upon. When the operator is compelled to go below the knee the juncture of the middle with the lower third should, if possible, be selected, since we are told that no advantage can accrue from leaving bone between this and the ankle, a mistake not infrequently made by the surgeon. The want of space preclude the possibility of constructing a suitable artificial limb.

Amputations through or below the ankle-articulation are performed in the main with the view of receiving the weight upon the plantar surfaces; this result is generally obtainable, and a limb capable of doing good service is left. But the question presents itself, whether the amputation should be made with reference to leaving this natural support or for the better adaptation of an artificial appliance. The financial and social standing of the patient will enter largely into the decision. If the conclusion to act with reference to the adaptation of an artificial limb is reached, then the surgeon must be governed by the suggestions of the manufacturers; since they tell us that amputation in this locality involves one of the most perplexing problems in prothetical science.

I cannot do better in this connection than to use the words of Mr. A. A. Marks, of New York, whose excellent pamphlet should be in the hands of every surgeon. Mr. Marks tells us that the amputations through the metatarsus, known as Hey's and Chopart's, leave the most troublesome stumps, and mainly for the following reasons, which to my mind appear good and sufficient: 1. The natural length of the leg from the knee to the heel is retained, thus allowing no space for attachments or mechanism in the appliance. 2. All dimensions of the stump from the end to the articulation are either normal or increased, and, as the appliance must encase the stump, the diameters about and below the ankle are necessarily very much larger than natural; this gives the apparatus an unsightly and clumsy appearance. 3. The stump will not permit a firm grasp, as the remaining bones and the nervous mechanism of the foot are such as to forbid continuous pressure. On account of this the ankle-joint articulation cannot be used; for, in order to secure an artificial foot to the stump, the pressure must be considerable. Among the most serious objections, however, that Mr. Marks urges, and which alone in his estimation should condemn the operations, is the disposition of the amputated surface to point downward, occasioned by the severance of the flexors, thus destroying all opposition to the extensors. The division of the tendo-Achillis to obviate this difficulty, he tells us, affords only a partial relief. The operations at the tibio-tarsal articulation, known by the names of Syme and Pirogoff, have so many advantages over all others, fulfilling, as claimed, the most important conditions and at the least cost to the wearer, that they should always, if possible, be chosen. It is well perhaps, in connection with this, for us to recall the fact that the Syme operation has grown somewhat into disrepute among some surgeons because the necessity for reamputation is greater by about three per cent. in this than in any other amputation. The cause recently assigned for this by some authors is the failure to appreciate the importance of making the plantar incision far enough forward, as recommended and emphasized by Syme himself, and of preserving the proper vascular supply to the posterior flap.

In amputations of the upper extremities one broad guiding principle should govern us, namely, extreme conservatism ; save everything possible, for the best devised substitute known to the art is here far inferior to nature's provisions and but a poor aid at best.

To recapitulate briefly, the most desirable points for amputation in the thigh and leg are the lower thirds. When the operation must be in close proximity to the knee, the articulation should be selected as more available than a position immediately above or below. In amputations near the ankle the tibio-tarsal, Syme's, or Pirogoff's method should be chosen. It is evident that the point of selection is not always within the power of the surgeon to decide, owing to the nature of the injured part. We are assuming that it is practicable ; that it is opposed to the former practice of saving in every instance "as much of the maimed limb as is consistent with the life of the patient," and that the decision conforms to the proper adaptation of the more perfect compensative appliances of the present.

The after-treatment of the stump comes in here for our attention. One of the principal objects to be attained in an amputation is a good stump. This ideal may appear to have been obtained when the wound heals, but with the lapse of time we may note changes in its integrity, the muscles, soft parts and bone to some extent atrophy, the latter may become necrosed and the extremity painful. Some recent researches by a Frenchman, whose name I do not recall, have thrown light upon this important point. He states that a stump is a distinct organ ; that it has its own life, its special innervation and vascularization. His studies have been mainly with the venous supply heretofore neglected, and he traces the anatomical relation of this system throughout its most minute ramifications and connections, showing wherein the superficial supply is feeble and deficient. An important element in the production of the venous circulation he finds wanting, namely, muscular compression, as the muscles about the cicatricial plexus are represented mostly by fibrous lamellæ. This condition explains how external agencies, such as cold, etc., bring about reaction in the end of the stump, forcing the blood from the superficial network into the deeper veins causing neuromata, congestion, pressure, and pain. It is within the power of the surgeon to crowd out the fatty tissues and to solidify and harden the stump, making it richer in blood-supply, by a systematic process of bandaging tightly, bathing, rubbing, etc. ; increasing and exciting the circulation and enlarging bloodvessels. It is highly important that this condition of the stump should be attained before our patient comes to the hands of the manufacturer for the fitting of an artificial limb. It is true that these changes will be brought about by the pressure of the apparatus, but with the shrinking of the stump the appliance becomes loosened, necessitating a second fitting.

The final question for us to consider and one with which we will be frequently confronted, is, How long after an amputation before an artificial limb can be properly applied ? Of course there are many determining conditions and circumstances, but as a rule the experience of both surgeon and manufacturer agree, that the apparatus should be applied as soon after perfect healing as possible. Among the theoretical and physiological reasons deduced to support this position by those in military practice and by government inspectors of artificial limbs, may be mentioned the well-known law that the muscles after an amputation become weak and undisciplined from the loss of that nice balance and coöperation that is natural between them and the will-power, and that in consequence the ability to control the movements of the stump and of the apparatus will be to a great degree lost.

The application of the substitute is the first stimulus that serves to arouse the muscles from a state of comparative inertia or inactivity. Increased tone and strength are imparted, the tendency to waste or atrophy is prevented and the disposition to the accumulation of adipose tissue is materially checked.

Is will be observed that I have purposely avoided entering at length into the many methods of amputating, which would be a wearisome repetition of unnecessary details with which all are perfectly familiar. I have merely attempted to give a brief outline.

Hospital Ships.—There are three floating hospitals in the North seas, designed to go from point to point among the deep-sea fishermen. The skippers of these vessels have been instructed to some extent in the principles of "first aid" in the accidents and ailments to which the fishermen are exposed.

MENTHOL IN DISEASES OF THE AIR-PASSAGES.[1]

BY SETH S. BISHOP. M.D.,
SURGEON TO THE ILLINOIS CHARITABLE EYE AND EAR INFIRMARY, ETC., CHICAGO.

MENTHOL, a peppermint-camphor, is a powerful antiseptic and a local anodyne. I have used it considerably in a variety of diseases, and believe that its remedial properties entitle it to an important place in the work of general practitioners and of specialists. To speak systematically concerning the effects of menthol on the upper respiratory tract I will begin with the nose. Acute coryza or influenza in the first stage can be checked by inhalations or sprays of the drug. If the attack is a light one nothing is necessary beyond smelling the crystals contained in a wide-mouth vial or tube. I have aborted colds in the head at their onset by such inhalations of thirty minutes' duration. This, of course, was before the nasal irritation had passed to the stage of inflammation. The sense of fulness and constriction about the nose and frontal sinuses and the flow of mucus disappeared, the nostrils opened for the free passage of air, and complete relief followed. The remedy is well adapted for inhalation on account of its being very volatile. In the later stages of a coryza, where an actual inflammation exists before treatment, it is necessary to use sprays of menthol dissolved in liquid albolene, in order to protect the membrane and to keep the medicine in contact with the diseased surface a long time.

The strongest solution I have used was one of twenty per cent., but that is too powerful for most individuals. Five- or ten-per-cent. solutions are as strong as most people will bear. The sense of heat is considerable at first, and it materially contributes to the comfort of patients to instruct them to take several prolonged inhalations of air directly after using the sprays. This converts the burning sensation into one of agreeable coolness. Even in chronic cases of nasal catarrh I have been able to open a closed nasal passage by one or two treatments with a fifteen-per-cent. solution, thus affording great relief to mouth-breathers. Whenever a patient comes with turbinate bodies so enlarged as to obstruct the passage of air, and to prevent the entrance of sprays through the nostril to the throat, I resort at once to this remedy, with the effect of shrinking the engorged tissue and restoring the natural air-channel.

It is advantageous to prescribe inhalations of menthol for patients who take cold easily, so that they can employ the treatment at home whenever a coryza is coming on. A drachm or two of the crystals in a wide-mouth vial, with a metallic screw-cap, or a glass tube, is a convenient device. A pledget of cotton should be pressed into the vial to prevent the menthol from escaping and coming in contact with

the nose, for it occasions smarting sensations wherever it touches the nostrils. If a large glass tube is used, both ends should be plugged with cotton-wool. As menthol does not melt at a temperature below 98° F., it can be carried in the pocket for ready and frequent use. When not in use, however, in should be tightly corked to prevent evaporation. In prescribing it for patients to use in atomizers it is best to use a solution not stronger than five or ten per cent., in oil. Albolene is preferable to fluid vaseline, for the latter alone often proves irritating to the mucous membrane.

In chronic hypertrophic rhinitis, with a foul-smelling discharge, menthol is sufficiently antiseptic and alterative to lessen the amount of discharge and to banish the odor. The peppermint aroma is usually agreeable, and more especially so when it supplants the stench of decomposition. In atrophic catarrh the stimulating properties of the drug, combined with the emollient and protective qualities of albolene, afford a means of speedy improvement.

Pruritus nasi yields to nothing, excepting cocaine, more readily than to menthol, and in connection with this, if it will not be too severe a tax upon our sense of continuity to pass from the upper air-passages to the seat of pruritus ani, I will remark, parenthetically, that menthol is vastly superior to cocaine in its effects here. I have seen the most exquisitely torturing itching and burning of the anus relieved in a few minutes by a twenty-per-cent. solution of this simple drug, after other ordinary and extraordinary remedies had utterly failed.

In laryngitis not dependent on a rheumatic condition menthol proves valuable. Even in rheumatic laryngitis it is an efficient adjunct to salicylate of sodium, iodide of potassium, etc. In simple acute laryngitis, if used in the early stage, it will relieve as it does in coryza, but the spray is the most effectual form in which to use it. When the soreness of the larynx and trachea, and hoarseness appear, a few inhalations of the spray often nip the attack in the bud. It relieves the hoarseness, and imparts a smooth, reed-like *timbre* to the voice. In advanced cases several inhalations of the spray should be used in the course of a day, and a continuous effect is often advantageous. This can be secured by keeping a saucer heated in the patient's room, and occasionally dropping a few of the crystals on it during the day and night. They melt readily at a low temperature, and fill the atmosphere with their penetrating fumes.

In whooping-cough I have directed patients to inhale constantly from a cloth saturated with a solution of menthol, and placed beneath the chin. Besides this I have sprayed the nose and throat daily, taking care to project the spray into the throat just at the beginning of inhalation. The

[1] Read before the Illinois State Medical Society, May, 1890.

paroxysms of cough were lessened in intensity and frequency, and the course of the disease appeared to be shortened. Bronchitis does better with this treatment than with other topical applications, or with internal medication alone. The spray should be inhaled after a forced expiration, and retained as long as possible in the bronchial tubes before the next inhalation. This brings the fine smoke-like vapor in contact with the diseased surface. It is best to have patients exhale it through the nose, and it can readily be seen the course of the nostrils for several seconds, after a forced retention, showing that the respiratory tract is thoroughly medicated. The effect is distinctly felt deep in the chest.

In catarrhal conditions of the Eustachian tube and middle ear I have employed menthol on account of its effect in relieving turgescence and stenosis in the nasal passages. I use the menthol in Buttle's inhaler as iodine crystals are ordinarily used, substituting cotton for sponges. If a stronger impression is desired I use the liquid albolene solution. Simply throwing the spray against the Eustachian orifices with the de Vilbiss' atomizer produces a thorough impression on the tube and tympanum.

Suppurative inflammation of the middle ear readily yields to the menthol treatment. Long-standing cases rapidly healed after the use of a twenty-percent. solution. I have just seen several cases of this kind in which the purulent discharge ceased after a few such applications. Furunculosis of the ear has been in my hands more amenable to this than to any other remedy. A pledget of cotton, moistened with a twenty-per-cent. solution, should be so placed that it will remain in contact with the centre of the furuncle. A warm or burning sensation follows, but soon gives place to one of coolness. The pain is relieved, the bacteria destroyed, and the swelling and discharge checked.

I have not yet used menthol in hay-fever, but have taken steps to give it a thorough trial during the summer by the members of the United States Hay-fever Association.

In corroboration of my account of the behavior of menthol in my practice I will briefly quote from a few authors on the subject. Mr. Lennox Browne says:

"Menthol contracts the capillary bloodvessels of the nose and throat, arrests sneezing and nasal discharge, stops pain and fulness of the head, and kills the microbe of infection. When the nasal discharge is excessive it is checked ; when deficient and thickened, as in hypertrophic rhinitis, its healthy character is restored ; and when it is arrested, inspissated, and malodorous, as in atrophic rhinitis, fluidity is promoted and the foul smell corrected."

William Hill, of London, claims to have found menthol an excellent substitute for cocaine in hay fever. Jones is authority for the statement that inhalations of menthol have proved useful in asthma. He used a twenty-per-cent. solution in olive oil, and relieved a case that had resisted all the common remedies. Nye says that these inhalations facilitate and diminish the expectoration in chronic bronchitis and relieve the cough. Potter and Knight have reported cases of improvement in laryngeal phthisis, and Rosenberg and others claim a large percentage of cures in this disease from the local application of menthol.

It is not my purpose to speak of the effects of this drug when administered internally, or when applied to the cutaneous surfaces for neuralgia, etc., but excluding these uses which are yet in the experimental stage, we are justified in according to menthol an important place in therapeutics.

70 STATE STREET.

FIVE SURGICAL CASES OF SOMEWHAT EXCEPTIONAL INTEREST.

BY CHARLES A. POWERS, M.D.,
SURGEON TO OUT-PATIENTS, NEW YORK HOSPITAL ; ASSISTANT SURGEON
TO THE NEW YORK CANCER HOSPITAL.

CASE I. *Compound, comminuted fracture of the os calcis ; partial resection, followed by primary union in the bone ; large attached skin-grafts used ; complete cure.*—A man, aged twenty years, was taken to the Chambers Street Hospital, October 11, 1887, with a history of having had the right foot caught between an elevator and its shaft a short time previous to his admission. In the absence of the attending surgeon, Dr. W. T. Bull, he fell under my care. He was found to have a compound fracture of the os calcis, it being broken transversely at about the juncture of its posterior third with its anterior two-thirds. The bone in the vicinity of this transverse lesion was severely comminuted, but there was no longitudinal fracture running through either its anterior or posterior surface. The posterior fragment hung dangling from the tendo-Achillis, which latter structure was intact. The interosseous calcaneo-astragaloid ligament was not broken. The soft parts were severely lacerated over an area which extended from the medio-tarsal articulation on the plantar surface of the foot to a point five inches above the insertion of the tendo-Achillis, and this area embraced the malleoli laterally.

The numerous small fragments of the os calcis were removed and the large fragments sawn transversely (Fig. 1), when by flexion of the leg and extension of the foot they could be approximated. A transverse hole was bored in each fragment and they were held together by heavy copper wire.

The lacerated and contused soft parts were freely cut away and the stripped-up plantar tissues were thoroughly drained. A large antiseptic dressing was applied and left in place for six days, when it was removed and reapplied. On the twentieth day there had been no pus formation. There was primary union in the bone, but there was a large open space at the heel about three inches wide by seven inches long. This was dressed with balsam of Peru, and by repeatedly applied small skin-grafts it was reduced to an area of two by three inches. This was over the posterior surface of the os calcis, a surface which was the seat of necrosis below the insertion of the tendo-Achillis. The

FIG. 1.

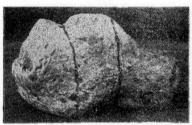

Postero-external aspect of an os calcis (right). Approximately, the amount of bone embraced between the black lines was removed in Case I.

wires were removed on the forty-fifth day. A tendency to talipes equinus was overcome by an elastic band which was stretched between the upper part of the leg and the front of the foot.

The necrosed tissue on the posterior surface of the bone came away in due time, but despite the frequent application of small grafts an ulcer persisted over an area a little larger than a silver dollar.

The cure of this was undertaken, at my request, by Dr. Robert Abbe, who, in October, 1888, applied a large attached graft, which was dissected from the posterior surface of the calf of the opposite leg and sewn to the freshened ulcer. Primary union followed the procedure.

FIG. 2.

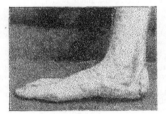

Result in Case I.

The young man now has a perfectly useful foot, the functions at the ankle being complete. Its antero-posterior length is seven-eighths of an inch shorter than that of its fellow.

The shortening in the os calcis has relaxed the

plantar ligaments and fasciæ, letting down the head of the astragalus, and a moderate degree of flat foot remains, but this is corrected by an appropriately constructed shoe. (Fig. 2 shows the foot as it appeared one month after the application of the last graft.)

CASE II. *Dislocation of the right humerus of long standing, accompanied by exceptional displacement.*— A man, twenty years of age, presented himself at the out-patient department of the New York Hospital, December 1, 1889, seeking relief for the disability attending a dislocation of the shoulder of three years' standing. He gave the following history: In October, 1886, while at work upon a brush-making machine, his arm and forearm were caught in such a way that he was thrown forcibly against the machinery, the forearm being violently wrenched and the shoulder receiving a severe contusion. This accident was followed by pain and disability at the shoulder-joint, and in the following January he was admitted to a hospital where efforts were made, under ether, to afford him relief. He says: "The doctors said that my shoulder was dislocated, but that they could not keep it reduced—they could not prevent it from slipping out of place." He resumed his work as a brush-maker and was able to perform his duties with fair success.

When seen by me the humerus was the seat of an anterior dislocation, the head of the bone resting above and in front of the glenoid cavity. The deltoid was extremely atrophied. On passive motion the humerus could be made to undergo complete internal rotation, external rotation being a little restricted. Abduction was possible to but forty-five degrees.

When the arm was lifted the head of the humerus could be made to undergo a very marked excursion forward and upward, resting without and above the coracoid process (Figs. 3 and 4), and could even be forced to lie entirely above the clavicle.

FIG. 3.

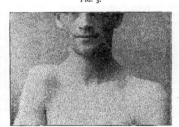

Dislocation of humerus, Case II.

On bringing the elbow to the side, twenty degrees in front of the mid-axillary line, the head of the humerus could be forced into the glenoid cavity, or rather to a glenoid position, but when the force was released it would at once fly forward. When the elbow was at the side, and the head dislocated forward, the right hand could easily be placed on the opposite shoulder. The axillary acromial measurement was three-quarters of an inch greater than that on the opposite side. The circumference at the middle of the arm and at the middle of the forearm was the same on both sides. The functions of the hand and forearm were excellent.

FIG. 4.

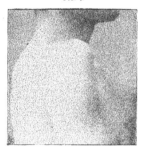

External aspect of shoulder, Case II.

The entire head, tuberosities, and neck of the bone could be intelligently palpated. At the inner side of the neck a prominent ridge could be distinctly felt, and the presence of this raised the question of longitudinal fracture at the time of the original injury.

Operative procedure for the relief of the disability was deemed inadvisable.

It would seem highly probable that the patient suffered, at the time of his accident, an anterior luxation, probably complicated by a longitudinal fracture through the upper part of the bone, and that constant use of the arm enabled the head of the humerus to make its wide excursion inward and upward. He states that in his work as a brush-maker he was obliged to draw the arm forcibly backward. In this motion the humerus would become a lever of the first class, the humeral head being the weight.

CASE III. *Specimen of a simple fracture through the carpal scaphoid.*—This specimen was brought to me by Mr. L. T. Mason, one of my pupils in medicine, who had discovered an anomaly in the bones of a cadaver, during his anatomical studies. It was taken from a man of about fifty years, of whose previous history nothing, of course, could be learned. The bones of the upper extremity are all of exceptionally large size, and very well marked. All are normal except the scaphoid. This is the seat of a fracture which runs from before backward, dividing the bone into two portions, of which the outer is somewhat the larger.

The fractured surface of the inner fragment is slightly concave from before backward, and is a little convex from above downward and inward. That of the outer fragment corresponds.

Each fractured surface is smoothly polished, and is covered with a thin layer of cartilage, which is distinctly lighter in color than that which invests the normal articular surfaces of the bone.

The lower articular surface of the radius presents three articular facets instead of two. Of these the inner is the normal quadrilateral surface for articulation with the semilunar. The outer two occupy the triangular space on which the scaphoid rests, this space being subdivided by an outer posterior ridge, which corresponds to the fracture in the scaphoid.

The plainly-marked differences in the articular cartilage investing the various surfaces of the fragments would indicate an acquired condition rather than a congenital increase in the number of the carpal bones. The absence of any evidences either of remote lesion in the soft parts or of inflammatory reaction warrants the assumption that the fracture was simple rather than compound.

The man, probably, suffered a traumatism inflicted upon the wrist, and did not allow the joint to be confined. The non-union was the result of constant motion.

I do not think it probable that this condition could be recognized without incision. Positive diagnosis could rest only on independent mobility of the fragments, and it would be most difficult to obtain this evidence.

The specimen is in the Museum of the New York Hospital.

CASE IV. *Angio-sarcoma of the humerus; amputation at shoulder; death.*—D. M., a man of twenty-one years, presented himself at the Out-patient Department of the New York Hospital, December 1, 1889, seeking relief for a swollen and painful shoulder.

He stated that he had fallen forcibly on the shoulder some four weeks previously, and that the accident was followed by pain, swelling, and disability, for the relief of which liniments had been applied.

Examination revealed a diffuse swelling of the left shoulder, extending from the origin of the deltoid half way to its insertion, and limited anteriorly and posteriorly by the axillary folds. The joint was the seat of almost complete disability. On pressing the thumbs well up into the axilla, the head and tuberosities of the humerus could be grasped. An assistant was asked to rotate the shaft of the humerus, and when this motion was made the head and tuberosities remained stationary. This rotation elicited a diffuse bony crepitus. There was no noticeable deformity other than that occasioned by the swelling.

Diagnosis of fracture through the surgical neck of the humerus was made, and the limb was enveloped in a plaster-of-Paris splint from the wrist to the shoulder, with a spica about the latter.

Three days after the application of the splint the patient complained of very severe pain in the shoulder. The splint was removed, and it was found that the swelling had considerably increased.

The splint was re-applied. but continuation of the swelling again necessitated its removal.

Two weeks after the patient came under my observation the enlargement of the shoulder was distinctly fluctuating. An exploring-needle was introduced and withdrew a fluid which microscopic examination showed to be pure blood.

During the following week the shoulder increased in size with considerable rapidity, and he was referred to the ward-service of the Hospital, where Dr. R. F. Weir, Attending Surgeon, made an exploratory incision, and found a large cavity filled with fresh and clotted blood, and fragments of bone loosely attached by periosteum. The upper extremity of the humerus, to the extent of about three inches, seemed to be wanting, a shell of bone alone representing the humeral head in the glenoid cavity.

The surfaces were thoroughly scraped with a sharp spoon, and fragments of tissue were subjected to microscopical examination, but no malignant elements were found therein.

During the week which followed the curetting the growth rapidly increased in size. The wound gaped, the skin was everted, and the protruding granulations bled profusely when irritated.

The patient developed a febrile movement, and the pulse became rapid and feeble.

On January 7th amputation at the shoulder-joint was decided upon, and was performed in the usual manner, but the patient succumbed to the shock of the operation and died shortly after its completion. The specimen was examined microscopically by Dr. F. Ferguson, pathologist to the hospital, who found it to be an angio-sarcoma of the humerus and surrounding tissues.

Upon the first study of the case I thought it probable that the man had sustained a fracture through the surgical neck of the humerus at the time of his original injury, and that the development of the sarcoma was consequent upon the traumatism; but after perusal of the literature of the subject, and especially after hearing the comments which followed the narration of the case before the Surgical Section of the New York Academy of Medicine, I think it more probable that the angio-sarcoma had existed for a considerable period without occasioning symptoms, and that the fracture took place through previously weakened bone.

CASE V. *Lympho-sarcoma of neck.*—F.E., a stoutly built, robust man of thirty-seven years, applied for treatment at the out-patient department of the New York Hospital, May 4, 1889, suffering from a swelling of the neck, which had existed for several months. His previous personal history was good. He had never suffered with serious illness, and there were no evidences of specific or of tubercular taint.

In his work as the driver of an ice-cart he had been in the habit of lifting heavy cakes of ice, and he remembered that seventeen months previously he had severely strained the muscles of the back and neck while attempting to lift an unusually heavy weight from the ground to his wagon. Shortly after this unusual exertion he noticed small lumps on either side of the neck. These were painless, and he gave them but little thought until their increasing size led him to consult a physician, who prescribed internal remedies.

The medication did not, however, effect a diminution in the size of the lumps, and they rapidly increased in extent until they reached the dimensions which they presented when he first came under my observation. At this time the neck was

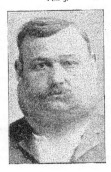

FIG. 5.

the seat of a hard, irregular swelling, which reached from the median line posteriorly to the symphysis of the jaw on the left side and to the middle of the body of the inferior maxilla on the right. It extended to the lobes of the ears above, and to the clavicles below (see Figs. 5 and 6).

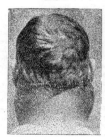

FIG. 6.

It was made up of nodular, rounded masses, fused and immovable. The skin over these was congested and adherent. Hearing was diminished on each side. The neck measured twenty-three and a half inches in circumference. The floor of the mouth was slightly invaded. The pharynx was free and there was neither dysphagia nor dyspnœa.

Examination of the body showed no other glandular enlargement. The spleen was normal in size. The specific gravity of the urine was 1035 and it contained a trace of sugar. Microscopical examination of the blood was negative in result.' His general health was good. The size and character of the growth precluded the thought of operative procedure. Arsenic and iron were administered internally.

The growth steadily increased, and on July 10th the neck measured twenty-seven inches in circumference. He began to lose flesh and strength and rapidly emaciated.

Hard nodules appeared on the shoulders and chest, he began to be troubled with cough and dyspnœa, and gastric disturbances developed.

He sank progressively, and died about September 1st, some four months after I first saw him. An autopsy was not obtained.

Although the diagnosis of lympho-sarcoma lacks microscopical confirmation, yet the clinical aspects of the case would seem to warrant the belief that it is a reasonable assumption.

CLINICAL MEMORANDA.

OBSTETRICAL.

A Case of Extensive Dropsy during Pregnancy.—The following case is reported because of its comparative rarity. A primipara, seven months pregnant, was suffering from dropsy of the lower extremities and of the external genital organs. The legs and feet were swollen to an enormous size. The vulva was extremely œdematous, particularly the labiæ minoræ, which were as large as a hand, translucent, and extremely tender on pressure. The urine was scanty and albuminous. Rest in bed and the internal use of Epsom salt and cream of tartar rapidly reduced the effusion in the legs but had not the slightest effect on the swollen genitalia.

After persisting for a few days I punctured the organs with excellent results, the labiæ diminishing to almost normal size. Patient was then put upon tincture of the chloride of iron, and was apparently doing well. About five days after this I was summoned, found her in labor and delivered her of twins, one of which died in a few hours; the other is still living. The patient made a rapid and complete recovery.

Lusk speaks of six cases of dropsy in pregnant women treated by him, in which miscarriage followed puncturing the labiæ. Whether labor was brought on by the reflex effects of the operation or by the condition that caused the œdema, is a question on which I desire an expression of opinion. J. E. COVEY, M.D.

LEXINGTON, ILLINOIS.

MEDICAL PROGRESS.

Treatment of Eczema.—According to PICK, in a recent paper before the German Dermatological Society (*Medicinische-chirurgische Rundschau*, July, 1890), the indications in the treatment of eczema are, first, protection of the skin from external irritants, and secondly, by means of antiseptics, prevention of local infection. In the earlier (dry) stages of the disease these indications are fulfilled by the use of sublimated gelatin prepared as follows:

> ℞.—Refined gelatin . . 7½ drachms.
> Distilled water, a sufficient quantity.

After standing for some hours this is heated until completely liquefied and is then evaporated to 2½ ounces. Then add,

> Glycerin . . . 6½ drachms.
> Corrosive sublimate . ¼ grain.

Before using, the gelatin must be melted by gentle heat in a water-bath, and it should be applied with a soft brush.

For the moist and vesicular, as well as the chronic form with more or less thickening of the skin, a permanent application of salicylic acid and soap should be used. The following is the formula used by Pick:

> ℞.—Liquefied soap plaster . 3¼ ounces.
> Salicylic acid . . . 75 grains.—M.
> Spread on soft cloths.

This may be rendered more adhesive by the addition of olive oil, thus:

> ℞.—Liquefied soap plaster . 2½ ounces.
> Olive oil . . . 5 drachms.
> Salicylic acid . . . 37 grains.

The plaster should be cut in strips so that it may be closely applied to the diseased parts. If there is much secretion the plaster should be removed on the third or fourth day, but the subsequent dressings may remain in place eight days or longer. After the amount of secretion has been reduced, the sublimated gelatin may be used as in the dry form of the disease.

Lysol; a New Antiseptic.—GERLACH writes ot the new coal-tar product, lysol, that it surpasses creolin and carbolic acid in germicidal powers; that it is less poisonous than either creolin or carbolic acid; that its composition is constant; that it is soluble in any proportion of water, and that even weak solutions are strongly antiseptic. For the treatment of wounds, Gerlach considers that a 1-per-cent. solution is sufficiently strong, and that for internal use solutions of half this strength are sufficient. —*Centralblatt f. d. Gesammte Therapie*, July, 1890.

Treatment of Chronic Hypertrophy of the Spleen.—DR. MOSLER, in the *Wiener med. Wochenschrift*, argues against extirpation of the spleen as a method of treatment in leukæmia. The chief danger is the tendency to hæmorrhage in such patients. The difficulty in deciding whether in any given case the condition is one of simple hyperplasia or a serious disease of the blood is also against the propriety of operation. In such cases Dr. Mosler first tries parenchymatous injections of a 2-per-cent. solution of carbolic acid, and then a mixture of one part of Fowler's solution and ten parts of distilled water. An ice-bag is applied to the spleen before injection, and owing to the contraction of the splenic muscles, the amount of blood contained in the organ is diminished. Ice-bags are also applied to lessen pain and prevent inflammation. This method, as well as injections of extract of ergot and sclerotinic acid, has frequently been employed by Mosler and others. In one case Dr. Mosler had the opportunity of examining the anatomical conditions of the spleen after injections of Fowler's solution. The capsule was found wrinkled and thickened, presenting patches over the thickened parts. The connection of those conditions of the capsule with the injections was indisputable. Dr. Mosler does not ascribe the diminution of the organ to the mechanical irritation produced by the injections, but rather to a direct influence on the spleen. He recommends great care in the use of the parenchymatous injections. Encouraged by these favorable results, Dr. Mosler tried these methods of treatment in the hypertrophy of leukæmia, and here also obtained considerable decrease of the organ. The subjective disturbances due to the hypertrophied spleen were thus lessened, and the moral impression made on the patient by the active treatment was also of value.—*British Medical Journal*, July 5, 1890.

Iodoform Emulsion in the Treatment of Cold Abscesses.— In the Polish journal *Gazeta Lekarska*, DR. R. JASSINSKI reports the results he has obtained in the treatment of cold abscesses with iodoform emulsion. He opens an abscess only when it has become "residual," that is, when the primary focus in the vertebral column has healed or is separated from the abscess cavity. He has used iodoform emulsion in eighty-six cases, with the following results : A certain number of abscesses healed after a single injection, others after two or more injections. In 11 cases the abscess burst spontaneously after injection, and much pus, mixed with emulsion, escaped. Healing occurred without further surgical interference. In 19 cases aspiration was impossible owing to blocking of the trocar ; the opening was therefore dilated, and the cavity washed out with a 3-per-cent. carbolic acid solution. Iodoform emulsion was then injected, and the wound stitched up. Occasionally a drainage-tube had to be inserted, and the injection frequently repeated. Dr. Jassinski has never seen symptoms of poisoning, though he has injected 180 grammes of a 10-per-cent. iodoform emulsion at once.—*British Medical Journal*, July 5, 1890.

Treatment of Lupus.—MR. H. G. BROOKE suggests a preliminary treatment in lupus vulgaris which he states (*British Journal of Dermatology*) considerably reduces the field in which operation is necessary, involves no pain, and requires, in most cases no suspension of work or of ordinary habits. The formula for the application he uses is as follows, this being the limit as to strength :

℞.—Oleate of mercury (2½–5 per ct.) 1 ounce.
Salicylic acid . . . 10 to 15 grains.
Ichthyol . . . . 15 minims.
Oil of lavender, a sufficient quantity.

In every case it is better to begin with the smaller proportions, and the skin must not be broken by the application. If it becomes sore and threatens to break, the ointment must be diluted with pure lard. The ointment should be rubbed in ten minutes in the morning and twenty in the evening, and kept on during the intervening time. The effects are claimed to be most excellent. In some few cases the above ointment has been curative, but it produces its best effects in those in whom there has been no previous surgical interference. Its action upon deeply embedded nodules, lying among the fibrous meshes of old sores is not so marked, although it prevents or retards further growth.—*St. Louis Medical and Surgical Journal*, July, 1890.

Application for Fissured Nipples.—The *American Practitioner and News* quotes the following prescription for the treatment of fissured nipples :

℞.—Salol }
Ether } of each . . ' . 1 drachm.
Cocaine hydrochlorate . . 2 grains.
Collodion . . . . 5 drachms.—M.

Prescription for Malaria.—The following is used by BACELLI in the treatment of malaria :

℞.—Sulphate of quinine . . 45 grains.
Tartrate of iron and potassium 105 "
Distilled water . . . 9 ounces.
Fowler's solution . . 24 minims.—M.
One teaspoonful from one to three times daily.
—*Centralblatt f. d. Gesammte Therapie*, July, 1890.

Nitroglycerin in the Treatment of Opium-habit.—In the Paris letter to the *Lancet* of June 14, is reported the success of DR. OSCAR JENNINGS in the management of the opium-habit. He presented to one of the medical societies a member of the profession who had been addicted to the drug for twenty years, and who had repeatedly failed in his efforts at self-cure. Dr. Jennings had him under treatment three weeks, and ten days had elapsed without a return to the use of the drug. There remained considerable prostration, but none of the craving that leads to the resumption of the habit. Dr. Jennings, in his treatment of such cases, relies largely on the heart-tonics, especially nitroglycerin, in the form of the compound tabloids, and galvanization of the head with baths of hot water and of hot air. The withdrawal of the opiate is gradual, oecupying a period of from two to three weeks, the latter period being commonly required in cases of long duration. The compound tabloids of trinitrine contain nitroglycerin $\frac{1}{100}$ grain, amyl nitrite ¼ grain, capsicum $\frac{1}{30}$ grain, and menthol $\frac{1}{30}$ grain each.

Fatal Case of Schoeler's Iodine-injection Treatment of Retinal Detachment.—DR. GELPKE (*Centralblatt f. Praktische Augenheilkunde*) reports a fatal result following Schoeler's injection-treatment of retinal detachment. The patient was a male of sixty-six years, of robust build, in whom the detachment took place in an eye, formerly perfectly healthy, without known cause. Three drops of the tincture of iodine were injected into the vitreous chamber, after the method described by Schoeler, with rigid antiseptic precautions at every step of the procedure. Despite these precautions an infectious purulent choroiditis sprang up in the eye operated upon, and two days later this was succeeded by a purulent meningitis. Death took place on the sixth day after the operation.

Therapeutic Uses of Aniline.—As is well known, PROFESSOR KREMIANSKI, of Kharkoff, has for some years advocated the employment of aniline as an inhalation in phthisis because of its great germicidal power. He continues to practise this method, as he says, with considerable success, and has just published a new brochure on the subject detailing an interesting recent case in which, he states, it proved most beneficial, and ˙he describes a new and more convenient form of inhaler. His methods have hitherto found but little general favor, it having been stated by some observers that the inhalation of aniline is very dangerous. Dr. Kremianski has, however, always denied this, declaring that aniline, if pure, is practically nọn-poisonous, and this view has been confirmed by the researches of Professor Stilling, of Strasburg, who has just published an important work on the subject of aniline colors as antiseptics and their employment in practice. He finds that the most antiseptic of these colors is the violet, which is known to microscopists as methyl-violet. A solution of this of the strength of 1 in 1000 can be injected under the skin of a guinea-pig to the amount of 5 drachms, or more, without harm to the animal. Half that quantity, ˙however, if injected into the peritoneal cavity, proves fatal, the viscera, and especially the kidneys, with the exception of the Malpighian corpuscles, being colored blue. A few drops of the solution instilled into the eyes of rabbits colored the conjunctiva, but left the cornea—if this were uninjured—unaffected, the coloration disappearing the next day. Professor Stilling then employed this solution with marked success for the treatment of many eye and other diseases, including scrofulous ulcers of the cornea, conjunctivitis, eczema of the lids, parenchymatous keratitis, serous iritis, disseminated choroiditis, sympathetic ophthalmia, whitlow, varicose ulcers of the leg, etc. A pure form of methyl-violet for surgical purposes is now manufactured under the name of pyoktanin. It is only right to add that Dr. Mauthner, of Vienna, has just published a statement that he has been quite unsuccessful in his trials of this substance in a number of eye cases similar to those in which Professor Stilling has recorded such favorable results.

Professor Ehrlich and Dr. Lippmann have found that methyl-blue, when perfectly free from chloride of zinc and all other impurities, is a valuable and safe remedy for relieving pain of various kinds. They have given as much as fifteen grains daily in gelatin capsules without producing any toxic symptoms. The usual doses were from a grain and a half to four grains internally, and one grain hypodermically. The remedy was employed in twenty-five cases of painful nervous affections, and rheumatism of the muscles, tendons, and joints, and in every case it proved more or less efficacious. In two cases of migraine, also, it was very successful. In many ways this substance appears to act similarly to antipyrine, over which it has the advantage of cheapness, and of being painless when given hypodermically.—*Lancet*, July 5, 1890.

Prescription for Constipation in Infants.—According to the Paris correspondent of the *Archives of Pædiatrics*, the following is a prescription used by DR. FERRAND :

R.—Manna . . . . 12½ drachms.
Calcined magnesia } of each, 2½ "
Sublimed sulphur }
White honey . . . 7½ " —M.
One or two tablespoonfuls in a cup of hot water.

Thymol Tooth-powder.—The *American Practitioner and News* quotes the following :

R.—Precipitated chalk . . 7½ ounces.
Powdered soap . . . ½ ounce.
Saccharin . . . . 5 grains.
Thymol . . . . 7½ "
Camphor . . . 15 "
Vanillin . . . . 2½ "
Oil of rose . . . . 3 drops.

Rub the camphor and thymol together in a mortar and warm gently until the mixture is liquefied. Then add the chalk in small portions, reserving about half an ounce. Next add the other ingredients, the perfumẹs having been mixed with the remaining half ounce of chalk.

The Transmission of Typhoid Fever by the Air.—DR. BORDAS (*La Revue Médico Pharmaceutique*) has instituted experiments to determine the relation between the humidity of the atmosphere and the transmission of the typhoid bacillus. A current of dry air, completely devoid of germs, was conducted through a vessel containing a beef-broth culture of the bacillus and into a second vessel containing sterilized beef-broth. The second vessel remained sterile. The result was the same when a dry atmospheric current was passed over pumice stone saturated with a culture of the typhoid bacillus. When moist air was passed through the same vessels a very different result was obtained. The sterile beef-broth culture was found, after the lapse of a quarter of an hour, to be thickly planted with the bacilli.

In nature this state of humidity is supplied by mist or fog, and statistics show an increase of typhoid fever in Paris during the months of October, November, December, and January. The most general mode of propagation of typhoid fever is by the contamination of the soil or water, but there are cases in which it is manifested by pulmonary localization. The germ may penetrate into the bronchial system in spite of every means of defence possessed by the organism. Metchnikoff's studies prove that the lungs are a phagocyte battle-ground. In typhoid infection, due primarily to pulmonary lesion, it would seem that the phagocytes of the lungs are ordinarily sufficient to prevent the development of the infectious germ, and that contagion by means of the air can take place only when the macrophagic cells cease to offer an obstacle to the invasion of the microbe.—*Abstract of Sanitary Reports*, July 11, 1890.

Nitrate of Cocaine in the Treatment of Urethral Diseases.—LAVAUX thinks that nitrate of cocaine should replace the hydrochlorate as a urethral anæsthetic previous to the application of nitrate of silver. The nitrate may be prepared by pouring a solution of the hydrochlorate into a solution of nitrate of silver. An insoluble precipitate of chloride of silver falls, and nitrate of cocaine remains in solution.

The following formula for an injection to be used in the treatment of gonorrhœa is given :

R.—Nitrate of silver } of each 15 grains.
Nitrate of cocaine }
✦ Distilled water . . . 1½ ounces.—M.

The injection of this solution is said to be painless.—*Journal of Cutaneous and Genito-urinary Diseases*, July, 1890.

THE MEDICAL NEWS.

A WEEKLY JOURNAL
OF MEDICAL SCIENCE.

COMMUNICATIONS are invited from all parts of the world. Original articles contributed exclusively to THE MEDICAL NEWS will be liberally paid for upon publication. When necessary to elucidate the text, illustrations will be furnished without cost to the author.

Address the Editor: H. A. HARE, M.D.,
1004 WALNUT STREET,
PHILADELPHIA.

Subscription Price, including Postage.

PER ANNUM, IN ADVANCE . . . . $4.00.
SINGLE COPIES . . . . 10 CENTS.

Subscriptions may begin at any date. The safest mode of remittance is by bank check or postal money order, drawn to the order of the undersigned. When neither is accessible, remittances may be made, at the risk of the publishers, by forwarding in *registered* letters.

Address,   LEA BROTHERS & CO.,
Nos. 706 & 708 SANSOM STREET,
PHILADELPHIA.

SATURDAY, JULY 26, 1890.

ANTIPYRINE IN OBSTETRICS.

THERE are but few painful conditions in which antipyrine has not been used, and while its haphazard employment has no doubt done much harm and has led to its indiscriminate use by the laity, yet this widespread use has brought to light many facts as to its therapeutic value. The well-known analgesic property of the drug naturally led to its employment to relieve the pains of labor, and it was not long before reports were published in various parts of the world which unfortunately have been of such contradictory character as to make it of doubtful value for the relief of the pains of childbirth.

In the *Revue Générale de Clinique et de Thérapeutique*, M. MISRACHI reports the results of his investigations to determine the indications for antipyrine in obstetrics, and by closely studying his cases has thrown much light upon the subject. An analysis of the facts offers a very satisfactory explanation of the numerous contradictory reports. It is well known that a certain amount of pain during labor is physiological and normal, and in the cases in which antipyrine has been employed with success it is noteworthy that the pains were invariably aggravated. Thus, its successful use has been reported in cases of miscarriage, accompanied "with most violent pains." Another observer gave it with suc-

cess to a primipara long in labor, who "screamed loud enough to be heard in adjoining rooms," and another to a patient "in labor for two days without any dilatation of the cervix." M. Misrachi administered antipyrine to thirty women during labor, and found it efficient for the relief of pain in only nine of the cases. In five of these the lumbar pains were intense; in one there was tetanic contraction of the uterus; in two excessive rigidity of the cervix, and in one great nervous excitability. In four of the cases premature discharge of the liquor amnii had occurred, and in all, the pains had lasted for a long time—six, seven, twelve, eighteen, and in some seventy-two hours, with only slight dilatation of the os. In these nine cases the drug acted most happily. The pains were relieved, the nervous excitability calmed and the tetanic contraction of the uterus and rigidity of the cervix disappeared. In the remaining twenty-one cases, which were normal in every respect and in which the drug was given merely as an experiment to determine its action upon normal labor pains, it gave no relief whatever.

These observations seem to prove conclusively that antipyrine should not be considered an obstetric anæsthetic to be used in all cases; that when labor is normal it is useless and not to be compared to ether or chloroform; but that it is of value in the treatment of certain painful complications of labor. Every obstetrician meets with cases in which the contractions of the uterus are vigorous but the accompanying pain so intense that it reflexly interferes with the contractions, rendering them inefficient and irregular, the patient meanwhile continuing in her struggling efforts. In such cases antipyrine is most efficient. It relieves the excessive pain and favors a return of effective uterine force. Its employment is therefore indicated when labor is tedious; when there exists an exaggerated nervous susceptibility to pain; when the liquor amnii has been prematurely discharged; when there is rigidity of the cervix, spasmodic contraction of the os or of the body of the uterus. There have been many such cases reported in which antipyrine has proved more efficient than the usual treatment with opium, belladonna, warm injections, chloral, or quinine.

M. Misrachi also confirmed by his observations a fact that had been noted before by others; namely, that antipyrine should not be employed to relieve the pain of the second stage of labor. At this time, when the pain is due to compression and to the great distention of the genital canal, antipyrine, like opium and chloral, is of no service. The anæsthesia of ether or chloroform is required. These limitations to the employment of antipyrine do not, however, entirely remove its usefulness in obstetric practice.

Besides the relief it affords to excessive pain during the first stage of labor, it has given very good results in the treatment of false pains, threatened abortion, and after-pains. A woman pregnant about eight months was seized with pains analogous to true labor pains. Examination two and three hours later revealing no dilatation of the os, antipyrine was given and the pains promptly disappeared.

In those cases in which throughout pregnancy there occurs at each presumed menstrual epoch a slight hæmorrhage and considerable pain, antipyrine has been used with great success. M. Misrachi mentions a case of this kind, in which it succeeded after opiates and prolonged 'rest had failed. Favorable results have been obtained from its employment in the treatment of threatened abortion and miscarriage, but they are, as would be expected, by no means constant. In any case of abortion or miscarriage it is usually difficult to decide whether it is avoidable or inevitable, and if the ovum is partially or completely separated antipyrine, of course, fails, just as every remedy uniformly fails. Nevertheless, M. Misrachi employed it with success in cases where the usual treatment failed and thus avoided the unfortunate necessity of converting a threatened miscarriage into an inevitable one. In connection with this it is interesting to note the results of the use of antipyrine in the treatment of a condition somewhat analogous to threatened miscarriage ; namely, placenta prævia. Of two cases reported, in one it controlled the bleeding three times, at the fourth, sixth, and seventh months, respectively. In the other a slight hæmorrhage had occurred at the sixth month, and at the end of the eighth month there were profuse hæmorrhage and uterine contractions, and the os dilated to the size of a silver dollar, the placenta being centrally implanted. Forty-five grains of antipyrine (fifteen grains every half-hour) diminished the contractions and arrested the hæmorrhage. The delivery was completed six hours later with no bad results. Although, as M. Misrachi remarks, these two cases prove nothing, since it is well known that the hæmorrhage of placenta prævia in the course of preg-

nancy often ceases spontaneously, especially when the head engages, yet it is interesting to note these results with antipyrine, as it would be a decided therapeutic advance if it could be shown to have uniformly so good an effect.

The very numerous favorable reports indicate that antipyrine is of undoubted value in the treatment of after-pains. M. Chauppe was the first to call attention to its value in cases when the pains are due to ergot. M. Negri announces that in his clinic it has replaced all other remedies for after-pains, and M. Misrachi concludes from his own observations and those of his colleagues at the Salonique, comprising hundreds of trials, that it succeeds in 95 per cent. of cases. In his large experience with the drug in obstetrics he has not met with a single case in which it has produced untoward symptoms. The numerous reported cases of antipyrine poisoning are doubtless due to personal idiosyncrasy, and in obstetrics, as elsewhere, this of course cannot be foreseen. M. Misrachi generally administers fifteen, thirty, or forty-five grains at intervals of one hour, decreasing the intervals to a half-hour in urgent cases. He found that ordinarily thirty grains were sufficient. When a tendency to vomiting exists he prefers enemata. Two or three may be given, composed of thirty grains of antipyrine dissolved in four ounces of water containing five drops of laudanum.

REVIEWS.

CYCLOPÆDIA OF THE DISEASES OF CHILDREN, MEDICAL AND SURGICAL. By AMERICAN, BRITISH, AND CANADIAN AUTHORS. Edited by JOHN M. KEATING, M.D. Vol. III. 8vo., pp. 1370. Philadelphia: J. B. Lippincott Company, 1890.

MANY of the remarks we had occasion to make in our reviews of the preceding volumes of this work are also applicable to Volume III. The same accurate judgment is shown by the editor in his selection of authors best fitted for the articles which they have contributed, and with few exceptions the contributors have done their work conscientiously and well.

Part I., on Diseases of the Digestive System, opens with a thirty-page article by Pepper on Functional Disorders of the Stomach. A large part of this is naturally devoted to a discussion of dyspepsia. Treatment is very fully entered into and numerous, somewhat conventional, prescriptions are given. Hare follows with a carefully worked-up paper upon Diseases of the Stomach, the most exhaustive portion of which is that upon dilatation of the stomach, a condition that, we have reason to believe, is frequently overlooked. An excellent cut taken from a photograph is given (unfortunately entitled a *distended* stomach) showing how great the dilatation may be.

Next are more than one hundred pages by Holt upon the Diarrhœal Diseases, Acute and Chronic. This is one of the longest papers in the volume, and is undoubtedly the most valuable contribution upon the subject in the English language. It is illustrated by sixteen "process "- and wood-cuts of the pathological anatomy of infantile diarrhœa. Pathologically, Dr. Holt divides diarrhœas into : (1) Acute desquamative catarrh, embracing the acute cases with no lesions except loss of the superficial epithelium ; (2) acute catarrhal inflammation, other lesions than the loss of epithelium being present ; (3) acute inflammation with ulceration of the lymph nodules ; (4) acute croupous inflammation ; and (5) chronic inflammation. We can see no reason why the first two divisions should be separated, Dr. Holt himself intimating that the second is only an advanced stage of the first. Clinically the author classifies the diarrhœas thus : (1) Simple diarrhœa ; (2) acute mycotic diarrhœa, including (a) acute dyspeptic diarrhœa and (b) cholera infantum ; (3) acute entero-colitis ; (4) chronic diarrhœa, including (a) primary cases due chiefly to depraved constitution and continued improper feeding, and (b) secondary cases in which the chronic disease follows acute entero-colitis. In the treatment of simple diarrhœa, Dr. Holt advises a full dose of castor oil followed by an opiate, and almost complete abstinence from food for twenty-four hours. In acute dyspeptic diarrhœa he gives castor oil or calomel, and when the bowels have been thoroughly cleared out he prescribes bismuth subnitrate, "two or three drachms daily to a child a year old." Naphthalin, after a thorough trial, he has concluded is greatly inferior to bismuth.

Booker contributes an interesting, though decidedly prolix, article upon the intestinal bacteria of children. Twenty pages devoted to this subject seem an unnecessarily large number, and a few illustrations would increase the value of the article. Excellent advice is given upon the management of constipation in children by Earle, who is evidently thoroughly familiar with the subject of which he writes. Tabes Mesenterica is discussed by Jacobi in his usual readable and instructive manner. Much of the article is devoted to showing that the pathological anatomy of tabes mesenterica "is by no means the same in all cases, and that the term itself should disappear from our indexes or be recognized as merely a convenient expression for a complex of more or less similar symptoms." To those who are not familiar with the etiology and life-history of intestinal parasites we commend the concise paper on the subject by Councilman. Hernia in children is considered in a very practical manner by William J. Taylor. Next follows a very valuable paper by Keen on Intestinal Obstruction, a subject on which he is eminently qualified to write. In the article on Peritonitis, by Ashby, we are surprised at the statement of the author that in a fair proportion of cases of tubercular peritonitis under medical treatment recovery may be looked for. To us, supposed recovery from tubercular peritonitis as from tubercular meningitis means in most cases error in diagnosis. Fenger's article on Perityphlitis, Paratyphlitis, and Perityphlitic Abscess, reveals a large amount of research, but is disappointing in that it is to a great extent a reflection of others' views with but few of the author's own opinions.

Congenital Abnormalities of the Intestines—Malformations, Injuries, and Diseases of the Rectum and Anus, are handled in a masterly manner by Wharton, and the same may be said of the articles by Packard on Colotomy and by Senn on Diseases of the Pancreas and their Operative Treatment. A brief article by Chapin, on Functional Disorders of the Liver, Jaundice, and Diseases of the Ducts and of the Portal Vein, is followed by sixty-six pages on Enlargements of the Liver in Children, by Musser. The latter paper includes a description of affections which simulate enlargement of the liver, namely, congestion, fatty infiltration, amyloid disease, hydatid disease, abscess, and tumors. Contractions of the Liver, including both hypertrophic and atrophic cirrhosis, are considered by Hatfield.

In Part II., Diseases of the Genito-Urinary Organs, the most valuable contributions are those of Goodhart, on Acute and Chronic Bright's Disease ; Hunt, on Vesical, Urethral, and Preputial Calculi ; Vander Veer, on Diseases of the Bladder ; the Editor of the *Cyclopædia*, on Diseases of the Uterus, Vagina, and Vulva ; and Kelly, on Diseases of the Ovaries and Tubes. Next follow eighty-four pages on Diseases of the Blood and Blood-making Organs, by Griffith. No pains have been spared by the author in making this article complete. Descriptions and illustrations of the various apparatus for estimating hæmoglobin and counting corpuscles are given with full directions upon the method of using. A somewhat original and very excellent classification is in itself evidence of the care given to his work by the author.

Part III., Surgery, contains four excellent articles— Minor Surgery and Emergencies in Children, by Dulles ; Plastic Surgery, by Morton ; Wounds, by McCann ; and Anæsthetics and Anæsthesia, by Allis. We regret that in the last-named article the author shows so strong a preference for chloroform as an anæsthetic. True, he recommends it with this qualifying sentence, "on the condition that it shall be properly administered." Doubtless chloroform administered carefully is safer than ether administered recklessly, but there seems no longer reason to doubt that, if given with equal care, fewer deaths will occur from ether than from chloroform. The very fact that the latter demands more care is an argument in favor of the former.

We have already so far exceeded the space allotted to us that we can only briefly mention Part IV., Diseases of the Osseous System and of the Joints. The most valuable of the articles in this part, perhaps because on the most important subjects, are those of Bradford and Brackett, on Club-foot ; A. Sidney Roberts, on Pott's Disease ; Poore, on Diseases of Major Articulations ; and Gerster, on Deformities of Bone—Osteoclasis and Osteotomy.

The volume deserves a much more extended notice than it has been in our power to give it. There is little or nothing to be said in criticism ; editor, authors, and publishers have done their work in a manner that disarms the critic.

Marine-Hospital Service.—The United States Senate has passed a bill increasing the salary of the Surgeon-General of the Marine-Hospital Service to $6000 per annum.

SOCIETY PROCEEDINGS.

NEW YORK ACADEMY OF MEDICINE.

Stated Meeting, May 15, 1890.

THE PRESIDENT, ALFRED L. LOOMIS, M.D.,
IN THE CHAIR.

DURING the past few years various efforts have been made to utilize the telephone and microphone in connection with the study of physical diagnosis, but without very flattering success; for, delicate as these wonderful instruments are, they have not been able, as yet, to differentiate those nice distinctions in the quality of sound, which are so full of meaning to the practised ear of the diagnostician. One of the latest attempts in this direction has been made by Dr. L. L. Seaman, who presented the result of his labors to the Academy of Medicine, in an instrument which he called

THE AUSCULTATORY PERCUSSOR.

The apparatus may be said to consist of the well-known Cammann's binaural stethoscope with a large wooden chest-piece, connected with a mechanical device for performing percussion simultaneously with auscultation. The percussor works through a slot in the side of the chest-piece, and strikes a thin metal pleximeter situated in the centre of the "field" of the stethoscope. The blow of the hammer is delivered vertically, and its force can be readily regulated, thus giving more accurate results. Another source of error is eliminated by having the pressure of the pleximeter against the chest constant. Permanent records of the examinations made with this instrument can be obtained by attaching it to Edison's phonograph; and these records when reproduced by the phonograph might be utilized for class instruction in physical diagnosis. Dr. Seaman gave a demonstration of its powers in this direction, by so attaching it to a phonograph that fourteen persons could listen simultaneously to the reproduced sounds.

The remainder of the evening was devoted to a discussion of the advances made in

SPINAL SURGERY.

It was opened by Dr. Robert Abbe, who reported eight cases. From a study of these cases, he concluded that the pressure of the displaced bone in fracture of a vertebra is of secondary importance, unless the arch is driven in by a blow. There is usually no marked deformity of the canal; and if the fracture occurs at or below the first dorsal vertebra, the crushing does not as a rule destroy the nerves. In efforts to relieve these cases by operative means, one is confronted by a difficult problem—*i. e.*, how to connect the lower segment of the spinal cord with the upper portion, when there is a gap of half an inch or more. Dr. C. L. Dana has suggested the ingenious expedient of transplanting the cut nerve-roots into lower roots, or into a lower segment of the cord.

In discussion, Dr. John A. Wyeth commented upon the frequency with which the injury occurs at the eleventh dorsal vertebra, and spoke of some of the difficulties he had encountered in this line of work. He related the history of one case of fracture of this bone,

in which paraplegia was instantaneous, and persisted for about eight months, when the speaker partially relieved the patient by operation. When the canal was opened the dura was so distended with fluid as to project through the wound, and when punctured by the operator a stream of spinal fluid was forced upward for a distance of six or eight inches. Two and a half inches of the cord was exposed, and inflammatory lymph was found between the dura and the cord. Adhesions were broken up and the wound closed. Sensation returned at once throughout the entire leg, and motion was restored to the two great toes. Dr. Wyeth thinks that the field of spinal surgery is just beginning to open up to us, and he believes that many of these unfortunate patients might be restored to usefulness, particularly those in whom the paralysis has been gradually produced by pressure in Pott's disease.

Dr. A. G. Gerster said that he had been particularly interested in those cases where the spinal marrow is divided in consequence of traumatism, leaving a more or less extensive gap. Reasoning from analogy, he thought that re-union of the divided ends of the cord would probably result in a restoration of function. These cases, he said, are so desperate that almost any measure which holds out any hope of relief is justifiable. He thought that in the future it might even be shown to be possible to remove the vertebra, and so enable the separated ends to be brought into apposition.

Dr. R. T. Morris was sceptical as to the benefits that would follow this procedure of suturing the cord, for experiments on animals have shown that ascending and descending degeneration begin immediately after section of the cord, and progress for days and even weeks. It is possible that the operation might prove successful if performed within a few hours after the receipt of the injury. The spinal cord cannot retract very much when divided, because of the spinal nerves. Nor does the proposal to remove the entire vertebra offer a solution of this problem; for even supposing it could be done, trouble would arise from the consequent crowding of the spinal nerves. In one case of gunshot injury to the spine at the level of the ninth dorsal vertebra, upon which he had operated, the patient suddenly found, about ten months later, that he could move the adductors of the left leg. This is an example of very late regeneration of the cord.

Dr. R. H. Sayre said that although many cases of Pott's paraplegia will recover without operation, he thought those cases which do not yield to other treatment within twelve months are suitable for operative interference.

Dr. B. Sachs said that the most suitable cases for operation are the recent ones, and those in which the symptoms subsequently improve, showing a probable obstruction to proper nerve conduction. Dr. Abbe, he said, deserves credit for showing that even tubercular cases might yield favorable results from operation. The speaker did not see any need of such extensive opening of the canal as had been described; for a careful diagnosis of the distribution of the paralysis in a given case would indicate the exact seat of the trouble, even to the very segment of the spinal cord which is involved. Although both of Dr. Abbe's cases of neuralgia were improved by operation, Dr. Sachs considered it an extremely radical measure to attempt operation upon the intervertebral spinal roots. Unless one has has good reason to believe that there is organic disease of the posterior spinal roots, it is well not to interfere.

Dr. Abbe, in closing, said that it is only in these exceptionally severe neuralgias that any sane man would think of operating. Mr. Bennett, of England, has recently reported a case in which he had divided the posterior roots of the lumbar and sacral nerves, intradurally, for intractable neuralgia of the leg. The wound healed and the patient was entirely free from pain for twelve days following the operation, when he died of apoplexy. The ascending degeneration which takes place after division of the posterior root, certainly obliterates the remnant up to the ultimate fibres of that root; and this, Dr. Abbe thought, should remove the pain. Operations on fractures of the spine are ordinarily useless; but he hoped that future experiments on animals would show us how to innervate the upper and lower portions—probably by transplantation of the roots, or some similar method. The removal of the entire vertebra, in view of its important surroundings, and the mechanical obstacles to be overcome, seemed too difficult a problem even for modern surgery.

CORRESPONDENCE.

VIENNA.

To the Editor of THE MEDICAL NEWS,

SIR: When the Vienna faculty called Professor Krafft-Ebing to the university from Graz last fall they showed their wisdom, for his clinics are well attended and are constantly growing in favor. On Mondays and Thursdays he holds clinics on Mental Diseases and Insanity at the Insane Asylum; on Tuesdays and Fridays he lectures on "Legal Psychiatrie," illustrating the points by cases; and on Wednesdays he demonstrates "Selected Cases of Nervous Diseases." He shows many cases of the same disease together, thus presenting the clinical picture in all its forms and varieties—for example, he recently showed some twenty cases of tabes dorsalis. Krafft-Ebing is not a believer in the syphilitic etiology of tabes, and some of the men who were the most ardent advocates of this theory last year are becoming very reserved. He uses the suspension treatment for tabes, and in several cases has seen excellent temporary results, yet he does not consider it by any means a specific.

Dr. Salzer, the son of Professor Salzer the gynecologist, the brilliant first assistant at Billroth's clinic, has accepted a professorship at Utrecht, Holland, and leaves Vienna at the close of the present semester. He is a fine operator, and gave excellent courses in atypical operations, so that he is popular among the Americans here. Dr. Eiselsberg now becomes Billroth's first assistant. Professor Kahler is very ill with some nervous disease, and his first assistant, Dr. Kraus, has been delivering the lectures on internal medicine with marked success.

A few days ago, at Albert's clinic, we saw a case of traumatic contusion and laceration of the right kidney. The boy had been severely injured, was very anæmic, and had been passing blood with his urine for several days. There were great pain and marked dulness over the region of the right kidney. Operation for removal was performed. Albert prefers a long incision at right angles to the spinal column, beginning at about the posterior axillary line; and he opens the peritoneum in order to have plenty of room and light for operating. The kidney was found to be severely injured, its lower end was considerably lacerated, and nearly two pints of blood-clot and urine were removed. Now, a week after operation, the case is doing very well.

The surgery of the liver is progressing rapidly, and they quite often remove the gall-bladder for cholelithiasis. In a case at Albert's clinic Hochenegg removed a gall-bladder containing fifty-two gall-stones, and as the walls were carcinomatous, he examined the liver carefully for metastasis. He found but one metastatic deposit near the anterior border, removed it with the knife, sewed the peritoneum all around the wound, and finally sewed up the abdomen in such a manner that the wounded liver could be seen from without. The extirpated portion was one by one and one-half inches in size. It is now over nine months since the operation, and there seems to be no recurrence. The case is interesting because it is believed to be the first where a neoplasm was removed from the liver with good result.

There is much tuberculosis in Vienna, and the disease has even received the name of *morbus Viennensis* among medical men. Sarcoma is also alarmingly frequent, and it is now taught here that when sarcoma affects a limb the best treatment is early amputation. An immense experience and all statistics prove, says Professor Albert, that in nearly every case where sarcoma is removed, even by a very thorough operation, recurrence takes place either in the scar or near it, and a second operation though more thorough can avail but little. Finally amputation of the limb becomes a necessity, and it would have saved the poor patient much suffering if this radical operation had been performed at once.

Dr. Jahoda, Professor Salzer's first assistant, gives an excellent course in gynecology, and though he has been teaching only a few months the demand for a place in his course is so great that a man must apply months ahead. He takes but four men in his class. In all the Vienna clinics gynecological examination is made almost exclusively by the bimanual method, two fingers in the vagina, the other hand on the abdomen; and the use of the speculum for diagnosis is unusual. Examination per rectum is resorted to very frequently, and bringing the uterus down with a bullet forceps introduced into the vagina, it can be felt by the finger in the rectum. Treatment of fibroids by electricity has found some followers here, though the general opinion is strongly in favor of operation for most cases, and when one speaks of the dangers of laparotomy for fibroids they quote their brilliant record—less than 10 per cent. of deaths. In Salzer's clinic they now use the Lawson Tait method of perineorrhaphy almost exclusively, and report most excellent results.

In Nothnagel's clinics two instruments are in constant use which should be in the hands of all physicians, for they make the differential diagnosis of leukæmia, leucocythæmia, chlorosis, and pernicious anæmia almost mathematically certain. With the hæmocytometer the blood-corpuscles are counted, and the proportion of red to white established, and with the

" Fleischl hæmoglobinometer " the relative amount of hæmoglobin in the blood is found. A few drops of the patient's blood are sufficient for the examination. Dr. Lorenz, Nothnagel's assistant, showed us a case of tetanus. A week ago the man was severely injured in his right eye by an iron splinter from the hoop of a barrel. The cornea was torn and the iris prolapsed, and he was treated for nearly a week at Fuch's clinic. On Thursday they noticed there a slight trismus, difficulty in swallowing, and some stiffness in the legs. He was transferred to Nothnagel's wards, and on Friday morning showed the following symptoms: His mind was clear, there were no marked symptoms in the face, and chewing was quite easy ; forward and backward motions of the head were limited, lateral motions free. It was hard for him to swallow liquids, and he took but little at a time, but the lips moved very freely. The muscles of the chest and arms were free, but a slight spasm could be detected in the pectorales and the muscles of the shoulder stood in more marked relief than normal. The diaphragm was movable and the breathing good. Attempting to raise the patient to a sitting posture at once produced opisthotonus. Sensibility of the entire skin was perfect, fever was absent, but there was profuse sweating on the face, chest, and limbs. Every few moments clonic spasms, in which the pains were intense, occurred. Two days later the patient died. There was no post-mortem rise of temperature. On section a broncho-pneumonia was found, but no changes in the nervous system save a few very small hæmorrhages in the cord, and the immediate cause of death was the pneumonia. In his lecture on Tuesday Nothnagel said : " Tetanus is an acute infectious disease, due to a bacillus, which has been thoroughly studied, has been cultivated in pure culture and inoculated, always producing tetanus. The bacillus can always be found in cases of true tetanus, and it is also frequent in garden soil and dust. It is probable that the disease is due primarily not to the tetanus bacilli, but to a toxine which is produced called tetanin or tetanotoxine, and this acts on the nervous centres. Frieder, of Berlin, has extracted tetanin from the bodies of cases of tetanus, and by its inoculation has caused the disease in lower animals even without inoculations of the bacilli. Death from tetanus occurs in 85 per cent. to 96 per cent. of the cases, and is brought on in one of three ways: by paralysis of the nerve centres, by suffocation from tetanic contraction of the muscles of respiration, or from complications, as in our case." Nothnagel's therapy is as follows : " Place the patient in a dark room, away from all irritation and noise, give large doses of morphine hypodermically, and great quantities of chloral and bromides by the stomach and rectum. Feed the patient well, by the stomach-tube if necessary." He considers physostigma less valuable than the bromides and chloral, and curara he thinks is useless, because it merely paralyzes the peripheral motor nerves, and does not affect the centres.

The system of promotion and of training men for didactic medicine in Vienna is peculiar. The student is required to give proofs of a thorough education, about equivalent to that of our colleges before he can be admitted to the medical school. The course in medicine is ten semesters or five years, and after graduation good scholars can serve for an additional two years in the various clinics, each of which admits about five men every year. During these two years they have splendid advantages, specially in surgery and gynecology, where they perform even capital operations. From the best of these operators or aspirants, as they are called, the professor selects his assistants, who may serve for six years. The assistant has almost complete charge of the clinic, can use the clinical material for teaching, and can thus gain valuable experience as a teacher, as well as make a good income. As the students are free to choose their instructors from a large number of assistants, of course merit and ability succeed best, and when the assistants become favorites their future is secure. They next become private docents, and then receive calls to other universities as extraordinary professor, and finally they reach the professorship " ordinarius." This thorough method of promotion is the secret of the fame of the Vienna teachers.

NEW ORLEANS.

Malarial Fevers. New Orleans Polyclinic. Medical Legislation. Arsenical Poisoning from Iced Sherbet.

To the Editor of THE MEDICAL NEWS,

SIR : The warm weather and the large area of overflowed land in the State have not yet had any perceptible effect in increasing the usual amount of malarial fevers treated in Charity Hospital during the summer. Strange to say, Dr. Bruno, the pathologist of that institution, has not had Osler's and Councilman's success in finding the hæmatozoön of Laveran in the blood of many cases that he has examined.

Speaking of this institution recalls the fact that the existing laws give the Tulane University the sole privilege of using the wards for clinical purposes. As soon, however, as the session has ended the clinical professors take a vacation until the commencement of the fall session, and during the summer their places are filled by younger men, most of whom are members of the faculty of the Polyclinic. In a former letter the brief spring session of this institution was referred to, and as the work is essentially practical, the course could not be continued in winter unless the State Legislature granted to the Polyclinic the privilege to use the wards.

With a singular monopolistic tendency the Tulane University is antagonizing such legislation. The law has passed the State Senate, but in the lower house it is meeting with active opposition from the administrators of Charity Hospital, who are acting in behalf of the University. It seems unfortunate that, for no valid reason, a worthy educational institution may be deprived of what seems as much a right as a privilege.

The action of a Legislature in medical matters is notoriously uncertain, often opposing the enactment of what would be excellent sanitary laws. Only recently the coroner of New Orleans urged the passage of a bill that would do away with a coroner's jury; that would permit the employment of an expert chemist in cases of suspected poisoning, and would require coroners to make annual reports to the Governor. There were other minor sections relative to fees to coroners. Yet the act was so amended that when it passed the Legislature it was practically emasculated.

Dr. Chassaignac, president, and a committee from the

Orleans Parish Medical Society, have been before the Legislature to urge the passage of an act to regulate the practice of medicine, and there is reason to believe that such a law will be enacted. The law recommended by the Society provides, in the first section, that no person shall practise medicine in the State unless he possesses the qualifications required by the act. The second section demands a diploma from some medical college in good standing, and an examination in the different branches of medicine before the State Board of Examiners, who—the third section provides—are to be appointed by the Governor from the six different Congressional districts. The fourth section allows the members to grant a temporary permit until the next meeting of the Board; and the fifth section provides that the members shall be appointed for twelve years. Other sections provide that the Board shall meet at least twice a year; that it shall elect officers, who are authorized to administer oaths; that the District Court of each parish shall keep a record of certificates issued, and send a copy thereof to the State Board of Health; that an annual list of registered physicians shall be published; that compensation and travelling expenses shall be allowed members of the Board; that itinerant quacks shall be fined; that persons practising without a certificate shall be fined; that licences may be revoked for unprofessional conduct; that officers of government medical services shall be exempted from the provisions of the act, and that the expenses of the Board shall be paid from its revenues. The law essays to be comprehensive, and has been carefully considered by its advocates.

An effort was recently made to separate the local and the State functions of the Louisiana State Board of Health, by depriving it of jurisdiction over sanitary matters in New Orleans, and creating a Board of Health for the city. This was not proposed on account of any inefficiency of the Board, but only to divest it of a dual character; and, if carried into effect, the change might have proved advantageous to each board. The State Board, however, vigorously and successfully resisted the proposed innovation.

On account of the failure of the United States Government to locate sanitary inspectors in Central America, where the existence of yellow fever is reported, the State Board will send one, and possibly two, experts to traverse that country from Bocas del Torro to Belize, including all places that ship fruit to this city. The fruit steamers are not allowed to carry any passengers unless they are willing to undergo detention at quarantine for the full length of time.

Recently a young lady was fatally poisoned by drinking some red sherbet, purchased from an itinerant confectioner, her companions who had drank some of the same delicacy also being made very sick. An examination of the viscera demonstrated the presence of about a grain of arsenic; and on analyzing the solution of aniline-red used to color the sherbet, one-fifth of a grain of arsenic was found in each ounce.[1] The chemist accounted for the presence of so large a quantity of arsenic in the viscera by the fact, that an acid fruit-juice in contact with the iron or copper of the freezer would dissolve a small quantity of the metal. When the arsenical coloring solution was added, an arsenite of the dissolved metal would be formed and fall to the bottom of the freezer Hence but a small portion of the contents of the freezer would contain arsenic. This accounted for the fact that other persons who had drank sherbet from the same freezer were not affected, and that only those who drank the last of the sherbet in the freezer were poisoned.

NEWS ITEMS.

International Medical Congress; Programme of the Section of Surgery. — The meetings of the Section of Surgery will take place in the chief building of the Exhibition close to the Station, "Lehrter Bahnhof." Entering by the main door, the room for the Surgical Section will be immediately to the left of the entrance hall.

The meetings will be held from 8.30 A.M. until 10.30 A.M. on the days when the general meetings of the Congress take place; from 9 A.M. until 12 P.M. on days when no general meetings take place.

Scientific reports will be made on each day of meeting, first by those surgeons who have accepted the request of the Committee on Organization to report on a certain subject. Only the names of these speakers will be put down in the programme.

The remaining time will be taken up with reports, communications, and demonstrations from other members.

As the opening of the Congress at the general meeting on August 4th may last until 2 P.M., the Surgical Section has agreed to assemble for their first meeting on Tuesday, August 5th.

First meeting, Tuesday, August 5th, from 9 A.M. until 12 P.M. The President of the Committee on Organization, Mr. Bardeleben, will welcome the members; after this he will request the election of the Secretaries and five Presidents for the five different meetings. The election being finished, Mr. Bardeleben will give the chair to the President elected for the first meeting.

Scientific reports will be made by : 1. Mr. Ollier (Lyon, France), On the Surgical Osteogenesis. 2. Mr. König (Göttingen, Germany), On Hydrops Tuberculosus of the Cavum Peritonei and its Treatment.

Second meeting, Wednesday, August 6th. 1. Mr. Jonathan Hutchinson (London, Great Britain): On the Surgical Treatment of Intussusception. 2. Mr. Billroth (Vienna, Austria): On his Experience in Resection of the Stomach and Intestines.

Third meeting, Thursday, August 7th. 1. Mr. Bottini (Pavia, Italy): On the Treatment of Enlarged Prostate. 2. Mr. Iversen (Copenhagen, Denmark): On Modern Operations for Cancerous Diseases of the Rectum.

Fourth meeting, Friday, August 8th. 1. Dr. Senn (Milwaukee, U. S. A.): On the Diagnosis and Treatment of Gunshot Wounds of the Stomach and Intestines. Illustrated by experiments. 2. Mr. Lewschin (Kasan, Russia): On Vesical Calculus in Russia.

Fifth meeting, Saturday, August 9th. 1. Mr. Rubio (Madrid, Spain): New Method of Decapitation of the Femoral Head. 2. Remaining undelivered reports.

Drs. Bernays, Biondi, Harrison, Keen, Morris, Marck, Newmann, Robson, Schede, Storrs, Wagner, Watson, White, Ziegel, and others, have announced up to the present, reports, presentations of patients, demonstrations of specimens, remarks, etc.

---

[1] The aniline itself contained 1.6 per cent. of arsenious oxide.

A list will be found in the meeting room for writing down the names and address of the members of the Section.

Any announcements of reports, etc., should be addressed to the Manager of the Committee on Organization for the Section of Surgery, Professor E. von Bergmann, Berlin, N. W., Alexander-Ufer 1.

On the afternoon of the first day of the Congress, Monday, August 4th, at 3 P.M., Dr. E. von Bergmann will be pleased to show to the members of the Section of Surgery the clinical hospital (Ziegelstrasse 5–9), as well as the methods of operating, and the aseptic treatment of wounds practised in the hospital.

The Alvarenga Prize.—The Alvarenga Prize, of the College of Physicians of Philadelphia, consisting of one year's income of the bequest of the late Señor Alvarenga, of Lisbon, has been awarded to Dr. R. W. Philip, of the Victoria Dispensary for Consumption and Diseases of the Chest, Edinburgh, for his essay on Pulmonary Tuberculosis, which will be published by the college.

Obituary.—Dr. Willis F. Westmoreland, one of the best-known surgeons of Georgia, died in Atlanta, on June 27th. Dr. Westmoreland in 1855 founded the *Atlanta Medical and Surgical Journal*, and continued as one of the editors to the time of his death. He was also Professor of Surgery in the Atlanta Medical College. He was graduated by the Jefferson Medical College in 1890.

Fifth District Branch of the New York State Medical Association.—The eighth special meeting of the Fifth District Branch of the New York State Medical Association was held at Kingston, New York, July 22d. Papers were read by Drs. T. H. Manley, J. G. Porteous, J. D. Sullivan, and others.

McGill University, Montreal.—Dr. G. E. Fenwick has resigned the chair of surgery at the McGill University, owing to impaired health. Dr. T. G. Roddick, one of the editors of the *Montreal Medical Journal*, will be Dr. Fenwick's successor.

A Students' Aid Organization at Paris.—M. Pasteur is the chairman of a committee, formed at the Sorbonne, for encouraging foreign students to enter the University of Paris. The committee proposes to assist strangers immediately upon their arrival in the city for the purposes of study, and to furnish gratuitously a kind of bureau of information and elementary advice.

State Board of Health Precautionary Circulars.—The Pennsylvania State Board of Health has issued a series of circulars entitled, "Precautions against Consumption;" "Precautions against Contagious and Infectious Diseases;" "Precautions against Typhoid Fever;" "Precautions against Scarlet Fever;" and "School Hygiene."

These circulars are written in a manner that makes them instructive both to physician and to the general public, and they should be widely distributed.

They will be mailed to any address upon receipt of a request and a two-cent postage stamp, by Dr. Benjamin Lee, Secretary of the Board, Philadelphia.

Bellevue Hospital.—It is stated that the Commissioners of Charities of New York City have obtained possession of real estate near Bellevue Hospital which will increase the depth of the hospital 150 feet, an extension that has been greatly needed for some years.

OFFICIAL LIST OF CHANGES IN THE STATIONS AND DUTIES OF OFFICERS SERVING IN THE MEDICAL DEPARTMENT, U. S. ARMY, FROM JULY 15 TO JULY 21, 1890.

By direction of the Secretary of War, leave of absence for three months, to take effect September 15, 1890, or as soon thereafter as his services can be spared, is granted to WILLIAM H. ARTHUR, *Captain and Assistant Surgeon.*—Par. 1, S. O. 160, A. G. O., *Washington, D. C.,* July 11, 1890.

By direction of the Secretary of War, the leave of absence on surgeon's certificate of disability granted LOUIS M. MANS, *Captain and Assistant Surgeon,* in S. O. 4, January 6, 1890, from this office, is extended six months on account of sickness.—Par. 16, *S. O. 160, A. G. O., Washington, D. C.,* July 11, 1890.

By direction of the Secretary of War, leave of absence for four months, on surgeon's certificate of disability, with permission to leave the Division of Missouri, is granted WILLIAM H. CORBUSIER, *Captain and Assistant Surgeon.*—Par. 4, *S. O. 162, Washington,* July 14, 1890.

PAGE, CHARLES, *Colonel and Assistant Surgeon-General,* Medical Director of the Department, is granted leave of absence for one month, to take effect the 30th instant.—Par. 3, *S. O. 91, Department of Missouri, St. Louis, Mo.,* July 14, 1890.

By direction of the Secretary of War, leave of absence for two months is granted JOHN F. PHILLIPS, *Captain and Assistant Surgeon.*—Par. 4, *S. O. 164, Headquarters of the Army, A. G. O., Washington,* July 16, 1890.

OFFICIAL LIST OF CHANGES IN THE STATIONS AND DUTIES OF THE MEDICAL CORPS OF THE U. S. NAVY FOR THE TWO WEEKS ENDING JULY 19, 1890.

AUZALL, E. W., *Assistant Surgeon.*—Detached from U. S. S. "Galena," and to await orders.

ECKSTINE, A. C., *Surgeon.*—Granted leave of absence for month of August.

PENROSE, T. M., *Medical Inspector.*—Granted leave of absence for two weeks.

CABELL, A. G., *Passed Assistant Surgeon.*—Granted leave of absence for the month of August.

ASHBRIDGE, RICHARD, *Passed Assistant Surgeon.*—Granted one month's sick leave.

HEYL, T. C., *Surgeon.*—Granted leave of absence for the month of August.

COOKE, GEORGE H., *Medical Inspector.*—Detached from Navy Yard, League Island, and ordered to the "Pensacola."

WHITE, C. H., *Medical Inspector.*—Detached from the "Pensacola," to proceed home and wait orders.

HOEHLING, A. A., *Medical Inspector.*—Detached from Naval Hospital, Washington, and ordered to League Island Navy Yard.

WELLS, H. M., *Medical Inspector.*—Detached from Museum of Hygiene and ordered to Naval Hospital, Washington, D. C.

WHITFIELD, JAMES M., *Assistant Surgeon.*—Ordered to the U. S. S. "Ajax" and other monitors.

WOOLVERTON, THERRON, *Medical Inspector.*—Ordered to the U. S. S. "Philadelphia."

LEVERING, P. A., *Passed Assistant Surgeon.*—Detached from the U. S. R. S. "Wabash," and ordered to the U. S. S. "Philadelphia."

BAILEY, T. B., *Assistant Surgeon.*—Detached from the U. S. R. S. "St. Louis," and ordered to the U. S. S. "Philadelphia."

WHITE, S. S. *Passed Assistant Surgeon.*—Ordered to the Marine Rendezvous, San Francisco, Cal.

THE MEDICAL NEWS *will be pleased to receive early intelligence of local events of general medical interest, or of matters which it is desirable to bring to the notice of the profession.*

Local papers containing reports or news items should be marked.

Letters, whether written for publication or private information, must be authenticated by the names and addresses of their writers—of course not necessarily for publication.

All communications relating to the editorial department of the NEWS *should be addressed to No. 1004 Walnut Street, Philadelphia.*

THE MEDICAL NEWS.
A WEEKLY JOURNAL OF MEDICAL SCIENCE.

Vol. LVII.	Saturday, August 2, 1890.	No. 5.

ORIGINAL LECTURES.

DIATHESES AS APPLIED TO SURGERY. GANGRENE IN ITS VARIOUS FORMS. REMOVAL OF A GANGRENOUS CANCER.

A Clinical Lecture, delivered at the Philadelphia Hospital.

BY ERNEST LAPLACE. M.D.,

PROFESSOR OF PATHOLOGY AND CLINICAL SURGERY IN THE MEDICO-CHIRURGICAL COLLEGE; VISITING SURGEON TO THE PHILADELPHIA HOSPITAL. ETC.

[Reported by W. A. NEWMAN DORLAND. M.D.]

GENTLEMEN: There is at present a dearth of surgical material in our wards, and in view of that fact I desire to speak, during a portion of my hour, upon the general question of diatheses, especially as applied to surgery. There are two words, "*diathesis*" and "*cachexia*," which are frequently employed by all of us, but which to many are very indefinite in their meaning. Especially is this so with students, and often it is long before they acquire an accurate knowledge as to what is understood by these terms. It is well here, as elsewhere, to possess always fixed ideas as to the meaning of technical terms. The word "diathesis" comes from two Greek words, and means "I dispose" or "predispose." The word "cachexia" also comes from the Greek, and means a "bad existence." Therefore, a diathesis is an inherited predisposition to a certain disease, while a cachexia is an acquired condition in which the body has lost its former normal state from having passed through some pathological condition. For instance, we speak of the malarial cachexia as existing in an individual who, though not suffering from malaria at the time, still has the appearance of having had that disease; while we know that a child the offspring of tuberculous parents is born with the so-called tubercular diathesis. From time immemorial it was evident that parentage had something to do with the condition of health and of disease as occurring in the offspring. Especially has this been marked among the lower animals, and if it be true here, how much more forcible must it be in man who is the paragon of animals! Also it is true that civilization is to man what domestication is to the inferior animals.

With this introduction let me say a few words regarding the various diatheses with which we are acquainted. The one we most frequently speak of is the tubercular diathesis, a term which is indiscriminately used with tuberculosis, scrofula, and scrofulosis. Let me establish here what we mean by the tubercular diathesis. A child born of parents who have had or who have inherited tuberculosis, need not have any evidence of the disease itself in order to possess the tubercular diathesis. The appearance of children with this diathesis is characteristic. Generally they are bright children. fair. with blue eyes and transparent skin, the marvel of the neighborhood, never very strong, and irritable in disposition. They are only waiting for the occasion to develop tuberculosis. Now suppose that two children receive a fall, the one a healthy child, and the other one of these bright children. The healthy child will suffer a contusion of his knee which will be well in two or three days. Not so the other child. The contusion is followed by a swelling in the knee-joint, and the child develops a "white swelling," or tuberculous disease of the joint. Both of these children had been breathing the germs of tuberculosis since birth, and the germs had not developed because there was not a suitable condition of the system. Now the one child falls, and from this slight cause the development takes place, and the disease manifests itself, whereas, in the healthy child the germ still resists development.

Now, what do we understand by scrofulosis? A child with scrofulosis is one with tuberculosis of its lymphatic glands. From the moment the symptoms of scrofula appear. the child is tuberculous, for the germs have begun to develop within the glandular system. There are no reliable cases on record to warrant the belief that a child is ever born with fully developed tuberculosis in its system. It must, therefore, be born with the tubercular diathesis, to develop sooner or later tuberculosis in one of its forms; either as scrofulosis, or tuberculosis of the lymphatic glands; as "white swelling," or tuberculosis of the knee-joint; as tubercular meningitis; as cold abscesses in various parts of the body; or finally, later in life as that most fatal development of tuberculosis, tuberculosis of the lungs. There are many among us who, if they lived according to the laws of hygiene, would never develop tuberculosis; but the most of us, if placed under improper hygienic conditions, would contract the disease from the development of the germs which we now breathe with impunity. It is possible, thus for a person who has not the tubercular diathesis to develop the disease if the proper soil is acquired, and this soil is called the cachexia.

Leaving, now, the question of tuberculosis, let us take up that of syphilis. Syphilis is also a condition in which a diathesis exists, but unlike tuberculosis the child may be born with the affection fully developed. Cancer is another affection exactly in the same condition, so far as development is concerned, as syphilis. There are cases on record of children who have been born with fully developed cancers of the mesentery. These cases, though extremely rare, are sufficient to prove the assertion. The malarial poison, the poison of syphilis, tuberculosis, etc., all starting as cachexiæ may manifest themselves as diatheses in our children. Suppose now that a person who is perfectly healthy acquires tuberculosis. He will very probably give the diathesis to his offspring.

What, then, is the difference between a person who has the tubercular diathesis and one who has not? It is purely a chemical difference, possibly modified by temperature. Since we know to-day that the tuberculous condition is due to a peculiar seed, the tubercle bacillus, falling upon a suitable soil, just as a certain seed falling into the ground will develop a particular plant, or as one soil is suitable for the development of wheat, and another for the development of corn, so, I say, in these cases the only difference is one of a chemical nature; the soil not being suitable to the development of the germ in the one, and being suitable in the other. There is a true chemical difference in the albuminoids of the two persons, a difference at present inappreciable to chemists, but which, judging from the present state of investigations, will shortly be discovered.

Gentlemen, this is no hypothesis, but we are speaking of something which can be demonstrated as clearly as that two and two make four. If we take a proper preparation of agar-agar and add to it four per cent. of glycerin, the tubercle bacillus will grow and develop; but if we add six or eight per cent. of glycerin, the tubercle bacillus will not grow. The agar-agar preparation with the four per cent. of glycerin is the tuberculous child, and the germ grows; the agar-agar solution with the eight per cent. of glycerin is us, on whom, though the germs fall, they will not grow. Therefore, since these things can be demonstrated in any bacteriological laboratory, cannot any logical mind draw the inference that the same thing will occur in the individual?

One more fact to illustrate this idea. Diseases are different because the germs which produce them are different, though the soil is the same. Eight years ago, in the Academy of Sciences of Paris, Pasteur had just discovered a method of inoculating for splenic fever in animals. It was known that splenic fever would not attack fowls, though it did attack both beasts and man. On the other hand, Pasteur had noticed that the germ of the disease at the temperature of the human body was deadly, while if the temperature was raised a few degrees higher the germ became inert. Then the thought occurred to him to investigate the temperature of fowls, and he found that it was 101°, the same temperature at which the germ became innocent. At once he reasoned that this was why the germ would not grow. He took the fowl and put it into cold water, and reducing the temperature in this way, he introduced the germ, which now grew and killed the fowl. What could be more conclusive than the effect of temperature in producing disease? Thus two men get a wetting; the one develops a pneumonia, because his temperature has become reduced, while the other escapes, his temperature remaining normal at the time of exposure.

Let us now see what is to be done from a remedial standpoint. What should be done to preserve ourselves against these conditions? The first one to turn our minds into the right direction was Jenner, the discoverer of vaccination, or the introduction into the body of a certain amount of a living chemical substance which when developed in the body causes the soil to become barren. This being the case with smallpox, what a great field lies before us, as many affections are due to microorganisms capable of development, but which may be prevented from developing by altering the condition of the soil! What great opportunities are afforded us for studying these germs and their processes of develop-

ment! The other conditions which are acquired from vices or alcoholic excesses may easily be removed, and the time may yet come when Addison's allegory, the Vision of Mirza, will prove indeed only a dream. Instead of the seventy broken columns, with the path beset with snares and pitfalls, there will be one hundred complete columns, and a perfect highway along which man may travel happy and healthy to the Elysian fields beyond.

The next patient shows a condition of gangrene—a very important subject. Gangrene is always due to some interference in the circulation, either arterial or venous, or often both. If arterial, we have the dry form of gangrene; if venous, the moist form; if due to interference with both arteries and veins, we have capillary gangrene, such as occurs in old age, or as a result of a severe bruise, or following that condition of the system produced by certain remedies, as ergot. Here is this old woman suffering from senile gangrene. Her circulation is too weak to afford proper nourishment to the toes. The patient came into the hospital three days ago in a pretty fair condition. Very often this disease is self-limiting, and so we waited; but there does not seem to be any tendency to self-limitation. The proper treatment in these cases is amputation, not close to the gangrenous area, but far from it. The amputation here should be just below the knee. The patient has developed septicæmia, and is now suffering from septic pneumonia, and operation would probably not be followed by success. Yet if she would give consent—which she positively refuses to do—I would operate. Gangrene always results from cessation of the circulation, and is a process of putrefaction and fermentation. The odor is due chiefly to sulphuretted hydrogen. There is also developed carbonic acid, which we can see coming in bubbles from under the skin.

Here is another patient who presented on entrance a condition of gangrene. She suffered a severe fall and, as a result, experienced great contusion of the parts around the anus, sufficient to impair the vitality and permeable condition of the bloodvessels. There is sloughing of the parts, which is nothing more nor less than gangrene. When this slough comes off we call it a sphacelus. The wound to-day looks very healthy.

The next case is the one I brought before you when I was speaking of metastasis in cancer. To-day I bring him here to show you another case of gangrene, and to operate upon him. The man is young, and the metastasis in his groin is rapidly progressing; therefore I shall try to remove most of the disease, and, by the application of proper remedies, endeavor to destroy the disease-germ as far as possible. Around the ulceration you will notice these large, dark spots, which are gangrenous in nature. The poison developing there is directly interfering with the circulation. Just as we see the chemical poison of a snake-bite, or the poison of ergot or of carbonic acid producing gangrene, so here we see the poison of disease causing his gangrene. Therefore, remember that microörganisms may also excite gangrene when growing in certain tissues, as may be seen in the case of a carbuncle, which is due to the staphylococcus pyogenes aureus.

While waiting for the case to be etherized, I will say that the cure of cancer should not be considered hopeless. At the recent Congress of Surgeons in Berlin there were reported six undoubted cures of epithelioma and sarcoma by the following treatment. About twenty years ago a French surgeon, still living, had a case of cancer of the breast which was too far advanced for operation. As the surgeon was not very cleanly, not being acquainted with our methods of antisepsis, the patient developed erysipelas, and after nearly dying, recovered. About a month later she had a second attack of erysipelas, after which the growth took on a benign appearance and progressed to recovery. Since then two surgeons have been inoculating cancerous patients with the germs of erysipelas, and now report the cure of six cases.

The patient now being ready I shall proceed to cut away with scissors as much of this gangrenous tissue as possible. The femoral artery is in this region, and is probably not far from the inroads of the disease. I shall therefore be very careful in the use of the curette.

ORIGINAL ARTICLES.

CIRCUMCISION.

BY E. R. PALMER, M.D.,
OF LOUISVILLE, KY.

In offering for consideration the subject of circumcision I am certainly not actuated by the idea of novelty. The veil of mystery of old that has never been lifted, that still enshrouds the reasons that impelled Abraham to institute this operation among the chosen people; the persistence with which the rite has been performed upon the males of that people in epochs of prosperity and in ages of adversity should have given us a definite literature of the subject from a surgical standpoint. That this is not the fact, and that crudities still cluster around the operation, whether done as a religious rite or as a surgical necessity, are among the reasons that have suggested this paper.

Before entering into a consideration of the purely scientific or surgical aspect of my subject, its relations to the laws of heredity and evolution may well be considered. The development of new species by the selection and cultivation of "sports" in the botanical kingdom is a common occurrence. In the animal world the once famous Ancon sheep of New England were bred from a bench-legged "accident of birth." The tailless and the hairless families of dogs still further illustrate the power of heredity by selection. Among men the transmission of supernumerary toes or fingers through generations, a transmission of tendency to redundancy, is probably the best of the few instances I can choose for illustration, unless the growing tendency to early baldness, which is clearly hereditary, may be pointed to as presaging a coming family of hairless humanity.

What of circumcision? Has this most venerable rite had any effect on the length of the normal Hebrew prepuce? In reply I will quote from two recent editorials in the *New York Medical Journal.*

"Are Mutilations Inherited? *The Lancet,* in a recent issue, discusses this subject and refers to some recent studies by Professor Weismann on the subject. The distinguished professor cut off the tails of nine hundred and one white mice of successive generations, but in no case was a white mouse born without a full-sized tail. It has always been something of a puzzle that jews should, after thousands of years of circumcision, still bear infants with long prepuces. Darwin refers to the fact, as noted by Gordon, that different races of men have from time immemorial knocked out their upper incisors, cut off joints of their fingers, made holes of immense size through the lobes of their ears or through their nostrils, tattooed themselves, made deep gashes in various parts of their bodies, and yet there is no reason to suppose that these mutilations have ever been inherited.

"It must be conceded that, in the higher mammals, at least, mutilations are rarely, if ever, transmitted."

"Dr. Levy, a dentist of Stettin, has written to the editor of the *Archiv für pathologische Anatomie und Physiologie und für klinische Medicin* an account of some occurrences in his own family that have a bearing, he thinks, on a question raised by Professor Weismann at the sixty-first 'Versammlung Deutscher Naturforscher und Aerzte' —that of the hereditary transmission of acquired peculiarities, such as the lack of a foreskin in jews. He states that, like his father before him, he was born without a foreskin—as he expresses it, '*regelrecht beschnitten'*— furthermore, that this was the case with his four brothers also, who died in childhood. An occasional natural *apelle* is to be met with among Gentiles, but this, of course, raises no question of heredity; such a group of them as Dr. Levy's communication mentions is a different matter, however, although not a very convincing evidence of evolution."

In my personal experience I can report a single case, that of a young man of Jewish lineage who came to me with a stricture. On exposing the penis an excessively redundant prepuce presented. In answer to my query, the young man said that when he was born his father lived in the country, in a sparsely settled region, where no one could be found to perform the rite. The cases in the Levy family raise another question whose answer I think readily explains the peculiarities. Do all baby boys left uncircumcised grow to man's estate with redundant foreskins? In my opinion the answer is. Not more than two-thirds. How is this to be explained? Boys are born with adherent prepuces as puppies are with closed eyes—a normal evolution of the parts should give a loose, freely retractable prepuce, covering about half the glans during rest. This is the typical evolution of these parts. Sometimes at one extreme the organ in the uncircumcised, except for the absence of scar marks cannot be told from one that has been operated upon, a condition that has by some surgeons been atributed to excessive masturbation in early youth. In others a prepuce closely adherent to the glans, or congenital stenosis of the preputial orifice may be observed. Probably each of us has seen adults presenting the latter condition where a ballooning of the preputial sac occurred on any attempt at free urination.

Should boy babies be circumcised? In most cases they should. But as done by the *mohel* the operation is needlessly painful, occasionally fruitful of permanent harm, and sometimes dangerous to life itself. In examining young men of Jewish families I have a number of times noted the removal of the tip of the glans itself, leaving behind not only a troublesome traumatic stenosis, but what is worse, possible barrenness, whilst cicatricial bands and disfiguring scars innumerable have been observed again and again. How should the operation be done?

In very early life it is an exceedingly simple operation. All that is needed is to assist nature in the normal evolution of the parts. The proper operation lies between two extremes. It is not necessary to remove tissue, nor will ordinary divulsion with forceps suffice. The operation of splitting the upper surface well back on a grooved director with a pair of scissors is all that is necessary, no stitching being called for, and only a simple antiseptic dressing is required. I grant with others that this is on the adult an exceedingly unsurgical procedure as a rule, leaving as it does useless and unsightly ears on either side. Not so, however, with the babe. In the adult the evolution of the parts is complete; in the babe the operation acts like the woodman's tree-belting. Beyond the base of the slit evolution ceases and a scarless *apelle* is the result. I first saw this operation done eighteen years ago, and I had occasion the other day to examine the babe, now grown. The result was all that could be desired. I have done the operation many times in later years, and am so far pleased with the outcome. As I said before, this method is usually an unsurgical procedure in the adult. Occasionally one presents with a scant but very tightly fitting cover, and here splitting may be indicated. I believe that were the ritualist, the *mohel*, to split freely only, and then thoroughly separate the adherent surfaces, giving proper directions to the nurse for keeping them so, he would accomplish safely, quickly, and almost painlessly all that reason and science at least could ask. In after years, I question if the subject would be distinguishable from one operated on by the old method, except by the superior beauty of the result.

It would consume too much time to go into a detailed account of the various neuroses of childhood that are attributable to a long foreskin. Their recognition makes it imperative that every doctor should examine all boy babies in his charge, whether sick or well, and see that the condition if existing be removed.

When should circumcision be performed in the adult? In what class of cases? First, in all men who, otherwise sound, possess a long, non-adherent prepuce that is so narrow at its orifice, or so glove-fitting in its nature as to prevent easy retraction while in a state of complete erection. Second, in cases of redundant prepuce, where only extreme cleanliness and care can prevent frequently recurring excoriations or ordinary balanitis; and, finally, in the group of cases where, notwithstanding that the prepuce is freely movable, full erection fails to uncover the glans.

The following conditions call for the operation in disease: First, preparatory to urethrotomy in gleet with stricture, where a long, close, and troublesome foreskin constantly projects itself into the operator's way. Second, in cases with chronic herpetic and balanitic tendencies. Third, *in syphilis*, where (*a*) the chancre may by such an operative procedure be removed, and where (*b*) syphilitic hyperplasia of a general and extensive type produces phimosis or furnishes in useless tissue a nidus for the further evolution of poison, it being a matter of frequent observation that extreme venereal syphilitic infiltration is no obstacle to ready union after operation.

Finally, shall we circumcise in phimosis complicated with chancroids? I confess that I have in the past been often at sea in such conditions. Influenced by the teachings of authorities I have again and again in spite of extreme care had chancroids escape control and do much harm under a tight phimosis. Now, in many cases, I have by operating early not only avoided this accident but cut short the disease.

When shall we operate in these cases? The answer is found in the condition of the groin. If the lymphatic glands are not involved the operation may be safely performed. If hot, rapidly advancing adenitis exists, to operate would be to assume a grave responsibility, yet even in such cases with our present increased knowledge of the laws and control of sepsis I would frequently fear the knife less than the disease itself, concealed deep beneath the fixed and swollen foreskin. In the last few months I have operated in such cases four times, using the extremest care in the matter of quick cauterization and antiseptic after-treatment, and in such cases the result has been all that could be desired. In the last case, a young Irishman of not over-cleanly habits or occupation, the excision showed a large, gray suppurating sore that had just destroyed the frænum. Cauterization with pure carbolic acid was done, the wound was washed with bichloride solution and dressed with iodoform. Two days later there suddenly appeared in the left groin a huge bubo—a so-called sympathetic bubo—which almost as suddenly disappeared under the pressure of a spica bandage. The healthy tissue of the cut united nicely, and though the sore was some weeks in healing, no new infection followed. This is typical of my other cases.

There is a group of cases that comes under this class about which there should not be a moment's hesitation. Every city practitioner meets with them. They present on the free edge of a long prepuce grayish ulcers or often, at first, fissures only, sometimes single, sometimes multiple, but with a marked tendency to extend and to resist treatment. When the foreskin is in place, they are usually concealed in a fold. To expose them it is necessary to retract the part partially, which tears them open and tends to increase their extent. I formerly wrestled with such cases for a month or two, but now by immediate circumcision the cases are not only at once cured but often the disease is forever afterward prevented from returning.

I shall not weary the reader with general details of operative procedure, but will emphasize only a few of the important points.

Immediately before operating in cases of gleet, wash out the urethra, by means of a Jacque's catheter, with a hot 1-to-15,000 bichloride solution. In cases of balanitis or excoriation dress the parts twice daily for several days before the operation, with cotton wet in saturated solution of boric acid. In case of chancroids, touch every visible sore with pure carbolic acid just before operating, and in *all cases* cleanse the parts and surroundings very thoroughly with hot 1-to-2000 bichloride solution, being especially careful to purify thoroughly the balano-preputial fold. Chloroform or ether need never be used; 4-per-cent. cocaine solution injected into and beneath the skin with a hypodermic syringe and incarcerated by the Corning method is sufficient. In applying your rubber for this purpose follow the Esmarch method. It will give a bloodless operation.

A familiar problem has been how to cut both skin and mucous membrane at the same time. It is an idle and fallacious problem. In some cases, for instance of chronic balanitis, very little mucous membrane and more skin is desirable. By trimming the mucous membrane after removing the skin one is enabled, looking always to the preservation of the fraenum, to prevent bridling at that point during future erections. Like a tailor fitting the sleeve to a garment the surgeon should cut diagonally, beginning close to the glans on the dorsum and shading out to a lengthy fraenum below. Speaking of cutting both layers at once, it is of especial importance to recognize that not two but three coats must be cut if a neat operation with speedy union is the aim. After trimming the mucous layer, and just before introducing the stitches, the connective tissue in the bottom of the wound should be seized with a pair of small dressing forceps, drawn

outward and then with scissors be carefully clipped away around the entire circumference of the floor. Where this is neglected the now useless tissue will push outward between the stitches and, later, leave a ring of induration that is a long time in finally disappearing. In the matter of stitching, having tried both the interrupted and continuous suture, I have found that after removal of connective tissue from four to six interrupted silk stitches are all that is needed. It is the rule with some excellent surgeons always to destroy the fraenum. Not only should this not be done, but, so far as possible, where it has by previous accident been ruptured, it should be restored.

What is the fraenum? What are its functions? In the mechanism of erection while the corpus spongiosum enlarges at its two extremities, its erection is chiefly characterized by *elongation*, carrying with it the cavernous bodies that at the same time expand laterally to give increased circumference to the organ. When the penis is flaccid the scrotum is in most cases pronouncedly pendulous. In erection the testicles hug closely to the region of the bulb, for the fraenum has done its duty and carried upward with the ascending glans the scrotal raiment of the now fully erect organ. To destroy wholly the fraenum entails inevitably a diminution in the size of the organ during erection. Nor is this the only office of the fraenum. In the introduction of the cocaine during the cutting, trimming, and sewing, one point is always painful—the fraenum. Why? Because it is the centre of penile sensation. Because, more than the entire surface of the glans does it possess that exquisite sensitiveness with which the bulbs of Krause endow these parts. During erection not only does it draw upward the lax scrotum as a covering for the organ, but its two edges acutely sensitive and now thoroughly tense, like vocal cords, voice the passion that overpowers. My first stitch looks always to the preservation or restoration of this part.

In former years, circumcision in the adult meant a week, perhaps more, of confinement in bed and room. Under modern methods not an hour need be lost from business. This is in part due to the substitution of local for general anaesthesia, but mainly to the antiseptic precautions used, including dressings, of which I shall in conclusion say a few words.

I spoke a while ago of the thorough use of a 1-to-2000 solution of bichloride in the preparatory cleansing. From a brilliant young Kentuckian, Dr. John Young Brown, I have learned the value of absolute dryness during the operation and in the after-dressing. Formerly I encountered frequent and annoying tumefaction of the adjacent parts, which I thought was due to the cocaine. At Dr. Brown's suggestion I operated and dressed dry, and have never encountered that trouble since. Even in case of hæmorrhage, which is, however, rarely a factor in the operation, the cotton should be absolutely dry. Like others I am not opposed to blood in dressings if it is *clean* blood. A little oozing all around the line is not objectionable. After stitching, a piece of dry, aseptic gauze, four inches long and an inch and a half wide, covered with iodoform and boric acid, and spread on a clean towel, is laid under the frænum, brought up around the cut, right and left, to the dorsum and trimmed with scissors. Over this a strip of absorbent cotton, three-quarters of an inch wide, is applied. Next, a Maltese cross of dry gauze, with a central hole for the meatus, is applied, and then a similar cross of rubber tissue, and the whole bandaged snugly in place. A waist belt, a jock strap, and a bunch of cotton, to cover the glans, well dusted with boric acid, complete a dressing that permits the subject to go to work at once at any ordinary vocation. By directing the patient to retract the dressing on urinating and to absorb the final drops with a soft cloth this original dressing may be left on five days. When the stitches are removed the parts should be dusted with boric acid, a loose pledget of cotton wrapped around them, and the patient discharged.

Occasionally, owing to oozing of blood, it may be found necessary to apply the dressing too tightly for permanency. In such cases an extra one-inch roller may be applied over the permanent dressing, to be removed some hours later without disturbing the dressing proper.

THE CAUSES AND TREATMENT OF PNEUMONIA.[1]

BY J. M. G. CARTER, M.D., Sc.D., PH D.,
OF WAUKEGAN, ILL.
FELLOW OF THE AMERICAN ACADEMY OF MEDICINE; MEMBER OF THE
AMERICAN MEDICAL ASSOCIATION, ETC.,

PNEUMONIA is one of the diseases best known to the medical profession, but that a disease is well known and easily diagnosed does not necessarily imply that it is thoroughly understood. When a disease is said to be thoroughly understood, it is meant that its etiology, its processes, or pathological modifications, its sequelæ, and its proper treatment are known and accepted as settled by the profession. It was formerly supposed that idiopathic pneumonia was due to some atmospheric influence which, by checking the peripheral circulation, turned the blood-current with greater force to the lungs, the result of which was congestion and inflammation. This is still considered the pathological process, but the question of etiology has given rise to some discussion, and, in many minds, to doubt.

---

[1] Read before the Illinois State Medical Society, May, 1890.

The germ theory, which is accepted as the explanation of many diseases, has been advanced to explain the origin of pneumonia. Since the discovery of the peculiar form of bacteria in the lungs of persons dead from pneumonia, a discovery made by Friedländer and Frobenius, much thought has been given to the bacterial theory of the disease. Six different varieties of bacteria have been mentioned by Bremner as causing this disease, and others have been mentioned by later writers. The diplococcus of Fränkel has lately been shown to be present in most cases of pneumonia, especially croupous pneumonia. Wolff found it in ninety-four per cent. of the cases examined by him, there being but a single negative result in seventy successive cases. Baumgarten thinks it is safe to assume a single cause for pneumonia. In Wolff's cases verification was established by cultures in more than half the cases.

The first investigations were made after death, but later authors have examined sputa and exudations from the lungs. Monti examined the exuded fluid in twenty cases, with but one negative result. Sometimes the Fränkel diplococcus was found in company with other bacteria. In these cases of Monti, Friedländer's micrococcus was not seen. Inoculation of fifty-nine rabbits, while universally successful, produced typical pneumonia only when the sputum was introduced into the trachea. Inoculation under the skin produces septicæmia; into the pleura, pleurisy; into the pericardium, pericarditis. Inoculation into the dura mater of a dog produced meningitis and lobar pneumonia. Fränkel, Foa, Whittaker, and others have shown that the cause of pneumonia is not confined to the lungs, but invades other organs and tissues. Weichselbaum, Netter, Mircoli, and others, have found the diplococcus, after pneumonia, in the ventricles of the brain, connective tissue of the mediastinum, and in that about the clavicle, in the cavities about the nose, and in the drum-cavity and labyrinth of the ear. It has been cultivated from the serum of the pericardium, before there were any visible signs of inflammation. It has been found, likewise, in inflammations of the spinal cord.

Emmerich found great numbers of bacteria of the varieties here referred to under the floor of a hospital ward where many cases of pneumonia had been treated.

Writing in regard to pneumonia proper, Weichselbaum sums up his conclusions as follows:

1. "The bacteria found in different forms of pulmonary inflammation are regarded as the cause of them. This conclusion is completely justified on the following grounds: Definite, well-characterized species of bacteria not only occur constantly in acute pulmonary inflammations, but can be demonstrated in greatest abundance and activity in the earlier stages of inflammations. They have been isolated, cultivated, and, when introduced into certain animals, have produced processes which,

taking them *in toto*, correspond to inflammation of the lung in man.

2. "The pulmonic virus is no unity, inasmuch as acute pulmonary inflammations, even croupous pneumonia proper, can be produced by different kinds of bacteria. In this the pneumonias recall acute inflammation of the connective tissue, in which several species of organisms occur.

3. "The separation of pneumonias into lobular and lobar, croupous and non-croupous, has an anatomical, but no etiological significance. Moreover, the so-called secondary pneumonias, etiologically considered, are not secondary.

4. "The diplococcus pneumonia is to be regarded as the most frequent exciter of inflammation of the lungs. Friedländer's bacillus but rarely causes croupous pneumonia. 'Catching cold' has only a possible predisposing effect."

This summary is, perhaps, a clear representation of the opinion held by the majority, of bacteriologists at least, at the present time. The opinions of general practitioners are universally more conservative than those of specialists, and many able physicians still hesitate to accept the theories and radical views of some bacteriologists. It is well known that there is much study devoted to this subject at the present time, and many investigations have been made during the past year, but, perhaps, nothing can be added to the stock of knowledge or opinions detailed above. Dr. F. S. Billings, of Chicago, informs me that nothing new has been discovered; and as his personal views correspond with those of most other bacteriologists, I will quote his own words: "Personally, I do not think either the Weichselbaum, Fränkel, or Friedländer organism has any specific relation to pneumonia in man." He gives, as a reason or basis for this opinion, "That they are present in the mouths of healthy individuals, and do not cause pneumonia, and have also been found attached to the bronchial mucosa of persons killed by accident or dying with intact lungs;" but he further states that, "When active and prolonged congestion with serous bronchial effusion is present, then they may cause pneumonia."

When an epidemic of a disease caused by bacteria occurs it is said that the air is filled with them. Professor Nussbaum has stated that during an epidemic of cholera the air is filled with cholera bacilli, and yet only one per cent. of the population is affected by the disease. Hence ninety-nine people in every hundred, though eating, drinking, and breathing cholera bacilli escape the disease. Such may well be believed to be the case with the bacillus of pneumonia, though it must be less powerful in its activities than that of cholera.

It is well known that pneumonia is more prevalent in some seasons than others, and that it occurs most frequently under certain atmospheric conditions. Perhaps most cases occur during the winter and spring months. The humidity of the atmosphere and the presence of ozone also seem to exert a causative influence. On October 12, 1889, at Waukegan, Ill., the wind was in the southwest; it suddenly changed to the northeast, the temperature fell from 70° to 50°, and the ozone in the atmosphere was increased. Several cases of catarrhal pneumonia occurred, the apparent cause being the change in the condition of the atmosphere. I noticed, however, that during the same period, many cases of pneumonia were reported in other localities. On February 15, 1890, the wind was in the southwest; the temperature rose from 30° to 65°; ozone was not marked; the atmosphere was humid, and there were several cases of pneumonia. From April 1st to 5th the wind was mostly from the east and southeast, it was rainy and warmer, the temperature varying from 40° to 65°. New cases of pneumonia developed. Such observations are prone to make one believe that atmospheric changes are causative of the disease. Jaccoud, while not denying the etiological influence of bacteria, holds that exposure to cold is also causative, and perhaps generally the exciting cause.

Dr. Baker demonstrated before the Brooklyn Pathological Society that the curve representative of sickness from pneumonia pretty regularly followed the curve of temperature. His studies extended over many years and included nearly fifty thousand cases of pneumonia. He showed, in all his references, "that the sickness curve follows the temperature curve, not only in pneumonia, but also in bronchitis. If pneumonia were due to bacteriological influence, this cause must certainly be influenced by the weather, and more than that, bronchitis would probably be caused by the same germ."

Sevestre considers that certain cases of endemic and epidemic broncho-pneumonia in children during the summer months are due to dietary indiscretion, the inflammation extending to the lungs from the intestines through the lymph-channels.

Tomasi, Golgi, and others believe pneumonia to be sometimes caused by malarial poison, and this view corresponds with that of the physicians in the southern part of Illinois and other malarial districts in the United States, where this form of the disease is called "winter fever."

Dr. Mosny reported to the Academy of Medicine of Paris a case of broncho-pneumonia in a woman who had been nursing a patient with erysipelas. The patient died, and the examination of the exudation in the lungs revealed the fact that the pneumococcus was not present, but that the streptococcus erysipelatis was, showing that the disease in this case was not caused by the bacillus of pneumonia.

At present it must be admitted that the cause of pneumonia is not fully determined, and probably the majority of physicians are not willing to accept the bacillus theory. It is unproven that the bacillus is not a concomitant rather than the cause of the disease. Future investigations must make the final decision, and probably we shall not wait long before the decision is made.

It has been hoped that the germ theory of disease might lead to specific medication, and it may justly be anticipated, if this theory is true, that absolute cure of many diseases may be promised as soon as germicides are discovered which will kill the germs without injuring the patient. Is this possible? At present we do not know. So far as pneumonia is concerned, the knowledge or lack of knowledge of the presence of pneumococci is of no importance in the treatment of the disease.

In the present state of our knowledge the following indications for the treatment are clear: (1) To equalize the circulation and diminish the determination of blood to the lungs. (2) To reduce the temperature of the body. (3) To sustain the patient's strength. (4) To assist the mucous membranes and organs of secretion and excretion in the performance of their functions. (5) To allay pain.

The first two of these indications are met by the same general treatment. The chief object is to control the high temperature, and this is largely accomplished by reducing the blood-pressure and allaying the excitability of an overworked heart. For these indications I use aconite, gelsemium, or digitalis, according to the grade of the fever and the condition of the lungs, the heart, and the stomach. In high fever, with strong, bounding pulse, I use aconite and add gelsemium if there is irritable stomach with or without headache. Petresco says that digitalis may check pneumonia at the outset. It is of value in asthenic cases and where the heart is weak. Convallaria is sometimes advantageously substituted when digitalis is not well borne.

I have not been favorably impressed with antipyrine nor with antifebrin, and of late have not given them. Dr. Humphreys remarks that antipyrine should not generally be given in catarrhal pneumonia nor in lobar pneumonia when there is œdema of the lungs.

Quinine is usually serviceable, and in malarial cases is essential, not only to reduce temperature, but also as a germicide and antiperiodic. But in some cases it has a bad effect upon the stomach and nervous system. Dr. Jacobi believes that quinine lessens pulmonary congestion and strengthens the heart's action. Alcohol, brandy or whiskey in large doses will help to reduce temperature and equalize the circulation. It has seemed to me that the alcohol secures this result by its action on the vaso-motor system. I have also seen most beneficial results from early blistering with cantharides, which not only alleviates pain but assists in controlling the congestion.

Liebermeister advises bloodletting when there is œdema of the lungs; but I believe this may be avoided by blistering and the use of digitalis. He is also much in favor of the cold bath, given preferably in the evening. There is no doubt that a wise use of the bath—tepid or cold, as circumstances may require—assists in reducing temperature and has a restorative rather than a debilitating effect.

In many sthenic cases tartar emetic seems to be of special value. Bruckner has reported over seventy cases treated with this drug, in which the success was so marked as to make him enthusiastically in favor of the remedy.

An ice-bag to the head and affected portion of the lung, as recommended by Angel Money, may be used with success, and often gives great comfort to the patient; but, like the baths, it must be used systematically. Money says that the ice-bag acts as a tonic to the heart, to the nervous system, to the muscular system, and to the respiratory centres. It thus aids in the third indication, maintaining the patient's strength. It soothes the motor and sensory systems, and in this way produces sleep.

For the difficult breathing likely to occur on the fifth day, with small and rapid pulse, perhaps nothing is better than camphor, benzoic acid, or valerian. Alcohol in large doses is also beneficial. The inhalation of carbonic acid in broncho-pneumonia, as recommended by Dr. Lamallerée, I have not used. The third indication—the maintenance of the patient's strength—is accomplished chiefly by nourishment. With Fräntzel I recommend absolute rest in bed and liquid nourishment. The patient should be well fed from the beginning. For thirst, lemonade, and mineral and vegetable acids are refrigerant and assist the digestive process. I generally use aromatic sulphuric acid, believing that it may have a salutary influence upon the stomach, liver, and pancreas, and that it aids digestion and assimilation of food.

The secretory functions should be carefully observed, and aid should be given to the mucous membrane of the lungs, to the liver, kidneys, pancreas, and alimentary canal. Ipecacuanha is an invaluable remedy as a stimulant to the mucous membranes and to the liver. Aromatic sulphuric acid is a stimulant to the pancreas, and is of especial value in cases with typhoid symptoms. Digitalis and potassium nitrate are excellent renal stimulants. Mercury, in some form and in small doses, as a stimulant to the liver and intestinal canal is very useful. I prefer the mercury and chalk mixture given for a few days, and then followed by muriate of ammonium.

Pain must be controlled, and for this nothing can

take the place of opium. I am in the habit, in uncomplicated cases, of giving the following prescription :

R.—Sulphate of quinine   .   . 30 grains.
    Dover's powder   .   .   . 40   "
    Mercury with chalk   .   . 20   "
Mix and divide in 10 capsules.

This dose is for an adult and is varied to suit the patient and his diseased condition. I give it at intervals of four hours. This prescription assists in controlling the congestion, acts as a heart tonic, aids the patient in expectorating, assists the liver and intestinal canal in the performance of their functions, alleviates pain, and, if the Dover's powder is made with the nitrate instead of the sulphate of potassium, stimulates the kidneys.

PERFORATIVE APPENDICITIS. WITH REPORT OF A CASE TREATED BY LAPAROTOMY.[1]

By SCHUYLER C. GRAVES, M.D.,
VISITING SURGEON TO ST. MARKS AND THE U. B. A. HOSPITALS,
GRAND RAPIDS, MICH.

THE search of the followers of de Soto in the land of flowers for the fountain of perpetual youth forcibly illustrates the yearning of human nature for continued health and happiness. The fountain of youth could not, and never can be, found ; but with the astonishing progress of the science and art of medicine and surgery within the past quarter of a century the search for health has become far less discouraging and its discovery very much more possible.

Theories may oft-times be interesting, but facts are always the great *desiderata* in the practice of the healing art.

It is needless to say that facts which have a direct bearing upon the'life or death of human beings are of the most vital moment to both patient and surgeon. The surgeon cannot learn too much in regard to them, and he should not fail to profit by the experience of other surgeons who are engaged in the same investigations.

The subject of appendicitis has, of late, attracted world-wide attention in the medical profession. Abdominal surgery in general, and intestinal surgery in particular, have made wonderful strides within the last decade, principally, we are proud to say, through the labors of American surgeons, notably those of Senn and of Parkes.

The terms typhlitis, perityphlitis, and paratyphlitis, although sometimes correctly applied to morbid conditions, have long been surgical misnomers, for what has seemed to be an inflammation *of. around* or *behind* the cæcum, has undoubtedly, in the majority of instances, been an inflammation of the appendix vermiformis. This little organ, rudimentary in its capacity for good, seems to be thoroughly developed in its capacity for evil. Often with slight provocation it takes on a destructive inflammatory activity—an inflammation with an ulcerative tendeney—which, very frequently and more or less rapidly, leads to perforation with subsequent intraperitoneal complications of the gravest nature. I say frequently, for we know that inflammation of a purely catarrhal type does occur, although, according to Musser, even this mild inflammation may at any time become ulcerative, subsequently perforating.

The substances which act as the immediate cause of the disease will almost always be found fæcal in character, although, as Musser states, foreign bodies, such as "buttons, bristles, worms, shot, pins, and gall-stones," have been observed. To this list might be added the seed of the grape, lemon, and orange, as well as that of other small-seeded fruit. In regard to the finding of these causative bodies, either before or after death, Greig Smith[1] says that " of 125 cases collected by Dr. Fenwick, in 55 a foreign body was found."

An obstruction of whatsoever nature having occluded the mouth of the appendix, irritation is set up. This is followed by increased secretion on the part of the mucous glands and by the constantly accumulating products of the inflammation which soon supervenes. Unfortunately ulceration is initiated, perforation takes place, and the distended organ gives up its burden of purulent fluid. While these destructive processes, however, are going on in the appendix, nature is busy with constructive processes with the evident aim of limiting the mischief and preventing infection of the general peritoneal cavity. Protective inflammation glues together the intestines in the region of the disease-focus and builds a wall of lymph to oppose and confine the septic matters soon to escape from the appendix. If now adhesive inflammation permits the discharge of the pent-up fluids through a neighboring hollow viscus, or if this protective process be carried to such an extent as to allow the " pointing" of the abscess externally we have a fortunate, natural termination of the trouble ; but, unfortunately, we have too often been called upon to witness the breaking of the protective wall and, a few hours later, the death of the patient from general septic peritonitis.

There are three types of the disease : First, the acute ; second, the subacute ; and, third, the chronic. The duration in all the types varies from one day to several years, and the subacute and chronic forms may undergo an acute termination at any time.

[1] Read before the Michigan State Medical Society, July 19, 1890.

[1] Abdominal Surgery, second edition, page 72.

The following are the chief symptoms: Pain, generally commencing and continuing in the right iliac region, and varying in intensity and area according to the condition within; tenderness, usually pronounced; rapid wiry pulse; temperature low—101°–102°; pinched features; decided sweating; occasionally vomiting; tympanites, generally marked; frequently œdema of the iliac region and inguinal tumefaction. These symptoms and signs vary with the type of the disease. Frequently no tumefaction can be detected, and I have seen well-marked cases, such as are mentioned by Pepper, which manifested no dulness on percussion.

The gravity of the prognosis depends upon the degree and kind of mischief present. But how can this be accurately determined? I maintain that it is practically impossible to make this all-important differentiation. Pepper has said that "if the prominence, induration and dulness are marked, delay is safe, especially if rectal examination does not indicate any fulness on the right side of the roof of the pelvis." "If this is present," he goes on to say, "it indicates an amount of exudation which will probably end in abscess and is a strong indication for operation." And yet in the case about to be reported rectal examination indicated absolutely nothing; but the operation revealed a condition of affairs amply justifying the procedure, and showed the location of the abscess to be approachable by the rectal route.

Rules for the employment of operative procedures, unless it be in the purely chronic forms, cannot be laid down. Our judgment, based upon personal experience and the results of other operators, must be the guide. The practice of using the aspirator needle in order to establish the presence or absence of pus cannot, in my estimation, be too strongly condemned.

There is one class of cases—the chronic—which should, perhaps, receive further notice in this paper: cases where successive attacks are followed by periods of immunity, frequently lasting for several months. These cases are associated with a chronic disorder of the appendix, without perforation, which undergoes exacerbations and remissions from slight and sometimes unaccountable causes, thus placing the life of the patient in constant jeopardy. This matter has been freely discussed and there is still a difference of opinion in the profession concerning it. Shrady is one of others who believe that each recurrence often, and perhaps generally, tends to remove still further the possibility of a rupture by adding to the mass of protecting inflammatory exudate already present. There is also reported a type of cases where, after repeated recurrent symptoms, the patients having died of other causes, post-mortem inspection has revealed nothing whatever

abnormal in the appearance or condition of the appendix.

But while such testimony cannot be gainsaid, there is plenty of evidence, on the other hand, in regard to cases where both ante- and post-mortem examinations have shown free appendices distended with pus and ulcerated in spots through the mucous to the peritoneal coat. No remarks are necessary in regard to the wisdom of operating in such instances. The question is: How are we to diagnose them? How to differentiate?

There is but one way open to us, and that is in cases of doubt to make an exploratory incision. It does not follow that because the abdomen has been opened in these chronic cases the appendix should necessarily be removed. In such cases as the above it is, of course, the only thing to do; but where the organ is firmly imbedded in a mass of adhesions, requiring difficult and tedious dissection, with imminent danger of tearing into a contiguous coil of intestine, it would be wiser to refrain from attempts at excision, and to be satisfied with flushing, and establishing proper drainage.

A history of two or three recurrences in any particular case would not justify operative interference; but repeated attacks, sufficient in number to embarrass seriously business obligations, or occurring in individuals whose duties frequently compel their sojourn in regions where surgical skill cannot be obtained, particularly if we realize the liability to hepatic abscess and phlebitis from the continued presence of a disease-nidus connected with the portal system, justify an intermediate operation. Such is the doctrine of Weir, Bull, and others, and I consider it sound philosophy.

The medical treatment of acute and subacute cases I leave untouched; but the operative, as well as the medical details will be mentioned in the report of the case which follows:

S. M., aged eighteen years; employed in a furniture factory; taken sick on the afternoon of April 13th. The next morning the family called Dr. H. E. Locher, who kindly furnished the following report:

"Was called to see the patient on the morning of April 14th, and found him suffering from severe pain in the right iliac region. Patient stated that the pain had come on suddenly after dinner the day before. Pulse 105; temperature 101° F. He had vomited frequently during the previous afternoon and evening. Examination located the pain in the ileo-cæcal region. I questioned the patient closely in regard to his actions prior to the seizure, whether he had done any heavy lifting, wrestling, etc.; but the only fact of importance was a history of having gone some distance from the factory during the noon hour, in consequence of which, fearing that he might be late in getting to his work again, he ran very rapidly part of the way back. Shortly after returning the pain came on and grew more and more intense until it compelled him to leave his work and go home in the middle of the afternoon.

"Judging from the history and circumstances of the case, the diagnosis pointed to some form of intestinal obstruction near the ileo-cæcal valve, possibly a volvulus, or to a commencing appendicitis from the lodgement and impaction of partially digested or other matter in the appendix.

"Treatment at that time was as follows: Bismuth subnitrate and Dover's powder in moderate doses every four hours and potassium bromide, gelsemium, and morphine oftener. Hot fomentations over right iliac region. Ordered a small dose of castor oil to be given if pain became markedly less.

"*April 15.* Patient considerably better; continned treatment as before; also ordered mustard poultice to affected region and more castor oil, inasmuch as the bowels had not yet moved. Patient suffered much during the afternoon and evening, which was thought might be due, in part at least, to the effect of the oil. Pulse at evening 110; temperature 101° F.

"*16th.* Was much better; bowels had moved three times during the night and tenderness in the affected region was considerably diminished. Pulse 96; temperature normal; tongue had been slightly reddened, but this morning had a white coating. Bismuth and Dover's powders continued and patient ordered to remain in bed, inasmuch as several attempts at getting up had materially increased the pain.

"Did not see patient again, but was told by a member of the family on the next day, April 17th, that the boy was much better."

On the evening of this day, April 17th, Dr. Eugene Boise was called to attend the case. He states that he found the patient with a temperature of 101.5° F. and a pulse of 110; dry tongue; abdomen swollen and tender; great pain in region of appendix; pinched features, etc. Morphine, quinine, hot fomentations, and general supporting treatment ordered. Appendicitis was diagnosed.

Matters ran along until the afternoon of April 19th, when the writer was called by Dr. Boise. The diagnosis of perforative appendicitis was confirmed and operation advised.

As the family desired the counsel of Dr. George K. Johnson before proceeding to such a measure, the matter was deferred and a consultation was not held until the afternoon of Sunday, the 20th. This consultation resulted in the opinion that if patient was not better by morning the abdomen should be opened. Morning came, the patient was no better, and preparations for the operation were made. Thus, valuable time had been lost, and the operation was undertaken without much hope of saving the patient's life. However, surgery offered a better chance than medicine, and hence was chosen in the dilemma.

Operation on morning of April 21st. The physicians present were Drs. George K. Johnson, Eugene Boise, D. M. Greene, R. H. Spencer, C. A. Johnson, and the writer, all of Grand Rapids, and H. Boss, of Zeeland, Mich.

Through the courtesy of Dr. Boise and with his valuable assistance, as well as that of the other physicians present, the writer operated.

Patient was anæsthetized with ether in his bed, and then transferred to a table in the adjoining room. The abdomen was cleansed with hydronaphthol soap, shaved, douched with bichloride solution (1 to 2000), and surrounded by towels wrung from hot sublimate solution. Chloroform was then substituted for ether. An incision three inches long (afterward increased to four inches) was made over the cæcum, a little external to the right linea semilunaris. The different layers of tissue were divided by shallow strokes of the knife or upon the director. Hæmorrhage was slight and was controlled before entering abdomen. Peritoneum nicked, carefully enlarged to admit the index finger, and then divided with a probe-pointed bistoury to the extent of the wound. Great thickening of the peritoneum was observed.

The small intestines and omentum were strongly bound together by inflammatory exudation, necessitating careful tearing with the fingers to effect separation. At this point a gush of pus indicated the proximity of the expected abscess.

A strong fæcal odor was manifest. The point where the pus had welled up was cautiously enlarged and the cavity of the abscess freely opened. Upon passing the finger into the sac a foreign substance, about the size of a small hazel-nut, and which afterward proved to be a fæcal concretion, was felt lying loose in the cavity.

Considerable difficulty was met with in the recognition of the various tissues on account of inflammatory deposits and the quite free oozing of blood, which resulted from the separation of adhesions in spite of the great gentleness with which this was done. All, however, was soon made clear, and the appendix was found lying upon the inner wall of the abscess, as is the rule in these cases. The distal half of the organ, as a result of destructive inflammation, was absent, and the fæcal concretion which had obstructed this portion of the appendix was free, as stated above, at the bottom of the sac. The proximal half of the appendix was freed from its adhesions, cut off close to the cæcum and the stump inverted and disposed of by the application of three Lembert sutures of fine aseptic silk.

Four gangrenous masses which had been observed, three of omentum and one of abscess-wall, were ligated with aseptic gut and removed.

Throughout the operation hot, boiled water was in almost constant use for flushing the sac and also the general peritoneal cavity, for a small portion of the appendix was within the abscess, thus communicating with the general cavity.

After tying a few vessels and flushing with hot water to check oozing, and to wash out any remaining débris, the boiled water returned quite colorless. Two rubber drains were then placed in position (one in abscess sac and the other in the general cavity) and the incision closed by a combination of aseptic silk and catgut sutures passed through all the layers of the abdominal wall, including the peritoneum. Several superficial sutures of catgut were taken. the cavities were once more flushed with boiling water, and the usual antiseptic dressings applied.

The patient's pulse, at the close of the operation, was 150. He was put in bed, hot bottles placed at his feet, and morphine, atropine, and brandy administered hypodermically.

When consciousness returned he was ordered fluid extract of digitalis, 1 minim hourly, a half-teaspoonful of Armour's Beef Extract in a little hot water, every half hour, and a teacupful of warm milk, with a tablespoonful of brandy, every two hours.

At 5 P. M., four hours after the completion of the operation, his pulse was 130; temperature not taken.

At 10 o'clock P. M. pulse the same; nourishment and medicine had been retained; his skin was warm; facial perspiration much diminished. When asked how he felt he replied: "Better."

April 22, 8 A. M. Temperature during previous night ranged from 102° to 103°; pulse remained at 130 in spite of full doses of digitalis. Nourishment and stimulants were still retained. Urine was passed involuntarily several times during the night. 12 M. condition unchanged. Catheter introduced and considerable urine withdrawn. Patient was under the influence of morphine and was somewhat "flighty;" wound had a bad odor; cavities washed out with hot Thiersch's solution and fresh dressings applied. Patient evidently sinking. Death occurred rather suddenly at 2 P. M.

There was one serious objection to the performance of this operation, and that was the necessity of using a stuffy, upper room which could not be made aseptic. The parents would not tolerate the thought of having their son removed to a hospital.

I have reported this case because I deem it the duty of surgeons to make known the results of their operations regardless of the results, for otherwise statistics would be worthless.

In conclusion:

Although cases of perforative appendicitis do occasionally terminate favorably by means of adhesions to and discharge through neighboring hollow viscera, or by external pointing, can this very fortunate turn of affairs be counted upon in any individual case of the disease? Is it not wiser, where the symptoms do not abate in three or four days, to give the patient the benefit of surgery in time by performing an early laparotomy?

The operation itself, under antiseptic details, although not devoid of danger, is quite safe, and if nothing more is needed than the flushing of the abdominal cavity with hot, boiled water good cannot but be accomplished.

On the other hand, if the condition be such as to show the probability of a fatal termination if left to medical treatment alone, we have the advantage of an early opportunity to attack the disease before inflammatory and septic shock have

so exhausted the patient as to render our endeavors to save him from death vain and ineffectual.

Consideration of the facts associated with the foregoing case have caused the crystallization, in my mind, of two salient ideas:

1. The patient should be treated in a well-equipped hospital, if possible.

2. The operation should be performed early.

SURGICAL AND MECHANICAL THERAPEUTICS IN DISEASES USUALLY TREATED BY MEDICINE ALONE.[1]

By GEORGE M. KREIDER, A.B., M.D.,
of SPRINGFIELD, ILL.

No fact is more patent nor more pleasing to the intelligent observer of our profession than the ever increasing use of surgical and mechanical appliances for the treatment of diseases formerly treated by medicines alone. The too great reliance which was placed on drugs in former years led to the most absurd theories concerning their action and influence, and resulted, after homœopathy and kindred dogmas had had their day, in a therapeutic nihilism quite as absurd and cruel as they. Mechanical methods of treatment are slowly but surely trenching on the domain of medicine, and together with that other benevolent giant, prevention, are destined to narrow down the effective use of drugs to a very small circle and to a very small number. Thorough knowledge of a disease simplifies the treatment of it. Scientific methods of investigation, and instruments for testing diseased organs and tissues supply this knowledge, and these methods and instruments are no longer ridiculed, but are the common property of all intelligent practitioners. One of the apparent dangers of practice now is, not that we are too conservative but are rather too prone to take up and laud new treatments before they have stood the all-important test of time.

All dropsies were formerly treated by diuretic or purgative medicines, later by palliative tappings, but now the wonders performed by the removal of the cause of many dropsies, ovarian tumors and kindred abdominal growths, are so common that they are no longer matters of discussion. I do not intend, in this paper, to touch on these well-known topics, but there are other methods of mechanical relief which are not so well known and of which I may be permitted to speak. For example, who would have thought a few years since of treating erysipelas by anything but large doses of drugs, or of relieving neuralgias of the fifth nerve by anything except hypnotics or sedatives. Hysteria was formerly the name given to all of the numerous nervous complaints of females, and was a term

---

[1] Read before Illinois State Medical Society, May, 1890.

of ridicule. It received no treatment, and its victim little sympathy, but now we find that mechanical treatment will remove most of the cases, and it becomes an interesting study to discover the cause and the methods of relief. It will be my object in this paper to give a *résumé* of the recent application of treatments other than medical which I have myself used and which I believe are too often overlooked and ignored.

First, let us take that most universal symptom of disease which we are called upon to treat—fever. The drug treatment of this has passed successively from quinine to antipyrine, from antipyrine to antifebrin, from antifebrin to phenacetin, and so on, aconite and veratrum included, to an unending number of aspirants for its complete conquest. For some years I have ceased to rely upon these drugs for the reduction of fever, or at least have only used them under protest and as adjuncts to the use of water, either by sponging, bathing, or the ice-coil. I need only mention here that my ideas on these methods have been fully detailed in other papers, namely: "The Treatment of Fever by the Ice-coil;" the "Treatment of Puerperal Fever by Disinfection of the Uterine Cavity and the Use of the Ice-coil;" and the "Treatment of Pneumonia by Tepid Baths." Since the reading of the last-named paper at Jacksonville I have treated all the cases of pneumonia coming under my care by bathing or sponging, and can reiterate with emphasis the conclusions then reached. I have also had renewed proofs of the value of the ice-coil in cases of fever in which it was either impossible or impracticable to use the bath. Up to the present time I have treated eighteen cases of puerperal fever by the method mentioned above, with two deaths.

At the last meeting of the Illinois State Medical Society the late lamented Dr. Alexander Darrah read a valuable paper on the prevention and treatment of summer diseases of children by cool baths, which confirmed me in my estimate of the value of baths. Other mechanical procedures in these cases of summer complaint may be used with good effect. For example, last June I was called to see a four-year-old child in the last stages of dysentery, which had been carefully and skilfully treated by the attending physicians. She had a dry tongue, bloody stools, high fever, and was greatly prostrated. Under these circumstances I suggested, and with the aid of her attending physicians carried out, thorough irrigation of the colon with a solution of boric acid, followed by a solution of tannic acid. From the time this treatment was commenced the child began to improve and made a perfect recovery. A case of more than usual interest where irrigation was effective in disease of another portion of the alimentary tract, is the following:

Mrs. B., aged sixty-nine, had suffered for some weeks with symptoms of gastric ulcer. For several months she had experienced burning sensations in the stomach, coming on a few hours after eating. Later she had repeated attacks of vomiting of alkaline mucus. These attacks became more and more frequent and protracted. Nausea was a constant symptom day and night unless she was quieted by medicines. Finally she vomited bloody mucus and clear blood, and her condition became extremely serious. She rejected all food, and life was sustained by enemata. To quiet the intense pains six ounces of chloroform were inhaled every twenty-four hours. At this time my advice was given by telegraph to irrigate the stomach. Irrigation was delayed by the fear of her attending physicians that she was too weak to endure the operation of passing the tube to the stomach. As a last resort lavage was finally made, and from the hour of its employment improvement in her condition began and continued, after repetitions of the lavage, to her complete restoration to health.

A return of the symptoms some eleven months later does not vitiate the value of the treatment. I have been urged by those acquainted with the history of this case to make known this treatment of gastric ulcer, cancer, or dilatation for the benefit of those members of the profession who are possibly not cognizant of its value. Dr. Bodman, of Toledo, O., who was acquainted with the history and treatment of this case, writes that it certainly saved her life.

The attention of the profession has been frequently called to the fact that a tight prepuce may so affect the nervous system as to produce reflex disturbances of a serious nature. I have had some interesting cases of nervous disturbances arising from this source, which were, of course, relieved by the operation of circumcision. In one case talipes varus existed, but disappeared within a week after circumcision. In another case there was partial paralysis of the lower extremities, which was recovered from soon after the operation. Slighter forms of irritation from this cause are so often overlooked and the patients treated for something else, that I make it a rule to examine all male children suffering from nervous disturbances, for this disability.

A frequent cause of nervous disturbance is to be found in errors of refraction. In a paper read at a meeting of the District Medical Society I detailed some of my experiences with this difficulty and its relief by properly fitted glasses. Since reading that paper I have had one case in which. apparently, spasm of the bladder was caused by eye-strain. or at least, this symptom has become less frequent since the proper glasses were used. In another instance chorea was cured by the same means.

Speaking of neuralgia reminds me of the numerous cases which I have seen, where suppuration of the middle ear was treated for neuralgia until the mastoid cells were invaded and dangerous complications existed. Of course these mistakes were due to ignorance or carelessness, but such ignorance is frequently shown and serves me to emphasize a point which should be made prominent, viz. : that all practitioners should be so familiar with the instruments for making exact diagnoses, and with the proper mechanical treatment, that such mistakes may become impossible.

Many of the diseases of the ear can be relieved by mechanical treatment only, and a majority of the operations are such as the general practitioner should be able to perform. Perhaps he may not operate so rapidly or skilfully as the specialist, but just as effectually.

A change in the treatment of erysipelas has already been hinted at, and the new method is doubtless well known to most of my readers. Instead of large doses of chloride of iron, an anæsthetic is given, the affected part is surrounded by slight scarifications, and an antiseptic lotion is applied. By this treatment the disease can usually be made to disappear within twenty-four hours.

Speaking of diseases of the skin recalls the importance of destroying all suspicious growths in their very incipiency. Every surgeon has had patients who have been advised by their family physician to refrain from having anything done with excrescences or tumors, which have afterward gone on to the formation of most painful and dangerous cancers. Very few growths can be said to be without danger, and even if they are harmless, they usually produce mental worry, which causes the patient to resort to all sorts of quacks and quack remedies for his relief. By a full statement of the possibilities of the case the ready consent of the patient to their removal can usually be gained, while at the same time any groundless fears may be calmed by the assurance of the lack of danger if removed early. At the present time cancers and similar growths can be best cured by being extirpated in the very earliest stage, and this possibility should not be denied to suffering humanity by such advice as "Do not hurt the growth until it hurts you," or "Let well enough alone."

Diphtheria, tonsillitis, and their results can usually be better treated with the assistance of mechanical methods than by internal medication alone. In tonsillitis the endeavor should be to disinfect each crypt by passing to its bottom a fine probe coated with antiseptic lotion, and, when a case is thus early treated, I believe much serious trouble can be prevented. After the early stage is passed I find that the steam spray can be used with great advantage. I have the record of one case of diphtheria

treated with success in this way. That it was genuine diphtheria was proven by the paralysis which followed. A most interesting case of this character was that of my colleague, Dr. O. B. Babcock, of Rochester. While attending a case of fatal scarlatinal diphtheria he himself became infected with the poison. In a very short time, despite the use of medicines, douches, syringes, sprays, and incisions, his condition became dangerous. The soft palate touched the pharynx, and the œdema of the tonsils was so great that, notwithstanding removal of the uvula, he was left without adequate breathing space. The incisions and the stump of the uvula remained perfectly dry, and the tissues were as tense and brawny as a board. In this extreme condition I secured a gasoline stove, a tea-kettle, and a piece of tin spouting. The stove was placed near the bed and the steam conveyed through the spouting in large quantities to the patient's mouth. So great was the resolving and relaxing effect of the hot vapor that very soon the exudate came through the cut surfaces in large quantities and in due time a cure was effected. By the use of medicines alone this case would undoubtedly have been fatal. I cannot leave the discussion of this region without referring to the excellent progress which has been made in the treatment of catarrhs and nasal diseases by the various modern operations and mechanical procedures. How many cases of deafness, scrofula, anæmia, and narrow chest can now be cured by the removal of adenoid vegetations in the pharynx and of hypertrophied tonsils which medicines will absolutely fail to relieve ? I have in several instances been called on to treat cases of chronic hoarseness which were due to growths on the vocal cords, and were, of course, curable by local treatment only, and yet had been treated for months and weeks by internal medicines. O'Dwyer's inventions, and the tracheal tubes used in tracheotomy, are modern mechanical improvements in the treatment of diseases which were formerly palliated by medicines alone.

Pleurisy which has gone on to effusion is now no longer treated experimentally for the reabsorption of the fluid, but the cavity is drained by surgical and mechanical means, and a failure to cure is the exception. Typhlitis and obstruction of the bowel are boldly attacked, and although my own record in this class of cases is not encouraging, I recognize the fact that my failures are due to too late operations, or to the difficulties in diagnosis or treatment which others have overcome and which I hope to conquer in the future.

The same statement may be made concerning my experience in the diagnosis and treatment of brain- and spinal-cord diseases. I have endeavored to apply the proper treatment in two cases of brain disease, one of which I here report.

CASE.—Mr. H. E., aged thirty-two years, clerk. Seen with Dr. Ryan. On rising from a stooping position in a cellar, his head struck a timber with great force, and he was stunned and nauseated by the jar. He continued at work for some days, but was obliged to stop for a part of each day because of pains and dizziness. About ten days after the receipt of the injury, at an early hour of the morning, we were called to see him. The family had been aroused by hearing him fall heavily on the floor, and when they reached him he was in a stupor from which he could not be awakened. No history of the injury could be obtained at this time, but later the history and symptoms made a diagnosis of abscess possible. The symptoms were headache on the right side of the head, vomiting, paralysis or weakness of the left side, hesitation in answering questions, involuntary passage of urine and fæces, and gradually increasing coma. There was a choked disk on the right side. As the paralysis of the side was general, we were unable to locate the abscess. The patient being in a state of profound coma, the cranium was trephined over the motor centres and a hollow needle passed in different directions. The pus was either not reached or else it was so thick that it would not flow, and the patient died unrelieved. The post-mortem examination on the following day revealed a large abscess in the region of the parieto-occipital fissure which had broken into the third ventricle and caused death.

Did time permit I might detail the benefits of suspension and other mechanical treatments of spinal and spinal cord diseases; the effects of hot water in gynecological practice; of early incisions in bone diseases, and of numerous other measures not less worthy of discussion, but I will conclude with the following summary:

1. That mechanical and surgical measures are the most certain in our armamentarium and are only now assuming their proper position.

2. That when called to see a case of disease the first aim of the practitioner should be to determine, by proper examination and research, whether some mechanical or surgical appliance cannot be used in conjunction with or in place of medical treatment.

3. That the "do something" which this action implies will be more uniform in its results, more successful in its curative effects, and more pleasing to the patient than the "think something" treatment, which tries every medicine by turns and nothing long, and hopes for beneficial results.

4. That the ability to use exact appliances for the examination of patients and treatment of disease should be possessed by every one attempting to practise, and that this ability is only to be obtained by preliminary training and clinical instruction.

5. That treatment of disease in this manner has a tendency to elevate the profession in the eyes of the public, and to dissipate nonsensical sects which divide the profession and waste its energies.

CLINICAL MEMORANDA.

OBSTETRICAL.

A Plea for the Term "Heart-failure," with Notes of a Case.
—Of late, registry bureaus, coroners' clerks, and closet pathologists, have refused to accept the term "heart-failure" as a sufficient cause of death, and the physician who dares to sign his certificates in such a manner is regarded as uncertain in his diagnosis and a stranger to modern pathology; but, on behalf of clinical experience, I venture to make a plea for the actuality of heart-failure, without pathological lesions sufficient to explain it, and I report the following somewhat unusual clinical history and result of autopsy, in support of the heresy.

Mrs. C., a multipara, aged forty years, who had not required the services of a physician in any capacity since her last confinement, found herself pregnant January, 1889, with her third child. On Wednesday, July 17th, I was called to see her, and found her with preparations made for a confinement, which she had expected to occur between the 15th and 20th. Questioning revealed that there had been a few very slight pains, active fœtal movement, abundant "show," and the passage of some clots. There had been œdema of limbs, but it had disappeared; there was no vertigo, nor vomiting; urine was passed freely; the pulse was 76, full and strong, and the respiration was clear and normal. Examination revealed obliteration of cervix; a closed but dilatable os; the fœtus presenting by the head, and the uterus well contracted upon its contents. With instructions to the patient to send for her nurse and for me, at the first appearance of actual labor, I left her, and was called again on Friday, about 6 P.M.

At this visit I found the os about the size of a silver quarter; head presenting; membranes intact, and I felt what seemed to be a thickened anterior lip of the os. The patient had felt some slight pains, and said she had had very profuse bleeding an hour or two before. Her color was good, and her pulse normal. Instructing the nurse to keep careful watch over the symptoms, and particularly for bleeding, I again left, to be re-summoned about 10 P.M., from which time I remained with the patient.

Patient had complained of faintness, profuse bleeding, and slight infrequent pains. Examination revealed several large clots about the os, which was dilated to the size of a silver dollar. Within the anterior margin of the os was found a soft, smooth mass, which was readily pushed up between the head and the anterior lip. Diagnosis: marginal placenta prævia.

Consultation was called, but on the arrival of the consultant the head had been descending upon the os, so that the thickened mass was not discoverable; and, as bleeding had stopped, and the patient's condition was good, it was not deemed expedient to enter the uterine cavity for purposes of exploration. Pulse 72 and strong; uterus conforming well to its contents. Fœtal movements felt by patient. I ordered fluid extract of ergot, one drachm, and tamponed the vagina. From this time, 12.30 A.M., labor progressed. Pains were of short duration, but increased in frequency and strength. No hæmorrhage; patient warm and comfortable. Complained of some faintness, but there was no "yawning."

and the pulse remained so full and slow, that we were inclined to regard the amount of hæmorrhage as having been exaggerated.

At 3 30 A.M. the patient was doing well, the pains increasing in power, and characteristic of the second stage of labor—patient somewhat hysterical. Fœtal head found descending. At 4 o'clock, on examining the patient, the head was found in the hollow of sacrum, and the perineum relaxed. About this time the pains suddenly ceased, the patient asked for a drink, and complained of feeling faint. Pulse fading, extremities cold, countenance distressed and pale. Patient put her hand over the region of the heart. Heat was promptly applied to the extremities and spine, the pillows were removed, and brandy and aromatic ammonia given. The first heart-sound could not be heard, the breathing became more rapid, and the patient suddenly died about 4.15 A.M.

To save the child, version by the feet was then speedily and easily performed, but the child was dead. The placenta was purposely left within the uterine cavity.

Autopsy, made at 4 P.M., by Dr. J. W. Brooks, coroner's physician. Heart normal. Uterus contained no more blood than would normally appear after abstracting a child from a non-contracting cavity. The placenta was still adherent, and the inferior margin stretched slightly across the anterior lip of the os. The only pathological lesion was an interstitial nephritis, the capsule being somewhat adherent to the kidney.

The physician who performed the autopsy, declared that the lesions were suggestive of either coma or convulsions, but the symptoms were against such a conclusion. The patient was conscious to the last, and not a muscle was at any time convulsed (unless it were the heart).

Now, of what did the patient die ? Not from bleeding, pure and simple, for the pulse remained good for two and more hours after bleeding had ceased. There were no evidences of blood-poisoning—nothing but giving out of the heart's power after a not excessive hæmorrhage. Respiration even continued after the radial pulse was lost to the touch. To elucidate our pathology, this patient ought to have had coma or convulsions, but three witnesses failed to observe either condition ; or she ought to have had some valvular lesion, but there was none. However, her heart *did* grow weak in its action, and she *did* die.   FRANK W. THOMAS, M.D.

6 MT. AIRY AV., GERMANTOWN, PENNA.

MEDICAL PROGRESS.

Thiersch's Method of Skin-grafting.—DR. IVAN FOMIN, of St. Petersburg, reports eighteen cases in which he used Thiersch's method of skin-grafting (*Vratch*, No. 11, 1890). The author carried out the method as follows: The surface of a crural ulcer, for example, is dressed with compresses wrung from a 1-to-5000 solution of corrosive sublimate until complete cleansing of the granulating surface has taken place—usually in from three to seven days. On the day of the operation the entire limb is washed with soap and water and an antiseptic lotion, after which a syringeful of a 4-per-cent. solution of cocaine is injected in the neighborhood of the ulcer, and the latter is carefully scraped away, with a sharp spoon,

down to the muscle or fascia. After this a bandage to arrest hæmorrhage is applied and left in place for from half an hour to two hours. Next, thin cutaneous strips, measuring about five or six inches in length and two and a half in width, are sliced, with a sharp razor, usually from the patient's arm, which should have been thoroughly disinfected. This step of the operation may be rendered painless by giving a hypodermic injection of cocaine. The strips are then moistened with a 1-per-cent. solution of carbolic acid and placed on the ulcer, not only the entire surface being covered, but the healthy skin slightly overlapped. The grafts are then carefully dried with absorbent cotton, dusted with a thin layer of iodoform, and covered with fenestrated strips of protective, which overlap each other like tiles. The whole is then dressed with antiseptic material and the limb immobilized.

The results obtained by Dr. Fomin are excellent—even most extensive and obstinate ulcers healing in a few weeks.—*Annals of Surgery*, July, 1890.

Diabetes following Resection of the Pancreas.—VON MERING and MINOWSKI have undertaken a series of experiments upon extirpation of the pancreas as a cause of diabetes (*Archiv f. experimentelle Pathologie*). The operations were performed under strict antiseptic precautions, and were followed by permanent diabetes, resembling the severest form of the disease in man. The animals became very hungry and thirsty, but, though well fed, emaciated rapidly. If even a small part of the pancreas was allowed to remain, diabetes did not follow, showing that the disease was not due to traumatism, but to the absence of the pancreas. The authors think that their experiments prove that one of the functions of the pancreas is destruction of sugar, either if introduced from without or formed within the body. As an additional proof of this, if grape sugar is given to an animal which has lost the pancreas, the whole of the sugar can be recovered from the urine.

DOMINICUS, of Italy, has also made a series of similar experiments, and with much the same results, but he concludes that the diabetes is caused only indirectly by the loss of the pancreas, the immediate cause being the disturbances of digestion produced.— *Centralblatt f. klinische Medicin*, June 7, 1890.

Prescription for Vomiting of Pregnancy.—According to the *Canada Medical Record*, M. HUBERT uses the following mixture to relieve the vomiting of pregnancy :

R.—Tincture of iodine . . 6   drops.
Potassium iodide . . . 1½ drachms.
Distilled water . . . 4½ ounces.—M.

One teaspoonful three times daily.

Treatment of Erysipelas.—The *Weekly Medical Review* quotes the following prescription used by KOCH in the treatment of erysipelas :

R.—Creolin . . . . . 1 part.
Iodoform . . . . . 4 parts.
Lanolin . . . . . 10 " "—M.

This ointment is painted on the diseased parts by means of a soft brush and covered with gutta-percha tissue.

HALLOPEAU applies compresses saturated with a 1-to-20 solution of sodium salicylate, and, to prevent evaporation, covered with impervious tissue.

WÖLFLER uses mechanical compression by means of adhesive-plaster straps, applied on the healthy skin and surrounding the diseased area.

The Treatment of Uterine Cancer.—MR. F. B. JESSETT writes (*British Gynecological Journal*, May, 1890) upon the treatment of cancer of the uterus as follows:

Palliative treatment is adopted in cases of advanced disease. By means of it much may be done to relieve suffering, to arrest the rapid progress of the disease, and to improve the general health. The vagina should be thoroughly syringed with "sanitas" or some other antiseptic lotion through a full-sized speculum; then, with pieces of cotton-wool, the cavity should be wiped out as far as possible, removing all débris and loose sloughs; a tampon of cotton-wool soaked in equal parts of pinus canadensis and glycerin, or smeared with an ointment composed of one ounce of sanitas oil, ten grains of chloride of zinc, and an ounce of vaseline, should be introduced into the cavity; this should be used night and morning, the vagina being syringed out each time, and the cavity wiped with cotton-wool before the insertion of fresh tampons. By adopting this simple plan of treatment the sloughs become dislodged and a clean ulcerated surface exposed. All offensive smell will disappear, and the pain and vesical irritation be much decreased. The disease will be considerably retarded in its growth, the patient's appetite returns and the general health improves, doubtless owing to the non-absorption of the poisonous discharge. Perfect rest should be insisted on, and the general health attended to by the administration of appropriate tonics; and if pain is present and prevents sleep, small doses of morphine may be advantageously given. It may be added that no success has attended the use of any drug given for the purpose of arresting the disease.

In attempting a *radical* cure the case must have been seen early, while the uterus is still freely movable, and before the vaginal walls have become involved. When the vaginal portion of the uterus is alone affected, amputation of the cervix by means of scissors is recommended. Caustics in this, and other forms, are unreliable.

When cancer involves the cervical portion of the canal, the disease should be removed by cutting away a conical portion of the uterus beyond the disease. This method the author prefers to the total extirpation of the organ—an operation which he cannot at present bring himself to adopt. Total extirpation may, however, be performed in suitable cases when disease in the body of the uterus has been early recognized. In removing the conical portion the operation closely resembles the high amputation of the cervix. The vagina around the cervix is snipped with blunt-pointed scissors, and the vaginal mucous membrane and tissues beneath pushed up as far as possible. The uterine tissues are then divided by short snips with the scissors, the part to be removed being, at the same time, firmly pulled down by a vulsellum. In this way the diseased tissues may be removed, even to the fundus.—*Medical Chronicle*, July, 1890.

India-rubber Iodoform Plaster.—The *American Druggist* quotes the following prescription for the preparation of a 20-per-cent. iodoform plaster:

R.—Dammar resin	.	.	.	.	15 parts.
Benzoated tallow	.	.	.	.	30 "
Lanolin	.	.	.	.	20 "
Caoutchouc	.	.	.	.	5
Glycerin	.	.	.	.	10
Iodoform	.	.	.	.	20 "

The resin is melted by heat, then the tallow is added, and the whole is strained through several layers of gauze. With this mass, while still liquid, the caoutchouc in solution and the lanolin are incorporated. The iodoform is triturated with the glycerin, and added after the mass has somewhat cooled.

The caoutchouc solution is prepared by dissolving flake India-rubber in five times its weight of benzine.

Hydronaphthol as an Intestinal Antiseptic. — DR. J. MITCHELL CLARKE (*Practitioner*, July, 1890) reports a series of experiments to determine the influence of hydronaphthol on digestion and its value as an antiseptic in the treatment of intestinal diseases. He concludes that to patients on an absolute milk diet the drug can be given without fear of seriously interfering with digestion; but that if gastric disturbances are produced they are probably due to retardation of peptic digestion and to the accumulation of curds in the stomach. Under the latter circumstances, perhaps under all, it is advisable to give the drug in pill-form coated with keratin in order that it will not be set free before reaching the intestine. For adults, Dr. Clarke thinks a dose of two or three grains given every two hours sufficient. In diarrhœas the intervals may be increased after the first few doses. For children under one year the dose is half a grain.

Five cases of typhoid fever were treated with hydronaphthol by the author. All did well, though two were severe, and at the beginning had profuse diarrhœa which ceased soon after the treatment was instituted. In two less severe cases diarrhœa was also quickly checked, and it was noticed that the stools soon lost their offensive odor. In the treatment of the summer diarrhœas of infants the drug also seemed to be of benefit. In one case of dysenteric diarrhœa which had lasted for five weeks with from twenty-five to thirty stools daily, a milk diet and the administration of hydronaphthol was followed in four days by great improvement, the stools being reduced to four daily. In thirteen days the patient was cured.

One case of tubercular diarrhœa and several cases of ordinary diarrhœa from indiscretions in diet also yielded to the administration of the drug.

[It is obvious that the observations are too few for positive conclusions, but the apparently good results certainly warrant a more extended trial of hydronaphthol as an intestinal antiseptic.—ED.]

The Treatment of Burns of the Eye.—DR. A. TROUSSEAU (*Recueil d'Ophtalmologie*, No. 8, 1890) recommends, in burns of the eye by acids, free irrigation with cold water, followed by compresses soaked in an alkaline lotion or Vichy-water, and placed over the half-closed lids. If the pain is severe the compresses should be alternated with ice-poultices, which give great relief and often prevent inflammation. In injuries caused by caustic alkalies, the cornea and conjunctival *culs-de-sac* must be thoroughly irrigated and foreign bodies carefully removed. The after-treatment should consist in copious instillations of a ½-per-cent. solution of carbolic acid. Lime burns are especially serious in their subsequent effects, as they rapidly destroy the corneal tissues, and by their escharotic effect on the conjunctiva are apt to produce contraction and symblepharon. These sequelæ may, to a great extent, be prevented by freely washing with a very dilute acid solution, or by Gosselin's method of syringing the eye with sugar-water, with the object of forming a soluble saccharate of lime.

Burns by molten metal are best treated by the removal of metallic fragments, which are usually firmly embedded in the tissues, followed by compresses soaked in boric or carbolic acid lotion. In every case a drop of atropine solution should be used.—*Medical Chronicle*, July, 1890.

The Treatment of Diphtheria.—In an interesting and able paper upon the treatment of diphtheria, DR. MANUEL HERRERA, of Guanajay, Cuba (*Revista de Ciencias Médicas*, Havana, April 20, 1890), strongly condemns the removal of the false membranes, even if the larynx is involved. For the treatment of the disease he relies on general and local measures, and advocates the following, as leading to the best results. He seldom uses ipecacuanha, but usually employs quinine and calomel continuously in doses of fifteen grains and one and a half grains, respectively, during the twenty-four hours, stopping the latter drug when the first symptoms of ptyalism appear. The use of calomel, however, is resumed; and should the mercurial effects return, they are checked with chlorate of potassium, internally; and thus a continuous mercurial saturation of the system is maintained, without the danger of a stomatitis that would, undoubtedly, aggravate the primary disorder.

Dr. Herrera particularly lays stress upon the local treatment proposed by him. For this purpose he employs iodoform, cocaine, hydrochloric acid, camphor, mercurial ointment, and extract of belladonna, with the best results. Thirty-four cases, of the worst type, reported in his article, entirely recovered under this local treatment. Dr. Herrera's prescriptions are as follows:

1. R.—Sulphate of quinine . . 30 grains.
   Calomel . . . . 3 "

Divide into ten powders, and give one every two hours until five are taken.

2. R.—Iodoform . . . . 75 grains.
   Saccharated lime . . 2½ drachms.
   Cocaine hydrochlorate . 4 grains.
   Camphor . . . 15 "

To be dusted over the membrane, by means of an insufflator, every five hours.

3. R.—Hydrochloric acid } of each 75 minims.
   Distilled water }

To be applied locally, three times a day, by means of a camel's-hair brush.

4. R.—Mercurial ointment . 7½ drachms.
   Extract of belladonna } of each 75 grains.
   Iodoform }
For external application.

The Modes of Administering Cardiac Tonics.—The therapeutics of cardiac affections has been greatly advanced recently, not only by the addition of numerous cardiac tonics to our list of remedies, but also by the acquirement of important details in the administration of the older remedies, by which their efficiency has been greatly advanced.

GAUTHIER, especially, has devoted himself to the study of this subject, and an analysis of his work, as published in the *Wiener medizinische Blätter* of May 22, 1890, is well worthy of notice.

As is well known, the administration of digitalis in the form of powder or pill is apt to produce vomiting or diarrhœa. The best form is that of an infusion made by macerating the digitalis leaves, and, when time permits, it is this preparation which should always be used as the one which gives the most prolonged and intense action on the heart, and which is most efficacious in producing diuresis. The infusion should be given in gradually decreasing doses. Digitalin is by no means a constant preparation, and it does not possess all the properties of the digitalis leaves. Nevertheless, the crystallized digitalin is of use where an extremely rapid action is desired, although ordinarily its action is too intense, and, therefore, dangerous, while its subcutaneous employment is extremely painful, and often produces abscesses.

Convallaria is also best employed in the form of an infusion, 8 to 10 parts being macerated in 1000 of water, to which syrup may be added, and administered the day in which it is made.

Convallarine, the active principle, may be employed in doses of ⅙ to ¾ or 1½ grains.

Strophanthus is best given in the tincture (the one officinal in the English Codex being the best) in 5-drop doses three times daily, although 10 to 20 drops may be given once or twice in the twenty-four hours in a single dose.

Adonis may be employed in the form of an infusion or decoction, or its active principle, adonidine, may be given. The infusion seems to be inconstant in its activity, and both of the watery preparations have an extremely bitter taste, which must be masked by syrup. Adonidine may be given in the quantity of from ⅙ to ⅓ grain in twenty-four hours. Its toxic action is ten times greater than that of digitalis. Caffeine is likewise a reliable remedy, provided it is given in sufficient dose, 15 to 30 grains being ordinarily required. This dose should, however, not be exceeded without great care, as in larger quantities it is not free from danger.

The salts of caffeine are nearly insoluble in water, and are, therefore, not suitable for subcutaneous injections, although the double salt—the benzoate of sodium and caffeine—is an exceedingly valuable preparation. Sparteine may be used, either in the form of an infusion or decoction of the plant; or its active principle, sulphate of sparteine, may be employed, the latter being especially valuable for its action on the heart in doses of from ¾ to 4 grains, while the infusion possesses marked diuretic properties.—*Therapeutic Gazette*, July, 1890.

THE MEDICAL NEWS.

A WEEKLY JOURNAL
OF MEDICAL SCIENCE.

COMMUNICATIONS are invited from all parts of the world. Original articles contributed exclusively to THE MEDICAL NEWS will be liberally paid for upon publication. When necessary to elucidate the text, illustrations will be furnished without cost to the author.

Address the Editor: H. A. HARE, M.D.,
1004 WALNUT STREET,
PHILADELPHIA.

Subscription Price, including Postage.

PER ANNUM, IN ADVANCE . . . . $4.00.
SINGLE COPIES . . . . 10 CENTS.

Subscriptions may begin at any date. The safest mode of remittance is by bank check or postal money order, drawn to the order of the undersigned. When neither is accessible, remittances may be made, at the risk of the publishers, by forwarding in *registered* letters.

Address,   LEA BROTHERS & CO.,
Nos. 706 & 708 SANSOM STREET,
PHILADELPHIA.

SATURDAY, AUGUST 2, 1890.

DIABETES MELLITUS.

ONE of the features that will mark the present era of medicine is the earnest endeavor to classify diseases with regard to their etiology and pathology rather than to their symptomatology. Constantly do we find ourselves able to apply a more fitting and accurate name to various groups of symptoms, and to assign to them a proper place in our nosological tables. Not merely this, but only by striking at the ultimate pathological cause can the true and rational treatment be properly conceived of and instituted.

The name diabetes mellitus has answered the purpose of designating a condition the most obvious and constant sign of which is the excretion of large quantities of saccharine urine; but the comfortable idea that in *all* cases this symptom is due to disturbance of the vaso-motor supply of the liver must give place to more definite views, and undoubtedly ere long we shall find that there are many lesions capable of producing, and having as a common symptom, the excretion of sugar in the urine. In that case diabetes mellitus may occupy the same position as a diagnostic term as do other symptomatic phenomena — albuminuria, convulsions, coma, and fever.

In the *Medico-Chirurgical Transactions* for 1833 Bright reported a case of jaundice in which fatty stools occurred and "the urine had a sweet taste," and at the autopsy there was found a scirrhous mass occupying the head of the pancreas. In 1877 Longstreth exhibited a specimen of cystic disease of the pancreas from a case of diabetes mellitus, while similar cases have lately been recorded by W. T. Bull and I. A. Nichols. Many authors speak of the presence of hypertrophy and sclerosis of the pancreas in these cases. In the Middleton-Goldsmith Lecture of 1889 R. H. Fitz quoted a case, reported by Frison (*Marseille Médicale*, 1875), of multiple pancreatic abscesses which presented sugar in the urine during life.

It is clear, however, that we have not as yet arrived at the precise conditions or lesions of the pancreas capable of causing or being frequently associated with the appearance of sugar in the urine. This is shown by the numerous cases of cystic and other pancreatic disease reported by Fitz in the lecture above mentioned, wherein glycosuria was not present, while Langenhaus has lately reported a case dying of necrosis of the pancreas without the presence of sugar in the urine.

Von Mering took the initial step in the way of experimental determination of the position occupied by the pancreas in the production of glycosuria. In dogs from which he had removed the pancreas he found an abundance of sugar in the urine. That this phenomenon was not due to the withdrawal of pancreatic digestion was shown by the negative result if but a small portion of the pancreas were allowed to remain. M. Lépine went a step further. On comparing the blood of a healthy dog with that from a dog whose pancreas had been previously removed, he found an excess of sugar in the latter, which excess was much more slowly broken up than in the blood from a dog whose pancreas had not been removed. On the addition of starch to the two specimens it was found that the blood from the dog whose pancreas had not been removed produced more glucose than did the blood of the dog so operated upon. From these experimental facts he deduces the theory that, owing to the absence of a ferment produced by the pancreas, and whose duty it is to destroy sugar in the blood, glycolysis takes place to a less extent than glycogenesis, with the result of the presence of an excess of sugar in the blood and the excretion of sugar in the urine.

There must still remain, however, many cases of diabetes mellitus independent of pancreatic disease. The frequent occurrence of glycosuria in various cerebral lesions is well known, while a sufficient number of cases of diabetes mellitus following prolonged anxiety or sudden shock are recorded to cause these to rank as etiological factors. Many authors have recognized the relation between the gouty diathesis and diabetes mellitus.

It is manifest that glycosuria may be a symptom of many conditions and of diverse lesions. To what number these may in time be limited cannot be premised, but by the studies of von Mering, Minkowski, and Lépine, our knowledge has been much broadened. By careful observation it may be possible in the future to recognize during life various causes for the symptom of saccharine urine, and undoubtedly different plans of treatment will be followed according to the causative condition. M. Lépine has already followed up his experimental work by administering pilocarpine, as a pancreatic stimulant, to a few cases of diabetes mellitus, and, although his cases have been too few to give reliable data, he has had enough success by its use to warrant further investigations in the same line.

CORRESPONDENCE.

THE AMERICAN OPHTHALMOLOGICAL SOCIETY.

To the Editor of THE MEDICAL NEWS,

SIR : Among almost one thousand guests now enjoying the 2700 feet of elevation and grand outlook of this mountain resort, the fifty members and others present to attend the meeting of the American Ophthalmological Society would attract little attention. At certain times they might be seen conversing in groups on the veranda or in the corridors of the hotel, but during the sessions there are but few absentees, and yesterday they held three sessions. To-day (July 17th) they have completed the consideration of the thirty-five papers brought before them, several of which started animated and prolonged discussions. This afternoon the Society concluded with the consideration of a fine salmon, sent by an absent member, and as his representative most cordially taken in by the Society as a whole, through its individual members.

In executive session, which seems to be guarded by as much secrecy as that of the United States Senate, we learn that three or four new members were elected, and that one name was stricken from the roll.

Of more general interest is the fact that the Society suspended the by-law fixing its time of meeting, and next year will hold its regular meeting in Washington at the time of the meeting of the Second Congress of American Physicians and Surgeons.

It will be remembered that in the year of the first Congress the Society held its regular meeting as usual in July, and a rather small special meeting for the Congress; being then unwilling even for once to give up its midsummer meeting in some cool, quiet summer resort.

This time more interest is exhibited in the Congress, and an effort is to be made to secure the presence of prominent European ophthalmologists, and their participation in the meeting.

Of general interest were two cases reported by Dr. William F. Norris, and one by Dr. C. A. Oliver, of brain tumor, recognized and located almost entirely by eye-symptoms, the diagnosis being in each case confirmed by autopsy.

Dr. George C. Harlan reported a transient amblyopia and bitemporal hemianopsia in a case of malarial cachexia, in which, other treatment failing, full doses of quinine quickly brought relief.

Cataract extraction is a subject of perennial interest to the ophthalmic surgeon. And an animated discussion was started by a paper on the so-called simple extraction, by Dr. Charles S. Bull, in which he re-affirmed his conviction that it was the best operation for the removal of the opaque lens in a large majority of cases of ordinary senile cataract. This opinion was shared by some of his fellow members, but was not held by quite a number of others.

Much has been said of the advantages of the small, mobile pupil secured by simple extraction. But the small *immovable* pupil, due to iritic adhesions, is of such frequent occurrence as to increase decidedly the risk attending the simple extraction, and to offset its other advantages. It is not claimed to be applicable to all cases; but when successfully performed in a proper case is an almost ideal surgical procedure.

Dr. H. Derby reported a family in which two brothers and a sister and eight out of ten of their children were affected with congenital zonular cataract. There was no history of convulsions in early infancy in any case.

Dr. T. R. Pooley and Dr. R. A. Reeve reported cases of removal of large ivory exostoses from the inner wall of the orbit: and Drs. William F. Norris and L. H. Taylor cases of large foreign bodies lodged for some time in the orbit.

Dr. C. E. Rider, under the head of the "Winking Test," called attention to the strong tendency to wink, or close alone, the abnormal eye, much more readily than the normal, where there was an appreciable difference between the visual acuteness of the two. This he proposed to have used as a test when it was desirable to ascertain which had formerly been the worse eye, as in advanced double cataract, or malingering, or when decided inferiority in the vision of one eye has been recently discovered. The test is, however, scarcely applicable to women, because very many, who have visual acuteness about equal in both eyes, are still unable to wink with either eye separately. No explanation was given of this sexual difference.

Disorders of the ocular muscles were discussed at length in connection with a paper by Dr. H. D. Noyes on the treatment of muscular asthenopia and its results. Graduated tenotomy seemed to be less in favor than in the past two years, and the use of prisms more generally relied on.

A committee on the prevention of blindness found that in this, as in other civilized countries, about 20 per cent. of all blindness is caused by ophthalmia neonatorum.

The general adoption was urged of a law recently enacted in New York, requiring midwives and others to notify in six hours some health officer, or legalized practitioner of medicine, should inflammation of the eyes of a newborn infant be noticed.

Several speakers testified to the value of the Credé method of dropping into the eyes a 2-per-cent. solution of silver nitrate immediately after birth.

Drs. W. F. Mittendorf and O. F. Wadsworth reported cases of embolism of the central artery of the retina, with the retention of good vision at the macula, by reason of its being supplied by cilio-retinal vessels quite unaffected by the embolism.

Dr. William H. Carmalt reported two cases of sarcoma of the conjunctiva, and two of glioma of the retina. In one of the latter both eyes were removed, and there had been no recurrence. In the other the growth was so soft, and pus-like in consistence, that its nature was not recognized until it recurred, after the enucleation of the affected eye. Death occurred from extension of the growth to the brain.

Cases of remarkably good vision in spite of age and hyperopia were reported by Dr. S. Theobald; and a group of cases of increasing hyperopic astigmatism by Dr. Edward Jackson. These latter cases are rare, but they do occur, and it should be borne in mind that astigmatism sometimes changes.

Dr. Harlan described a new operation for keeping the lid free in symblepharon, by replacing its conjunctival surface by a sliding flap of skin.

Dr. B. A. Randall argued that we have no evidence that hyperopia can be healthfully outgrown ; the prevalent idea that it is generally outgrown being quite incorrect and unsupported by facts.

Dr. F. M. Wilson exhibited three specimens of filaria oculi humani, taken from just beneath the skin of the lids of a missionary who had acquired the parasite on the West Coast of Africa. The worm is very frequent on a certain limited portion of the coast. It is most frequently seen just beneath the ocular conjunctiva, and not, as has been asserted, in the anterior chamber of the eye.

Dr. C. W. Kollock reported two cases of a new form of xerosis occurring in colored children, marked by an elevated ring around the margin of the cornea, and quite amenable to general tonic treatment. He also reported two anomalous cases of glaucoma, in one of which the tension quickly rose after an iridectomy, and though unaffected by weak solutions of eserin was promptly reduced by a strong solution. The other occurred in an eye the seat of monocular hæmorrhagic albuminuric neuro-retinitis.

The Society, in accordance with its custom, continues in office its officers, viz. : President, Hasket Derby, M.D., of Boston; Vice-president, G. C. Harlan, M.D., of Philadelphia; Secretary and Treasurer, S. B. St. John, M.D., of Hartford.

HOTEL KAATERSKILL, July 17, 1890.

"THE ETIOLOGY AND TREATMENT OF MIGRAINE."

To the Editor of THE MEDICAL NEWS.

SIR : Having been very favorably impressed with the exhaustive and scholarly article by Dr. Wharton Sinkler upon "The Etiology and Treatment of Migraine" in THE MEDICAL NEWS of July 19th, and believing that, when considered as a disease, too much attention is given to its treatment, I should like permission to offer some suggestions calculated to throw a different light upon the subject, treating it rather as a symptom than as a disease. In the closing paragraph of Dr. Sinkler's paper migraine as a symptom is merely referred to, and, for the most part, the treatment is confined to the exhibitiou of drugs, or the use of local measures, such as electricity. That my views are entitled to consideration will be apparent from a quotation from the paper, which runs as follows: "Most authors now agree as to the prime importance of hygienic measures in connection with any remedy used for the relief of this disease. Removal from care and work, with fresh air, good food, and change of climate, will do more to relieve the frequeney of the attacks than any drug."

Taking this quotation as a text, together with the assumption that migraine is a symptom of disease, the general practitioner will be interested in knowing the methods to be pursued for the purpose of removing the underlying cause of these derangements of the nervous system ; and, by way of introduction, I may repeat the time-worn maxim that such attacks are generally due to an impoverished condition of the system, and that neuralgia is the cry of the nerves for pure blood. We not infrequently meet with cases of anæmia with neuralgia, which we have learned to speak of as the anæmia of plethora, and, in these it has been found empirically tbat purgatives are useful. Still, I doubt if a very large proportion of the physicians who come to this decision and who successfully follow this practice, could give a rational explanation of the *modus operandi* by which the good results are secured. The modern practitioner regards the success of the doctor of a generation ago as somewhat enigmatical, considering the liberal use of purgatives which was the custom of that period; and in calling attention to the treatment of migraine as a symptom of disease, I hope to be able to clear up this matter, so that hereafter purgatives may be used intelligently and in accordance with well-known scientific principles.

The question will be better understood by the presentation of cases in which the cause of the disorder is made apparent, and from which appropriate deductions can be drawn, and the matter settled beyond dispute. For example, does any modern physician doubt the causative relation existing between derangements of the digestive apparatus and attacks of cholera morbus ? The disease known as cholera infantum is so closely related to cholera morbus that it ought to be included in the same category, and, without undue stretch of the imagination, the list might be extended bv including such specific diseases as typhoid fever, anæmia, and chlorosis, and, in not a few instances, consumption. In regard to the latter disease, I cannot accept the modern theory that the bacillus tuberculosis bears a direct causative relation, but is rather in the nature of an incidental complication. In proof of this assumption, I have but to point to the very large number of persons who suffer for years from what is termed " general debility." but finally the bacilli, finding a suitable nidus for their development. take possession of the tissues. With the rapid multiplication of the germs, and the distribution of the poisons derived therefrom, the patient begins to sink, and is accordingly treated for pulmonary tuberculosis. No one doubts, now, that many of these patients, if properly treated in time, or, in other words, if those "measures of prime-importance" had been adopted, would have recovered, and consumption have been avoided. Without going further into this question, my impression is, that these diseases are, for the most part, due to disorders of digestion, and that by proper attention to diet, including, of course, hygienic measures and climatic treatment, a fatal issue may be indefinitely postponed, if not altogether avoided.

It will be argued that migraine occurs too frequently to be placed in this classification, and that if the proposition is true, other nerves should show derangements of a like character; but upon reflection, and the elimination of those direct causes pointed out by Dr. Sinkler, which may easily be traced, I think the point will be conceded as well taken. In the case of typhoid fever, for example, what observing physician has not witnessed patients who *walked* themselves into the disease? How many patients can the active country practitioner recall, within the period of a year, who have persistently violated his advice and have finally contracted the disease? On the other hand, he is able, at the same time, to point out a number who have carefully complied with his directions and have escaped.

As a rule, it will be found that those who suffer from migraine are under-fed. Notwithstanding that they take a seat at the table three times daily, and apparently enjoy their food, something is wanting either in the primary or secondary assimilation, and this peculiar pain is the result. When there is a rheumatic tendency, it may appear in the form of intercostal neuralgia, or sciatica, or one or more of the joints may be affected. At other times these manifestations will be in the form of fugitive pains, which appear to have no local habitation. The number of persons who suffer from rheumatic tendencies is daily increasing, and it would be difficult to find one of these who does not suffer more or less from indigestion and from acidity of the stomach.

To meet these demands, quite a number of remedies suggest themselves. The most natural conclusion is, that all our troubles will vanish after the introduction of alkalies into the system, but a more specious fallacy was never promulgated, and yet many physicians cling to it with wonderful persistence. Others believe that the difficulty may be overcome by the introduction of acid into the stomach shortly before meals, on the theory that this will lessen the secretion of the acid juice of the normal stomach, and notwithstanding the scientific basis for its employment, the results have been anything but satisfactory. The advocacy of the digestive ferments, together with the temporary benefits which they confer when judiciously used, has furnished employment to hundreds of men, and large manufacturing establishments have sprung up for the exclusive manufacture of these products. Unfortunately, these measures furnish but transient relief. The general use of pancreatic ferments has had a tendency to enable us to locate with more certainty the real causes which combine to produce this abnormal condition, and for this reason I have to suggest that the diet is of the utmost importance.

A few words in relation to the diet will suffice to start the reader in the proper channel of investigation, as it will be impossible in this letter to touch upon the details which naturally present themselves to the thoughtful physician. Attacks of migraine should always be regarded suspiciously, owing to their dependence upon an unhealthy condition of the alimentary tract. While the tongue may offer no indications of mal-assimilation, the history of the onset of the attacks will frequently point to intestinal indigestion, and the most certain method consists in cutting off all foods which have a tendency to cause fermentation after reaching the small intestine. All starchy foods, sweets, and pastry, must be eliminated from the dietary, and the patient compelled to subsist entirely upon properly cooked beef or mutton, to which may be added a little stale bread or toast. When not specially contra-indicated, a little tea, coffee, or cocoa may be permitted with meals. The results of treatment will be manifest in the course of a week or ten days, providing that the patient is not compelled to work too hard, and is placed under favorable hygienic conditions. Without attention to food, clothing, air, and exercise, medication of whatever sort is but palliative.

For the emergency, to relieve the pain and place the patient in a favorable condition, I cannot speak too highly of an assayed preparation of cannabis indica, and in order to present the method of administration in practical form, will record the following illustrative case:

About two months ago, while on professional business in the country, thirty miles from the city, I was compelled to remain during the night, and in the evening was requested to prescribe for a housemaid, aged thirty-five years. This patient had been suffering for nearly three weeks from a most stubborn attack of migraine, which had obstinately resisted the domestic remedies, as well as drugs. The pain was persistent both night and day, and for many nights she had not been able to obtain any rest until four or five o'clock in the morning. The condition of the digestive apparatus was unfavorable, although she had eaten but little food during the time of her illness. There was no history of uterine trouble, and no indications of decayed teeth to account for the persistence of the attack.

At ten o'clock this patient was placed upon the following mixture:

R.—Extract of cannabis indica (Normal Liquid)   .   .   .   . 5 drops.
    Water   .   .   .   .   .   . 4 ounces.

One teaspoonful was given every ten minutes for one hour. At the expiration of the hour the patient returned to say that she began to feel better after taking the second dose, and that now she felt quite well and perfectly free from pain. As a result, she had a good night's rest, and experienced no symptoms of a return until after sunrise next morning, when there was slight pain on the affected side She was instructed to take one teaspoonful of the mixture at intervals of an hour during the day, and a restricted dietary was ordered. In addition to this treatment, she was advised to take $\frac{1}{100}$ grain of the arsenite of copper after each meal for five days, and it affords me pleasure to add that the patient rapidly recovered, and has had no further symptoms of migraine.

The circumstances connected with this case were somewhat peculiar. She was living in the country, where the air was especially bracing; her food was well cooked, and she had an abundance of everything that was wholesome; the work was neither hard nor confining, and apparently there was no earthly reason why she should suffer when all the others in the house enjoyed perfect health. Having seen so many cases of this character yield promptly to this treatment, it would be a waste of time to describe others. I should add, in conclusion, that the arsenite of copper was exhibited for its supposed alterative and antiseptic effects, especially where we have to deal with an unhealthy condition of the alimentary canal, a suggestion which will be appreciated by many who have difficulty in getting patients to take drugs with a disagreeable taste. Clinical observation warrants me in saying that it is a remedy of great utility in this class of cases.

JOHN AULDE, M.D.

1910 ARCH STREET, PHILADA.

ATLANTA vs. CHATTANOOGA.

To the Editor of THE MEDICAL NEWS,

SIR : I have just read Dr. Baird's polite communication in THE MEDICAL NEWS of July 5th, under the title of "Typhoid Fever in Chattanooga," and feel constrained to make the following reply:

Notwithstanding Dr. Baird's gratuitous interpretation of the "official records of the Chattanooga Board of Health," and his abiding faith in the old saying that "figures won't lie," the remarkable immunity in this city from enteric or typhoid fever, diphtheria and scarlet fever, is precisely as stated in my paper read before the Association of American Physicians, and published in THE MEDICAL NEWS of June 7th.

I submit, in much kindness, that Dr. Baird's own experience as Health Officer of Atlanta should have thoroughly convinced him by this time of the unwelcome truth that the average death-certificate is an unknown quantity, and of all things in this world the most unreliable. Health officers cannot "go behind the returns," no matter how doubtful the correctness of the certificate may be, they must, *nolens volens*, report accordingly.

Dr. Baird has fairly stated that 107 deaths from typhoid fever represent, probably, more than 1000 cases of the disease in any given community where it prevails; yet I doubt if any physician could be found in Chattanooga who would venture the statement that there have been 100 cases of typhoid fever in this city "during the last four years." The occurrence of 50 cases, or less, would have furnished enough *seed*—if the situation were not a sterile soil—to cover the ground, and make the disease so common that there could be no difference of opinion concerning its presence. And is it possible for one to believe that 1000 cases of the disease could have occurred, within four successive years, without attracting the special attention of the local medical profession, and alarming the whole community ?

When the population of Chattanooga is alluded to by the Health Department, the thriving suburban communities of East Lake, East End, Ridgedale, St. Elmo, Hill City, Sherman Heights, Highland Park, etc.—aggregating a population of 15,000 or 16,000—are not included. In fact the census just completed show that in the city's limits proper, the population does not exceed 32,500; and it is upon this basis that the Health Department must begin the new decade. The correction as to population makes the "official records" all the more unreliable ; for who, indeed, can believe that within the limit of such a population typhoid fever could be so common, yet unknown clinically to such an extent that there are several physicans of large experience in practice in Chattanooga who have not seen a case ?

But however disappointing to the pride of enthusiastic Chattanoogans that our boasted "60,000 population," including the suburban centres, has been reduced to less than 50,000, the happy truth remains that the city is remarkable for its almost entire immunity from typhoid fever, diphtheria, and scarlet fever, thus maintaining a most wholesome contrast with all other American cities in public health, and holding, especially, its advantage over Atlanta.

Very soon after my return from the meeting of the Association of American Physicians, the Chattanooga *Daily Times* gave notice of the presence of typhoid fever in some of the outlying districts, with two deaths from the disease ; whereupon, at the next meeting of the City Medical Society, I called attention to the newspaper report, and said, if it was true, it flatly contradicted the statement I had made in my paper. In the interest of medical truth, I urged a closer study of the question, if possible, than had hitherto been given it, asserting that it was not complimentary to the medical profession of Chattanooga that there should exist a difference of opinion on the subject.* In the same spirit, I addressed the President of the City Board of Health, calling his attention to the newpaper reports above named, and asked for the facts. Here is his reply :

CHATTANOOGA, TENN., June 12, 1890.

DR. JAMES E. REEVES, M.D.,

DEAR SIR : Your kind note of yesterday received. Allow me to say that the *squib* in the *Times* of yesterday was without my approval, and quite a surprise to me. Since my residence in Chattanooga, I have been very sceptical as to the existence of typhoid fever in the city.

Very respectfully,　　J. L. GASTON.

The question of the infrequency of typhoid fever in Chattanooga is not a new one, but has, again and again, been discussed in the City Medical Society—called up usually by the report of a "rare case." Within the last few weeks, the "official figures"—for which Dr. Baird has so much respect—barely escaped recording another death from "typhoid fever." The case was, at first, thought to be one of "meningitis ; " after a consultation, "typhoid fever." The patient expired suddenly and unexpectedly, and the post-mortem revealed a large hepatic abscess as the cause of death.

The "one physician, in active practice for more than thirty years," who has seen "only three or four cases within that period," is Dr. P. D. Sims, member of the State Board of Health and secretary of the City Board of Health. No one who knows Dr. Sims will doubt his ability to speak positively on this or any other subject connected with medical practice in Chattanooga. His professional standing, large experience in general practice, every quality to make his opinions and utterances command respect, outweigh the "random estimates of individuals," and sufficiently attest the fact that typhoid fever is but rarely met with in Chattanooga ; but why the immunity no physician is wise enough to tell.

Respectfully,   JAMES E. REEVES.
201 McCALLIE AVENUE, CHATTANOOGA, TENN.

NEWS ITEMS.

Orthopædic Surgery at the Berlin Congress.—Dr. Newton M. Shaffer, Chairman of the Orthopædic Section of the New York Academy of Medicine, announces that a Section of Orthopædic Surgery has been formed by the Committee of Organization of the approaching Berlin Congress. Members of the profession interested in this department of surgery are requested to be present at the Congress and to become members of the Section.

Medico-legal Society of Chicago.—At the annual meeting of the Medico-legal Society of Chicago, held June 7, 1890, the following officers were selected for the ensuing year: *President,* Dr. E. J. Doering ; *Vice-Presidents,* Dr. B. Bettman and Judge O. H. Horton ; *Treasurer,* Dr. L. L. McArthur ; *Secretary,* Dr. Edward B. Weston.

Case of Beri-beri.—A case of beri-beri has recently been received at the Long Island College Hospital, to which institution it was removed from the Quarantine of New York Harbor. The disease is a very unusual one here, and this case presents itself in the person of a sailor on the German ship " Warns."

Burial Reform in London.—The dangerous overcrowding of the London cemeteries has been often commented on by the medical press of that city, but the evil remains almost wholly unabated. The Sanitary Committee of the London County Council has reported that no time should be lost in closing burial grounds such as the Brompton, which contains 155,000 bodies ; and the Tower Hamlets Cemetery, with its 247,000 bodies crowded into only seventeen acres. The average grave is seven by three feet, and contains eight adults and fourteen children, the covering of earth being about one foot. In one instance, a committee of inquiry regarding this cemetery found eighty infants interred in a grave or trench of less dimensions than that of the average grave. There are twenty-one burial places, with a total extent of less than 300 acres, holding a million and a quarter of bodies. The soil in most of these places is clay, and the process of decomposition goes on so slowly that bodies buried for a dozen years remain remarkably well preserved. This unfortunate state of affairs, especially as seen in the overcrowding that takes place wherever the bodies of the poor are buried, is universally acknowledged to be a serious menace to the public health and to demand the prompt attention of the government.

The Antisepsis of Oath Administration. — The *British Medical Journal* states, under the title of " Kissing the Book," that the old-fashioned greasy book so often tendered in the law courts to a witness about to be sworn, is a source of danger that is fully recognized by some officials. For example, when the Duke of Fife appeared lately at Stratford in a prosecution, the book on which he took the oath was enveloped in a piece of clean, white paper for his use, a precaution that might with advantage be more generally adopted. The *British Medical Journal* proceeds to ask, " Why should not the formula of the oath taken in our courts of justice be altered—possibly in imitation of the method in vogue in Scotland, which is that of raising the hand—in lieu of kissing the book ?" Not long since a woman was a witness in a court in Philadelphia, and when taking the stand to testify refrained from kissing the dirty volume presented to her by the court officer, whereupon a juror objected to her testimony because, as he said, it was invalid and incomplete by reason of her omission of this time-honored ceremonial ; but the judge ruled that an oath was valid without the kissing of the sacred volume, and that the kissing itself was a relic of idolatry that should be abolished. " I think," he said, " that this witness has refrained from kissing the book, not because she has any intention of giving false testimony, but because it is a dirty book. I respect her regard for her person and her health."

In almost every civilized country, people who have scruples against swearing are relieved from that formula by the simpler " affirmation " to the truth of their proposed testimony. Affirmation may be less impressive to certain classes, but it commends itself as a clean and safe method.

Antivivisection Bitterness.—The Society for the Protection of Animals from Vivisection recently held its annual Spring conference in London. The war-cry this year was " Pasteurism and Crime," and Canon Wilberforce is reported to have rejoiced in the fact that the movement to found a Pasteur Institute in England had been defeated by the society's method of placarding the city with large posters, containing the list of those who had died after treatment by the Pasteurian system. Many others indulged in bitter denunciation of both vivisection and Pasteurism, as being the means of brutalizing the otherwise honorable and useful profession of medicine. One speaker likened vivisection to the liquor traffic, and said that inasmuch as it would be impossible to regulate either by laws, they must be torn out root and branch. Other speakers said that they could prove by competent medical testimony that humanity had been injured by the attempt to apply the results of investigations made on the inferior animals. Altogether, much zeal, though but little knowledge, was exhibited by these people, who are friends to every animal but man.

OFFICIAL LIST OF CHANGES IN THE STATIONS AND DUTIES OF THE MEDICAL CORPS OF THE U. S. NAVY FOR THE WEEK ENDING JULY 26, 1890.

STONE, L. H., *Assistant Surgeon.*—Ordered to the U. S. Receiving-ship " New Hampshire."

URIE, J. F., *Assistant Surgeon.*—Detached from the U. S. Receiving-ship " New Hampshire," and ordered to the U. S. Receiving-ship " Wabash."

NORTON, OLIVER D., *Passed Assistant Surgeon.*—Granted leave of absence for the month of August.

BABIN, H. J., *Surgeon.*—Granted one month's leave of absence from July 23d.

THE MEDICAL NEWS.

A WEEKLY JOURNAL OF MEDICAL SCIENCE.

VOL. LVII.   SATURDAY, AUGUST 9, 1890.   NO. 6.

ORIGINAL ADDRESSES.

ANÆSTHESIA.

An Address delivered before the International Medical Congress, Berlin, August 6, 1890.

BY H. C. WOOD, M.D., LL.D.,
PROFESSOR OF THERAPEUTICS IN THE UNIVERSITY OF PENNSYLVANIA.

THE most brilliant modern achievements, in the direct saving of life, of the science and art of medicine are connected with surgery. These great achievements have been rendered possible by two epoch-making discoveries, antisepsis and anæsthesia. The long array of fatal cases of poisoning by carbolic acid, by iodoform, by corrosive sublimate, and by other antiseptic agents; the hundreds of deaths from chloroform, ether, and other anæsthetics, all bear witness to the verity of that strange law, in obedience to which the progress of the human race is so often at the sacrifice of the individual. Antisepsis has outgrown the dangers of its youth, and to-day the measures that are meant to save, very rarely kill. On the other hand, the death-roll of anæsthesia is daily added to; added to, according to my belief, at a rate that has not changed in forty years. Though this be true, from far-off Australia comes the news that jury and judge have condemned to heavy penalty a chloroformist who had lost his patient; and in Old England itself, the leading medical journal lends support to such a verdict by affirming that " deaths from chloroform are preventable, that with due care they may be avoided," and that, therefore, when they occur, they are the result of ignorance or carelessness. Five hundred deaths and more—the result of ignorance or carelessness ! Five hundred surgeons, including such names as Billroth, Jaeger, Simpson, McLeod, Agnew, Hunter McGuire, and others of equal rank, guilty of manslaughter! And still the carnage goes on. Surely under such circumstances the subject of anæsthesia is worthy of the attention of even this, the most learned medical gathering of the nations that the world can furnish. Antisepsis, the gift of the Old World to humanity: anæsthesia, the gift of the New World, which made the fruits of antisepsis possible : surely it is fitting that I, standing here to-day before you all, as the representative of the newer civilization, should be the chosen mouthpiece for the renewed discussion of this old but pressing theme.

In attempting a fresh study of a well-threshed-out subject, I propose to take advantage of the modern physiological methods, and to endeavor to discover by experiments upon the lower animals how anæsthetics kill, and what drugs or measures are most powerful in putting aside their lethal effects. This brings us face to face with the question—How far is it possible to adapt experiments to the needs of practical medicine, and to reason from the dog to the man? A full discussion of this subject would not be opportune, but it does seem necessary for our purpose to devote a few minutes to the pointing out of certain general guiding principles.

It ought to be acknowledged as a fundamental axiom, that no amount of experiments can overthrow a clinical fact; although when a contradiction between experimental and bedside observation seems to arise, such contradiction challenges the correctness of the alleged clinical and experimental facts alike, and should lead to a careful reëxamination. No amount of failure to purge a dog by elaterium proves that elaterium does not purge man ; whilst, on the other hand, the discovery that digitalis increased the blood-pressure in the lower animal very properly led to doubt as to the correctness of the, at the time, general belief that digitalis acts upon man as a cardiac sedative, and finally to the recognition of the falsity of the clinical observation upon which such belief rested.

Whatever difficulties may beset the path of the experimental therapeutist, it is certain that law is throughout the universe supreme : that man, at least in his physical nature, is only an especially developed animal : and if drugs act differently upon different animals, such action must be in obedience to certain laws, to us known or unknown.

Any attempt to discuss fairly these laws would lead us too far afield for the present. One law, however, treads so closely upon the matter at hand this morning, that it requires statement. This law is, that when an apparatus or system is of similar function and of similar functional activity in different animals, the difference in the action of remedies is very rarely, if ever, in kind, though it may be in degree. Throughout mammalia the heart has one general structure, and one general function ; the heart of the dog responds to the touch of digitalis precisely as does the heart of the man. The human brain is so much more highly developed than the brain of the lower mammal, that it is, in fact, a new organ or apparatus, and its relation to drugs changes with the change of structure and of function. The scope of this law in regard to anæsthesia is not far to seek. The functions especially compromitted in lethal anæsthesia are respiration and circulation. Surely these functions are similar throughout mammalia, and surely we ought to be able to reason safely concerning them, from the dog to the man.

Recently, however, alleged clinical facts have been challenged by high authority, upon the strength of experimental results. Under these circumstances, nothing must be at once abandoned, everything must be reexamined. These reëxaminations I have made, and I may be pardoned, perhaps, if I affirm that a complete study of the clinical and experimental evidence brings out, not a discord, but a most beautiful concord—that concord between experimental and practical medicine which so often fails to appear simply because we cannot fit together the fragments of truth in our possession.

Although numerous substances have been tried, there are to-day in use, practically, only three anæsthetics—nitrous oxide, ether, and chloroform. Of these, nitrous oxide stands apart, because it produces loss of consciousness not by virtue of any inherent properties, but simply by shutting off from the nerve-centres the supply of oxygen.

It has been asserted that the changes of circulation produced by the inhalation of nitrous oxide are essentially different from those of mechanical asphyxia, and that therefore nitrous oxide does not act as an asphyxiant. It must, however, be borne in mind that the phenomena of mechanical asphyxia are largely due to the presence of an excess of carbonic acid in the blood, whilst in the asphyxia produced by nitrous oxide there is no excess of carbonic acid, so that the phenomena present are simply the outcome of a lack of oxygen. It is, therefore, *a priori*, to be expected that the phenomena of mechanical and of nitrous oxide asphyxia should differ to a certain extent. To determine the way in

FIG. 1.

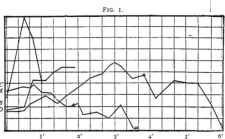

Plot showing effects of inhalation of nitrous oxide upon blood-pressure. *A*, first inhalation. *B*, second inhalation. *C* and *D*, inhalations in different dogs.

which nitrous oxide inhalation affects the circulation, I have, during the past winter, in connection with my assistant and friend, Dr. David Cerna, made a long series of experiments. The result has been to show that usually the inhalation is followed by a rise of the arterial pressure, accompanied by a great disturbance of the pulse; the pulse at first becoming irregular and tumultuous, but by and by settling, so that when anæsthesia is complete the pulse-wave is remarkably large and full, and the rate very slow. The rise and fall of the arterial pressure in nitrous oxide anæsthesia was found to vary remarkably, not only in different inhalations, but in different periods of the same inhalation. Sometimes the rise was sudden, sometimes it was slow and gradual: sometimes it was maintained until near death, sometimes it was interrupted very early: sometimes it was not very well marked, sometimes it was enormous. As illustrating it, I have the accompanying diagrams, accurately showing the curve of the blood-pressure obtained in four inhalations practised on three different dogs. (Fig. 1.)

In all our experiments respiration ceased while the heart was still in full activity. Indeed, instead of the gas acting as a cardiac depressant, it appeared to act as a cardiac stimulant, although it paralyzed the vaso-motor apparatus. Thus, during complete anæsthesia, faradic irritation of the sciatic nerve always failed to register itself in an increase of the blood-pressure, although the heart was beating very powerfully, and although the pneumogastrics had been previously severed: whilst late in the poisoning—at a time when the respiration had absolutely ceased, and the animal was in this respect dead, and without the power of self-recovery, and when the arterial pressure also had fallen almost to zero—the pulse-waves were frequently still nearly three times the norm. In evidence of this I append a reproduction of a tracing (Fig. 2).

We made but few experiments as to the action of artificial respiration upon the animal dying from nitrous oxide, but these experiments proved that even after complete paralysis of the respiratory function, artificial respiration is capable of rapidly bringing the animal

FIG. 2.

Figure showing the relative size of the pulse waves in nitrous oxide anæsthesia. Tracing *A*, before inhalation. Tracing *B*, after breathing had stopped.

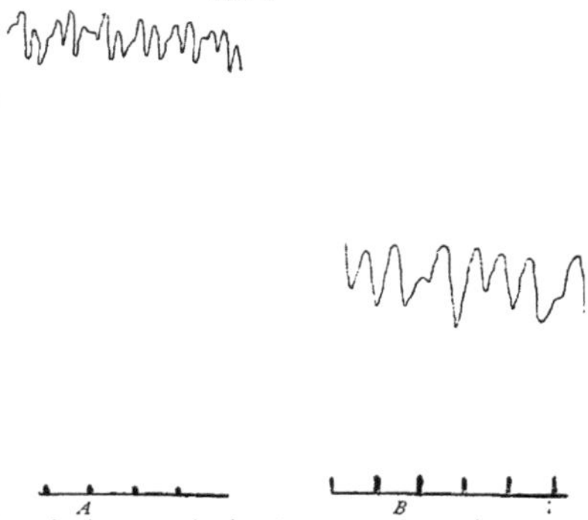

back to life. The heart lives on through nitrous oxide anæsthesia long after the respiratory function has been abolished, and even when the strong, full pulse fails, and the heart has almost ceased to quiver, recovery is still hopeful, because the loss of function has been caused, not by the presence of a poison, but by the absence of oxygen; and although the paralysis may be complete, the life-power sleeps before it dies, and is ready to awake at the touch of fresh oxygen.

These experimental results are in strict accord with clinical observations. The S. S. White Dental Manufacturing Company supply a very large, if not the largest, portion of the apparatus and material used for the administration of nitrous oxide in the United States; and, in answer to my inquiry, Dr. J. W. White, their President, writes me that a computation based upon their own sales, and a knowledge of those of their rivals, has reached "the somewhat appalling result, that anæsthesia by nitrous oxide gas is probably effected in three-quarters of a million of cases annually in the United States." Most of these inhalations have been given, not by trained physicians, but by comparatively untrained, and often very ignorant dentists; have been given to patients in a sitting or semi-sitting posture: have been given apparently without thought or care to the general community, as the units presented themselves, to the healthy and to the diseased alike; and the result is, out of many millions of inhalations only three deaths recorded as directly due to nitrous oxide! Could anything be safer?

A suggestive and very practical fact which came out in our experiments, is that sometimes during an inhalation of nitrous oxide the rise of the arterial pressure is extraordinary and abrupt. Not long since, in the city of Philadelphia, a gentleman arose from the dentist's chair after an inhalation of nitrous oxide, staggered, and fell in an apoplexy. Is it not easy to perceive that when the arterial system is diseased, the great strain of a sudden rise of blood-pressure may produce rupture?

Some years since, Dr. Kenderdine, a Philadelphia surgeon of local note, died of diabetes, which he insisted was produced in him by the inhalation of nitrous oxide. This is in accord with the researches of the French physician Dr. Lafont, who reported a case in which sugar appeared in the urine twice in a patient, after inhalation of the gas; and who also caused in himself, and in dogs, temporary glycosuria by such inhalations. Further, Dr. Lafont noticed in a case of mitral insufficiency temporary albuminuria.

I am not aware that these very suggestive statements of the French physician have given rise to any research, except five experiments made recently upon healthy men, with negative results, by two medical students of the University of Pennsylvania, Messrs. George S. Woodward and Alfred Hand, Jr. I do not believe that ordinarily the inhalation of nitrous oxide is followed by sufficient disturbance of the circulation to register itself in the urine, but the negative evidence of Messrs. Woodward and Hand is not sufficient to render it improbable that in exceptional cases the inhalation of nitrous oxide may produce albuminuria or glycosuria. Such phenomena, if they occur, are in all probability not directly produced by the nitrous oxide, but are due to the disturbances of capillary circulation caused by it.

However these facts may be, it seems to me that great caution should be used in the administration of nitrous oxide to persons the coating of whose arteries is diseased, and it is probable that when widespread atheroma exists, ether is a safer anæsthetic than nitrous oxide.

When respiration has been suspended in nitrous oxide anæsthesia the overwhelming indication is certainly for the employment of artificial respiration.

Notwithstanding the great safety and the many advantages which attend the anæsthetic employment of nitrous oxide, the gas can never be used for the general purposes of the surgeon, on account of the excessive fugaciousness of its influence.

The perfect anæsthetic will be a substance which has the power of paralyzing the sensory nerve-trunks without affecting other functions of the body. If such drug exists, it yet awaits the coming of its discoverer. Probably until such a sensory nerve paralyzant is found, chloroform and ether will maintain the complete supremacy which they now have; and in the further discussion of my subject I shall confine my remarks to them. Lack of time limits this discussion to:

First. The method in which these two drugs kill, both in man and in the lower animal; that is, whether they destroy life through the circulation or the respiration.

Second. The comparative fatality attending the use of these two agents, and the reasons for the difference.

Third. The comparative disadvantages between the two agents, and the best method of securing the desired results.

Fourth. The treatment of accidents occurring during ether or chloroform anæsthesia.

In regard to the method in which anæsthetics kill, my own teaching hitherto has been: first, that although ether in moderate doses acts as a stimulant to the circulation, yet in overwhelming amount it is capable of depressing the heart, but that such depression of the heart is always less than the depression of the respiration, and therefore, ether kills always through the respiration; second, that chloroform may produce death by paralysis of the respiratory centre, or by a simultaneous arrest of respiration and circulation, but that primary paralysis of the heart may occur, and is especially prone to do so when the chloroform vapor has been given in concentrated form.

I think that these views are in accord with general professional belief, but it has recently been alleged that they are at variance with experimental evidences, so that a reëxamination is necessary. What then are the clinical facts?

If any credence is to be attached to the statements of competent witnesses, who have recorded human deaths during anæsthesia, it is certain that in some cases, under the influence of chloroform, the pulse and respiration have ceased simultaneously; whilst in other instances the respiration has failed before the pulse; and in still other cases the pulse has ceased its beat before the respiratory movements were arrested.

Usually ether arrests respiration in man before it paralyzes the heart, but the collection of records made by Dr. J. C. Reeves certainly shows that the fatal result may be produced by syncope. Thus Dr. Ernest H. Jacobs, in a report of a fatal case, asserts positively "the pulse ceased, the breathing continued." It would seem that we must admit that ether in the human subject may cause death in the same methods as does chloroform.

Such then are the clinical facts; or in other words, such are the results of observations made upon the human subject. What are the results of observations made upon animals?

The general teaching in regard to chloroform has been recently challenged by Dr. Lauder Brunton, who, as the result of 450 experiments made by himself upon the pariah dogs of India, has reached the conclusion, published in the London Lancet, that however concentrated the chloroform may be it never causes death from sudden stoppage of the heart. In the physiological laboratories of the University of Pennsylvania, for some years, several hundred dogs have been annually used, and a very large proportion of these dogs have been, at the end of an experiment, killed by chloroform. The observations of Dr. Reichert, Professor of Physiology in the University, Dr. H. A. Hare, Demonstrator of Therapeutics, and myself, have been concordant in showing that chloroform is a cardiac paralyzant, and often does kill dogs by a direct action upon the heart or its contained ganglia. The statements made concerning the Hyderabad Commission, however, led Dr. Hare and myself to a thorough and careful restudy of the subject. Some of our experiments were made by injecting chloroform into the jugular vein; others by administering it by inhalation in the usual way.

The action of the chloroform seems to be not seriously modified by the method of administration. We definitely proved that in the dog chloroform has a distinct, direct, paralyzing influence on both respiration and circulation; that the respiration may cease before the heart-beat, or the two functions be simultaneously abolished; but that in some cases the heart is arrested before respiration, We have several times seen the respiration continue as long as one, and even two minutes after the blood-pressure has fallen to zero, and the pulse has completely disappeared from the carotid artery.[1]

The correctness of our experiments, we claim, must be acknowledged. The experiments have not only been witnessed by a number of persons, but I have with me to-day tracings which I will gladly show anyone especially interested in the subject. I do not desire to express any doubt whatever as to the correctness of the experimental data of Dr. Brunton; I simply claim that both sets of experiments, although they have yielded different results, have been correctly and properly performed. It may be that the high heat or other climatic conditions surrounding the pariah dog make his heart less sensitive to the action of chloroform than is the heart of the dog bred in Northern climates. That the thought of the different constitutions of animals in different climates is not absurd, is shown by the fact that some years ago, after I had affirmed before the Physiological Section of the International Medical Congress at London, that if certain asserted results were obtained upon European dogs, said dogs must differ from those of America, and had been met with a smile of incredulity, Dr. Brown-Séquard rose and stated that he had experimented upon hundreds of dogs on both continents, and that there was a distinct difference between the animals, the vascular system of the European dogs being much more developed, and operations upon them being, therefore, much more bloody than was the case with the American dog.

A very curious parallel might be traced at this point between the experimental and clinical evidence in regard to the effect of climate upon the action of chloroform. In the Southern United States chloroform is used with great freedom, and with great alleged safety; and as long ago as 1878, Dr. Landon B. Edwards, editor of the *Virginia Medical Monthly*, wrote: " It is one of the most peculiar facts I have ever known in medical practice—the difference of experience in Europe and the North, with chloroform and ether, as compared with that of the South— the high rate of mortality in the North, and the low rate in the South.

In a series of experiments which I have recently made to determine the changes in the circulation produced when ether anæsthesia is carried on to death, I have found that in the first periods of anæsthesia the blood-pressure is usually elevated, and that it is usually quite high at a time when the respirations are very shallow and imperfect, and the dark color of the blood shows that

[1] No tracings showing these facts are here given because they have been previously published in THE MEDICAL NEWS (February 22, 1890).

it is heavily charged with carbonic acid. It is not, however, very rare for the blood-pressure to remain near the norm, and I have seen the blood-pressure begin to fall in the very first stages of ether anæsthesia; moreover, in at least two experiments death occurred from syncope, the respiration continuing for one or two minutes after the complete cessation of the circulation. In an experiment in which the fall of blood-pressure was most pronounced, and the arrest of the heart most complete, the dog was sick from the mange, and it is possible that the weakened heart was more susceptible than is the normal heart to the depressing influence of ether.

FIG. 3.

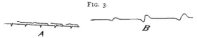

Tracing showing respiratory movements, *B*, registered one and a quarter minutes after circulation had fallen as shown in *A* during death from ether in the dog.

So far, then, as concerns the method in which ether and chloroform kill, I claim most urgently that there is no contradiction between the results as obtained by the bedside and in the physiological laboratories, and that a complete, broad study of the clinical and experimental evidence leads to one conclusion, namely, that chloroform and ether are capable of paralyzing the respiration and the circulation; that in some cases one function, in other cases the other function, is primarily arrested; but that ether is less prone to produce a primary arrest of the heart than is chloroform.

In the discussion of the second point which I have raised, namely, the comparative fatality attending the use of ether and chloroform, I shall not occupy time with any elaborate setting-forth of the clinical evidence. In regard to the number of recorded deaths, I shall content myself with accepting the latest statistics at hand, namely, those collected by Dr. Laurence Turnbull, who has found 375 deaths reported from chloroform, and 52 from ether. I do not believe that these figures nearly represent the total mortality; I doubt very much whether one-third of the deaths from anæsthesia are reported; certainly not one-third of the cases I have had personal knowledge of have been publicly recorded. Moreover, the pressure to conceal deaths from chloroform is greater than when the lethal result is due to ether. The surgeon who uses ether feels that he has employed the safest anæsthetic, and that he will receive no blame if a death occurs from it, and feels also that he has a rare case to put on record, which will give his own name a permanent place in anæsthetic literature; whereas the surgeon who uses chloroform knows that if death occurs from the anæsthetic, a very large proportion of the profession, at least in the United States, will condemn him either in public or secret for the use of this drug, and that he will be fortunate if he escape being publicly condemned by a coroner's jury. Moreover, deaths from chloroform are only too common, so that the surgeon has nothing to gain and much to lose by publication of a chloroform death, and if possessed of the average human nature, holds his peace. The Coroner's Physician of Philadelphia, Dr. Formad, informs me that he has made autopsies in 15 cases of ether death, only 3 of which have been reported in medical journals: how many chloroform deaths have been lost in eternal quiet?

It seems to me impossible to get at the exact number of anæsthetic deaths, or the proportionate fatality of ether and chloroform. Lyman considers that in regard to chloroform, the ratio of deaths to inhalations is 1 in 5860; Richardson, that it is 1 in 2500 to 3000. Andrews puts it for ether, at 1 in 23,204; and Lyman, at 1 in 16,542.

Without claiming strict accuracy for any of these figures, I think it can be asserted that the ratio of deaths from chloroform is probably at least four or five times that of deaths from ether.

When we come to study the effects of chloroform upon the lower animals, we find that it varies very distinctly in its action on the different species. The cat seems to withstand the fatal influences of chloroform with a power worthy of its reputed "nine lives." Many years ago, Professor Schiff called attention to the fact that the use of chloroform as an anæsthetic in the dog is usually attended with the loss of many animals. Professor Martin, of the Johns Hopkins University, writes me that the margin between complete chloroform anæsthesia in the dog, and chloroform death, is a very narrow one. This certainly is our experience in the University of Pennsylvania; we have never been able to use chloroform as an anæsthetic without losing a very large proportion of our dogs.

Clinical and experimental results—i. e., the results of experiments made in the physiological laboratory upon the lower animal, and the results of experiments made in the amphitheatre upon the higher animal, Man—are again concordant. Chloroform is much more inimical than ether to animal life. The cause of this singular fatality is not, however, chiefly the cardiac action of chloroform. Chloroform is more apt to cause cardiac arrest than is ether, but it is also much more prone than is ether to cause death by failure of the respiration. Almost invariably, when ether is withdrawn before the dog is absolutely in the grasp of death, recovery occurs; but over and over again I have noticed that although the chloroform was taken away whilst the respirations were still being maintained with regularity, the arterial pressure much above zero, and the pulse very apparent, yet the symptoms of cardiac and respiratory failure continued to increase until the fatal issue was reached.

It seems to me that certain general facts or principles in regard to anæsthesia must be considered as established:

First, that the use of any anæsthetic is attended with an appreciable risk, and that no care will prevent an occasional loss of life.

Second, that chloroform acts much more promptly and much more powerfully than ether, both upon the respiratory centres and the heart.

Third, that the action of chloroform is much more persistent and permanent than is that of ether.

Fourth, that chloroform is capable of causing death either by primarily arresting the respiration, or by primarily stopping the heart, but that commonly both respiratory and cardiac functions are abolished at or about the same time.

Fifth, that ether usually acts very much more powerfully upon the respiration than upon the circulation, but that occasionally, and especially when the heart is feeble, ether is capable of acting as a cardiac paralyzant, and may produce death by cardiac arrest at a time when the respirations are fully maintained.

Chloroform kills, as near as can be made out, proportionately four or five times as frequently as does ether; partly, no doubt, because it is more powerful in depressing the heart, but largely because it lets go its hold much less rapidly than does ether when inhalation ceases. Is it not possible that this "holding on" is because it is less volatile than ether, and can we not here get a hint why chloroform is less deadly in the South than in the North? The diffusibility of vapors or gases is in inverse proportion to the square of their densities, and the vapor of chloroform would certainly diffuse itself with far greater rapidity at 90° F. than at 70° F.

The comparative advantages and disadvantages of the two anæsthetics in practical medicine, are so well known, that only one or two points seem to force themselves upon our present attention. I cannot see that the surgeon is justified in putting the life of the patient to the unnecessary risks of chloroformization, except under special circumstances. I believe, moreover, that much of the unpopularity of ether is due to its improper administration. It is so easy to embarrass the respiration seriously by the folded towel, as commonly used, that not only are the struggles of mechanical asphyxia almost invariably produced, but probably death itself is sometimes caused. Especially is there danger of death being thus caused mechanically in the advanced stages of etherization, when the patient is too thoroughly etherized to struggle, and when the attention of the etherizer is, it may be, attracted by some novel and difficult operation. I myself confess to having once nearly killed a patient in this way.

A proper apparatus is certainly preferable to the folded towel. Various apparatus have been invented, but as the time is short I shall only mention one—one which seems to me a practically perfect mechanism, although it is probably little known this side of the Atlantic.

The inhaler invented by Dr. O. H. Allis is based upon the theory that the patient to be etherized should be supplied with a full abundance of air, saturated with the vapor of ether. It consists essentially of a series of foldings of muslin on a wire framework, arranged almost like the gills of a fish, so as to allow the air to pass freely through, but everywhere to come in contact with ether. It should be placed upon the face of the patient dry, and the ether gradually poured on from a bottle with an especially prepared cork, known in Philadelphia as the "polyclinic" bottle. When properly used the Allis inhaler practically does away with the sense of suffocation, and the consequent struggles which have made etherization alike so repulsive to patient and surgeon.

In order to determine the rapidity with which etherization can be produced by this inhaler, Dr. M. H. Williams kept for me notes of thirteen consecutive cases in the clinic of the Jefferson Medical College Hospital in Philadelphia. The average time required for the production of complete unconsciousness was eight minutes. The average time during which anæsthesia was fully maintained was thirty-two minutes; and the average amount of ether used during this time was 7½ ounces. In 21 surgical cases occurring this spring in the clinical service of Professor J. William White, of the University of Pennsylvania, the average time for the production of complete anæsthesia with ether, used through Allis's inhaler, was seven and nine-tenths minutes. The results arrived at in these two clinics are so close that eight minutes must be considered the average time required for full etherization by this apparatus.

In discussing the treatment of the accidents of anæsthesia, the results obtained at the bedside naturally press forward for careful consideration, but in going over the subject from this point of view, I have found so little that was novel, and so little that was satisfactory to myself, that I shall not occupy the time of this Congress with any conclusions drawn from reported cases, or personal experience in chloroform accidents. I do not think myself that the problem can be solved by any such study of cases. Death is so near and so terrible, time is so absolute, moments so important, that no surgeon would be willing or justified in waiting for the effect of any one remedy; and when a man is dosed with alcohol, nitrite of amyl, hypodermic injections of ether, digitalis, atropine, and other powerful agents; faradized, slapped, douched, stood on his head, subjected to chest movements for artificial respiration, and to various other measures too numerous to mention; who can tell, if by chance he recover, why he has done so? or who can point out, if by chance he die, what is the remedy whose omission or commission has led to the fatal result?

The problem is a very complex one, not to be worked out amidst the excitement and responsibilities of the amphitheatre. Only in the physiological laboratory can its various elements be separated and studied each by itself, without regard to the individual life which is at stake.

In the physiological laboratory two distinct paths open, each promising to lead to some positive knowledge. We may, on one hand, enter upon the study of the minimum fatal dose of the anæsthetic, and of the results by the concurrent or subsequent administration of its supposed physiological antagonist; or we may investigate the effect of remedies upon functions that are failing under the influences of the anæsthetic.

The objections to the first of these methods have been, in the present instance, overwhelming. The accidents seem to be independent of the amount of anæsthetic inhaled; and such a method of investigation would have required far more time than was available after I had had the honor of being asked to address this body. Death is produced by chloroform and ether through paralysis of the respiration and the heart, and the method of experimental study which I have employed consisted in a study of the action of powerful agents upon these functions when oppressed by chloroform. I have selected chloroform chiefly because it is the more powerful agent of the two anæsthetics, and the more certain in its lethal results.

The experiments have all been made upon dogs, by one plan. The carotid artery and also the trachea, having been connected with a recording drum, so that the movements of the circulation and the respiration could be consecutively recorded, the animal was anæsthetized, and when the blood-pressure had fallen almost to zero, and the respiration had ceased, or nearly ceased, as the case might be, the remedy to be tried was injected into the jugular vein, through a canula which had been previously inserted.

The more important remedies which have been used by clinicians for the averting of threatened death during anæsthesia are ether, alcohol, ammonia, nitrite of amyl, digitalis, atropine, and caffeine, alterations of position, and artificial respiration.

Although, at least in America, hypodermic injections of ether have been frequently employed even in ether accidents, such use is so absolutely absurd that it does not seem to me to require any experimental evidence of its futility. Ether in the blood acts as ether, whether it finds entrance through the lungs, through the rectum, or through the cellular tissue; and the man who would inject ether hypodermically into a patient who is dying from ether, should, to be logical, also saturate a sponge with the ether and crowd it upon his unfortunate victim.

Instead of simply stating the results obtained in my experiments, I have thought it would be more interesting to show reproductions from some of my tracings. The first drug that I shall report upon is caffeine. I have injected it during the cardiac failure produced by chloroform, in doses varying from 3 to 7½ grains, and have never been able to perceive any distinct alteration in the arterial pressure, and no consistent distinct change of the pulse either in number or force. So far as the experiments go, they certainly indicate that the drug has no influence upon the heart that is being overpowered by chloroform. I may also state here, that it is not possible in any of my tracings to make out any influence exerted by caffeine upon the respiration.

FIG. 4.

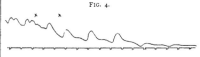

Anæsthesia complete. Dog still breathing. ½ gramme of caffeine injected at X X, each.

With atropine, I have made a few experiments, the results being almost as negative as with caffeine. Ten c. c. of a 2-per-cent. solution of atropine injected into the jugular vein of a chloroformed animal, altered the rate of the pulse-beat, but had no apparent effect or influence upon the arterial pressure, or upon the respiration, and in no wise prevented final cardiac arrest.

Of all drugs, that which I think is usually most relied upon by clinicians as a cardiac stimulant in anæsthesia, as in other cases of heart-failure, is alcohol. The chemical and physiological relations of alcohol to ether and chloroform are, however, so close, that many years ago I became very doubtful of the value of this drug as a stimulant to a heart depressed by anæsthesia.

These doubts continually grew stronger from what I saw and read as to the effects of the administration of alcohol during anæsthesia, and were finally changed into conviction by the experiments of R. Dubois (*Progrès Médical,* 1883, xi. 951), who found that in the animal to which alcohol has been freely given, much less chloroform is required than in the normal animal, to anæsthetize or to kill; or in other words, that alcohol intensifies the influence of chloroform and lessens the fatal dose.

In my own experiments with alcohol an 80-per-cent. fluid was used, diluted with water. The amount injected into the jugular vein varied in the different experiments from 5 to 20 c. c.; and in no case have I been able to detect any increase in the size of the pulse, or in the arterial pressure, produced by alcohol, when the heart was failing during advanced chloroform anæsthesia. On the other hand, on several occasions, the larger amounts of alcohol apparently greatly increased the rapidity of the fall of the arterial pressure, and aided materially in extinguishing the pulse-rate.

FIG. 5.

1.

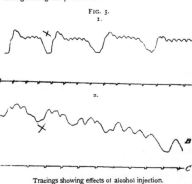

2.

B

C

Tracings showing effects of alcohol injection.
No. 1. four cubic centimetres of 80 per cent. at X.
No. 2. five cubic centimetres of 80 per cent. at X.

FIG. 6.

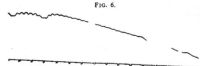

Experiment showing effect of injecting twenty cubic centimetres of alcohol in advanced chloroform anæsthesia. Injection made at beginning of tracing between X and X.

The effects of ammonia upon the failing heart of chloroform anæsthesia, has been in my experiments uncertain; sometimes distinct, although very fugacious,

FIG. 7.

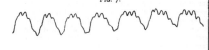

Injection of twenty cubic centimetres of a 10-per-cent. solution of aqua ammoniæ fortior. Injection given just after beginning of tracing.

and sometimes imperceptible Twenty cubic centimetres of a 10-per-cent. solution of aqua ammoniæ fortior (U. S. Pharmacopœia), in some cases produced an immediate rise in the arterial pressure, and even fugaciously registered itself in the respiratory rate, but perhaps more frequently it failed in its influence.

The influence of injections of digitalis has been, in a number of experiments, very pronounced in producing a persistent gradual rise of the arterial pressure with an increase in the size of the individual pulse-rate In several instances, death was apparently averted by its injection, and I saw in one or two cases, where large amounts of the digitalis had been employed, sudden systolic cardiac arrest, indicating that digitalis, if in sufficient amount, is able to assert itself victoriously in opposition to chloroform. Moreover, when I have given chloroform to dogs whose hearts were already under the influence of digitalis, there has seemed to be a peculiar steadying or sustaining power combating the circulatory depression naturally produced by the anæsthetic, and I believe that in all cases of weak heart in man a full dose of digitalis before the administration of chloroform would greatly lessen the danger of cardiac collapse.

FIG. 8.

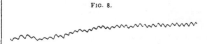

Tracing showing effect of five cubic centimetres of tincture of digitalis in advanced chloroform anæsthesia. Injection given at X.

With the nitrite of amyl four experiments were made; in some of these from 4 to 10 drops of the nitrite of amyl were injected in the jugular vein; in others the nitrite was used by inhalation. No distinct effect upon the arterial pressure was in any instance produced, and usually no alteration in the size of the pulse-waves, although sometimes the pulse did appear to be a little fuller.

FIG. 9.

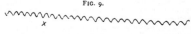

X

Tracing showing effect of nitrite of amyl, given freely by inhalation, upon the circulation. Inhalation begun at X.

Of all my experimental results, those which have been reached with strychnine have been the most surprising. The injection of strychnine into the jugular vein usually produced a gradual rise of the arterial pressure, and always caused an extraordinary and rapid increase in the rate and extent of the respiration. Thus I have seen the respiration, which had practically ceased for ten seconds, suddenly, under the influence of an injection of two-tenths of a grain of strychnine, become at once very large and full, and reach a rate of 130 a minute.

A series of elaborate experiments made upon the effect of the position of the animal on the blood-pressure in the carotid and other arteries, has very clearly proven that the body of the animal whose circulation has been paralyzed by chloroform, acts in a measure like a tube filled with fluid. Thus, if the feet of the dog were raised vertically above the head, whilst the latter remained upon the table, an immediate rise of pressure occurred, even though the heart had entirely ceased beating; provided that the head of the animal was kept upon a

FIG. 10..

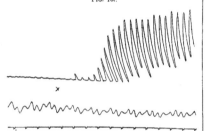

Tracing showing effect of injection of strychnine, after breathing had ceased, in an advanced chloroform anæsthesia. 0.193 grain of the sulphate was injected at X.

level with the table. If, however, the head of the animal was depressed below the level of the table for a distance equal to, or greater than the length of the body of the animal, a decrease of the arterial pressure occurred at once, although the animal was in a vertical position. The phenomena observed were precisely such as would have been produced if the canula had been inserted into a tube filled with fluid, instead of into the carotid artery, and the elevation and depression of this tube had registered itself on the recording drum, in obedience to the ordinary laws of hydrostatics. The phenomena were entirely independent of any beat of the heart, and were readily produced when the animal was dead, provided the death had not occurred too long previously. Sometimes, even a very few minutes after the cessation of the heart-beat, it was impossible to produce the changes of pressure upon the drum. This I believe to have been due to coagulation of the blood, occurring very early after death to a sufficient extent to interfere with the liquid properties of the fluid. In no case was any effect upon the respiration produced by change in position of the animal. In a number of cases, however, when the feet were elevated, the heart, which had entirely ceased beating, recommenced its work, and I have several times seen a pulse entirely disappear when the animal was taken from the vertical to the horizontal position. On the other hand, very frequently it was impossible to affect the cardiac action by changing the position of the animal. Nevertheless, the phenomena spoken of occurred too frequently to be a mere outcome of chance, though I several times noted that the heart was usually more affected by alternately elevating and depressing the feet of the animal, than by keeping it in a steadily elevated or horizontal position.

When the circulation has practically ceased, under the depressing influence of an anæsthetic, inverting the body must cause the blood which has naturally collected in the enormously relaxed vessels of the abdomen, to flow into the right side of the heart and distend·it, and this distention—this increase of pressure—appears at times to have a sufficient momentary influence to stimulate the failing organ.

The theory which has been advocated by some therapeutists, that inversion of the body is of value in the accidents of anæsthesia, because it causes the vital centres of the brain to be supplied with blood, is proba-

FIG. 11.

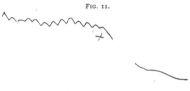

Tracing showing effect upon the heart of a dog which had been vertical, with his head on level of the table, of bringing him into horizontal position. Feet dropped at X.

bly incorrect. The respiration in anæsthesia fails, not through want of blood in the respiratory centres, but because the blood contains a poison which paralyzes these centres.

The most remarkable results which I have reached in bringing about recovery of animals to all ordinary intents and purposes dead, were obtained through the use of artificial respiration. Thus, I have seen an animal, in which no respiratory movements whatever had taken place for two minutes, and in which, during that time, no movements of blood had occurred in the carotid artery, and in which, therefore, the heart had ceased to beat, rapidly and permanently restored by artificial respiration.

At one time in these researches, it appeared as though after any dose of chloroform by inhalation the animal could be resuscitated by artificial respiration, even though heart and lungs were completely paralyzed by the drug; but finally I did find a case in which artificial respiration failed.

The results of my experiments with the lower animals may be summed up: that nitrite of amyl, caffeine, and atropine are of little or no use in chloroform-poisoning; that alcohol, when given in small amounts, has no influence, but that when given largely materially assists in paralyzing the heart and producing fatal results; that ammonia has some little influence upon the heart, but that of all substances tried, digitalis is by far the most powerful in stimulating the failing circulation; indeed, my experimental results indicate that it is the only known drug which is of any real practical value in such cases. Next, or perhaps even before digitalis, strychnine seems to be of value in the accidents of anæsthesia, because, whilst having some influence on the circulation, it powerfully affects the respiration. For many years chloroform has been used in practical medicine as the physiological and practical antagonist to strychnine, and it seems rather odd that strychnine should never have been employed as the practical antagonist to chloroform.

The one measure which in practical value far surpassed all others for the restoration of the dying animal was artificial respiration, and I have no doubt that a great majority of the deaths which have occurred in man from anæsthesia might have been avoided by the use of an active artificial respiration. The difficulty with artificial respiration as it has been hitherto practised upon man, after the Sylvester or other methods, is its inefficiency; whereas the artificial respiration which I used on animals was very active—indeed, much more efficient than natural breathing in causing circulation of air through the lungs, and therefore in removing excess of the anæsthetic from the residual air in the lungs, and from the blood.

The use of what may be called "forced" artificial respiration by the physiologist, so naturally suggested a similar practice in man, that the celebrated John Hunter invented for the purpose an apparatus which consisted of a bellows so constructed that when it was extended one compartment drew in air from the lungs, whilst the other drew air from the atmosphere; and when it was closed the process was reversed, the fresh air being thrown into the lungs, the foul air into the atmosphere. In 1867, Richardson, of London, invented an apparatus more elegant and portable, although identical in principle with that of John Hunter's; but I have not found that either Hunter or Richardson treated by forced artificial respiration an actual case of disease or poisoning. In 1875 (*Boston Medical Journal*, vol. xxi.), Dr. John Ellis Blake reported a successful case of aconite-poisoning, in which life was apparently saved, although there was no pulse for over three hours, by artificial respiration, with the use of oxygen. In this case Marshall Hall's method was at first used, but later, a small rubber tube was connected directly with a copper reservoir of condensed oxygen, the other end of the tube terminating in a small nozzle, which was inserted in one nostril. Four hundred gallons of oxygen were thus used, but how far the force of the compressed gas was employed to dilate the lungs is not very clear; and it is somewhat doubtful whether this case should be considered as one of forced respiration. The first physician to use forced respiration in actual human poisoning, with a clear idea of its value and power, so far as my reading goes, was Dr. George E. Fell (*International Medical Congress*, Washington, 1887).

It is plain that the bellows constructed by John Hunter and by Richardson are unnecessarily complex and faulty in principle. There is no need whatever of drawing the air out of the fully filled lungs. Every physiologist knows that when the muscular system is completely paralyzed by woorari or even by death, that the chest-walls have sufficient elasticity to force air out of the lungs, and all ordinary laboratory apparatus for artificial respiration is based upon this fact. For forced artificial respiration in man an ordinary bellows of proper size is all that is required for the motive power.

The real difficulty—the point to be especially investigated and studied—is as to the connection between the bellows and the lungs. Hunter and Richardson simply placed a tube in one nostril, closing firmly the other nostril and the mouth of the subject.

6*

Dr. Fell at first used a tracheal tube, the insertion of which, of course, necessitated the performance of tracheotomy. In one case, however, a simple mask covering the mouth and nostrils was a perfect success. I have had no opportunity of trying the apparatus on the living, but have made a series of experiments upon dead bodies, which have demonstrated that usually a face mask is all that is necessary for the performance of artificial respiration. Before using the mask the tongue should be well drawn forward, and, if necessary, fixed in this position by an ordinary piece of suture silk run through it, which can be held in the hand of the operator. If in any individual case the mask fails, an intubation tube may be introduced into the larynx. I do not believe that it is ever necessary to perform tracheotomy.

Dr. Fell's apparatus consists of a pair of foot-bellows by which air is forced into a receiving chamber, which is connected with an apparatus for warming the air, and a valve which can be opened and shut by a movement of the finger. This valve in turn leads to the tracheal tube. When the valve is opened the air rushes through the chamber into the lungs and expands them; the finger is lifted, the valve shuts, the lungs contract; and so the respiration goes on. I have no doubt that this apparatus is very efficient in practice, but it is open to the serious objection of being unnecessarily complex and costly.

A much simpler, cheaper, and probably equally efficient apparatus may consist simply of a pair of bellows of proper size, a few feet of India-rubber tubing, a face mask, and two sizes of intubation tubes; there should also be set in the tubing a double tube, with an opening similar to that commonly found in the tracheal canula of the physiological laboratory, so that it is in the power of the operator to allow for the escape of any excess of air thrown by the bellows. I suppose this whole apparatus could be prepared at the expense of less than five dollars, and it seems hardly necessary to point out the probable value of this simple apparatus in various narcotic poisonings, and other accidents in which death is produced by a paralysis of the respiratory centres, of temporary nature. The proper use of it could be taught to persons without special medical skill, so that it not only ought to form a part of the surgeon's outfit, but might be of great service in life-saving stations, about gas-works, etc.[1]

In conclusion, I may be allowed to state, that if the results and deductions arrived at in this address are, as I believe, correct, the rules for the proper treatment of accidents during anæsthesia can be summed up in a very few words:

Avoid the use of all drugs except digitalis and ammonia.

Give the tincture of digitalis hypodermically.

Draw out the tongue, and raise up the angle of the jaw, and see that the respiration is not mechanically impeded.

Invert the patient briefly and temporarily.

Use forced artificial respiration promptly, and in protracted cases employ external warmth and stimulation of the surface by the dry electric brush, etc., and above all,

---

[1] Messrs. Charles Lentz & Sons, Philadelphia, can furnish the apparatus for artificial respiration at a cost of $8.50.

remember that some at least, and probably many of the deaths which have been set down as due to chloroform and ether, have been produced by the alcohol which was given for the relief of the patient.

INTERNATIONAL UNIFORMITY IN ARMY MEDICAL STATISTICS.

An Address delivered before the Section of Military Hygiene, Tenth International Medical Congress, Berlin, August 7. 1890.

BY JOHN S. BILLINGS, M.D., LL.D.,
SURGEON UNITED STATES ARMY.

" CAN the sick-lists and sanitary reports in the different armies be made up after a pattern uniform at least in essentials, in order to obtain statistics which may furnish data of scientific worth for comparing diseases, wounds, and deaths occurring in the different armies in times of peace and war?"

In attempting to comply with the request with which I have been honored, that I should prepare a paper in answer to this question, I propose to consider the subject under the following heads :

I. What are the most important data which can be obtained for the preparation of such statistics?

II. What are the principal combinations of these data which have been given in army medical statistics heretofore published?

III. Which of these data, or combinations of data, are most important to the individual command or army, or country, for purposes of military administration?

IV. What are the most desirable combinations of these data for publication for the purpose of increasing our knowledge of the laws of health and disease by comparison of the mortality and morbidity statistics of different armies in times of peace and war?

V. What forms of returns and reports are best calculated to secure the data desired, as specified under III. and IV., *supra*, with accuracy, promptness, and completeness?

VI. Will it probably be possible to induce the different Governments to agree to a uniform system of publication of the data and combinations of data recommended as desirable in answer to question IV. ?

Let us consider these several points in the order stated, and for the sake of brevity and simplicity I shall first speak with regard to diseases only, and as to those occurring in times of comparative peace.

The data given in the reports of army medical officers relating to individuals taken sick or injured, relate to

1. Locality of the post.
2. Arm of the service, as $\begin{cases} \text{Artillery.} \\ \text{Cavalry.} \\ \text{Infantry, etc.} \end{cases}$
3. Rank—*i. e.*, $\begin{cases} \text{Commissioned officers.} \\ \text{Non-commissioned officers.} \\ \text{Privates.} \end{cases}$
4. Occupation prior to enlistment.
5. Length of service.
6. Age of the individual.
7. Race or nationality (including color distinction).
8. The date of occurrence of the disease or injury.

9. The nature of the disease or injury.
10. Complications and sequelæ of the disease or injury.
11. Results, including length of time of treatment required :
   a. Returned to duty.
   b. Transferred.
   c. Discharged.
   d. Invalided.
   e. Died.
   f. Otherwise disposed of.

Of these the most important in the order named are the nature of the disease or injury ; the result ; age ; date of occurrence of affection ; the number of days of treatment ; locality of the post or station ; the period of the year ; the length of service ; the arm of service ; rank ; race ; and occupation prior to service. To permit of comparisons and the calculation of percentages, there is also needed information as to the mean strength of the command during the period under consideration, with distinction of arm of service, rank, and color, and for some purposes with distinction of age, race, or nationality, length of service, and previous occupation.[1]

The following are the formulæ of some of the tables occupying the greatest amount of space in the published medical statistics of different armies. The data indicated by the letters are shown in the foot-note, the exponential figures after certain letters show the number of subdivisions of that item, thus : C (199) indicates that the figures are given for 199 different causes of admission to sick report. L (53), that they are given for 53 different localities, etc. The symbols to the left of the perpendicular line indicate the headings in the first or left-hand column of the table, while those to the right of the same line show the headings at the top of the remaining columns :

Austrian Army.

C. (194) $\begin{cases} \text{T. t.} \\ \text{D.} \end{cases}$ | L. (16) + A. S. (11).   4 pages quarto.

C. (194) $\begin{cases} \text{T. t.} \\ \text{D.} \end{cases}$ | $\dfrac{\text{A. S.}}{\text{L.}}$ 36 pages quarto.

---

[1] The following are the abbreviations used to designate these data in the formulæ of tables given hereafter :

A.	Age.
Ad.	Admission.
A. S.	Arm of Service : Infantry, Cavalry, etc.
C.	Cause of admission to treatment.
Col.	Color.
D.	Deaths.
Di.	Discharged.
D. t.	Days treated.
Du.	Returned to duty.
I.	Invalided.
L.	Locality.
L. S.	Length of Service.
M.	Months.
M. S.	Mean Strength.
O.	Occupation prior to enlistment.
O. d.	Otherwise disposed of.
R.	Remaining on hand.
Rnk.	Rank : Commissioned Officers, Non-commissioned Officers, Privates.
S.	Seasons.
T. d.	Total disposed of.
Tr.	Transferred.
T. t.	Total treated.

Bavarian Army.

C. (199) $R + \dfrac{Ad.}{M.} + \dfrac{T.d.}{Du. + D - O.d.} + R. + D.t.$
36 pages quarto.

L. (53) $M.S. + Ad. + D. + \dfrac{C.(37)}{Ad. \cdots D.} + Di. + I.$
10 pages quarto.

Belgian Army.

C. (24) $Ad. + T.d. + D. + D.t.$ For 22 localities in separate tables.
11 pages octavo.

C. (185) $Ad. + T.d. + D + D.t.$ 5 pages octavo.

British Army.

{ M.S.
{ C.(39) $Ad. + D. + (Di. + I.).$ Separate tables for 29 principal localities and many subdivisions of localities.
62 pages octavo.

A. (7) $M.S. + Ad. + D. + I.$
L.S. (8) $M.S. + Ad. + D. + I.$
A.S. $M.S. + Ad. + D. + I. + L.$ 40 pages octavo.

French Army.

M.S. $L. (377).$
C. (27) $\dfrac{L. (377)}{Ad. + D.}$ 45 pages quarto.
D.t. $L. (377).$
A.S.(10) $\dfrac{M.S.}{Rnk. (3) + L.S. (2) + A.} + Ad. + D.t. + I. + D.$
46 pages quarto.
C. (27) $R + \dfrac{Ad.}{Rnk. (3)} + L.S.(2) + T.t. + D.t. + A.S.(24).$
2 pages quarto.

German Army.

C (199) $R + \dfrac{Ad.}{M.} + \dfrac{T.d.}{Du. + D. + O.d.} + R. + D.t.$
15 pages quarto.

L. (319) $M.S. + A.d. + D. + \dfrac{C.(37)}{Ad. + D.} + Di. + I.$
53 pages quarto.

M. $M.S. + \dfrac{Ad.}{C.(37)}$ for each of 16 army corps.
46 pages octavo.

Italian Army.

A.S. $M.S. + Ad. + D. + Di. + D.t.$ 30 pages octavo.
C. (102) $L (93) + Ad.$ 12 pages octavo.
C. (102) $L. (93) + Ad.$ 12 pages octavo.

Netherlands Army.

L. (37) $\dfrac{C. (24)}{Ad.}$ 2 pages octavo.

U. S. Army.

C. (46) $\dfrac{L. (182)}{Ad. + D. + Di.}$ 74 pages octavo.

L. (182) $M.S. + \dfrac{C. (2)}{Ad.} + Di. + D.$ 20 pages octavo.

The principal combinations of data heretofore used in regular periodical reports, including both those relating to the sick and injured, and to all men of the command, are shown in the following tables, which indicate the data, and combinations of data, given in medical statistical reports of the Austrian, Bavarian, Belgian, British, French, German, Italian, Netherlands, and United States armies in recent years :

	Austrian army.	Bavarian army.	Belgian army.	British army.	French army.	German army.	Italian army.	Netherlands army.	U. S. army.
Mean strength									
×Age	0	0	0	0	0	0			0
×Arm of serv.			0	0					
×Length of serv.			0	0					
×Localities									
×Months									
×Occupation									
×Race									
×Rank						0			
×Age ×Arm of serv.									
×Age ×Localities									
×Arm of serv. ×Length of serv.									
×Arm of serv. ×Localities									
×Arm of serv. ×Rank									
×Length of serv. ×Localities									
×Months ×Race									
Admitted									
×Age	0	0	0	0	0	0	0	0	0
×Arm of serv.			0						
×Cause	0		0	0		0		0	0
×Length of serv.			0						
×Localities				0	0	0		0	
×Months	0					0			0
×Occupation	0								
×Race									
×Rank									
×Age ×Cause									
×Age ×Localities									
×Arm of serv. ×Cause									
×Arm of serv. ×Cause									
×Cause ×Length of serv.									
×Cause ×Months	×	×			×	0		0	
×Cause ×Occupation	×								
×Cause ×Race									
×Cause ×Rank									
×Length of serv. ×Localities									
×Localities ×Months									
×Months ×Race									
×Cause ×Localities ×Months									
×Cause ×Months ×Race									
Died	0	0		0	0	0	0	0	0
×Age		0		0	0	0			0
×Cause									
×Cause				0	0	0		0	0
×Length of serv.	0	0			0	0			0
×Localities	0	0			0	0		0	
×Months	0	0			0	0			
×Quarterly periods.									
×Rank									
×Religion	0	0	0		0	0	0		
×Age ×Arm of serv.	0								
×Age ×Cause									
×Age ×Localities									
×Arm of serv. ×Cause	0								
×Arm of serv. ×Length of serv.									
×Arm of serv. ×Localities									
×Arm of serv. ×Quart. periods									
×Arm of serv. ×Rank									
×Arm of serv. ×Religion									
×Cause ×Length of serv.									
×Cause ×Localities	0								
×Cause ×Months									
×Cause ×Quart. periods									
×Cause ×Race									
×Length of serv. ×Rank									
×Localities ×Localities									
×Localities ×Months									
×Localities ×Rank									
×Cause ×Cause ×Localities ×Months									
Discharged or invalided	0	0	0	0	×	0	0	0	0
×Age			0		×				0
×Arm of serv.	0				0	0	0	0	0
×Cause	0				0	0	0	0	0
×Length of serv.	0							0	0
×Localities									
×Months									
×Quart. per.									
×Race									
×Rank									
×Religion	0								
×Age ×Cause	0								
×Age ×Localities									
×Arm of serv. ×Cause									
×Arm of serv. ×Length of serv									
×Arm of serv. ×Localities									
×Arm of serv. ×Quart. periods.									
×Arm of serv. ×Rank									
×Arm of serv. ×Religion									
×Cause ×Length of serv.									

Left table

	Austrian army.	Bavarian army.	Belgian army.	British army.	French army.	German army.	Italian army.	Netherlands army.	U. S. army.
Discharged or invalided									
×Cause ×Localities				×					×
×Cause ×Months							×		×
×Cause ×Quart. periods.									×
×Cause ×Race					×				
×Cause ×Rank				×					
×Length of serv. ×Localities				×					
Returned to duty									
×Arm of serv.	o				o	o	o		
×Cause	×				×		×		×
×Localities						o			
×Months						o			
×Localities ×Months						×	o		
Total treated	o	o			o	o	o		
×Arm of serv.	o	×			×	×	o		×
×Cause	o	×		×	×	×			
×Localities	o						×		
×Months	o								
×Arm of serv. ×Cause	o								
×Arm of serv. ×Localities	o								
×Cause ×Localities	o								
×Cause ×Months									
×Arm of serv. ×Cause ×Localities	×								
Total disposed of									
×Cause	×				×				
×Localities							×		
Causes									
×Admitted	o	×	o	o	o	o	×		o
×Admitted ×Age		×							
×Admitted ×Arm of serv.									×
×Admitted ×Length of serv.							×		×
×Admitted ×Localities	×	×	×	×	×	×	×		×
×Admitted ×Months	×					×	o		
×Admitted ×Occupation	×								
×Admitted ×Race									o
×Admitted ×Rank					×				
×Admitted ×Localities ×Months							×		
×Admitted ×Months ×Race									
×Died	o	×	o	o	o	×	×	o	o
×Died ×Age	o	×			×	×	×		
×Died ×Arm of serv.		×			×	×	×		
×Died ×Days treated					×	×	×		
×Died ×Length of serv.	o	×			×	×	×		×
×Died ×Localities	×	×	×	×	o	×	×	×	×
×Died ×Months	×								×
×Died ×Quart. periods									
×Died ×Race					×	×	×		
×Died ×Rank									×
×Died ×Arm of serv. ×Localities	×								
×Died ×Localities ×Months		×							
×Duty: cured	o	o		o	o	o	o	o	o
×Disch. or inv.	o	o			o	o	o		×
×Discharged, etc. ×Age	×						×		
×Discharged, etc. ×Arm of serv.	×								×
×Discharged, etc. ×Length of serv.	×				×	×	×		×
×Discharged, etc. ×Localities				×					×
×Discharged, etc ×Months									
×Discharged, etc. ×Quart. periods							×		×
×Discharged, etc. ×Race					×				
×Discharged. etc. ×Rank	o				×				
×Total treated	o								
×Total treated ×Arm of serv.	o								
×Total treated ×Localities	×								
×Total treated ×Months	×								
×Total treated ×Arm of S ×Loc.									
×Days' treatment	×	o		×	×				×
×Days' treatment ×Localities									
×Total disposed of	×					×			
Ages									
×Mean strength				o	o				×
×Mean strength ×Arm of serv.				o	×				
×Mean strength ×Localities				o					
×Admissions									o
×Admissions ×Cause									×
×Admissions ×Localities				×					
×Died	o	o	o	o	o	o			×
×Died ×Arm of serv.				×					
×Died ×Cause	×				×	×	×		×
×Died ×Localities	×	×		o		×	×		o
×Disch. or inv.				×					o
×Disch. or inv. ×Cause	o	o			o	o	o		o
×Disch. or inv. ×Localities	×	o		×	×	×			×
Days' treatment	o	o		o	o	o	o		o
×Arm of serv.	×	o			×	×	×		×
×Cause	×	o		×	×	×			
×Locality		×							
×Months							×		
×Race							×		
×Cause ×Localities		×							×
Occupation									×
×Mean strength	×								
×Admitted	×								

Right table

	Austrian army.	Bavarian army.	Belgian army.	British army.	French army.	German army.	Italian army.	Netherlands army.	U. S. army.
Occupation									
×Causes	×								
×(Died, invalided, and discharged)	×								o
Length of serv.									
×Mean strength			o	o					×
×Mean strength ×Arm of serv.			o	o		×			
×Mean strength ×Localities							×	o	
×Admitted									o
×Admitted ×Cause									×
×Admitted ×Localities							×	o	
×Died	o	o	o	o			o	o	o
×Died ×Arm of serv.	×								
×Died ×Cause		×					×	×	×
×Died ×Localities	o	o		×	×	o	o	o	o
×Disch. or inv.		×							
×Disch. or inv. ×Arm of serv.	×								
×Disch. or inv. ×Cause		×					×	×	×
×Disch. or inv. ×Localities				×					×

In the above tables the cross indicates that the special data, or combination of data, indicated in the left-hand column, are given in the statistical reports of the medical department of the army indicated in the heading of the perpendicular column. The circle indicates that the data, though not given directly, are given in some other combination indicated by a cross in the same column. It will be seen, for example, that the important datum of age is only given for the mean strength of the commands in the periodical reports of the French, British, and United States armies, and that, therefore, it is impossible for all other armies to make comparisons as to the proportion of soldiers of each group of ages who are affected with disease or injury. The age-grouping of those taken on sick report is given only in recent annual reports of the British and United States armies; it is given for those discharged or invalided in the German, Italian, Bavarian, British, and American reports only; for those who died, in the German, Bavarian, French, Belgian, British, American, and Italian reports, and it is not given at all in any army medical report in relation to the average number of days of treatment. Moreover, the age-groupings used in different army reports do not correspond to each other, nor, which is more important, to the age-groupings used in published vital statistics of civil life, as will be seen by the following table:

TABLE SHOWING AGE-GROUPINGS IN DIFFERENT ARMY MEDICAL REPORTS.

Ages.	Bavar'n army.	Belgian army.	British army.	French army.	German army.	Italian army.	U. S. army.
11-15		×					
15		×					
16		×					
17	×	×	×	×	×	×	×
18							
19	×	×				×	
20	×	×				×	×
21	×	×				×	×
22	×	×	×	×		×	×
23	×	×				×	
24	×	×				×	
25-30	×	×		×	×	×	×
30-35		×		×		×	×
35-40		×		×			×
40-45		×	×		×	×	×
45-50	×	×		×		×	×
50-55	×	×		×		×	×
55-60		×					×
60 +		×					×

Keeping before us this bird's-view of what has been attempted in published military medical statistics, let us proceed to our third question, viz.: Which of these data, or combinations of data, are most important for local military administration?

Evidently they are those which show the actual effective strength of the command, and the causes of its diminution. The actual number on sick report, the number returned to duty, died, discharged or transferred must be given on the daily, weekly, and monthly reports for the immediate information of commanding officers. We need only consider the tables to be published, which will, for the most part, be yearly summaries relating to the total treated or excused from duty during the period to which they relate. The distinction between the "number admitted," the "number treated," and the "number disposed of" must be borne in mind, for these are not the same—they have different statistical uses and values—and cannot be directly compared with each other. The "number treated" includes the number remaining under treatment at the beginning of the period and the number admitted during the period. Those remaining under treatment at the end of the period are, of course, included in this sum. It is, therefore, greater than the "number admitted," and in most cases greater than the "number disposed of." The number of admissions may be either equal to, or greater or less than the "number disposed of," depending on the difference between the number under treatment at the commencement and the number remaining under treatment at the close of the period. The form of table most useful for these administrative statistics is one like the following, which

Station _____ Period _____
Mean strength of the command:
Officers _____ Enlisted men _____ Total strength _____

TABULAR LIST OF DISEASES. The names of diseases not printed below, and the number occurring during the month, will be written under the class to which they belong.	Remaining under treatment from last report.	Admitted.	Total treated.	Number of days' treatment.	Returned to duty.	Discharged or invalided.	Died.	Otherwise disposed of.	Remaining under treatment.
Smallpox Other acute contagious fevers									
Diarrhœa Dysentery Typhoid fever									
Malarial fever									
Venereal { Primary syphilis Secondary " Gonorrhœa									
Septic diseases									
Pulmonary phthisis Other tubercular diseases									
Etc.									

shows for the command the mean strength, number taken on sick report, number died, number discharged, number transferred or otherwise disposed of, average number of days sickness to each soldier, with distinction of certain causes or groups of causes.

Such tables may be given in more or less detail, for each month or year, for different localities, regions, ranks, arms of service, for those under and over one year in service, or for other units of military administration. The death-rates and discharge-rates may be given for these units, but for most individual causes of sickness or death the numbers are too small to make it worth while to calculate ratios except for groups including 25,000 men and upward, or for periods of five or ten years. The ratios derivable from half a dozen cases, or less than half a dozen deaths, are, for the most part, of little value, owing to the law of probable error in relation to number of individual data, although it would be easy to indicate possible exceptions to this rule. It appears to me that it is sufficient to publish details as to causes for separate posts and garrisons, and for months or seasons, by periods of five or even of ten years. The statistics of principal causes of disease in relation to locality would certainly have more scientific value if compiled for the longer period, in connection with the information derived from sanitary reports as to soil, climate, altitude, drainage, water-supply, buildings, duties of troops, etc.

The particular forms of disease of most interest in the administrative point of view, can best be discussed in connection with my fourth question, viz.: What combinations of these data are most desirable in publication for the purpose of making reliable and useful comparisons of the medical statistics of different armies in times of peace and war respectively?

These are the statistics which are to be published a long time after the events with which they are concerned have occurred, and whose importance, for the purpose of international comparison, is in proportion to the possibility of increasing by them our general stock of knowledge of the laws of health and disease.

We have to consider death-rates and sick-rates, mortality, and morbidity. As regards general or gross death-rates, they depend so much upon the proportion of discharges for disability, which in turn depend upon whether service is voluntary or compulsory, and for long or short terms, that for armies which differ in these respects no useful comparisons can be made. The death-rates from acute forms of disease in armies are much more valuable for purposes of comparison with each other and with the corresponding rates in civil life, but for the latter purpose they should be given by age-groups. The special value of army medical statistics for scientific purposes lies in the sick-rates, for these are our chief source of information with regard to the number of cases of disease occurring in a given number of adult males in a given time under different conditions of climate, locality, etc. General or gross morbidity rates in armies are not valuable for purposes of comparison unless they include substantially the same class of facts. Where the soldier is officially taken up on the sick report whenever treated by the medical officer, no matter for how short a time, or for how trivial a cause, or whether excused from all duty or not, the sickness-rate will, of course, be higher than where this is not the case. It is in the special sickness-rates and death-rates, due to certain diseases or groups of diseases, and in the relation of these to age, nationality, race, season, and conditions of environment, that the scientific value of army medical statistics chiefly consists.

What are these diseases or groups of diseases which are thus specially important, and the data for which should be rendered comparable in the published reports of different armies?

As regards individual forms of disease, the most important, and those for which the data are in most of the published reports given in more or less detail are the following, viz., smallpox, typhoid fever, diarrhœa, dysentery, malarial fevers, syphilis, gonorrhœa, pulmonary phthisis, pneumonia, acute bronchitis, tonsillitis, scurvy, alcoholism, diabetes, rheumatism, malignant tumors, mental disorders, and suicides.

Let us consider these briefly. The statistics of smallpox in an army indicate the relative completeness with which vaccination and revaccination are thus carried out among the men, and thus furnish a test of the administrative efficiency of the medical department, and a demonstration of the importance of these measures in civil life; but there is no probability that the army statistics of this disease will add materially to our knowledge of its causes, pathology, or treatment. It is useless to give details with regard to the cases. All that need be stated is the total number of cases, number of deaths, and the condition of the command, and of those affected, as to vaccination. The number of cases of typhoid fever, diarrhœa, and dysentery, form the chief test as to the character of the water supplies. Recent advances in bacteriology have made it improbable that the most elaborate statistics of these affections will materially increase our knowledge as to their causes or pathology, though the field is still open for the collection of data as regards sequelæ and treatment. Here again, then, the statistics must be considered to be chiefly useful as a means of measuring local efficiency of administration, and of testing results obtained in the laboratory.

With regard to typhoid fever there is one important question which might be answered from army medical records, and that is as to the amount, or proportion, of immunity conferred by the first attack of this disease. What proportion of men subjected to the influence of the specific cause of typhoid are attacked a second or a third time by this disease, at what ages, and at what length of time from the previous attack? To answer this question it will be necessary to make a special inquiry with regard to each man serving at a post in which typhoid fever prevails, noting whether he states that he has or has not had this disease, in case of an affirmative answer, when and where, and the duration and severity of the attack, his present age, and his length of service.

In many cases the answers would no doubt be vague or unreliable in themselves, but in many such cases, by referring to previous army medical records, or by correspondence with the physician who is said to have attended him, it would be possible to ascertain whether the disease was really typhoid or not. The results of such an inquiry can only be approximate, but they would certainly be interesting and valuable. By the system of card records, which will be described hereafter, the results of a series of years of experience on this point would be brought together.

The statistics of malarial fevers are chiefly interesting in their relations to locality and as contributions to geographical pathology. Differences of race, and especially of color where they occur, should be indicated in such statistics, but elaborate combinations of rank, length of service, previous occupation, etc., cannot be expected to increase our information with regard to these diseases.

The statistics of venereal disease in armies are of general as well as of local importance, since they furnish data from which to judge of the merits of various schemes which are proposed for their diminution in civil life. The statistics of scurvy, like those of smallpox, are merely a test of the efficiency of the administration of an army, and cannot be expected to add to our knowledge of this disease, except, possibly, as regards methods of treatment. The statistics of alcoholism, while chiefly important as bearing on local administration, have also a considerable value from a sociological point of view, and should be given in some detail by groups of ages, with distinction of rank and of arm of service, and, as far as possible, the results observed. The distinction between acute and chronic alcoholism should be insisted on.

For pulmonary phthisis, and, in fact, for tubercular diseases in general, the recent advances in our knowledge as to the essential cause enables us to put more definite questions than was heretofore possible, which may be answered, to some extent, at least, by army medical statistics. The prevalence of this disease in a body of troops taken in conjunction with the statistics of cases of inflammatory affections of the throat, such as tonsillitis, affords a very good test as to the efficiency of the ventilation of the barracks and quarters of the men. It is not meant by this to assert that defective ventilation is the only cause of these affections, but, whenever they are found to prevail in unusual proportions, it will usually be found that the men have been unduly exposed to a defective and impure air supply.

The number of cases of insanity and suicide attempted or effective which occur in an army are of special interest when the data are given in connection with distinctions of age, race, rank, and length of service. If given for comparatively short periods, as for a single year, the numbers are usually insufficient to do more than indicate points to be especially attended to in administration. It. is for periods of five or ten years that statistics of these affections are the most likely to be of scientific value and interest. The same may be said with regard to statistics of tumors of all kinds, and especially of the malignant forms of the sarcomas, myxomas, and true epitheliomatous growths. It is known that these occur in different proportions in different races and at different groups of ages. But there are many points in regard to this class of affections in relation to which an international statistic, derived from the records of the large armies of different countries for a period of years, indicating their relative frequency in different parts of the body, etc., would be of great interest.

(To be continued.)

ORIGINAL ARTICLES.

CLINICAL OBSERVATIONS ON DIPHTHERIA AND DIPHTHERITIC PARALYSIS, WITH SPECIAL REFERENCE TO TREATMENT.[1]

BY JAMES HENDRIE LLOYD, M.D.,

PHYSICIAN TO THE HOME FOR CRIPPLED CHILDREN, PHILADELPHIA.

DURING the last winter and spring diphtheria prevailed quite extensively in Philadelphia. It was probably not as virulent and fatal a type of the disease as has prevailed at some other times, but it nevertheless caused many deaths. Variations in its severity make it difficult to estimate with accuracy the merits of different plans of treatment, and may also have something to do with variations in the prevalence of one of the most formidable complications of the disease, namely, paralysis. Observation and inquiry have led me to believe that this particular sequela (or as I prefer to call it, complication) has been noted rather more frequently of late than in former years; but I do not infer from this fact that paralysis is a more common result than formerly, but, rather, that the complication in minor degrees is more readily recognized by the practitioner, because of the more general cultivation of neurological science.

Although more than twenty years have passed since Oertel announced that a micrococcus was always present in the membrane and in the blood of diphtheritic patients, and broadly stated that "without micrococci there can be no diphtheria," the time has not yet come for us to abandon the clinical for the bacteriological study of this important disease. The weight of opinion seems to be that the specific poison of diphtheria is either a bacterium or the ptomaine generated by it. This gives us at least a working theory, upon which we can hope to establish, if not a specific, at least an active and even aggressive treatment. For the rest we must be content to leave the, perhaps yet unsolved, problem of the exact form and habits of the specific microbe to the numerous workers in this field of medical research.

The pathology and morbid anatomy of diphtheria, especially in the cerebro-spinal system, while a question of great interest, is not one which will especially detain me. The action of this poison, whatever it is, upon nerve-tissue is so distinctly like that of other morbific agents whose action is fairly well known, that there is little doubt that it acts especially upon what Gowers calls the "lower segment" of the nervous system; that is, the large cells in the anterior horns and the nerve-fibres running out from them to form the nerve-trunks. That some observers have located the lesions in the horns and others in the nerve-fibres only furnishes additional evidence that these two parts form really one anatomical organ, and that the diphtheritic poison acts probably upon the whole. It might even be claimed on good clinical evidence that it is a general protoplasmic poison, which does not confine itself to one group of cells, just as arsenic, alcohol, and some other substances, whose effects upon nerve-tissue are not unlike those of diphtheritic poison, are known to attack many tissues of the body.

The similarity of action upon the peripheral nervous system of these several poisons seems to me to furnish some important indications not only for treatment, but, what is of equal importance, for prevention, and finally for prognosis. The clinical picture of a peripheral neuritis—with perhaps also an associated anterior poliomyelitis—is perfectly delineated in post-diphtheritic paralysis, and associates it at once with the general peripheral neuritis which in recent years has been so successfully studied. From this association we gain additional insight into pathology and some important hints in therapeutics.

If, in the first place, we may assume that a violent protoplasmic poison is being generated in the body, we have the first and I believe the most important indication, viz., to prevent its generation, as far as possible, by early local treatment. Secondly, having the lesions of a peripheral neuritis, we have some ground upon which to base an intelligent prognosis, and an efficient, although somewhat expectant, treatment.

As this scheme includes of necessity the treatment of the primary disease, I desire to offer a few observations on the subject.

Chlorate of potassium seems to be losing the confidence of the profession in the treatment of diphtheria, because it is known to have, in large doses, an injurious effect upon the kidneys. Some therapeutists even say that it is responsible for some of the deaths in this disease. It is probably a safe drug if given in doses aggregating less than a drachm a day to young children—the condition of the urine being watched. I speak of it now only to recommend as a substitute the chloride of ammonium. I have observed the use of this remedy in diphtheria for twelve years, and know of its successful use by another practitioner for a much longer period. Our knowledge of the effects of chloride of ammonium, as of chlorate of potassium, in a specific disease like diphtheria is mostly empirical, and on this basis I feel justified in saying that the former will do all that the latter drug can do and without its injurious effects. The physiological action, however, of chloride of ammonium[1] indicates, to a certain extent, its therapeutic use. It

---

[1] Read at the annual meeting of the American Neurological Association, Philadelphia, June 5, 1890.

[1] See Ringer's Therapeutics.

acts as a stimulant to the mucous membrane, increasing the normal secretion and so diluting and dissolving thick, tenacious mucus and fibrinous masses. That it has any true antiseptic action, either locally or in the blood, cannot be affirmed, and the same must be said of the chlorate of potassium in safe therapeutic doses. It is eliminated unchanged in the urine,[1] and without any apparent irritating effects upon the kidneys. The chloride of ammonium makes an admirable mixture with the tincture of the chloride of iron, and in combination with this invaluable drug constitutes a remedy for diphtheria in which experience has taught me to place an unusual degree of confidence. The tincture of the chloride of iron is in itself the one remedy which seems to hold its place in the esteem of every practitioner. Such universal testimony cannot be without great weight. It is most important that this remedy should be applied locally and thoroughly to the membrane. A mixture of one-half drachm each of the iron and of the chloride of ammonium to one ounce of a thick syrup (preferably of tolu) may be administered internally every two hours in teaspoonful doses, and at the same time a soft camel's-hair throat-brush is to be used to apply the mixture thoroughly to the diseased parts. It is not enough to direct the patient to hold the dose in the throat against the soft parts before it is swallowed. Many patients are too young to do so, and no one can do it efficiently. Internally it may be given every hour in bad cases, but the application by the brush every two hours, if done properly, is sufficient. It is very probable that the tincture of the chloride of iron is antiseptic when thus directly applied to the exudate, which we have reason to believe swarms with pathogenic organisms, while the chloride of ammonium, by increasing the mucous secretions of the throat and mouth, assists to dissolve and loosen this mass and promotes its expectoration. All evidence of value furnished by modern research tends to prove that diphtheria begins—and often continues for a long time—as a local affection. It is from this focus that the living germs of the disease gain admission to the lymph-spaces and bloodvessels. It is here that the distillation of protoplasmic poison probably begins, and it is here, reason teaches, that the disease must be combated with vigor at the very outset.

During the past winter I frequently tried the calomel treatment and have confidence in it, but I cannot say that I have seen as prompt results as from the treatment above described. I have usually given a fractional dose (¼ to ⅛ of a grain) every hour or two, according to the severity of the case. I do not believe it necessary or desirable to give the heroic doses recommended by some—5 grains every one or two hours. Such doses weaken the patient by the violent cathartic action almost always excited, and it is doubtful if more constitutional impression is made by these giant doses, as much of the substance is probably not absorbed. It is not certain that calomel acts thus locally as a germicide, and I am positive that its administration should be accompanied with an antiseptic wash or spray to the throat and nose. The substances which are useful for this purpose are boric acid, oxide of lime, sulphur, oil of eucalyptus, and carbolic acid, variously combined. The extract of pancreatin may be added on theoretic principles. In the use of the spray it is of the utmost importance that the nasal chambers be cleansed. To neglect this is to neglect half the field. Although I believe this treatment by calomel is good, I must say that I have seen an obstinate diphtheritic membrane which did not yield to it for a week melt away rapidly under the treatment by iron and ammonia above described.

The corrosive chloride of mercury appears on some accounts to be the model remedy for diphtheria, and it can be used both locally and internally. As an antiseptic spray it probably has no superior. It can be used as strong as 1 to 4000 (and in some cases stronger). The amount which thus enters the stomach is small and promotes the cure. It can be combined for internal use with the tincture of the chloride of iron ($\frac{1}{18}$ to $\frac{1}{12}$ grain in three to eight drops of the iron) and given every two hours. I think that the exceedingly small doses ($\frac{1}{96}$ to $\frac{1}{32}$ grain) recommended by some are of little use unless in the case of very young children. It is necessary, of course, to watch for symptoms of stomachic irritation.

It is not within the scope of this paper to present a complete statement of all forms of treatment which are approved by different authorities. Other germicidal agents than those mentioned are salicylic and carbolic acids and turpentine. The recent researches of Roux and Yersin[1] demonstrate again how important is the local, disinfecting treatment. As between the spray and the brush, I think that the latter is often the more effectual for the fauces, while the spray is necessary for the nasal cavities. Some object that local applications by the brush are irritating and alarming to very young children. In my experience they are not as much so as is the spray through the nose, and can generally be managed with a little tact. Medicated vapors in the room are too dilute to be of any importance.

---

[1] Parkes, quoted by Ringer.

[1] Revue Mensuelle des Mal. de l'Enf., abstracted in Arch. of Pædiatrics, April, 1890.

The recognition of diphtheritic paralysis as a toxic neuritis, caused by poisonous products of the local disease, demands that this set of symptoms be no longer regarded as a rare sequela of only special interest, but as part of the general symptom-group, some evidence of which may be found in very many more cases of diphtheria than is generally supposed. Bernhart, for instance, pointed out that the knee-jerk is abolished in many cases of diphtheria which do not exhibit distinct paralytic symptoms. This, as Gowers says, is only part of a broader fact. This fact, it must be emphasized, is that a toxic agent begins *early*, and probably in *all* cases, to threaten the integrity of the peripheral nervous system.

Another, and much more alarming symptom, is the heart-failure which so suddenly and with little warning sometimes terminates life. This is probably due to involvement of the vagus—at least, all the symptoms indicate such involvement. It is usually observed earlier than other paralytic symptoms, but it is a mistake to suppose that it never appears after them. I once observed the symptom in a case of multiple neuritis of alcoholic origin ; the patient, a woman, suddenly collapsed, and died in a few minutes of heart-failure. The following case illustrates this complication :

A boy, aged seven. The disease began with a chill and sore-throat. In a few hours a membrane began to form on one tonsil, and in two days had spread over both tonsils and the back of the pharynx. There were great enlargement of the glands, earache, and a purulent discharge from the nose. The calomel treatment was actively pushed, the throat and nose frequently sprayed, and careful attention given to his nutrition. By the end of the tenth day the membrane had disappeared, the glandular swelling was gone, the pulse was between 90 and 100, and the patient was convalescent. On the eleventh day he suddenly became sick and began to vomit ; had pain in the epigastrium, and grew deadly pale, while his pulse increased in frequency and was very small. Nerve and heart stimulants had not the least effect upon the symptoms. On the twelfth day he was inclined to play with his toys ; his vomiting had ceased, but the pallor and the feebleness of the heart continued. He suddenly screamed out with pain in his leg along the great vessels, and in a few moments was dead. I think the pain in his leg was caused by a dislodged embolus from the enfeebled heart.

Another case was seen by me for a fellow-practitioner who said that the child was convalescing from diphtheria. A change had occurred during the day, and when I saw the child she was almost pulseless, although the mother had noticed nothing. The patient died in a few hours.

In another case, in a rural district, as soon as the child was apparently well, the parents most unwisely took it out for a ride. When they brought it home it expired soon after being taken into the house:

In these cases there were no other paralytic symptoms. The force of the poison seemed to be exerted upon the cardiac apparatus, and, most probably, upon its nerve-supply. If these children had lived it is possible that some of them would have had paralysis of other parts.

In the general multiple neuritis of diphtheritic origin the prominent symptoms are often not noticed for several weeks after the disappearance of the primary disease. It is thus customary to say that they appear suddenly, and that the poison, whatever it is, has lain dormant in the system for a long time, but the observation of Bernhart, already alluded to, that the knee-jerk is absent in many cases, must make us cautious about accepting this opinion as final. I have had reason to believe that these symptoms have often been insidious in their approach, and hence unnoticed. If a child has only an abolished knee-jerk, and continues listless, the actual state may readily be overlooked ; even a slight nasal twang in its voice might escape notice ; until at last regurgitation of fluids, head-drop, and an ataxic gait force attention. I had a case recently which illustrates some of these facts :

A boy, aged five years, had extensive pharyngeal diphtheria, with swollen glands. He was treated with the chloride of ammonium and tincture of the chloride of iron internally, and the same remedies were thoroughly applied with a brush to the throat at frequent intervals. He made a good recovery, and had no nerve symptoms, unless it was the weakened patellar reflex. After an interval of five weeks he was again brought to me in a bad condition. He could not articulate clearly ; the soft palate was flaccid and rather anæsthetic ; the left eye had convergent squint (paralysis of sixth nerve). There was no paralysis to light or of accommodation, although the latter was not tested by near objects, as the boy could not read. He had head-drop, caused by paralysis of the muscles at the back of the neck ; there was loss of power in the forearms ; the patellar reflexes were abolished ; cutaneous sensibility was difficult to test. This child was admitted at once into the Home for Crippled Children, and under care and treatment recovered. On inquiry I found that the symptoms had been coming on very gradually. These were strangling, regurgitation of fluids, dropping of the head, and a staggering gait. When strabismus became marked the parents were alarmed and sought advice. There was probably no time after his supposed recovery from the diphtheria that nerve lesion in some minor degree, shown by abolished patellar reflex, ataxia, and nasal speech, could not have been detected by a more careful examination.

The lesson to be drawn from this case is obvious. The physician should not think his duty done when he has cleared away the membrane and established convalescence. If he remembers that he has had to combat a nerve poison, which in many cases shows its effects almost from the start, he will be guarded in his prognosis and more expert in detecting early symptoms.

The treatment of diphtheritic paralysis itself is mainly expectant. The nerve lesions demonstrated in the autopsies of these cases are degenerative—destructive; they are the lesions especially of parenchymatous neuritis—*i. e.*, destruction of the axillary fibre, segmentation of the medullary substance, and proliferation of the cell-elements in the nerve-sheath. The repair must be by a gradual and rather slow nutritive process.

The effect of drugs upon this process is at least problematical. Strychnine has been recommended, apparently because it acts as a violent excitant upon healthy motor-nerve cells, but why this endows it with a power to build up degenerated cells, both motor and sensory, has not been explained. Our knowledge of it is therefore empirical, and justifies its use in moderate doses. We may theorize that as an excitant to nerve tissue it excites nutrition, somewhat as a mechanical irritant will determine blood to a part, or as increased functional activity promotes structural increase. Clinical observations confirm the use of the drug. It has been used hypodermically with advantage, but I have seen ugly abscesses follow, which must be guarded against by careful antisepsis. Digitalis appears to be indicated in failing heart-power. I have used it in large doses when the pulse became feeble; but I doubt if it has the power to support a heart which is failing because of ptomaine poisoning of the nerve-elements. To do so effectually it would have to be antidotal to the noxious agent, and of this there is no evidence. I have not seen it act advantageously when cardiac collapse was sudden and marked. If digitalis acts upon the heart chiefly through the nerve-supply, as seems to be the fact, it may be that a depressed or degenerated state of these nerves in such cases hinders its proper action. Alcohol, as a more diffusible stimulant, is better than digitalis. The most important indication is to feed; or, as has been said, "to keep the bloodvessels and lymph-spaces full." There is some reason to believe that full bloodvessels are the best antidote to the infectious diseases and the best remedy for many of their sequelæ. The phosphates, especially the old formula of Parrish, are invaluable in the treatment of diphtheritic paralysis.

Electricity holds, I think, a rather uncertain position at present in the treatment of the acute degenerative paralyses which have a tendency to recover. The faradic current will not act at all upon a degenerated nerve, such as I have briefly described above; and it is worse than useless, because it deceives the patient and tends to bring reproach on a valuable therapeutic agent. And yet it is the one remedy to which the majority of laymen, and even physicians, naturally turn. It is not uncommon in the several forms of paralysis in children for the family to buy a small faradic battery, and, with the physician's encouragement, use it upon a flaccid limb which gives no response. It is a sort of talisman. To be sure, in mild cases, in which the nerve-fibres are not completely degenerated, a response may be had, but it is difficult to see how, even then, an agent which acts by such a momentary shock can advance nutrition. The same objection does not apply to galvanism, which acts upon both degenerated nerve- and muscle-fibre, and probably promotes nutrition, although we do not know just how. It is the current which should be used, but only by the physician, as, indeed, is apt to be the case, because it requires a more expensive plant, which is more difficult to use and to keep in order than the faradic machine.

In conclusion, I desire to call attention to the fact that diphtheritic paralysis can be mistaken for locomotor ataxia. As this is a grave error, especially affecting the prognosis of the case, and as it might reflect seriously upon the reputation of the practitioner, it is evident that the distinction should be emphasized more than is customary. I recently saw a case of diphtheritic paralysis in a man, in the practice of a friend, in which the resemblance to locomotor ataxia was so marked as to deceive one observer. In this case there was a history of a precedent "sore-throat." The man had numbness of the extremities, slight ataxia, abolished patellar reflexes, and some suspicious change in the pupils. The principal points of distinction were the loss of muscular power, flabby muscles, absence of fulgurant pains, ability to stand firm with closed eyes, and the history of his precedent diphtheria.

The changes in the pupils in diphtheritic paralysis are the opposite of those occurring in the "Argyle-Robertson" phenomenon of locomotor ataxia—*i. e.*, in diphtheritic paralysis the power of accommodation is lost to near objects and not the reflex to light. The onset of locomotor ataxia is more gradual than that of the other disease. In children the resemblance of the two affections is not so great, and locomotor ataxia in them is, of course, very rare, but in adults the symptoms may be confusing.

A CASE OF PORRO-CÆSAREAN OPERATION.[1]

BY J. F. BALDWIN, M.D.,
OF COLUMBUS, OHIO.

MRS. I. F. W., aged twenty-four years, weight 100 pounds, height 47½ inches. I was called to see the patient by her attending physician,

[1] Read at the meeting of the Ohio State Medical Society, june 5, 1890.

Dr. J. F. M. Heeter, July 12, 1889, and found a typically rhachitic dwarf, who was, according to her account, at about the full term of gestation. External and internal examination showed a uniformly contracted pelvis, with an antero-posterior diameter of about one and one-fourth inches. The case was manifestly one for the Cæsarean section, or some of its modifications, and it was agreed that the Porro operation was the best under the circumstances. The patient was quite intelligent, and placed herself unreservedly in our hands. Her hygienic surroundings were bad, as she lived with her husband in a cellar basement.

July 16, 10 P. M., I was called again and found her in labor. The pains were short and frequent and the os just beginning to open. Labor had commenced about five hours before. We ordered full doses of morphine, hoping thus to delay labor so as to operate by daylight. But in this we were disappointed. The pains continued to increase in frequency and severity, and by 2 A. M. of the 17th it was evident that longer delay would diminish the chances of recovery. The pains at that time recurred every three minutes, and the os was dilated to about the size of a twenty-five cent piece.

Accordingly, the operation was commenced as soon as the necessary assistants could be secured. Dr. W. H. H. Nash administered the chloroform, Dr. E. J. Wilson assisted directly, Dr. J. Leeper watched the pulse, Dr. S. L. Kistler held the rubber tube, and Dr. Heeter took charge of the infant.

The operation was performed after the method of Tait. While I had with me, for any emergency, my regular laparotomy case of instruments, I laid out: Two scalpels (one for shaving the pubes), a few hæmostatic forceps, two feet of pure rubber tubing, two knitting needles, ligatures, sponges, a drainage-tube and sutures.

As soon as the parts were cleansed and shaved an incision was made in the linea alba down to the womb, the incision being barely long enough to enable me to introduce my hand. The rubber tube looped between two fingers was then carried over the fundus and pulled down to the cervix, the fingers being carried around at this point to ascertain that no bowel had been caught. Everything then being in readiness, this tube was quickly tightened, a single hitch made, and the ends given to an assistant. The uterus was next incised, this small incision torn by the two index fingers to the full extent of the abdominal incision, a leg grasped and the child promptly delivered. Dr. Heeter at once seized the cord with compression forceps, cut it and proceeded to resuscitate the child. The placenta was then extracted through the wound, the womb lifted out of the abdomen, the rubber tube tightened and secured by a second hitch, the cervix transfixed by the knitting needles in the form of a St. Andrew's cross, and the body of the womb with the ovaries

and tubes cut off. There was no hæmorrhage from the stump, but there was some from the left broad ligament, which seemed to have been cut by the pressure of the tube. This hæmorrhage was easily controlled, though, owing to the poor illumination, it caused considerable delay. The bleeding point being finally secured, the abdomen was thoroughly washed out, a drainage-tube inserted, the incision closed in the usual way, and the stump treated with perchloride of iron. There was no perceptible shock, and the patient came out from the anæsthetic nicely. There was some discharge, for a few hours, from the drainage-tube, which was removed on the second day.

Convalescence was prompt and unmarked by any special occurrences. The highest temperature was 101°. The rubber ligature came away with the slough on the thirteenth day. Her milk came in small quantity at first, but soon became ample for the support of the child. In three weeks she was permitted to be removed to a distant part of the city and the case was virtually dismissed.

The child was a female and weighed at birth seven and a half pounds. Although inheriting the peculiar deformity of the mother, it thrived very well until April 6, 1890, when it became affected with angina Ludovici, of which it died two days later.

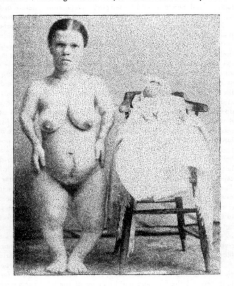

Remarks.—The fortunate result in this case is to be attributed almost entirely to the promptness with which operative procedures were instituted. As soon as it is determined that an operation is necessary and that the parts are in a proper condition, further delay is fraught with danger, and every hour of suffering and consequent exhaustion inflicted on the woman diminishes the chances of recovery. A very few hours of delay may suffice to turn a glorious success into a disastrous failure.

According to the statistics of Dr. R. P. Harris, of Philadelphia, this case ranks ninth among American Porro operations, and is the third successful one. It is the first in Ohio.

Tait is a strong advocate of the Porro-Cæsarean section, and under many circumstances, as when the operation has to be done at night, it is certainly the operation to be elected.; but when the circumstances are favorable I regard the Sänger-Cæsarean section as preferable, for two reasons : First, because its death-rate is lower ; and, second, because it does not in any way unsex the woman. But she should not be subjected to the risk of again becoming pregnant, and hence the Fallopian tubes should be ligated and cut across before the abdomen is closed.

But the Porro operation is easier of execution. Tait says it is as easy as the application of the long forceps, and hence should be selected by operators not familiar with abdominal work.

The technique of the operation, as given by Tait, is as follows :

"The first step is the abdominal incision, four inches in length, involving first the skin and then the muscles down to the sheath of the rectus, all of which ought to be divided by a sharp knife at one blow ; then the tendon of one or other of the recti is opened, the muscular tendons fall aside, the posterior layer of the tendon is nipped up by two pairs of forceps and divided between them. The extraperitoneal fat is treated similarly, then the peritoneum is raised again by two pairs of forceps, a slight notch being made between them, and the moment this is effected air enters and all behind falls away. No director is required, nothing but an observant pair of eyes, lightly applied forceps, and a delicately applied, sharp-cutting knife. The finger is then introduced into the peritoneal cavity, and the relations of the uterus and bladder exactly ascertained. The peritoneum is then opened to the full extent of the four-inch incision, and the cut edges of the peritoneum are seized on each side by a pair of forceps and are pulled severally to the respective sides. No better retractors can be employed.

"The piece of India-rubber drainage tube, about eighteen inches or two feet long, is now held as a loop between the fore and middle finger of the left hand, and is by that means slipped up over the uterus and pulled down over the cervix, passing the fingers behind the cervix to see that coils of intestine are not included in it. One hitch is then made on the tubing when it has been got as far down as possible, and it is pulled as tight as is consistent with safety. The second hitch may be made in it, but what is far better an assistant keeps the tube on the strain, so that one hitch will be quite enough to effect the most efficient clamping.

"A small hole is then made in the uterus, just large enough to admit the finger. If it is possible, the position of the placenta may then be ascertained ; if not, the right forefinger follows its colleague, and between the two, by gentle rending, an aperture is made in the uterus and the leg of the child is seized. The fœtus is then carefully delivered feet first, and this, despite all the authorities to the contrary, is by far the best proceeding ; less blood is lost, and it requires but very gentle manipulation to release the head.

"As soon as the fœtus is removed, the placenta is sought for and removed similarly ; the uterus itself, being completely contracted by this time, is then pulled out of the wound and the elastic ligature is tightened once more and finally arranged round the cervix, and the second hitch is applied. The main details of the operation are now completed ; all that is required is to pass the needles through the flattened tube and through the uterus and out at the other side, forming a St. Andrew's cross, or two parallel bars, to support the weight of the uterus and the stump and keep it outside the wound. A complete toilet of the peritoneum is then made, not forgetting the anterior vesical *cul-de-sac;* stitches are passed in the ordinary way to close the wound accurately round the uterine stump.

"The uterus is now removed close down to the needles and strangulating rubber tubes, so as to leave a little tissue above. It does not do to run any risk of the ligature slipping off, though this is hardly possible after the needles have been passed carefully through the structure of the tube. A little perchloride of iron is then rubbed gently over the surface of the stump ; it is dressed with dry lint and some dry cotton gauze, an ordinary obstetric wrapper is put on, and the operation is at an end. The operation really takes very much less time to perform than it takes to describe, and, as I have said before, because the details must always be the same, it is an operation in which there can never arise any unforeseen or unexpected difficulty."

In connection with this I may be allowed to state that during the last year, and in addition to this Porro operation, I made three other laparotomies.

One for adherent ovary and Fallopian tube. The parts were torn loose, but not removed. The patient made a prompt recovery, the temperature never rising above 98.6° nor the pulse above 80. Drs. Wilson, Nash, and Adams assisted me.

A second for chronic salpingitis, with retroversion and universal adhesions. The operation was exceedingly difficult, great force being required to tear up adhesions. The tubes and ovaries were removed, the uterus, which was adherent in its abnormal position, was torn loose and stitched to the anterior abdominal wall. There was free hæmorrhage, which was with difficulty controlled. Patient made an excellent recovery. I saw her about six months later and found her in robust health and the uterus in normal position.

The third case was one of uterine fibroid with general adhesions, following repeated attacks of pelvic peritonitis. The relative dangers of hysterectomy and of removal of the appendages were fully presented to the patient, and she preferred the latter operation. The operation was quite difficult owing to the adhesions, but was successful. The patient made an excellent recovery, and reports, four months after the operation, that there has been no menstruation; that she is free from attacks of pelvic inflammation, and that the tumor is perceptibly reduced in size.

I was assisted in these last two operations by Drs. Walker and Morehead, of Plainfield, Ohio, and in the last by Dr. F. F. Lawrence, of Columbus.

A CASE OF PRURITUS UNIVERSALIS PRODUCED BY THE PASSAGE OF A BOUGIE.

BY ORVILLE HORWITZ, B.S., M.D.,

DEMONSTRATOR OF SURGERY IN JEFFERSON MEDICAL COLLEGE; CHIEF OF OUTDOOR SURGICAL DEPARTMENT, JEFFERSON MEDICAL COLLEGE HOSPITAL; SURGEON TO THE PHILADELPHIA HOSPITAL, ETC., ETC.

RECENTLY a case of pruritus universalis, produced by the passage of a bougie for the cure of a lesion in the urethra, presented itself to the writer, and so far as can be ascertained it is the only case reported to the profession where the passage of an instrument has been the cause of this most distressing disease.

The writer in the course of a large experience in urethral work has seen many cases of general and local, motor, sensory and secretory neurosis dependent upon lesions of the urino-genital apparatus; but he did not believe it possible, nor did he accept it as a fact, until repeated experiments with passing a bougie produced after each operation an attack of pruritus universalis, that it was due to the instrument.

E. B., aged thirty; single; merchant. Began to masturbate at fifteen years of age and continued to do so until his eighteenth year, when he discontinned the habit and indulged in frequent sexual intercourse. This he practised three or four times a week, cohabiting twice and often four or five times a night. States that he never had any venereal disease, has not indulged in the use of intoxicating liquors, and is not a smoker.

About one year before presenting himself for treatment he began to suffer from pain in the back and nucha; later, there was burning pain on passing water, the burning sensation lasting a considerable time after each effort at micturition. He lost flesh, became morbid, irritable and restless, and sleep was unrefreshing and unsound. Heart, lungs, and urine normal.

On examination a contracted meatus and a stricture, calibre 20 F., just back of the orifice, were found. The most intense hyperæsthetic condition prevailed throughout the entire canal, especially in the prostatic portion.

The pain caused by the passage of the exploratory bougie was so intense as to produce slight epileptiform convulsions. The patient states that he had never before been similarly affected.

The meatus was enlarged and the stricture divided so as to admit the passage of a 35 F. meatus-bougie. The patient was directed to take a hot hip-bath every night before retiring; to pass a 35 F. meatus-bougie daily; to refrain from sexual intercourse, and to take sulphate of atropine, $\frac{1}{50}$ grain, with sodium bromide, 1 drachm, at bed-time.

At the end of three days he again presented himself. The burning pain after urination was much relieved; he was still suffering from pain in the back and head.

At this visit a bougie, 31 F., was passed into the bladder. Three days later the bougie was again introduced.

On the following morning an urgent message was received from the patient requesting the writer to call as soon as possible. On visiting the invalid's house he was found in bed, suffering agony from general pruritus, which had begun on the penis and scrotum and had gradually spread over the body.

To relieve the suffering every remedy recommended by the most reliable authorities was tried without any immediate benefit. Within the space of eight or ten days the pruritus gradually subsided, when a bougie was once more introduced, and the pruritus returned. A trip to Atlantic City was now recommended, and the patient remained at that resort for two weeks, when he returned, much improved in general health.

Up to this time no connection between the pruritus and the passage of the bougie had been suspected; it was presumed to be merely a coincidence. A bougie was therefore again introduced, when the terrible itching on all parts of the body returned in full force. At the end of five days, the pruritus having disappeared, the bougie was once more introduced, when the itching returned with undiminished vigor.

It now became manifest that the pruritus was entirely due to the passage of the bougie, and that the plan of treatment must be changed. A 6-per-cent. solution of cocaine was injected into the urethra, and having passed a Winternitz psychrophor, water at the temperature of 57° F. was introduced into the instrument, reducing the temperature of the water at the end of five minutes to 52° F.

A spinal ice-bag was applied to the lumbar region every night before retiring for the space of one hour, massage used every morning, and a Turkish bath once a week. Later, after the patient began to convalesce, the following remedies were prescribed: Sulphate of quinine, sulphate of iron, of each 2 drachms; phosphate of zinc, 2 grains; sulphate of strychnine, ⅔ grain: divided into 40 pills, of which 1 was taken morning and evening. Under this treatment the patient rapidly recovered. He has since married.

It would seem at first glance to be difficult to explain the sympathy that evidently existed between the irritability of the urethra and the irritability of the cutaneous surface, but reflection naturally leads to the conclusion that inflammatory lesions of the prostate gland bear the same relation to nervous affections of the male that lesions of the uterus do to allied disorders in the opposite sex.

The prostate and the structures intimately associated with it are largely supplied by nerves derived from the hypogastric plexus of the sympathetic, the several plexuses of the spinal nerves, and from the lumbar plexus through the lumbo-sacral trunk, and by reason of this free interchange of nerve fibres between the sympathetic and the cerebro-spinal system of nerves that the component parts of the genitalia are not only in intimate connection with one another, but, through the agency of the cord, with remote parts; hence it is that hyperæsthesia and inflammation of the prostate gland and its included structure, give rise not only to essential symptoms, but occasion various signs in other organs and tissues which are of a reflex or functional nature.

EARLY OPERATIONS IN PURULENT PERITONITIS.[1]

By JOSEPH PRICE, M.D.,
OF PHILADELPHIA.

In operations for purulent peritonitis, the results have been almost uniformly satisfactory. Dr. Bantock, in a late discussion, said that in opening the abdomen for these cases, he has been very much disappointed with the results. Possibly, he says, *he operated too late*, but *always* with unsatisfactory results—drainage did not seem to make any difference for *all* the patients died. Such an experience from such an operator, is a most telling argument for the early interference which he has advocated in other abdominal troubles.

No case of *general* puerperal peritonitis will recover without operation. Where there are simple inflammatory signs without localized mischief, which is the focus of the general trouble, recovery will follow general treatment. If there is pus in these cases, the necessity for early operation is as much

¹ Read before the American Medical Association, Section of Surgery, May, 1890.

to be recognized as in any other case or set of cases in abdominal surgery. There is but one treatment for suppurative peritonitis—section, irrigation, and drainage. Postponement is more dangerous than the operation, and at the worst only hastens a result which is certain to follow without operation.

In the *Medical Mirror*, May, 1890, is reported a case of general peritonitis, from appendicitis, in which the patient died on the thirty-first day. The results of delay are here too evident, when we take into consideration the numerous cases of appendical trouble, now relieved by prompt operation.

The late Lexington disaster, in which Colonel Goodloo lost his life, by a delay in operating of twenty-four hours, followed by another case in the same city, in which prompt intervention saved the patient, who is now active and well, is also a lesson in cases of this kind.

Further, to illustrate the subject, I introduce the following cases of my own. Other recent illustrations could easily be cited, but these are sufficient:

CASE I.—Mrs. B., aged twenty-eight years. Seen five weeks after labor. High temperature; rapid pulse; rapid progressive emaciation; profound sepsis. Abdominal section revealed, thickened omentum adherent over entire pelvis; right pyosalpinx and abscess the size of an orange in the ovary; universal adhesions; six inches of ileum cheesy and disorganized to the mucous coat along the line of adhesion on the right side. A knuckle of bowel was opened in enucleating the appendages; it was trimmed and stitched; there was purulent peritonitis, and one pint of pus free in pelvis, from leakage; appendages removed; cavity irrigated and drained; recovery.

CASE II.—Mrs. M., aged twenty-four years, seen twenty one days after labor. Abdominal section showed acute puerperal pyosalpinx on the left side, and general purulent peritonitis; bowel, omentum, and pelvic organs matted together by friable adhesions; left tube gangrenous; right tube congested, but showed no evidence of pus; only the left tube removed; irrigation and drainage; recovery.

CASE III.—Mrs. W., aged thirty-six; seen twelve days after labor; most profoundly septic. At the section universal friable adhesions were found; both appendages absolutely gangrenous; uterus large and soft, with cheesy walls; removal of both appendages; irrigation and drainage; recovery.

CASE IV.—Mrs. F., aged twenty-three; seen four weeks after labor; removal of both appendages for left pyosalpinx and ovarian cyst; right tube occluded, adherent, and acutely inflamed; adhesions universal; general peritonitis; irrigation and drainage; recovery.

CASE V.—Mrs. S., seen two years after labor. She had puerperal fever and was in bed nine months; since then has been a hopeless invalid, with loss of locomotion, constant agonizing pain, great emaciation, constant nausea and recurring attacks of peritonitis. I removed a left psyosalpinx and ovarian abscess; dense bowel adhesions; omenteum, bladder, and uterus glued together ; irrigation and drainage ; recovery from the operation and cure.

It should be noted that :

1st. All were cases of true puerperal " fever. "

2d. All were saved by section, after well-directed medical treatment.

3d. The operations were undertaken to save life, not to demonstrate ideal surgical procedures.

CLINICAL MEMORANDA.

MEDICAL.

Cancer of the Pancreas and Stomach in a Woman aged Twenty.—Clara L., single, was admitted to Dr. Morris Longstreth's wards at the Pennsylvania Hospital, February 20, 1890.

For the following notes of the case I am indebted to Dr. F. B. Gummey, the resident physician :

Patient's mother died of abscess of the liver, and one uncle of phthisis contracted during the war. Her family history was otherwise negative. She had never been robust, and after a wetting, four months before her admission, menstruation ceased, and since then she has suffered greatly from pains at the epigastrium, flatulence, and constipation. The pain had been so severe as to prevent her from sleeping. It was sometimes most severe beneath the left nipple, at others, on a level with the seventh dorsal spine. At other times she had severe lancinating pain along the fifth and sixth left intercostal spaces, but it was, for the most part, worse at the epigastrium than elsewhere. There had also been progressive emaciation and loss of strength. Tongue dry and coated. Patient very anæmic. Examination of heart and lungs negative. Urine normal.

Treatment.—Calomel and soda, and milk diet.

February 24. Vomiting and flatulence relieved, but pains unabated. No tumor can be felt in the epigastric region.

March 5. Passages chalky and liver dulness apparently diminished, but there is no jaundice.

7th. Cannot retain more than an ounce of milk at a time, which is given every hour; pain radiates to the right as well as to the left hypochondriac and lumbar regions.

15th. Passages somewhat more natural after taking chopped meat and a more liberal diet.

On March 28th it was noted that she had been taking one-quarter of a grain of codeine for the relief of her pains.

On April 14th it was noted that codeine, and even morphine, in doses of one-sixth of a grain, relieved the pain only slightly. The dorsal pain was intense, patient saying " that she felt as if some one were scraping her backbone with a knife." A distinct bruit was heard over the abdominal aorta close to the cœliac axis. No thrill nor excessive pulsations could, however, be detected. The left rectus muscle very tense, and sore to the touch. Peptonized milk was ordered, but, as it induced vomiting, it was discontinued.

April 15. Ordered peptonized beef, reduced iron, and Fowler's solution, three drops three times a day, on

account of the progressive anæmia. A systolic murmur was heard over the aortic cartilage.

22d. Pains unabated. At 2.15 o'clock this morning patient vomited about five ounces of blood. Up to this time she had neither vomited blood nor passed it by stool. Her pulse immediately became small and frequent, and she became dizzy, and had marked hallucinations of sight and hearing. She was given fluid extract of ergot one drachm, opium one grain, and ten minims of aromatic sulphuric acid, which she retained. Ten minutes later twenty grains of tannic acid were administered, which induced vomiting. Vomiting of blood recurred twice during the night.

While visiting the wards about noon of the following day, I was called in to see her, and found that she had another rather copious hæmorrhage from the stomach, and that her pulse was almost imperceptible. Whiskey was given hypodermically, and champagne was given by the mouth, and she soon rallied a little ; her pulse returned, and she was able to swallow and to retain milk in teaspoonful doses. Enemata of peptonized milk were ordered.

23d. She was a little stronger. Nutritive enemata and hypodermic injections of whiskey and of tincture of digitalis continued. Her stomach, however, retained nothing, so the champagne was stopped.

24th. Three more hæmorrhages to-day ; pulse imperceptible, somewhat delirious.

25th. Died, after a hæmorrhage, early this morning.

Autopsy showed that the head of the pancreas was firmly adherent to the greater curvature of the stomach, and presented distinct carcinomatous infiltration. In the greater curvature of the stomach, about midway between the pyloric and cardiac orifices, was a circular excavation, about three inches in diameter, the sides and floor of which showed carcinomatous infiltration. The liver was adherent to the stomach, and presented on its under surface one or two points of carcinomatous infiltration.

HENRY M. FISHER, M.D.

HOSPITAL NOTES.

LUPUS AND INFLAMMATORY NODULES ON THE FACE — DIFFERENTIAL DIAGNOSIS OF A CHRONIC INFLAMMATORY NODULE FROM EPITHELIOMA—INCIPIENT SCABIES— AND OTHER CASES.

Abstract of a Clinical Lecture delivered at the New York Post-Graduate Medical School.

BY ROBERT W. TAYLOR, M.D.,
PROFESSOR OF DERMATOLOGY AND SYPHILOGRAPHY.

CASE I.—The first case was that of a girl, seventeen years old, with a good family history. The eruption from which she was suffering followed a mild attack of scarlet fever at the age of nine years. "Blisters" first made their appearance, and subsequently developed into abscesses of the post-cervical glands. One or two of these abscesses were treated by incision. This history, Dr. Taylor said, was not uncommon. For eight years there had been a warty incrustation at the site of the original incision on the left side of the neck. On pinching up the patch of skin situated about three inches in front of the right ear (the " naso-labial zone "), it was found decidedly indurated and thickened; the skin was reddened, and the epithelium was shiny and cracked. This patch was oblong, and about one and a half inches long; and on its upper part were crusts composed of serum, epithelium, and sebaceous matter. The disease evidently involved the whole thickness of the skin.. The lesion pointed either to a late syphilide, or to lupus; but the history, and the absence of all concomitant symptoms, excluded syphilis; while the age of the patient, and the history, pointed indisputably to lupus. Lupus, Dr. Taylor said, usually begins before puberty, either at quite an early age, or between nine and twelve years. Formerly, lupus was considered as a scrofulous trouble, but modern medicine demands a more exact nomenclature; and since the discovery of the tubercle bacillus, clinical observations have furnished some reasons for believing that lupus is a localized tuberculosis. It is reasonable to suppose that the debilitated state of the system existing after scarlet fever, especially if complicated with cervical suppurative adenitis, offered a favorable opportunity for the entrance of such bacilli into the system; and clinical experience shows that the scars or unhealed wounds left after such an adenitis are prone to degenerate into lupoid tubercles. It has been claimed by some that the tubercle bacilli have been found in lupoid nodules, but equally competent observers emphatically deny this. These discrepancies might be explained by the well-known fact that the skin is not a favorable habitat for the bacilli, and that, consequently, they are not found in this tissue in large numbers.

Treatment.—Only external remedies are indicated. The crusts should be removed, and the underlying portions well curetted under cocaine, after which an ointment, consisting of one drachm of balsam of Peru to the ounce of vaseline, should be applied. Carbolic acid ointment might be substituted for this; or, if the patient were in bed, cotton soaked with a five-per-cent. solution of carbolic acid should be applied until the inflammation subsides, when the balsam of Peru could be employed.

CASE II.—The next case, a woman, thirty-three years of age, had on the tip of the nose an irregularly round, infiltrated, and ulcerated patch, which had existed for nine years, during which time she had enjoyed otherwise perfect health. The history, together with the non-destructive character of the lesion, excluded both syphilis and lupus; and the diagnosis rested between an inflammatory nodule resulting from the long-continued irritation of a pustule, and an epithelioma. The ante-auricular glands were slightly enlarged, but the cervical glands were normal.

Epithelioma, Dr. Taylor said, usually begins either as a minute crack, as a small wart, as a slight brownish discoloration of the skin, or as a small papule at the side of the nose, which bleeds freely upon irritation. The disease is sometimes of very slow growth, and exists perhaps for many years before showing its malignancy; but when this becomes manifest, the growth is found surrounded by a wall of distinctly thickened and slightly nodular tissue. In epithelioma of the face there is very slight glandular involvement. In this case there seemed to be no good grounds for believing that the lesion was more than a chronic inflammatory condition of the skin.

Treatment.—After thoroughly cleansing the part, it should be well curetted under chloroform or cocaine anæsthesia, and then irrigated with a five-per-cent. solution of carbolic acid. The subsequent process of healing should be treated on general principles; usually the balsam of Peru ointment is quite satisfactory.

CASE III.—The next patient was a man who, at first, appeared to have only a few patches of thickened skin in the interdigital spaces of the right hand; but other similar patches were found along the left wrist and forearm, with a few scattered papules on the abdomen. The eruption caused much itching. The lecturer said that the case was one of incipient scabies, and still in the papular stage.

Treatment.—His bedding should be entirely renewed, and clean clothes provided. After a thorough soaking in an alkaline bath, consisting of one pound of sal-soda to thirty gallons of water at 100° F., he should receive a thorough inunction with the following ointment:

Naphthol }
Balsam of Peru }   .   . of each 1 drachm.
Vaseline .   .   .   .   .   . 1 ounce.

This, in so mild a case, will probably be all that is required.

CASE IV.—The next case afforded an excellent study in diagnosis. The patient, a man twenty-four years of age, had had a hard chancre five months before, and still had a cervical adenopathy, with the remains of a roseola upon the body and shoulders. On the forearms were to be seen the lesions of psoriasis which had existed as long as the patient could remember; while, by a peculiar coincidence, the outer aspect of the arm was the seat of a syphilitic papular eruption of recent development. In the absence of such a clear history, one would have been inclined to consider the entire disease psoriasis. Another point of interest was the epithelial hyperplasia found on the sides of the tongue; for a few authors claim that psoriasis occasionally affects the mucous membranes.

Treatment.—This patient should receive the usual antisyphilitic treatment by baths and inunctions.

CASE V.—Another manifestation of syphilis, alopecia, next received attention. The man, thirty years old, was in the fifth month of his syphilis. The spots of alopecia were quite small, and did not present the shiny appearance of alopecia areata. There were papules and pigmented patches on the hands; round, ulcerated, and exfoliated patches upon the tongue; the throat was filled with ulcers, and the tonsils were much enlarged.

Treatment.—The patient was cautioned about conveying contagion by means of cups, tobacco-pipes, and similar utensils, and directed to spray and gargle the throat frequently. In severe cases of syphilitic sore-throat in hospital, Dr. Taylor directs the patient to gargle for fifteen minutes with a drachm of table salt to a tumbler of water, as hot as can be tolerated, and then to use the following strong gargle:

Bichloride of mercury .   .   . 8 grains.
Tincture of myrrh   .   .   . ½ ounce.
Water .   .   .   .   .   . 8 ounces.

When the ulcerative process begins to subside, the quantity of bichloride should be gradually reduced. The patches on the hands should be rubbed every night with mercurial ointment, and gloves worn during the night.

CASE VI.—Another patient, a Chinaman, forty-seven years old, who had had a chancre four years before, and had been pretty thoroughly medicated with the mixed treatment, presented himself with a non-ulcerating tubercular syphilide on the left side of the neck, showing decided thickening of the skin, and extending at the periphery in an irregular manner. This lesion belonged to the tertiary period.

Treatment.—Dr. Taylor directed the continued application of mercurial ointment, with frictions of the part, and the administration of the following:

Biniodide of mercury	. . .	3 grains.
Potassium iodide	. . .	6 drachms.
Comp. tinct. of cinchona .	. .	4 ounces.

One teaspoonful three times, increasing to four or five times, daily.

CASE VII.—A young woman was then shown with condylomata near the anus, which, if not treated, would extend and lead to ulceration, fissure, and stricture of the rectum.

Treatment. — The treatment should consist in the judicious use of mercury, if possible by inunction, and the careful washing of the patches with carbolic soap, followed by dusting with calomel and the application of cotton.

MEDICAL PROGRESS.

The Administration of Creasote in Phthisis.—From observations made on seventy-three cases of phthisis treated with creasote, DR. WILLIAM H. FLINT (*New York Medical Journal*, July 26, 1890) draws the following conclusions:

1. That intrapulmonary and intratracheal injections of creasote are of doubtful utility, and may be positively injurious.

2. That, for administration by mouth or rectum, solutions and emulsions of creasote are preferable in most cases to capsules, pills, or wafers.

3. That milk is an excellent vehicle for the administration of creasote in solution or in emulsion.

4. That each method of administering creasote used by the author—viz., by inhalation, by mouth or rectum alone, and by both the latter channels simultaneously—is useful, and may each be particularly adapted to individual cases. In suitable cases the most rapid progress seems to be made when all these methods are utilized.

5. That the best results for each individual attend the administration of the maximum quantity of creasote which this patient will bear.

6. That the average patient will not easily tolerate more than ten to fifteen minims of creasote *per diem* for any great length of time, and that many will only bear two or three drops *per diem*, continuously administered.

7. That it is very important that the treatment be uniform and uninterrupted.

8. That, consequently, an effort should always be made, if intolerance of creasote is shown by any one mucous surface, to employ some other channel of introduction, in order that the continuity of the treatment be not interrupted.

The solution used by Dr. Flint for inhalation was composed of equal parts of creasote, alcohol, and chloroform. The inhalers used were Dr. Robinson's and that of the Brompton Hospital. In mild cases the inhalations were given for fifteen minutes, every two or three hours, in severe cases every hour during the day, and every three hours during the night. Internally he at first used Jaccoud's mixture (creasote, 6 minims; glycerin, 1 ounce; whiskey, 2 ounces), but found that the creasote could not be given in large dose without administering at the same time more whiskey than, in many cases, was desirable. In some cases, too, it was not well borne. For these reasons he finally adopted an emulsion of cod-liver oil, 40 parts; mucilage of acacia, 60 parts; with 2 minims of creasote to each drachm. This was well tolerated, especially if given after food. In suitable cases the emulsion was given every two hours and increased up to the point of toleration. To patients who could be persuaded to adopt temporarily an exclusive milk diet the creasote emulsion was administered in the milk, being thoroughly mixed with the latter by energetic shaking. Dr. Flint succeeded in giving more creasote in this manner without exciting gastric disturbances than by any other method. In several cases twenty-four minims of creasote were daily given for several consecutive days.

Iodoform-emulsion in the Treatment of Tuberculous Joints and Cold Abscesses.—At the recent meeting of the German Surgical Association (*Centralblatt f. Chirurgie*, June 21, 1890), BRUNS of Tübingen, and KRAUSE of Halle, reported their results in the treatment of tuberculous joints and cold abscesses by means of injections of mixtures containing iodoform. Bruns uses a sterilized mixture containing 1 part of iodoform to from 10 to 20 of olive oil or glycerin, which is injected into the abscess cavity after the pus is evacuated. The operation may be repeated, if necessary, and usually within a few weeks or months the abscess diminishes, and finally disappears. Bruns has treated in this manner over 100 cold abscesses, among them 10 cases of psoas abscess, with 80 per cent. of cures. He has also used the method in the treatment of tubercular pleuritis, and in 50 cases of tubercular joint-disease, with surprisingly good results, even in cases of long duration. If there are fungoid, tuberculous granulations in or around the joint he inserts a hollow needle, breaks them up and injects in one or more places from 30 minims to 1½ drachms of the emulsion. If there is an abscess, the pus is withdrawn and the cavity filled with the emulsion.

Nearly all the surgeons who discussed this paper were in accord with the author. Trendelenburg said that he had treated 135 cases in this manner. Von Eiselsberg said that Billroth had practised the method with satisfaction in the treatment of cold abscesses and other tubercular diseases since 1881.

Krause reported 60 cases of joint disease treated by injecting a 10-per-cent. emulsion of iodoform in glycerin, or a mixture of iodoform in water of the same strength. In 36 cases of knee-joint disease there were 15 cures, in 15 of hip-joint disease 4 cures, in 6 of disease in the tarsus 1 was cured, and in 5 of disease in the joints of the hand 3 were cured. All of these cases were far advanced when the treatment was commenced. If there are abscesses around the joint, Krause evacuates them and washes out the cavities with boric acid solution before injecting the iodoform. The injections are made every two, three, or four weeks, according to the severity of the case.

Extemporized Surgical Gauzes. — HELBING gives the following recipe for the rapid preparation of surgical gauzes: Select a good material, free from oily matter, weighing about ten drachms per square yard, and having not less than thirty threads, running each way, in the square inch. Weigh out as much of the gauze as is required, and take a corresponding weight of the antiseptic. The material should be saturated with ether or with a mixture of ether and alcohol, in which the antiseptic has been dissolved, one ounce of the gauze requiring thirty ounces of solution. The gauze is wrung out several times and resaturated. In drying the gauze, it should simply be unfolded and shaken a few times. All the different gauzes may, in this manner, be prepared, as carbolic acid, corrosive sublimate, eucalyptol, iodoform, or thymol.—*Pharmaceutical Era,* June, 1890.

Injection of Filtered Air in the Diagnosis of Ruptured Bladder. — PROFESSOR KEEN suggests the following method (*Annals of Surgery,* July, 1890), which he has not yet used in practice, of determining the presence of a rupture of the bladder :

1. Introduce the catheter and empty the bladder of any urine that may be present.

2. Connect the catheter with an ordinary Davidson's syringe. This should have been disinfected. Over the distal end of the syringe a moderately large mass of absorbent cotton is tied. If the operator prefers, he can connect the distal end by a rubber tube, which has been padded with absorbent cotton, which may itself have been made antiseptic. The cotton in either case acts as a bar to the entrance of germs, as in the tubes of bacteriologists. Air is then pumped into the bladder. Should no rupture have occurred, the rounded, elastic, tympanitic bladder will appear in the hypogastrium. Should there be a rupture, the air will escape through the rent into the general peritoneal cavity, and distend the entire belly. It is, perhaps, even a needless precaution to have the air free from germs in carrying out this procedure, for, should the bladder be ruptured, laparotomy, of course, would be done, and the unfiltered air of the room would gain free access to the peritoneal cavity from the abdominal wound. If the bladder is not ruptured, the air pumped in would, of course, escape at once by the catheter, and have done no harm ; but it would be better to filter the air, and so exclude any possibility of infection.

Ear Reflexes.—DOWNIE (*Archiv f. Kinderheilkunde*) describes various reflexes having their origin in the ear, which are familiar to otologists, but, perhaps, not so well known by general practitioners. Cough, this writer says, may be excited by introducing unwarmed specula

into the meatus, and may also be produced by inspissated cerumen, especially if the mass is loose and changes its position during the movements of the lower jaw. This cough is often falsely called " stomach cough." Foreign bodies in the ear may produce similar phenomena. The author reports an example in which a phthisis-like cough with pulmonary symptoms disappeared after removing a plug of cerumen. Irritation of the external canal may cause gastric reflexes, such as vomiting. Aural polypi, as well as cerumen plugs, may excite irregular cardiac action, which rapidly disappears after removing the local trouble. Epileptiform convulsions may be due to the same causes, in proof of which the author cites a series of cases observed by himself.—*Archives of Gynæcology and Pædiatry,* July, 1890.

Violet Mouth-wash.—The following is said to be an excellent mouth-wash :

R.—Tincture of benzoin	.	.	7 parts.
" " rhatany	.	.	30 "
" " myrrh	.	.	60 "
" " orris root	.	.	500 "
Rose water	.	.	.	250 "
Alcohol	.	.	.	250 " —M.

—*American Practitioner and News.*

Treatment of Anal Fissure.—*L'Union Médicale* for June 28th gives the following formula for the treatment of anal fissure ;

Boric acid	.	.	.	.	45 grains.
Hydrochlorate of cocaine	.	.	15 grains.
Lanolin	.	.	.	.	1 ounce.

This is to be made into an ointment and applied to the fissure, after which the spot is to be touched with a solid stick of silver nitrate.

Lactic Acid Treatment of Diarrhœa. — HAYEM has recently reported before the *Société Médicale des Hôpitaux* the success which has attended his employment of lactic acid in diarrhœa. He prescribes the acid in the dose of 2 drachms in the form of a lemonade, made as follows :

Lactic acid	.	.	.	.	2 drachms.
Simple syrup	.	.	.	.	½ ounce.
Water	.	.	.	.	3 ounces.

To be drunk during the intervals between meals.

HAYEM thinks this particularly useful for the diarrhœa of typhoid fever, and in that form of lientery dependent upon *hypo*-acidity of the stomach. The same observer also recommends it as a cure, and prophylactic in epidemic cholera.—*L'Union Médicale,* June 28, 1890.

Salve for Alopecia.—MORWIN recommends, in *L'Union Médicale* for June 28, 1890, the following salve for alopecia :

Gallic acid	.	.	.	.	45 grains.
Essence of lavender	.	.	.	15 drops.
Vaseline	.	.	.	.	1½ ounces.
Castor oil	.	.	.	.	6 drachms.

This is to be well rubbed in at night over the part affected.

THE MEDICAL NEWS.

A WEEKLY JOURNAL
OF MEDICAL SCIENCE.

COMMUNICATIONS are invited from all parts of the world. Original articles contributed exclusively to THE MEDICAL NEWS will be liberally paid for upon publication. When necessary to elucidate the text, illustrations will be furnished without cost to the author.

Address the Editor: H. A. HARE, M.D.,
1004 WALNUT STREET,
PHILADELPHIA.

Subscription Price, including Postage.

PER ANNUM, IN ADVANCE . . . . $4.00.
SINGLE COPIES . . . . 10 CENTS.

Subscriptions may begin at any date.   The safest mode of remittance is by bank check or postal money order, drawn to the order of the undersigned.   When neither is accessible, remittances may be made, at the risk of the publishers, by forwarding in *registered* letters.

Address,   LEA BROTHERS & CO.,
Nos. 706 & 708 SANSOM STREET,
PHILADELPHIA.

SATURDAY, AUGUST 9, 1890.

THE TENTH INTERNATIONAL MEDICAL CONGRESS.

RECOGNIZING the interest which every member of the profession must feel in the proceedings of the Tenth International Medical Congress, now holding its meetings in Berlin, THE MEDICAL NEWS presents in this issue two of the most important papers read by Americans, and also a detailed account by cable of the meetings of August 4th, 5th, and 6th. The paper by Dr. Wood not only possesses a value of its own, but a peculiar interest in that it was the only address delivered before this representative body of medical men as the contribution of American medicine to the general fund of knowledge, while that of Dr. Billings is noteworthy because of its scientific bearing upon questions which are of peculiar interest to the Germans, and to all countries forced to maintain large armies.

The use of the cable also places in the hands of each reader of THE NEWS a report of the three most important days of the meeting almost before the Americans who attended the Congress have had time to digest the information to which they listened; and in the issue of August 16th we hope to present the proceedings of the closing days of the meeting in an equally readable form.

PERFORATION OF TYPHOID ULCERS.

IN the treatment of typhoid fever no danger is so much dreaded as hæmorrhage from the ulceration of a bloodvessel in a Peyer's patch, or the collapse which is sure to follow perforation of the intestine through the same morbid process. Everyone who has seen much of typhoid fever must have met with cases in which during advanced convalescence or in a mild period of the attack one of the accidents named above has occurred, and has felt that at last the case had been taken entirely beyond his control and that the patient was doomed almost without a single hope. Very recently before the Association of American Physicians, at their meeting in Washington, DR. JAMES E. REEVES, of Chattanooga, expressed the belief that he had seen recovery take place after perforation had occurred in enteric fever, and although others of wide experience, notably Dr. Loomis, of New York, expressed a doubt if any such cases were *bona fide* perforations, and if recovery ever followed perforation, several instances confirming the assertions of Dr. Reeves have been recently reported.

In the *Deutsche medicinische Wochenschrift* of December 26, 1889, DR. REUNERT reports three cases, all occurring in women under forty-eight years, in which during the course of enteric fever the classical symptoms of perforation occurred, such as collapse, violent pain in the belly, and a rapid, feeble pulse, with a great fall of bodily temperature. The vomiting was incessant, and palpation revealed a swelling in the right iliac fossa of considerable size, while constipation was present. In all these instances opium, small pieces of ice taken by the mouth, and the general measures devoted to the treatment of peritonitis occurring in a feeble subject were resorted to, and recovery ultimately occurred, the patients, after some weeks of convalescence, leaving the hospital entirely well. It would appear, therefore, that perforation of the intestine in typhoid fever is not necessarily fatal, although the vast majority of cases do not survive the accident.

Aside from the question which we have just been considering, another point of interest, of a surgical character, is not to be overlooked. Already surgeons have reduced the mortality of intestinal perforations arising from traumatic causes to a very low percentage, and a few of them have been bold enough to attempt such measures in the perforations we are considering. Although the results reached in most instances have not been encouraging, in certain picked cases we believe an operation to be perfectly justifiable, and, if the accident occurs during advanced convalescence from indiscretions in diet, to be absolutely indicated. Indicated, because the escape of pieces of hard food into the abdominal cavity places the patient beyond all hope of recovery, and because his physical state at such a time is sufficiently good to give a skilful surgeon at least a chance of saving the patient's life.

THE RECENT ELECTRICAL EXECUTION.

THE revolting details of the recent electrical execution have been so fully reported in the newspapers that more than an allusion to them in our columns is unnecessary. The results of this, the first execution under the guidance of science, will give the opponents of the method a powerful weapon, and, we fear, it is not improbable that the law requiring the execution of condemned murderers by electricity will be in consequence repealed. The enemies of capital punishment, too, will use the reports to endeavor to prove that no form of execution can be painless, and that the maximum penalty for murder should be imprisonment for life. From the daily papers we learn that our esteemed contemporary, the *Medical Record*, will editorially take this opportunity of denouncing all forms of capital punishment.

It must be remembered that the entire proceeding was in the nature of an experiment; that those in charge were nervous and apprehensive of failure, and thereby incapable of carrying out the verdict of the court with proper precision. Furthermore, it is probable that after the first shock the contortions of the victim were as painless as the legendary spasms of the frog's legs on Volta's copper railing. Sickening and revolting as the spectacle was, there is reason to believe that the death was less painful than is ordinarily that by hanging, after which muscular spasms often continue for many minutes. It has been claimed by the opponents of electrical execution that this method of punishment is brutal, but the measure of brutality should be the suffering of the victim, and no proof is available that death was not painless in this instance. We believe that the death penalty should be effected by electricity. Hanging has become so familiar to us that its brutality is forgotten. We forget that many a man on the gallows dies from *slow* asphyxia—than

which probably no form of death is more horrible. Electricity is a substitute not only better from the standpoint of simple humanity, but, as shown by Professor J. William White in a letter to this journal (April 26, 1890), is more likely to prevent crime. Dr. White's belief is that the criminal classes are influenced more by the probability of conviction than by the severity of the punishment, and that the number of convictions increases in direct proportion to the mildness of the penalty. The New York Commission to Investigate the Most Humane and Practical Method of Carrying into Effect the Sentence of Death reached the same conclusion, and reported that "any undue or peculiar severity in the mode of inflicting the death penalty neither operates to lessen the occurrence of the offence, nor to produce a deterrent effect."

It is, therefore, clearly evident that upon other grounds than pure humanitarianism capital punishment should be as painless as it can be made.

That electricity can be so applied as to cause instant and painless death no one can doubt who reads of the too frequent fatal accidents with broken "live wires."

One object of the new law, and a laudable one, is to limit the publication of the details of an execution to a simple statement of absolute fact. This has been entirely ignored—horrible, disgusting, and exaggerated descriptions were spread broadcast, descriptions that no one can read without a sense of degradation. For this publicity unfaithful servants of the law and the reportorial desire for the sensational are responsible.

It is greatly to be hoped from the standpoints of humanity, and for the checking of crime, that the State of New York will not hastily abandon the advanced position she has assumed in this matter, and equally desirable that before a second execution by electricity takes place, competent and cool-headed officials will be selected to carry into effect the verdict of the law.

The autopsy showed that the changes in the floor of the fourth ventricle were sufficient to cause death, and it cannot be doubted that death would have taken place without delay but for the too early order to stop the current. The misfitting of the head electrode was no worse than the misplacing or slipping of the hangman's noose, and the slight burning of the body of no more moment than the awful parchment-like blue line of the rope with the exophthalmic eye and swollen face.

(*By Cable.*)

SPECIAL CORRESPONDENCE.

INTERNATIONAL MEDICAL CONGRESS.

Tenth Annual Session.
Held at Berlin, August 4th–9th, 1890.

(*From our own Correspondent.*)

THE International Medical Congress was called to order in the Circus Renz, on Monday morning, August 4th, by the President, Professor Virchow. The beautifully decorated hall held 5000 representatives from all parts of the world, to whom Professor Virchow extended a most hearty welcome. In his opening address he called attention to the great advances in medicine, and to the value of international meetings in uniting the medical world in the struggle against disease and death. He further said that the object of medical associations should not be to get more pay or shorter hours, but to increase our ability for research, and to diminish the dangers that surround humanity. He expressed the Emperor's sympathy with the objects of the Congress, and said that Germany would devote herself to science and humane efforts.

Secretary Lassar reported that 5000 delegates were present, 2500 of whom were foreigners. Of all countries the United States takes the lead, with 500 delegates. England follows with 300. It was announced that there were 700 papers to be read in the three official languages, namely, English, German and French. This report was followed by addresses of welcome by Herr von Boettscher, German Minister of Education, and the representative of the Chancellor; Herr von Gossler, Prussian Minister of Ecclesiastical Affairs; Herr von Fordensbeck, the Mayor of Berlin, and by Dr. Graf, President of the German Medical Association. On behalf of the American delegation, Surgeon-General Hamilton thanked the Germans for their great hospitality; Sir James Paget tendered the thanks of the English delegates, Dr. Bouchard those of the French, and Dr. Bacelli then spoke for Italy, in a delightful Latin oration, that charmed the hearers and demonstrated that the dead language united all scientists. Tremendous applause proved how well the oration was appreciated.

The following Honorary Presidents were then announced: From the United States, John S. Billings, M.D.; Austria, Professor Billroth; England, Dr. Stokes; France, Professor Bouchard; Italy, Dr. Bacelli; Germany, Carl Theodore, Duke of Bavaria, who, though of royal blood, is a distinguished surgeon. Professor Virchow was made the permanent President and Dr. Lassar, the permanent Secretary.

Sir Joseph Lister then read a paper entitled "The Present Position of Antiseptic Surgery," in which he referred to Metschikoff's brilliant experiments in regard to the destruction of bacteria by the amœboid cells of living tissue, and showed how small particles of septic material are destroyed by leucocytes. He said that the work of Tait and Bantock is not opposed to the principles of antisepsis, but, on the contrary, that their cleanliness, and care in the preparation of instruments, sponges, and dressings show how well they follow the laws of antisepsis.

He believed in the use of strong antiseptic washes in all surgery except that of the peritoneum, where we should use solutions not stronger than 1 to 10,000, and in synovial membranes, where 1-to-4000 solutions are proper. The spray, he said, has no real value, and he hopes that the day may come when we will need little irrigation and no drainage. Floating particles in ordinary air, he thinks, can be disregarded. He recommended the double-cyanide gauze as the best dressing.

Dr. Robert Koch, the famous discoverer of the tubercle and cholera bacillus, followed with a paper on "The Present Status of Bacteriological Science." He thinks that the future will give us fixed ideas of the etiology of all infectious diseases, be they bacterial or not. He believes that species of bacteria are fixed and that one form cannot develop into another. In bacterial examinations he said that we must never depend on one characteristic, but should exhaustively test all the qualities. He described a new bacillus, very similar to that of tuberculosis, but showing slight differences, and though it had puzzled the author of the paper, it is now established that this new form is a distinct species which causes chicken tuberculosis. It seems now that the exanthemata are not due to bacteria, but, perhaps, to some organism similar to the plasmodium malariæ; but long and patient work and culture experiments must decide this point. The results of bacteriology are comparatively slight so far, but if the apparent results of his present work are true, bacteriology will be a greater science in the future. He has a new remedy by which he can check tuberculosis in the guinea pig, and can prevent even inoculations from affecting the animal; he did not say, however, what the remedy is.

Tuesday was devoted to the work of the sections. In the section of Internal Medicine the treatment of chronic nephitis was the main theme. An absolute milk diet and the administration of little medicine seemed to be in the opinion of all present the proper treatment.

The treatment of tubercular peritonitis by laparotomy was discussed very fully. No one seemed to have a clear idea of how a cure takes place after abdominal section, although according to the reports cure results in 30 to 60 per cent. of the cases. It was therefore thought that laparotomy is the best therapy if a diagnosis can be positively established. In the acute miliary form operation was, of course, considered of little value.

Terillon reported his results in resection of the stomach and intestine for carcinoma. His present position is that although so far no operation has resulted in preventing a recurrence of carcinoma, the patient's comfort is so much increased and his days so much lengthened that it is our duty to give him the benefit of an operation.'

At the second general session, Sir James Paget and Dr. John S. Billings presiding, it was decided to hold the next meeting of the Congress at Rome. The official records show an attendance of 5561 members. Of these there are 623 Americans, 421 Russians, 353 English, and 171 French.

Professor Bouchard, of Paris, then spoke for two hours on the "Mechanism of Infection and Immunity, and was followed by Axel Key, of Stockholm, on The "Relation of Puberty to the Diseases of School Children." Key has found that the year of greatest growth in boys is the seventeenth; in girls the fourteenth. While girls reach full height in their fifteenth year they acquire full weight at the age of twenty. Boys are stronger than girls from birth to the eleventh year; then girls become superior physically to the seventeenth year, when the tables are again turned and remain so. He stated that from November to April children grow very little and gain no weight; that from April to July they gain in height but lose in weight, and that from July to November they increase greatly in weight but not in height. These are the result of over 6000 observations. During the school months children suffer far more from disease than in the vacation, and during school years far more than before or after. Key thinks that usually school work is far too hard in the lower classes and that the children do not get sufficient muscular strength. Less school work and more physical training until the twelfth year are necessary to make our coming generation strong; and a child should not undergo any severe mental labor.

There is a splendid exhibition of medical and surgical appliances, in which all nations are represented. The place of the special sessions is the famous Art Exposition buildings, and no International Congress ever met in more beautiful quarters. The arrangements are perfect, and one hears nothing but praise from all foreigners. Very differently were the Americans treated who attended the British Medical Association, in Birmingham — over fifty withdrew their credentials on the second day, and nearly every American member resigned. The Americans are intensely indignant, especially so at

Mr. Lawson Tait. Further details concerning the action of these delegates will be sent in time for your next issue. Tuesday evening the city of Berlin gave a magnificent banquet to the foreigners in the city hall, and Wednesday evening there were banquets by the different sections. The delightful weather adds not a little to the enjoyment of the meeting.'

CORRESPONDENCE.

LONDON.

Nurses and Nursing. Operative Treatment of Pyæmia following Ear-disease. Legislation for Infant Life Insurance. The Amended Scheme for the new University of London.

Nurses and nursing have lately been much discussed. A few days ago the National Pension Fund for Nurses was formally inaugurated by a most successful gathering under the direct patronage of the Princess of Wales, when about a thousand nurses who have already enrolled themselves as members were present. The institution has made a most excellent start, a sum of something like £70,000 having been already accumulated, largely owing to the munificence of four donors of £10,000 each. Started almost contemporaneously with this is the Jubilee Institute for Nurses, which also has the advantage and benefit of royal patronage, for the Queen has graciously handed over the money received from the women of England in commemoration of her jubilee to found an institution for supplying trained nurses to the sick poor in their own homes. A very representative committee has been appointed to carry the scheme into effect, the medical element on it being Sir James Paget and Sir Dyce Duckworth, whilst at least two of the ladies on the council have had some years' practical experience in nursing. For several years past a private association has been carrying on work of this kind as successfully as its limited means would permit, so that the new undertaking starts with every prospect of a career of great usefulness and success. The profession of sick-nursing has become so popular in late years that almost all the leading hospitals have started nursing homes, and advertise their willingness to send out nurses to private cases. The fact is that this is a very satisfactory way of making money, as from one to two guineas a week are charged, which, of course, leaves a good margin for profit. Of course, the thing will soon be overdone, and there are indications that before long the market will be overstocked, but we have not yet quite reached that point.

In a former communication I alluded to Mr. Arbuthnot Lane's work on the subject of pyæmia consecutive to ear-disease and thrombosis of the lateral sinus. He has followed up his former paper with a note on pyæmia from otitis without thrombosis of the lateral sinus, and apparently his remedy is to ligature the internal jugular vein and occlude the sinus. He does not give the line of reasoning which led him to adopt the treatment, but it appears to have been successful. His patient was a child of three years, admitted for a left otorrhœa of three weeks' duration, and facial paralysis of that side for about the same length of time. A week before the patient came under observation the discharge ceased, the mastoid area became tender, and he had a rigor every day. On admisssion to the hospital there was a fluctuating swelling over the mastoid, some discharge from the meatus and facial paralysis; there was no optic neuritis. His temperature was 104°. Under an anæsthetic the mastold antrum, which was distended with pus, was obliterated by levelling down its edges, and the middle ear was freely opened, so that the dura of the middle fossa was exposed. It was thickened and inflamed, but there was no pus on it. On the evening of the following day he had a rigor, and the next morning the dura of the posterior fossa was fully exposed, and a collection of pus discovered between the lateral sinus and adjacent dura and temporal bone. Though the wall of the sinus was soft and doughy, there was no evidence of thrombosis. The child had a rigor that day and on the following day, and Mr. Lane then determined to ligature the internal jugular vein, and to open and plug the lateral sinus. The vein was thereupon ligatured, but the child became so collapsed that the subsequent steps of the operation were deferred. On the following day he had a rigor, and on the succeeding day Mr. Lane reopened the wound, and found that the sinus was firm, having evidently quite recently undergone thrombosis. From this time up to the date of the report, sixteen days later, the child did well, and his condition was, in all respects, satisfactory. Mr. Lane is certainly to be congratulated, for in the hands of a less courageous operator it is more than likely that the disease would have run its usual course to a fatal termination.

Two schemes are at present before the Legislature with a view to the better protection of infant life. That which is though to have the most chance of becoming law is the one introduced into the House of Commons, which makes more stringent regulations respecting baby-farming. The other is the bill of the Bishop of Peterborough introduced into the House of Lords, and at present passing through the ordeal of a preliminary committee. The bishop, who is certainly one of the greatest orators of the day, did not mince matters when introducing his bill, and did not hesitate to say that children were killed for the sake of the insurance money notwithstanding all the supposed safeguards of a medical certificate of the cause of death, or even a coroner's inquest. His proposals strike at the root of the whole matter, and, in my opinion, no scheme will be efficacious which does not follow pretty closely the lines he has laid down. The pith of his proposal is that the parents shall not directly or indirectly receive any money on account of the death of a child; they may insure its life as at present, but the amount insured shall be paid solely to the undertaker, and shall not exceed that necessary for the funeral expenses. It is rumored that there is very little chance of such a bill getting through the House of Commons, but I am quite sure that nothing else will really check the present great and growing evil.

The University of London, or rather the senate of that university, have promulgated their revised scheme for the re-constitution of the university, and it seems to be meeting with considerable support. University and King's Colleges have already accepted it, and it remains to be seen what the College of Physicians and Surgeons will do. Whatever they do must be done jointly. On the whole, the scheme seems to be as favorable to them as anything they are likely to get in any other way, for it provides that they shall conduct the examinations in conjunction with the university, but it is not made clear in what way the new examination is going to be more accessible than the old one. Two great causes of complaint against the existing scheme are the severity of the preliminary examination in scientific subjects, and the fact that a man cannot count any medical study toward his degree till he has passed this examination. These two facts do not seem to be in any way remedied, so I doubt very much whether the student will really be much better off. The scheme has not, however, yet been approved by all parties concerned.

NEWS ITEMS.

The Nova Scotia Medical Society.—The twenty-second annual meeting of the Nova Scotia Medical Society was held July 2d, 3d, and 4th, at Granville Ferry, Annapolis County. The following officers were elected for the ensuing year: Dr. J. A. Coleman, of Granville Ferry, President; Drs. Stephen Dodge, of Halifax, and G. E. Buckley, of Guysboro, Vice-presidents; Dr. W. S. Muir, of Truro, Secretary and Treasurer. Delegates were chosen to meet delegates from the New Brunswick and Prince Edward Island associations, with a view to a union of forces under the guise of a Tri-provincial or Maritime Medical Association. If such a union is effected, the membership will be not far from six hundred.

Mississippi Valley Medical Association.—The Mississippi Valley Medical Association will hold its sixteenth annual session at Liederkranz Hall, Louisville, Kentucky, October 8, 9, and 10, 1890. The medical profession is cordially invited to attend. Papers are solicited, the titles of which should be sent to the Secretary, Dr. E. S. McKee, 57 W. Seventh Street, Cincinnati, as soon as possible. The social arrangements are to be in keeping with Kentucky's well-known hospitality. The programme is already assuming proportions of magnitude and interest, and is still growing. The annual meeting of the American Rhinological Association will be held at the same place, October 6, 7, and 8, 1890. The Secetary, Dr. R. S. Knode, National Bank Building, Omaha, Nebraska, will receive titles to papers. Dr. John A. Wyeth, of New York, and Dr. Frank Woodbury, of Philadelphia, have consented to read papers.

Medical Missions.—At a recent meeting in London the subject of medical missions was discussed. One of the speakers, a veteran official from India, stated that among the Asiatics no mission can be regarded as fully equipped unless it has a medical department. Medical skill is extremely important as a pioneer influence, and a physician will be able to establish a mission where others would fail to obtain a footing. The Indian government highly appreciates the work that has been done by the medical men who have gone among the wild tribes along the northern frontiers. Traders know of all these posts, and frequently travel a long distance to obtain medical assistance. In January, 1879, a very warlike tribe on the frontier made a raid on Tonk, which is in

British territory. The place was sacked and burned; but the hospital and the house of the medical missionary were spared, because half of the patients that had been treated there were members of the attacking tribe.

An Aboriginal Method of Preventing Over-population.— An editorial in the *Weekly Medical Review* describes the following curious method of preventing over-population as practised by the aborigines of Australia. The method, called the " mika " operation, consists in making an incision into the urethra, near the scrotum, with a flint knife, cauterizing the wound with hot, stones, and inserting wooden pegs to prevent closure during cicatrization. In some tribes it is said that all but about five per cent. of the male children are compelled to undergo the operation. In other tribes the operation is postponed until just before marriage.

Medico-Chirurgical College.—W. C. Hollopeter, M.D., has been elected Lecturer on Diseases of Children ; and Ernest B. Sangree, M.D., Director of the Histological Laboratory.

The Climax of Quackery.—An infamous example of quackery was recently brought to light in Milwaukee, in the prosecution of the " Gun Wa Medical Company." The supporters of this fraud have branches in several cities, in which they advertise that they have an eminent Chinese physician, Gun Wa, who is versed in the medical lore of the Oriental schools, and who has a remedy for every disease to which flesh is heir. This " physician " is generally some ignorant laundryman, who knows too little English to be able to communicate with those who would consult him. He therefore has an interpreter—in Milwaukee this was " Doctor " Jansen—and this " interpreter " does not know a word of Chinese. During the active operations of this swindle in Milwaukee, this alleged famous Chinese physician, Gun Wa, was personated by three different laundrymen. It is not easy to conceive of a more barefaced and impudent imposture than this, which has been practised with considerable success in several Western cities.

A Summer Camp for Boys.—On the southern border of Lake Asquam, in New Hampshire, midway between Centre Harbor and Plymouth, is a camp for boys who require out-door life. The camp is on high and dry ground, with fine views of mountains. The exercises embrace boating, swimming, tours of exploration, base ball, tennis, and other summer sports, always under competent supervision. The physical needs of each boy are studied, with a view to instruct him in the proper manner of breathing, walking, running, jumping, and other forms of athletics in his critical formative period. The plan was originated by Mr. William T. Talbot, of Boston.

The Medical Department of the University of New York.— The Medical Department of the University of New York has just issued its semi-centennial catalogue ; an interesting pamphlet, well illustrated with photogravures of all the new laboratory improvements. Our medical college annual announcements are too often not at all descriptive of their respective institutions, and this is a welcome departure from the old rule.

The New York Hospital Sunday Fund.—The collections on behalf of this fund in New York City, in 1889–'90, amount to $57,079, being the largest yet received. In the previous year the fund received $52,039 ; while in 1879, the year of the first collections, the receipts were $24,465.

OFFICIAL LIST OF CHANGES IN THE STATIONS AND DUTIES OF OFFICERS SERVING IN THE MEDICAL DE-PARTMENT, U. S. ARMY, FROM JULY 29 TO AUGUST 4, 1890.

With the approval of the Acting Secretary of War, leave of absence for ten days is granted CURTIS E. PRICE, *Captain and Assistant Surgeon.*—Par. 3, *S. O. 175, A. G. O., Washington, D. C.,* July 29, 1890.

OFFICIAL LIST OF CHANGES IN THE STATIONS AND DUTIES OF THE MEDICAL CORPS OF THE U. S. NAVY FOR THE WEEK ENDING AUGUST 2, 1890.

BLACKWOOD, N. J., *Assistant Surgeon.*—Ordered to duty in the Bureau of Medicine and Surgery.

WALES, P. S., *Medical Director.*—Ordered to duty in charge of the Museum of Hygiene.

OFFICIAL LIST OF CHANGES OF STATIONS AND DUTIES OF MEDICAL OFFICERS OF THE U. S. MARINE-HOSPITAL SERVICE, FROM JULY 5 TO JULY 26, 1890.

BAILHACHE, P. H., *Surgeon.*—Granted leave of absence for seven days, July 26, 1890.

HUTTON, W. H. H., *Surgeon.*—To proceed to Chicago, Ill., on special duty, July 24, 1890.

GODFREY, JOHN, *Surgeon.*—Granted leave of absence for thirty days, July 21, 1890.

PECKHAM, C. T., *Passed Assistant Surgeon.*—When relieved at Memphis, Tenn., to proceed to St. Louis, Mo., and assume command of the Service. July 9, 1890

DEVAN, S. C., *Passed Assistant Surgeon.*—Granted leave of absence for twenty-five days, July 15, 1890.

KALLOCH, P. C., *Passed Assistant Surgeon.*—Orders of July 5th, to St. Louis, Mo., revoked July 8, 1890.

WILLIAMS, L. L., *Passed Assistant Surgeon.*—Relieved from duty at Baltimore, Md., and to assume command of Service at Memphis, Tenn., July 8, 1890.

PERRY, T. B., *Assistant Surgeon.*—To proceed to Baltimore, Md., for temporary duty. July 17, 1890.

STONER, J. B., *Assistant Surgeon.*—Granted leave of absence for thirty days, July 21, 1890.

HUSSEY, S. H., *Assistant Surgeon.*—To proceed to Pittsburg, Pa., for temporary duty, July 18, 1890.

YOUNG, G. B., *Assistant Surgeon.*—Granted leave of absence for fifteen days, on account of sickness, July 12, 1890.

STIMPSON, W. G., *Assistant Surgeon.*—To proceed to Buffalo, N. Y., for temporary duty, July 12, 1890.

HOUGHTON, E. R., *Assistant Surgeon.*—To report to the medical officer in command New York Marine Hospital, for temporary duty, July 14, 1890.

PROMOTION.

MAGRUDER, G. M., *Passed Assistant Surgeon.*—To rank as such from July 12, 1890.

APPOINTMENTS.

HOUGHTON, E. R., *Assistant Surgeon.*—To rank as such from July 12, 1890.

BENEDICT, A. L., *Assistant Surgeon.*—To rank as such from July 24, 1890.

THE MEDICAL NEWS *will be pleased to receive early intelligence of local events of general medical interest, or of matters which it is desirable to bring to the notice of the profession.*

Local papers containing reports or news items should be marked.

Letters, whether written for publication or private information, must be authenticated by the names and addresses of their writers— of course not necessarily for publication.

. All communications relating to the editorial department of the NEWS *should be addressed to No. 1004 Walnut Street, Philadelphia.*

THE MEDICAL NEWS.
A WEEKLY JOURNAL OF MEDICAL SCIENCE.

| VOL. LVII. | SATURDAY, AUGUST 16, 1890. | No. 7. |

ORIGINAL ADDRESSES.

INTERNATIONAL UNIFORMITY IN ARMY MEDICAL STATISTICS.

An Address delivered before the Section of Military Hygiene, Tenth International Medical Congress, Berlin. August 7, 1890.

BY JOHN S. BILLINGS, M.D., LL.D.,
SURGEON UNITED STATES ARMY.

(Concluded from page 134.)

IT is impossible to publish the data for each individual form of the thousand and more varieties of disease which medical officers are called on to record, since to do so would occupy far more space than the amount of information thus obtained by the public would justify. We must, therefore, group the great majority of them according to some nosological system of classification ; and herein lies one of our greatest difficulties. There is no uniformity in the system of classification in use in different armies, and there is no system which is satisfactory to one who is familiar with the recent advances in pathology. Even as regards the nomenclature of causes of death, the terminology of which is much more limited than that which must be used by the army medical officer in recording cases of disease, there is no uniform classification adopted in different countries. That it is very desirable to secure uniformity in nosological arrangement is admitted by every one ; but is it possible to accomplish it ? In attempting to answer ·this question we must fully recognize the difficulties which exist in each country in the way of changing its present methods.

In the first place, it is desirable that the classification for each army shall be such that its results can be compared with those given in previously published medical statistics of the same army, and also, with the published mortality statistics of its own country. Any changes, therefore, which render such comparison impossible are undesirable.

In the second place, it is admitted that no system of nosology at present in use is satisfactory. and, therefore, if an absolutely uniform system is to be prepared and adopted it will require a change in the form of statistics of every country, and these changes should affect the forms in which the mortality statistics of civil life are published, as well as those of armies and navies.

Taking all these facts into consideration, as well as the general characteristics of human nature which lead a man to think that his own plans, or the system of his own country is the best—which characteristics affect those having charge of the organization of army medical departments very much as they do other men—and also the fact that in view of recent discoveries it would be unwise at present to attempt to classify from the etiological point of view quite a number of forms of disease, it seems evident that it is not worth while now to attempt

to secure a uniform and rigid system of nosological classification. When, however, we come to consider the forms of disease which are of the most frequent occurrence and which cause the greatest amount of disability and loss of life in armies, we find that it is not so difficult to suggest a system which will permit of comparison of the more important facts in the statistics of different armies.

If the data are given for each of the individual forms of disease above specified, we shall find that most of the more important difficulties have been practically overcome. For example, diarrhœas are included under one classification of diseases of the digestive organs, and in others in one of the sub-groups of the general diseases. In one classification phthisis pulmonalis is given under diseases of the respiratory organs, in another under the group of tubercular diseases, which in turn are classed with rheumatism. Tetanus is usually given under diseases of the nervous system, but if a new nosology were now to be constructed it would probably be placed with specific infectious diseases. Diabetes, or glycosuria, appears in one classification under diseases of the digestive system, in another under diseases of the urinary organs, in another under diseases of the nervous system, and in still others under the heading of general diseases. But if the data for each of these forms of disease are given separately it is possible to make all the comparisons which are desirable between the statistics arranged in these widely different forms of classification. The chief difficulty, of course, occurs in the class of what are termed general diseases. If we can agree upon the groups into which these are to be divided, and as to what each group shall include, there is little difficulty in arranging a scheme for the classification of the local diseases. Among these general diseases the statistics of the following should be given separately from any system of classification whenever they occur among the troops, viz., cholera, yellow fever, plague, spotted typhus, relapsing fever, cerebro-spinal fever, diphtheria, tetanus, and specific influenza, or grippe. Excluding these from the grouping in addition to the specially important individual forms of diseases previously considered we should have groups of the so-called general diseases something like the following :

1. Acute contagious fevers, including more especially the ordinary eruptive fevers, such as measles. scarlet fever, and rötheln.

2. Septic diseases, due to pyogenic bacteria or their products.

3. Tubercular diseases, including all forms, with the exception of phthisis pulmonalis, which is to be given separately.

4. Diseases due to animal parasites. such as trichinæ, worms, etc.

5. Diseases derived from animals or so-called zoögenous diseases—glanders. anthrax. etc.

6. Tumors and new growths.
7. Debility and other unknown or vague causes.

The classification of the local diseases would then be the usual one, excluding as before the individual diseases of special statistical interest. It would include diseases of the nervous system, of the respiratory system, of the circulatory system, of the digestive system, of the genito-urinary system, of the absorbent system, of the locomotor system, of the eye, of the ear, of the nose and throat, and of the integumentary system.

Let us now see how far it would be possible to obtain data, in accordance with the individual items and groups of this classification, from the army medical statistics heretofore published. This is shown by the following table:

DISEASES AND GROUPS OF DISEASES GIVEN IN DIFFERENT ARMY MEDICAL REPORTS.

	Austrian army.	Bavarian army.	Belgian army.	British army.	French army.	German army.	Italian army.	Netherlands army.	U. S. army.
Smallpox	X	X	X	X	X	X	X		
Enteric or typhoid fever	X	X	X	X	X		X	X	X
Acute contagious fevers		X	X	X		X		X	X
Diarrhœa			X					X	X
Dysentery	X	X		X	X	X		X	X
Malarial fever	X	X	X	X	X	X	X	X	X
Venereal diseases	X		X				X	X	
Primary syphilis			X						
Secondary syphilis		X	X	X	X				X
Gonorrhœa		X	X	X	X	X			X
Septic diseases						X			X
Pulmonary phthisis	X	X	X		X	X	X	X	X
Tubercular diseases							X		
Rheumatism		X	X	X	X	X	X	X	X
Diabetes and glycosuria						X			
Scurvy				X	X		X		
Alcoholism		X	X	X	X				X
Tumors and new-growths	X				X				
Malignant tumors	X				X				
Diseases due to animal parasites	X					X			X
Diseases from animals (zoögenous)									
Debility and other unknown or vague causes									
Mental disorders	X		X						
Suicide	X								
Diseases of the nervous system	X	X	X		X	X			
Tonsillitis		X				X			X
Bronchitis	X	X	X			X			X
Pneumonia		X				X		X	X
Diseases of the respiratory system	X	X	X	X	X	X		X	
of the circulatory system						X			
of the digestive system	X		X	X				X	X
of the genito-urinary organs			X			X			X
of the absorbent system			X	X					
of the locomotor system	X	X		X		X			X
of the eye	X	X		X	X	X	X	X	
of the ear			X		X	X			
of the integumentary system		X		X			X	X	X

The Belgian, British, Italian, Netherlands, and United States reports give only the number "admitted;" the Bavarian, French, and German reports give the number "admitted" and "total treated;" the Austrian report gives the "total treated" only.

Thus far, for the sake of simplicity, we have been speaking of the statistics of diseases only, not including injuries, and of those used in regular periodical reports in time of peace and not of those employed in setting forth the medical history of a campaign or war. As regards the general class of injuries and wounds of all kinds, the classification used in the regular periodical reports of the different armies is shown in the following table, the combinations with other data being substantially the same as those used in connection with the different diseases.

TABLE SHOWING INJURIES REPORTED FOR ARMIES IN REGULAR REPORTS IN TIMES OF PEACE.

	Austrian.	Bavarian.	Belgian.	British.	French.	German.	Italian.	Netherlands.	United States.
Burns		X							
Contusions									
Contusions and lacerations						X			
Contusions and sprains									X
Dislocations	X	X	X			X			X
Excoriations									
Fractures (not gunshot)		X				X		X	X
Fractures (including all)			X				X		
Frostbite	X	X	X			X			X
Heatstroke									X
Incised, lacerated and contused, and punctured wounds									X
Incised, punctured, and bit wounds						X			
Injuries					X				
Injuries, general				X					
Injuries, local				X					
Injuries, received in action									
Lacerations			X				X		
Luxations								X	
Shot wounds	X	X				X			X
Sprains		X				X			
Wounds (not including injuries)			X					X	
Sore from riding or walking		X				X			
Other injuries			X						X

The forms of statistics of wounds and injuries occurring in a campaign or war which have heretofore been given on the most extensive scale, are contained in the reports of the French Army in the Crimea, 1854–56, the British Army in the Crimea for the same period, War of the Rebellion, United States, 1861–65, and the statistics of the Franco-German war published by the medical department of the German army, for 1870–71. The data or combinations of data given in these reports with regard to wounds and injuries are indicated in the following table:

WOUNDS AND INJURIES.

	French in Crimea.	British in Crimea.	German army 1870–71.	U. S. army 1861–5.
Injuries of head	X	X	X	X
of face		X	X	X
of eyes	X		X	
of lower jaw				
of neck	X	X	X	X
of back and spine			X	X
of chest	X		X	X
of abdomen			Data beyond *abdomen* not yet published.	X
of pelvis				X
of sacro-lumbar region				
of iliac region and buttocks				
of inguinal region				
of perineum and genito-urinary organs		X		
of genital organs		X		X
of ano-perineal region	X	X		
of shoulder	X			X
of arm	X	X		X
of elbow-joint		X		X
of forearm		X		X
of wrist-joint		X		X
of hand and fingers	X	X		X
of hip-joint		X		X
of thigh	X	X		X
of knee-joint				X
of leg		X		X
of ankle joint		X		X
of foot and toes				X

Each group subdivided according to nature of weapon: 1, punctured and incised wounds; 2, shot wounds; 3, other injuries. And, again, according to parts injured, in: 1, flesh wounds; 2, fractures.

Giving for each class also—complications, sequelæ, and operations.

The statistics with regard to disease given in the above mentioned reports of campaigns, vary greatly in fulness and form of combination. In the United States report of the war of 1861-65, the figures are given for the total admitted for each of 152 causes, for each month, for each color, for each of twenty-four localities or regions with the corresponding number of deaths and discharges.

In the report of the British Army in the Crimea the data are given for the total admitted for each of 101 causes, for each month, with the corresponding number of deaths. The total deaths are also given by age-periods, and for each arm of service by months, and the discharges are given by causes and arm of service.[1]

In the report of the German army in the campaign of 1870-71, the data are given for twenty-seven diseases or groups of diseases, for each month, for each arm of service, with the corresponding deaths.

In the report of the French army in the Crimea, the data are given by months for the total admitted and treated for each of seven forms of disease, with the corresponding number of deaths and transfers.

TABLE SHOWING SPECIAL DISEASES AND GROUPS OF DISEASES GIVEN IN MEDICAL REPORTS OF CAMPAIGNS.

	British in Crimea. 1854-57.	U. S. army. 1861-65.	German army, 1870-71.
General diseases			
Infectious diseases			
Smallpox			
Diphtheritis			
Typhus			
Dysentery			
Cholera morbus			
Malarial fevers			
Fevers			
Rheumatic diseases			
Acute rheumatism of joints			
Consumption			
Scurvy			
Parasitic diseases			
Debility			
Other general diseases			
Diseases of the nervous system			
Diseases of the respiratory system			
Pneumonia			
Pleuritis			
Diseases of the circulatory system			
Diseases of the digestive system			
Diseases of the genito-urinary system			
Venereal diseases			
Diseases of the eyes			
Diseases of the ears			
Diseases of the integumentary system			
Diseases of the locomotor system			
Sore from walking or riding			
Other unknown or undefined diseases			

In statistics of disease and death an exceedingly important factor is age, and unless the data for certain individual causes are given by age-groups it is impossible to make such comparisons with the corresponding data relating to persons in civil life, or in other occupations, as are now required by scientific students of these subjects. We have no reason to hope that any substantial increase of our knowledge will come from mere gross sick-rates or death-rates, or from the proportion of deaths to cases for individual causes of disease. We

[1] The report also gives for each arm of service the length of treatment of fatal cases for six selected causes and the deaths by rank.

have already a vast amount of statistics of this kind, which have been and will be useful, but it is improbable that more tables of this kind will open any new paths to knowledge. If, however, we can obtain data of this kind with age and race groupings, I think that they will indicate some new fields of investigation, and furnish valuable information.

TABLE SHOWING THE NUMBER OF SPECIAL DISEASES, WITH COMBINATIONS, GIVEN IN MEDICAL REPORTS OF CAMPAIGNS.

	British in Crimea.	U. S. army, 1861-65.	German army 1870-71.
Number of causes	101	152	27
Admitted	0	0	0
Causes	0	0	0
Causes × Arm of serv.			0
Causes × Color		0	
Causes × Localities		0	
Causes × Months		0	
Causes × Rank			0
Causes × Arm of serv. × Months			0
Causes × Arm of serv. × Rank			0
Causes × Color × Localities		0	
Causes × Color × Months		0	
Causes × Localities × Months		0	
Causes × Months × Rank			
Causes × Arm of serv. × Months × Rank			
Causes × Color × Localities × Months			
Died	0	0	0
Causes	0	0	0
Causes × Arm of serv.		0	
Causes × Color		0	
Causes × Localities		0	
Causes × Months		0	
Causes × Rank			
Causes × Color × Months		0	
Causes × Color × Localities		0	
Causes × Localities × Months		0	
Causes × Color × Localities × Months			
Discharged			
Causes	(		
Causes × Color			
Causes × Arm of serv.			
Invalided	0		
Causes	0		
Causes × Arm of serv.			

Another factor in medical statistics the effects of which it is desirable to study in connection with certain forms of disease, is race. In armies which contain both white and colored troops, such as the British in India and the United States army, it is usual to give separate tables for each, and the only special precaution required is to give separately the data relating to white officers serving with such troops.

With regard to white troops, the regimental and corps organizations in most armies are such that the different races are to a great extent classed by regiments, as for example the Irish and Scotch, the Saxon and Hanoverian, the Hungarian and Bohemian, etc. In the United States army, men of all nationalities are mingled in each regiment, and being thus exposed to the same conditions as to locality, food, climate, nature of service, etc., the race data may become especially valuable when collected for considerable periods of time—say ten years—as indicating for certain races a tendency to, or comparative immunity from, certain forms of disease.

Statistics of previous occupations are of much more importance when applied to the results obtained in those countries where military service is compulsory for a certain period of time than in those where it is not. For the latter, as in England and the United States, the

only value of such statistics in times of peace is in connection with the data relating to recruits, and is sociological rather than medical. Where military service is
compulsory, if not on all adult males, at least on a certain proportion of them, the data of previous occupation,
although still chiefly valuable when taken in connection
with the data relating to recruits, have some value in
connection with the data relating to certain forms of disease such as phthisis pulmonalis, rheumatism and gout,
malignant tumors, and diseases of the circulatory system and locomotor apparatus. Such statistics are given
only in the reports of the Bavarian army so far as I have
seen, and in these reports the data of age are not given,
so that it is not possible to compare them with corresponding data obtained from civil life.

For scientific purposes it appears to me desirable that
the tables should deal chiefly with the total disposed of
and not with the total number treated. For administrative purposes it is, as I have said, desirable to know the
total loss of effective strength, which can only be done
by taking into account those remaining under treatment
at the end of the period for which the report is made, and
in the study of causes of disease in relation to season,
locality, etc.; the number of admissions for each cause is
the most useful factor, but the data to be used for advancing our knowledge of the effects of certain forms of
sickness in their relation to locality, season, age, race,
etc., should be derived solely from the completed cases.
For such completed cases, then, I would suggest that the
following combinations of data be given in the tables,
viz.:

Table A., showing for the total number disposed of by
certain causes and groups of causes, the number returned
to duty, the number died, the number discharged, the
number invalided otherwise disposed of, and the average
duration of treatment, with ratios per thousand of mean
strength for the total disposed of, and the ratio per thousand of all disposed of, for the deaths, discharges, and
invalided. This table should be made out for the whole
army for each year; it should also be made out for such
subdivisions of locality as may seem desirable in each
country for the total period under consideration; for the
total troops in each arm of service, and for each of not
less than five groups of ages. For each individual disease, and for each group of diseases adopted a table
should be given, showing, with distinctions of five groups
of ages and of under and over one year of service, the
total number of cases disposed of and the number of
deaths for each.

This table to be prepared:
1. For the whole army.   2. For each arm of service.
3. For selected localities.   4. For color and nationalities.

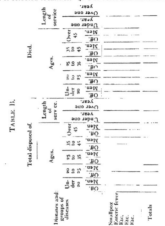

This table to be prepared:
1. For the whole army.   2. For each arm of service.
3. For selected localities.   4. For color and nationalities.

Table C.

Arm of service.	Mean strength by ages.					Mean strength by months.												
	Under 20	20 to 25.	25 to 35.	35 to 45.	Over 45.	All ages.	January.	February.	March.	April.	May.	June.	July.	August.	September.	October.	November.	December.	Total.
Infantry																		
Cavalry																		
Artillery																		
Etc.																		
Etc.																		
Total command																		

This table to be made for selected localities and for
the whole army.

Table D.

Diseases and groups of diseases.	Total admitted.	Admissions by months.											
		January.	February.	March.	April.	May.	June.	July.	August.	September.	October.	November.	December.
Smallpox.													
Enteric fever													
Etc.													
Etc.													
Totals													

Table A.

Diseases and groups of diseases.	Disposed of.													Average duration of treatment.	Total disposed of per 1000 mean strength.
	Total disposed of.		Re-turned to duty		Died.		Dis-charg-ed.		Inva-lided.		Other-wise dispos-ed of.				
	Off.	Men.	Off.	Men.	Off.	Men.	Off.	Men.	Off.	Men.	Off.	Men.			
Smallpox.															
Enteric fever															
Etc.															
Etc.															
Totals															

We now come to the question of the mode of obtaining the data for such statistical reports as must be prepared at the central office of the medical department of an army, whether these are intended only for the information of the central office and for that of the War Department, or for publication. There are two essentially different ways of obtaining this information. The first is to throw a large part of the work of statistical compilation upon the medical officers of the several posts or commands, requiring them to transmit periodical forms monthly, quarterly, or annually, on which forms are given the medical statistics of their commands for the period in question in greater or less detail.

The other is to require the medical officers to furnish the complete data with regard to each case to the central office, where the work of compilation is chiefly done, leaving to the medical officer of the post or command the duty of preparing such statistics only as are required for the information of his commanding officer or of the commanding officer of the department. The conclusion which has been arrived at in the Surgeon-General's Office at Washington is, that the second method is preferable, and our present forms are, therefore, prepared upon this basis. They are large sheets on which are given the name, rank, company, regiment, age, race, birthplace, length of service, cause of admission, date of admission, complications and sequelæ, result and date of disposal (specimen submitted) of each person taken on sick report during the period for which each report is made, and the name and identification data for each name remaining on sick report at the beginning of the period, without attempting to sum these up in all the various combinations of which the data are susceptible—merely the gross morbidity and gross death-rate being stated. When these sheets are received at the central office, the individual data are copied off on cards which are then assorted in all the different combinations which are desired. I see no good reason why all this information should not be furnished by the medical officers of posts and commands upon cards—one for each individual case, when completed by return to duty, transfer, death, discharge, etc. At the end of the year cards should be forwarded for all cases then under treatment, and subsequent cards should be forwarded for these cases when completed. Cards of different colors, or printed with different colored inks, might be used for classification in various ways. The use of individual cards or slips is now recognized by all experienced in such work as the most convenient means of securing all the various combinations desired in vital and medical statistics, with the least amount of skilled labor. If desired, much of the sorting of the cards can be effected by mechanical devices, or they can be punched, and any combinations counted by means of the Hollerith electrical apparatus for that purpose. When not required for statistical uses, these cards can be filed in the alphabetical order of the names of the men to whom they relate, and in this way the medical and surgical history of each case in which there have been successive admissions on sick report will be brought together.

From much practical experience with this card system of records, I can confidently recommend it as the best method of securing and compiling medical and surgical statistics, and of preserving in convenient form the

original data upon which such statistics must be based, and from which new combinations may hereafter be desirable. Herewith are presented the form of card used in the statistical division of the Surgeon-General's Office at Washington, and also the form upon which cases of injury or surgical operation are reported, together with forms of cards used in the Vital Statistics Division of the United States Census.

The great objection to relying exclusively on forms of reports compiled by individual medical officers, on which the detailed data for each individual are not given, is that they do not permit of numerous combinations which the statistician may desire to make when he has large numbers at his command, but which it is not worth while to provide space for in a form which is to be used for a single post or regiment.

For example, the form of monthly report of sick and wounded for administrative purposes proposed by Surgeon J. R. Smith, U. S. A., and approved by the Washington International Congress,[1] gives the data for individuals only for those dead or discharged, and it is, therefore, impossible to obtain from it with regard to those who do not die or are not discharged—i. e., the great majority of cases—the data relating to age, race, duration of treatment, rank, etc., in their various combinations, with different forms of disease at different seasons of the year, which it may be desirable to compile for scientific purposes. It appears to me best to use forms of this kind for administrative purposes, and in addition to use the card system, combined with detailed reports of the more important cases, as the chief reliance for the collection of data to be compiled for scientific purposes.

We now come to the last subdivision of the problem under consideration, namely: Will it probably be possible to induce the different governments to agree to a uniform system of publication of the data and combinations of data which are required to increase our knowledge of the causes and results of disease and injuries? It appears to me that the answer should be "Yes." It is not likely that uniformity can be secured in the forms of returns of sickness and injury which are chiefly valuable for administrative purposes, since these must depend largely upon the organization and mode of administration of the individual armies, upon the duties of the chief medical officers of corps or departments, upon the amount of centralization in administration, etc., and it is not worth while to lose the substance by grasping too insistently at the shadow. But if the central office can obtain, by some such simple method as the card system above referred to, the statistical data for each completed case, and can at the same time obtain the data with regard to the whole body of men among whom the sickness and injuries have occurred—the mean strength data, in other words—for the purpose of computing ratios, it can then make careful studies of individual forms of disease or injury for long periods in all their various relations, and this without in any way interfering with administrative statistics, or being fettered by rigid forms adopted without sufficient prevision of the points which future discoveries may show to have been of scientific importance.

[1] See Transactions Ninth International Medical Congress Washington, D. C., 1887, vol. i, p. 71, and vol. ii. p. 29.

To sum up then, Army medical statistics of scientific value relate mainly to individual forms of disease and not to nosological groups, and are to be derived from individual records of completed cases; they should cover longer periods than one year to give valuable results in medical geography, and should be given with more details as to age, race, length of service, and average duration of cases than have heretofore been supplied in published statistics of this kind. Absolute uniformity is not to be expected nor is it desirable, but such statistics of different armies can be made comparable with each other and with the morbidity and mortality statistics of civil life to a much greater extent than has been done heretofore. The object of this paper is to establish a few general principles upon which we can agree and in accordance with which we may work in the future, rather than prescribe precise forms or to criticise the details of those heretofore employed.

ORIGINAL ARTICLES.

SOME NEW BACTERIAL POISONS; THEIR CAUSAL RELATION TO DISEASE AND THE CHANGES IN OUR THEORIES SUGGESTED BY THEIR ACTION.

By VICTOR C. VAUGHAN, M.D.,
OF ANN ARBOR, MICHIGAN.

IN a paper[1] read in May, 1888, before the pædiatric section of the New York Academy of Medicine, I stated, as my belief, that the ordinary summer diarrhœa of infancy is not due to specific pathogenic microörganisms, but that it is due to putrefactive or saprophytic germs, which induce disease and death by the elaboration of chemical poisons in the intestines.

Able and skilful bacteriologists, among whom Booker in this country and Escherich in Germany deserve special mention, have made diligent search for the specific bacterium of summer diarrhœa, but no such organism has been found, and the probabilities are that it does not exist. The failure to find a specific germ has not arisen from the absence of bacterial species. On the contrary, the number of varieties and species has been confusingly great; but there is no constancy in the presence of any of them. In his first communication Booker reported the isolation of eighteen species, and he has subsequently added fifteen new ones to the list. Forms which appeared frequently one summer were wholly wanting the next. The large number and the great variety were not due to contamination, for the work was done with unusual care, the cultures being taken directly from the intestines of the sick child. Thus, it will be seen that in the case of this diarrhœa, which is so frequent during the hot season, and which has been diligently studied by a number of the best bacteriologists, the very first of

[1] THE MEDICAL NEWS, June 9, 1888.

Koch's rules has not been substantiated. In view of these facts the following question quite naturally suggests itself: "Are there not two or more germs which are capable of inducing this disease?" With the hope of answering this question I asked Dr. Booker to send me some of his cultures. This he did last February, and with three of these species I did the following work. The germs used are the X, a, and A, of Booker.

Flasks of sterilized beef-broth were inoculated separately with these germs and kept in the incubator at 37° C. for ten days. At the expiration of this time the contents of the flasks were filtered twice through heavy Swedish filter-paper, and during the second filtration the filtrate was allowed to drop into a large volume of absolute alcohol, which had been feebly acidified with acetic acid. A voluminous flocculent precipitate resulted in the filtrate from each of the cultures. After subsidence of the precipitate the supernatant fluid was decanted and the precipitates from the cultures of X and a were dissolved in water and reprecipitated with absolute alcohol. The precipitate from A proved to be so sparingly soluble in water that, after thorough agitation with water, it was caused to subside by the addition of a large volume of absolute alcohol.

The precipitates were then collected and speedily transferred to a vacuum and allowed to dry over either sulphuric acid or caustic potash. They are proteid in character, yet differ in character from ordinary proteids and from one another. That from a forms on the porous plate a scaly, dark substance, which is easily soluble in water. From its aqueous solution it is not precipitated by heat or nitric acid, alone or combined. It is not precipitated by saturation with sodium sulphate or by a current of carbonic acid gas, and, therefore, cannot be a globulin. It is precipitated by saturation with ammonium sulphate, and, consequently, we cannot call it a peptone. It gives the xantho-proteid and biuret reactions, and on the application of heat gives off the odor of burning feathers. The proteid from X is lighter in color and less readily soluble than that from a, but in the other reactions the two agree. That from A is practically insoluble in water. The chemical properties of these substances will receive further attention.

All are highly poisonous. Small quantities injected under the skin of kittens and dogs cause retching, vomiting, purging, collapse, and death. Ten milligrammes of the dried proteid from a killed a large guinea-pig within twelve hours. A much smaller amount proved equally fatal, but the time required was much longer. When very small, but unweighed, quantities were used, many days (from ten to thirty) passed before death followed. A small percentage of the animals experimented upon with the very small doses have remained permanently unaffected.

The post-mortem appearances in all the cases have been practically the same. The small intestines are pale throughout and tightly constricted in places. The heart is in diastole. Marked changes in other organs have not been observed.

These experiments show that three germs, which differ morphologically from one another sufficiently to be classified as different species, form poisons which also differ in their chemical properties, but which produce the same symptoms and post-mortem appearances. It must be remembered that no one of these germs is constantly present in summer diarrhœa. Sometimes X is found almost in pure culture, while in other cases this is absent and a or A abounds, and in a still greater number of cases no one of these three can be found and we have in their stead another or others of Booker's long list. These three were taken at random from the number which Dr. Booker has isolated, and it is probable that many more are equally powerful.

While X, a, and A differ morphologically, physiologically they are near akin. All are capable of producing powerful poisons. I propose that such germs be called *toxicogenic*. Not only do X, a, and A resemble one another in producing poison, but their poisons cause similar effects.

Germs, in their causal relation to disease, cannot be classified simply from their morphology; we must also understand their physiology; we must know something of the chemical changes which they cause by their growth.

Bacteria are divided into the parasitic and the saprophytic. The obligate parasite can live only on living matter; the obligate saprophyte can feed only on dead matter. The bacilli of leprosy and of syphilis are probably obligate parasites. They have not been grown on artificial media. True parasitic germs do not prove speedily fatal to their hosts. Their own continued existence depends upon the continued existence of their host, or on their transference to another host. Bacteriologists have taught that the true parasitic germs are the most deadly. This cannot be true. On the other hand, it is for the well-being of the saprophytic germ to destroy life, for in so doing such a germ furnishes itself with more nutriment and improves the conditions of its own existence. But, it will be asked, How can a saprophytic germ live in the human body and how can it prove fatal? The bacterium growing in the intestines of man does not necessarily feed upon living matter. The food before absorption is not endowed with vitality. Saprophytic germs will grow in the peptone preparations in the test-tube; why should they not feed upon peptones in the small intestines? The excretions passed into the intestines are not living, and upon these also, saprophytic germs may feed. Growing in the intestines saprophytic germs induce disease and death by producing chemical poisons which are absorbed.

These facts, if they be true (and their truth seems to me to be demonstrated by the facts shown above, that three different saprophytic germs produce poisons capable of causing the symptoms of summer diarrhœa, and death), materially alter the teachings of the bacteriologist. The tendency of such teachings has been for the past few years toward the belief that filth in and of itself cannot cause disease. That filth must be infected with some parasitic or specific germ in order to cause disease. is a doctrine which has met with acceptance. If my deductions from the above experiments be true, there is no specific germ in summer diarrhœa. All toxicogenic germs are dangerous when introduced into the intestines. They will there find an abundance of dead matter to feed upon. Not only is this true, but they will find that kind of dead matter which is best suited for their growth. It is generally conceded that saprophytic germs can only feed upon, or at least thrive best only in the presence of, diffusible proteid material. For this reason peptone is an important constituent of the nutritive gelatin which we use in our culture-tubes. In the intestines these diffusible proteids abound. Many of the saprophytic toxicogenic germs are anaërobic, and in this respect also, the conditions prevailing in the intestines favor their growth.

Again, if these deductions be correct, we have, in the question of the prevention of the intestinal diseases of childhood, quite a different problem from that presented by those who believe in a specific germ. We have to guard against the introduction into the child's stomach not of a single germ which abounds in certain localities, but we must protect the child from a whole host of toxicogenic germs which are widely and abundantly distributed. Milk infected with any one of a dozen different organisms may cause disease and death.

But, says one, if this be true. if there are so many possible causes of these diseases, how is it that so many children manage to live? The mortality must be admitted to be great, when we remember that more than one-fourth of the children born in the United States die before they reach five years of age. However, nature has not placed about infancy so many dangers without making some provisions to protect the child. In the first place, as has been shown by numerous experiments, the infant taking its food directly from the clean breast of the healthy mother gets its food wholly free from germs of all kinds. Moreover, both in infancy and in adult life at least one of the digestive secretions, the gastric juice, is a powerful germicide, especially destructive to those organisms which infect by the way of the intestines. So far as experiments have been made, there is no germ which is known to have a causal relation to an intestinal infectious disease and which is not destroyed by the action of a healthy gastric juice, when exposed to such action for only a few minutes, or for half an hour at most. As Escherich has shown, one of the great dangers in artificial feeding lies in the greater power of cow's milk to neutralize the acid of the gastric juice. Overfeeding is also an important factor in the production of the intestinal diseases of infancy. I believe with Bunge[1] that the chief office of the acid of the gastric juice is to protect us against infection through the intestines. Certainly every step in the process of digestion could be carried on without the presence of acid in the stomach. Even the digestion of proteids proceeds much more rapidly in the alkaline secretion of the pancreas than in the acid one of the stomach.

Again, we are probably to a large extent protected from the injurious effects of these poisons formed by the saprophytic germs in the intestines by the absorbing mechanism of the intestinal walls. We know that in health we are thus protected from the injurious effects of certain products of normal digestion. The proteids of our foods are converted into peptones, but there are no peptones in the blood, even in the portal blood. If peptones are injected into the blood they are poisonous. In health they are changed into serum-albumin and globulin while they are being absorbed. Now, these new bacterial poisons are proteid in character, as has been shown, and when formed in the intestines the only way in which we can be saved from their deleterious effects is by the action of the absorbing mechanism of the intestines upon them, converting them into harmless proteids. Right here lies the explanation of the greater susceptibility of the infant to these poisons formed by the saprophytic germs in the intestines. The rapid absorption from the intestines of the infant renders the passage of these poisons into the blood unchanged more easy and certain. In this is also to be found the explanation of the favoring influence of constitutional disease, and of prostration from heat, on the frequency and fatality of summer diarrhœa. Anything which lowers the general vitality of the child diminishes the normal resistance of the living cells to the proteid poison.

To conclude this part of the discussion, we may say that any germ which is capable of producing a poison in a flask containing a proteid material is not a safe one to introduce into the intestines. It is not necessary, in order to show the dangerous char-

acter of a germ, to prove its pathogenic property by inoculating an animal through the blood. In the blood the bacterium meets with very different conditions from those existing in the intestines.

The same general statements which I have made concerning the summer diarrhœa of infancy will, I believe, hold good in the case of enteric fever. I have recently reported the isolation of proteid poisons from cultures of two germs found in drinking-water supposed to have caused typhoid fever.[1] But, says one, the specific germ of typhoid fever has been found, and is the well-known Eberth bacillus. It is true that this organism is found in the spleen practically in every case of death from typhoid fever, and this is the sole evidence that we have of its relation to the disease. Continued fever with ulceration of the small intestines can be induced in the lower animals by a number of saprophytic germs. The great diversity in the symptoms and course of the continued fever in different sections of the country, and in the same locality at different times, seems to me quite an argument against the specific character of the disease. There is now fair promise of a satisfactory explanation of the true relations between the Eberth bacillus and typhoid fever. The bacterium coli commune is an organism which is constantly present in the healthy large intestine. In certain diseased conditions it finds its way into the internal organs. Typhoid fever is one of these diseases, and Rodet and Roux[2] conclude from their studies that Eberth's bacillus is only a degenerative form of the bacterium coli commune. Just what rôle this germ, by altering its place of residence, plays in the causation of the disease we do not know. But practically this observation is of great importance, because, if it be true, filth, in and of itself, may cause typhoid fever.

The fact that these new bacterial poisons may cause death, when injected under the skin in small amounts, after from ten to thirty days, is of great interest. We cannot believe that chemical poisons increase in amount in the body. They probably have a catalytic action, setting up a series of changes from which death results. The great majority of catalytic changes consist in the splitting up of complex molecules into simpler ones. Such a conversion is accompanied by the liberation of heat. In this we may have an explanation of the causation of fever in the infectious diseases. Some of the proteid of bacillus a was injected under the skin on the backs of two dogs. Retching, vomiting, and purging began within half an hour and continued for two days, after which the dogs slowly recovered. During these two days the dogs were much exhausted, and lay for the greater part of the time with their heads on

---

[1] Physiologische Chemie.

[1] THE MEDICAL NEWS, June 14, 1890.
[2] Comptes Rendus, February 21, 1890.

the floor, and shivering; but the rectal temperature during this time varied from 102.5° to 103.5°.

The following experiment was made with great care, but must be repeated before any positive conclusions can be drawn:

Two guinea-pigs were treated with hypodermic injections of one of these poisons. Within twelve hours both were dead. Plate-cultures made from the liver, spleen, blood, brain, and spinal cord remained sterile. Small quantities of the brain and spinal cord were rubbed up in a sterilized Petri dish with sterilized water, and a Pravaz syringeful of this emulsion was injected under the skin of each of four guinea-pigs. These animals seemed to be very excitable the next day, throwing themselves about violently in the cages when slight noises were made about them. Three out of the four have died, the first after sixteen, the second after eighteen, and the third after twenty days. This would indicate to me that the poison accumulates in the brain and spinal cord. However, similar experiments must be made with the blood and with emulsions similarly prepared from other organs of the body.

The following question has arisen in my mind: If these small cellular organisms, the bacteria, are capable of converting the ordinary proteids into such powerful poisons, why is it not reasonable to suppose that the glandular cells of our own bodies may under abnormal nervous stimulation or excitement also convert the ordinary proteids into similar poisons? Is the story of the nursing mother's milk becoming poisonous to the infant after great fright altogether unreasonable and wholly unexplainable? May not the hunted dog, when pursued and stoned, become rabid on account of the improper action of the cells of the salivary glands? These and other questions of a similar character quite naturally present themselves, and I have no doubt that in time a satisfactory answer will be found for them.

The discovery of these new bacterial poisons promises materially to alter our views of the nature of disease in many important respects.

Some four years ago Mitchell and Reichert[1] announced the discovery of poisonous proteids, a globulin and a peptone, in the venom of serpents. At that time their work was criticised, notably in Germany, on the ground that poisonous proteids were not believed to exist, but there can no longer be any such doubt. In 1888 Christmas[2] obtained from cultures of the staphylococcus aureus a proteid which, when injected into the anterior chamber of the eye or under the skin, caused suppuration. Haskins[3] has isolated from cultures of the bacillus anthracis a poisonous albumose. Very recently

Brieger and Fränkell have obtained from cultures of Löffler's bacillus of diphtheria a poisonous albumin which induces the paralysis and other symptoms of the disease, and which, when used in small quantity, produces death, sometimes after a period of twenty or thirty days. The same investigators have shown that similar bodies are produced by the germs of cholera and tetanus, and by Eberth's germ. Baginsky and Stadthagen[2] have found a poisonous proteid in growths of the summer diarrhœa bacterium, discovered by the former. These numerous investigations leave no room for doubt as to the existence and importance of these bodies. I have no doubt that they will prove to be the active agents in some cases of milk- and cheese-poisoning. Indeed, in the article which I read two years ago, referred to in the beginning of this paper, I predicted the discovery of new chemical poisons which would prove to be the active agents in the causation of the catarrhal diarrhœas of infancy. The new poisons which I have isolated from growths of the germs of Booker make good this prediction.

This paper would be incomplete if we did not look at another side of the question. While the harmful proteids play such an important part in the causation of disease, there are other proteids which serve to protect us against disease. The germicidal properties of the blood have recently attracted much attention. These properties have been shown to reside, not in the white corpuscles or other formed elements, but to be due to the presence and activity of certain proteids. This has been satisfactorily demonstrated by Büchner, Sittmann, and Orthenberger;[3] also by Fodor.[4]

Thus, it will be seen that the study of the proteids of the body and of those altered by bacterial growths promises to throw much light upon the causation, prevention, treatment, and nature of disease.

We may formulate the conclusions which are apparently justified by the present state of our knowledge, in the following propositions:

1. Man is attacked by the infectious diseases either through the alimentary canal or through the blood (or lymph).

2. The gastric juice is a physiological guard against infection by the way of the intestines.

3. Additional guards against infection by the intestines are probably to be found in the absorbing cells of the stomach and intestines.

4. Susceptibility to the intestinal infectious diseases is increased when for any cause these physiological guards are defective.

[1] Researches upon the Venom of Serpents, 1886.
[2] Annales de l'Institut Pasteur. 1888.
[3] British Medical Journal, 1889.

[1] Berliner klinische Wochenschrift, Nos. 11 and 12. 1890.
[2] Ibid., No. 13. 1890.
[3] Archiv für Hygiene. B. 10. H. ii., 1890.
[4] Centralblatt f. Bacteriologie u. Parasitenkunde. B. 8. No. 24. 1890.

5. All toxicogenic germs are dangerous when introduced into the intestines, and their capability of doing injury lies in their production of chemical poisons.

6. Many of these poisons are proteid in character.

7. These poisonous proteids most probably act by catalysis.

8. In the splitting up of complex molecules into simpler ones heat is liberated and fever manifests itself.

9. The physiological guard against infection through the blood or lymph lies in the germicidal action of the proteids of these fluids.

10. Susceptibility to infection through the blood or lymph is increased by impoverishment of these fluids.

11. We can continue to treat consumption and other systemic diseases by the employment of liberal diet, exercise in the open air, and constitutional remedies without being unscientific in our practice.

12. Filth, without being the bearer of a specific germ, is a cause of disease.

13. Wherever man pollutes the soil about him, the air which he breathes, and the water which he drinks, with his own excretions, there enteric fever will be found.

14. In their causal relation to disease, germs cannot be classified without a knowledge of the chemical changes which they induce.

15. While certain bacterial poisons can result only from the growth of certain germs, other poisons similar to one another in their action, though probably not identical, may result from any one of a number of organisms. In the former case we have such diseases as anthrax and smallpox, with their practically constant symptoms and well-marked course; in the latter case we have such diseases as the summer diarrhœa of infancy and enteric fever, with their varying symptoms.

PERMANENTLY GOOD RESULTS OF EXCISION OF THE MEMBRANA TYMPANI AND MALLEUS IN A CASE OF CHRONIC AURAL VERTIGO; ALSO IN A CASE OF CHRONIC SUPPURATION OF THE TYMPANIC ATTIC.[1]

BY CHARLES H. BURNETT, M.D.,
AURAL SURGEON TO THE PRESBYTERIAN HOSPITAL, PHILADELPHIA.

As two years and more have elapsed since the first of the two cases I narrate was operated upon and a year in the second case, I have considered the results as worthy the attention of this Society; because, no matter how good the immediate result of any operation may be, a just estimation of the

[1] Read at the annual meeting of the American Otological Society, Hotel Kaaterskill, July 15, 1890.

operation and its results can be formed only after the lapse of considerable time.

The case of chronic aural vertigo was operated upon in May, 1888, and a report of the case and the operation was read at the meeting of this Society, in July, 1888. Briefly recapitulated, the case was as follows:

Miss D., aged thirty-one, was first seen by me in November, 1881, the case being diagnosed as one of chronic catarrh of the left middle ear, attended with annoying tinnitus and with hearing of only six inches for isolated words. All known methods of treatment for such cases failed to relieve the deafness and tinnitus.

There was no aural vertigo at that time. I lost sight of the case for six years, when I received a letter from the patient stating that she was suffering greatly from tinnitus in the left ear and frequent attacks of severe vertigo, which at times obliged her to cling to a lamp-post or a similar object when she was attacked by vertigo in the street. Upon inspection of the ear in May, 1888, it was found that the malleus was adherent to the promontory, and the constant retraction of the chain of ossicles thus produced was deemed the cause of the tinnitus and vertigo.

The patient was etherized and the membrana tympani and malleus excised. The tinnitus and vertigo immediately ceased and have never returned. A new membrana tympani formed in this case in the course of two months and has persisted to the present time. The hearing has remained unchanged.

A letter from the patient a few weeks ago informs me that her health and strength, previously impaired, are now excellent, that the ear remains free from subjective noise, and that the vertigo has never returned. More than two years have elapsed since the operation which gave the relief. As far as I can discover, this is the first case of chronic aural vertigo (so-called Ménière's symptoms) reported as cured by an operation such as I have described. The case furthermore proves the mechanical origin, and not a neuropathic one, of many cases of so-called Ménière's disease, a point I have long contended for.

The second case was a typical one of that inveterate class, known as "attic disease," in which a chronic suppuration in the tympanic attic has its only outlet through the membrana flaccida, and in my experience always bids defiance to all modes of treatment heretofore proposed for its cure.

This case came under my observation two years ago, and gave the following outline of history:

The patient, a lady of twenty-three, stated that she had had some catarrhal symptoms in her nose, throat, and ears in childhood, and that the tonsils were deemed worthy of excision, and this was followed by earache and dulness of hearing in both ears. These symptoms soon wore off and were forgotten, excepting that the right ear, the one now suppurating, never heard well after the excision of the tonsils.

In 1882, six years before first consulting me, suddenly, and without previous warning of any kind, the right ear felt *stopped*. She says that examination by her physician at that time revealed a polypus in the right ear. The polyp was removed, and since then there has been a slight, nearly constant, offensive discharge from this ear, but hardly enough to flow from the meatus. In the meantime numerous polypi have been removed from this ear, probably from the region of the perforation in the membrana flaccida, by surgeons in this country and in Europe, but no permanent relief has followed these operations. This want of success was due to the fact that the treatment had been one of symptoms and not of the disease itself, which in reality was a necrosis of the head of the malleus, as shown by the operation I performed.

At the time I first examined the case the hearing in the affected ear was *nothing*. The membrana vibrans was found intact and dry, retracted, white, and shining; in the membrana flaccida there was a large perforation, through which the white neck of the malleus could be seen, and from which a scanty, sticky, offensive discharge came, clinging mostly to the upper wall of the external auditory canal. I, too, then proceeded to treat symptoms, as my predecessors in the case had done, and for one year I applied all known rational means of treatment to the case, by antiseptic injections into the attic cavity with the tympanic syringe, and by snaring off small polypi from time to time as they appeared around the perforation; but all without any good result, simply because I had not reached and could not get at the true disease in the attic, so long as the membrana tympani and the malleus barred the way.

Therefore, on July 29, 1889, the patient was etherized, and under illumination of the auditory canal by means of the electric head-lamp, as devised for Dr. Sexton by the River and Rail Electric Light Company of New York, the membrana tympani and the malleus were excised. The head of the malleus was found half destroyed by necrosis in its free anterior portion, its articular surface with the incus being normal. The other ossicles were not seen, but as far as could be decided by the probe, there were no necrotic spots anywhere else within the tympanic cavity—an opinion which was strengthened by the speedy healing of the diseased region after the operation.

Here, then, was the cause of the previously incurable purulent discharge from the attic space. The ligaments about the neck of the malleus were very tough and broad, and had acted as a diaphragm between the attic and the atrium, and also as the floor of a sinus running from the diseased malleus to the perforation in the membrana flaccida.

The steps of the operation of excision consisted in :

1. An incision behind the short process, with a slender blade.

2. Through this initial incision a round-pointed blade, curved in the plane of its broad surface, was introduced, and being kept close to the manubrium, below the insertion of the tendon of the tensor tympani, was pressed upward against the latter, and the tendon thus severed.

3. Then a straight blade, with rounded blunt end, was used to cut around the membrana tympani in the annulus tympanicus, thus entirely detaching it, and severing the hammer ligaments at the neck of the bone.

4. Instead of forceps the polypus snare was now used to seize the malleus, being passed around the manubrium, and the malleus with the membrana tympani was removed from the ear.

The slight hæmorrhage was controlled by mopping the fundus of the ear with a 4-per-cent. solution of cocaine muriate. During the operation the fundus of the ear was mopped frequently with a 2½-per-cent. solution of carbolic acid. After the operation the meatus of the canal was lightly tamponed with cotton sprinkled with iodoform, and left in place for twenty-four hours.

The next day the patient went about the house. The cotton tampon was slightly discolored on its inner end with a pinkish serum. There was no purulent discharge and there has not been any since the operation, nearly twelve months ago.

The iodoform tampon in the auditory canal was discontinued in four or five days, and one containing powdered boric acid sprinkled over it was substituted and worn for a week longer. Then simply a little cotton pellet was worn in the meatus, in the open air, to protect the exposed tympanic cavity. On some days the tampon was a little moistened with a serous fluid, but this soon ceased to appear. The absence of any reaction and the tendency to rapid healing in this case I am disposed to attribute largely to the antiseptic measures during and after the operation.

By August 12th there was no discharge of any kind from the ear. The hearing was found to be a little improved ; about a foot for loud words.

Aug. 19. Still no discharge. The mucous membrane of the promontory is pale and rough, but entirely dry. The region of the membrana flaccida is narrowing. Hearing equals a whisper at six inches.

The patient now went on a tour to the Adirondacks, *free, for the first time in seven years, from the annoyance of a running from the ear and the care it demanded.*

The patient was not seen again until September 25th, when it was found that a new membrane had formed from the segment of Rivinus, the region of the membrana flaccida, down to the promontory. There was no discharge. The hearing for whispered words, was two to three feet.

October 11. The delicate membrane, bluish and transparent, rises and falls under gentle suction with the pneumatic speculum. The hearing is *nine feet* for isolated words in ordinary conversational tone.

At the present time the hearing is fifteen feet for whispered words.

Here, therefore, is offered an account of a case of chronic purulency and deafness, caused by necrosis of the head of the malleus and altered tension and conductivity in the ossicles, cured of the discharge and the deafness by excision of the useless membrane and a necrotic malleus. The cure of the purulency is easily explained, but the improved hearing is not as easily explicable. I venture to suggest that the conducting power of the ossicles was interfered with by the presence of pus about the ossicles in the attic, and by the pathological bands about the malleus already mentioned, which prevented ready vibration. Also the diseased condition of the head of the malleus loosened its articulation with the incus, and impaired its leverage on the latter. Hence, a wave of sound falling on the membrana and malleus could not transmit its inward oscillations to the incus and thence to the stapes and the labyrinth.

When the membrana tympani and the necrotic malleus-head were removed from the attic, waves of sound fell directly upon the incus and the stapes and were conveyed to the labyrinth. As the new membrane formed and rested against the ossicles remaining, its expansion offered a broader surface to the waves of sound, and possibly helped to increase their leverage on the remaining ossicles, thus transmitting more sound and increasing the hearing. The continuance of this normal stimulus to the movements of the stapes in the oval window gradually overcame the partial ankylosis which had ensued at that point, from disuse, and the hearing, in consequence, has *steadily improved* since the operation from nothing to *fifteen feet* for whispered words.

Let us suppose that the chronic purulency of the attic had been, or could have been, cured by injections through the perforation in the membrana flaccida into the attic cavity. The hearing would not have been improved, because the impaired malleus-head and the pathological bands around the neck of the malleus would not have been removed, and hence the impaired mobility of the incus and stapes would still have remained as a hindrance to hearing.

We see, therefore, that the operation of excision of the membrana tympani and the malleus offers not only a great means of curing chronic purulency, especially of the attic, but also of relieving deafness due to a stiffened membrana and ossicles, by the removal of pathological bands prohibiting free oscillations in the ossicles, and by thus permitting sound-waves to fall directly upon the stapes in the oval window.

Longevity in Norway.—A recently published government report from Norway shows an increased average longevity for that country. The average duration of life there for males is 48.3 years, and for females 51.3 years.

FISTULOUS ESCAPE OF LIGATURES AFTER PELVIC OPERATIONS.[1]

BY MARIE B. WERNER, M.D.,
OF PHILADELPHIA.

As the science of abdominal surgery advances, we feel that it is not a report of successful operations alone, but the number of absolute cures, which establishes a reputation and makes the successful surgeon. Since the days when Lister first laid down the rule for antisepsis, which in turn gave birth to the crowning aid to surgery, thorough asepsis, the rate of mortality has diminished remarkably. The number of abdominal sections for various lesions increased, and with the number of recoveries the dread of such surgery diminished. Those earnestly engaged in effecting lasting cures soon began to see that it was not always recovery from an operation which meant a cure. The patient was not yet always safely landed; fistulæ, secondary adhesions, painful stumps, or unfinished operations, marked the shoals upon which the hopes for a perfect cure might be wrecked. It becomes our duty to study, like the successful navigator, these shoals in detail, and, if possible, to place the danger signal conspicuously in our minds, in order to be able to avoid a second exposure to similar dangers.

The reports of the most successful operations prove that rapid aseptic work, with as few instruments and sponges as possible, a clean stump, light ligatures applied closely to the uterus and with the ends cut short, and thorough irrigation prevent many of the complications. If there is much oozing from torn adhesions, or if pus is present, the drainage-tube becomes a valuable aid, provided it is properly cared for, cleaned at intervals of twenty or thirty minutes with a syringe, and removed as soon as the effusion becomes serous and less than a drachm at each removal.

Last but not least, comes the importance of including muscle and fascia in closing the abdomen. The fact that various gynecological societies have taken up the discussion of the behavior of ligatures after the removal of diseased uterine appendages induces me to record the following cases. The first was my own operation; the second case placed herself under my care three months after operation.

Knowing full well that there must always be a cause for unexpected happenings, I was anxious to satisfy myself of the cause in these cases, and I think that I succeeded.

CASE I.—Operation in March, 1887. Right ovarian cyst; cyst-walls friable, and adhesions present. The ligature was of Chinese twisted silk and of

---

[1] Read before the American Medical Association, May, 1890.

Operator.	Operation.	Ligature.	Drainage.	Remarks.	History of Fistulæ.
Dr. W. H. Parrish, 2 cases, personal communication.	Double ovariotomy.	Black silk figure-of-8, one side; shoemaker's knot on the other.	No.	Both ovaries cancerous, one presenting a large tumor of about twenty pounds, the other the size of a large orange. General condition poor.	Fistula: two months later shoemaker's ligature discharged and fistula closed spontaneously.
	Removal of appendages on both sides.	"Rather large Chinese ligature," figure-of-8.	Yes.	Syphilitic negress; confirmed drunkard; unruly, and walked across the ward on second day, the glass tube in situ. Fistulous opening in lower angle of wound.	Nine months after operation removed one ligature with hooked end of small probe. Subsequently a counter opening was made, per vaginam, by another gentleman; no avail. Later, laparotomy by a third resulted in death.
Dr. Charles M. Wilson, personal communication.	Ruptured ectopic gestation of six months.	Staffordshire knot.	......	....	Six months later one of the ligatures ulcerated its way out through the abdominal cicatrix.
Dr. H. M. Weeks, personal communication.	Ectopic gestation, November, 1888.	Twisted silk No. 3, figure-of-8.	Prolonged drainage; tube cleaned by irrigation and the long syringe with distilled water.	....	Ligature came away five months after the operation.
Dr. H. T. Hanks, reported to the N. Y. Obstet. Soc., Jan. 7, 1890.	Ruptured ectopic gestation.	......	Yes; irrigation twice daily.	"The right broad ligament through which the hæmatocele had ruptured was very friable, and the suture had a strong tendency to cut through."	Ten days after operation two ligatures were removed from the sinus. Patient made a good recovery.
Dr. Ashton, Annals of Gynecology, April, 1890.	Jan. 1888, abscess of right ovary and tube.	......	Yes.	Track of drainage-tube did not close. October, 1888, second section resulted in finding one ligature after flushing out the abdomen; no drainage, yet a fistula resulted, necessitating a third operation in February, 1889, with complete closure. The following August, however, the fistula reopened and discharged a ligature.	
Dr. B. F. Baer, personal communication.	Ovariotomy.	Chinese twisted figure-of-8.	Yes, for two days; tube cleaned with syringe every half hour.	There were intra-ligamentary adhesions to descending colon and small intestine; fæcal fistula resulted.	Fæcal fistula caused by thinning of bowel and the drainage-tube. Ligature came away two weeks after operation.
Dr. J. M. Baldy, personal communication.	Ectopic gestation; local peritonitis.	Twisted silk, figure-of-8.	Yes, 8 to 12 days; tube cleaned with syringe every hour.	Intestinal adhesions, beginning gangrene of sac, fistula at site of drainage-tube, refused to heal by usual methods.	Ligature came away thirteen weeks after operation; fistula healed spontaneously.
Dr. H. Beates, Jr., 4 cases, personal communication. Dr. Beates has had three cases of fistulæ from other operators, in which "fishing out" resulted in a cure. Ligatures, twisted No. 4 in one, smaller in two.	Salpingitis.	Twisted silk No. 3, Staffordshire.	Yes, 1 to 2 days; injections of bichloride (1:10,000) cotton capillary dressing.	General adhesions.	Fistula at site of drainage-tube. Ligature came away in twelve weeks; healed.
	Pyosalpinx.	Same.	Same as above.	General adhesions; patient in bed five weeks.	Fistula. Ligature came away in eleven weeks; healed.
	Pyosalpinx.	Same as above.	Same as above.	General adhesions; patient in bed five weeks.	Ligature came away in fourteen months.
	Ovariotomy; multilocular cyst.	Same as above.	Same as above.	No complications.	Ligature expelled through abdominal fistula in ten weeks.
Dr. Hannah T. Croasdale, personal communication.	Removal of tube and ovary of one side; local peritonitis.	Cable twist No. 3. Staffordshire knot.	8 hours.	Extensive adhesions prevented removal of appendages of other side.	Patient in bed from June 2d to February 9th. Ligature discharged January 31st; rapid improvement afterward; the wound entirely healed February 4th.
Dr. Joseph Hoffman, 2 cases, personal communication. One case from his practice, the other under his observation.	Pyosalpinx.	Chinese twisted No. 3, figure-of-8.	Yes; tube cleaned with syringe at short intervals.	General intestinal adhesions; local peritonitis.	Ligature discharged in about three months. Patient remained in bed six weeks.
Dr. H. A. Kelly, reported in the British Gynecological Society, by F. B. Jessett, October 23, 1889.	Pyosalpinx.	Same.	Yes.	General intestinal adhesions; general peritonitis; pus.	Ligature discharged in about three months. Patient in bed two months.
	Left ovarian dermoid cyst.	Chinese silk.	......	Dr. Kelly reports that "in her convalescence she had a large ante-uterine hæmatocele which is slowly undergoing contraction."	Mr. F. B. Jessett finds, five months after operation, an abscess in the anterior wall of the vagina; opens, drains, and finds a Chinese silk double ligature. Negative history regarding rigors and high temperature.

Operator.	Operation.	Ligature.	Drainage.	Remarks.	History of Fistulæ.
Dr. D. Longaker, personal communication.	Hydrosalpinx, puerperal; local peritonitis.	Plaited silk medium size, figure-of-8.	Yes; 36 hours	Extensive adhesions; sinus following drainage track.	After a few months one ligature was thrown off; at the end of the sixth month the second came away. Fistula failed to heal for one year; was finally curetted and injected with nitrate of silver and healed.
Dr. Charles B. Penrose, personal communication.	......	Twisted silk No. 3, figure-of-8.	......	....	Has had two cases in which a sinus lasted several months: one due to syphilis, the other to tuberculosis. Never had a case of discharged ligatures in abdominal section.
Dr. Wm. Goodell, reports in the Phila. Obst. Soc., March 7, 1889, the following 3 cases.	Removal of intra-ligamentary cyst.	......	......	Compelled to re-open wound for bleeding; five days after a fistula resulted.	One and a half years after operation fistula still remains; the only annoyance to the patient is an escape of gas.
	Pelvic abscess.	......	Prolonged.	A counter-opening may yet be necessary per vaginam.	Fistula caused by the prolonged use of the drainage-tube.
	Recurrent intra-ligmentary cyst lying in a large abscess cavity.	......	Yes.	Fistula resulted from a previous operation in which a clamp had been used many years ago.	Fistula still present at the time of the report; was then trying to heal with iodine applications along the entire track.
Dr. B. C. Hirst, 2 cases, personal communication.	Pyosalpinx.	Twisted silk, figure-of-8.	No.	Patient was easily managed; out of bed three weeks. Excessive hæmorrhage necessitated passing two strong ligatures at the base of the right broad ligament	Fistula of a year's standing. After discharge of ligatures, fistula healed.
	Removal of former stump one-quarter ovary, and four ligatures.	.....	......	The ligatures were not surrounded by lymph; accessible to sight and touch. Pain, which had followed previous operation, disappeared after their removal.	
Dr. John B. Deaver, 2 cases, personal communication.	Double pyosalpinx.	Twisted silk, figure-of-8.	Yes.	Many adhesions.	Fistula at site of tube track. Ligature was expelled four weeks after operation.
	Ovariotomy for large multilocular purulent cyst.	......	Yes.	Patient had been tapped a number of times, making dense adhesions.	Fistula in tube track. Ligature was expelled six weeks after operation.

medium size. A Staffordshire knot was used. Drainage for five days; recovery good. With the exception of an occasional pain in the region of the stump the patient was well and attended to her household duties. Fifteen months later, however, the patient brought the ligature, claiming to have discharged it from the urethra after much tenesmus at micturition. She gave a history of much previous pain over the right side of the bladder and frequent desire to urinate. Examination showed slight tenderness of stump and a tendinous cord leading to bladder. After a few weeks all tenderness disappeared and the patient was well.

CASE II.—Operation in May, 1887, by Dr. R. S. Hunt. I was present at the operation. There was a cyst of the left broad ligament. The ligature was braided silk, No. 9, tied in a Staffordshire knot; no drainage. Aside from several stitch abscesses recovery was good, and patient was up in four weeks.

During the latter part of August of the same year the patient experienced great pain in the scar, shooting toward the right side. A small abscess formed in the scar, was lanced, washed, probed, and found to extend down toward the stump. In about two weeks the ligature was expelled, and in a short time all had healed.

The first case presents two factors, each of which may account for the discharge of the ligature. First, the friable condition of the cyst-wall, part of which helped to form the stump, the surrounding tissues from want of vitality failing to encapsulate or absorb the ligature. Second, the length of time the drainage-tube was left *in situ*, owing to my inexperience, this being my first case in which drainage was used. I left it in long enough to become an irritant, and had some difficulty in healing the track.

The trouble in the second case was undoubtedly due to the size of the ligature; the tumor being small and the pedicle in consequence short, the ligature slipped over the button the moment shrinkage of the stump took place.

In connection with this subject I have endeavored to collect as many cases as possible, with a brief history of each. It is only by concentrating our forces that we are able to win the battle, hence the study of cause and effect becomes most necessary.

Dr. Thomas Keith, in his little book entitled *Contributions to the Surgical Treatment of Tumors of the*

Abdomen, relates his experience with catgut ligatures.   He says:[1]

"Twice I have had hæmorrhage happen in ovariotomy, and on both occasions catgut ligatures were used; in one some thick catgut ligatures had been used on very thick omentum. Several of the knots came away through the wound, and after weeks of horrible suffering from cystitis, a thick knot of catgut, with the loop but little absorbed, was passed by the urethra."

Dr. Matthew D. Mann tells us in his report of 160 abdominal sections[2] that fistulæ are due either to an abscess in the pelvis from some foreign substance, or the use of the drainage-tube, and he cites an experience in which a fistula resisted all attempts at healing for four years.   He is confident that this case was due to a silk ligature.   This induced him to use catgut, which proved more satisfactory.   Indeed, he feels so sure of its harmlessness that he was comparatively at ease when he found a fistula and discharge of pus follow the use of the drainage-tube, knowing that there was no infected silk at the bottom of the sinus.   Later, two knots of catgut came out of the sinus, after which it readily closed.

In a communication from Dr. H. A. Kelly he writes the following:

"I have had a number of cases in which the ligatures have all been cast off through the abdominal walls. In one case of hydrosalpinx and ovarian tumor, the patient afterward had a cellulitis. This suppurated and was drained through the vagina and the ligature discharged. It has frequently happened in cases of pyosalpinx, where long-continued drainage was necessary. I have observed it very constantly in cases in which the pyosalpinx has already ruptured, or been on the point of rupturing into the bowel, these cases always requiring prolonged drainage.

"Ligatures of twisted silk, doubled figure-of-eight, were used. These have been cast off from two months to a year after operation. I never use heavy strands of gut, as there is considerable doubt as to our ability to disinfect them satisfactorily. In all cases there has been drainage from four to five days. I clean the tube at intervals not longer than twelve hours. No sort of antiseptic injections are ever used in any of my abdominal sections."

Dr. Kelly's remark regarding the use of heavy strands of catgut seems of importance. We are never sure of healthy membrane, hence in spite of antiseptic precautions we may often use septic gut. Dr. Matthew D. Mann's statement that gut shrinks one-tenth its length when wet with water should be considered in tying, since too much pressure may cause some necrosis of the stump.

The causes of fistulæ may be summarized as follows: (1) Adhesion to the bowel which, in being loosened, may cause thinning and subsequent sloughing. (2) Heavy ligatures on small stumps. (3) Ends of ligature left too long. (4) Ligatures not thoroughly aseptic. (5) Part of the stump consisting of unhealthy tissue. (6) Prolonged use of the drainage-tube, which may cause localized inflammation, resulting in abscess of the stump or surrounding tissue.

Drainage, however, seems too valuable an aid to discard lightly, for we may meet with serious difficulties in closing the abdomen where there is danger of oozing of blood, which may accumulate and decompose, giving rise to troublesome secondary symptoms.

Among the secondary adhesions most commonly found may be mentioned omental and intestinal adhesions with the stump or abdominal incision as a focus. Such a case was reported by E. Sinclair Stevenson before the British Gynecological Society, April 24, 1889. In this case intestinal obstruction called for a second operation, the omentum was found twisted like a loose rope, dipping into the abdominal cavity, glued to coils of intestine, and its extremity firmly attached to a deeply-seated coil. The importance of carefully inspecting torn surfaces of omentum or peritoneum and obviating adhesions by stitch or removal, spreading out the omentum toward the left just before tying the abdominal sutures, becomes at once manifest.

Omentum caught in the holes of the drainage-tube, is another unpleasant complication, but can be avoided by using tubes of small calibre with small perforations, as advocated by Dr. Joseph Price.

Intestinal adhesions to the stump or to surfaces of torn adhesions are best overcome by free purgation and the avoidance of opium.

Painful stumps may be due to an uncovered ligature, to unhealthy tissue left in the stump, or, as Dr. B. C. Hirst has shown us, by too much ligature and an unfinished operation.

This brings us to the last point of importance, namely, unfinished operations. With this I had an unpleasant experience in two cases some years ago, and have profited by it. In one case a pus-tube was so tightly adherent to the pelvic walls and uterus that my courage failed me, and contenting myself with removal from one side I closed the abdomen. Three months later my patient had a sharp attack of septic peritonitis, and she died five months after this, her abdomen literally filled with multiple abscesses. The second unfinished case was of a similar nature, though not so far advanced: the adhesions again intimidated me; the patient recovered promptly, and in spite of hot July weather was temporarily relieved. The following winter I was called to treat a localized peritonitis on the side where I left the pus-tube. She recovered, but has since passed out of my hands. I have learned that to open an abdomen and leave pus there, is as harmful as to know of the presence of pus and not

[1] On page 17.
[2] Buffalo Medical and Surgical Journal, April, 1890.

attempt its removal. I have since endeavored to remove the cause of sepsis, even though the ideal operation was out of the question, and the results have been more satisfactory.

This leads me to an important question which has agitated my mind of late, and which is best illustrated by a brief account of two cases from my practice, both unilateral hydrosalpinx. In both I removed the affected tube and ovary—one in March, 1887, the other in February, 1888, the remaining appendages being apparently normal. Both recovered promptly and improved in health. But in each the former symptoms returned on the other side in eighteen and six months respectively.

The first case reported again three months ago, and I found a painful mass on right side. She at once made preparations for a second operation, which was performed in March, 1890. Some omental adhesions to the incision were found ; the tube and ovary were adherent and cystic ; the stump was healthy. Patient recovered promptly, and it is now seven weeks since the operation ; no pelvic pains ; intestinal functions normal.

In the second case operation was performed on May 9, 1890. There were omental adhesions to the abdominal wall and intestinal adhesions to the stump. The uterus, abdominal wall, ovary, and tube were adherent. There was decided constriction of the 'tube near the ostium internum. I removed the tube and cystic ovary and separated all adhesions except those to the stump.

May 18. Patient doing well.

This leads to the question : Is it the proper course to remove an apparently normal ovary and tube when there is hydrosalpinx on one side, or shall we let the patient run the possible risk of a second operation ?

Is there the same danger as in pyosalpinx ? Should this last question receive an affirmative answer it certainly behooves us to explain such dangers fully to the patient and gain her consent to remove, if necessary, even an apparently healthy ovary and tube, so that she may not be exposed to the dangers of a second operation.

REMARKS ON THOMSEN'S DISEASE, WITH REPORT OF A CASE.[1]

BY HAROLD N. MOYER, M.D.,
PROFESSOR OF PHYSIOLOGY IN RUSH MEDICAL COLLEGE, CHICAGO.

IT is scarcely necessary to enter upon an extended consideration of the literature of this subject, as all that was previously known of this disease was admirably summarized in the monograph of Professor Erb, published in the early part of the year 1886.[2] In this article Professor Erb states that he

believes the disease to be a tropho-neurosis of the muscles, forming a definite clinical group with characteristic symptoms. In January, 1886, an article by Dr. Allan McLane Hamilton[1] denies this conclusion and states that the peculiar symptom-complex termed Thomsen's disease is frequently found in other diseases, particularly in hystero-organic disorders, and in the third stage of posterior spinal sclerosis, and is by no means uncommonly associated with coarse cerebral lesions. He regards it as in most cases a purely psychic disorder, which depends first upon inhibitory insufficiency, and secondly, upon an unstable emotional state, which interferes with the origin of proper volitional mandates. In support of his views Dr. Hamilton describes several cases, in two of which the symptom of muscle stiffness was present, associated with other nerve lesions. The third case was evidently one of hysteria complicating a fairly well marked case of paralysis agitans.

That the symptom of spasm at the inception of voluntary impulse does not alone constitute Thomsen's disease will hardly be denied, and that it may be occasionally associated with other organic lesions, would seem to be attested by Dr. Hamilton's cases ; that it occurs as frequently as he thinks it does, I am inclined to doubt, as it has never come to my notice in a not inconsiderable neurological practice.

Erb divides the cases so far reported into typical, doubtful, and symptomatic. In typical cases the lesion is always confined to the voluntary muscles, begins in early childhood, and probably in many cases is congenital. It is usually hereditary or appears in families with a strong neurotic taint. The majority of cases so far reported have one or more relatives affected with the same disease. The disease is characterized by a peculiar stiffness and cramp in the muscles, which comes on with the inception of voluntary motion and which, after a time, gives way and permits the performance of the contemplated movement. After a certain number of repetitions the movements become easier, and the cramp, which is painless, disappears. The contractions are always increased by cold and mental excitement. The muscles are commonly well developed, and elastic, but they do not contract as strongly as in health. The electrical reactions are changed and, according to Erb, consist in an increase in the excitability of the muscles and a response, normal or diminished, to the stimulation of the nerve, with both currents. The galvanic current gives a qualitative change, in that the ACC is prompter and stronger than CCC. All contractions last several seconds after the stimulus is withdrawn. Erb found in several of his cases considerable hypertrophy of the muscular fibres, with increase in the nuclei, changes in the

---

[1] Read before the Chicago Medical Society, June 16, 1890.
[2] Die Thomsensche Krankheit (Myotonia Congenita) Studien von Prof. W. Erb, Leipzig 1886.

[1] Medical Record. 1886, vol. i. p. 85.

finer structure, and a slight increase in the interstitial connective tissue.

While the histories of these cases are sufficiently clear to warrant us in assuming that we have here a pathological entity, yet I am not sure that the disease does not also occur later in life, in the so-called adult forms. It is possible that at least some of these cases can be classed as true examples of the disease, particularly those of Schonfeld's, Seligmüller's and Engel's.

The following is perhaps the most clearly marked of all the adult cases thus far described :

W. H., of Arkansas, aged twenty-five, presented himself in January, 1884. Notes made at that time are as follows : The family history shows that his father died of consumption at the age of thirty-two, and that his mother was killed by an accident at about the same age. The paternal grandparents are still living at an advanced age, and are in good health. Maternal grandfather still living, aged seventy-eight. Maternal grandmother died of erysiplas at an advanced age. Patient is the second child. He has one brother and two sisters living and well. They have never been affected with any disease similar to that of the patient, and no neurotic trouble has ever been observed in the patient's family. He has always had the best of health. Has used tobacco excessively, but alcohol only occasionally and in small quantities. Is married and has one child. There is no evidence of venereal disease. Has worked hard since his seventeenth year as a sailor, fireman and an engineer, and in these occupations was exposed to varying and extreme temperatures.

About two years ago he was employed in a nail factory, and at that time he noticed the first symptoms of his present trouble. The work required him to stand in front of his machine and to make constant and rapid flexion and extension of the forearms, at the same time stepping from side to side. The first symptom noticed was a slight stiffness, first on one side, then on the other. For a time these symptoms would cease only to recur again at varying intervals of from a few days to a couple of weeks, but with ever increasing severity. Finally the patient had to give up his employment, owing to the lessened control over his muscles. When grasping anything it was impossible for him to loosen his hold promptly, and he experienced great uncertainty in attempting to walk, as he was likely to fall on his face owing to the flexion of the legs. He now rises very slowly from the chair, and walks with a hesitating gait until he has taken a few strides. The contractions often persist for ten or fifteen seconds, and are always aggravated by cold and mental excitement. The patient has a fine physique and the muscles are exceptionally well developed; indeed, from their volume and firmness he would be considered quite an athlete. The peculiar condition is absent on rising in the morning, but after he has been up for a few minutes the contractions begin and seem to increase until after working a few hours, when they decrease. Since changing his

work to that of a night watchman, the disease has not been so severe. All the nervous functions except motility are perfectly intact. The reflexes are normal, and the patient eats and sleeps well and has not the slightest pain. The muscles of the face and of mastication are intact. The voice and mental characteristics are unchanged. Electrical excitation of the muscles is followed by a long contraction which persists some seconds after the current is broken. The qualitative reactions described by Erb had not at that time been pointed out, but it is possible that they might have been found had they been looked for. The size and appearance of the muscles also indicated that the peculiar muscular changes had come on ; and while they appeared strong, they were not actually so, as their voluntary contractions were much weaker than would be expected.

The fact mentioned by this patient that immediately after leaving the bed in the morning he gets about much more easily than later in the day, was also observed in one of the typical cases described by Bernhardt.[1]

While we cannot draw definite conclusions from a single case, yet the history of this patient teaches that Thomsen's disease may occur in adults without special neurotic heredity, and from causes competent to produce other forms of nervous disorder. Unfortunately, this individual was only a short time under observation. All possible means have been used to learn his subsequent history, but thus far without success.

MEDICAL PROGRESS.

The Treatment of Injuries of the Urethra.—DR. HAEGLER has made a series of experiments on dogs to elucidate the proper method of dealing with wounds of the urethra (*Deutsche Zeitschrift f. Chirurgie*). His conclusions are as follows :

1. After extensive rupture of the urethra external urethrotomy should be done at once, and the ends of the torn urethra sutured. The edges of the wound cannot, however, be always closely united.

2. The suture should be introduced as far as possible into the submucous tissue, and during the first twenty-four or forty-eight hours a catheter should remain in the urethra, the perineal wound being open.

3. Bougies should not be used until the wound has completely healed.—*Annals of Surgery*, july, 1890.

Rhinoscleroma.—WOLKOWITSCH defines rhinoscleroma as a disease localized in the mucous membrane of the nose and surrounding skin, characterized by hard proliferations, by an exceedingly chronic course, and by being absolutely incurable (*Centralblatt f. Chirurgie*, june 7, 1890). Cases have been reported from Austria, Italy, Russia, Central America, Cairo, Switzerland, and Sweden. The disease begins with few symptoms, most frequently in the nasal cavities, but occasionally in the

---

[1] Centralblatt für Nervenheilkunde, 1885, p. 124.

fauces and larynx, and one case is reported in which it began on the hard palate. Wherever the disease begins the nasal cavity is soon involved. The macroscopic alterations are the formation of more or less circumscribed nodules, tubercles, and plates, involving the deeper layer of the skin and mucous membrane, and with marked swelling around them. Occasionally the nodes atrophy, the connective tissue contracting in consequence and causing distortion, and sometimes interfering with respiration. The swellings never ulcerate unless antisyphilitic treatment is used. The symptoms are few; pain is almost entirely absent; there are the usual symptoms of nasal catarrh; and if the larynx is involved, dyspnœa may become a prominent and serious symptom. The course of the disease is very slow, lasting in one case for twenty-six years. No treatment save excision of the nodules seems of the slightest use. Histologically the growth consists chiefly of a small-cell infiltrate. Microörganisms resembling the pneumococcus are invariably found.

Treatment of Sciatica and other Neuralgias.—MORD-HORST (*Therapeutische Monatshefte*, June, 1890) states that the diagnosis of sciatica is not always easy, and that inflammatory thickening of the rectus femoris and vastus externus may be mistaken for this condition. It may also be confounded with rheumatic affections of the trochanter major and the muscles covering the hip-joint, especially the tensor vaginæ femoris, in the tendon of which may be found small masses varying in size from a lentil to a bean. These may be mistaken for true *punctata dolorosa*, as they are painful upon pressure. In many of these cases the author has found an excess of free uric acid in the urine, and so concludes that these masses are urates deposited in the tissues.

With these few remarks on diagnosis, the author takes up his special methods of treating sciatica, which he has employed for the past four years, and for which he claims the best results. In cases of neuritis—most of these cases belong to that class—it is well, he says, to begin with a hot bath of from fifteen minutes to one hour's duration, followed by rest in bed of at least one hour, after which electric massage is to be used after the author's method. This consists of the application of the cathodal electrode having a surface area of at least 100 square cm. to the sciatic notch, while a revolving cylinder connected with the anode is passed down the limb along the course of the nerves. Deep pressure is made when the electrode is drawn downward, but it should only touch the skin lightly when returned, to prevent a break in the current. The author says that strong currents (from 5 to 10 milliampères) can be used in this manner, with a corresponding rapid absorption of inflammatory exudate.

Of 36 cases of sciatica treated in this way, 30 recovered, and 6 were improved. One case was cured in eight days, but the average length of treatment was from three to six weeks. Of 13 other neuralgias, 10 were cured and 3 improved.—*Journal of the American Medical Association*, July 26, 1890.

Incompatibilities of Antipyrine.—The *American Druggist* gives a list of drugs with which antipyrine is incompatible. Among them are the following : Carbolic acid

in strong solution, hydrocyanic acid, nitric acid, tannic acid, iodide of arsenic, chloral, sulphate of copper, decoction and fluid extract of cinchona, sulphate of iron, bichloride of mercury, infusion of uva ursi, solution of potassium permanganate, sodium salicylate (liquefies), spirit of nitrous ether, syrup of iodide of iron, tincture of chloride of iron, tincture of cinchona, tincture of catechu, tincture of iodine, tincture of kino, and tincture of rhubarb.—*Therapeutic Gazette*, July, 1890.

Intestinal Antisepsis.—CANTANI believes that the best method of applying antiseptics in the treatment of intestinal diseases is by rectal injection (*Wiener med. Blätter*, No. 22, 1890), experiments having shown that fluids given in this way reach not only the upper part of the intestines, but may even reach the stomach. If necessary, the reservoir may be raised two or three yards above the level of the rectum. If there is fever, the temperature can be reduced by using the solution cold ; if collapse, as in cholera, the patient can be stimulated by using the solution warm or hot.

Cantani thinks the best antiseptic to use in this manner is tannic acid, which not only checks the multiplication of bacteria, but destroys the ptomaines. The solution should contain not more than one per cent. of tannic acid. In diarrhœa and dysentery this solution acts not only as a disinfectant, but also as an astringent. In typhoid fever, Mosler has found it very efficient in reducing tympany and checking diarrhœa.—*Medical Chronicle*, July, 1890.

Treatment of Snake-bites.—PROFESSOR KAUFMANN contributes to the *Revue Scientifique* a paper describing his recent researches and experiments regarding the bites of poisonous snakes. He advises that in the treatment of a bite the injured limb should be tightly bound above the bite, as quickly as possible, with a handkerchief or any other available constrictor, and that then a 1-to-2 solution of chromic acid should be injected deep into the wound, making several similar injections in the neighborhood of the wound. If these directions are carefully followed, the poison will be destroyed before being absorbed. If there is already much swelling of the wound, more injections should be made in various parts of the swelling, which should then be manipulated to bring the acid thoroughly in contact with the poison. The swelling should then be freely lanced and as much as possible of the fluid squeezed out. The skin should be washed with the chromic acid solution, followed by the application of compresses saturated with the solution. If the swelling returns, these procedures should be repeated.

This local treatment should be supplemented by the internal administration of alcoholic stimulants and aqua ammonia. Professor Kaufmann, however, strongly condemns the use of large quantities of alcohol, which, he thinks, paralyze and depress the nervous system.—*Indian Medical Gazette*, May, 1890.

Œdema Pulmonum.—GROSSMAN (*Zeitschrift für klinische Medicine*, Bd. 34, H. 1, 2, 3, 4, 1889; *Wiener klinische Wochenschrift*, April 2, 1889), in his remarkable experiments concerning œdema of the lungs, which have been carried out in the laboratory of Professor v. Basch, in Vienna, has made some important discoveries. An acute general pulmonary œdema occurs in dogs, and not as hitherto supposed in rabbits alone, from obstruction of the left auricle and compression of the left ventricle. He has learned that the transudation plays but a secondary *rôle* in the causation of the dyspnœa, and that the most important obstruction to respiration is the inflexibility of the lung on account of the œdema. In consequence of the vascular engorgement there occurs an enlargement of the alveolar spaces, that is, an enlargement of the lungs. He considers transudation a factor of no importance in dyspnœa. We not only have congestion and œdema through muscarin intoxication, but also swelling and stiffness of the lungs and bronchial cramps. He thinks that his investigation prove the primary cause of the congestion of the lungs to be the narrowing of the left side of the heart, contrary to the theory of Conberm-Welch, who considers it due to paralysis of the left side of the heart.

Moyer (*Medical Standard*, September, 1889), in a recent discussion in the Chicago Pathological Society, took the stand against the majority of the members regarding the indications for pilocarpine in pulmonary œdema. His views meeting with scant support, he determined to try the drug in the first case that offered, where there were no heart complications or threatened coma. A case recently came under his care presenting these conditions, and the drug was administered with the most happy effect.

Fothergill's Anti-rheumatic Pills.—The late DR. FOTHERgill used the following combination in a large proportion of his cases of chronic rheumatism :

R.—Arsenious acid . „ 3 grains.
    Powdered guaiac . . . 3 drachms.
    Powdered capsicum . . 30 grains.
    Pill of aloes and myrrh . . 3 drachms.

Mix, and divide in 120 pills. One pill was ordered three times a day, in connection with a diet rich in fatty foods. Also, a general tonic treatment was in most cases found advisable at the outset.

Treatment of Tympanites.—

R.—Naphthol)
    Carbonate of Magnesia ⟩ of each 1½ drachms.
    Charcoal)
    Essence of peppermint . . 10 drops.

Make into twelve powders, and take one every two hours until relief is obtained.—*Revue Obstétricale et Gynécologique*, July, 1890.

Creolin for Pruritus Vulvœ.—

Creolin . . . . . 3 to 5 parts.
Linseed oil . . . . . 100 parts.

Apply with friction to the affected parts every four or five hours.—*Revue Obstétricale et Gynécologique*, July, 1890.

Formula for the Administration of Creasote in Phthisis.—

R.—Creasote . . . . 30 grains.
    Rum . . . . . 1½ ounces.
    Syrup of tolu . . . . 1 ounce.
    Distilled water . . . 2 ounces.

A dessertspoonful twice or thrice a day in a wineglassful of water, to persons having a tubercular tendency.—*L' Union Médicale*, July 3, 1890.

Mercurial Fumigation in Pseudo-membranous Laryngitis.—DR GEORGE E. LAW (*Brooklyn Medical Journal*, August, 1890) enthusiastically advocates mercurial fumigations in the treatment of pseudo-membranous laryngitis. His opinions are based on the results of treatment in seven cases, six of which recovered. Of the six, three had diphtheritic membrane in the pharynx in addition to that in the larynx, and paralysis followed in one.

The apparatus used by Dr. Law consists of a tent, and an alcohol lamp with arms to support a piece of sheet-iron. The tent may be improvised by fastening a bed-slat to each post of the child's crib, connecting them by cross-pieces, and throwing a sheet over this frame-work. The lamp is then lighted, and, when the sheet-iron plate is hot, thirty grains of calomel are dropped upon it, and the apparatus quickly placed in the tent. The duration of the fumigation should be about ten minutes. The procedure should be repeated at first every two hours, increasing the intervals as the symptoms diminish. Attendants must be cautioned not to inhale the fumes, as there is danger of mercurial poisoning, though this danger does not seem to exist in patients suffering from pseudo-membranous laryngitis.

Hot Enemata in Typhoid Fever.—Following the suggestion by Professor I. T. Tchüdnovsky, DR. THEODOR K. GEISSLER, of St. Petersburg (*Vratch*, No. 22, 1890), has undertaken an experimental inquiry into the action of hot enemata on patients suffering from enteric fever. In all, five cases (males, aged from fifteen to twenty-nine years) were selected for the purpose, each experiment lasting eight days, and being divided into two periods of an equal duration, during one of which the patients received daily (at 11 A.M.) an enema of one quart of water at 108.5° F. The essential results of the researches are as follows : (1) Hot enemata manifest a very favorable influence on the intestinal tract in typhoid fever. In cases of diarrhœa, they markedly diminish the frequency of stools and improve their quality, the fæces becoming less fluid. The injections also relieve abdominal pain, and produce a beneficial action on constipation when present. (2) Immediately after an enema, the bodily temperature, as a rule, slightly rises. When examined an hour later, the temperature proves to be the same as, or even lower than, the temperature before the enema. (3) In the long run, the injections seem to promote defervescence, or, at least, the transformation of a continuous fever into a remittent or intermittent one. (4) Immediately after an enema, the frequency of the pulse commonly somewhat decreases, to increase at the end of an hour. At the same time, the pulse becomes firmer and fuller, its dicrotism less pronounced, and the cardiac contractions more vigorous. (5) The respiration usually quickens, but becomes slower in an hour or two. (6) The blood pressure distinctly rises. (7) The daily amount of urine increases, while the specific gravity sinks. (8) The enemata are invariably perfectly well borne, the patients being rather pleased with them, and a sensation of well-being always follows. As a rule, the injection is retained by the patient from twenty to thirty minutes.—*London Medical Recorder*, July, 1890.

THE MEDICAL NEWS.

A WEEKLY JOURNAL
OF MEDICAL SCIENCE.

COMMUNICATIONS are invited from all parts of the world. Original articles contributed exclusively to THE MEDICAL NEWS will be liberally paid for upon publication. When necessary to elucidate the text, illustrations will be furnished without cost to the author.

Address the Editor: H. A. HARE, M.D.,
1004 WALNUT STREET,
PHILADELPHIA.

Subscription Price, including Postage.

PER ANNUM, IN ADVANCE . . . . $4.00.
SINGLE COPIES . . . . 10 CENTS.

Subscriptions may begin at any date. The safest mode of remittance is by bank check or postal money order, drawn to the order of the undersigned. When neither is accessible, remittances may be made, at the risk of the publishers, by forwarding in *registered* letters.

Address,   LEA BROTHERS & CO.,
Nos. 706 & 708 SANSOM STREET,
PHILADELPHIA.

SATURDAY, AUGUST 16, 1890.

DELAYED LABOR FROM PROLAPSE AND OCCLUSION OF THE CERVIX.

A VERY frequent cause of delay during normal labor is prolongation of the anterior lip of the cervix produced by the presenting part, and its impaction between the head and the symphysis pubis. This minor complication is generally readily detected by the examining finger, and may be remedied by placing the woman upon her side, employing an anæsthetic if her suffering is severe, and, in the intervals between the pains, pushing the head a little upward and backward and carrying the projecting lip above the head with the finger until the commencement of the next pain. A few efforts in this way will generally result in the retraction of the cervix over the head and labor will go on naturally. It is sometimes observed with primiparæ that the cervix becomes excessively distended and that the external os remains very slightly dilated. The cervical tissue may become so thin as to resemble closely the membranes, and we recall a case in which the attending physician punctured this tissue with a probe, supposing that he was rupturing the membranes. In such a case the os uteri will be found near the posterior wall of the pelvis and can usually be dilated by the fingers or by a Barnes' bag.

It occasionally happens, however, that so firm is the tissue about the external os that the cervix containing the head becomes excessively thin, and projects between the woman's thighs. Such a case is described by Jentzer (*Archives de Tocologie*, May, 1890). The patient had been in the care of a midwife, but labor had been delayed. The physician was summoned with the statement that the cervix was dilated and obliterated; that the head was presenting, but that neither the cervix uteri nor the neck of the child above the head could be felt by the examining finger. On examination a tumor as large as the head, reddish in color and containing an opening about a third of an inch in diameter, was found projecting from the vulva. The occiput of the child had descended toward the mother's left side, rotation not having occurred. The patient was anæsthetized, the tissues at the borders of the os uteri were incised and dilatation was rapidly performed by the fingers, and the membranes were ruptured, but the child was found dead. While the midwife made counter-pressure upon the sides of the cervix, the child was delivered by traction without great difficulty. The cervix was easily replaced. Under antiseptic precautions the patient made an uninterrupted recovery. It is interesting to note that no history or evidence of prolapse occurring during pregnancy, or of endocervicitis, or any inflammatory disorder, could be obtained, and the cause for the complication remained unknown.

Martin, Latz and Auvard have reported similar cases. Quite recently in examining a patient seven months pregnant, we found great elongation of the cervix with prolapse and ulceration. It was necessary to replace the cervix and to maintain its position by antiseptic tampons renewed every second day.

It is not infrequent to find, in women giving a history of specific infection, such deposit of syphilitic tissue about the os and cervix as to make dilatation excessively difficult. In these cases profound anæsthesia, manual dilatation, and elastic dilators may be employed to advantage. As soon as a narrow-bladed forceps can be introduced the head may be brought down and dilatation completed, under anæsthesia, by the forceps. In a case of labor in which the first stage lasted seventy-two hours, it was necessary to complete delivery in this manner, and under antiseptic precautions mother and child recovered well.

Dührssen has recently advocated multiple incisions in the cervix in delayed labor. While this procedure can hardly be thought devoid of danger, yet if caution be exercised to incise in many places but not deeply in any one, and if strict antiseptic precautions be observed, the lives of children can doubtless be saved by this expedient which otherwise must be lost through delay. The tampon of iodoform gauze furnishes a safe and reliable method of checking hæmorrhage should serious bleeding follow such dilatation.

REVIEWS.

TERMINOLOGIA MEDICA POLYGLOTTA: A CONCISE INTERNATIONAL DICTIONARY OF MEDICAL TERMS. Compiled by THEODORE MAXWELL, M.D. Camb.; B. Sc. Lond.; F.R.C.S. Edin. 8vo., pp. 459. Philadelphia: P. Blakiston, Son & Co., 1890.

THIS work represents an enormous amount of labor on the part of the compiler and his assistants, comprising, as it does, the French, Latin, English, German, Italian, Spanish, and Russian synonym of every medical term, and it is only owing to an exceedingly ingenious arrangement and the avoidance of descriptive definitions that the volume is not as large as an "Unabridged." French is selected as the key-language, but this fact in no way interferes with the usefulness of the book to a student who cannot read French. Suppose, for example, that an Italian in reading German comes to the word *zunge*, of which he wishes to know the meaning. Turning in this work he finds the English, *tongue*, and French, *langue*. If, now, he is unfamiliar with the English and French words, he must turn to *langue*, under which he will find the synonyms in six languages, including that of his own. Again, suppose that an Englishman wishes the synonym for the Italian *malattia*. Turning to this word, he finds the English, *disease*, as well as the French, *maladie*, while a Spaniard would have to turn to the French heading, *maladie*, where he would find among the other synonyms his own word, *mal*. In other words, every medical term in seven languages has a separate heading (excepting the Russian, which has no separate headings) with the synonym of at least two other languages; and under the French heading the word is repeated in six languages.

The book is well bound and clearly printed, and, while we believe it will be welcome to a few students of foreign medical literature, and especially to medical editors, the number of physicians who are interested in the language of more than one country besides that of their own is so small, that we doubt if the compiler or publisher will ever be repaid for the labor and expense of preparation.

"*The Lesson in Anatomy.*"—Referring to Rembrandt's celebrated picture, "The Lesson in Anatomy," the *Lancet* describes a curious anatomical error which is certainly not generally known. The pronator radii teres is drawn as if it ran from above downward and *in*ward from the radius to the ulna, instead of downward and *out*ward from the ulna to the radius.

SOCIETY PROCEEDINGS.

PHILADELPHIA COUNTY MEDICAL SOCIETY.

Stated Meeting, June 25, 1890.

THE PRESIDENT, JOHN B. ROBERTS, M.D., IN THE CHAIR.

DR. EDWARD JACKSON read a paper entitled

THE RECOGNITION OF EYE-STRAIN BY THE GENERAL PRACTITIONER,

in which he dwelt on the futility of attempting to give relief from the symptoms of eye-strain by drugs, though they are frequently persisted in until the patient deserts his so-called medical adviser, and takes his chances with the specialist or the charlatan.

From time to time, he said, efforts have been made by ophthalmologists to secure a more general recognition of eye-strain on the part of the mass of the profession; but usually these efforts consist in a recommendation of some special instrument or procedure of diagnosis, as the refraction ophthalmoscope, or the shadow-test, or a set of trial lenses, reduced in size and price to the supposed needs of the mass of the profession. If it were really necessary to apply such special means of diagnosis in order to recognize the presence of eye-strain, there would be little prospect of its early general recognition. But the condition is frequently recognized by the patient himself, and the ophthalmic surgeon finds in the general rational symptoms sufficient grounds for a provisional diagnosis; and if the mind is clear from preconceived hypotheses as to the causes of the symptoms there is no reason why any one reasonably qualified for practice of general medicine should not be able to make a provisional diagnosis, in the great majority of cases, with sufficient certainty to serve for the basis of further investigation and treatment, without resort to any special method of examination. The speaker did not wish to underestimate the value of the ophthalmoscope to the general practitioner, for he did not regard anyone who is unable to use the ophthalmoscope as properly qualified for general practice, but he meant that inability to measure refraction with the ophthalmoscope is no reason for failing to recognize eye-strain.

The patient suffering from eye-strain comes with a certain history and certain complaints, which, carefully considered by the light of a very moderate knowledge of the subject, usually clearly indicate the cause of the trouble. The symptoms in question are:

(1) *Impairment of vision*, either quite temporary, more prolonged, or permanent. A very characteristic form of temporary impairment of vision is that due to sudden relaxation of the accommodation. This occurs when the ciliary muscle has long been overtaxed, and especially in the latter hours of the day, when the muscle is tired out. The patient notices that the print or other near object on which the attention is fixed suddenly becomes blurred, compelling the cessation of the eye-work. After a moment, however, the power of again focussing the object returns, and work can be resumed. The patient is apt to close his eyes for an instant, and, perhaps, rub them, and then finds the sight again restored. If the eye-work is continued, the failure of ac-

commodation recurs, to again rapidly pass away; and keeping on with the work, these periods of inability to see become more and more frequent, until, finally, they greatly interfere with the continuance of the work or quite prevent it. This form of impairment affects only the vision for near work.

Another form of temporary impairment is that due to spasm of the accommodation; it affects distant vision only, and is noticed chiefly by those whose distant vision is otherwise pretty good. It comes on after prolonged straining of the eye, usually for near vision, and lasts until the eye is rested. It is a valuable danger-signal, and should secure cessation from the work causing it until the symptom has disappeared. Permanent impairment of vision is brought about when eye-strain causes myopia or decided permanent damage of the choroid and retina.

(2) *Headache and aching of the eyes.* Eye-strain should be the first thought suggested by any complaint of headache, for in our day and civilization it is by far the most common cause of that symptom. It enters as a factor into the causation of nearly all headaches not due to pyrexia, toxæmia, or diseases of the brain or its membranes. Often it comes on whenever the eyes are used, and is absent when they have a proper period of rest. Very often a chronological connection between the use of the eye and the occurrence of the headache, although perfectly certain after it has been once observed, was not noted by the patient until his attention was directly called to it. Even when the headache is constant and apparently uninfluenced by variations in the amount of eye-work, it may be due wholly to eye-strain.

In hyperopia in young people the accommodation is in excessive use so long as the eyes are open and the attention fixed on any visible object; and hyperopia is the most common cause of constant headache. Dr. Jackson said that he himself was formerly subject to headache whenever confined to the house, and he believed it was caused by breathing vitiated air, until cured by the correction of his hyperopic astigmatism. Many persons have the same idea as to the causation of the headaches they experience when attending the theatre or other place of public amusement, and which are really due to eye-strain. Others ascribe these headaches, and those experienced in travelling or shopping, to exhaustion. This is nearer the truth, only they commonly have in mind a condition of general exhaustion, whereas it is largely one of local exhaustion of the special nervous apparatus concerned in the act of seeing.

The *location of the aching* is of some significance. Generally it is frontal, often described as beginning in the eye, or just back of the eye, or through the temples. Frequently it extends to the occipital region, and may sometimes be felt principally or wholly in that region. Headache most severe in the vertex or confined to that region is probably not very common from any cause, but from eye-strain it is almost unknown. Often the headache is more severe on one side of the head than the other. Sometimes it is entirely confined to one side, but usually it is bilateral.

Those more or less regularly periodical headaches, known as nervous or sick headaches, migraine, or, when confined to one side of the head, hemicrania, are in many cases caused by eye-strain and relieved by its removal. Attacks of this kind are frequently ushered in by certain interferences with vision and subjective sensations of light, affecting a part or the whole of the visual field, and known as ophthalmic migraine. These visual disturbances are simply a part of the general " nerve-storm," and it is not certain that they especially indicate eye-strain.

(3) *Congestion, irritability, or inflammation of the eyes and their appendages,* should always cause the suspicion of eye-strain. A single attack of this kind has no special significance, but repeated attacks of inflammation, or prolonged congestion or irritability, are exceedingly suggestive of a continuing cause; and the most common cause is eye-strain. Every case of chronic inflammation of the margins of the lids, or of recurring conjunctivitis, or repeated styes, should be carefully investigated for eye-strain. Persons when they begin to feel the effects of loss of accommodation in presbyopia or absolute hyperopia, suffer from repeated attacks of conjunctivitis, which they commonly ascribe to "taking cold in the eye," but which are cut short by use of the appropriate lenses, and which, if unchecked, would tend to establish a chronic catarrhal condition which is a constant discomfort to many elderly people.

Of course, these conditions of ocular congestion and inflammation will be recognized by the usual symptoms of redness, swelling, and itching, smarting, or burning pain. It should be noted that headache and these local inflammatory conditions are not usually presented by the same case. They may co-exist, but, more commonly, if one is decidedly present, the other is absent.

So far nothing has been mentioned of the diagnosis of eye-strain, but only the facts ascertained by questioning the patient, and from simple inspection of the eye. If, now, the physician's office contains—what every general practitioner's office should contain—a card of test-letters for accurately ascertaining the distant vision, and a card of fine print for ascertaining the near point of the eye, additional valuable evidence is easily obtainable. The trial of the distant vision will give indication of any considerable degree of myopia or astigmatism. But it must always be borne in mind that troublesome ametropia may be present without preventing perfect distant vision. The position of the near point, if farther from the patient's eye than his age would indicate, is pretty good evidence of strain of the accommodation. Evidence of strain of the external muscles of the eye, heterophoria, can be obtained by simply getting the patient to keep his eyes fixed on some object, near or distant, and covering one eye; then noting whether the covered eye deviates from its position of fixation, and especially whether it makes a quick movement to return to that position when it is uncovered.

To recapitulate briefly, the common symptoms of eye-strain are:

(1) Certain forms of impairment of vision.

(2) Headache, which is to be studied with reference to the times of its occurrence, and the parts of the head to which the aching is referred.

(3) Chronic or repeatedly recurring congestion or inflammation of the eye or its appendages.

And if to these symptoms are added the results of the simple tests of near and distant vision, and the evidence of tendency of the eyes to deviate from their normal position when covered, a very good basis is furnished for the probable or provisional diagnosis of eye-strain, without recourse to any special apparatus or unusual diagnostic procedure. And in view of these facts there is no justification for the general practitioner who fails to recognize most of the numerous cases of eye-strain with which he is brought in contact.

In the discussion which followed, DR. GEORGE M. GOULD referred to other symptoms the result of eye-strain; namely, sleepiness after persistent reading ; anorexia and dyspeptic symptoms; nervousness, choreic movements, and even true chorea, and car-sickness when travelling. All of these symptoms he has observed in his practice. With reference to testing the eyes by the general practitioner, he suggested the following simple plan: Have two test-cards, so that the patient will not learn and remember the letters. Let the physician first test distant vision with one of the test-cards; then instil homatropine. This will give perfect paralysis in three-quarters of an hour. Then retest with the other card. If vision has decreased, there is eye-strain, due to astigmatism or hypermetropia. Another practical point is, that if the patient is suffering with headache, he will be relieved by the application of the mydriatic.

DR. MARY E. ALLEN asked if, in these cases, the condition of the recti muscles has not something to do with the symptoms. In her own case she had suffered from eye-strain for a long time, with insufficiency of the recti muscles. She frequently had a feeling as though a blow had been struck against the eye. Her explanation of this was that, by a spasmodic contraction of the straight muscles, the elastic eyeball was suddenly drawn with force against the back of the orbit, giving the sensation of a blow.

In closing the discussion, DR. JACKSON said that his paper simply dealt with the *recognition* of eye-strain, and that he purposely considered only those symptoms most generally present, and had in mind the great mass of cases, not the exceptional ones, which, though in the aggregate many, still are proportionally few.

In his experience, myopia sometimes caused severe eye-strain. There is also the strain of convergence, and any inequality between the two eyes in the amount of myopia—and myopia is usually unequal—is very likely to cause eye-strain. The discovery of myopia should not, he thought, rule out the existence of eye-strain.

CORRESPONDENCE.

MEDICAL LAW IN THE STATE OF WASHINGTON.

To the Editor of THE MEDICAL NEWS,

SIR : The subject of medical legislation is one that has been considered, more or less, by all of our States, and when the framers of the Constitution of the new State of Washington met they designated as one subject for special legislation the practice of medicine. But before that there was a Territorial enactment to the effect that a physician, before entering practice, must register his diploma with the county auditor ; or, if he had been practising for five years before the passage of the law, he should make a statement of the fact to the auditor in writing. This law became a dead letter, as no one paid any attention to its enforcement. As to all new and promising countries, a large flock of all kinds of quacks and itinerants came here.

When the Legislature of the new State met, a bill, known here as the "Powers bill," was introduced, which virtually left all in the hands of a board to be appointed by the Governor. But the bill provided that the board should be chosen from the ranks of the regular profession only, which was considered by the homœopaths, who are about one-eighth of the entire number of medical men in the State, a manifest injustice. After the passage of the bill, the Governor returned it with his veto attached.

Another bill, leaving out the objectionable features, was prepared, and provided that all persons, before practising medicine here, should be examined and licensed by a State board. The meetings of this board are held every six months only—July 1st and January 1st—and no provision is made whereby one entering the State between examinations can practise; he must wait for periods varying from one to six months.

According to his previously announced intention of giving the regular profession a minority representation, the Governor appointed on the board four regular practitioners, three homœopaths, a "physio-medic," and an eclectic. It was no more than was to be anticipated that a portion of the board should be composed of homœopaths, but now the profession consider that a burning insult has been committed against them in the appointment of a "physio-medic." It is difficult to learn what that class of men represents, and no one here knows. At the board meeting a homœopath was elected president, and, without reference to his medical beliefs, it must be said that a better president could not have been found. Although the proceedings of the board were conducted in harmony, the hearts of the "regulars" burned with a feeling of disgust, while the "irregulars" were, of course, well satisfied. With a little stratagem the latter gained their point, by a combine with the "physio-medic" and eclectic members, which enabled them to elect their candidate president of the board, and to place such other members as they pleased in office. The whole scheme was "cut and dried" before the board met, and the opening of the session was delayed so that the "irregulars" could perfect their plans.

The board adopted rules to the effect that a general average of 65 must be made by all but old graduates (of at least five years' standing), who need not average as high in chemistry, physiology, or anatomy as graduates of less than five years' standing. At this meeting each man was given subjects to prepare questions upon.

The examinations were held July 1, 1890, at Walla Walla, when ten men presented themselves, among them your correspondent; and but one man, a homœopathist who graduated in March of this year, failed. The examination was entirely a written one, and was a perfectly fair test of our medical knowledge. There were one hundred and fifty-six questions—viz.: five each on Diseases of the Eye and Ear ; ten each on Medical Jurisprudence, Surgery, Histology, Preventive Medicine, Practice, Diseases of the Nervous System, Anatomy, Materia Medica and Therapeutics, Diseases of Women, and Diseases of Children. On Obstetrics there were eleven questions; on Chemistry fifteen, and on Physiology twenty. On Materia Medica there were two sets of questions, one for the homœopaths and one for the regular practitioners, and the other schools would have had the same privilege had any candidates applied. Two days were consumed in this work.

Laying aside all prejudices, a perusal of some of the questions of the "physio-medic" and eclectic members will show the injustice of having men of that class on the board. During the examination the writer carefully copied the questions, and, in some instances, the spelling—for the question-sheets came to us in the handwriting of the members by whom they had been prepared. The "physio-medic" asked, "What is *pertusses?*" and also the very comprehensive question, "What does delayed dentition prognosticate?" To this last I could not answer, nor could the two or three members of the board, to whom I afterward repeated the question. In Diseases of Women he questioned upon "*leucarrhœa,*" "*amenarrhœa,*" and "*dysmenarrhœa.*" Other questions of his were, "Define *mammary absess,*" and "What is pelvic *absess?*" while the last question was upon "lacerated *peroneum.*"

The eclectic prepared questions on anatomy and physiology, one of which read as follows: "Name the divisions of the abdominal *aorta,* large branches, and from where *does* the lower extremities derive *there* blood-supply?" Another asked, "What's the *peremtory* condition of pepsin in the stomach?" to which we afterward discovered he wished us to answer "Hydrochloric acid." Another question was, "What's the effect of *too much* red corpuscles in the blood?"

Under the heading of Preventive Medicine, in the list of questions prepared by a homœopath, we found two as follows: "What means would you take to resuscitate from an overdose of chloroform?" and "How would you treat a case of poisoning from opium or morphia?" He evidently looks at the subject broadly, and thinks that any means of preventing death should be placed under the head of preventive medicine.

The examination, as a whole, was rigid, and a good test of a man's ability to practise medicine. I was recently informed by a member of the board that the examinations would be made still more severe.

Of all classes of practitioners we have a superabundance, and had the Legislature framed this law so that all men practising medicine in the State of Washington at the time of the passage of this act must come up for examination, the effect would have been excellent.

When I first came to Seattle, a place of 35,000 people, I was told that there were two hundred and fifty physicians here, which is about twice as many as the actual number. Both here and in Tacoma some homœopaths have the largest practice.

It seemed to me ridiculous that we should be required to go before a board in which the representation of the so-called schools was so unequal, but still more when I read the list of questions of the "physio-medic."

There is a class who refuse to pay attention to this law, and another class who were here in sufficient time to register, but neglected to do so, and are inclined to cause trouble.

SEATTLE, WASHINGTON.

NEWS ITEMS.

Surgeon Parke on Vaccination.—At the great banquet of welcome given in London to Surgeon Parke, he briefly referred to the inestimable benefit of vaccination. Before the expedition started for Africa he vaccinated nearly every man in Stanley's little army, with the result that when they were surrounded by smallpox there were only four cases among the members of the expedition, none of which proved fatal. But among the camp-followers and irregulars, who had not been vaccinated, smallpox was almost universal, and large numbers of them died. It is probable that, without the precaution of vaccination, the expedition would never have had strength to complete the march across Africa.

A New Method of Advertising.—According to the *Boston Medical and Surgical Journal,* for some time past complaints have made to the Health Commissioners of Brooklyn, New York, of the persistence with which mothers of very young infants are besieged by agents of the manufacturers of infant-foods. Most of the complainants were physicians who said that they had been requested by their patients to take measures to prevent the annoyance. Investigation resulted in the discovery that one of the clerks of the Bureau of Vital Statistics had been communicating the name and address to the manufacturers of the infant-foods, of every recently confined woman. The clerk was, of course, well paid for his information.

OFFICIAL LIST OF CHANGES IN THE STATIONS AND DUTIES OF OFFICERS SERVING IN THE MEDICAL DEPARTMENT, U. S. ARMY, FROM AUGUST 5 TO AUGUST 11, 1890.

By direction of the Acting Secretary of War, WILLIAM STEPHENSON, *Captain and Assistant Surgeon,* now on duty at Columbus Barracks, Ohio, is assigned to temporary duty at Jefferson Barracks, Missouri, during the absence on leave of Daniel G. Caldwell, Major and Surgeon, and will report accordingly. On the return to duty of Major Caldwell, Captain Stephenson will rejoin his proper station.—Par. 2, *S. O. 176, A. G. O., Washington, D. C.,* July 30, 1890.

By direction of the Acting Secretary of War, leave of absence for one month and fifteen days, to take effect about August 15, 1890, is granted to DANIEL G. CALDWELL, *Major and Surgeon,* —Par. 1, *S. O. 176, A. G. O., Washington, D. C.,* July 30, 1890.

By direction of the Secretary of War, the ordinary leave of absence granted to JAMES P. KIMBALL, *Major and Surgeon,* in S. O. 152, July 1, 1890, from this office, is changed to leave of absence on surgeon's certificate of disability, with permission to leave the Division of the Missouri.—Par. 7, *S. O. 182, A. G. O.,* August 6, 1890.

OFFICIAL LIST OF CHANGES IN THE STATIONS AND DUTIES OF THE MEDICAL CORPS OF THE U. S. NAVY FOR THE WEEK ENDING AUGUST 9, 1890.

WALES, P. S., *Medical Director.*—Ordered in charge of the Museum of Hygiene, Washington, D. C.

BRIGHT, GEORGE A., *Surgeon.*—Ordered to the U. S. S. "Constellation."

MACKIE, B S, *Surgeon.*—Detached from the U. S. S. "Constellation," and ordered to Naval Hospital, Philadelphia, for medical treatment.

DERR, E. Z., *Surgeon.*—Ordered to the U. S. S. "Minnesota."

WAGGENER, J. R., *Surgeon.*—Detached from the U. S. S. "Minnesota," and ordered to the U. S. S. "Kearsarge."

MOORE, A. M., *Surgeon.*—Detached from the U. S. S. "Kearsarge," and granted three months' sick-leave.

THE MEDICAL NEWS.

A WEEKLY JOURNAL OF MEDICAL SCIENCE.

VOL. LVII.   SATURDAY, AUGUST 23, 1890.   No. 8.

ORIGINAL ADDRESS.

THE RELATION OF EYE-STRAIN TO GENERAL MEDICINE. [1]

BY GEORGE M. GOULD. M.D.,

OPHTHALMIC SURGEON TO THE PHILADELPHIA HOSPITAL.

LADIES AND GENTLEMEN: In response to your kind invitation to speak to you concerning some of the relations of Ophthalmology to general medicine, I have chosen one aspect of the subject that is at once most neglected, least understood, and important—to me, indeed, the most important. Other subjects may be more interesting, promise more brilliancy of treatment, or illustrate better one's special knowledge, but in your practice you will have a hundred cases of eye-strain to one of optic neuritis; a hundred of anorexia and malassimilation due to ametropia, to one of contraction of the field of vision; a hundred of nervousness and hysteria to one of hemianopsia or albuminuric retinitis. Moreover, without special training you will not be able to diagnose pathological changes in the fundus of the eye, whilst the recognition of an irritational eye-strain is relatively an easy task.

The essence of what I shall say to you to-night will consist simply in pointing out a few classes of patients, to whom, if you do your duty, you will say, "Go to the oculist." Upon my part this may seem to you a bit of somewhat cunningly selfish advice; but I protest that the matter has certain very unselfish phases, and must, by both of us, be taken very seriously. I have, truly, had in my practice hundreds of patients who have had years, and even a life of daily anguish, because their physicians had not known enough to give them this advice.

The moral of my sermon, therefore, is that eye-strain is an enormously frequent, fertile, and nnsuspected source of non-ocular disease. I beg of you not to let any long-eared prejudice blind you to this fact. Fact it is, and he who soonest recognizes it will do himself the more honor and the world the more good. I purpose speaking directly and solely from my own experience, and no fact has been so frequently and emphatically borne in upon me by every day's practice as that eye-strain is a great promoter and producer, first of functional systemic

[1] An address to the Philadelphia Hospital Medical Society, July 9. 1890.

disease, and even, finally, indirectly of organic disease. And the correlate of that truth is this other, that the general physician makes no more frequent and bitter mistake than his indifference to or ignorance of it. To help you to avoid such errors let us try to answer these questions:

1. What is eye-strain?
2. What is its etiology?
3. How is it diagnosed?
4. What are its effects?

This is in accordance with the wise, old advice, that prior to curing an evil we must know its nature, cause, extent, and results.

The term eye-strain is usually applied to the irritational incoördinations and abnormal exertions of the intra-ocular or extra-ocular muscles. The function of the eye is to form a perfect image of an object upon the retina in precisely the same way as a photographic camera does upon the sensitive plate. Strain arises when the eyeball is abnormally long, short, or curved, or when the muscles are not dynamically balanced. The term may be applied to the results of abusive use of the perfect eye, but that is not the common meaning. As defined above, the words need two criticisms. The first relates to an extension of the meaning so as to include nervous and centrally located phenomena. As commonly used the emphasis—indeed, the sole thought—concerns the muscles. But, the simple muscular over-use or strain is, if not entirely absent, at least often, and, I doubt not, generally, a small factor. Where else in the body does one find undue muscular exertion producing such effects as are the rule in eye-strain? The nearest analogy of so hard-worked a set of muscles consists of those implicated in scrivener's and piano-player's palsy. But the ciliary muscle is more over-worked than the muscles of the hand, whilst the effects are dissimilar. In other parts of the body you may have exhaustion, paralysis, localized soreness, myositis, etc., but never the mental, cerebral, and distant reflexes that are the rule in eye-strain. This is an indication, proved by other considerations, that the central neural. or cerebral, elements are predominant, and that the muscular element *per se* is subordinate and *post hoc*. Failure to see this has led to the woful error of those extremists who cure all the ills that eyes are heir to by tenotomies—graduate and undergraduate. It is, indeed. a noteworthy fact that the patient complains little or not at all of ocular symptoms. In the greatest eye-strain the patient will heartily aver that the eyes themselves are perfect, and give no trouble. There are no pains, no soreness of muscles, no local symptoms whatever. This is an anomalous and interesting, but genuine, fact. I have partially tried to explain it elsewhere, and must pass it by at this time.

The second criticism refers to the origin of insufficiency, or lack of muscular balance in the external muscles. It is too commonly supposed that this is, as it were, congenital, or a positive cause of eye-strain. But it is certainly usually true that the insufficiency is a mere consequence of the ametropia. Correct the latter, and the muscle equilibrium is generally soon restored. Tenotomy, before a lengthy trial of this procedure, is no less than surgical barbarism. This, indeed, is a corollary of the fact that the insufficiency is a phenomenon of nerve centres and nerve forces, rather than of strengths or strains of muscle fibre. The acknowledged etiology of much insufficiency is the disturbance produced by ametropia of the normal relation between accommodation and convergence. But, this is patently a nervous phenomenon, pure and simple. The muscle chiefly strained in eye-strain, if any, would assuredly be the ciliary muscle. But, despite the Herculean tasks and torsions it often has to undergo, it does not from these causes inflame, is not paralyzed, or weakened, but actually develops *de novo* a new set of fibres, almost a new muscle, called the Müller ringmuscle. Thus, from a variety of considerations we conclude that in eye-strain we have chiefly to do with nervous, not muscular forces. The facts to fix attention upon are dynamic, not static ; neurological, not muscular ; central, not peripheral.

As to the ametropia that produces eye-strain, it is almost entirely limited to two varieties, hyperopia and astigmatism. Simple myopia, unless widely differing in degree in the two eyes—anisometropia—produces no eye-strain. For other reasons it may be well to correct near-sightedness, but when you are simply trying to establish a differential diagnosis, you may be assured that if your patient is myopic to only a moderate degree, there will be no reflex neurosis for you as a general practitioner to combat. The danger from following this rule consists in the easy and terrible blunder made by opticians every day, of mistaking a so-called spasm of the accommodation, an astigmatism, or even a high degree of hyperopia, for myopia. As general physicians, however, you will not thus ruin eyes, because you will not prescribe spectacles.

Let us now examine more closely the mechanism whereby hyperopia and astigmatism produce eye-strain.

When the eyeball (antero-posteriorly) is too long—or, what amounts to the same thing, when the refracting powers of the ocular media are too strong—the natural focus of the entering light-rays is in front of the retina. This condition constitutes *myopia*, and from the above explanation it becomes evident that there can be no strain, since the effort, if one may so speak, is to reduce strain. There is already too much refraction, and hence there can be no strain by the eye in attempting to overcome the condition. The rays need to be further dispersed, not more gathered together, and it is the greater gathering that requires an expenditure of nerve or muscular force.

When the eyeball is too short (or the media too weak in refractive power) the retina is in front of the natural focus, and the accommodative apparatus is put to an excess of effort to bring the focus forward, so that it shall be upon the retina. This is hyperopia. All good definition, as the photographers say, depends upon an accurate focalization of the rays from an object, whether upon the sensitive plate of the camera or upon the retina. In hyperopia the definition is only obtained by unceasing over-exertion. It is a Sisyphian task. The focus slips back from its proper position with every instant of inattention. When the object is near, as in reading and writing, the need of greater refracting power is increased or multiplied. This is because rays from near objects are more divergent than from more distant ones. Hence the greater strain in this condition, from near work, and the more marked increase of the whole train of pernicious symptoms when the hyperopic eye is forced to undertake it. The eye being naturally hyperopic, the task set for it by civilization becomes the more glaringly contrasted and severe. Upon the principles of American politicians the oculists and opticians should erect the highest statue in the world to the inventor of printing.

Suppose, now, the cornea unsymmetrical, that is, unequally curved in different meridians, like the bowl of a spoon, the rays of the entering beam of light will be brought to a focus more quickly in the more curved meridian, and the retinal image proportionally blurred. This is *astigmatism*, and, of course, may complicate either myopia or hyperopia. If coexisting with hyperopia it produces the greatest strain.

We understand this by remembering that the ciliary muscle is a sphincter muscle, normally acting equally upon all sides by a common innervation. But with astigmatism, this muscle, or the central nervous system controlling it, seeks to neutralize the effects of the corneal asymmetry by unequal contraction, or excessively straining certain fibres in such a way as to cause the lens to react upon the traversing rays, so as to counteract the unequal influence of the corneal asymmetry. This action of the ciliary muscle is unphysiological, and as is readily seen, productive of a peculiar irritation.

Besides myopia and hyperopia, complicated or not with astigmatism, we may have presbyopia superadded. This consists of a growing inelasticity of the crystalline lens, or failure in the power of accommodation, which, increasing all through life, reaches in emmetropic eyes such a degree, at about forty-five years of age, that the artificial help of biconvex lenses is required for near work. If hyperopia be also present, presbyopia becomes apparent earlier, and proportionally to the amount of such hyperopia. If myopia be present, then presbyopia comes on so much later.

In passing it may be asked why hyperopia and astigmatism, or eye-strain, seems so much more frequent now than formerly. The answer is clear, but apparently contradictory. It is this: hyperopia and astigmatism are probably less common now than ever before, and yet the direct result of these same defects, that is, eye-strain, is immensely more common. The explanation of this paradox is that the eye of animal, savage and child, is naturally hyperopic. Up to the present century the work of the eye has been adapted to the mechanism. But now, printing, schools, cities, sewing and commercialism have suddenly given the eye tasks for which it was never made, or to which it was never habited. The deity of natural selection never foresaw civilization. Great interest attaches to the inquiry how the eye is to react and adapt itself to meet the duty thrust upon it. One fact is evident: when the recognition of the enormous body of ill-results from eye-strain finally succeeds in battering down professional and popular prejudice, spectacles will be almost as common as noses. Nearly every one would be the better, intellectually, morally and physically, from the proper use of proper spectacles. There are extremely few emmetropic eyes. If from his occupation the farmer may be able to do without correction of ametropia, the farmer's child, if he goes to school, will not be able to do so. The greatest good of spectacles will be prophylactic. Thousands all about us are to-day suffering multiform and irremediable injury, directly or indirectly, because of unsuspected eye-strain. The day will sometime come when a conscientious parent will never permit a child, however apparently healthy, to grow to puberty without a scientific examination of the eyes having been made, and repeated at intervals thereafter. The consequences of eye-strain are so subtle, so varied, so remote, so peculiar, so unforseeable, and so harmful, that only by this plan can they be obviated.

How is the existence of hyperopia and astigmatism to be diagnosed—their existence, I say, not their amount? That either exists to a harmful degree is all you desire to know, but knowing this you also know that, until corrected, it is a permanent source of mischief, and that all remedies other than spectacles are palliative or useless. Many plans are advocated, but every one is objectionable. I take it for granted that you will not use the ophthalmoscope. For twenty years the general practitioner has been urged to do so, and for twenty years medical students have bought instruments that they never used after "swinging their shingles to the breeze." I think their advisers gave bad, or at least useless advice. To use an ophthalmoscope properly requires much and continuous practice. The general practitioner soon finds he has not the time nor the patience, and the specialist who can do it better is close at hand. Whether the growth of specialism generally be for good or bad, it is quite certain to grow, and ophthalmology, of all the specialties, has always been pointed to as a model. The wise man accepts and makes the most he can of the inevitable.

Retinoscopy is a popular fad among my brethren: my advice to you is that you would better let us make mistakes with it. If you try to rely upon it you will utter either many falshoods or many objurgations—probably both. Proficiency in its use, as in that of the ophthalmoscope, requires special aptitude and training, and I do not believe that it is to be relied on as an accurate method even in the hands of its best friends.

Of many devices I shall recommend but one to you. Get two differently lettered cards of Snellen test-letters for distance, and hang them in your office, in a good light, fifteen or twenty feet from your patient. With every patient complaining of headache, neuralgia, or dyspepsia, with nervous, hysterical, choreic or anæmic symptoms, test accurately by one card, each eye separately, the ability to read. Keep a record of the lines read in each case. Then paralyze the accommodation with a six-grain solution of homatropine. Half a dozen instillations within three-fourths of an hour are sufficient, but it will be better to give the patient the drops, to be used every hour for a day. When he returns in one or two days, if the headache has in the meantime been better or has disappeared, you may be quite sure you have an eye-strain reflex. This, in fact, is the best method of differential diagnosis between headache due to eye-strain and that due to other causes. Since the great majority of all headaches is due to eye-strain it is a point worth bearing in mind. But now, when your patient returns with thoroughly functionless accommodation, you will retest the acuteness of distant vision, using a different test-card, to avoid the error arising from remembrance of the other letters. If this acuteness is markedly less than it was before using the mydriatic, that is, if only larger letters can now be read, you are convinced that hyperopia or astigmatism, or both exist. The amount of the defect is roughly estimated by the extent to which the visual acuity has fallen off. If originally normal, *i. e.*, if the twenty-foot line was read with each eye, and after paralysis of the accommodation it remains the same, you have a rare case of emmetropia. If originally subnormal, and after the mydriatic it remains the same, you have simple myopia. If you wish to tell whether the diminished acuity is due to hyperopia or to astigmatism, you can do so roughly by an astigmatic test-card. But this is a dangerous road, and for your purposes, one that you do not have to travel.

This plan seems to me the simplest and easiest of all for ascertaining the existence of eye-strain. It may be relied on absolutely, it demands no special training or superfine observation, no costly instruments or appliances. It tells you precisely what you need and want to know, and with little or no trouble. You should remember to warn your patient of the symptoms of mydriasis. Moreover, do not forget that with patients over fifty years of age, Time, that conquers all things, has pretty effectually paralyzed the accommodation, and other mydriatic is unnecessary. Before this age pathological reflexes have mostly subsided.

There is one aspect of this question that we must not overlook: How much lessened acuity, or how much hyperopia or astigmatism is sufficient to set up eye-strain and pathological reflexes? This depends entirely upon two things, the nature and the occnpation of your patient. If the patient be one of civilization's hot-house plants, a neurotic, sensitive, nimble-witted girl, the smallest defect is sufficient to play havoc with such a quivering bundle of nerves. If with such a case there is the slightest falling off of distant acuity under the mydriatic, if the same line of the test-type cannot be read just as easily, pack her off quick!

Between such a case and the rugged, phlegmatic out-of-door-living farmer there are a thousand degrees to tax the best judgment of the best oculist as to what to do. In general the young have less "leeway" than the older, girls and women less than boys and men, the educated less than the uneducated, those doing much reading, writing, sewing, or other near-work, less than those not so busied. A farmer can safely carry for a lifetime five or ten times the defect that a city girl could endure for only a day.

One word more, despite your smile. Never send or allow your patient to be prescribed for by an optician. This disgrace to medicine and sin against humanity should be forbidden by law. Ruined eyes and inexpressible sufferings daily turn up in every oculist's office as the direct result of this execrable habit. If the oculist's fee is frightful, there are in every hospital ophthalmic departments where outpatients may be treated, free of charge, by competent hands.

I fear I have left myself too little space to speak of the essential or vital part of my subject. The heart of the whole matter is as to the effects of eye-strain.

These may be divided into two chief classes, those limited to the eye itself, and those presenting systemic or extra-ocular results. The first class concerns particularly the ophthalmic specialist, but it is well to note them as we pass by. Some of them serve as pointers, or clear indications of the ametropia. In children, especially boys, styes, blepharitis, and conjunctivitis, often mark the deep-seated trouble. The most common ocular symptom is accommodation-failure. The ciliary muscle temporarily relaxes under the strain, and the words of the printed page blur, and run together, and the eyes must be closed for a moment. Such failures occur more frequently if near-work be persisted in, and may be accompanied with conjunctival injection, pains, flow of tears, spasmodic blinking, or "tic" of the lids, face, etc. Among the organic changes produced by eye-strain is myopia. This may sometimes be caused by changes induced by ametropia, whilst insufficiency and strabismus are almost certain proofs of this cause. A still more profound injury is one that I have pointed out to the profession — a chronic macular choroido-retinitis, with pigmentary changes about the posterior pole, lessened visual acuteness, etc. Thus the eye itself may be irremediably injured by uncorrected eye-strain. It is not true that so long as none of the palpable symptoms appear the condition of the eyes may be ignored. Many of these symptoms are so subtle as not to be noticed until the disastrous result is accomplished. It is doubtless true that eye-strain plays an etiological *rôle* in the production of cataract.

Turning now to the more widespread systemic abnormalism and disease produced by eye-strain, we are struck by the awful, discouraging, exasperating slowness with which even the most glaring consequences are ignored, with what intolerable difficulty this knowledge pounds its way through prejudice and ignorance, both lay and professional. Take headache as the best example. The "common people" are to-day more alive to the fact of its true causation than their doctors. Most medical articles on the subject, and books on practice, either ignore the eye-strain or allude to it as a minor factor. The fact, of course, is that it is far more frequently the cause than all others put together. I do not doubt that ninety cases out of one hundred are due to eye-strain In my first series of one thousand refraction cases in private practice a chief complaint in more than eight hundred was of headache. The failures to cure or greatly relieve were not over half a dozen. Eye-strain headaches, or neuralgias, as they are sometimes called, may usually be diagnosed by the following considerations:

1. The patient, nine times in ten, is a girl or woman.

2. In the great majority of cases the patient locates the pain in the forehead or temples, or says it starts there.

3. If the headache is not continuous it is usually brought on or made worse by near-work—is greater, for example, during the school season than in vacation, during school-hours than holidays, etc.

4. The headache is frequently associated with anorexia, fickleness of appetite, malassimilation, or some other digestional abnormality, all these being common eye-strain reflexes.

Sick-headache, there can be little doubt, is very often, if not generally, due to eye-strain, though it, like any other functional abnormality, may not be quickly curable by stopping the cause after continuance for half a lifetime.

Fits of nausea and vomiting are not infrequently produced, and I have now had six or eight cases of pronounced "car-sickness," which never returned after getting spectacles. I had one patient last week who was intensely sick with vomiting, dizziness, etc., for twenty-four hours following every street-car ride. She walked twenty squares to see me. I sent her home, with paralyzed accommodation, upon the street cars, without a return of the usual effects. One wonders if sea-sickness is not more or less connected with ocular functions. A physician wrote me from the West that he could produce giddiness and nausea in himself by rolling his eyes upward in a peculiar manner. One of my patients can read without trouble while sitting up, but gets sick at his stomach at once if he reads lying down.

But the cerebral evidences of irritation and disorder, however marked and clear, are of less importance than others that strike at the nutrition and welfare of the whole organism. The war must be carried into Africa! *Delenda Carthago!* Despite all disbelief, prejudice, and the smiles of superior wisdom, it is my well-proved and deep-rooted conviction that eye-strain very frequently produces digestive troubles of various kinds, all resulting in malnutrition. Those who ten or twenty years ago preached the ocular origin of headache, encountered the same wall of prejudice as one does now in reference to this aspect. I shall not attempt to explain the mechanism of this reflex neurosis, that of any such reflex is not wholly clear, but it is certainly as easily understood as a metastatic orchitis in mumps. Whether understood or not, if you will bear the fact in mind you may save yourself much

8*

vexation and your patient much suffering by testing the eyes of many an anæmic, nervous, dyspeptic girl, whose trouble you cannot account for or cure. I have had very many such patients freshen up at once upon getting spectacles, and in a month or two gain ten or twenty pounds in weight, without any medicine, and after years of other treatment. It seems at first sight the extreme of absurdity to say that anæmia may be due to eye-strain, yet such is the fact, because nothing can shake my conviction that malnutrition may be caused by it, and anæmia is only the consequence of persistent malnutrition. In girls and young women with severe eye-strain, fickle and poor appetite is almost always an emphatic complaint. Their mothers nickname them " pickers." I know well enough the tricks of *post hoc propter hoc* logic, but if such patients return in a month or two with better health patent in every feature, and now eating three meals a day, I trust my conclusions. The iron on their noses in the form of spectacle-frames has done the red blood-corpuscles more good than it would have done in pills.

It is by thus producing continued anorexia and malnutrition that eye-strain may indirectly lay the foundation for other evils that else had not existed. The headache, hyperæsthesia, or nervous exhaustion, brings the organism just to such a degree of weakened vitality that further resistance is impossible, and the upspringing of latent or inherited diseases of many kinds and of differing degrees of fatality is permitted. No lesson is more clear now-a-days than that disease germs find a nidus only where vitality is subnormal.

Two indirect proofs of the power of spectacle lenses to prevent these results are at hand: First, put a pair of spectacles before your normal eyes that will create an eye-strain such as others have without glasses. Headache, dizziness, and vomiting will in a few hours teach a very practical lesson. Second, note this: A spectacle gets broken, and in twenty-four hours the patient returns with a terrible recurrence of the old but long unknown trouble, the headache, the nausea, the unrest, etc. If an astigmatic lens gets bent a small fraction of an inch out of its proper place, there is the same phenomenon. A visit to the optician is all that is needed.

All the reflexes of eye-strain are primarily phenomena of increased nervous action. They are peculiarly central in character, and may perhaps be considered as a struggle of the ocular and optical centres to translate into sensations imperfect retinal stimuli or optic-nerve messages, as well as to react upon the eye itself so as to perfect its function. With hyperopia and astigmatism present this becomes an irritating and harassing labor. disturbs the equilibrium of the cerebral centres. and liberates large excesses and incoördinations of nerve force.

These unregulated discharges overflow the normal outlets, and produce results varying according to the somewhat accidental routes, and the commissural fibres over which the superabundant discharges pour upon centres incapable of resistance. If the phrenic-nerve centre is flooded, the diaphragm is stimulated to excessive action, and vomiting or other disturbance follows. In connection with this I may mention the case of one of my patients, Mrs. G., who had suffered for twenty years with a persistent and harrowing flatulent dyspepsia, for which many physicians had been consulted, and limitless quantities of medicine had been taken. I speak advisedly when I say that the minute proper glasses were applied the frightful eructations and discomfort stopped. If the glasses are left off a minute or two the diaphragm begins its spasmodic action. If the innocent overflooded centres happen to be inhibitory centres the results are in accord with the function of those centres. Possibly the digestive torpor and malassimilation are explainable as an unregulated stimulation of the pneumogastric. I reported a case last year in which violent rapidity of the heart's action came on with outrageous abuse of hyperopic eyes, and persisted despite all treatment until correcting spectacles were found, then suddenly subsided. Another noteworthy illustration was that of Miss U., who had suffered from periods of aphonia for years. The mydriatic brought the voice back, and the glasses have assured the cure. I have had several cases of non-appearance of menstruation, amenorrhœa, and dysmenorrhœa, in which the proper function was established at once upon the use of spectacles. Two patients had periods of partial paralysis and anæsthesia of the limbs prior to coming to me. These instances of derouted reflex action are characterized by appearing at more or less regularly recurring periods with increasing headache and sometimes with "blind-spells," or other ocular symptoms.

Generally speaking, the excess of irritational stimulus results in positive overstimulation of motor centres. In a large class it will manifest itself as a diffuse abnormal activity. The child or young person is simply "nervous," restive, cannot keep still, will not stick to studies, etc. If the derouted reflex take more specialized channels certain muscles or groups are acted upon, and simple chorea follows. One girl wore out the right shoe in a few weeks by excessive scraping of the foot. A boy was always snuffing or making grimaces with the lips. Tics of the cheek muscles and jerking of the hand or arm are also met with. I have had quite a number of cases of pronounced chorea cured at once by correction of ametropia. I have had no experience with epilepsy or insanity. If I had a case of *petit mal* I would try prolonged mydriasis. Very frequent symptoms of eye-strain are insomnia and night-

terrors. The child rolls, cries out in its sleep with fright. The surcharged cerebral centres after the day's warfare are for a long time unable to reach a condition of normal equilibrium. I have more than half a belief that enuresis may sometimes be traceable to the same irritation.

It may be thought that the reports of many of such cases as the above are to suffer revision in the light of one error common to all—hysteria. The old pianoforte tuners swept all the discords into one octave that was called *the devil*, and this was avoided as much as possible in playing. There was a time when, whatever was not understood, or not easily curable in female nervous disease, was called hysteria. It was a convenient cover for professional failure in therapeutics. I have no doubt that many, very many such cases needed, and still need, a pair of proper spectacles, instead of sneers and pilulæ asafœtidæ.

One final illustration and I have done. The common-school system as now carried on is largely responsible for a deal of suffering such as I have described. Children are forced to needless and unhealthful study, and manufactured into sorry examples of intellectual *pâte de foie gras*, namby-pamby mimics and memorizers when they should be in training to make of them healthy young animals. Under this system of over-pressure and sham education the civilized eye, like many another product of civilization, is a poor and pitiable thing. Its little possessor, sadly unconscious of what is the matter, goes on with high pressure, and ambition, and tonics, until one after another the strings of life snap under the high tension. If not so, he finds study becoming irksome, and the parents grieve as they painfully watch intellectual capacity slowly and persistently renounced and life shunted into the world's humdrum and routine. Eye-strain has thus derouted many a natural genius, subtly turning him from intellectual culture to physical but less painful outlets for his activity.

The multiformity and apparent exaggeration of the effects of eye-strain indicated above may seem less extravagant if we remember how vital the function of vision is to every act, how necessary to every minute's safety of the organism, how uninterruptedly active during every instant of waking life. Not only every act, but every emotion and thought—intellect itself, and imagination, are born of or bound up with visual acts and results. The very letters of the alphabet are conventionalized pictures of things. Mind is incarnate and concentrate seeing. The visual centres of the brain are in the closest and most vital connection with all other brain centres. How easily, therefore, must a disturbance of the peripheral mechanism send a jarring and discordant thrill throughout the entire motor, sensory, and psychic being. At once the microcosm is aroused to correction and adjustment; subordinate and commissurally connected centres feel the challenge and the overflow according to the accidents of weakness, diathesis, disease, and their varying powers of resistance. The result of this overflow, or switching, is a reflex neurosis, and from the supreme importance of the function of vision and the unusual strain that civilization puts it to, the eye becomes the greatest originator of these disturbances.

ORIGINAL ARTICLES.

ON HYPEROSTOSIS OF THE PRÆMAXILLARY PORTION OF THE NASAL SEPTUM, AND A DESCRIPTION OF AN OPERATION FOR ITS RELIEF.

BY HARRISON ALLEN, M.D., .
OF PHILADELPHIA.

IN a well-defined group of cases there exists at the lower part of the septum, anteriorly, between the triangular cartilage and the floor of the nose, a disposition to hyperostosis which may so far encroach upon the vestibule (as this passage is seen just within the plane of the nostril) as to create an obstruction. The triangular cartilage itself, in these cases, though it may remain straight, is usually deflected to the side occupied by the main portion of the hyperostosis. Fully one-third or one-half of this osseous growth lies below the plane of the nostril, and the obstruction which it causes is not removed by any of the means for correcting deviation of the septum. The existence of the hyperostosis can be demonstrated by passing a curved probe within the nasal chamber, placing its free end on the floor, and drawing the instrument forward. The probe is felt to touch a resisting mass at a distance, on an average, of one-half inch from the anterior edge of the nasal aperture. It is evident from such a conformation that the mucus which trickles to the floor of the nose cannot be easily removed, and that when inspissated it will excite irritation, and lead to insufficiency of nasal respiration.

Careful dissection shows that the growths can be best exposed by separating the upper lip from the jaw at the region of the nasal spine. The lip being elevated, an incision is made through the frænum, and a chisel is employed to break down the resisting mass of bone at the præmaxillary portion of the septum. In some cases a metacarpal saw is preferred, or a gouge can be used with advantage. A hand-drill is sometimes very effective. The single object in view is to remove as much bone as may obstruct the chambers. The bone is of great hardness, and rapidly dulls the sharpest instrument. It thus becomes necessary to have a number of freshly sharpened instruments for each operation. After the parts have been sufficiently reduced the triangular cartilage, if it be deflected, may be separated from the lower border of the notch, and set in a favorable position by the use of either pins or plugs.

It is hardly necessary to state that many phases of distress are relieved by less interference than is described above; but it is nevertheless true, that some patients who have had all the resources at my disposal exhausted without obtaining relief, were promptly cured, or greatly improved, by the supra-labial operation. I have operated many times, and in no instance have I observed any rise of temperature. I believe the procedure to be free from risk. The after-treatment is exceedingly simple. The lip being allowed to fall into position makes perfect adaptation, and closes the oral wound. Until the septum is attached in its new position, ivory or cotton plugs are used as splints. These must be removed daily for a week, at the end of which time the parts are entirely healed. The lip remains slightly swollen for a very short time, but I have never seen any inflammation.

CASE I. *An inveterate, chronic, nasal catarrh greatly relieved by the supra-labial operation, after all other means had failed.*—W. J., twenty-eight years old, reported to me for catarrhal difficulties, arising from obstruction to the nasal respiration, of four years duration. I found hypertrophy of the right turbinated bone, and a sharp spur on the nasal septum at the junction of the anterior part of the vomer and the perpendicular plate of the ethmoid bone; the septum was deviated to the left. The anterior end of the left middle turbinated bone was the seat of a chronic hyperplasia. The quantity of discharge in this case was exceptional. It was constantly flowing, both day and night. The largest part passed backward, and greatly interfered with sleep and appetite. Its presence did not excite any reflex symptoms.

In January, 1885, under ether, I loosened the triangular cartilage from its inferior attachment, at the same time removing the hyperplastic membrane from the left middle turbinated bone, and the hypertrophied tissues from the right turbinated bone. The spur which was formed at the junction of the vomer and the perpendicular plate of the ethmoid was ablated with a saw, as originally recommended by me. Great relief followed this manipulation, but the triangular cartilage, in time, resumed its old position. In September, 1888, he reported a second time. Since, in this long interval, much of the original distress remained unrelieved, he had been under the care of leading laryngologists, and all had been done for him that was possible to do. Examination revealed no cause for interference with either the turbinals or the septum. I detected, however, that the præmaxillary portion of the septum was unusually thick, and, with the object in view of reducing its size. I proposed to him the supra-labial operation. which. up to that time, I never performed.

On December 1, 1888, I performed the operation under ether. Separating the under lip from the jaw, at the junction of the labio-alveolar mucous membrane, the nasal spine was exposed and freed from periosteum. A stout chisel was then used, which measured about two-thirds of an inch on its cutting surface. The instrument was pushed firmly against the junction of the spine with the triangular cartilage, thus separating the cartilage from the maxillary portion of the septum, and was thence directed downward and inward. It soon met with the hyperostosis, and could not be urged forward without the aid of a mallet. The chisel, being slightly wedge-shaped, increased the interval between the septum at the place of division and the floor of the nose, so that some relief of the strain under which the part had before suffered was to be expected. The sides of the mass were reduced by the saw.

The patient was greatly relieved by the operation, although not to the extent that I desired. There is still a disposition for the triangular cartilage to return to its old position, which, however, is, in great measure, under control.

CASE II. *Chronic nasal catarrh, pharyngitis, deafness, vertigo, and impairment of memory; relief by intra-nasal treatment; a return of the pharyngitis in an obstinate form cured by the supra-labial operation.*—S. S. D., aged forty-nine; reported May 14, 1887. The patient had received a severe injury on the left side of the face when a boy. Nothing appeared to have followed the direct effect of this injury until the patient was thirty-seven years old. At this time he suffered from attacks of "sore-throat," and conditions connected with ineffective nasal respiration. In time nocturnal mouth-breathing was established; a headache of high grade was developed on the right side of the brow; the memory became impaired; the patient became dyspeptic, and was greatly annoyed with vertigo. The distress arising from these symptoms gradually increased until, at the time he reported for treatment, he was contemplating, on account of his ill health, retirement from business. Chronic aural catarrh supervened in 1884. The hearing distance on the right side was seven inches, and that on the left side four inches. The vibrations of the tuning-fork were referred to the left side. The handle of the malleus was retracted on each side.

The nasal septum was so far deflected to the right, directly within the nostril, as to prevent any view being obtained of the interior of this chamber. On the left side the parts were open anteriorly; but, at the junction of the middle and anterior third, the septum was thickened, and hyperostosed in the præmaxillary portion, and greatly deflected to the right at the line corresponding to the juncture of the vomer and perpendicular plate of the ethmoid bone. The inferior meatus at the upper part was thus completely obliterated. Posterior rhinoscopy showed the septum to be uniformly thickened. The left choana was markedly smaller than the right in all its proportions. Lateral swellings on the vomer were conspicuous, the swelling of the left side being much the larger, nearly obliterating the choana.

The left middle turbinated bone was nearly vertical; the turbinals were nowhere enlarged. The walls of the oropharynx were infiltrated, of a red color, and the entire region was excessively irritable. Quantities of tenacious mucus were seen occupying the pyriform sinuses.

On May 16, 1888, I advised that the patient be etherized, and the nasal chamber explored, the object being to determine its condition on the right side, and to remove the septal ledge on the left. The little finger being passed into the right nasal passage, I found to my surprise that the triangular cartilage readily yielded to gentle pressure, and permitted the finger to pass well into the chamber. The inferior turbinated bone was atrophic. A moderate amount of hyperplasia was detected at the anterior part of the middle turbinal. The only surgical measure at this time resorted to was the removal of the septal ledge on the left side, which was easily accomplished with a saw.

The patient returned to his home a week after the operation, and was not seen until November 5, 1888, when he presented himself with the following report. The pain over the right brow and the vertiginous symptoms had disappeared; digestion and the habit of mouth-breathing were improved; the hearing distance on the right side had increased to eleven inches, and that on the left side to seven inches; the tuning-fork was referred to the vertex; the memory was not improved.

The patient reported again in a fortnight, complaining that the pain had returned, the other symptoms remaining the same. I did not see him again until March 7, 1889, when the improvement recorded under note of November 5, 1888, was found unchanged. He had greatly increased in weight—before the operation he weighed 185 pounds, and at this date 224 pounds. The only symptom of which he complained was a slight discharge into the nasopharynx, which annoyed him in the early morning. He remained in this condition until May 3, 1889, when he reported with the statement that the throat had remained perfectly comfortable for a year, then gradually became uncomfortable, and, at the date of report was about the same as before the operation. The headache, vertigo, and oral breathing had not returned; the hearing distance remained the same. A slight degree of fetor was noticed on the breath. I again advised another examination under ether, with the object of placing the triangular cartilage in a better position, and diminishing the thickness of the septum at the præmaxillæ.

Accordingly, on June 21, 1889, I performed the supra-labial operation. There was more oozing of blood than usual, and reflex neuralgic pains followed. The patient, however, made an entirely good recovery, and reported on October 8, 1889, with entire relief of all his symptoms, save the impairment of hearing and of memory.

November 13, 1889, the patient reported with a slight recent catarrhal pharyngitis, which excited anxiety. There was no return of the nasal difficulties. The hearing distance on the right side remained at eleven inches, but on the left side it had improved, the distance being eight inches.

REMARKS.—This case is of interest on account of the acquired habit of mouth-breathing in an adult exciting chronic pharyngitis and aural catarrh. These symptoms were either greatly relieved or entirely removed by operative procedures within the nasal chambers. It is also interesting to observe that while considerable comfort was derived from the reduction of the septal spurs, which were placed far back within the nasal passages, entire relief from the nasal and pharyngeal symptoms was not acknowledged until the hyperostosis of the præmaxillary portion of the septum was removed.

CASE III.—A. H. D., a lawyer, thirty-seven years of age, was sent to me by Dr. Lewis Taylor, of Wilkesbarre, Pa., October 4, 1888. The patient complained that from his seventh year he had suffered from nasal catarrh associated with attacks of spasmodic asthma. He was peculiarly susceptible to the odors arising from horses. These odors increased the secretions, including those of the lachrymal apparatus. The odors of the seashore had a similar effect, but were less constant and not so severe. Independent of these serious distresses, the catarrhal attacks were irregular, and were often dependent upon systemic causes as well as those of climate. Aggravated forms of the attacks were sufficiently common to interrupt seriously his professional engagements. A physician had, a short time previously, amputated the uvula, but without effecting relief. In 1880 symptoms of lachrymal obstruction appeared.

Examination showed that the nasal chambers were normal in all respects, except the præmaxillary portion, where the septum was enormously thickened anteriorly, and the floor of the left side elevated considerably above the level of the right. Both chambers were large anteriorly, just above the plane of the nostril. The pharynx presented the ordinary signs of chronic inflammation. Both lachrymal punctæ were small. I recommended that the supra-labial operation be performed. This was accordingly done October 18, 1888. The patient made a prompt recovery, and was immediately relieved of all his symptoms, excepting those which pertained to the lachrymal ducts. I last heard from this patient June 18, 1889. He remained perfectly free from all his catarrhal and asthmatical symptoms, and had been much improved by treatment, at his home, of the lachrymal obstructions.

REMARKS.—This case is an illustration of the long-standing effects which can arise from irritations excited by the hyperostosis of the anterior part of the septum, and of the necessity of a surgical operation.

CASE IV.—F. G., a machinist, aged twenty-four years, was sent to me by Dr. C. A. Wirgman. Since childhood he had suffered from nasal obstruction and catarrh. The anterior portion of the nasal chamber was obstructed by thickenings of the nasal septum over the præmaxillæ.

On June 3, 1889, I performed the supra-labial operation. The parts were exceptionally dense; the nasal spine was long, with a broad base; the triangular cartilage was bent far over to the right, completely occluding the nasal chamber at this point. To remove this occlusion the cartilage was separated from the vomer and anterior nasal spine by means of my septum knife. It was then pushed over toward the left side and was held in position by cotton pledgets. I did not see the patient again for a week, as he was placed under the care of Dr. Wirgman. He had returned to his work—that of a laborer in an iron mill—the third day after operation. He was instantly and entirely relieved from all his distress, which has not since returned.

CASE V.—D. S. W., twenty-four years of age, reported, June 10, 1887, at the recommendation of Dr. C. H. Spooner, suffering from attacks of epistaxis. The disposition to hæmorrhage was hereditary, being transmitted by the father. The subject's brothers and sisters possessed the same peculiarity. One sister died of consumption, and he said that all his family had weak lungs. Attacks of bleeding occurred about every month or two. The patient complained of sensations of heat and dryness within the nostrils, and he was constantly disposed to pick the right nostril, and to wake up in the morning from unrefreshing sleep to find the mouth and throat parched. Nasal respiration was normal except at night, when oral breathing was established. He was treated in early life for attacks of stomatitis by Dr. Spooner, who believed the patient to be strumous.

Inspection of the nasal chambers showed great thickening of the præmaxillary portion of the septum. The deflection of the triangular cartilage to the right was sufficient to effect contact with the anterior end of the inferior turbinal. In almost its entire extent the cartilage was the seat of a superficial ulceration which bled upon the slightest touch. A peculiar odor was detected about the parts which I have noticed with the subjects of chronic bleeding. It is apparently caused by the decomposition of mucus containing blood-clot.

The left choana was very much smaller than the right and possessed a nearly vertical middle turbinated bone. I treated the ulcerated surface with applications of nitrate of silver, but without success. I saw the patient every week or fortnight until October of the same year, when he was attacked with an acute coryza followed by pharyngitis and a great deal of œdema. This attack greatly increased the difficulties attending nasal respiration. On the sixth day a spontaneous hæmorrhage occurred which appeared to be from both nostrils. I saw him at noon of the same day of the attack, and plugged the nostrils. The hæmorrhage was arrested for seven hours, but returned at eight o'clock in the evening of the same day, when the parts were again plugged, this time permanently stopping the bleeding.

The inferior turbinals were subject to great alterations in size, but, as a whole, they were normally proportionate, the left being slightly larger than the right. The masses in the naso-pharynx were seen to vary in size at different times, and occasionally to project from the choana into the naso-pharynx, but without exciting, at such times, any distress.

Believing that the unrelieved ulceration was a constant exciting cause of hæmorrhage, and the condition of mouth-breathing a predisposing cause to laryngeal or pulmonary phthisis, I operated on him, February 19th, to relieve the strain of the triangular cartilage, trusting by this manipulation to cure the ulcerated surface. The patient did well until June 25th, when a profuse bleeding occurred. This was controlled by pressure from without, proving that the bleeding-point was near the nostril. A week later a second bleeding occurred, which was promptly checked by the patient pressing the alæ of the nostril firmly against the septum. He made a good recovery.

Six months after the operation he reported, saying that all the symptoms had disappeared, and that he had had no bleeding since the attacks immediately after the operation. The alæ was entirely healed.

REMARKS.—In this case an intractable ulcer of the triangular cartilage, in an hereditary bleeder with a strumous history, was cured by relieving the nasal septum from strain at its anterior part. Owing to the constitutional peculiarities the operation was essayed under difficulties, but none of these interfered with a good recovery and correction of an annoying and dangerously diseased condition.

The operation of resetting the triangular cartilage, as performed by myself, consists in separating the lower border of the cartilage from the triangular notch, pushing it toward the larger cavity of the nose, and fixing it in its new position. Should the spur on the smaller side be very prominent, it may be sawed off. In the absence of hyperostosis of the præmaxillary portion of the septum, this little procedure is often all that is required to give comfort. In all operations on the septum it must be remembered that no radical increase of diameters is to be sought for. A tendency for the parts to return to their original positions is in constant operation. The surgeon must not be disappointed to find the triangular cartilage disposed to return to its primal place; but while the parts often look as though little had been accomplished, the reports of the patient are encouraging. Something in the way of relief has been accomplished and in the great majority of cases sufficient to warrant acceptance of the procedure as a safe means of curing the symptoms attending nasal obstruction. Occasionally, after healing is completed, small fibroid or cartilaginous nodules are seen occupying the inferior meatus. These result from the process of cicatrization, and they must be removed by the knife or the scissors.

Simple Method of Curing Obesity.—A French journal announces a cure for obesity which is as simple as it is said to be effective (*Weekly Medical Review*). The method consists in never eating more than one variety of food at a meal, without any restriction in the amount taken. Two cases are reported illustrating the effects of the treatment.

MITRAL STENOSIS IN CHILDHOOD.[1]

BY WILLIAM A. EDWARDS, M.D.,

OF SAN DIEGO, CAL.

FELLOW OF THE COLLEGE OF PHYSICIANS OF PHILADELPHIA, AND OF THE AMERICAN PÆDIATRIC AND PHILADELPHIA PATHOLOGICAL SOCIETIES; FORMERLY INSTRUCTOR IN CLINICAL MEDICINE IN THE UNIVERSITY OF PENNSYLVANIA; PHYSICIAN TO ST. JOSEPH'S HOSPITAL: AND ASSOCIATE PATHOLOGIST TO THE PHILADELPHIA HOSPITAL, ETC.

THE constant advance in medical knowledge is in no way better illustrated than by the fact that the mitral stenotic murmur is again tossed into the arena of controversy, and that the object of this paper is partly to defend its existence.

First referred to by Gendrin in 1841, and differentiated by Fauvel in 1843, it had a somewhat checkered career until 1862, when Gairdner so ably described its characteristics that its position in the nomenclature of cardiac disorders seemed to be assured. Very recently, however, the old dispute, opened by Barclay, has been renewed by Dickinson (1887), who does not accept the statement that the presystolic murmur is indicative of mitral stenosis; but Balfour, Gairdner, Bristow, and more recently Sansom, have most vigorously re-asserted the diagnostic importance of this murmur. It is the object of the writer of this paper to add his testimony to the value of this sound in interpreting conditions of obstruction at the mitral orifice. It is my opinion that obstruction at the left auriculo-ventricular orifice presents a most characteristic sound.

Having stated the position we occupy in regard to this controversy, we will proceed to a consideration of the murmur *seriatim*. By mitral stenosis we understand an alteration in the histological structure of the left auriculo-ventricular orifice which causes an obstruction to the passage of the blood from auricle to ventricle.

The accompanying Table (p. 187) presents a series of cases of mitral stenosis taken from my case-book.

Etiology.—This condition is probably never congenital, although some observers have stated the contrary. The most recent and most authoritative communication upon the subject, that of Osler in Keating's *Cyclopædia*, dwells upon the condition of tricuspid stenosis with atresia of the orifice, but does not make any reference to a similar condition on the left side, although illustrations are appended of an irregular differentiation of the segments and of numerical anomalies of the curtains of the valve. Furthermore, it is not at all likely that fœtal endocarditis would produce this condition, for endocarditis in the fœtus is, almost without exception, confined to the right side; and again, the murmur has perhaps never been recorded during the very early years of life. In

---

[1] Read before the Medical Society of the State of California, April 16, 1890.

No.	Age.	Sex.	Murmur.	Concomitant disease.	Results and remarks.
1	Observed from 8 to 12 years.	Male.	First, presystolic; later, regurgitant; thrill. Early reduplication of second sound disappeared later.	Rheumatism and anæmia.	Child under careful observation for four years. Dilated hypertrophy for last two years. Œdema, dyspnœa, and death from exhaustion. Autopsy: Buttonhole mitral. A photograph of the boy in his eighth year is pictured in Bruen's Physical Diagnosis. He died under my observation in the Hospital of the University of Pennsylvania.
2	12 years.	Female.	Loud, rasping, presystolic murmur, followed by low purring, systolic bruit; thrill.	None; she and her friends can recollect no attack of acute disease, and state that the child has hardly been sick a day in her life. Sought advice for shortness of breath.	Case is fully reported in Diseases of the Heart and Circulation in Infancy and Adolescence, by Keating and Edwards, 1888, p. 110. Alive at report.
3	13 years.	Female.	Pronounced presystolic, with low systolic.	Coxalgia: enuresis; some hypertrophy; heart acting well.	Observed in consultation with H. W. Yeamans, M.D., San Diego. Alive and well at report.
4	7 years.	Female.	Presystolic; thrill.	Anæmia and deficient personal hygiene.	Observed in Children's Hospital, Philadelphia, with C. W. Kollock, M.D.
5	9 years.	Male.	Pronounced presystolic; apparent reduplication of second sound.	Ill-defined rheumatism, not articular.	Private practice, Philadelphia. Alive at report.
6	12 years.	Male.	Presystolic.	Ill-nourished. Died during a severe epidemic of measles. Heart was hypertrophied, but auricle dilated.	Death. Stenosis marked, orifice irregular, and valve segments fibroid; funnel-shaped. Private practice, Philadelphia.
7	7 years.	Male.	Presystolic, with slight systolic thrill.	Bulging præcordium; emaciated; pale; anæmic; no rheumatism; hemiplegia and aphasia.	Death. Post-mortem: Buttonhole mitral; stenosis marked; clots fibrinous and organized; anterior and middle cerebral arteries of left side contained emboli. Observed in Third Outdoor District, Philadelphia.
8	11 years.	Female.	Typically presystolic; thrill.	Bulging præcordium; top-heavy appearance, due to auricular dilatation. No rheumatism. Aphasia; hemiplegia.	Death. Post-mortem: Funnel-shaped mitral; clots fibrinous; middle and anterior cerebral plugged. Observed in the Third Out-door District, Philadelphia.
9	6½ years.	Female.	Presystolic.	Anæmia; ill-nourished and poorly developed; slight rheumatism; frequent attacks of diarrhœa.	Alive at report. Heart-beats irregular; apparent reduplication of second sound. Private practice, Philadelphia.
10	9 years.	Male.	Predominant, loud presystolic, with low systolic thrill.	No symptoms; sought advice on account of nightmare.	Alive at report. Private practice, Philadelphia.
11	12 years.	Female.	Loud presystolic thrill.	No rheumatism; few symptoms; short breath most exacting.	Alive at report. Private practice, Philadelphia.
12	5½ years.	Male.	Presystolic.	Ill-defined rheumatism; dyspnœa; præcordial bulging; anæmia.	Died from asthenia. Auricle dilated; contained clots; ventricle dilated; hypertrophy. Observed in the Third Out-door District, Philadelphia.

most instances the child has reached or passed its fifth year, although occasionally cases are recorded at a younger age, as, for example, Chapin's[1] case of two years, and Sansom's[2] case of four years and three months. The latter observer has also recorded the case of a baby two months old who presented a ring of granulations of endocarditis with thickening of the mitral valve; so that, on the whole, we can conclude that the congenital origin of mitral stenosis is not proven. Not so in regard to rheumatism; the association between the two conditions is, as we all know, as definite as

that which exists between regurgitation at the same valve and the rheumatic diathesis. An analysis of the recent literature shows that the association is apt to be with a rheumatic condition that is not marked or acute, but latent and insidious, in contradistinction to the severity of the attack in which the regurgitant murmur is usually produced. For example: in Chapin's series of 31 cases, 20 presented rheumatic involvement, as follows: In 6 there was a history of rheumatism in the immediate family, but none in the patient; in 4 cases there was rheumatism in the family, and the child had also been rheumatic. In 10 instances the patient alone presented a rheumatic history. Sansom most aptly remarks that the stenosis is rarely associated with

[1] New York Medical Record, January 4, 1890, p. 5.
[2] American Journal of the Medical Sciences, March, 1890, p. 284.

the explosive varieties of rheumatism. Of his 40 cases, 26, or sixty-five per cent., were rheumatic. Cheadle has noted an even more intimate association—that is, seventy-nine per cent., or 44 cases out of 57, being rheumatic. This, as we see, leaves a small proportion of cases which occur independently of any rheumatic taint, cases whose etiology has been the cause of much speculation, and not infrequently of the advancement of somewhat improbable hypotheses in endeavoring to unravel the problem. Sansom, indeed, loath to relinquish the rheumatic taint as a causative factor, states that even in cases in which there was no history of rheumatism obtainable the changes in the endocardium were identical with those that occur in association with the d athesis; in fact, he was unable to differentiate these cases from those that were known to be rheumatic; and Chapin, in an earlier paper (1886), presented notes of 26 cases of heart-disease in rheumatic children, in which only 4 presented evidences of mitral obstruction, and in 3 instances it was associated with other murmurs. Of the remaining moiety of cases, the etiology has been placed in one or other of the accepted causative agents of valvular derangement.

Duroziez, Landouzy, and Schnell[1] testify to the possibility of a so-called idiopathic origin of mitral stenosis, more particularly in women and children, an illustration of which would seem to be a case recorded by Sansom,[2] in which there were signs of wasting and long-continued malnutrition. The girl, aged nine, whose general appearance and condition suggested tuberculosis, wasted rapidly and had nightsweats. The physical signs, however, were "a typical presystolic murmur, with sharp, loud impulse, and the signs of considerable cardiac hypertrophy."

Another series of cases seem to arrange themselves naturally under a derangement of the nervous system. One of Chapin's cases had chorea but not rheumatism, and nine of Sansom's cases manifested chorea, two were right and two were left hemichorea; in several of his cases hemiplegia, paresis, and epilepsy were associated with the vascular lesion. Then, again, a mitral stenotic murmur may be heard in association with other valvular murmurs; particularly is this the case when the aortic leaflets are incompetent, allowing regurgitation at this orifice, with a constant damming back of blood in the ventricle, which perhaps might float the mitral curtains out into the current, and thus produce an obstruction in the direct mitral current —a mechanism by which Guitéras has endeavored to explain the cases of what he terms direct functional murmur. A small number of cases are no

doubt due to the fact that a valve which was primarily incompetent and which permitted regurgitation, may undergo further change, and become stiffened, indurated, and stenosed, thus giving rise to the murmur of stenosis.

Diagnosis.—The peculiar percussion outline in this affection was well illustrated by two cases, one of which was under my observation for about four years in Philadelphia. The heart was secured at autopsy in the Hospital of the University of Pennsylvania. The other case I have fully reported elsewhere.[1] The increase in the size of the auricle gives the heart a top-heavy appearance, and in the first case an auricular impulse was many times demonstrated to the class. This pulsation, seen in the second and third left interspaces, always preceded the apical impulse, and, to our mind, clearly demonstrated the presystolic impulse of an hypertrophied auricle dependent upon mitral stenosis, and, in consequence, the presystolic time of the murmur. It is granted, of course, that an auricular impulse is not a constant concomitant of mitral constriction (in Sansom's series it was present in 4 of 35 cases); but, when it does exist, its significance is evident. Not so, however, with a thrill, which is a much more constant attendant, and was present in 7 of our cases and absent in 5. This thrill was always presystolic—that is to say, it ceased abruptly with the occurrence of the apex beat.; it was usually felt best by the tips of the fingers placed somewhat above and to the right of the apex. The thrill may not be constant in a given case; it may exist at one examination, and be absent at the next.

It is more particularly, however, to the murmur that we desire to call attention. A murmur heard above and within the apex; that ceases abruptly with systole, immediately upon the apex striking the chest-wall, or, with the finger upon the carotid, as soon as the pulse is felt; a murmur which in a child is usually harsh or rolling in timbre, and may commence immediately after the second sound and occupy the entire long pause, or may be audible only at the termination of this pause (the presystolic period or according to some the post-diastolic) is, as we understand it, diagnostic of mitral stenosis.

But to assist us in our diagnosis there are certain concomitant signs, such as accentuation of the pulmonary-artery second sound, and seeming reduplication of the second sound, explained by some by the fact that the unfilled right chambers cause a right ventricle and pulmonary artery systole to precede the same act upon the left side, as Da Costa remarks in illustration of the fact that practically two hearts exist in the chest. Sansom, however, considers this an example of what has been recorded by Henry

[1] Annual of the Universal Medical Sciences, 1888.
[2] American Journal of the Medical Sciences, March, 1890, p. 234.

[1] Diseases of the Heart and Circulation in Infancy and Adolesence. Keating and Edwards, 1888.

as a case of asynchronous contraction of the cardiac ventricles.[1] Reduplication may be due to a sudden tension of the mitral valves following the normal second sound and preceding the presystolic murmur. We have already called attention to the thrill, which may be associated with the murmur, or may exist independently. It must be borne in mind that the presystolic murmur of mitral stenosis is not constant, it may be present one day and absent the next. The largest proportion of cases is accompanied by the murmur of regurgitation, but in 7 out of the 12 above cases the murmur of stenosis alone existed. In differentiating it is well to remember, with the other differential signs, that systolic murmurs fade away, whereas a presystolic murmur ends abruptly with systole.

Reference must be made to the careful work of Dickinson,[2] although we are unable to accept his deductions. He concludes that the murmur we are considering usually runs into the systole about as far as the carotid beat and then ends with the terminal knock. He, however, concedes the little murmur which follows the second sound and occurs in the mid-diastolic period to be the true murmur of mitral stenosis; this he terms the old direct mitral murmur, made from auricle to ventricle through a much-contracted valve. It is, however, not granted by this observer that the murmur which begins after this has ceased (the presystolic murmur of this paper) is correctly termed presystolic. He prefers to consider it really a regurgitation, or a direct mitral murmur which rumbles up to near the end of the ventricular systole. This effort of Dickinson to prove the systolic nature of the murmur that we are pleased to call presystolic, concludes in this wise—"Does the lifting of the chest-wall, as felt with the fingers, indicate the systole? Does the murmur accompany the lifting? Does the carotid beat follow the murmur without an interval? If these do so, the murmur is systolic." We, of course, concede that the chest-lifting indicates the systole, but do not believe that the murmur accompanies this lifting, nor can we reconcile our answer in the affirmative in regard to the last proposition. Indeed, it would be still harder to concede these propositions after a careful study of Fenwick and Overend's paper.[3] The cardiograms of these observers demonstrate beyond peradventure that the murmur commences immediately before the ventricular contraction, and that the bruit is both presystolic as regards sound and contraction. Gairdner has suggested, and we are heartily in accord with him, that the auricular systole gives to the blood column an additional

impetus, thus increasing its rate of flow through the constricted valve, causing the fluid to vibrate and the sound thus produced becoming audible to us as the presystolic murmur.

We quote two conclusions from the above observer, the application of which will be obvious to all.

"1st. The auriculo-ventricular valves occupy a horizontal position during the systole of the ventricle, while the papillary muscles contract simultaneously with the rest of the ventricular wall. The ventricle does not empty itself completely, there being a certain amount of residual blood.

"2d. The mid-diastolic mitral murmur in mitral stenosis owes its existence to the influence of the high pulmonary tension. The latter also plays an indirect part in the production of the early and late (presystolic) mitral murmur; but the immediate exciting cause of the early diastolic is the negative pressure of the left ventricle, while the late diastolic is usually due to the force of the auricular contraction. The murmur and the thrill coincide with each other in the cases we have examined."

The affirmative view of the diagnostic significance of presystolic murmur in mitral stenosis has been most ably defended by Reynolds,[1] but space forbids further reference to it. One has but to read the little work of Davies[2] on the mechanism of the circulation of the blood through organically diseased hearts, to be further convinced of the fallacies of the statement of those who consider that the murmur indicative of mitral stenosis is systolic in rhythm.

Clinical Symptoms.—As a rule, these resemble somewhat closely those of regurgitation at the same valve. There are dyspnœa, cough, and later, general or local dropsy, delirium cordis and tachycardia, or cardiac distress. Some of our cases, as we have already stated, have been very insidious in their onset; indeed the first physical signs were, apparent reduplication of the second sound followed in a variable time by the typical presystolic murmur; in other children who had presented a systolic murmur, a presystolic murmur would be found at a subsequent examination, either replacing the former or appearing as a concomitant. Other cases, which, however, are in the minority, may present evidences of lesions in the nervous system as the most evident symptoms of mitral stenosis. But two of our cases presented such an association; that is, hemiplegia and aphasia in connection with a buttonhole mitral; though Sansom in thirty-eight cases has observed quite a number with manifestations of nervous disorders, such as chorea, epilepsy, hemiplegia, and localized palsies from emboli. As this observer remarks, it is a fact worth noting that, with the exception of chorea, not one of these severe lesions of the nervous system

[1] Archives of Medicine, August, 1881.
[2] Lancet, October 19, 1889, p. 779.
[3] Ibid., October 26, 1889, p. 843.

[1] Lancet, November 9, 1889, p. 976.
[2] London, 1889. H. K. Lewis, Publisher.

occurred in children who presented mitral insufficiency.

Prognosis.—In the child, unlike the adult, we do not fear the absence of compensatory hypertrophy, but rather do we fear the known liability to recurrences of rheumatic endo-pericarditis; and superadded to this danger is the ever-present liability to embolism.

As we have stated elsewhere the inherent power of the growing heart is usually sufficient to allow the organ to accommodate itself to the organic alteration, and, in the absence of new invasions of the disease, to permit the child to attain maturity with a fair degree of health. On the whole, however, in early life, mitral stenosis probably more often proves fatal than does regurgitation at this orifice.

1855 Fourth Street, San Diego, Cal.

PERFORATING ULCER OF THE STOMACH, WITH THE REPORT OF A CASE.[1]

By U. O. B. WINGATE, M.D.,
OF MILWAUKEE, WIS.

THAT the early diagnosis of ulcer of the stomach, which may perforate the gastric walls and end the life of the victim, is, often beset with the utmost difficulty, I believe cannot be gainsaid. With the object of calling attention to this difficulty, I venture to report the following case and to make some observations:

B. G., female, five and a half years of age, gave the history of a weak stomach from birth. Has passed through a severe attack of membranous croup and several gastro-intestinal attacks of varying severity. During the past summer has been quite well—occasionally, however, complaining of some pain in the stomach, and has had diarrhœa at times, but which was not sufficiently severe to require medical treatment—so thought the parents.

On Friday, October 12th, she came home at noon, after having been playing with other children, complaining of feeling ill, and soon vomited freely. Of what this ejecta consisted I was unable to learn definitely, but the mother was quite sure that it contained nothing remarkable or unusual. She could not find that the child had eaten any unusual food while out; at home her diet was always carefully regulated. She passed a restless night and was no better in the morning. In the afternoon of this day, Saturday, when I saw her for the first time, she appeared very ill. Pulse 140; temperature 102° F.; tongue furred with quite a heavy yellowish-white coating; stomach tender on pressure; bowels constipated; abdominal walls retracted and muscles rather rigid. No cardiac or pulmonary symptoms. The next day, Sunday, she was no better, and was still inclined to vomit everything swallowed. I saw

[1] Read before the Milwaukee Clinical Society, May 13, 1890.

her twice this day, and after several enemata given by the mother, an evacuation of the bowels was obtained, but nothing unnatural was observed in the matter evacuated. After this she seemed better, passed a good night, and on the next morning, Monday, her pulse was 120 and temperature 99° F. She still vomited occasionally, and was quite irritable, but the latter symptom was not unusual to her. On Tuesday and Wednesday nothing was noted and she appeared to be improving. On Thursday morning at my visit her pulse was 115; temperature normal; she was retaining lime-water and milk, and a little wine whey. She wanted to get up, but this I advised against, though I fear my advice was not heeded. That evening the father called at my office, and stated that the child's hands were cold, but that she seemed bright and strong, and he did not think it necessary for me to see her. I asked him to call me on his return if she appeared worse. I heard nothing until early the next morning, when I was telephoned for, and responded at once, to find the patient in complete collapse; pulseless; feet and hands cold and purple; eyes sunken; mind clear; stomach and abdomen tympanitic; stomach somewhat prominent. The liver dulness could not be made out. There was paroxysmal pain, and at times regurgitation of thin, greenish fluid. The parents, when told that the child was past hope could not believe me, and called in another physician who resided near, and who in my presence concurred in my diagnosis and statements. The patient died in a few hours.

An autopsy could not be obtained; however, I do not think there can be any doubt about the diagnosis.

Up to the time of the collapse I had considered the case one of mild gastritis, and though the idea of an ulcer was present, it did not make much impression on my mind. I now believe that an ulcer had existed for a long time and that the gastritis hastened the perforation.

There are some points of interest connected with this class of cases to which I desire to refer briefly. Brinton was able to collect two hundred and thirty-four cases of perforation from ulcer of the stomach, and, of course, many cases are not reported. The largest number of perforations occur between the ages of fourteen and thirty years. The ulcers which perforate are found about twice as frequently in females as in males—corresponding about to the ratio of ulcers generally in the sexes.

The location is important, from a surgical point of view, as well as interesting. Thus, according to Dreschfeld's report, 85 per cent. of ulcers situated on the anterior wall of the stomach, 2 per cent. of those on the posterior wall, and about 10 per cent. of those located at the pylorus, perforate. The history is also interesting and important. In many cases where perforation takes place the symptoms of gastric ulcer are wanting. Profuse hæmatemesis, excessive and constant pain, and symptoms of dilatation of the stomach are, as a rule, absent. This is accounted for by the location.

Sudden pain, often of a paroxysmal character, is said to be almost always present. Sudden collapse is present if the perforation be at all extensive. Epstein has called attention to an important symptom, viz., rigidity of the abdominal muscles, or walls of the abdomen. This is present whether the walls are retracted or distended, is probably due to irritation of the peripheral nerves, and gradually subsides with the progress of the case. Tympanites is always present—in some cases the region of the stomach will bulge, while the abdomen is retracted. An important diagnostic point in connection with tympanites is the absence of liver dulness, due to the presence of air in the abdominal cavity. Vomiting is reported to be usually absent in cases of perforation. After perforation, death is almost invariably the result. Some cases of recovery are reported, but in them there is the possibility of an incorrect diagnosis.

The question of surgical interference is an important one. The difficulty of diagnosis immediately after perforation perhaps is an objection, but when seen early, even if in doubt, where collapse is advancing, and the pulse present, but increasing in frequency, I believe that abdominal section should be performed at once.

In the case which I report there was so little life left when seen after the perforation, that an operation was out of the question. Had I seen the patient the night before, when the father reported the cold extremities, perhaps something more could have been done.

204 BIDDLE STREET.

CLINICAL MEMORANDA.

MEDICAL.

Case of Purpura Hæmorrhagica Rheumatica. (Peliosis Rheumatica; Morbus Maculosus Werholfii.)[1]

EDDIE D., aged thirteen years. Previous health good. His first attack was in March, 1889, and began with swelling of all the joints, pain, especially in the knees and ankles, a purpuric eruption over the entire body, and pain in the stomach and vomiting .

The pain in the knees and ankles was excruciating. He was put on a diet of milk and Mellin's food, and recovered in two weeks. This attack followed prolonged exposure and excitement at the base-ball grounds —the boy being infatuated with the game was frequently all day without food, except ginger cakes, pie, and peanuts, and sat on the rough benches of the ball grounds in cold winds, in rain, or in heat.

The second attack was in September, 1889, and was

[1] Patient was presented to the Association of American Physicians, May 14, 1890.

similar in character, except that the swelling and eruption were confined to the right half of the body. He had then been exposed to scarlatina.

The treatment up to this time had been acids, iron and quinine, and, to relieve pain, morphine.

The third attack was on November 15, 1889, and was similar to the preceding, but more severe. Pain in the abdomen and left side of chest was intense. In addition to the purpuric eruption there were hæmorrhages from the bowels and bladder, and, in large patches, into the skin. No hæmorrhage from the nose or lungs.

There had been very little fever during the attacks, the temperature seldom rising above 100°.

In the third attack he was delirious, and had dyspnœa, swelling of the forehead and conjunctivitis. Arsenic, which he had been taking for several weeks, was discontinued.

On December 17, 1889, and on February 27, 1890, he had relapses. After this to the present time relapses recurred at intervals of a month or six weeks, but were less severe.

During the intervals he is not perfectly well, though comparatively comfortable and free from pain. Since the beginning of the disease the purpuric eruption has never been absent.

The urine was examined from time to time, and, excepting the presence of blood, was found normal. On one occasion, however, there was a greatly diminished amount and much albumin, evidently due to acute nephritis.

Dr. Theobald Smith, Bacteriologist to the Government Agricultural Department, was kind enough to examine the blood, but discovered nothing abnormal, as will be seen by the accompanying report :

"*January 21, 1890.* The blood from the finger was dried on a cover-glass, and stained with methylene blue. Some of the preparations were decolorized in one-per-cent. acetic acid. There was no change in the size or form of the red corpuscles. Occasionally isolated corpuscles were observed, which retained the stain faintly. These forms are probably young corpuscles. The leucocytes were slightly increased in number ; otherwise the blood elements appeared normal."

Dr. Smith also sent the following interesting note of a hæmorrhagic disease that occurs among guinea-pigs :

"Among guinea-pigs, kept for experimental purposes, a disease occasionally appears which usually ends fatally and may carry off the greater number of those living together. The disease seems to be due to the exclusive use of dry food, such as grain of various kinds. When the food is changed, and vegetables, fruits, etc., are given, the disease is checked and disappears. That it is a food disease I feel quite certain. The examination of the dead animals reveals, as a rule, extensive subcutaneous and intra-muscular ecchymoses, limited chiefly to the limbs. Occasionally they are found on or in the muscles of the chest and abdomen. The internal organs contain no bacteria."

The characteristic symptoms in this case of peliosis rheumatica are :

Swelling and pain in the large joints, closely resembling rheumatism, but coming and going sometimes within a few hours.

The characteristic ecchymoses of true purpura are

present. There are hæmorrhages into the bladder and bowels, but none from the nose or lungs.

Of particular interest in this case was a peculiar hæmorrhage into the true skin—apparently between the epidermis and the true skin—which destroyed the skin by gangrene. The most marked of these ecchymoses were in the skin of the abdomen—two patches, each the size of the palm of the hand, one on the left, the other on the right of the navel. These ecchymoses appeared within half an hour, and were at the beginning perfectly black and painless patches of true gangrene. In a few days a line of demarcation formed, and in due time the dead tissue sloughed, leaving a granulating surface which healed slowly, forming scars which can still be seen.

The boy formerly had a tight phimosis, for which I intended circumcising him, but one of these sloughs appeared on the under surface of the prepuce and cured the phimosis.

Among the symptoms were frequent vomiting and violent pains in the abdomen.

The abdominal pain at times was so violent that I thought there was a peritonitis from a hæmorrhage into the peritoneum, but the absence of tenderness and the rapid disappearance of the pain rendered this view improbable.

The attacks, as stated, are remittent in character; exacerbations occurring at intervals of one or two months. The later attacks have been less prolonged than the earlier.

As to treatment, the medicine that appears to have done the most good is arsenic—and possibly salol given for relief of the rheumatic symptoms.

D. W. PRENTISS, M.D.

WASHINGTON, D. C.

MEDICAL PROGRESS.

Craniectomy.—The Paris correspondent of the *Lancet* (july 19, 1890) writes that at the last meeting of the Academy of Sciences Professor Verneuil called attention to an operation just performed by PROFESSOR LANNELONGUE on a nearly idiotic girl four years old, whose skull was about one-third the normal size. She could not walk or stand without support. M. Lannelongue attributes this condition—microcephaly—not only to the insufficient capacity of the skull but to cerebral lesions caused by pressure, and in the case of the child above referred to he believed that if more space were given to the brain the condition would disappear. Acting on this hypothesis, he made along the median line of the cranium an incision corresponding to the sagittal suture and extending from the frontal to the occipital suture. On the left of the incision he removed a piece of bone about three and a half inches long by half an inch wide and including the entire thickness of the skull. The dura was left intact and the superficial wound was united without drainage. Union took place by first intention. The operation was performed on May 9th, and on June 15th a change in the condition of the child was apparent; she walked, smiled, and had lost much of her previous apathy. M. Lannelongue has quite recently performed a similar though more extensive operation on another child.

Hypodermic Injections of Ether in the Treatment of Neuralgia.—The parenchymatous injection of ether for the relief of neuralgia is by no means a new method of treatment, though it has had but few advocates, and has been practised to only a limited extent. KUMPS (*Revue de Thérapeutique*, June 15, 1890) again brings the method forward as a valuable addition to the therapeutics of neuralgia, and cites a number of cases in which relief followed the injection of equal parts of alcohol and ether into the neighborhood of the affected nerve. Among other cases reported by him are the following : A neuralgia of the shoulder which for two weeks had prevented sleep and had resisted a variety of other methods of treatment, was cured by a single injection. Two cases of sciatica, both of which were much relieved after the first injection. Two cases of facial neuralgia, and three of rheumatic neuralgia of the head were also relieved.

Kumps uses the injections not only in cases of true neuralgia but in rheumatic pains and in torticollis. Two cases of the latter disease were cured by the method, only one injection being required in each case. The amount of the mixture used by the author is 30 minims, and he states that though the pain of the injection is considerable it soon passes away. There is also often some local swelling which can be dissipated by gentle manipulation.—*London Medical Recorder*, July, 1890.

Keen's Methods of Compressing the Subclavian Artery.— All surgeons know the difficulty of maintaining steady and effectual occlusion of the subclavian artery by pressure above the clavicle where the third part of the vessel crosses the first rib, and will welcome the following simple plans devised by PROFESSOR KEEN (*Annals of Surgery*, july, 1890) :

A rolled bandage two inches wide is placed above the clavicle over the position of the artery, as ascertained by the finger. The strong rubber strap which accompanies Esmarch's bandage is then passed over the roller above the clavicle, then down the back, between the thighs, and up in front of the chest. The ends can then be held by an assistant, or, better, tied or hooked together. If it is desired to release the artery, the rubber strap is slipped off the bandage : pressure can be renewed as easily. An assistant should stand on the side of the patient opposite to the side of the operation, to steady the strap and bandage.

The advantages of this method are, that it is reliable, that the compression will be maintained, even though the patient should struggle, and that not only is the assistant not tired out, but he has one hand free for other purposes. An Esmarch bandage can, of course, be applied to the arm before compressing the artery.

With the elastic strap of the Esmarch apparatus, Professor Keen found some difficulty in retaining the roller in place over the artery. To obviate this, he has resorted to the elastic *bandage* of Esmarch, which is applied as follows : The tendency to displacement of the roller downward below the clavicle is counteracted by laying the free end of the elastic bandage on the chest, then passing the unrolled end over the shoulder and down the back. If the *strap* is used the natural tendeney, when it is placed in position, is to pull on both ends at once, and the upper end being drawn downward tends to displace the roller in the same direction. If the elastic *bandage* is used, traction being made with the unrolled part of the bandage, over the shoulder *from front to back*, this subclavian displacement is prevented. To prevent outward displacement, the alternate turns of the bandage should be carried under the opposite axilla. By these means the roller is held in place fixedly, and requires no care from an assistant.

The Faradic Current in Uterine Hæmorrhage.—DR. EUGENE

BOËR writes (*Lancet*, july 19, 1890) that though iodo-form-gauze tampons, if carefully applied, will usually arrest the flow in menorrhagia, still, cases occur in which this plan does not succeed, probably because the hæmorrhage is due to atony of the uterus. In one case of this kind, that of a girl of eighteen, having tried all the usual internal and local remedies, and the patient having become unconscious from loss of blood, he used the faradic current, which arrested the bleeding in ten minutes. When, three days later, there was a return of the hæmorrhage the method was again used with success. The effect was permanent, for, though the faradization had to be resorted to at the next period, the subsequent one was normal. A similar plan of treatment proved equally successful in the case of a multipara with profuse and intractable menorrhagia. Dr. Boër at first applies the negative electrode directly to the cervix, and, after the arrest of the hæmorrhage, to the perineum, the positive pole being applied with some little pressure to the abdominal wall over the fundus of the uterus.

An Enormous Nasal Polyp.—SCHMIEGELOW (*Medicinske Selskob i Kjobenhavn*)

demonstrated, at a recent meeting of the Copenhagen Medical Society, a nasal mucous polyp which was five inches in length and extended through the entire right nasal cavity, prolongations reaching to the edge of the soft palate. The growth was removed with a wire loop, and its point of origin found on the posterior end of the lower turbinal.—*Annals of Surgery*, july, 1890.

Treatment of Chancres by Creolin.—In the *Bulletin Générale de Thérapeutique*,

july 15, 1890, BUSQUE, of Brazil, writes a note to Dujardin-Beaumetz detailing his experiences in the treatment of chancres by this means.

His custom is to apply to the sore a solution of the strength of from 12 to 20 parts to 1000, and he believes that the progress of the malady is shortened and relief speedily obtained. Compared to iodoform Busque thinks these solutions of creolin equally serviceable. The best treatment, however, is to combine these drugs, using the creolin solution as a wash and then iodoform as a dressing.

Nephrectomy for Pyonephrosis. — WISHART (*Montreal Medical Journal*,

july, 1890) reports two abdominal nephrectomies for hydronephrosis, and draws the following conclusions:

1. That in a large proportion of cases of advanced hydronephrosis, where the tumor fills the abdomen, it is impossible for the average operator to say whether the growth is a cyst of the kidney or an ovarian tumor.

2. That supposing hydronephrosis is suspected, it is not possible to say which kidney is the diseased one.

3. The last two propositions being admitted, it follows

that, in all advanced cases, incision in the loin and drainage cannot be advocated, as the surgeon is unable to say which side should be incised.

4. In view of these difficulties in diagnosis, it would seem preferable to make an incision in the linea alba, completing the diagnosis with the hand. If the case be a cyst of the kidney, carry the incision upward and complete the operation by enucleating the tumor.

5. This operation is suitable alike for hydro- or pyonephrosis, the danger, of course, being greater in the former.

6. That abdominal nephrectomy by the median incision is a difficult operation, owing to the high position of the tumor and the close relations of the aorta and vena cava, the large size of the renal vessels, and the fact that the tumor is behind both layers of the peritoneum.

7. If a correct diagnosis could be made, abdominal nephrectomy by incision along the linea semilunaris is probably the best operation, but it is not possible to remove very large cysts by incision in the loin.

8. In the case of a weak patient, or one advanced in years, supposing the abdomen to have been opened, the safer procedure might be to open the cyst and drain from the loin. This operation is safer than nephrectomy, but it usually leaves a permanent fistula.

9. It is advisable, in completing the operation of abdominal nephrectomy, to secure drainage by making an opening in the loin.

Prescription for Bronchitis.—According to the *Southern Medical Record*,

the following is used by JANEWAY in the treatment of bronchitis:

R.—Syrup of tolu . . ⎱
　　Syrup of wild cherry . ⎱
　　Tincture of hyoscyamus ⎰ equal parts.
　　Compound spirit of ether ⎰
　　Water . . . ⎰
Dose, a teaspoonful.

Prevention of Linea Albicantes of Pregnancy.— F. W.

LANGDON (*Cincinnati Lancet-Clinic*, August 9, 1890) believes that the linea albicantes of pregnancy can be prevented by daily inunctions of the abdomen with olive oil, followed by gentle friction with the hand. The inunctions should begin at or before the fourth month of pregnancy, bearing in mind that prevention, not cure, is the object.

[This method of treatment, while by no means new, is not used to the extent that it should be. It adds to the comfort, particularly of primipara, diminishing the sense of distention which is frequently very annoying.—ED.]

Sarcoma of the Breast.—DR. JOSEPH SCHUOLER

has published a valuable contribution (*Basle Inaugural Dissertation*) to our clinical knowledge of sarcoma of the female breast. The following are the most important of his conclusions, based on a study of forty-one cases of the disease:

1. Sarcomata constitute about 10 per cent. of all new growths of the female breast.

2. The tumors make their appearance most frequently between the ages of thirty and fifty years.

3. Hereditary influence cannot usually be detected, and there is apparently no causal relation between the function of the gland and the growth.

4. Traumatism, however, seems to play some part in causation.

5. The left mamma is more frequently attacked than the right.

6. As a rule, the first symptom noticed is gradual enlargement of the organ; pain in the early stages is very exceptional. The consistence of the tumor varies from hard to semi-fluid, and it may reach the size of an adult head.

7. Medullary sarcoma cannot be distinguished from medullary cancer until after extirpation.

8. The treatment should be complete excision. Of forty cases operated upon, recurrence took place in 25 per cent. Recidives usually occur within a year after operation, but have been observed as late as nine years after excision.—*Provincial Medical Journal*, Aug. 1890.

Etiology of Tuberculosis of the Intestine.—DR. MARIN ROUSSEFF (*Dublin Journal of Medical Science*, August, 1890), after an exhaustive study of the post-mortem condition of the stomach and intestines in cases of phthisis, formulates the following:

1. Intestinal tuberculosis in chronic pulmonary tuberculosis is caused by the state of the stomach. This organ modified in its structure by interstitial inflammation or by amyloid infiltration can no longer discharge its functions normally, and hence does not act as a barrier against the invasion of the tubercle bacilli.

2. A capital point in the treatment of phthisis should be attention to the state of the stomach; preventing pathological alterations if possible, or treating them if they are present, for intestinal tuberculosis hastens the course of pulmonary tuberculosis.

3. Men more frequently than women are attacked by intestinal tuberculosis, probably because they lead less natural lives, and in consequence are more prone to gastric derangements.

4. The age of the patient, the amount of pulmonary involvement and its duration have but little influence in the causation of intestinal tuberculosis.

5. Pulmonary tuberculosis *per se* cannot excite a gastritis which would lead to tuberculosis of the intestine.

Iodoform and Creasote as an Inhalation in Phthisis.—The following inhalation is recommended by BRUNTON in the treatment of phthisis:

℞.—Iodoform	.	.	24 grains.
Creasote		.	4 minims.
Oil of eucalyptus	.	.	8 "
Chloroform	.	.	48 "
Alcohol }			
Ether }	equal parts to make ½ ounce.		

To be used in a Robinson's inhaler.—*Virginia Medical Monthly*, August, 1890.

Suppository for Cystitis.—

℞.—Iodoform	.	.	.	2 grains.
Extract of belladonna		.	.	½ grain.
Cacao butter	.	.	.	45 grains.

Pass this well into the bowel, and morning and night inject into the rectum hot water. If any inflammation

of the urethra occurs or is present 1 grain of terpine or salol may be given in pill twice a day.

Permanganate Treatment of Smallpox.—GAWALOWSKI reports the successful employment of baths, colored rose red by the addition of potassium permanganate, in the cure of the eruption of variola and for the reduction of excessive high temperature. The general state under these circumstances was found to improve, the pustules looked better, and the progress of the case went on rapidly toward recovery without any relapses.

Treatment of Laryngeal Phthisis.—HUNT, in the *Annales des Maladies de l' Oreille* for December, 1889, considers the treatment of laryngeal phthisis briefly, as follows: In the early stages, which are always accompanied by anæmia, he prescribes inhalations of oil of tar or creasote, and local applications of chloride of zinc or iron, believing that nitrate of silver is useless at this period. When the catarrhal process is active he uses sedatives or stimulants, as may be indicated, inhalations of mineral astringents, perchloride of iron or an atomized spray of a 1-to-2000 of corrosive sublimate. For the quieting of the cough he thinks the oil of eucalyptus is the best remedy and prefers iodol as an insufflation to all other substances, such as iodoform and lactic acid. The latter he thinks produces pain and inflammation, and increases the cough. When stenosis and œdema of the larynx come on he believes in scarification of the mucous membrane, and also in curetting the surface which is diseased. When stenosis threatens life tracheotomy may be needed.

Ointment for Pityriasis Versicolor.—

℞.—Acid salicylic	.	.	1 drachm.
Precipitated sulphur	.	.	5 drachms.
Vaseline	.	.	3 ounces.

Make into an ointment, and before using place the affected part in hot water for several hours, adding one ounce and a half of powdered borax to each gallon of water used. The skin should be well dried before the salve is applied.—*L' Union Médicale.*

Suprapubic Puncture of the Bladder.—According to DR. DENEFFE (*Journal de Médecine de Paris*), the dangers of suprapubic puncture of the bladder in retention of urine are exaggerated, and the operation should not be considered a last resort. He describes a case of retention due to enlarged prostate, and in which the catheter could not be passed, that was punctured seventeen times without harmful effects. After the seventeenth puncture the canula was permitted to remain in place, and ten days later micturition took place through the urethra. Nevertheless the canula was not removed for twenty-nine days. The fistula closed in four days and the patient permanently recovered. Dr. Deneffe has performed the operation on 301 patients with a mortality of 2½ per cent. He believes that sudden retention in cases of stricture or of enlarged prostate is due to spasm of the posterior part of the urethra, that the spasm can be relieved only by removing the urine, and that catheterizing increases the spasm.—*Provincial Medical Journal*, August, 1890.

THE MEDICAL NEWS.

A WEEKLY JOURNAL
OF MEDICAL SCIENCE.

COMMUNICATIONS are invited from all parts of the world. Original articles contributed exclusively to THE MEDICAL NEWS will be liberally paid for upon publication. When necessary to elucidate the text, illustrations will be furnished without cost to the author.

Address the Editor: H. A. HARE, M.D.,
1004 WALNUT STREET,
PHILADELPHIA.

Subscription Price, including Postage.

PER ANNUM, IN ADVANCE . . . . $4.00.
SINGLE COPIES . . . .   10 CENTS.

Subscriptions may begin at any date. The safest mode of remittance is by bank check or postal money order, drawn to the order of the undersigned. When neither is accessible, remittances may be made, at the risk of the publishers, by forwarding in *registered* letters.

Address,   LEA BROTHERS & CO.,
NOS. 706 & 708 SANSOM STREET,
PHILADELPHIA.

SATURDAY, AUGUST 23, 1890.

THE EDUCATION OF LAWYERS AND PHYSICIANS.

THE MEDICAL NEWS has just received a copy of an address delivered by GEORGE GLUVAS MERCER, LL.M., J.C.D., before the Alumni Association of Haverford College, Pennsylvania, in June, 1889, which is entitled the "American Scholar in Professional Life." In this address its learned author, by a series of quotations taken haphazard from various medical writers, attempts to show that the average medical man of to-day is a mental nonentity possessing so rudimentary an education as to make him little better than a laborer. He also adds his voice to the old cry, that the medical schools of this country are at fault in that they permit men to graduate who do not possess degrees in arts, and fail to insist on a four or five years course, quoting the schools of Germany and England as instances where preliminary study and a course of four or five years are required. While the entire address is most pessimistic in tone we cannot let it pass without at least pointing out some of its faults and fallacies.

No one denies that medical education in the United States is, in the majority of cases, utterly inadequate, and while it is not half so careless in many cases as is that of the law. the greater responsibility of human life, perhaps, makes the teaching worse than the informal courses taken by aspirants for legal honors. Many years have elapsed since a man has been admitted to the ranks of the medical profession simply because he had practised or studied in another man's office; yet in the law this is a most common thing, even in the great cities, where students learn how to draw up a deed or will and little of the real nature of the law. Lawyers' offices are generally notorious loafing-places for young men whose only aim is to learn enough law to pass an entrance examination to the bar. Such individuals perhaps "read law," but never obtain instruction concerning it from a lecturer or teacher. In this much the position of the law to medicine, so far as education is concerned, is that of the individual who must "first cast out the mote in his own eve." In regard to the assertion that a longer time is required abroad than in this country for medical education, qualifying information should have been given. In the best schools in America the student often attends lectures for seven, eight, or nine hours a day, while in England he rarely hears more than four lectures, and most commonly attends but one or two, amusing himself as he pleases during the rest of the 'twenty-four hours. In Germany the same condition of affairs exists, and in most cases the first two years of so-called study are spent in the beer-garden, or in the pursuit of some still less intellectual enjoyment.

These are mere comparisons, however, of little importance. The question which Mr. Mercer has raised he has failed to answer, or even to offer an idea as to the remedy for the iniquities which he asserts are present. And this is not surprising, in view of the fact that he has not been a teacher in a medical school, and in consequence has but little idea of the expenses connected therewith, independent of the professors' salaries. We doubt if any more expensive educational institution can be found than a well-equipped medical school, pursuing the highest course possible, and in consequence money must be had. The State and nation will not give it, as they do in Germany, nor has America reached an age in which by the accumulations of years the hospitals and universities are richly endowed, as in England. Educational institutions are generally the result of private enterprise, or are so meagerly fed from the State treasury as to be on the verge of inanition. There are, in consequence, but two changes which will remove all ignorance from the medical profession—namely, an improvement in mental calibre throughout the race, with the elimination of all stupid persons, or, what is more practical, the arousing of the people to the fact that their lives are dependent upon proper medical attendance, which can only be obtained by State contributions to support the medical schools, or by insisting that no one who cannot afford to spend at least four years at college shall attempt to enter the ranks of the profession. If physicians as a class are ignorant, it is because the supply of knowledge, like coal and iron, is always largely governed by demand, and the country doctor can no more invest five years' income in medical centres than the owner of a country store can carry the finest silks instead of the cheapest calicoes.

Mr. Mercer repeats the time-worn assertions that we have an excessive growth of doctors as compared to other countries, but neglects to state that the doors of the law are equally wide open, and that the proportion of lawyers to the population is largely in excess. The one-sided character of the legal mind is, however, thoroughly represented by the closing words of the lecturer in his attack on medical illiteracy, for he asserts that medicine does not necessarily train the mind, in that it is not a science, because "the physician can never know beforehand the precise effect which a drug will produce in a given case, or whether a particular complication will occur in the course of a familiar fever." This lack of knowledge on our part can only be excused when the learned gentleman remembers that as God did not make us all alike, the same rules cannot apply with equal force to each individual. The "uncertainty of the law" depends upon the same variations in mental qualities as the uncertainty of medicine, with the addition that the perverted mental activity of an ignorant judge may give birth to a decision which will at least stand as an important precedent a thousand miles away, or years afterward in a similar case.

Last of all, we are accused of "narrow-mindedness" if we fail to consult with homœopaths, and the author of the paper here loses sight of the very first principle which the law is supposed to uphold, namely, honesty and equity; for if a regular physician consults with a true homœopath the result must be barren, or if the homœopath be one in name only and not in deed, he is a fraud and charlatan with whom a reputable physician has no more right to confer than has a respectable lawyer a desire to take as his colleague a member of the bar whom he regards as devoid of honesty and a disgrace to his profession.

The law deals with facts, medicine with the ever-varying personal equation, an equation generally utterly unknown. Is it not time for the pot to stop calling the kettle black, and for both professions to unite in an effort which will arouse popular feeling to such an extent that our educational institutions will not be dependent upon the whim of a few individuals who may be too lazy, too stupid, or too poor to enter the sacred precincts of any learned profession except through a side door. The people of the United States have provided every child with schooling, and enacted laws preventing illiteracy among those who deal in stoves, or wood, or food, yet they calmly turn their backs, and utterly ignore a lack of knowledge in the individuals who are the only barriers between their dear ones and the grave. The endowment of a hospital is a noble charity, but the endowment of a medical school not devoted to the filling of the professors' pockets, but to the advancement of medicine, is far nobler, since for every moment of suffering saved in a ward, hours of grief, pain, and poverty may be avoided by the skill of thoroughly qualified physicians scattered here and there among the millions of people inhabiting this continent.

IODINE IN OBSTINATE VOMITING.

EVERY physician who treats his cases intelligently must recognize that he meets with vomiting arising from two opposing states of the stomach or general system. In one case inflammation or irritation of the gastric mucous membrane may exist, while in the other depression and a depraved functional activity prevent the organ from retaining food by some nervous reflex which we do not understand. The vomiting of inflammation may be controlled by aconite in full dose; the vomiting of depression by small or stimulating doses of ipecacuanha.

Within the last few months the tincture of iodine has been highly recommended by a number of writers in the current journals, and they have one and all pointed out that its sphere is in the forms of vomiting due to depression of the stomach. Thus ROQUES (*Gazette médicale de Liège*) has employed this drug in the vomiting of tuberculosis in its early stages with good results, and recommends its use in chronic gastritis and simple gastric ulcer. He also thinks it of value in the vomiting of pregnancy, and in chlorosis. The drug is not very disagreeable to take, and produces a sensation of warmth in the stomach which, in some cases, is pleasant to the patient. The tincture should be given, adding ten drops to four ounces of water, one-third of which should be taken immediately after the meal which produces the nausea. Very rarely does this use of the drug produce disagreeable after-effects, but its persistent employment may cause coryza or iodism.

REVIEWS.

ESSENTIALS OF ANATOMY AND MANUAL OF PRACTICAL DISSECTION. By C. B. NANCREDE, M.D. Third edition, revised and enlarged. Colored plates and woodcuts. Philadelphia : W. B. Saunders, 1890.

THE third edition of Nancrede's Anatomy which has just appeared, is a manual of usefulness and value. The publisher has greatly added to the book by the introduction of a large number of beautifully executed plates, which were selected by Dr. Edward Martin, owing to the author's absence from Philadelphia. We have never before seen a book which contained so much in a small space, and yet served as an atlas, quiz-compend, and text-book at one and the same time, which was not so far removed from the grasp of the ordinary student by its cost as to be useless as an aid to general anatomical study. Three editions in less than two years is a success to be envied, and we doubt not that the sales will be doubled during the next year.

CORRESPONDENCE.

"MENTHOL IN DISEASES OF THE AIR-PASSAGES."

WE have been requested to publish the following remarks made by Professor E. Fletcher Ingals in the discussion of Dr. S. S. Bishop's paper on " Menthol," read before the Illinois State Medical Society (see THE MEDICAL NEWS, July 26, 1890):

"I have had some experience with menthol in the last four or five years, having used it considerably, but I am sorry to say, I cannot corroborate Dr. Bishop's statements in all respects. He recommends strong solutions of menthol, whereas, if I should use such solutions, I would find that, as with any other irritant, the patient would be made worse. I find that hardly more than two or three grains of menthol to the ounce of liquid albolene will be tolerated by the majority of patients. Of course, some patients will stand more, just as one will tolerate bichloride of mercury better than another. I fear you will not obtain the good results from the use of this drug that would be expected from a consideration of the paper of Dr. Bishop, although the author's results have been excellent.

"The use of menthol vapor, as an inhalation, is a different matter, and used in this way others may have results similar to those recorded by the author. I presume this drug does not act very differently from other irritants, such as iodine, sulphate of zinc, or anything

else that stimulates the parts. The result is essentially the same whatever drug is employed, providing we get just the right amount of stimulation. Occasionally, perhaps once in four cases, menthol, properly applied, will relieve congestion of the mucous membrane for a considerable length of time, but in the majority of cases it will not do so. In the cases relieved, the swelling disappears and the nose remains comparatively free for an hour or two, but it subsequently stops up, just as it would if cocaine had been employed. In nearly all cases, if used in the strength, even of one and a half or two per cent., the patients are made worse ; at least this has been my experience.

"Dr. Bishop spoke of menthol as a good remedy for stopping discharge, and so it is in some cases, but if used a little too strong, the discharge is increased by it, as by other remedies.

"I was glad to hear him speak of the use of the drug in affections of the Eustachian tube and middle ear. I see but little of these affections, as I do not treat diseases of the ear except when they come directly from throat trouble that requires my attention. But in those cases that I do treat I have latterly used about a 2-per-cent. solution (ten grains to the ounce) of menthol in liquid albolene, thrown up behind the palate. I have no difficulty in most cases in getting this directly into the Eustachian tubes. For this purpose I use the spray tubes which are known as Davidson's No. 66, with a tip half an inch long, which can be carried above the point where the palate is drawn firmly against the pharyngeal wall, though with a shorter tip this cannot be done. With a pressure varying from fifteen to forty pounds, which can be regulated at pleasure, the menthol solution can be forced directly into the Eustachian tube, if the nose is held during the application. This pressure, however, is not applied to the middle ear, for the palate will not resist any great force, and the vapor passes backward into the mouth before the pressure gives the patient discomfort. For this application I regulate the pressure according to the sensitiveness of the ear.

" In hay-fever the vapor of menthol gives a little relief to some patients, but, unfortunately, it is not much.

"In laryngeal phthisis this drug has been used for a number of years with the same enthusiasm that has characterized the use of iodoform and many other drugs; and we find reports of many cases of this affection said to have been benefited by menthol. But when we apply it in laryngeal tuberculosis, we find that although there is a little relief at first, an hour or so afterward the patient feels as badly as ever. There are a few cases of laryngeal tuberculosis that are benefited while menthol is being used, but any remedy that we may apply to the larynx, be it menthol or what not, makes very little difference in the actual condition of the parts, unless, by some means, the constitutional disease be checked. Then, and only then, the larynx may be expected to heal ; though local applications often appear to hold the disease in check for a short time, and, in so far as they render deglutition easier, they are beneficial.

"Several years ago, at a meeting of the American Laryngological Association, some gentleman spoke of wonderful results obtained in laryngeal tuberculosis from the application of iodoform, which was said to have a specific influence in healing ulceration. At that time I questioned this so-called specific influence and doubted whether the drug accomplished much, if any, good. To-day, I think, all laryngologists are in accord with the views I then expressed. Menthol in the treatment of this disease has had a history similar to that of iodoform, but thus far it has been found much less useful than the latter."

LONDON.

A Medical Degree for London Students; the Hospitals Committee; the Grievances of Army Medical Officers; Infant Life Insurance; Transplantation of the Thyroid in Myxœdema.

To the Editor of THE MEDICAL NEWS,

SIR: The scheme for the reconstitution of the University of London is still the burning question of the hour, though only a comparatively small number of people take an interest in it, and fewer still really understand it in all its bearings. The agitation originated with the teachers in the Metropolitan schools, who felt that the great majority of students in London had not as fair an opportunity to obtain a degree as they would have in any of the other centres of medical education in the United Kingdom. The original idea was to found a new university on a different plan from the University of London. When the agitation had reached a certain pitch the Government appointed a commission to investigate and report on the subject. Before this body all who objected to the creation of a new and separate university were well represented, and were successful in their efforts, for the Commission reported in favor of altering the regulations of the existing university so as to meet the demands of those who desired a new university. A scheme, with several subsequent modifications, was submitted by the Senate of the University of London, to the licensing bodies, and met with support as well as opposition, and on the whole it seems likely that the latter will prevail.

There are several reasons why it should fail. As at present constituted the degree of the University of London is open to any candidate, no matter in what part of the country he has been educated. Under the new scheme, education *in London* would be compulsory, which is manifestly unjust to the provincial schools, and yet absolutely necessary if the existing university is to satisfy the essential features of the demands of those who originated the agitation. This creates a deadlock which is quite certain to upset the whole scheme, and the sooner the Senate of the University of London recognizes this fact and gives up its opposition to the creation of a new university the sooner will this question be settled. There are other very thorny problems connected with the subject, but the most important matter is that there should be a degree for the attainment of which a certain amount of study in London should be compulsory, and this difficulty can only be met by the establishment of a new university.

The Special Hospitals Committee of the House of Lords is probably by this time thoroughly ashamed of itself and wishing to be released from its undertaking. About twenty meetings have now been held, and, as far as can be judged, the only function of the Committee is to afford one hospital an opportunity to reveal mistakes in management, a proceeding which cannot possibly have any useful effect. Thus far none of the leaders have come forward to give evidence, but inasmuch as there is no likelihood that the meetings of the Committee will have any practical result, this is perhaps not a matter of much moment. The two grievances which have been chiefly aired are, that the hospital appointments are mostly restricted to men who have passed the higher examinations at the College of Physicians and Surgeons here, and are not open to similar qualifications from Scotland or Ireland, and that the out-patient departments damage the general practitioners. In regard to the former point there is not the least likelihood of any change being made, and in regard to the second, the grumblers have not at present made out a case.

The grievances of army medical officers have been much debated of late, and at the instance of the Royal College of Physicians all the leading medical corporations sent a deputation to the Secretary of War, Sir Andrew Clark acting as spokesman. He defined the chief grievance to be the vexed question of rank; it was, he said, that the medical officers of the army having military duties, military responsibilities, and living in a military atmosphere, had not a definite military rank, and that men in other departments of a like constitution had that rank. He made a strong point when he remarked that military rank had, not long since, been granted to the conductor of one of the regimental bands, as this act proved that combatant duties were not essential qualifications for the possession of a military title. He also mentioned the fact that military titles were given to army medical officers in some countries, notably in America, and that no difficulties had been found to arise in consequence. It remains to be seen whether anything will result from the meeting; it is well known that the military authorities are strongly opposed to it, and further, medical officers in the army have hitherto declared that they did not want military titles. I confess it seems to me hardly possible that the granting of a title will have the effect of converting the service from being very unpopular to a position of popularity, and that some more real change will have to be made if good men are to be attracted to it.

The Bishop of Peterborough's well-meant efforts to reform the law upon the insurance of children do not seem likely to meet with the success which, in my judgment, they deserve. We are told that we must not discourage thrift, and that if we place obstacles in the way of parents putting by something for a rainy day, we will tend to discourage thrift. But it seems to me that until a child is old enough to become a breadwinner there should not be any insurable interest in its life, beyond the amount necessary for funeral expenses, for which purpose insurance is most proper. But this does not meet the views of certain self-constituted philanthropists in the House of Commons, and is in consequence not approved, so that this direct incentive to infant murder will be allowed to go on uncontrolled, and one might almost say directly sanctioned. It is no mere fancy that infants are murdered for the sake of the insurance money, for it was proved beyond doubt a year or two ago by some very gross instances, but the chief culprit died before she could be brought to trial.

Mr. Victor Horsley advocated some few months ago

transplantation of the thyroid in cases of myxœdema and sporadic cretinism. He has returned to the subject lately, and has discovered that a Dr. Bircher anticipated him, at any rate so far as a practical experiment is concerned. In Dr. Bircher's case symptoms of myxœdema having supervened upon removal of the thyroid, he transplanted a portion of a normal thyroid into the abdominal cavity, with the result that the myxœdematous symptoms in great measure disappeared. Some months later a second transplantation was made, again with distinct improvement.

NEW YORK.

To the Editor of THE MEDICAL NEWS,

SIR: As the season in which typhoid fever is most prevalent is at hand, I am reminded of an epidemic of that disease which occurred some time ago in the City Insane Asylum on Ward's Island. All the ordinary sources of infection were quickly excluded, and considerable investigation was necessary before it was discovered that the disease was confined to those patients and their attendants who were permitted to spend much of their time roaming about the northern end of the island. Further inquiry elicited the fact that these people had been accustomed to quench their thirst at a stream situated but a short distance from, and at a lower level than, a small cemetery which had been used at one time for the burial of the typhoid-fever patients from the Emigration Hospital. Such burial places are a constant menace to health, and the question—"How can the city best dispose of its dead? is one of growing importance. The Potter's Field has been removed from place to place: at one time it was on the site now occupied by the Woman's Hospital; at another time it was on Ward's Island; and still later it was transferred to a much more remote point—Hart's Island. The latter place has already a large almshouse population contiguous to this vast resting-place of "the unclaimed dead;" and very little digging on Ward's Island will furnish ample proof of the use formerly made of the land. Certainly the sanitary science of to-day calls for a better state of things, and Dr. A. E. Macdonald, the Superintendent of the City Insane Asylums, recognizing this need, is urging the introduction of cremation as a means of disposing of at least a large number of the bodies now sent to the Potter's Field.

The increased water-supply following upon the completion of the Croton aqueduct has made it possible this summer for many a filthy water-closet in our high tenements to be properly flushed; and if some of this large quantity of water could only be used in sprinkling our dusty streets, there would probably be much less pharyngitis and conjunctivitis among us.

The Board of Health has just published its report for the last year. Among other items of interest I notice that over six thousand quarts of adulterated milk were destroyed, and over one million pounds of fruit and food were condemned and seized. This is a good showing for the Board of Health, but "Little Italy" must have groaned in spirit at being thus ruthlessly deprived of its staple articles of diet. The death-rate for 1889 was 25,13 per 1000, not including stillbirths; and among the 122

deaths reported as resulting from surgical operations, 33 followed laparotomy.

There has been much talk during the last few years about the bad effect upon the public health of the frequent digging up of the streets, required to lay the electric subways and steam-heating pipes, and it has been pretty generally believed, both by the laity and the profession, that such disturbances of the soil are accompanied by malarial manifestation in the neighborhood. If by "malarial" we mean only *bad air*, it is certain that the term is correctly applied, for the freshly uncovered earth, saturated with illuminating gas, gives out a most unpleasant stench. But Dr. Charles N. Dowd, of this city, who has been making a careful bacteriological study of this subject, tells us there is very little reason to believe that genuine malaria is materially increased in this way. He found no marked difference in the bacteriological contents of a gaseous and non-gaseous earth, and the effect of the upturning of the earth without reference to the gas, was to increase markedly the amount of dust, but to augment only moderately the spread of bacteria. He believes that the organism which causes malaria belongs to a different class from those which he studied. The result of uncovering so much ill-smelling earth is chiefly impaired digestion and a feeling of malaise. Although Dr. Dowd's bacteriological research undoubtedly leads to this conclusion, clinical evidence is not wanting to show that malaria is more common after such upturning of the soil; and since the railroads have been making some changes in Morrisania the people there have become painfully aware of this relation between digging and malaria.

NEWS ITEMS.

Medical Examiners of New Jersey.—Governor Abbett, on August 19th, appointed the following physicians, who are to constitute the New Jersey State Board of Medical examiners:

Regular physicians: Dr. William P. Watson, Hudson County, to serve for two years; Dr. George W. Brown, Monmouth County, for three years; Dr. W. L. Newell, Salem County, for one year; Dr. Henry S. Wagner, Somerset County, for one year; and Dr. Hugh C. Hendry, Essex County, for one year.

Homœopathists: Dr. A. Uebalacker, Morris County, to serve for three years; and Dr. A. H. Worthington, Mercer County, for one year.

Eclectic: Dr. Eugene Tiesler, Essex County, to serve for one year.

The Board will meet for organization on Tuesday, September 2d.

A Supposed Case of Cholera in London.—According to Press dispatches from London, a sailor on the steamship "Duke of Argyle," from Calcutta, was landed with Asiatic cholera, on August 17th.

Virchow's Welcome to American Physicians.—Virchow is reported to have extended the following cordial welcome to the American delegates to the International Congress: "We in Germany have great admiration for the American medical world, which to-day excels in surgery, midwifery, and dentistry. I can say for myself and colleagues that the American contingent will be honored and heartily welcomed. We admire their scientific zeal and begrudge them their extraordinary skill, and shall try to imitate their push and energy. I find these latter virtues in the American student as well as in the finished scientist. My German students generally spend a few semesters deciding what line of medicine they shall follow, while the American student walks into the arena with a fixed purpose and an indomitable determination to accomplish it. This is why your men secure the laurels before their hair turns gray. My friend, Dr. H. Wood, of Philadelphia, will be the speaker for the Americans at the coming Congress. He is sure to do himself and the great city and country from which he comes high credit."

American Public Health Association. — The American Public Health Association will hold its eighteenth annual meeting December 16, 17, 18, and 19, 1890, at Charleston, S. C. The following topics for discussion have been selected by the Executive Committee: Sanitary Construction in House Architecture, including heating, lighting, drainage, and ventilation; Sewage Disposal; Maritime Sanitation at Ports of Arrival; Prevention and Restriction of Tuberculosis; and Isolation Hospitals for Contagious and Infectious Diseases. Papers on various sanitary and hygienic subjects will also be read.

Obituary. — Dr. WILLIAM BRODIE, of Detroit, who died July 31st, was a man of national reputation, having been president of the American Medical Association in 1886, as well as of his State Medical Society in 1875. He was born at Frawley Court, England, of Scottish parentage, July 28, 1823. He received his education in this country, graduating in 1850, from the College of Physicians and Surgeons of New York. He settled in Detroit nearly forty years ago, and became one of the best known of its citizens, winning high esteem both socially and professionally.

——Dr. J. W. HERON, one of the most prominent medical missionaries in the East, died at Seoul, Korea, August 1st, from dysentery. He was the superintendent of the Royal Hospital at the Korean capital and enjoyed the confidence of the king and of the foreign community.

——GEORGE PIERCE BAKER, M.D., died at Providence, R. I., August 2d, of cancer of the neck and throat. Dr. Baker was born in 1826, at Rehoboth, Mass. He entered Amherst College in 1846, but remained there only two years. His degree in medicine was received from the Harvard Medical School in 1851. He began practice at once in Providence, where he remained throughout the remainder of his life. He was a Fellow of the Rhode Island Medical Society for thirty-nine years, and of the Providence Medical Association nearly as long. He was for two years a vice-president of the former Society, and for nine years a member of its Board of Censors. For several years he was a visiting physician to the Rhode Island Hospital, and more recently one of its consulting staff. During the War of the Rebellion he served as Surgeon on the Peninsula, until prostrated by congestive chills which permanently impaired his health. Dr. Baker was an unpretentious but very thoughtful

man. He was a close observer at the bedside, and his wise and kindly advice to the many younger men who called him in consultation was always most valuable. In 1859 he married Miss Lucy D. Cady, of Providence, who died in 1883. He left an only son, who bears his father's name, and is an instructor at Harvard College.

OFFICIAL LIST OF CHANGES IN THE STATIONS AND DUTIES OF OFFICERS SERVING IN THE MEDICAL DEPARTMENT, U. S. ARMY, FROM AUGUST 12 TO AUGUST 18, 1890.

McCREENY, GEORGE, *Captain and Assistant Surgeon.*—The leave of absence for seven days, granted by order No. 84 (Fort Warren, Mass.), August 13, 1890, is hereby extended fifteen days.—*S. O. 193, Headquarters Division of the Atlantic, Governor's Island, New York City,* August 15, 1890.

OFFICIAL LIST OF CHANGES IN THE STATIONS AND DUTIES OF THE MEDICAL CORPS OF THE U. S. NAVY FOR THE WEEK ENDING AUGUST 16, 1890.

WALES, P. S., *Medical Director.*—Detached from Medical Examining Board and will resume present duty at the Museum of Hygiene.

AMES, H. E., *Passed Assistant Surgeon.*—Ordered as member of Medical Examining Board in addition to present duty.

SAYRE, J. S., *Passed Assistant Surgeon.*—Detached from Navy Yard, New York, and ordered to the U. S. S. "Ranger."

NORTH, J. H., Jr., *Assistant Surgeon.*—Ordered to the Navy yard, New York.

BARBER, GEORGE H., *Assistant Surgeon.*—Detached from the U. S. Receiving-ship "Vermont," and ordered to the "Pensacola."

VON WEDEKIND, L. S., *Assistant Surgeon.*—Detached from the U. S. "Pensacola," and ordered to the "Vermont."

AUZAL, E. W., *Passed Assistant Surgeon.*—Ordered to temporary duty at the Naval Academy to examine candidates.

FITTS, H. B., *Passed Assistant Surgeon.*—Detached from the U. S. S. "Pinta," to proceed home and wait orders.

STINE, E. P., *Passed Assistant Surgeon.*—Detached from the U. S. S. "Independence," and ordered to the "Pinta."

WHITFIELD, J. M., *Assistant Surgeon.*—Detached from the Monitors, and ordered to the Naval Hospital, Norfolk.

AYERS, JOSEPH, *Surgeon.*—Ordered to the Naval Academy, to examine candidates for admission.

BRIGHT, GEORGE H., *Surgeon.*—Ordered to the Naval Academy, to examine candidates for admission.

SMITH, GEORGE T., *Assistant Surgeon.*—Detached from the Naval Hospital, Norfolk, and ordered to the U. S. S. "Independence."

WHITE, S. S., *Passed Assistant Surgeon.*—Detached from Marine and ordered to the Naval Rendezvous, San Francisco, Cal.

OFFICIAL LIST OF CHANGES OF STATIONS AND DUTIES OF MEDICAL OFFICERS OF THE U. S. MARINE-HOSPITAL SERVICE, FROM JULY 26 TO AUGUST 12, 1890.

SAWTELLE, H. W., *Surgeon.*—Granted leave of absence for fifteen days, August 8, 1890.

WHEELER, W. A., *Passed Assistant Surgeon.*—Granted leave of absence for thirty days, August 5, 1890.

CARMICHAEL, D A., *Passed Assistant Surgeon.*—Granted leave of absence for thirty days, August 2, 1890.

PECKHAM, C. T., *Passed Assistant Surgeon.*—Granted leave of absence for thirty days, July 28, 1890.

AMES, R. P. M., *Passed Assistant Surgeon.*—Granted leave of absence for fourteen days, August, 1890. To proceed to Shreveport, La., as inspector, August 5, 1890.

KALLOCH, P. C., *Passed Assistant Surgeon.*—Granted leave of absence for seven days, July, 1890.

PERRY, J. C., *Assistant Surgeon.*—To proceed to Wilmington, N. C., for temporary duty, July 31, 1890.

SMITH, A. C., *Assistant Surgeon.*—Granted leave of absence for thirty days, August 11, 1890.

YOUNG, G. B., *Assistant Surgeon.*—Leave of absence extended twenty days on account of sickness, August 2, 1890. Upon expiration of leave, to proceed to New Orleans, La., for temporary duty, August 8, 1890.

STIMPSON, W. G., *Assistant Surgeon.*—When relieved at Buffalo, N. Y., to proceed to Norfolk, Va., for temporary duty, August 5, 1890

THE MEDICAL NEWS.

A WEEKLY JOURNAL OF MEDICAL SCIENCE.

| Vol. LVII. | Saturday, August 30, 1890. | No. 9. |

ORIGINAL LECTURES.

LUPUS ERYTHEMATOSUS, ACUTE VESICULAR ECZEMA OF THE HANDS, AND OTHER DISEASES OF THE SKIN.

A Clinical Lecture
delivered at the Hospital of the University of Pennsylvania.

By LOUIS A. DUHRING, M.D.,
PROFESSOR OF SKIN DISEASES.

GENTLEMEN: This patient is a well-nourished, rather stout woman, with brown hair and eyes, who has a remarkably extensive development of lupus erythematosus, occupying the nose and both cheeks, and extending as far back as the ears. The greater portion of each cheek is involved, and, as is usually the case in this disease, in a symmetrical manner. The well-known "butterfly" form, the body being represented by the nose and the outspread wings by the cheeks, is here not so striking as usual, because of the widespread extent of the disease. The diseased skin is uniformly infiltrated, and is everywhere surrounded with a sharply defined, distinct, very slightly raised, red border. The skin is of a deep red, somewhat violaceous color, with a faint brownish tinge; is harsh and rough with scales, and is also the seat of scanty, dirty-yellowish, adherent, sebaceous crusts, which are less abundant than usual. The skin is manifestly much inflamed, slightly puffed, and warm to the touch. The process is active, and is evidently encroaching on healthy skin, as shown especially by the bright-red, raised border. And yet, nowhere do we find signs of superficial, whitish, atrophy of the skin, usually so characteristic of the disease, but this will probably appear later. The patient states that the affection began two years ago, and, as we see, has made rapid progress. The patch on the cheeks consists of a continuous sheet of disease. Ordinarily the patches are multiple, with more or less sound skin between them. There is considerable burning, which is markedly worse during the period when the process is most active. In almost all cases the disease inclines to spread more or less rapidly for a few weeks, and then to become quiescent for a variable period, and in the patient before us we have that history. The color and the sharp outline, here, suggest the appearance of vascular nævus, but the diagnosis presents no difficulties. Lupus vulgaris is eliminated because of the acutely inflammatory state of the skin and of the uniform distribution of the pathological process, which shows no disposition to form foci.

Where the disease is active and spreading, and the skin sensitive and hot, local treatment is generally attended with difficulties, for the reason that applications of any kind or strength are apt to disagree with the skin. Remedies that are useful in the subacute or chronic stage are here not tolerated, and the list of available applications is small. It must be kept in mind that, in the acute stage, the disease is readily aggravated by injudicious treatment. We must first endeavor to control and reduce the active hyperæmia, and a valuable remedy for this purpose is composed as follows:

℞.—Potassium sulphide	.	.	5 to 20 grains.
Zinc sulphate	.	.	5 to 20 "
Water	.	.	.	4 ounces.
Alcohol	.	.	.	½ ounce.—M.

Apply as a wash, and shake before using.

The strength may be augmented or reduced to suit the skin. It should be dabbed on lightly for fifteen or twenty minutes two or three times a day, the sediment being allowed to remain. In the course of a few weeks this will probably prepare the skin for more energetic remedies, such as sulphur ointment or a tarry tincture. The prognosis, in such an extensive and virulent case as the present, is not favorable—at least a cure cannot be expected until after a long period.

PAPULO-SQUAMOUS SYPHILODERM.

This woman, about twenty years of age, exhibits an eruption of large, broad, sharply-defined maculo-papules, of a cherry-red color, some of them covered with slight scales, situated around the neck from ear to ear and extending into the scalp in the form of ill-defined, scaly patches. The lesions are a manifestation of syphilis, being a secondary eruption, the infection (of which there is no history) having occurred probably four or six months ago. The papules are linearly arranged around the neck, so as to resemble a necklace. About the angles of the mouth are syphilitic fissures, and about each ear there is a large, painful, fissured papule. There is also some glandular engorgement, post-auricular and epitrochlear. The general health is beginning to fail. The protiodide of mercury, one-quarter of a grain in pill-form, three times a day, and five-per-cent. oleate of mercury ointment to the lesions, will be ordered.

ACUTE VESICULAR ECZEMA OF THE HANDS.

The man before us, aged fifty, a street-car conductor, is suffering with an acute attack of vesicular eczema of the forearms, back of the hands, fingers, and sides of the face and neck, everywhere symmetrical. It began a week ago, and is now fully developed, showing vesicles, some ruptured and oozing, others intact; yellowish crusts; blood-crusts and scratch-marks, seated on a slightly puffed, inflamed skin. One of the best forms of treatment for such a case is a salicylic acid plaster, as the following:

℞.—Salicylic acid	.	.	.	15 grains.
Powdered starch	.	.	.	2 drachms.
Zinc oxide	.	.	.	2 "
Cosmoline	.	.	.	4 " —M.

This should be freely applied three or four times daily, the parts being well covered with the paste, to protect the skin and exclude the air. Should this not prove decidedly beneficial in a few days, black-wash, followed by oxide of zinc ointment, will be advised. Internally, a tonic, saline aperient mixture will probably prove of value. A drachm and a half of sulphate of magnesium and one grain of sulphate of iron in a gobletful of water, to be taken a half-hour before breakfast, daily, may be prescribed for the next week or two.

VESICULAR ECZEMA OF THE HANDS AND FINGERS.

This youth, seventeen years of age, has a similar form of extensive vesicular eczema upon his hands and fingers, and symmetrically developed. It is subacute, and he states that it is of eight years' standing. During this period he has never been free from it, although, as is almost always the case, the disease has been better and worse from time to time, and it incapacitates him for any manual labor or occupation. Here a more stimulating form of treatment is indicated, and a calomel ointment, twenty or thirty grains of calomel to the ounce of oxide of zinc ointment, will be ordered. In three or four days, should no improvement take place, an ointment of resorcin, thirty grains, and salicylic acid, ten grains to the ounce, will be substituted, to be followed later by a tarry wash of one drachm of the alcoholic solution of coal-tar to eight ounces of water.

DRY SEBORRHŒA OF THE SCALP.

The young man before us complains of excessive dandruff, and upon examination of the scalp we find typical dry seborrhœa—the common variety of this disease. In mild cases, such as are usually met with, the diagnosis is easy; but in severe cases the affection may resemble squamous eczema or psoriasis. The treatment is generally followed by satisfactory results. An ointment of precipitated sulphur, one or two drachms to the ounce, which is the simplest and at the same time one of the most efficacious remedies, will be prescribed. Resorcin, as an ointment or as a lotion, is also useful, and may be ordered in the strength of from ten to twenty grains to the ounce. Lotions are often more convenient to apply than pomades, and a formula like this may be employed:

R.—Resorcin . . . . . 15 grains.
    Glycerin . . . . . 10 minims.
    Alcohol . . . . . 15 "
    Water . . . . . 1 ounce.—M.

PUSTULAR ECZEMA.

The baby before us is suffering with a chronic, extensive, highly developed pustular eczema, involving the whole face, the greater part of the scalp, and the forearms and hands. The face is covered with brownish and greenish crusts, together with flat, yellowish pustules and excoriations. Upon the scalp the crusts are greenish. The crusts are to be loosened by soaking with a boric acid solution, after which a salicylic acid ointment, ten grains to the ounce, may be applied three times a day, to be followed in a few days by a mild tarry ointment, one drachm of tar ointment to the ounce. Should this not agree with the skin after a few days' trial, a calomel ointment, fifteen or twenty grains to the ounce, will be ordered. Directions will be given to the mother, who is nursing the babe, as to the general care of the patient.

The digestive tract must be watched, and any disorder corrected, for in many cases of infantile eczema the disease will be found to vary with the state of the alimentary canal.

ORIGINAL ARTICLES.

CLINICAL OBSERVATIONS ON THE HEALING OF ASEPTIC BONE CAVITIES BY SENN'S METHOD OF IMPLANTATION OF ANTISEPTIC DECALCIFIED BONE.[1]

BY WILLIAM MACKIE, M.A., M.D.,
ASSISTANT SURGEON TO THE MILWAUKEE HOSPITAL, MILWAUKEE, WIS.

IN a paper entitled, "On the Healing of Aseptic Bone Cavities by Implantation of Decalcified Bone," published in the *American Journal of the Medical Sciences*, September, 1889, Dr. Senn first called the attention of the profession to this method of hastening the repair in defects of bone, the result of either disease or trauma. In this article Dr. Senn gives a complete review of all that had been previously done in this direction, the result of his own experimental research on animals, and the record of ten clinical observations on the treatment of suppurative and of tuberculous osteomyelitis. Since then he has had under treatment, in the Milwaukee Hospital, eleven similar cases. These he has kindly placed at my disposal. Dr. O'Keef, of Oconto, Wis., at a recent meeting of the Brainard Medical Society, reported one successful case; and Dr. Jones, of Red Wing, Minn., has furnished me with an interesting case. These, with one from my own practice, make in all fourteen cases. In literature, as far as I am aware, only two cases are recorded, one by Deaver, of successful secondary implantation, and one by Weir, which resulted in failure. Professor Esmarch, in a letter to Dr. Senn, states that he has used decalcified bone-chips in two cases. In the first some suppuration occurred, and a few of the chips came away; and in the second, a case of necrosis of the shaft of the tibia, he obtained definite healing by the fourteenth day under one dressing.

Before proceeding to give these cases in detail, it would be well to consider briefly the structure of decalcified bone, and the changes which it undergoes when placed in the peritoneal cavity and in bone; also the preparation of the bone for implantation, the operation, and the after-treatment.

Structure of Decalcified Bone.—Decalcified bone is soft, flexible, and elastic, and by boiling can be reduced to gelatin. It constitutes about one-third part of bone, the other two-thirds consisting principally of phosphate and carbonate of lime. Histologically, it is made up of variously arranged lamellæ, apposed and bound together by fibres of white con-

---

[1] Read before Wisconsin State Medical Society, June 5, 1890.

nective tissue (Sharpey's fibres). The lamellæ at the periphery and around the Haversian canals have a concentric arrangement, and are irregular between the different systems. Interposed between and hollowed from the opposite surfaces of the lamellæ are the Haversian spaces, in which, in the intact bone, are situated the osteoblasts, and from these spaces extend the canaliculi through which they intercommunicate. Thus, decalcified bone is, histologically, an admirable framework for delicate granulating tissue, and this with a minimum amount of material to be removed by absorption.

In order to ascertain the changes undergone by decalcified bone after implantation, I chiselled out a rectangular opening, 8 by 4 millimetres, in the compact layer of the tibia of a young dog, and removed the medulla with a sharp spoon. After opening the medullary cavity the hæmorrhage was very free, but was effectually arrested by plugging the cavity with a solid piece of decalcified bone, over which the periosteum was sutured with catgut and the skin with silk.

Fourteen days after this the animal was killed. Examination showed a formation of new bone under the periosteum, where it had been separated from the bone. This was most marked above the opening, where it was 3 millimetres thick, and was entirely absent immediately around the margin. The periosteum was firmly adherent to the implanted bone. On longitudinal section, through the margin of the opening in the compact layer, the implanted bone was found softened, and of a delicate pink color. The medullary cavity was filled by a solid cylinder of new bone below the point of implantation; complete at the upper margin of the opening, and gradually diminishing in thickness in an upward direction and on the side remote from the opening. A transverse section through the middle of the implanted bone showed that about one-third of it remained in the form of a wedge, the base of the wedge corresponding to the opening in the compact layer, and its apex reaching the centre of the medullary cavity, one-third of which had been obliterated by new bone. Immediately surrounding this remnant, and separating it from the new bony formation in the medullary cavity, was a thin layer of granulation-tissue, on the medullary side of which could be detected filiform processes of new bone. Microscopical examination showed infiltration of the decalcified bone by small round cells,—osteoblasts, —most numerous at the periphery and gradually diminishing in number toward the periosteal side. At the margin the structure is composed of granulation-tissue; toward the periphery of the implanted bone the cells are arranged in rows between the lamellæ, and in circles around the Haversian system.

The changes observed are, removal of the decalcified bone, wholly or in part, by the action of the osteoclasts, and regeneration of the bone by osteoblasts, with or without the formation of granulation-tissue. Similar changes were observed in a thin piece of decalcified bone sutured to the serous coat of the intestine, and examined fourteen days later.

Preparation of Bone-chips.—The bones to be preferred are those with a thick, compact layer, such as the tibia and femur of the ox. They should be fresh, and after removing the periosteum and the medullary tissue, they are to be cut longitudinally into strips about 3 millimetres in width, and placed in a 10- to 15-per-cent. solution of hydrochloric acid. The fluid should be used in large quantity, and changed every twenty-four hours until the process of decalcification is complete, which requires from one to four weeks. The acid is removed by running water, or, better, by a weak solution of caustic potash. The decalcified bone is next cut into small chips, which are placed for twenty-four hours in a 1-to-1000 solution of corrosive sublimate for forty-eight hours, and finally preserved in a saturated solution of iodoform in ether. Before using they are taken from this solution, placed in a piece of aseptic gauze, and the ether and excess of iodoform dissolved out by alcohol. They should then be immersed in a 1-to-2000 sublimate solution, where they should remain until required for implantation, when the surface moisture is removed by rubbing them in iodoform-gauze. If the alcohol be not thoroughly removed, the chips, by imbibition of fluids after implantation, may swell and produce undue tension on the sutures. For the repair of cranial defects, plates of a thickness corresponding to that of the cranium are used. These are prepared by sawing the compact layer of bone into large, thin plates, and decalcifying them as above. Multiple perforations should be drilled in them to permit drainage of the space underneath, and the size and outline of the plate should correspond exactly to the bony defect.

Operation.—As stated by Dr. Senn, "The most essential condition for success in the treatment of bone defects by the implantation of decalcified bone is a perfectly aseptic condition of the tissues to be brought in contact with the implanted bone." These conditions are attained as follows: The field of operation is shaved, and washed with soft-soap and warm water, and then with 1-to-1000 sublimate solution. If time allows, this is done on the day prior to that fixed for the operation, and the parts are meanwhile kept covered by a moist sublimate compress. After the patient is anæsthetized the limb is elevated, the elastic constrictor applied, the field of operation surrounded by towels wrung from a 5-per-cent. solution of carbolic acid, the compress, if present, is removed, and the final disinfection is always made with alcohol. The seat of the disease is exposed by a free incision down to the bone, and the periosteum with the attached soft parts is reflected. If a sinus exists it serves as-a guide ; if absent a new bony formation under the periosteum will answer ; and in the absence of either the point of greatest tenderness must constitute the guide. The next step consists in exposing the seat of the bone-lesion by chiselling away the outer compact layer, sufficient of which should be removed to allow inspection and direct treatment of the whole cavity. All granulations and diseased tissue are to be removed by a sharp spoon or chisel, during which frequent irrigation with a 1-to-2000 sublimate solution (in cases of tubercular disease, a sherry-colored solution of tincture of iodine in water) should be used, in order to diminish the risk of traumatic diffusion of pathogenic microbes.

All unhealthy and undermined skin or cicatricial tissue should be excised, even at the risk of leaving a defect in the soft tissue covering the bone ; and sinuses in the soft tissues should be cleared of granulations by the sharp spoon and thoroughly disinfected and iodoformized. A final irrigation is then made, the cavity is dried and freely dusted with iodoform. Into the cavity thus made, the chips are firmly packed until the level of the periosteum is reached ; a catgut drain is introduced at the most dependent point (viewed from the recumbent position) of the cavity, and the periosteum sutured with fine catgut. If hæmorrhage from the soft tissues is expected, the constrictor is at this stage removed ; if hæmorrhage is not probable, it is allowed to remain until after the dressing has been applied. If necessary to secure accurate coaptation of the soft parts, buried sutures of catgut are introduced, and the skin is sutured with silk.

Dressing.—The wound is dusted with iodoform, and covered with oiled silk and several layers of iodoform-gauze, which should encircle the limb. The margin of the gauze is guarded by plenty of salicylated cotton, and over this is placed a cushion of sublimated moss and common cotton ; the whole being retained in position by a firmly and evenly applied bandage. To secure rest the limb is fixed on a splint and kept in the elevated position for from six to twelve hours.

When there exists a defect in the soft tissues, the chips are firmly retained in the cavity by the pressure of an iodoform-gauze tampon, and if the parts remain aseptic healthy granulations will encroach on the defect and fill it up.

After-treatment.—During the first twenty-four hours the dressing is frequently inspected, and if the discharge has soaked through, those points are covered with salicylated cotton. If, at the end of

that time, the dressing is still moist, it is changed ; but if dry, it is allowed to remain and infection guarded against by iodoformization and the application of several layers of salicylated cotton. The first dressing, in the absence of any complications, is made between the tenth and fourteenth day. when the sutures are removed. Union will generally be found complete, except a few granulations at the point of drainage. Future dressings are made at intervals of two to three weeks. The patient is confined in the recumbent posture until the site of the bony defect feels firm and is free from pain. This varies from one to four months, in accordance with the extent of the defect, age of the patient, and the regenerative power of the bone.

CASE I. *Circumscribed central osteomyelitis of the tibia.*—L. S., aged eighteen years, male, was admitted into the Milwaukee Hospital, March 13, 1889. For the past three years the patient had suffered from pain in the region of the left ankle ; the diagnosis of sprain and rheumatism had been made by different physicians, and treatment adopted accordingly, without any benefit. He had been able to walk until within the last few weeks. The symptoms present on admission were swelling and œdema over the lower epiphyseal line of the tibia, with local increase of temperature, and point of greatest tenderness immediately above this line.

Operation : Making a linear incision over the point of greatest tenderness and reflecting the thickened periosteum with the attached soft tissues, the bone was here explored with a drill, and pus found. This exploratory opening was enlarged by a chisel and an abscess-cavity, containing half a drachm of pus, surrounded by osteoporotic bone, was exposed. The removal of all the pus-infiltrated, cancellated tissue necessitated the exposure of the upper surface of the articular cartilage. and a central cavity remained, twice the size of a hazelnut. This was firmly packed with bone-chips.

First dressing at the end of a week ; incision healed, except at drain-opening. A week later, on changing dressing, superficial suppuration was present, and, despite daily change of dressing, the infection extended, so that about six days afterward some of the bone chips came away. Repair was complete by the tenth week from operation, the site of which was indicated by a slight depression in the bone.

CASE II. *Diffuse osteomyelitis of os calcis.*—J. G., female, aged forty years ; admitted into the Milwaukee Hospital, May 10, 1889, with the following history :

About one year ago she stepped hurriedly from a street-car, and alighted upon the rail with her left heel ; to this she paid no attention, considering the resulting pain only a simple bruise. The pain, however, continued to increase, and at last, calling in medical aid, treatment for sprain was adopted. This was continued for months, but the pain remained on throwing her weight on the heel. On admission, inspection revealed nothing ; there was no local increase of temperature; the point of greatest tenderness was located in the middle line on the posterior aspect of the os calcis, above the insertion of the tendo-Achillis, and, on comparing the heels, a nodular prominence could also be detected at this point.

Operation : The nodule was exposed by a linear incision which divided the tendo-Achillis longitudinally in the middle line; the thickened periosteum was reflected, with the soft tissue, and the compact layer of bone removed by a chisel, thus disclosing an extensive osteomyelitic focus. After removing all infected tissue, there remained a cavity one inch deep, one-fourth of an inch wide, and three-fourths of an inch long, which was packed with bone-chips. The periosteum and tendo-Achillis were sutured with fine silk and the superficial incision with medium silk. The relief from pain was prompt. The patient left the hospital at the end of three weeks, when firm pressure on the previously tender point did not give the slightest pain, and there has been no return of the disease.

CASE III. *Tuberculosis of the knee-joint; resection.*—M. L., a strong, apparently healthy female. twenty-six years of age, with no family history of tuberculosis, has, for the past eight years, suffered from knee-joint trouble. One year ago a layman undertook to effect a cure. This treatment was followed by an acute synovitis, which, after four months' rest in bed, subsided so that the patient was able to get around again. A second attack occurred during the past winter, leaving the knee permanently enlarged. Since March she has been walking on crutches. On admission to the hospital, November 5, 1889, there was found fibrous ankylosis of the knee and uniform enlargement of the joint, which to the examining finger felt firm. No glandular enlargement in the groin.

Operation : Complete resection of the knee-joint, patella included. On section of the tibia, the bone was found highly osteoporotic, and in the inner tuberosity a triangular sequestrum surrounded by granulation-tissue and encased by sclerosed bone. Corresponding to this there was present a caseous deposit in the inner condyle of the femur. Both these were eliminated, and there remained in the condyle a cavity the size of a pigeon's egg, and in the tibia one of half that size. After complete extirpation of the capsule, thorough iodoformization of the wound and ignipuncture of the tibia, both cavities were firmly packed with decalcified bone-chips before bringing the resected ends into apposition. A catgut drain was introduced at either angle of the incision, which was closed by deep sutures of catgut and superficial of silk. The quadriceps and patellar tendons were united by a strong catgut suture. A large antiseptic dressing was applied, and retained by a plaster-of-Paris bandage, in which was incorporated a posterior iron splint extending from the middle of the thigh to the toes. The limb was kept in an elevated position for two weeks. The highest temperature, 101.5° F., was reached the evening of the second day; the following morning it was reduced to 99° F.

No rise in temperature after this date. At the
9*

first dressing, on the sixteenth day, the incision had completely healed, except at the points of drainage; sutures removed and plaster-of-Paris dressing reapplied. Twelve days later, the dressing was removed and the incision found completely healed; examination at the end of the sixth week showed well-advanced consolidation, with only three-quarters of an inch shortening. Fixation dressings were dispensed with twelve weeks after operation, and the patient ordered to walk on crutches. This she refused to do until two weeks later, when, to her surprise, she could bear her weight on the limb without pain or inconvenience.

CASE IV. *Penetrating wound of the elbow-joint ; secondary suppurative synovitis and osteomyelitis of the humerus.*—C. P., male, seventeen years of age; admitted into the Milwaukee Hospital, July 20, 1889, suffering from suppurative synovitis of the right elbow and osteomyelitis of the lower end of the humerus, following a penetrating wound of the elbow-joint four weeks previously. The wound in the soft parts was situated immediately above the external condyle. On the day of admission thorough drainage of the joint was established, and all the infected medullary tissue removed by the chisel and sharp spoon. Everything progressed favorably until the middle of September, when the central osteomyelitis began to extend upward. Toward the end of November two abscesses developed in the upper portion of the arm, one opposite the middle of the humerus anteriorly, the other opposite the surgical neck on the outer aspect. These were incised and drained. In January, the elbow and the lower fourth of the humerus having recovered, the patient assumed the duties of the hospital choreman. The drainage-openings continued to discharge, and for the cure of this chronic central osteomyelitis the following operation was undertaken, November 26th : The shaft of the humerus was exposed at the superficial openings, and two corresponding cloacæ communicating with each other through the medullary cavity were found in the bone. Between these two points the medulla was exposed by chiselling away the outer lamella of sclerosed bone. The disease was limited above by the epiphyseal line to which the upper opening corresponded, and extended downward in the middle of the shaft to the point where the first operation terminated—at the upper boundary of the lower fourth of the humerus. To remove this, more of the outer lamella was chiselled away, so that when all the diseased tissue had been removed there remained a cavity half an inch wide, and spiral in direction, extending from the upper epiphyseal line on the outer aspect, downward and inward, and terminating anteriorly at the upper border of the lower fourth of the humerus. The cavity was filled with decalcified bone-chips, a catgut drain was introduced at the upper angle of the incision, and the wound sutured. The dressing was renewed on the second day, as it had become saturated with blood ; weekly dressing thereafter. The arm was kept in the elevated position for four weeks, and everything being healed, the patient was allowed to leave his bed. At the end of six weeks he resumed his duties as choreman. and left the hospital in the latter part of March. Examination at this time showed general atrophy of the whole upper extremity from non-use; cicatrix perfectly free, and painless throughout; the gutter represented by a very shallow groove, about one-fourth of an inch in width.

In this case implantation of decalcified bone was not practised at first, because the proximity to the suppurative process in the elbow-joint rendered it impossible to keep the parts aseptic. Even in the presence of this condition the osteomyelitis did not begin to extend upward for six weeks, and it is reasonable to infer that the extension was due to incomplete removal, or to latent microbes becoming again active from some unknown exciting cause, and not to reinfection, because repair in the lower fourth of the humerus was complete at the end of the fifth month. It also affords a comparison in regard to the time necessary for repair, with or without the implantation of decalcified bone. In the former, five months were necessary, and in the latter, six weeks sufficed, although there remained throughout the whole extent of the gutter only three-fourths of the compact layer of the humerus.

CASE V. *Chronic central osteomyelitis, secondary to compound fracture.*—C. L., male, thirty-eight years of age, sustained, five months ago, a compound fracture of the left leg, in the lower third. Sloughing of the soft tissues over the anterior surface of the tibia occurred about the end of the second week. Union advanced slowly, and at the point of sloughing there remained a small opening, surrounded by granulations and communicating with the medullary cavity of the bone.

Operation, December 31, 1889: The point of fracture was exposed by a linear incision, the periosteum reflected, and the medullary cavity opened by enlarging the opening in the bone by a chisel. Sufficient of the outer lamella was chiselled away to permit complete removal of all the diseased medulla by the sharp spoon. When completed there remained a cavity two inches in length, and half an inch in width, centrally located in the lower fragment. This was packed full of decalcified bone-chips, a drain inserted at the lower angle, and the wound closed in the usual manner.

At the end of the first week the dressing was changed, and sutures removed, when union was found complete, except at the lower angle, where some of the sutures had cut through. Eleven days later, on changing the dressing, some of the bone-chips came away while irrigating; those that remained were firmly embedded in granulation-tissue. This defect healed by granulation, and four weeks later the patient left the hospital cured, the upper part of the cicatrix being free. Where healing by granulation had taken place the cicatrix was adherent with but slight depression in the outline.

CASE VI. *Tuberculosis of the ankle-joint; resection.*—W. C., male, nineteen years of age; was admitted into the Milwaukee Hospital, January 21, 1890, with the following history : Father died of asthma,

and two sisters of phthisis. At the age of seven patient had measles, followed for three years by sore eyes. As the eyes improved trouble developed in the left ankle, which compelled him to use crutches for three years more. He continued well until about four months ago, when the same ankle began to swell. There was no pain except when stepping hard on the heel. Patient very anæmic; ankle ankylosed and enlarged; no fluctuation; swelling most marked behind the external malleolus; thickening of the lower end of the tibia.

Operation : Resection, with a chisel, of the external malleolus and articular surface of the tibia, and complete removal of the astragalus through a linear incision behind the external malleolus. The primary depots were found in the tibia, from which the disease had extended to the articulation and the astragalus. After removing these depots two cavities remained, one the size of a marble, and the other half that size. These were filled with decalcified bone-chips, and the bones brought into apposition; the incision closed; and the foot placed on a rectangular splint, and retained by plaster-of-Paris. On the third day a change of dressing was necessitated because of saturation with bloody serum; seventeen days subsequently the sutures were removed. Union was complete except at the points of drainage. With the exception of the formation of a small connective-tissue abscess on the inner side of the tendo-Achillis, recovery was uninterrupted. Patient walked on crutches at the end of the second month, and left the hospital two weeks later, greatly improved in general health, and with advancing bony ankylosis of the ankle.

CASE VII. *Tubercular osteomyelitis of the tibia.*—A. A., male, twenty-two years old, with no hereditary history of tuberculosis. An abscess developed over the lower half of the tibia twelve years ago. This opened spontaneously, and several small sequestra came away in the discharge, followed in several weeks by cure. Ten years later pain began in the middle of the tibia. This gradually increased, and finally poultices were applied. Two weeks ago, under this treatment, a small abscess opened, the site of which is now indicated by a small sinus on the inner side of the crest of the tibia, and a little below the middle of the bone. Below this point there is a general thickening of the bone with rounding of the crest.

Operation, January 30, 1890: On reflecting the soft tissues a small pin-hole opening leading to the medullary cavity was found in the middle of the anterior surface of the tibia, at the same level, but not corresponding with the opening in the skin. With this as a guide the medullary cavity was opened by a chisel, and found filled with fungous granulations, in which was embedded one small sequestrum. The disease extended upward, and when completely removed, there remained a cavity four inches in length and one in width, centrally located. This was packed with bone-chips, and treated in the usual manner. On the tenth day, when the dressing was renewed, the incision was completely healed, except at the point where the catgut drain had been introduced, and fourteen days later, on the second change of dressing, this also had closed. The new tissue in the cavity at this point felt firm, and was painless on pressure, and the cicatrix was almost on a level with the old bone. On the thirty-second day the patient was allowed to walk on crutches.

CASE VIII. *Osteomyelitis following compound fracture.*—J. L., male, aged twenty-four years, sustained a compound fracture of leg near the middle, ten months ago. Infection occurred; one small piece of bone was discharged; union was slow and accompanied with considerable thickening at the seat of fracture; a sinus surrounded by large œdematous granulations leads to the point of fracture.

Operation, February 5, 1890: After reflecting the soft tissues, the medullary cavity was opened by chiselling away anteriorly the exuberant callus around the sinus. Three small sequestra were found, and after removing all the osteomyelitic tissue a central cavity four inches in length and one in width remained. Bone-chips implanted in the usual manner. On the eighth day the sutures were removed, some of which had cut through at the site of the excised sinus-opening. This healed by granulation and left a slight depression, otherwise the contents of the cavity, in five weeks, were firm and on a level with the surrounding bone. At this time he resumed the use of his crutches, and one week later left the hospital.

CASE IX. *Osteomyelitis of the tibia and of the seventh rib.*—E. V., male, eleven years of age, had in the fall of 1888 an acute attack of osteomyelitis in the lower third of the right tibia. This was treated by hot and cold applications without avail; an abscess developed six months later and was opened. The seventh rib was simultaneously involved and treated similarly. From each, several small sequestra came away in the discharge, but the sinuses remained. Since then the patient's general health has greatly improved.

Present condition: Thickening of the lower half of the tibia and undermining of the cutaneous tissue on the inner and anterior surface of the bone in the lower third, over a circular area one and a half inches in diameter, with a central sinus communicating with the medullary cavity.

Operation, March 3, 1890: All of the undermined tissue was excised and the periosteum with the soft parts reflected. The outer compact layer, which was thickened and sclerosed, was chiselled away in an upward direction for a distance of four and a half inches from the epiphyseal line. This gutter, one inch in width, was packed with decalcified bone-chips. After suturing the soft parts a triangular defect remained where the soft tissues were undermined. Here the chips were firmly forced into the cavity by a small compress of iodoform-gauze and the ordinary antiseptic dressing was applied. Two inches of the rib were excised at the same time. Eleven days later the dressing was changed; some of the sutures had cut through, and the chips, left uncovered by soft tissues, were found firmly embedded in a blood-coagulum. The sutures were all removed and a similar dressing reapplied. The chest incision had completely healed.

At the second dressing, one week later, some of the superficial chips came away, when those underneath could be seen firmly fixed in the granulation-tissue and partly covered by the same. At the end of the tenth week repair was complete, and there remained a slight depression where healing took place by granulation.

CASE X.—*Tuberculosis of the knee; arthrectomy.*—E. K., four and a half years old; child of healthy parents, and with no family history of tuberculosis, was admitted to the Milwaukee Hospital, March 10, 1890, for knee-joint trouble secondary to an injury six months previously. At present the joint is uniformly enlarged, painless, and doughy on palpation. A typical arthrectomy was made on the same day, and the primary depot of infection found in the intercondyloid notch, where limited sequestration had occurred. When this depot was removed there remained a cavity the size of a hazelnut, which was packed with bone-chips. Recovery was retarded by an acute attack of catarrhal icterus, which developed the second day after the operation and lasted about a week. Some suppuration occurred in the superficial incisions, which had completely healed by the end of the twelfth week. There was also at this time some movement in the joint.

CASE XI.—*Tuberculosis of the knee; resection.*—J. H., male, seventeen years old, was admitted into the Milwaukee Hospital, April 5, 1890, with the following history: At the age of six he fell from a tree and injured his left knee; some stiffness of the joint remained, but not such as to inconvenience him. About one year ago he sustained a second injury to the same knee, which was followed by a painless enlargement of the articulation. Later the joint became painful on walking, and for the past month the pain has been constant. No hereditary history of tuberculosis.

Present condition: Patient very anæmic; slight rise of temperature at night; pulse small and weak; knee ankylosed and enlarged, with a point of fluctuation on the inner side of the patellar tendon, which is also the point of greatest tenderness.

Operation: Linear incision over the point of fluctuation was followed by the escape of tubercular pus. Digital exploration of the cavity showed that it communicated with the joint, which was opened by the usual transverse incision for resection. An atypical chisel-resection of the ends of the bones was made, during which three tubercular depots were found in the head of the tibia and one in the condyle of the femur. Of those in the head of the tibia, two were situated in the inner half and one in the outer. In the former, tubercular necrosis had occurred, and in the latter the triangular sequestrum was surrounded by sclerosed bone. When these had been removed, two cavities remained, each the size of a walnut, that on the inner side being divided into two parts by a septum of sclerosed bone, and extending downward for about one and a half inches into the shaft to opposite the lower angle of the vertical incision. That in the condyle was the size of a hazelnut. All these were packed with bone-chips before the bones were brought into apposition, provision being made for drainage by strands of catgut introduced at the angles of the transverse incision and at the lowest point of the vertical. Incisions closed by deep sutures of catgut and superficial of silk. On the following day, the dressing, having become saturated by sero-sanguineous discharge, was changed. The second dressing was made twenty-four days thereafter, when the incisions were found completely healed; the drain-opening at the lower angle of the vertical incision was closed by an aseptic blood-clot; the site of the cavity in the head of the tibia was firm, level with the surrounding bone, and painless on pressure, and consolidation of the bones had commenced. The sutures were removed and a light fixation-dressing of plaster-of-Paris applied, which, at the date of this report, has not been renewed.

CASE XII. *Osteomyelitis secondary to compound fracture of the femur.*—J. M. H., aged twenty-nine years, came under my care in May, 1889, for compound fracture of the femur, with extensive comminution of the bone immediately above the condyles. The periosteum was intact posteriorly. The wound in the soft tissues was on the inner side of the thigh about three inches above the epicondyle. Infection followed; a small shred of the underclothing and several small pieces of the bone came away with the discharges. In three months union had progressed so far that the patient could walk with the aid of crutches, and by the end of the sixth month a cane sufficed, yet the sinus at the site of the original wound in the soft parts did not close. On March 10, 1890, he was re-admitted into the Milwaukee Hospital for operation. The point of fracture was exposed by a linear incision on the anterior and inner aspect of the thigh. A small opening was found in the callus, and enlarging this by a chisel, a centrally located sequestrum, surrounded by granulations, was revealed. The sequestrum was extracted and the granulations removed by a sharp spoon, as were also those from the sinus. The cavity was the size of a walnut. This was packed with bone-chips; a small rubber drain was introduced through the sinus at the site of the original wound in the soft parts, and the incision closed by deep sutures of catgut and superficial of silk. A rise of temperature occurred on the fifth day, and on removing the dressing, superficial suppuration was found in the incision. Daily dressings were made, and on the ninth day some of the chips came away. Notwithstanding this the contents of the cavity at the end of the fourth week felt firm, and the incision had healed. The patient was now allowed to walk around, and two weeks later the sinus closed.

CASE XIII. *Compound comminuted fracture of the skull* (Dr. Jones's case).—A boy twelve years old. While coasting down a steep incline which crossed a railroad he came in collision with an express train, and sustained a compound comminuted fracture of the skull at the junction of the right parietal and occipital bones. Under the strictest antiseptic precautions the point of injury was exposed by a semilunar incision extending down to the bone, and the periosteum with the soft tissues was reflected. All the fragments of bone were removed,

leaving an irregular defect two and a half by three and a half inches. This was accurately closed by three pieces of partially decalcified bone; periosteum sutured with catgut and skin with silk. A small drain was introduced at the lower angle of the incision down to the implanted disks, and a large antiseptic dressing applied. On the second day the drain was removed and on the eighth the sutures, when union was found complete. Eleven weeks after the receipt of the injury the defect was so firm as to justify the boy's return to school. Four months have now elapsed since the accident, and the defect is still as hard and unyielding to pressure as the surrounding bone, with which it is on a level, and is, Dr. Jones believes, ossified. The use of partially decalcified bone was purely accidental, the bone having been taken from the decalcifying fluid at too early a date. The doctor suggests that the partial decalcification may account for so rapid ossification. This is not tenable, for the viability of all the osteoblasts must of necessity have been destroyed and the undecalcified portion of the bone was so much more foreign and inert material to be removed by absorption.

A parallel case to the above, where viable bone-grafts were used, is reported by R. Jaksch :[1]

"A soldier, aged twenty-two years, had a depressed' comminuted fracture of the right parietal bone. The opening was cleared, leaving a hiatus of three centimetres in diameter. It was dressed antiseptically. In eight days the skull of a living goose was laid bare, the head was cut off at a single blow, the skull disinfected with ether and sublimate solution, and the whole placed in a 2-per-cent. solution of carbolic acid at a temperature of 38–40° Cent. The calvarium was removed while in the solution and divided into eight pieces, which were laid upon the granulating dura. An iodoform dressing was applied and retained for ten days, when it was removed, and the bone-plates looked pink. Eight days subsequently they showed granulations on their upper surface. A week later the whole surface was granulating, and cure was complete in less than two months."

Contrasting these two cases, the first point to attract attention is the simplicity of Senn's method as compared with the course pursued in the latter case —a very complicated and time-consuming process, with multiple opportunities for accidental infection. Decalcified bone is always ready, or should be so, just as catgut is. There is no gain in time where viable grafts are employed. In the case of Jaksch's patient repair was complete in less than two months and in that of Jones's, in eleven weeks. In the former the time necessary for repair seems shorter, but in reality was not, for the defect there was only 3 centimetres (1⅕ inches) in diameter, and in the latter it measured 2½ by 3½ inches, nearly three times as large, and this had closed in about four weeks longer, so that the question of time is in favor of decalcified bone. The result was equally good in both cases.

CASE XIV. *Osteomyelitis of the head of the tibia.* (Dr. O'Keef's case.)—A young, healthy male, who,

[1] Wiener med. Wochenschrift, September 21, 1839.

while suffering from gonorrhœa, fell and contused the head of the fibula. This was followed by pain in the region of the knee, causing inability to walk. Point of greatest tenderness over the head of the fibula. Tentative drill-exploration of the head of the fibula revealed the presence of pus in the cancellated structure. Part of the compact layer was removed by a chisel, and the medulla by a sharp spoon, leaving only a shell of compact bone. This cavity was packed with bone-chips. Definite healing occurred in thirteen days, under two dressings, and three weeks later the head of the fibula was firm, painless on pressure, without depression, and the cicatrix non-adherent. The patient at this time could walk as well as ever.

The case recorded by Deaver[1] was one of secondary implantation in chronic central osteomyelitis of the lower end of the femur, with sequestration. His colleague, Dr. White, removed the sequestrum and all the infected tissue, leaving a cavity five inches in length and one in width. This was treated in the ordinary manner for seven weeks, but the progress of the regeneration was so slow that Dr. Deaver resolved to try the implantation of decalcified bone-chips. He modified Senn's method somewhat, by placing the bone-chips in successive layers with intervening layers of sterile iodoform. His patient suffered from iodoform intoxication, but this he considers no objection to the method, believing that the beneficial effects of absolutely sterile iodoform, especially in tubercular and syphilitic subjects, more than counterbalance any danger from this source.

This may be questioned by some, but as repair in the soft tissues progresses most rapidly where hæmostasis is absolute, is it not possible that the hæmostatic properties of iodoform may hasten the desired result in cases of implantation? Repair was complete in one month, one-half the time already consumed in treatment without implantation.

Weir's case[2] was one of necrosis of the lower end of the tibia. At the end of two weeks on making the first change of dressing he found that "although everything had apparently gone well, every one of the pieces of decalcified bone had dissolved and come away in the discharge from the wound, and that notwithstanding this there had been some organization of the blood-clot." In none of the above recorded cases did this happen. Even where some of the chips did come away, they were only softened and not dissolved, and if dissolved, how could they be distinguished in the discharge? It is more likely that there was faulty preparation of the chips, probably maceration, or imperfect packing of the cavity. Dr. Weir doubts the success of the operation for two reasons: First, the difficulty of securing a perfectly aseptic condition of the cavity, and, second, because

he fails to see how decalcified bone, catgut, or any similar material, can be converted into new bone. He believes that they may serve as a framework—and this is all that Senn claims for decalcified bone; a blood-clot can do no more, and the organization (so called) of this, Weir evidently believes in. He will try by preference the transplantation of viable bone-grafts from the bones of young animals taken from the neighborhood of the epiphyseal line; but to this procedure his first objection—the difficulty of securing an aseptic cavity—is much more applicable than to the use of decalcified bone-chips. In the viable grafts we have, at best, only an aseptic substance, while in the decalcified bone-chips we have a strongly antiseptic one. The latter is surely the more preferable to introduce into a cavity the sterility of which is doubtful; and, further, viable bone-grafts will retain their vitality and grow in an aseptic medium only.

A careful study of the foregoing cases conclusively demonstrates the advantage to be derived from the implantation of decalcified bone in hastening repair in bone cavities. It has been seen that decalcified bone is a porous substance; an aseptic blood-coagulum, as shown by Schleich, is nothing else; and neither is the sponge-graft, as introduced by Hamilton. Hamilton, in his experiments on sponge-grafting, found that the layer of organizing tissue varies from one-eighth to one-tenth of an inch in thickness, and that, when it exceeds this, the granulations become œdematous and flabby. When an artificial framework, such as a blood-coagulum, sponge, or decalcified bone, is introduced, this does not occur, because the advancing granulations find a temporary support until the embryonic tissue becomes sufficiently organized. One strong objection to the method of Schede is the introduction into a cavity, which is at all times difficult to render aseptic, of a substance which is the best culture for pathogenic microörganisms. In decalcified bone we have a strongly antiseptic substance which will tend to destroy any pathogenic microbes that may remain; it is, as Senn terms it, "an antiseptic tampon." Further, the hæmostasis is rendered as complete as possible, only enough blood remaining in the cavity to fill the small spaces between the chips, and thus is met Bergmann's great objection to Schede's method.

The use of viable bone-grafts in pathological processes of bone is unnecessary and objectionable. They are unnecessary because there is no lack of osteogenetic material; the irritative action of the trauma is a great stimulus to the regenerative process, and it has been found, both experimentally and clinically, that if a framework be supplied the defeet will become ossified just as soon, if not sooner, than where viable bone-grafts are used. They are also objectionable because sufficient aseptic bone-grafts can never be obtained from the site of operation to fill the defect remaining after the removal of all the diseased bony tissue, and there is always the risk of reintroducing a septic graft. Any attempt made to render the grafts aseptic would necessarily destroy the osteogenetic power of the osteoblasts, and would entail the removal by absorption of the inorganic portion of bone, which amounts to two-thirds of the whole. Consequently, there would remain in every case a depression at the site of operation. This objection can be met by the use of viable grafts obtained from other sources, such as the bones of young animals, in the neighborhood of the epiphyseal line, as advocated by Poncet. This is a very complicated process, and consequently opens up many avenues for infection, with a remote possibility of the transmission of some other disease, such as tuberculosis, which has been transmitted by skin-grafts taken from limbs amputated for joint-disease; and if true of skin, why not of bone? Further, in all inflammation of bone accompanied by the formation of new bone, the first change is absorption of the pre-existing bone prior to the osteogenetic process being established. Take, for example, a plastic osteomyelitis: there is first osteoporosis, then osteosclerosis. In other words, bone, before it can be regenerated, returns to its embryonic condition. The same may be safely said of bone-grafts—they must return to their embryonic state before their osteogenetic power can assert itself. Such being the case, in the use of decalcified bone two-thirds of the material implanted —the inorganic part of bone—is removed artificially, and nature is aided to this extent. The osteoblasts are wanting, but, so far, those in the surrounding bone, under the irritative action of the trauma, have sufficed to repair the defect completely, when the framework remained; in short, the absence of the osteoblasts is more than counterbalanced by the diminished absorption rendered necessary.

MEDICAL SCIENCE IN CHINA.[1]

BY EDWARD PAYSON THWING, M.D., PH.D.,
OF CANTON, CHINA.

THE aim of this paper is to describe some of the Chinese ideas of the nature of disease and the theory of treatment, then to sketch briefly the changes wrought in the past fifty years by the introduction of Western medical and surgical science.

The Chinese Empire has been fitly compared to Lot's wife: ever looking backward; wedded to the past. Confucius taught the nation that its work was not to create but to conserve and transmit. The usages of centuries have crystallized into unvarying forms. Life and thought move on through ancestral grooves, and that which is inquisitive,

[1] Read at a meeting of the Academy of Anthropology. New York, April, 1890.

inventive, progressive, is viewed with suspicion, if not at once rebuked as seditious. In its exact, comprehensive sense, science has no existence here. Theories, speculations, traditions, and superstitions abound, and are seen in astrology, geomancy, and medicine; but that cautious, candid, thorough investigation of facts, which we call scientific study, does not find an ally in the Chinese mind. The people are, moreover, fettered by a language pronounced by Professor Williams to be "the most meagre and tedious of all tongues." Though the most ancient, it is probably the most intractable of all spoken languages, making the Chinese scholar indifferent to other tongues, because it is impossible for him to study them through the medium of his own. All the terminology of chemistry, medicine, and natural history remains in Greek and Latin, but how to adapt technical Western science to the genius of this language is not easy to decide. Professor Williams also points out the indistinctness by which time is expressed; the confusion of common and proper names; the absence of punctuation, paragraphs, sentences, capital letters, and other helpful signs of speech which native conceit forbids and ridicules. Prejudice and ignorance, however, are greater obstacles than linguistic difficulties to the spread of modern science. This will be seen as we turn to the subject of medicine.

The literature, such as it is, is very copious. During my residence in Canton Hospital, I have had access not only to libraries but to other sources of information upon native medicine. One is amazed at the patience and industry of Chinese scholars in collecting observations in various departments of research. One work in materia medica and therapeutics appears in 40 volumes, and 756 authors are quoted on the same theme. Another work on the medical and agricultural uses of plants is printed in 60 volumes with 1715 engravings.

Dissection of the body being forbidden, the most absurd notions concerning anatomy and physiology have prevailed. Food is supposed to pass from the spleen into the stomach. The larynx leads into the heart; the soul is in the liver; and the pit of the stomach is the seat of breath and the source of joy —perhaps true in some cases. The skull is one bone, so are the arm and the pelvis. The right kidney is the gate of life. Each organ is related to one of the five elements: earth, air, metals, fire, or water. Fire rules the heart; metals rule the lungs; water rules the kidney; and so on. There is not a square inch of the body that is nameless. Applications to each region are made according to the guiding dual theory, of action and reaction—*yin* and *yang*. Heat and moisture are the vital principles. The blood and spirits are their vehicles. There are twelve channels of distribution.

The study of the pulse is the most important part of the physical diagnosis of disease. In the Peking Medical Museum is a copper model of a man pierced with many holes, and marked with the names of the pulse. There are three wrist-points and twenty-four kinds of pulse at each point of each wrist, so that the native doctor has 144 pulses to study, by which the condition of the body and even the sex of an unborn child are said to be determined. Of these twenty-four varieties, there are the slow and rapid pulse, the rough, the soft, the strong, the weak, the vibrating, the hidden and the impeded. If we find the latter at the first point of the left wrist, we may expect sudden death. If at the second point of the right wrist, water in the stomach is indicated. Seven cautions are given to the practitioner regarding his own quiet breathing and presence of mind, and manipulations. George Barrow, the traveller, was taken ill with cholera morbus, and a celestial Esculapius was called. Solemn as an undertaker, he fixed his eyes on the ceiling. Beginning at the wrist, he proceeded to the elbow, pressing hard with one finger and lightly with the other, as one plays a violin. After ten minutes' fingering, he pronounced the trouble to be gastric and caused by injudicious diet—a pretty good guess.

In taking the temperature of the body, I noticed that a native physician (whom I recently accompanied through the wards of his elegant hospital at Hong Kong) laid the back of his hand, as we do, on the cheek or carotid region. He also showed me the method of preparing the decoctions used internally and externally. Every fire-pot where the liquids simmer is marked, as are the scores of wooden boxes into which the dregs of the mixtures are put for inspection, whether from the animal, vegetable, or mineral kingdom. In one standard work there are 78 substances from the first and 314 from the vegetable kingdom. Mercury and arsenic are used in specific diseases. Ginseng is greatly prized. It is held as a governmental monopoly and gathered by detachments of soldiers. Opium, camphor, rhubarb, and other medicines used by us are found in the Chinese *Pharmacopœia*. There are many inert substances used. One author commends 132 substances from metals and stones, 99 from reptiles, shell-fish, and the like, and from parts of the human body and its exuviæ a great number of things. The entire catalogue numbers 1012.

The land is overridden with quacks. The extravagant street-signs show it, on which the adventurer announces himself as a "physician and surgeon by descent for several generations." Necromancy and fortune-telling are combined with medicine. I have seen many of these impostors sitting out of doors at their divining tables with their credulous dupes about them. It is also believed that the spirits sniff the refuse of the decoctions referred to, and so these are exposed in the streets. Good food and fruit are also spread on tables in-doors to appease the spirits, and mirrors to frighten them away. Burnt charms are taken in tea for cardiac disorders, and in pure water for ulcers and all fevers. Prayer-healing and casting lots in a bamboo tube with 100 sticks; rubbing a part of an idol, corresponding to the part of the body affected, and a multitude of other methods of treating disease cannot here be described.

At the hour of death, the Chinese, like the ancient Egyptians, believe that good and evil spirits seek the departing soul. I heard an attendant calling by the hour to a dying girl in a ward opposite my room in the hospital, a few weeks since, and was told that it was an appeal to the departing spirit to come back. The beating of gongs is common in Chinese homes in which death is near. So it is at fires. I have had evidence of this in two large conflagrations near us. The din was something dreadful.

Anybody can be a doctor here. If you read the books prescribed by the college at Peking and follow the pulse-points of the copper model, you are "a regular." If not, you are an irregular practitioner and may be convicted of homicide if your patient dies. If you prolong or aggravate the disease to increase your fee, the law says that the money is stolen, and if you lose your patient you must lose your head. I saw a pile of bloody heads on the execution grounds the other day, but did not identify any as belonging to doctors. Indeed, the law is dead, and thousands of mischievous heads remain on medical shoulders. Stranger still, the Chinese race increases, in spite of irrational medicine and the utter absence of those sanitary conditions on which we predicate health. The oldest nation on the earth shows no sign of physical decay.

As to surgery, there is none. Acupuncture may be an exception, and also the terrible emasculation practised at Peking, often with fatal results, in connection with the imperial harem, which is described in the papers of the North China Asiatic Society. Surgical interference is opposed by the superstitious notion that dismemberment or mutilation here will remain in the other life a permanent disfigurement. Furthermore, the rarity of drunkenness and the absence of railways and machinery diminish the number of cases requiring treatment by the surgeon. That there is no natural inability on the part of the Chinese to become first-class surgeons is a fact shown by notable examples. Dr. Wong, a classmate of mine, forty years ago, was the first Chinese on whom a foreign medical diploma had been conferred. He was a graduate in medicine of the Edinburgh University, twenty years a successful practitioner, in charge of the Presbyterian Hospital, Canton, part of the time, and died in 1878. Dr. Ato, a colleague, was the first Chinese to acquire at home a knowledge of Western medicine. He performed, in 1847, at this hospital, the first operation with ether, and soon after, with wonderful dexterity and success, removed an enormous tumor, three feet in circumference, from the back, and another as large as the patient's head from the axilla. This latter operation involved careful dissection and the tying of three arteries. The whole was finished in four minutes. He was an ambidexter, excelled as an oculist, acquired a large fortune and was a man of commanding influence.

The changes wrought in the past half-century by Western medical and surgical science are marvellous, and constitute a powerful argument in behalf of medical missions. Dr. Peter Parker opened here in 1835 the first medical mission hospital in China. It has been remarked of him that "he opened the gates of China with a lancet when Western cannon could not heave a single bar!" Thousands of patients flocked to him from seventeen provinces, some consuming months in the journey, and going home with the voice of gratitude uttering his praise. His patients were found from the beggar in rags to the Emperor's household. The popularity of the Presbyterian Hospital was a guarantee of its safety in time of war, so that a British Consul said that he would regard himself securer in this house where I am now writing than in a gunboat on the river.

Dr. J. G. Kerr, now in charge of the Canton Hospital, has seen thirty-five years of toilful service, and stands at the head of the profession in this country. He has had a medical class, male and female, who pay $20 annually for tuition, and study three years. The instruction is wholly in Chinese. He has published many original works and translations of foreign authors. We are working together now for the establishment of an asylum for the insane, something unknown in China. Dr. Swan and Dr. Mary Niles are physicians here, the latter attending more than a thousand of her sex yearly. There is an unlimited field for women physicians, for Chinese females will endure prolonged suffering rather than be attended by men.

I have visited the medical school connected with the Alice Memorial Hospital at Hong Kong, and heard Dr. Thomson lecture in English. At Formosa there is another school where a knowledge of English is a condition of entrance. The course is four years. There has been a great deal of dispensary work ever since Drs. Robert Morrison and Livingstone opened a dispensary for the poor in Macao, seventy years ago. Drs. Colledge and Brad-

ford, of Philadelphia, should also be mentioned as pioneers, as well as Dr. Pearson, Surgeon of the East India Company, at Canton, in 1805, who introduced vaccination into the Empire—an unspeakable blessing in arresting what before had been an annual epidemic of a most loathsome and fatal character. Asiatic cholera has been another fearful scourge, more than 100 deaths a day occurring in a single town, Amoy, for nearly two months, in 1842. Thousands of lives have been saved by the missionaries.

The expressions of gratitude to Christian doctors by their heathen patients are novel and often pathetic. Gratitude is shown, not only by the *Kow-kow—i. e.*, prostration and bumping the head on the earth—but by other acts, as at Foochow, where Dr. Kate Woodhull, a successful operator for cataract, some months ago received a handsome memorial tablet, which was hung up amid the explosion of firecrackers. The inscription read: "She has given her whole heart." One of Dr. Parker's patients requested leave to send a painter to make a portrait, that he might daily bow to it. Dr. Parker's pecuniary gifts were liberal, for he was an official secretary; and he composed an eloquent poem in praise of the medical missionary.

A sufferer from lupus at Kiang-Si, who had spent her all on native doctors and Buddhist priests, seeing the disease spreading over face and neck, went to the temple and told them that they and their gods were frauds. The priests were horror-stricken, and frightened her into the payment of $7.50 in gold, to get which she sold a few remaining personal effects. The failure of their incantations exhausted the last ounce of patience she had. She and her husband returned to the temple, and cursed the gods and the Buddhists to their hearts' content. On their way home they fell in with a former patient of Dr. Douthwaite, whose body and soul had been saved by this kind physician. Three days by wheelbarrow brought them to Dr. Douthwaite, who not only prayed and read the gospel to them, but gave potassium iodide internally and iodine ointment externally. The disease was arrested, and in a month cured. They returned home, renounced idolatry, and led many of their neighbors to do the same. A Christian teacher was sent for; many more of the villagers threw away their idols; a church was organized where the true God was daily worshipped, and the members became missionaries, sending from their own number an evangelist to preach the gospel, which had done so much for their own village, to regions beyond their borders.

There are about sixty mission hospitals and eighty foreign physicians connected with them in this Empire, besides clergymen and assistants who have acquired a practical acquaintance with medicine after years of service in isolated districts in the country.

In these far-away neighborhoods a knowledge of simple remedies in sickness and emergencies will save many lives, and invest a man with supernatural influence in the eyes of the priest-ridden and quack-denuded people. Shanghai, which I hope to visit shortly, and many other large cities and towns have hospitals, and natives are being taught Western science. Dr. Eldridge, who, under imperial patronage, has sent out more than thirty Japanese practitioners, said to me when in Yokohama, that in nothing had the recent intellectual advance been more satisfactory than in medical science in Japan. The more conservative Chinese are slower to welcome us with our Western ideas, but the leaven is surely working. Ever since Dr. Lockhart, who was a pioneer of 1843, went with Her Majesty's legation to Peking, at the close of the second war, princes of the palace and officers of highest rank have been applicants for relief at the hands of these "foreign devils," as we have hitherto been regarded.

A few weeks ago I was in an inland city, eighteen miles from Canton, where the chief manager of a native hospital came to the missionary physician, confessing the inutility of his own methods. He paid $15 to be rid of hæmorrhoids, and went his way rejoicing. A pagan teacher, speaking of doctors, said recently, in substance, "When you find a thief on his way to your money-drawer do you pray with him? No, you call the police! So, if you are really ill, you want a foreign doctor." A few days ago a message came to the hospital here for help for a woman who was dying in labor. Dr. Kerr promptly responded, and saved both mother and child. (In an arm presentation the mother is left to die.) Again, yesterday, he had a similar call. The ignorant midwife was doing nothing, and held one dead child. Two more unborn, and the mother as well. would have died but for Dr. Kerr. A fortnight since, the naval admiral, General Fong, a high mandarin, came to us for relief for his aged mother, hundreds of miles away. One of our skilled woman physicians responded. A long journey and several weeks' absence are involved. It was a suggestive sight as I saw this stately officer and his attendants, in silken robes and gracious speech, soliciting the aid of foreign science, which their own wealth and boasted civilization failed to furnish. It was a type of Asia, herself, waking from the sleep of centuries to feel the flush and throb of a new life. When an elaborate manikin was shown, and certain medical and surgical methods explained, their wonder and admiration were something interesting to study.

But, I have not time or space to recite further incidents, or to record other data as to the introduction of Western science into this long-sealed, hermit-like nation. My time is crowded, and postage is twenty cents an ounce! A long, *heavy* article is, therefore, out of the question. The Chinese Hippocrates of the second century, contemporary of Galen, gave medicine in doses of a pound, and the system which he founded was so popular that it continued one thousand years. I have ventured to give the reader an *ounce* dose, or less, promising more at another time, in reference to the special work in my hands, namely, the establishment, if possible, of an asylum for the insane. No such institution is to be found in the Empire. Such a humane and beneficent enterprise would fitly crown the history of Western medical science, which the last half-century has made so illus'rious in this vast Empire of the oriental world.

PRESBYTERIAN HOSPITAL, CANTON.

CROTON-CHLORAL IN NEURALGIA.[1]

BY H. A. HARE, M.D.,
DEMONSTRATOR OF THERAPEUTICS AND CLINICAL PROFESSOR OF THE DISEASES OF CHILDREN IN THE UNIVERSITY OF PENNSYLVANIA.

THE use of butyl-chloral hydrate in the treatment of insomnia due to neuralgic pain is resorted to. in my belief, so rarely in this country that I have thought it worth while to call attention to its interesting action and relative value and safety.

Physiological experiment coupled with practical experience has convinced us all that chloral, while it is the best hypnotic for the majority of cases, is not one which will give sleep in painful affections or relieve neuralgias unless it is given in full doses, so full as to be dangerous. At the same time it is very desirable that we should have some preparation at hand which will both produce sleep and relieve pain. At present we use chloral and morphine together—the first for its somnifacient effects: the second to relieve the pain, and also to cause sleep. A very great advantage of butyl-chloral hydrate is its safety. The active dose for many cases of neuralgia is only 5 grains, given in pill-form. yet as much as 40 grains may be used without producing any more noteworthy effects than 20 grains of ordinary chloral so far as the heart and respiration are concerned.

The following case is of interest, as showing its advantages:

M. G., aged thirty-five years, has had. for over two years, a severe supra-orbital neuralgia, varying in intensity, and accompanied by roaring in the ears and loss of appetite and sleep. The cause of the neuralgia rests in the presence of middle-ear disease, with varying amounts of discharge. The Eustachian tubes are widely dilated and relaxed. The neuralgia is always worse when the discharge becomes in

[1] Read before the American Medical Association. Section of Practice of Medicine. Nashville, May. 1890.

any way suppressed, and the branches of the entire trifacial nerve become involved in the painful neuralgic shootings. At this time it is impossible for the patient to go to the front door, as the noise of the street hurts her head so much as to make the pain unbearable. The loss of strength and flesh was considerable, owing to the decrease in appetite and loss of sleep. Five grains of butyl-chloral hydrate were ordered every two hours in pill-form. Six pills were taken, with entire relief of all the symptoms and the attaining of good sleep and a better appetite. The effects of each dose lasted twenty-four hours, and then the pain required another six pills. She had no attacks for some weeks after this, although the ear was not discharging.

Functional insomnia resting upon no known cause also yields to this drug very well, but insomnia due to any advanced systemic lesion, as in phthisis, is not relieved in every instance under its use. The history of cases of phthisis who use the drug is that they sleep well the first night, and lie awake the second night to cough the lungs clear of mucus which has accumulated during sleep and while the nerves are obtunded by the drug. This second sleepless night can be quieted by a large dose, 20 grains, if desired, but I have never wished to run the risk of choking up the lung by preventing expectoration. In the neuralgia of phthisis and anæmia the drug is very serviceable.

Neuralgias of other nerves than the cranial are rarely benefited by butyl-chloral; but it is worthy of note that it may sometimes give relief in such cases by using with it 10 to 15 drops of the tincture of gelsemium.

In migraine, sick headache, and bilious headache, Ringer has recommended it, and in true migraine with hemianopsia it is certainly one of the most useful remedies along with antipyrine and caffeine, cannabis indica and gelsemium.

Curiously enough, while it cures the neuralgia due to a carious tooth, it does not cure toothache.

A great advantage possessed by croton-chloral is the applicability of moderate doses in cases of heart-disease.

A SUCCESSFUL VAGINAL HYSTERECTOMY.

BY J. T. BINKLEY, M.D.,

CONSULTING SURGEON TO THE FANNIE PADDOCK HOSPITAL; SURGEON TO THE HOSPITAL OF THE SISTERS OF CHARITY; ETC., TACOMA, WASHINGTON.

ABOUT the first of May I was called to see Mrs. E. S., aged forty-seven years, a hard-working, fleshy, but cachectic woman, weighing 175 pounds, the mother of four children, of whom the oldest was twenty, and youngest seven years of age.

She was suffering from constant pain, was confined to her room, and had a muco-sanguineous discharge from a cauliflower mass on the posterior lip of the cervix uteri. Her mother had a cancer of the breast removed at the age of forty-five years, and died of

recurrence three months later. Her sister, aged thirty-six, now has cancer of the breast. Two physicians had previously examined the case, and declined to treat it. I concluded that I had to deal with a recent cancer, and thought at once of operative measures. Before expressing my opinion, however, I decided to consult my partner, Dr. McKone, who was at the time out of the city. On his return, two weeks later, we examined the case, and he concurred in my opinion. We removed a fragment of the mass, had our diagnosis confirmed by microscopical examination, and decided to do a vaginal hysterectomy, as the uterus was freely movable, and the cervix so much involved that an amputation would not be radical. Her menstrual periods were occurring about once in twenty-three days. June 8th, about two weeks after the next period, was the date decided upon for operating.

The patient was taken to the Fannie Paddock Hospital, and put under preparatory treatment for a few days, Miss Gray, of the Philadelphia Hospital Training School, executing my orders.

We decided upon the method outlined by the late lamented Dr. Hunter in his excellent monograph, "The Technique of Vaginal Hysterectomy."

The excellent coöperation of the hospital officers, and the skill of the nurse made the most thorough antisepsis and asepsis possible. The pubes and vulva of the patient were carefully shaved and scrubbed. She was etherized, and placed in the lithotomy position by the hospital staff, at 10 A.M., June 8, 1890. The parts were again thoroughly washed with a 1-to-2000 bichloride solution; the instruments, previously boiled and immersed in carbolized solution, were conveniently placed, and presided over by Dr. J. J. McKone, and Dr. T. F. Smith, Surgeon of the Northern Pacific Railroad. Dr. Grant S. Hicks, Surgeon of the Marine Hospital, held the limbs and retractors. Dr. Myles gave the anæsthetics. Dr. E. G. Stratton, of Orting, and the nurses, attended to the sponges.

A broad Simon's blade in the vagina exposed the vault of the vagina, which I mopped out with strong carbolized solution, and then curetted the growth, and touched it with pure carbolic acid. After this I grasped the anterior lip of the cervix with vulsella forceps, drew it down firmly, passed a stout silk ligature high up, and made traction downward and backward, both with the forceps and ligature. A semicircular incision was then made in the anterior vaginal vault, after which I carefully dissected with my finger through the cellular tissue between the bladder and wall of uterus, until the peritoneum was reached. An antiseptic plug of absorbent cotton was pushed into the cavity. The cervix was then drawn down and forward against the bladder, and a similar incision made in the posterior vault. The two incisions, however, did not meet, a small isthmus being left on either side of the neck. The posterior attachments were severed with the finger as before. An assistant then made forcible traction on the suture and forceps, while I applied a long-jawed Tait's hæmostatic forceps close to the cervix and body, avoiding the ureters, and severed the uterine arteries and tissues of the right side nearly to the point of the forceps. A second pair of forceps were similarly applied, and the tissue severed on the opposite side. Two other pairs of forceps were applied higher up, between the first forceps and body of uterus, on either side, embracing all of the tissues up to the broad ligaments, which were then severed. Firm traction failing to bring down the uterus, I decided to retrovert it, which was accomplished by passing a curved, male, urethral sound into the cavity of the uterus, and rotating the point backward, bringing the fundus out through the posterior incision. This brought the upper borders of the broad ligaments within easy reach. I hooked them down with my finger, brought them within the jaws of the forceps, and severed the tissues on either side, making a clean cut up to the point of the second forceps, and entirely freeing the uterus, which was then easily delivered. But one bleeding point presented, and this was readily controlled by the seventh pair of forceps.

The cavity was then carefully sponged, the forceps were supported by iodoform gauze, lightly packed around them in the vagina, and by absorbent cotton about the handles externally. Each pair of forceps was firmly tied with silk to prevent slipping, and the patient was transferred to bed.

The time occupied by the operation, including anæsthetization, was one hour and thirty-one minutes. The patient rallied well from the anæsthetic.

The following is a condensed daily report of the case :

June 8. Small portions of lime water and milk, and of water given. At 5 P. M. she had a little pain. Seven ounces of urine drawn, and a suppository of opium and belladonna inserted in rectum. Temperature 98¾°, pulse 96. Has had several refreshing naps. 10 P. M., pulse 110, temperature 98¼°.

9th. 4 A. M. Four ounces of urine drawn. Temperature 98¾°, pulse 112. Restless. Was given a suppository. At 9 A. M. four ounces of urine drawn ; face flushed ; thirsty ; "starts" in her sleep. At 4 P. M. five ounces of urine drawn. At 11 P. M. temperature 101½°, pulse 135. Pain in abdomen ; tympany. Ordered one drachm of whiskey hourly. Rectal tube gave exit to considerable gas, followed by much relief. Cold to abdomen increases pain.

10th. Temperature 99¾°, pulse 116. Gas escaping freely through rectal tube. A little nausea. Forceps removed at noon, forty-eight hours after the operation. The gauze came with them, and the vagina was repacked. Patient much relieved, but tympany persists. Passed twenty-three ounces of urine during the twenty-four hours. Turpentine stupes to abdomen.

11th. 1 A. M. Vomiting. Umbilicus protruding. Tympany enormous ; much pain. Gave one-fourth grain doses of calomel every half-hour for four hours, followed by two-drachm doses of Epsom salts. Turpentine internally, glycerin suppository, and turpentine enema, all failed to produce a passage. Temperature and pulse remain the same. Urine a little increased in amount.

12th. Tympany and severe pain in abdomen. Feels as if bowels would move, but continued doses

of calomel and sulphate of magnesium fail to produce a passage. Gave a dish of corn-meal gruel and molasses, and in one hour the faradic current to the abdomen. A small, semi-liquid movement followed in about an hour, and two more free passages during the day. Temperature and pulse somewhat reduced.

13th. Tympany disappeared ; patient much improved.

14th. Patient very comfortable. Quite natural passage from bowels. A slight burning sensation on urinating. Appetite good. Diet : Mush and milk, beef-tea, crackers, tea, and coffee. Slept well.

15th. Temperature 99¾° to 100⅓°, pulse 91 to 100. More pain on urinating. Removed tampon, gave a douche, and repacked the vagina with iodoform-gauze. Eats and sleeps well.

16th. Appetite good, but cystitis increasing, and bowels loose. Rests fairly well. Temperature and pulse improved. Gave vaginal douche.

17th. A small bedsore appeared on left hip. Cystitis more severe. Bowels loose. Gave an alkaline diuretic.

18th. Eats and sleeps well. Cystitis and bedsore improved. Two grains of quinine every four or five hours. Temperature 98¾° to 99¾°. pulse 84. Sat up in bed.

19th. Much improved. Temperature and pulse nearly normal.

Gradually improved up to June 22d, when she sat up about four hours, in an invalid's chair.

On the 29th she was walking about the room, writing to friends, receiving visitors, etc.

She desired to go home, but we thought it wise to keep her in hospital another week. On July 3d, she had two hard chills (the second, I think, was increased by the nurse—a new one—who exposed the patient for her evening douche directly after the first chill) followed by a temperature of 104¾°, entire loss of appetite, and one of the most violent cases of cystitis I ever saw. She begged to go home "to die." I had her removed, on a stretcher, on July 9th, to her home, where she rapidly improved under the usual treatment for cystitis until July 12th, when I discharged her.

She is now going about, free from pain, but has a slight serous discharge from the vagina. She eats and sleeps well.

FOUR CASES OF DISEASE OF THE MASTOID.[1]

BY ROBERT TILLEY, M.D.,
OF CHICAGO.

BARKER, of London, in a study of abscesses of the brain, states that three-fourths of brain abscesses are in the temporo-sphenoidal lobes, and that nine-tenths of subdural abscesses are found in a circle one inch and a half in diameter, with its centre one inch and a quarter behind and one inch and a quarter above the centre of the bony auditory meatus. It might further be said that nearly all these abscesses originate from disturbances in some

[1] Read before the Illinois State Medical Society, May, 1890.

part of the external auditory apparatus. As long as facts substantiate this statement the study of mastoid affections will not cease to be interesting.

I desire to submit the following brief notes of four cases of mastoid affection which have recently come under my care:

CASE I.—Mr. J. M., thirty-eight years old, first seen, February 25, 1888. Recommended to my care by Dr. H. T. Byford. The patient had been suffering great pain on the right side of the head, and great sensitiveness, expressed by rigors, when the ear was touched. There was some discharge from the external meatus, and granulation-tissue extended from the meatus to the membrana tympani. The temperature varied from 99° to 101°, and the pulse from 100 to 120. There was not severe pain on pressure over the mastoid region, but a good deal of pain was complained of over the whole of the temporal bone, and extending to the right eye. The distress associated with the eye gave him great concern. No proof of hearing could be elicited on the right side. He was delirious at times, and talked of being poisoned by his family. Though advised to do so, he refused, for some time, to go to the Hospital. With the use of cathartics, and by attention to the external meatus, his condition was somewhat relieved.

On the 17th of March, the following month, he entered St. Luke's Hospital for operative measures. But I determined to wait a day or two, and give him the benefit of the advantages the Hospital possessed over his own home during the interval. I explored anew the external meatus, but found nothing promising there. I explored the nose more thoroughly than was possible in his home, and I was a little less sensitive to his expression of pain. I found the cartilaginous septum eroded on both sides, and in the posterior and upper part of the nose a vast quantity of muco-purulent material. I will add here that I could elicit no history of syphilis. It was denied, and he offered no objective indications of its previous existence. He had a large family, and his wife had had no miscarriages. There was a history of a blow on the head, which I could in no way connect with the existing affection. From the condition of the nose, however, I concluded that constitutional treatment would probably be advantageous. This treatment was begun at once, and his nose was washed out three times a day. Two days later, Monday, his condition was so much improved that the operation was no longer justifiable, and by the following Saturday, seven days from the time of the proposed operation, he was dismissed from the Hospital, and continued under treatment as an office patient. The pulse and temperature became normal. The pain in the eye and in the head over the region of the temporal bone, and the distressing dizziness, disappeared. Still later, the discharge from the middle ear ceased, and the hearing became practically normal. The ulcerated spots on the septum of the nose were healed. The process of cure extended over four months. He has had no return of the difficulty.

The interesting points in this case are the severe pain in the head, requiring confinement to bed for six weeks, the extreme sensitiveness of the ear, and the confusing dizziness, all of which yielded, without operative measures, to intra-nasal treatment, and to persistent constitutional measures, notwithstanding the impossibility of obtaining any specific history.

CASE II.—Mr. A. C., aged thirty-three years. Admitted to Hospital, February 10, 1890. About six weeks previously he lost the hearing in right ear; no pain. Two weeks later, ear began to discharge. During the last week pain had been very severe. No evidence of hearing on affected side, and the mastoid region was tender, red, and swollen; there was some discharge from the external meatus, and the membrane was perforated. There was no delirium. The throat gave evidence of previous cauterization, which the patient said was done with nitric acid in London. The pulse averaged 100, and the temperature varied from 99° to 100° F. Fomentations and palliative measures were used for three days without effect.

On February 13, 1890, the usual mastoid operation was performed. The external part of the bone was not rough, and no pus was encountered in reaching the bone. The only variation from the usual proceeding was in the instruments used for perforating the bone. I used for this purpose a modified farrier's knife. The chisel is, in my judgment, much better than the drill for perforating the outer tables of the mastoid. The cut is clean, and the operative field is open to view, which is not the case when we use the ordinary drill devised for that purpose. With the use of this knife, however, the advantage of the chisel is obtained without the sudden blow associated with the chisel, which should certainly be avoided. If the knife is held firmly, and the patient's head kept steady, and a good support be secured for the elbow, the outer plate is very readily perforated. In the present case the antrum of the mastoid was rapidly reached, pus appeared in the field of operation, and water passed in through the opening readily came through the external meatus.

The wound and external meatus were irrigated with 1-to-2000 bichloride solution, and dressed with iodoform-gauze. In the evening of the day of operation the patient was reading the newspaper; the second day after the operation the temperature and pulse were normal, and discharge from the middle ear had ceased.

This was a typical case of simple abscess of the mastoid cells, uncomplicated by any marked necrosis; and one month from the time of his admission to the Hospital he was discharged, the wound completely healed and the hearing normal. The history is taken from the notes of Dr. J. E. Perekham, then interne in charge of the department at the Hospital. The reason of rapid recovery in this case was the absence of necrosed bone, the suppurative condition being confined to the soft tissues in the antrum mastoideum and the middle ear.

CASE III.—Mr. M. M., aged thirty-three years, bank clerk. Entered the Hospital, March 28, 1889. There was a history of protracted catarrhal affection of the nasal passages with impairment of hearing on each side, but worse on the left. Two weeks previously to his admission he complained of a "cold in the head." Severe pain, worse at night, was experienced in the right ear, and impairment of hearing was marked. There was some muco-purulent discharge from the right ear, and tenderness over the region of the mastoid, extending also in spots over the whole temporal bone. The swelling was insignificant; the pain was considerable, but there was no delirium. Temperature varied from 90° to 100° F., the pulse did not exceed 100.

During the interval between March 28th and April 14th, various emollient applications, constitutional treatment, and free paracentesis of the membrana tympani were tried without relief. The nose received attention, but beyond a puffiness of the inferior turbinated bones there was no disturbance in that region.

On April 14th, with the assistance of Dr. Robert Locke, interne in charge, from whose notes the case is reported, an incision was made in the usual position behind the ear. The bone was rough, and the periosteum was easily separated. The antrum was penetrated with the knife, previously described, making a gutter-like groove just on a level with and a little behind the external bony canal. The penetration of the cells gave exit to a small amount of muco-purulent discharge, and the solution used for the irrigation came from the external meatus. The wound was dressed with iodoform-gauze.

There was no marked relief from the pain over the temporal bone, nor was the temperature influenced. During the first few days after the operation, by closing the external auditory canal, the patient could force air through the opening in the mastoid. The same constitutional remedies were continued for about two weeks after the operation with no satisfactory result. There then appeared a swelling above and somewhat anterior to the ear; May 4th, about three weeks after the opening of the mastoid cells, the patient was again anæsthetized, a deep incision, parallel to but about an inch and a quarter anterior to the primary incision, was made, and the bone was found rough. The lower part of this incision began at the juncture of the upper part of the auricle with the integument of the scalp, and extended upward about an inch. This incision was connected with the wound of the first operation beneath the periosteum, and a strip of gauze was placed under the periosteum to facilitate the passage of irrigating fluids over the rough bone. Both wounds were irrigated with a 3-per-cent. solution of hydrochloric acid. There was no pus found in the second operation, and a steady but somewhat slow improvement followed, discharge from the external meatus ceased, and hearing improved. The pain was less severe, and gradually subsided. The irrigation was continued twice a day, and both wounds were kept open for three weeks. It was not, however, before June 3d—about a month after the second operation—that the temperature became normal, and even then slight elevations occurred regularly every evening till June 12th. June 15th, a little more than ten weeks after his admission to the Hospital, he was discharged. The wounds were completely healed. The perforation in the membrana tympani was healed, and the hearing was better than on the other side; not, however, so good as before the existence of the affection.

I am convinced that irrigation with hydrochloric acid solution rendered very good service here. In fact, I think it was the chief element in the cure. The swelling which appeared in front of the ear disappeared after its use, and no marked improvement was previously obtained. The use of hydrochloric acid solution for irrigation was, I think, first brought prominently before the profession by Dr. Edmund Andrews, of Chicago, in 1887.

CASE IV.—Mr. A. P., aged thirty-seven years. Saw the patient for the first time, March 22, 1890, when he was referred to me by Dr. D. T. Nelson. The left ear had been discharging for about two months. He had been in bed during that time, and was very weak. There was no cerebral disturbance. There were distinct redness, swelling, and tenderness over the left mastoid, extending in the direction of the sterno-cleido-mastoid; temperature ranged about 100° F. Examination of bony external meatus showed necrosed bone. He was recommended to the Hospital for operation, but he did not follow this advice until April 3d. At this time, when he entered the Hospital, the tissues extending downward from the level of the external meatus were greatly infiltrated, but gave no clear indication of the presence of pus. The breath was very offensive, and the tongue heavily coated.

On making the primary incision the bone was felt to be decidedly rough; the periosteum was easily separated, and exposure of the denuded bone showed rather a concave instead of a convex surface over the mastoid process, as though some operation had previously been performed there. On pulling the ear forward the sharp spoon slipped readily into the external canal, where the greater part of the diseased bone was located. It was not thought desirable, under these circumstances, to penetrate the cells, as the principal focus of necrosis was in the external meatus. The necrosed bone was thoroughly scraped with a sharp spoon, which was passed into the external meatus from the opening behind the ear. The infiltrated tissues in the neck were explored for pus, but none was found. The patient felt better, slept better, and ate better, after the operation, but it soon became manifest that some outlet would be necessary to relieve the inflamed tissues lower down. About ten days after the operation it was found necessary to make an incision in the tissues of the neck to give vent to a well-defined pocket of pus.

The original wound over the mastoid process and the necrosed tissue in the external meatus, as well as the wound in the neck, were freely irrigated twice a day with 1-per-cent. hydrochloric acid solution. His mouth was cleaned several times daily with 2-per-cent. chlorate of potassium solution.

The patient rapidly, improved so that on the 27th of April he was discharged from the Hospital, to be treated as an out-patient. Apart from the scraping of the bone and the incision to relieve the infiltrated tissue, the irrigation with hydrochloric acid solution was the chief feature of the treatment in this case. I should add that some preparation of mercury was administered, but my conviction is that the benefit obtained was rather due to the hydrochloric acid solution. He is still under observation, but, apparently, no modification of the treatment will be needed beyond the application of a little burnt alum to any fungoid growths which may appear.

MEDICAL PROGRESS.

Cannabis Indica in Gastric Disorders.—GERMAIN SÉE, in *La Médecine Moderne*, has published a long communication upon the action of cannabis indica in dyspepsia and gastric neuroses. His conclusions may be summed up briefly, as follows:

The drug, when employed in the form of the fresh extract, in doses of one grain divided into three equal parts for administration during the day, does not produce toxic symptoms, but is of value in the non-malignant forms of gastric trouble. These may be divided into two groups, namely, those in which there are alterations in the chemical character of the gastric juice, as, for example, hyper- or hypo-acidity; and those in which neuroses of the gastric or intestinal walls are present without modification of the gastric juice. In all these affections, whether dyspeptic or neurotic, we may find painful sensations, localized or radiating, spontaneous, or provoked by the contact of food. The troubles of movement are due to atony and dilatation, or the anti-peristaltic state may be due to neurotic disorders. We may have, too, the formation of gases with eructations, and with vertigo, migraine, and similar affections. Under these circumstances Sée finds that cannabis indica does good with extraordinary constancy, diminishing the pain, reëstablishing the appetite, and increasing digestion. Where there is hyper-acidity, Sée considers that the use of full doses of bicarbonate of sodium should be invariably administered in addition to the hemp, and that it should be taken after the ingestion of the meal.

Where atony is marked, cannabis indica does little good alone, but is useful if combined with lavage and hydrotherapy. Where spasmodic gastric movements occur, it is, however, very valuable by itself, and particularly so in the vomiting depending upon nervous disturbance. While it does not prevent the formation of gases in the stomach, nor stop eructations by any direct influence, cannabis indica prevents the uncomfortable distress accompanying this state, generally called pyrosis or "heartburn."

Sée asserts very strongly that gastric digestion is favored by the drug, and that it quiets hysteroidal tendencies, as well as removes melancholia.

In many cases it is necessary to administer other remedies at the same time, such as alkalies in full dose; purgatives, if constipation be present; and, finally, antiseptics to the alimentary canal. Finally, Sée concludes that in this drug we have a veritable gastric sedative devoid of unpleasant narcotic effects.

Treatment of Pulmonary Tuberculosis.—The late DR. BREHMER, who treated cases of phthisis so successfully in his sanitarium at Goerbersdorf, was a strong advocate of the treatment of the disease in sanitaria. Such institutions, he believed, should be situated among the mountains, as the elevation increases the heart's action through diminished atmospheric pressure, and improves nutrition by stimulating the appetite. The locality should be immune from phthisis, and well sheltered from winds, which are especially injurious. Patients may be allowed considerable exercise in the open air, but upon the least fatigue rest is exceedingly important. Dr. Brehmer, believing nutrition to be of great importance, provided his patients with five meals daily, vegetables occupying a prominent place in the dietary. Every patient should also take three pints of milk daily, increasing to four pints if anorexia is pronounced. Wine is useful because it increases the power of the heart and economizes nutrition.

In the symptomatic treatment, dry, irritative cough should be controlled by "psychical influences," and by the drinking of cold water or of hot milk with seltzer. Morphine is indicated only when the cough is accompanied with expectoration and interferes with sleep. Moderate hæmoptysis is checked by the hypodermic injection of morphine, and an ice-bag to the cardiac region. Ergotin may be used if necessary. In profuse hæmoptysis violent coughing is often necessary to dislodge the clots, but if insufficient they may be removed by a finger introduced into the larynx. If there is much weakness and dyspnœa champagne is a useful stimulant. Fever may be reduced by cold to the præcordium, but if this is not effectual antipyrine or antifebrin may be employed. Night-sweats can often be prevented by the ingestion of a glass of milk containing one or two teaspoonfuls of cognac.—*Occidental Medical Times*, August, 1890.

Sterilization of Catgut Ligatures.—DR. GEORGE R. FOWLER (*Medical Record*, August 16, 1890) has had a series of experiments made to determine if boiling in alcohol will sterilize catgut. The results were positive, and, using them as a basis, Dr. Fowler recommends the following method of sterilization: The catgut is wound on ordinary wooden spools which have been boiled in soda solution. The spools are then placed in a fruit-jar, or in a bottle with a glass stopper, alcohol is poured in, and the stopper loosely inserted. The jar is then placed in a water-bath and boiled for an hour. As bacteria will not develop in strong alcohol, the catgut may be kept indefinitely in the fluid, which can be again boiled should there be a suspicion that the gut has become infected.

The Spirometer in Diagnosis.—M. JOAL, of Mont Dore, has made a number of observations in spirometry that lead him to the conclusion that many nasal and pharyngeal affections produce a distinct diminution in the capacity of the lungs. Thus, in cases where hypertrophic rhinitis, adenoid tumors of the naso-pharynx, chronic coryza, etc., have been cured, the capacity of the lungs, as measured by the spirometer, is frequently increased by one-fourth, and occasionally even doubled. M. Joal has frequently found that public singers, when they complain of fatigue of the voice, or of diminution in its power or range, are suffering from some, perhaps quite unsuspected, disease in the nose or pharynx, and that if this is cured the normal condition of the voice is restored.

He suggests that professional singers should know their own respiratory capacity, and that this should be occasionally tested, so that any diminution may serve to give a warning of possible disease in the nose or pharynx, which may be the more easily cured because discovered early.—*Lancet*, August 9. 1890.

The Treatment of Ruptured Uterus.—In the treatment of ruptured uterus, DR. D. BERRY HART writes, that when the presenting part of the child is still in the genital tract, we must deliver in such a way as to avoid upward tension on the uterus, and, therefore, craniotomy or decapitation should be performed. If the rent is not extensive, he recommends either irrigation with weak sublimate solution, drainage, and abdominal pressure; or tamponade of the uterus, vagina, and rent with iodoform gauze, the edges of the rent being approximated by tenacula while the tampon is being applied. If the tear is extensive, and the fœtus or placenta has escaped into the peritoneal cavity, abdominal section is imperative. With regard to the treatment of the rent, suturing is condemned, as it is both tedious and ineffective. The choice is between Prevôt's operation and tamponing, both through the vagina and the peritoneum, with iodoform gauze. Dr. Hart is in favor of the former method, but mentions two cases in which the latter was successful. In conclusion, he expresses the opinion that even in apparently hopeless cases we should give the patient the chance that operative treatment offers.—*Medical Chronicle*, August. 1890.

Errors in the Diagnosis of Specific Fevers.—In a short paper based upon his report to the Glasgow Health Committee, DR. J. B. RUSSELL (*Glasgow Medical Journal*, July, 1890) calls attention, first, to the frequency with which an incorrect diagnosis is made in fever cases; and, secondly, to the cause of such errors, viz., the lack of proper training of medical students.

To show the frequency of mistakes in the diagnosis of infectious diseases, Dr. Russell has prepared a table of cases sent into the Belvidere Hospital during seven months of 1889. Of the 1499 cases admitted with the diagnosis of one of the various infectious diseases, in 114 the diagnosis was incorrect, and 85 were not suffering from any infectious disease whatever. The greatest number of errors occurred in the cases admitted as enteric and typhus fevers. Of the 42 cases sent in as enteric fever, 14 were cases of pneumonia, and 10 were absolutely non-febrile. Having pointed out the serious results of such mistakes in diagnosis, Dr. Russell shows how imperfect, in the majority of cases, is the student's training in the study of fevers [A fact no less true in this country than in Great Britain.—ED.], and that many

students have never even seen the rashes and other signs and symptoms of specific fevers.—*Medical Chronicle*, August, 1890.

Partial Removal of Diseased Ovaries.—DR. MARTIN, of Berlin, only partially removes ovaries not entirely diseased. In some cases he has also resected part of the tube, and made, by suture of the mucosa to the serous coat, a new ostium. Dr. Martin, as the result of his experience, published in Volkmann's *Klinischer Vorträge*, came to the following conclusions: Patients recover perfectly after partial removal of ovaries for localized chronic inflammatory changes, hydrops folliculi, and oöphoritis. Recovery is also complete, in most cases, after the resection of obstructed and otherwise diseased tubes. The after-histories of seventeen patients operated upon by Dr. Martin prove that women with resected ovaries and tubes are not more exposed than other women to further disease of the parts left behind. Menstruation continued in all cases, and some patients conceived. Dr. Martin states that in 1864 Sir Spencer Wells emptied some dropsical follicles in one ovary of a young girl, having just removed its fellow. The girl afterward married and had children.—*British Medical Journal*, August 9. 1890.

Antiseptic Vaginal Injection.—

R.—Bichloride of mercury	.	.	4 grains.
Sulphate of copper	.	.	15 "
Chloride of sodium	.	.	15 "
Tartaric acid .	.	.	8 "
Indigo .	.	.	a trace.
Distilled water	.	.	2½ drachms.
Glycerin	.	.	2½ " M.

This is to be added to one quart of water, and used after labor, if an injection is required.—*Gazette de Gynécologie*, August 1, 1890.

Treatment of Puerperal Convulsions.—In the treatment of puerperal convulsions, DR. R. T. TRIMBLE (*American Journal of Obstetrics*, August, 1890) advises the administration of veratrum viride, if the patient is plethoric, until its physiological effects are produced. This, if necessary, may be followed by morphine. If the patient is anæmic, it is better to commence with morphine. These remedies should be given hypodermically: the veratrum in doses of from 2 to 5 drops of the tincture, the morphine in doses of from ⅙ grain to ½ grain. If these drugs fail, give potassium bromide and chloral by the rectum in doses of from ½ to 1 drachm each. Chloroform is useful, and should be given during the convulsion to all cases. Delivery as early as the safety of the mother will permit should be the rule. Forceps-delivery is preferable, if it can be accomplished safely, but turning is better practice in some cases. Venesection is rarely required, as veratrum will accomplish all that can be expected from bloodletting, and more safely. One serious objection to bleeding is that we cannot know how much blood a woman in labor may lose from the uterus.

Bi-hydrochlorate of Quinine for Hypodermic Use.—In the *Bulletin Générale de Thérapeutique* of July 30, 1890,

BEURMANN and VILLEJEAN recommend the following preparation for the hypodermic use of quinine :

R.—Bi-hydrochlorate of quinine . 70 grains.
Distilled water . . . 2 drachms.—M.

This solution holds 7 grains in each 10 drops, so that 20 drops, or an ordinary syringeful, would give a good dose of the drug.

As the bi-hydrochlorate of quinine is not generally to be had, it is to be made by taking ordinary chlorate of quinine, as it is found in commerce, and preparing the bichlorate in a few minutes by the following process: Add to distilled water enough hydrochloric acid to give it a specific gravity of 1.045 at 60° F. Then take 1 drachm of this acid solution and add to it 1 drachm of the chlorate of quinine. Finally, add to this enough distilled water to make 2 drachms, and filter. This solution is not caustic, since the acid is neutralized by the basic chlorate of quinine, so that the bi-hydrochlorate is not irritating.

Mixture for Diarrhœa.—The following formula is quoted by the *Canada Medical Record* :

R.—Wine of opium . . . . 1 ounce.
Tincture of valerian . . 1½ ounces.
Ether . . . . . ½ ounce.
Oil of peppermint . . . 60 minims.
Fluid extract of ipecacuanha 15 "
Alcohol, sufficient to make . 4 ounces.—M.
Dose, for an adult, 30 drops every three hours.

Antipyrine in Cutaneous Affections.—One of the symptoms which is most disagreeable in a large number of skin diseases, is the intense itching or soreness which causes scratching, with consequent injury to the parts involved. Many remedies are now added to the applications usually ordered to allay this troublesome state. Chief among these are carbolic acid, menthol, chloral hydrate, and cocaine, but even these often prove inefficient. According to BLASCHKO, of Berlin, antipyrine proves a most valuable remedy under such circumstances, and he recommends that for infants the following be given internally :

R.—Antipyrine . . . . ½ drachm.
Simple syrup . . . 1 ounce.—M.
Dose, half a teaspoonful at night before going to bed.

Sometimes larger doses are needed, but excellent results are to be obtained by this means in eczema, urticaria, strophulus, pemphigus, lichen ruber and planus. Not only does it prove palliative, but often curative, probably by preventing scratching. Antipyrine may also be used for hysterical pruritus with advantage, but in adults must be given in full doses and frequently.

Prescription for Cardiac Dropsy.—FÜRBRINGER uses the following in cases of dropsy from valvular insufficiency :

R.—Infusion of digitalis . . 5 ounces.
Citrate of caffeine . . 30 grains.
Tincture of strophanthus . 75 minims.
Solution of potassium acetate 15 drachms.
Extract of glycyrrhiza . . 75 grains.—M.

This amount is to be taken in two days.—*Medicinische-chirurgische Rundschau,* August, 1890.

Treatment of Eczema in Children.—According to the *Centralblatt f. d. gesammte Therapie,* DELAPERT uses the following in the eczema of children :

R.—Boric acid . . . . 80 grains.
Balsam of Peru . . . 8 "
Vaseline . . . . 1 ounce.—M.

Atypical Whooping-cough.—DR. EIGENBRODT, of Darmstadt (*Zeitschrift für klinische Medicin,* Bd. xvii. No. 6), believes, (1) that in addition to the typical form of whooping-cough there is an atypical or abortive form; (2) that the abortive form differs from the typical, only in the absence of the whoop during the paroxysms of coughing; (3) that abortive whooping-cough can be distinguished from bronchitis only by the fact of its contagiousness; (4) that the typical form of the disease may be contracted from the atypical, but, (5) that an attack of the latter does not confer immunity from the former. In support of these conclusions Dr. Eigenbrodt cites a number of cases in which attacks of true whooping-cough were clearly traceable to other cases of prolonged cough without the characteristic whoop.

Saccharin Tooth-wash.—The following prescription is quoted by the *Internationale klinische Rundschau :*

R.—Tincture of myrrh ⎫
   " " benzoin ⎬ of each 13½ drachms.
   " " cinchona ⎭
Oil of cloves . . . . 15 minims.
Saccharin . . . . ¾ grain.—M.

The Acarus Folliculorum in the Eyelids.—In the *Centralblatt für prakt. Augenheilkunde,* July, 1890, PROFESSOR STEIDA, of Königsberg, notes the occurrence of this parasite in the hair follicles of the human eyelids as a point of scientific interest, but of little probable importance. They have been found on almost all parts of the body, and seem to give rise to no pathological condition. In a postscript he questions the latter point, since in the lower animals a similar parasite does lead to follicular inflammation ; and he cites a case where Burchardt found a living acarus in the contents of a Meibomian cyst, and a case of blepharitis in which Majocchi found a whitish secretion on the lid-margin, which contained numerous eggs and led to the discovery of numerous specimens of the acarus in the Meibomian glands. It is altogether probable, therefore, that they are by no means innocuous in the Meibomian and sebaceous glands, and that they may be found to be the cause of many of the obstinate and unexplained cases of inflammation of the lids. The subject seems well worth careful study.

Butyl-chloral in Trigeminal Neuralgia. — According to LIEBREICH, trigeminal neuralgia may be relieved by the internal administration of butyl-chloral (croton-chloral), which he prescribes in the following formula:

R.—Butyl-chloral . . . 40 to 75 grains.
Alcohol . . . . 2½ drachms.
Glycerin . . . . 5 "
Distilled water ⎰ sufficient
         ⎱ to make ⎰ 4 ounces.—M.

The dose of this is from two to four teaspoonfuls.—*Therapeutic Gazette,* July, 1890.

THE MEDICAL NEWS.

A WEEKLY JOURNAL
OF MEDICAL SCIENCE.

COMMUNICATIONS are invited from all parts of the world. Original articles contributed exclusively to THE MEDICAL NEWS will be liberally paid for upon publication. When necessary to elucidate the text, illustrations will be furnished without cost to the author.

Address the Editor: H. A. HARE, M.D.,
1004 WALNUT STREET,
PHILADELPHIA.

Subscription Price, including Postage.

PER ANNUM, IN ADVANCE . . . . $4.00.

SINGLE COPIES . . . .   10 CENTS.

Subscriptions may begin at any date. The safest mode of remittance is by bank check or postal money order, drawn to the order of the undersigned. When neither is accessible, remittances may be made, at the risk of the publishers, by forwarding in *registered* letters.

Address,   LEA BROTHERS & CO.,
Nos. 706 & 708 SANSOM STREET,
PHILADELPHIA.

SATURDAY, AUGUST 30, 1890.

THE PROPER PLACE FOR FOREIGN STUDY FOR AMERICAN MEDICAL MEN.

HUMAN beings are so much like sheep in their habit of following where their predecessors have led that it seems almost useless to attempt to divert their course from the clinics of Vienna or Berlin to those of London, Liverpool, or Edinburgh; yet anyone who has studied both on the continent of Europe and in England must have been impressed with a number of advantages possessed by English study over those offered in still more foreign lands. Very few medical men in this country recognize that the city of London, with its many millions of inhabitants, must possess a corresponding number of cases of disease and injury, and that the number of its hospitals, the thoroughness of its teachers, and the character of the people, all tend to aid in the pursuit of instruction in the cure of disease. There are other advantages, too, which are even more important. First and foremost is the fact that we all use the same language, and call things by the same names; second, the materia medica list is closely allied to our own, and the preparations are almost identical; third, the disease-processes seen in England resemble those seen in America more closely than do the diseases of other parts of Europe, and we can study morbid conditions in our own race instead of in races possessed of different temperaments and habits, as well as food and drink.

The advantage of the mother-tongue is inestimable. Very few Americans who do not possess German blood know enough of the German language to understand the terms used by a rapid lecturer in the Fatherland, and, if they do not, they lose that which they chiefly desire, namely, the minute points of the subject before them. The average American going to one of the Continental clinics receives most of his instruction from docents, or other instructors of a comparatively low grade, simply because he is one of hundreds who throng, not only around the chief, but overflow to the subordinates; while in England, notably in London, the number of eminent men is so great, and the percentage of foreign students so small, that each and every one can sit at the feet of the teacher whose writings are known everywhere in the civilized world. While the student in Berlin or Vienna becomes imbued with the views of the single individual governing a given course, in London he may go from hospital to hospital and obtain different views, and in consequence become a man of broader ideas and greater resource. The fees at the various hospitals are no higher than in Germany, and the student has the privilege of being in the healthiest city in the world, and eating food resembling that which he receives at home, instead of placing himself in the notoriously bad surroundings of a Continental *pension-loge*, and living on food which only a Teuton can withstand.

So infinite are the advantages of London as a medical centre to Continental centres that it seems almost absurd to sing its praises, were it not that so many of our countrymen fail to go there, and the establishment of a post-graduate course, with Jonathan Hutchinson at its head, renders our lack of recognition of our own Fatherland the more culpable.

THE RELATION OF FILTH TO TYPHOID FEVER.

ONE of the most interesting features connected with the development of what is known as the germ-theory of diseases is the ever-varying opinions expressed, by those best qualified to judge, of the relation of filth to the formation of a specific ailment. At one time, quite in the memory of comparatively recent graduates in medicine, it was taught that the presence of filth alone, without any specific virus, might provoke this disease. Thus, a very eminent teacher would freqently detail an instance in which some miners who had been killed by an accident, were buried in a lot so situated that·the water-supply of several houses became impure, and in these, in consequence, an epidemic of typhoid soon developed. Later than this we were taught that there was no typhoid fever without the presence of a typhoid-fever germ; and now we are informed by Dr. Vaughan, in his able and interesting article, published in the number of THE MEDICAL NEWS for August 16, 1890, that "wherever man pollutes the soil about him, the air that he breathes, and the water that he drinks. with his own secretions, there *enteric fever* will be found." Whether this conclusion is a correct one or not, only further study and wide experience can determine; and so many difficulties stand in the way of its proof that a distinct and positive result cannot be expected while our methods of experimentation are so crude. One of the chief difficulties connected with the study of the subject consists in the sterilization or preparation of the intestinal contents in such a manner as to prevent typhoid germs from growing, while others are allowed to thrive. This is necessary, since it is highly probable that these various germs may so alter the intestinal state that a few typhoid bacilli taken into the mouth in dust or water, and swallowed, may at once find a favorable place for growth. Doubt must always exist, in a case of typhoid fever where nothing but ordinary filth was ingested, as to whether that filth did not by means of the wind, or by other method of contamination, receive typhoid poisons. While it is true that ulcerations of the intestines, and fever, have been produced in man and animals, without the apparent presence of a typhoid bacillus as we know it, or are supposed to know it, we cannot help believing that the mere pollution of water or other ingesta with non-typhoidal filth will not produce this disease, and that the specific cause must be present. No better experiment to prove this can be cited than the epidemic of typhoid fever at Cumberland, Maryland, last winter and spring, which was especially reported to THE MEDICAL NEWS by a correspondent sent to the spot. As will be remembered by most of our readers, the entire drainage of the town was carried directly into the water-supply, and in consequence, for many months, dysentery and diarrhœa prevailed among the population who drank the water supplied by the city, but no typhoid

fever was present until an individual came to the town sick with this disease, when it speedily showed itself in an outbreak of a widespread character. The theory of the development of this disease must, therefore, be considered as represented in the following aphorism: No typhoid fever without infection from a previous case of typhoid fever. The ingestion of filth does not cause typhoid fever, but predisposes the patient to the disease by decreasing the vital resistance and affording a field for the growth of the peculiar germ.

CORRESPONDENCE.

TENTH INTERNATIONAL MEDICAL CONGRESS.

To the Editor of THE MEDICAL NEWS,

SIR: The fourth day of the International Medical Congress, Thursday, was devoted to the work of the different Sections. In that of Internal Medicine, diabetes was the main topic, and of course the question of diet was thoroughly discussed. Heart-disease and anæmia were also taken up, and the differential diagnosis between chlorosis, pernicious anæmia, and leukæmia were dwelt upon. In fact, diabetes, tuberculosis, nephritis, and empyema were the subjects to which this Section gave most of its attention.

On Friday morning, Dr. Senn, of Milwaukee, read his paper, "The Diagnosis and Operative Treatment of Bullet-wounds of the Stomach and Intestines." He illustrated it by three experiments on dogs. His claim, as many of your readers know, is that hydrogen gas should be used in all cases of gunshot-wounds of the abdomen to determine whether the gastro-intestinal canal is injured, and that unless it be injured, or unless collapse from bleeding is threatened, abdominal section should not be done. His first experiment proved that hydrogen can be forced from the rectum, through the ileo-cæcal valve, and small intestine, and can be ignited at the mouth. His second, that in case the intestine is wounded the gas will pass through the wound, and can be recognized by the tympany and by ignition at the orifice of the wound. In his third experiment, he shot a dog so as to make a number of intestinal wounds, and then by inflating through the rectum with hydrogen, he found each wound, no opening being overlooked. However, though he found the holes in the intestine, the dog died from hæmorrhage.

On Saturday morning the third and last general meeting was held. It was called to order by President Virchow, who read a telegram from Chicago, inviting the Congress to hold its next meeting at the time of the World's Fair in 1893. As Rome had already been decided on the thanks of the Congress were voted to the generous Americans for their kind invitation. Professor Wood, of Philadelphia, read the first paper, on "Anæsthesia," which was published in the THE MEDICAL NEWS August 9th. It was enthusiastically received and the thanks of the Congress were voted to the author. Professor Wood, as your readers know, comes to the conclusion that, in some cases, death from either ether or chloroform is due to heart-paralysis, in others to respiratory paralysis, and that in still others death results from a combination of both.

Professor T. Lauder Brunton, in another paper read before the Congress, decided that in every case of chloroform narcosis resulting in death, respiratory paralysis was the cause, and that if the respiration be closely watched, and if at the first sign of failure artificial respiration be resorted, to no deaths would result. Thus both Professor Wood and Professor Brunton agree that artificial respiration is of the greatest importance as a remedy in collapse during anæsthesia.

Professor Cantani, of Italy, read a paper on " Antipyresis." He said that it has been positively shown that fever may be due to many different causes and is the general reaction of the system to some poisonous material, probably bacterial. In the different kinds of fever we must, of course, look for agents to destroy primarily the cause. In malaria we have such a remedy in quinine. In the cases where we cannot reach the cause we reduce temperature in one of two ways : 1, by abstracting heat, by cold baths, etc. ; 2, by diminishing the production of heat by the antipyretic drugs. The object of the system in reacting by a high fever is threefold: 1. The high temperature actually destroys many of the pathogenic bacteria. 2. It increases the resistance of the tissues and the activity of the leucocytes in destroying bacteria. 3. It changes the tissues, making them an unsuitable soil for the growth of pathogenic organisms. If these conclusions are true, fever is a necessary reaction and must not be repressed, for it is better than artificial methods of killing the invading germs. The danger is not from the fever itself, save very rarely, and we should not give internal remedies which prevent the formation of heat. When, however, the temperature rises too high, the cold baths and sponging will greatly relieve the patient, while they will not check the reaction at all—in fact if anything will increase it ; thus helping the system in its struggle against the enemy and aiding it in its own exertions. Cantani, therefore, believes that unless we can attack the germ which causes the fever, by an internal medicine, the best therapy is cold applications ; and that all the antipyretics are dangerous, because they depress the already struggling system and stop the natural and best method of cure.

Professor Meynert, the famous neurologist of Vienna, read a very able paper on " The Synchronous Action of the Different Parts of the Brain," which, though valuable to the psychologist and specialist, is of little importance to the practising physician.

Professor Stokvis, of Amsterdam, followed with a paper on "Comparative Racial Pathology and the Capability of Resistance of the European in the Tropics." Long-extended study has convinced him that Europeans can be perfectly acclimatized to tropical climates, and that though the dangers to his life then are very great, he can, by close attention to hygiene, reduce the mortality there to the same percentage as at home. Professor Stokvis's studies have shown that the danger lies in the fact that Europeans do not always adjust their mode of living to the climate, but that when they do the results show that the European race is far more resistant to harmful climatic influences than even the natives. On these grounds he prophesies a complete control of all parts of the globe by the European.

Professor Virchow then made his closing address, in which he said that the world has never before seen such a medical meeting as this, in numbers or in the brilliancy of the members. He paid a glowing tribute to the visitors, and described the benefits of such international meetings. He closed with these words : "And now, my dear friends, let us part in the memory of eternal friendship ; let us forget all personal feelings, and remember that this is a league of true workers in truth and peace. May we meet in the same spirit in the Eternal City of Rome in 1893."

In the absence of Dr. Guyon, Dr. Billings, of the U. S. Army, responded on behalf of the Americans. He expressed the high appreciation and the thanks of our country for the splendid reception.

The Congress having finished its work, the members are fast leaving the city. At present it is difficult to judge the value of the work of the Congress, and not until the proceedings have been carefully studied is a complete résumé possible. Nearly 800 papers were read ; some were excellent, a few were poor, and many were mediocre.

Socially, the Congress was a grand success. The great reception in the Park on Monday, the reception by the city authorities in the Rathhaus on Tuesday, were events never to be forgotten. The Section dinners, the balls, and the closing festivity on Saturday, all tended to make friends of strangers, and to impress the minds of the visitors with the beauty of German hospitality. The French were highly flattered when the sound of the Marseillaise rang through the halls of the Rathhaus of Berlin ; the Americans were electrified by Yankee Doodle in the same magnificent building, and good-fellowship abounded everywhere. Not an American found the slightest flaw in the social arrangements.

As far as arrangements are concerned, the Executive Committee may well be proud, for they received nothing but praise, and every wheel in the enormous machinery of the Congress worked smoothly. The Circus Renz was a fine place for the general meetings, and the numerous rooms of the Art Exposition furnished excellent quarters to the twenty-two Sections. The rooms were adorned with the finest productions of modern art. Every Section looked more like a palace than the hall of a scientific meeting.

In regard to the benefits to the profession, every member goes home more ambitious and energetic.

If Koch's work, of which he gave us merely a glimpse, stands the tests of further study, we may look for a revolution in the treatment of tuberculosis, and we must be prepared for new discoveries in the exanthemata. Lister indicated the course of surgery : that the utmost cleanliness is our motto, and that the less we interfere and irritate the better, that the air is not a dangerous septic element, and that drainage is only a substitute which we must try to dispense with.

BERLIN, August 10, 1890

THOMSEN'S DISEASE.

To the Editor of THE MEDICAL NEWS.

SIR : In your issue of August 16th appears a paper by Dr. Harold U. Moyer, of Chicago, upon Thomsen's Disease, in which he takes exception to my views of this malady, expressed in a paper published in 1886, in the New York *Medical Record*. The author gives, I think, a wrong impression of what I then said, for the existence of the affection, described by Erb, and one or two others, has never been disputed. I still adhere to my original idea, however, that Thomsen's disease, as an entity, is a rare malady, but that in many forms of coarse disease of the brain there are salient motor expressions which are not strictly "hysterical," but belong to what has been called the "Thomsen symptom-complex." In this conclusion I am supported by such observers as Buzzard, of London, C. L. Dana, of New York, and others. I may say, finally, that the interesting case presented by Dr. Moyer is an example of what I mean, and from the symptoms detailed I think it may as well be assumed to be one of those vague conditions of hyperkinesis as anything else. If in my original paper, or now, I have appeared to be conservative, or even hypercritical, it is because I was, and am, heartily opposed to the growing tendency to redundant and uncertain nomenclature, and to the use of meaningless proper names for the designation of varying and erratic groups of symptoms and uncertain pathological states.　　　ALLAN McLANE HAMILTON, M.D.

NEW YORK, August 19, 1890.

NEWS ITEMS.

Cholera Intelligence.—According to the *Lancet*, the somewhat ominous silence in official quarters as to cholera in Spain has been broken by the announcement that the disease is still prevalent in Valencia, that it has undergone a recrudescence in that province, that there are also cases in the province of Alicante, and, lastly, that the disease has appeared in the province of Badajoz. Badajoz being one of the frontier provinces, the occurrence has led to great activity on the part of the Portuguese authorities, who have always put their main trust in quarantine restrictions, and who have already gone so far as to stop the entrance of Spanish trains into Portugal until the lazarettos and quarantine establishments are fully equipped. They have also stopped the mails, and letters from England intended to be shipped at Lisbon for the Cape have failed to reach that port. Between May 13th and August 2d, 1100 cases of cholera are stated to have occurred in Valencia and Alicante, 56 per cent. of the attacks having terminated fatally. France is still free from the disease, notwithstanding a recent assertion that a case had occurred in Paris. The attack in question was ultimately decided to be one of acute gastro-enteritis. The outbreak of cholera which has occurred in connection with the Mecca pilgrimage seems likely to be one of considerable importance. Stringent measures have been taken at the various ports and quarantine stations on the Arabian coast of the Red Sea to prevent the departure of the pilgrims except after they have undergone quarantine; but this part of the world is, above all others, the one where quarantine restrictions have exhibited their "leakiness"; and it has now been decided to employ a large number of troops to prevent exit from Arabia, and also entrance to Egypt, except by the recognized routes where lazarettos have been established. But the occurrence may come to have very serious significance for Europe,

for a number of Bosnian pilgrims will be returning to Austrian ports, and others will endeavor to reach Malta, and even get as far west as Marseilles. It is impossible to form any correct opinion as to the number of deaths which have as yet occurred. Whilst from one source of information it is stated that the largest daily mortality has reached 155, another source gives 500 as the diurnal number of victims.

Legacy to the Medical College of Indiana.—Dr. William Lomax, of Marion, Indiana, has given his estate, valued at $100,000, to the Medical College of Indiana. The desire of the donor was to make the school a department of the Depauw University, at Greencastle, Ind. Failing in this, however, he determined to give the estate directly to the medical school

Obituary.—Dr. J. Adams Allen, of Chicago, Ill., died August 15th, aged sixty-five years. For many years he held the chair of the practice of medicine and the presidency of Rush Medical College, having removed from Kalamazoo to Chicago, in 1859, in order to assume the former position. He edited the *Chicago Medical Journal*, in conjunction with Drs. Davis, Byford, and others, for ten or more years. He was surgeon-in-chief to the Chicago and Quincy Railroad. He published a work on medical examinations in life insurance that ran through several editions, and that was translated and published in Germany.

OFFICIAL LIST OF CHANGES IN THE STATIONS AND DUTIES OF OFFICERS SERVING IN THE MEDICAL DEPARTMENT, U. S. ARMY, FROM AUGUST 19 TO AUGUST 26, 1890.

With the approval of the Acting Secretary of War, leave of absence for four months, to take effect about September 1, 1890, is granted WALTER REED, *Captain and Assistant Surgeon.*—Par. 17, *S. O. 192, A. G. O., Washington, D. C.,* August 18, 1890.

By direction of the Acting Secretary of War, a Board of Medical Officers, to consist of: JOSEPH V. D. MIDDLETON, *Major and Surgeon;* CLARENCE EWEN, *Major and Surgeon;* and WILLIAM E. HOPKINS, *Captain and Assistant Surgeon,* will assemble at the U. S. Military Academy, West Point, New York, at 11 o'clock A.M., August 27, 1890, or as soon thereafter as practicable, to examine into the physical qualifications of the candidates for admission to the Academy.—Par. 1, *S. O. 192, A. G. O., Washington, D. C.,* August 18, 1890.

By direction of the Acting Secretary of War, CHARLES F. MASON, *First Lieutenant and Assistant Surgeon,* is relieved from further temporary duty at Fort Logan, Colorado, and will report for duty at his proper station (Fort Washakie, Wyoming).—Par. 3, *S. O. 191, A. G. O., Washington, D. C.,* August 16, 1890

By direction of the Acting Secretary of War, the retirement from active service, this date, by operation of law, of JOHN MOORE, *Brigadier-General and Surgeon-General,* under the provisions of the Act of Congress approved June 30, 1882, is announced. General Moore will repair to his home, Bloomington, Indiana.—Par. 2, *S. O. 191, A. G. O., Washington, D. C.,* August 16, 1890.

PROMOTION.

KENDALL, WILLIAM P., *First Lieutenant and Assistant Surgeon.*—To be Assistant Surgeon, with rank of Captain, after five years' service, from August 12, 1890.—*Headquarters of the Army, A. G. O., Washington,* August 18, 1890.

IVES, FRANCIS J., *Assistant Surgeon.*—To be Assistant Surgeon, with the rank of Captain, after five years' service, in accordance with the Act of June 23, 1890.—*Headquarters of the Army, A. G. O., Washington,* August 11, 1890.

RETIREMENT.

MOORE, JOHN. *Brigadier-General and Surgeon-General.*—August 16, 1890 (Act of June 30, 1890).—*Headquarters of the Army, A. G. O., Washington,* August 16, 1890.

THE MEDICAL NEWS.

A WEEKLY JOURNAL OF MEDICAL SCIENCE.

VOL. LVII.　　　SATURDAY, SEPTEMBER 6, 1890.　　　No. 10.

ORIGINAL ARTICLES.

ONE HUNDRED CASES OF TYPHOID FEVER.[1]

BY R. L. MACDONNELL, B.A., M.D.,

PROFESSOR OF CLINICAL MEDICINE IN MCGILL UNIVERSITY, MONTREAL; PHYSICIAN TO THE MONTREAL GENERAL HOSPITAL.

THE following remarks are based upon an experience of one hundred cases of typhoid fever which came under my observation in the wards of the Montreal General Hospital. The histories have been taken from my case-books, working backward from the present day. No selection has been made, except that I have put aside all incomplete histories, as well as those in which there was any doubt of the diagnosis. Such a plan of selection necessarily raises the mortality-rate, since all fatal cases were fully recorded, while many non-fatal cases escaped mention.

The period covered by these one hundred cases extends over part of the summer services of 1884 and 1885, part of 1886, all of 1887, part of 1889, and the winter service of 1889–90, and includes the severe epidemic of 1886–87, when the hospital authorities placed a large number of fever patients in tents, a necessity to which they had not been forced since the typhus fever visitations of the last generation. In the summers of 1888 and 1889 the number of typhoid cases in hospital at a time was limited to twenty. The one hundred cases, therefore, represent a selection of severe cases: 1. Because the Montreal General Hospital performs the duties of a city hospital, a marine and an immigrant hospital, and admits all sorts of men in all conditions of poverty and exhaustion. 2. Because, being always overcrowded, and the number of admissions latterly being limited, mild cases and those occurring among the fairly well-to-do are refused admission. For the same reason, children whose parents have homes are not often found among the patients, and in children the mortality is lower than in young adults. 3. A cause for high mortality lies in the fact that in the summer a patient is enabled to work longer with the disease in him than he would be able to do in the severe winters of Canada.

Age.—The mean age was 24.8 years. The extremes were 5 and 45. The age of 77 patients was between 20 and 30 years, and but 9 patients were

over 30 years. I wish to lay great stress upon the narrowness of the age-limit, for it explains how the disease fails to communicate itself among persons of different ages. I shall refer to this point again.

Mortality.—Sixteen patients died.

Infection.—Is typhoid fever directly communicable? I believe it is, and my reasons for so thinking are as follows:

1. That a large number of house-officers of the Montreal General Hospital have contracted typhoid fever while on duty. During the last twenty years 39 have served on the house-staff, and of these I have been able to ascertain that 4 had typhoid fever before entering. We have, therefore, 35 left; of this number, 7 had undoubted fever in the hospital, and in 2 other cases the diagnosis was not absolutely certain. This makes it plain that 7 out of 35, or 20 per cent. of the house-staff, took fever —a larger number than took diphtheria, with which at one time they were constantly in contact, for of the 39 but 4 took that disease during the period in question. As for nurses, a large number have fallen victims too, though I have not been able to obtain satisfactory information on that point.

2. That not many nurses of experience have escaped contracting the disease at one time or another. The fact that the disease does not usually affect more than one member of a family at a time may be explained by the narrow limits of the age of susceptibility. In a household the fever is likely to pass over the parents and the young children, and attack those members of the family whose age is between twenty and thirty, whose number must necessarily be limited.

3. There are instances of the disease being communicated to patients in hospital suffering from the effects of accidents and from other diseases, as for example the following:

CASE I.—A Swedish sailor, aged twenty-six years, with a cavity in one lung, but no febrile symptoms, was in constant attendance upon the sick in the epidemic of 1887. He took the fever and went through its regular stages, convalescing in the fifth week. Rose rash was well marked.

This coincidence of typhoid fever and pulmonary phthisis as in the preceding case is rare.

CASE II.—A patient, aged sixteen years, who was completely bed-ridden, and whose case was diagnosed as acute anterior poliomyelitis, after being

[1] A paper read before the Medico-Chirurgical Society of Montreal, June 13, 1890.

some months in hospital contracted typhoid fever in a typical form.[1]

CASE III.—One of my fatal cases was that of a girl who was admitted to hospital for ulcer of the leg.

CASE IV.—A surgical patient in Dr. Shepherd's wards, who had been some months in hospital, contracted typhoid fever. There were cases of fever in the same ward.

Many other examples might be brought forward. These four came under my immediate notice.[2]

Now it might reasonably be asked, If typhoid fever is communicable, why do not more patients in general wards take the disease? and the answer is simple. Because (1) many are protected by age. We see in my 100 cases how the fever stops at the line of forty-five years, while many are younger than the average typhoid age. (2) Many have other diseases, tuberculosis, for instance, which is rarely met in conjunction with typhoid fever. (3) A certain number of cases may have been protected by previous attacks of fever, and a certain number may not be susceptible. (4) Fever is not as likely to spread in a hospital as it is in a private house, because the ventilation is better, the excreta are more carefully disinfected, and better appliances for counteracting infection are at hand.

Typhoid fever would be much more prevalent amongst hospital nurses, were it not for the fact that a certain proportion of them are protected by previous attacks, and that nearly all of them are over twenty-five years of age (the average of my hundred cases) when they begin nursing.

The Skin eruption.—Rose rash was noted in but 51 per cent. of the cases. This is a low figure, and I have no doubt that the rash was more frequently present, and escaped being noted. The rash was present in 11 of my 16 fatal cases, and in 40 of the 84 non-fatal cases. In 6 of the 11 fatal cases in which rash was present it was noted as being very copious. In one case where death resulted from the exhaustion of diarrhœa, the rash closely resembled the eruption of measles.[3] A delicate, uniform, scarlet rash was present in one case, that of a girl of twenty-five.[4] At first I was under the impression that antipyrine was the cause, but I find, on looking up the subject, that these scarlet rashes have been fully described by Jenner, Murchison, and others. Urticaria was present in 3 cases. In one it followed the administration of antipyrine. An outbreak of several pustules on the wrist and arms occurred in a fatal case. This was in 1885, when smallpox was epidemic, and the appearance of the pustules gave rise to much alarm. The autopsy showed that the case was one of true typhoid fever.

The tongue.—Of all the symptoms of typhoid fever the appearance of the tongue is one on which the utmost reliance can be placed, both for diagnostic and prognostic purposes.

Meteorism must be regarded as of the most serious import. It was present in 10 of the 16 fatal cases, and in one of them it seemed to be the direct cause of death, causing upward displacement of the thoracic viscera and direct embarrassment of the respiration.[1] Murchison noted meteorism in 20 out of 21 fatal cases, and Jenner observed it in 18 out of 19 fatal cases.

It was a surprise to me to find that abdominal distention was noted in but 4 of the 84 non-fatal cases. Probably my house-physicians have not thought it necessary to note. mere slight fulness of the belly. All observers are agreed, however, that tympanites is a symptom of most serious import.

The treatment of this dangerous complication is most unsatisfactory. I have never been able to convince myself of the efficacy of the customary turpentine stupe, and internal medication has never yielded me satisfactory results. Charcoal, so constantly prescribed is, I believe, perfectly useless. Nor has the passage of a tube given as much relief as might reasonably be expected. Dr. Bell, in my case which was fatal from tympanites, dissuaded me from puncturing through the abdominal wall with an aspirating-needle, on the ground that when, in abdominal sections, the bowel is so punctured gas and fæcal matter escape through the openings for some time after the needle is withdrawn. Cases illustrating the soundness of this advice have been recorded by Curtis.[2]

Enlargement of the spleen.—Since the summer of 1887 I have paid special attention to the observation of this change. The spleen was found during life to be enlarged in 5 of the 16 fatal cases, but in only 7 of the 84 non-fatal cases. I was under the impression that it was clinically demonstrable in a larger proportion of cases. The fact is, that enlargement of the spleen is more often found by the pathologist than by the clinician, and is by no means constantly present. Small enlargements cannot be readily demonstrated, and even when the organ has attained a considerable size a distended abdomen may interfere with its being recognized.

---

[1] See Montreal Medical Journal, vol. xviii. p. 445.

[2] This is not the experience of others. Liebermeister boldly makes the statement that physicians and nurses who take care of such patients are not more frequently attacked with the disease than are persons who have never seen such cases. "Up to 1865 I have never seen in the hospitals which I visited (Griefswald, Berlin, Tübingen) a single hospital patient, physician, or nurse, attacked with typhoid fever, although such cases are placed in the general wards"

[3] Montreal Medical Journal, vol. xviii. p. 444.

[4] Ibid., p. 205

---

[1] Ibid., vol. xviii. p.444.

[2] Annual of the Universal Medical Sciences, 1890.

Dr. Frederick C. Shattuck, of the Massachusetts General Hospital, in his paper on typhoid fever, which is based on an analysis of 129 cases, comes to a similar conclusion.[1]

Fagge, too, states that he believes the organ may be many ounces heavier than the normal without there being any appreciable percussion-dulness over it; and he has discovered that the spleen is not always found swollen after death, even in young subjects who have succumbed when the disease was at its highest.

Diarrhœa.—It would seem that diarrhœa is the exception, and constipation the rule. Diarrhœa was present in but 27 per cent. of all cases, and of these 27 cases 14 were fatal. Only two patients died without diarrhœa, one of pneumonia, and the other of the effects of a miscarriage.

Murchison notes diarrhœa in 93 per cent. of cases in England, M. Barth (quoted by Murchison) in 96 of 101 cases in France, and Shattuck found it in 51 per cent. in Boston. The difference between these figures is remarkable.

Diarrhœa always means danger, and I have become more and more disposed to regard a patient as safe so long as the bowels remain confined.

Intestinal hæmorrhage occurred in 2 of the 16 fatal cases, but in neither was it severe, nor did it appear to be the cause of death. On the contrary, in all the severe cases of hæmorrhage the patient recovered, so that the opinion expressed long ago by Graves to the effect that hæmorrhages were rather beneficial than otherwise seems not far from the truth. Trousseau was also of the opinion that this symptom was less dangerous than was commonly supposed.

Taking all cases together, severe hæmorrhages occurred in 9 patients. Louis reported hæmorrhages in 8 of 134 cases; Jenner in 7 of 21 fatal cases; Murchison found copious hæmorrhages in 3.77 per cent. of his cases; Shattuck found hæmorrhage in 5.4 per cent.

Our high percentage shows the general severity of the cases admitted. It is remarkable from what very severe hæmorrhages a typhoid fever patient can recover.

H. B., aged twenty-four years; admitted under my care on the sixth day of an attack of fever. History of intemperance. Usual fever-symptoms present. Previously to admission there had been a very severe attack of epistaxis. No abdominal pain or distention. On the ninth day there was retention of urine. On the fourteenth there was a sharp attack of diarrhœa, which soon ceased. On the fifteenth day there were severe tremors. Hæmorrhage was predicted, and turpentine and opium mixture[2] or-

dered to be given as soon as bleeding occurred. On the seventeenth day blood came in gushes from the bowel, and during the next twenty-four hours several pints must have come away. The patient's condition became very low, but he eventually made a good recovery in spite of the fact that on the thirty-sixth day an immense bedsore formed which exposed nearly the whole of the sacrum.

Headache and delirium.—Headache is nearly always present during the first half or the first third of the disease, and disappears spontaneously. Hence, I have very rarely had occasion to direct any special treatment against it, owing to the fact that the headache period has nearly gone by before the patient has arrived in hospital.

I have not been able to verify the statement of Broadbent, in Quain's *Dictionary of Medicine*, that severe and persistent headache is the forerunner of intestinal hæmorrhage.

Delirium generally means danger, yet it is not necessarily a very unfavorable symptom. Fierce delirium was present in several instances, notably in that of a Hungarian, whose case is already recorded,[1] and who was at first thought to be suffering from acute mania. Delirium was a prominent symptom in 8 of the 84 non-fatal cases, and in 7 of the 16 fatal cases, and in 2 of the latter it was very furious.

Duration.—The duration of a fever can only be estimated by the number of days spent in hospital, and this depends upon the season of the year, the climate, and the character of the hospital. The average duration of non-fatal cases was 40.8 days. The longest case lasted 80 days. The shortest stay in hospital was 7 days. This last patient had been ill for some days before admission, and came from a house where there were three other cases of fever.

Retention of urine occurred in 7 of the 84 non-fatal cases, and in 4 of the 16 fatal cases, or in 11 per cent. of all cases. Incontinence of urine and fæces was noted as being urgent and troublesome in but 2 cases, neither of which was fatal.

Epistaxis was not serious in any case.

Venous thrombosis occurred in but 2 cases, both non-fatal.

Relapse.—It was a surprise to me to find the history of but one relapse, for I was under the impression that relapses were of much more common occurrence. Experiences upon this differ within very wide limits, owing to a diversity of opinion as to what constitutes a relapse. Thus, Murchison recorded 80 relapses in 2591 cases in the London Fever Hospital, or in 3 per cent.; Griesinger (quoted

---

[1] Boston Medical and Surgical Journal, vol. cxxi., No. 10.
[2] Tannic acid, 10 grains; tinct. of opium, 10 minims; spirits of turpentine, 15 minims; mucilage, 2 drachms; compound tinct.

of chloroform, 20 minims; peppermint water, 1 ounce, every two hours. This formula is borrowed from Murchison's work on the Continued Fevers.
[1] Montreal Medical Journal, vol. xviii. p. 444.

by Murchison) in 6 per cent. ; Human in 8 per cent.;
Maclagan in 10 per cent.[1]

I accept Dr. Murchison's definition of a relapse
as being " a second evolution of the specific febrile
process, after convalescence from the first attack is
fairly established," and a relapse includes such symptoms as rise of temperature, rigors, chilliness, headache, pains in limbs, loss of appetite, furred tongue,
nausea and often retching, diarrhœa, enlarged spleen,
and a fresh eruption of rose spots. The number of
relapses would be much increased were we to take
into account those cases in which the relapse began
before the original disease terminated. On this
point my cases have not been examined.

Recrudescences, or what are commonly called relapses, were not frequent, owing, I believe, to the
rule carried out that no change in the diet was to be
made until the patient had shown a normal night
temperature for a week.

Perforation was found at the autopsy of one
patient, but in the Montreal General Hospital the
occurrence is more frequent than my figures would
indicate. Dr. Wyatt Johnston, the present pathologist, tells me that in 18 autopsies since 1886 he has
found perforative peritonitis in 3, and Dr. Osler,
who was his predecessor in the same office, found it
11 times in 53 autopsies. These figures are much
higher than are elsewhere given. Autopsies are very
difficult to obtain in cases of fever. The friends
cannot understand why, if the doctors are satisfied
that fever was the cause of death, they should wish
for further examination.

Pregnancy.—The one pregnant woman with typhoid fever died. Murchison reports 10 recoveries
in 14 cases, and in 2 of the 10 recoveries the patients
carried the child through the fever.

Strümpell, in his *Practice of Medicine*, makes the
observation that when abortion occurs in the course
of typhoid a marked fall of temperature takes
place. In my case the result was different; the
temperature ran steadily up after abortion, reaching
108° in twenty-four hours, when the patient died.

Syncope.—In three non-fatal cases severe syncopal
attacks occurred. I have seen sudden fatal syncope
occur in convalescence from typhoid fever.

Complication with other diseases.—The following
complications were noted—all in non-fatal cases :
whooping-cough, old thickening of one pleura,
diseased mitral valve with cardiac hypertrophy,
periostitis of the superior maxillary bone, multiple
abscesses, parotitis, and acute anterior poliomyelitis.
One patient was a "jumper" from a lumber camp
in Maine. He "jumped" consistently all through
the fever and convalescence.

Pulmonary tuberculosis after typhoid fever.—I have
never seen phthisis occur after typhoid fever, but
upon several occasions I have made the mistake of
regarding cases of tuberculosis as being typhoid
fever.[1]

In connection with this, Fagge says that "it is a
remarkable circumstance that, after searching the
records of post-mortem examinations at Guy's Hospital, I have failed to find a single case in point."

Mortality.—The recorded mortality of my 100
cases represents neither remarkably good nor remarkably bad success. It must be remembered that
the average age was twenty-four years. The London
Fever Hospital has an aggregate mortality of 17.61
per cent., but a large number of the deaths occurred
in the young. The mortality of Homerton Fever Hospital is 17.83 per cent., and that of Stockwell Fever
Hospital 22.90. Shattuck's mortality in the Massachusetts General Hospital is but 8.37 in 129 cases,
but it must be remembered that that hospital is not
like ours, which is a city, marine, and immigrant
hospital combined. A certain not insignificant
proportion of cases were brought to the hospital
practically moribund.

1 patient died on the 3d day after admission.

1	"	"	5th	"	"
3 patients	"	"	6th	"	"
2	"	"	7th	"	"
1 patient	"	"	9th	"	"

Nearly all these had been transported from outlying villages.

I refuse to acknowledge the fairness of any comparison with figures taken from the experience of
private practice. Medical men, unless they are most
careful in noting cases, are apt to deceive themselves,
and to think in a vague and uncertain way of their
success or non-success, principally of the former.
Private patients of the well-to-do classes have every
possible point in their favor. They are not obliged
to go on working as long as possible, and they are
likely to meet with sensible treatment. Moreover,
they have no transportation to undergo,—a very
strong point in their favor. Only one-half of my
fatal cases came from the city.

General treatment.—I have no faith whatever in
the effect of medicines on the fever. Antiseptics
are unpleasant to take, and in my opinion no more
effective than so much water. To talk of disinfecting an abdomen full of typhoid excreta with small
doses of carbolic or sulphurous acid seems to me as
absurd as homœopathy.

Though all my patients have taken small doses of
the mineral acids, I have prescribed these merely as
a *placebo*, and I do not believe they have any action
whatever.

---

[1] Murchison on the Continued Fevers. Third edition, London,
p. 552.

[1] See Canadian Practitioner, June, 1888.

To purge at the outset, if constipation is present, is good practice, and I have frequently given 2 grains of calomel every two hours until the bowels moved. After that I follow Todd's advice, and when the bowels are fairly locked up I keep them so, merely ordering an injection every two or three days.

Diarrhœa itself seems to be dangerous, and no one can watch the course of many cases without being struck with the fact that it does not tend in any way to mitigate other symptoms whether abdominal or cerebral. Diarrhœa accompanies the worst cases of tympanites, and in hæmorrhagic cases it is often present.

Antipyretics.—Cold sponging was practised in all cases in which the temperature went above 102°. I have had no experience with the use of cold baths.

On the medicinal antipyretics I do not place any reliance. I remember well the days when no typhoid-fever patient could die without heavy doses of quinine. And where are they who now advocate quinine? A case in which temperature alone is killing the patient calls for antipyretics, but such cases are rare. Looking over my 16 fatal cases, I see that but 4 died with no other formidable symptom than high temperature. In Osler's 53 autopsies there were but 16 cases in which some such definite lesion as perforation, hæmorrhage, etc., was not present[1]—that is, but 16 cases on which antipyreties might have exerted a beneficial influence.

It would appear in some cases that, if we could overcome the hyperpyrexia, the patient would get well. Take, for example, the case of Matilda R.[2] This was a very severe case, and there were no symptoms beyond those which might have been attributed to the effects of heat. Now in this case there were found most extensive lesions in the bowel which were evidently keeping up the temperature. It seems to me that the use of antipyretics can have no better effect in typhoid fever than they would have in the fever of an internal abscess. In cases where other symptoms are bringing about the fatal result, symptoms such as extreme meteorism, exhausting diarrhœa, or severe brain symptoms, they are more than useless.

Some of the best recoveries from hyperpyrexia have taken place in cases in which no antipyretic was given. As, for example, the following case:[3]

A sailor who on the tenth day showed a temperature of 105.6° at 8 P. M., reaching 106° at 5.30 in the early morning of the twelfth day and dropping suddenly to 99° before 8 A. M.—a fact which shows the necessity of taking the temperature during the night as well as in the morning and evening. The next

rise, to 105.5°, took place in the afternoon of the same day, the temperature falling to 101.8° before 8 P. M. The highest point was reached, however, on the thirteenth day, when, at 2 A. M., it was 107°, but, as on the preceding day, a drop to 99° occurred, and the patient gradually recovered. This case occurred in 1884, and I have only to repeat what I said then, that I have lost faith in medicinal antipyretics.

We have come to regard confidently a morning fall and an evening rise as of regular occurrence—*e. g.*, in a private patient we have the temperature taken at 8 P. M., and if it be normal then we assume that it has been normal for the preceding twenty-four hours. This is a great mistake. If the temperature is taken hourly it will be found to vary greatly. In the case already described, as an instance of genuine relapse, the temperature was found very high when registered every four hours; being higher in the early part of the afternoon than in the evening, so that had we depended merely upon observations at 8 A. M. and 8 P. M. it would have entirely escaped our notice that hyperpyrexia was present. The truth is that remissions and exacerbations take place at any period in the twenty-four hours. "Generally the minimum temperatures occur between midnight and noon, and the maximum between noon and midnight."—*Colley.*

And in this way we deceive ourselves in the matter of antipyretics. For example, the case is running smoothly until we find that the temperature at 8 P. M. is too high; we accordingly give, say antipyrine, and then, and not until then, we begin making observations every four hours. Cousequently it is just possible that our observation after 8 P. M. may show a fall which we hasten to ascribe to the effect of our medicine.

I have found antifebrin more satisfactory than antipyrine. It has been given in 3-grain doses every three hours.

CEPHALHÆMATOMA.

A Case of Sub-pericranial Blood-tumor in the Newborn Child.

BY HOWARD A. KELLY, M.D., GYNECOLOGIST AND OBSTETRICIAN TO THE JOHNS HOPKINS HOSPITAL, BALTIMORE.

My desire in reporting a case of this interesting disease is not so much to place on record another example of a rare affection, but rather to call the attention of the profession to one of the most important, and as yet but rarely recognized diseases of very early childhood, as well as to prepare the way for a discussion of this subject at the meeting of the American Gynecological Society, to be held on September 16th of this year. Few men outside of the ranks of the pure specialists are aware that such a disease as cephalhæmatoma (cephalohæmatoma)

---

[1] Canada Medical and Surgical Journal, vol. xiv.
[2] Montreal Medical Journal, vol. xviii. p. 203.
[3] Reported in full in the Canadian Practitioner.

exists. Cases which occur in the practice of the general practitioner are diagnosed and treated by him upon "general principles."

The information which he possesses upon this subject is fairly comparable to that of a physician practising early in the last century.

A well-defined disease appearing soon after birth, running a brief, definite course, tending, as a rule, to resolution, but capable of seriously affecting the health, or even of implicating the life of the child, must be a matter of interest to every medical man; and the interest is heightened by the relative frequency of the disease (probably one in 250 obstetric cases), with the certainty that even a moderate obstetrical experience will sometime surely bring one or more cases under observation, and demand decision as to their nature and the course to be pursued.

Our curiosity is still further aroused, and our interest enhanced, when we learn that we have here also one of those curious examples of the tendency, felt even in scientific matters, of an important discovery to remain for a long time in the almost exclusive possession of its original promulgators, while, in the face of the clearest demonstrations and the most numerous writings, surrounding nations long seem to ignore its existence.

Thus the discovery of cephalhæmatoma dates from the close of the last century, when Dr. Michaelis, of Harburg, wrote in the second volume of *Loder's Journal*, "upon a peculiar kind of blood tumor,"[1] giving a full, clear account of the affection. This able article provoked within the succeeding thirty years a host of other writings, and abundant records of cases, in various German journals, and since that time cephalhæmatoma has been regularly registered among the more important diseases to which the newborn are liable.

In the following brief description of the disease, before illustrating my subject with the report of a case, I will make free use of the language of Michaelis.

Cephalhæmatoma (the name given to the disease by Naegele[2]) is a circumscribed effusion of blood between the periosteum and one of the flat cranial bones, appearing usually the day after birth, and gradually increasing in size until it forms a tense, prominent, rounded, or ovoid swelling. Its commonest seat is over one or both parietal bones. It is always lateral, never crossing a suture. The skin over the tumor remains movable and unaltered in appearance. The tumor is not painful, and does not decrease in size upon pressure. After two or three weeks, as a rule, it gradually disappears by absorption.

One of the most important diagnostic signs of the disease is the existence of a bony wall, one or two millimetres in height, which surrounds the whole outer circumference of the tumor. This can be distinctly felt through the skin, and gives at once the impression of a depressed fracture.

Injury usually has no apparent connection with the origin of this tumor, which often appears after natural, easy, and short labors, and upon a part of the head which was not prominent in the birth. Instead of being absorbed the collection ·of blood may undergo suppuration, perforating the cranial cavity, or rupturing externally.

The earlier observers frequently incised the tumor, cleaned out the blood, and put on a compress. The best treatment to-day is to wait for two or three weeks for resolution by absorption, and, if this should not take place, to incise and empty the sac under strict antiseptic precautions, and apply an antiseptic dressing. Whenever signs of suppuration arise the tumor should be freely opened at once, well washed out, and drained.

This, in brief, is the outline of the disease to which I desire to call attention by this preliminary note, in advance of a more formal, elaborate article upon the same subject, prepared for the meeting of the American Gynecological Society. The following case recently came under my observation :

I was called early one morning last June to attend Mrs. A., primipara, forty-one years old. She was of medium height, had a normal pelvis, and the uterus contained a living child.

She had had pains with great regularity during the preceding night, with the effect of bringing the head well into the pelvis, with the occiput to the left and anterior. The waters had already discharged through the os, which was dilated to about 2 centimetres. By noon the strong, regular pains had brought the head to within an inch of the floor of the pelvis—well flexed, and the flat bones extensively overlapping. At this point the head became firmly wedged. From 1.38 to 7.25 o'clock in the evening she had 106 pains, without bringing the head a half inch nearer the pelvic floor. The child was in good condition, but the mother seemed so exhausted that I then gave her benumbing doses of chloroform by inhalation, and applied Naegele's forceps. By assisting each pain I delivered her after an hour, with a slight tear, entirely within the vagina and in the left sulcus. The child was a female, weighing about 3000 grammes. At the outer angle of its right eye was a slight indentation in the skin from the pressure of the forceps, which disappeared in two days.

A large caput succedaneum covered the occipital region. No other deformity or evidence of injury was visible. On the second day I observed a reniform swelling over the most prominent portion of the right parietal bone, 6 cm. in length by 2.5 in breadth, lying entirely within the border of the

[1] "Ueber eine eigene art von Blutgeschwülsten."
[2] V. Zeller: De Cepha'hæmatomate seu sanguineo cranii tumore recensnatorum. Heidelberg, 1822.

bone, which could be felt on all sides around the swelling.   The concavity of its circumference looked downward toward the right ear, while its convexity was more or less parallel with the sagittal suture.

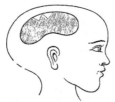

Showing the position of the cephalhæmatoma. Its relative size is greater than natural. The dotted triangles represent the bony plates which formed in the pericranium as the tumor disappeared.

At first slightly elevated, the tumor distended in two or three days, until it formed a prominent, rounded, tense sac. Its circumference did not appear to increase.   Elasticity and fluctuation were distinct.   There was no pulsation.

Pressure was painful only upon being prolonged when the child became restless.   It did not reduce the size of the tumor.   The scalp over the tumor was movable and unchanged in appearance.   Surrounding the whole margin of the tumor a distinct sharp ridge could be felt, and within this craterous orifice palpation at first conveyed the sensation that the bone was wanting.   Deeper palpation, however, touched the bony floor, removing the deception.

The tumor thus formed resembled in shape a potato cut in half lengthwise and laid flat on the head.   It thus made a very conspicuous deformity, giving the head an extraordinary lop-sided appearance.   The treatment was a policy of inactivity.

I did absolutely nothing to the tumor.   In about ten days it began to diminish in size, and in three weeks and a half it had almost entirely disappeared. At this time there was still a slight elevation, and on pressure the fluid seemed to shoot under a parchment-like membrane.   The borders felt rough, and from the upper margin two triangular plates projected over the denuded bone, apparently lying in the periosteum.   Later no trace of the tumor could be detected.

THE TOXIC PRODUCTS OF THE BACILLUS OF HOG-CHOLERA.

BY FREDERICK G. NOVY, Sc.D.,

INSTRUCTOR IN HYGIENE AND PHYSIOLOGICAL CHEMISTRY IN THE UNIVERSITY OF MICHIGAN, ANN ARBOR.

THE fundamental researches of Löffler, Schütz, Lydtin, and Schottelius, in Europe, and of Salmon and Smith, in America, have demonstrated the existence among swine of at least three distinct infectious diseases.   These are:

1. Hog-erysipelas, or *rouget* of France, and *schweincrothlauf* of Germany.

2. Swine-plague, or *schweineseuche.*

3. Hog-cholera, or *schweinepest.*

The first of these, hog-erysipelas, is exclusively a European disease, and has not, so far as known, been observed in this country.   In the course of this disease only general symptoms of infection, as in anthrax or septicæmia, are manifested.   The most important anatomical changes are as follows : The spleen is markedly swollen and dark-colored ; the mucous membrane of the stomach and intestines is inflamed and infiltrated with blood ; a parenchymatous inflammation of the liver, heart, and muscles is present, as well as some reddening of the skin.

The second disease, swine-plague, appears to be common to both continents.   It may be characterized as an inflammation of the lungs and skin, accompanied with death of the lung tissue and slight symptoms of infection.   When the disease becomes chronic, a caseous condition of the lungs results which may excite a similar condition in the lymphatic glands and the joints.

The third, hog-cholera, is preëminently a disease of the digestive tract, and the large intestine is especially involved.   It is the great swine-disease of this country, and is very probably present in England associated with other forms of disease under the name of swine-fever.   On the European Continent this disease was unknown until 1887, when it suddenly appeared in France, Sweden, and Denmark.

Apart from this sudden visitation of hog-cholera in the above-mentioned countries of Europe, it may be said that on the Continent there are two prevalent diseases—hog-erysipelas and swine-plague.   In this country the former is entirely absent, and appears to be replaced by hog-cholera, so that the two swine-diseases in America are hog-cholera and swine-plague.

A very careful bacteriological study of these three diseases has shown their microbic origin.   The researches of Löffler demonstrated the etiological importance of the bacillus of hog-erysipelas ; those of Schütz accomplished the same with reference to the bacillus of swine plague ; and lastly, Salmon and Smith have demonstrated that hog-cholera owes its origin to a specific bacillus.

But even when the causal relation of a germ to a disease has been shown, it does not follow that all the problems connected with the production of the disease have been settled.   Rather the reverse.   The first question that then arises is : " How does the germ produce the disease ?"   To answer this question briefly, without taking up discarded theories of only historical importance, consider the growth of the simple yeast-cell, an organism closely related to the bacteria proper.   The saccharine solution in which the yeast-cell is grown may produce, when ingested, marked toxic symptoms—*i. e.*, intoxication. The effects are not due, as is well known, to the yeast-plant directly, but to the chemical products formed by its growth—in this case, to the alcohol. And such is the explanation of the manner in which bacteria produce disease. In the body, whether of man or animal, these small disease-producing microorganisms find all the material necessary to their growth and multiplication. Like all living beings, they consume material which enables them to grow and multiply, and at the same time they secrete or give off products of cell-metabolism which may or may not be injurious—*i. e.*, toxic. Analytic as well as synthetic changes are constantly carried on during the lifetime of the simple bacterial cell, corresponding thus in every respect to the more highly organized members of the vegetable and animal kingdoms.

Among the products resulting from the growth of these microörganisms none have received more attention up to the present day than those which are known under the generic name of ptomaïnes. The word ptomaïne, first applied by Selmi to designate the basic or alkaloidal compounds which he found in decomposing cadavers, has been enlarged in its significance so as to embrace all basic products formed by bacteria in general. We, therefore, may have ptomaïnes produced by the activity not only of disease-producing bacteria, but also by the engenderers of putrefaction. With respect to their physiological action, it is customary to speak of toxic and non-toxic ptomaïnes. Quite recently, however, Brieger, of Berlin, who has done more than anyone else to bring light into this heretofore obscure field of knowledge, has proposed to restrict the word ptomaïne to only the non-poisonous basic products generated by the activity of bacteria, and to designate the poisonous basic bacterial products by a corresponding generic term, *toxine*. It is unnecessary at this point to consider the merits or faults of this classification, and beyond the mere statement of the fact it will receive no further attention. The term ptomaïne has at present such a well-accepted significance that it seems undesirable to restrict its meaning, and for that reason it is retained in this paper in its original sense.

In the light of very recent investigations, however, it seems that the noxious functions of bacteria can be manifested in the production of toxic bodies other than ptomaïnes. The latter may be considered as the final products of the action of bacteria on the proteid molecule; but intermediate between the complex harmless proteid and simple but toxic ptomaïne we may have one or more cleavage-products closely related to and apparently undistinguishable from the parent proteid molecule, except in physiological action. These new poisonous products generated by bacteria have been designated as *toxalbumins* by Brieger and Fränkel.

A brief *résumé* of the work of these two investigators will not be out of place at this point. Its great importance from a chemical standpoint, and the influence that it will undoubtedly exercise in the future, bringing forth as it does a great, if not the greatest, etiological factor in microbic diseases, will be readily recognized.

In studying the poisonous products generated by the growth of Löffler's diphtheria bacillus, Brieger and Fränkel found that the culture, liquid-freed from its bacteria by filtration, possessed a high degree of toxicity, which was partially lost when the liquid was kept at 60° C. for a short time, and completely destroyed by an exposure of ten minutes to a temperature of 100°. It could, however, be evaporated at 50°, or less, even when acidulated with hydrochloric acid. This showed that the poisonous substance was readily decomposed by a temperature exceeding 60°. A careful examination for basic products yielded absolutely negative results. The poisonous principle was found to be insoluble in absolute alcohol, but soluble in water, and thus could be obtained in a condition of purity. Its reaction showed it to be related to the serum-albumins, while chemical analysis indicated relationship with the albumoses or peptones. Even in very small quantities it causes in rabbits fatal results, which may not supervene until after an extraordinarily long time—weeks, and even a month.

From cultures of the same bacillus, after it had lost its virulence, a similar proteid body was obtained, which, however, was wholly inactive. Cultures of the bacillus of typhoid fever, of the bacillus of cholera, and of the staphylococcus pyogenes aureus yielded toxic globulin-like bodies; whereas, those of the tetanus and anthrax bacilli give toxic albumin-like bodies, resembling that obtained from diphtheria cultures.

Independently of Brieger and Fränkel, and at about the same time, Baginski and Stadthagen found that cultures of a common saprogenic inte-tinal bacillus, similar to, if not identical with Finkler-Prior's bacillus, produced, in addition to a moderately poisonous base, a toxic proteid substance related to the peptones.

The existence of poisonous proteid bodies formed by the growth of microörganisms, was shown by Christmas and by Hankin, some time previously to the investigations just referred to. From cultures of the staphylococcus pyogenes aureus, Christmas (1888) isolated a proteid substance which, when introduced into the anterior chamber of the eye, or into the subcutaneous tissue, produced suppuration. Hankin, in 1889, obtained immunity in mice and guinea-pigs against anthrax by first inoculating the animals with an albumose-like body, which he obtained from cultures of the anthrax bacillus.

In the following pages the results obtained from a study of Salmon's bacillus of hog-cholera will be given. The work at first was made to cover a search for the ptomaïnes generated by this microörganism, but subsequently has included an examination for toxalbumins. The methods pursued in this investigation were in general an adaptation of the methods of Brieger. The culture of the microörganism employed was obtained from the Agricultural Department at Washington, and before use was passed through a number of rabbits in order to secure maximum virulence.

Methods and results of analysis.—As a culture-medium pork broth was employed, and was prepared as follows: The finely-bashed pork was treated with distilled water, in the proportion of one litre of water to 500 grammes of meat. The mixture was then placed in tin pails, and heated in a steam sterilizer two hours daily for several successive days, in order to remove the excess of fat. This done, the material was poured into a number of half-litre and litre flasks, which had been previously cleaned, closed with a tight-fitting plug of cotton, and efficiently sterilized by heating for two or three hours at about 175°. The flasks, thus equipped, were sterilized in a Koch's steam-sterilizing apparatus by heating, two hours each day, for three consecutive days. When cool the contents were inoculated with the above-mentioned virulent culture of the hog-cholera bacillus, and the flasks then set aside in incubators, at a temperature of 35–37° C., where they remained nearly eight weeks.

At the expiration of that time the flasks were taken out and the contents subjected to examination. They were found to possess a strong alkaline reaction and an amine odor. A portion when heated on a water-bath gave off alkaline vapors, and the odor was more marked. Only those flasks were reserved for further study which were found to contain pure cultures of the hog-cholera bacillus.

Several preliminary examinations were made to ascertain the presence or absence of phenol, indol, and related bodies. For this purpose about 100 c. c. of the clear culture-liquid were acidulated with sulphuric acid, a marked effervescence resulting, and then subjected to distillation. A number of such distillations were made, but at no time was any reaction obtained on addition to the distillate of bromine water, or of hydrochloric or nitric acid, showing the entire absence of phenol, skatol, and indol.

The remaining contents of the flasks were then acidulated with hydrochloric acid and filtered through muslin. The filtrate, amounting to about six and a half litres, was neutralized with sodium carbonate solution, and evaporated on a water-bath. The residue of meat-fibre was extracted with about three and a half litres of five-per-cent. hydrochloric acid solution, filtered, and the filtrate evaporated separately, taking care, as before, to keep the liquid neutral.

In both cases thick, syrupy residues were obtained, which were taken up with successive portions of absolute alcohol, the extraction being markedly facilitated by the use of a pestle, whereby the material was reduced to a fine granular condition. The alcoholic solutions thus obtained were then combined and filtered, and the clear solution was precipitated with an alcoholic solution of mercuric chloride. An abundant, white, amorphous precipitate was obtained. This was filtered off, washed with absolute alcohol, then suspended in distilled water, and decomposed by a current of hydrogen sulphide. After removing the sulphide of mercury by filtration the filtrate was concentrated, taking care to keep the liquid near the neutral point, and finally again treated with hydrogen sulphide to remove the last traces of mercury.

The filtrate, now perfectly free from mercury, was neutralized and evaporated to dryness on a water-bath. A yellowish-brown syrup, containing some needle-shaped crystals and some crystals of salt, was obtained. This was taken up in 100 c. c. of distilled water, neutralized, and small quantities were injected into rats. One-fourth c. c. produced death in a very short time, preceded by spasmodic contraction of the limbs. The animal died on its side, with the feet extended. One-eighth c. c. produced marked excitement at first, but subsequently the animal assumed a fixed position, and the eyes were half-closed by a thick secretion. It was found dead thirty-six hours later, lying on its side, with the feet extended. Post-mortem examination showed bright-red lungs; heart in diastole; liver dotted with minute hæmorrhagic spots; spleen very light in color; kidneys mottled with superficial necrotic spots; and intestines reddened along the entire length, and with swollen, inflated patches.

These experiments demonstrated that a substance of marked toxic properties was present in the residue from the mercuric chloride precipitate. The solution was again evaporated to dryness on a water-bath, and the residue again extracted with a considerable amount of absolute alcohol. The alcoholic solution was in turn precipitated with alcoholic platinic chloride. A rather large flesh-colored precipitate was obtained, which was transferred to a filter and washed well with absolute alcohol.

The filtrate from the platinic chloride precipitate was diluted with water, and decomposed with hydrogen sulphide, and the filtrate thus obtained gave a small quantity of a sticky syrup, apparently identical with the syrupy salt obtained from the platinum precipitate. It may be mentioned at this point that the mercuric chloride filtrate was decomposed in like manner. It gave a considerable amount of ammonia, but otherwise no toxic substance was present.

The platinum chloride precipitate was then treated with cold distilled water, which readily dissolved all but a very small portion. The solution was filtered off, and the filtrate on standing gave a yellow deposit of a platinum compound, which under the microscope appeared perfectly homogeneous, and in the form of clear, yellow, oil-like globules. This deposit was filtered off, well washed with water, then dried at 75°C. The filtrate, on standing forty-eight hours, gave a second deposit, which was likewise removed by filtration, washed and dried as before. This deposit was subjected to elementary analysis, and the results obtained were tabulated (Table I.). The

TABLE I.

	Per cent. found.		Average.	Calculated per cent. for $C_9H_{14}N_4PtO_4$.
	I.	II.		
C =	20.19	19.49	19 84	19.66
H =	2.66	3.14	2.90	2.87
N =	11.65	......	11.65	11.47
Pt =	39.64	39.90	39.77	39.80
O =	......	......	......	26 20

addition of alcohol to the solution of the platinum precipitate, after removal of the last deposit, gave a light-yellow granular precipitate, which was found to consist almost entirely of the same compound as before. The alcoholic filtrate from the original platinum chloride precipitate, on standing some days, likewise gave a deposit of the same characteristic bright-yellow oil-like globules, which were likewise separated by filtration, well washed with water, then dried at 75°, and analyzed. The substance was not found to contain chlorine or sulphur. The results obtained are given in Table II.

In the dry condition this compound, which, perhaps, is closely related to creatin, forms a dull-yellow powder. When completely dry, it is insoluble in hot and in cold water; soluble in acids and alkalies, from which solutions it gives precipitates with barium chloride and silver nitrate. Owing to the small quantity at my disposal it was not possible to free the substance from platinum.

The dilute alcoholic filtrate from which the preceding compound was obtained was found to contain a platinum salt, crystallizing in long needles. In order to isolate this substance the filtrate was diluted with water, and the platinum removed by hydrogen sulphide. The filtrate from the platinum precipitate was concentrated on a water-bath, taking care to keep the solution near the neutral point. The small amount of platinum which was still in solution, and had not been precipitated before

owing to the presence of free acid, was now entirely removed, and the neutralized solution free from platinum was evaporated to dryness, or, rather, to a thick, dark-yellow syrup. The residue was taken up in distilled water, and decolored as much as possible with animal charcoal. The light-yellow solution thus obtained was again evaporated to dryness, and, in order to remove the salt, the residue was extracted with cold absolute alcohol, in which the syrupy portion was found to dissolve quite readily. The alcoholic solution in turn was evaporated to dryness, the light-yellow syrup again taken up with cold absolute alcohol, and this operation repeated until all the salt was removed.

In this manner a light-yellow syrup was finally obtained, which showed no tendency to crystallize, even when kept for a week at a temperature of 37°. It was soluble in water and alcohol, and proved to be the hydrochloride of a new base. In order to prepare it in a form suitable for analysis it was taken up in cold absolute alcohol, and the clear solution precipitated by an alcoholic solution of platinum chloride. The finely granular, light flesh-colored precipitate thus obtained was thoroughly washed with alcohol, dissolved in a small quantity of water, filtered, and from the filtrate the platinum salt was again precipitated by the addition of absolute alcohol. This precipitate was transferred to a filter, well washed with alcohol, and finally dried at 75°. On elementary analysis it gave the following percentage composition: C=20.40, H=4.67, N=4.99. These figures agree very closely with the calculated percentages in the formula $C_{10}H_{26}N_2 \cdot 2HCl \cdot PtCl_4$, in which C=20.57, H=4.79, N=4.79. The per cent. of platinum in the substance, however, varied in the several determinations, and from the theoretical value, so that it will be necessary to re-determine the composition of this new base as soon as new material is obtained.

The free base appears, therefore, to be a diamine, and future examination will prove whether it possesses the formula $C_{10}H_{26}N_2$. It exhibits marked, though not very strong, toxic properties, as will be seen from the experiments to be described. Moreover, it appears to be the only basic compound present which possesses such properties. On this account it is named, temporarily, *susotoxine*, from the Latin *sus*, a hog. The quantity obtained did not suffice for the isolation and study of the free base, and such examinations as were made were, therefore, confined to the hydrochloride.

The hydrochloride was obtained by decomposition of the platinum salt as a light-yellow, perfectly clear syrup, which showed no tendency to crystallize or harden, either on standing at the ordinary temperature or when kept for a week in the incubator at 35°. It is somewhat hygroscopic, and is readily soluble in water, as well as in cold absolute alcohol. When heated with a fixed alkali it gives off a strong amine odor, such as is perceived on evaporating the original culture fluid, if it happens to be alkaline in reaction. The following table gives a synopsis of its reactions with reference to the common alkaloidal and other reagents:

TABLE II.

	Alcoholic solution.	Aqueous solution.
Alc. HgCl₂	Heavy, white precipitate, soluble in water.	Slight cloudiness.
Alc. PtCl₄	Whitish precipitate, soluble in water.	Addition of alcohol produces precipitate.
Alc. AuCl₃	Slight cloudiness.	" " "
Alc. picric acid . . Phosphotungstic acid	Heavy, white precipitate.	Heavy, white precipitate, soluble in NH₄OH.
Phosphomolybdic acid	Heavy, yellowish precipitate.	Heavy, yellowish precipitate. soluble in NH₄OH. producing faint blue color.
Sodium tungstate . .	Flocculent precipitate.	" " "
I + KI	Addition of water produces precipitate.	Dirty-brown precipitate.
Bromine water . .	Addition of water produces precipitate.	Abundant yellow precipitate.
NH₄OH		" " "
(NH₄)₂CO₃		" " "
NH₄CyS		Slight cloudiness.
KOH	Amine odor on heating.	Volatile amine on heating.
Fe₂Cl₆		" " "
AgNO₃ + NH₄OH .		" " "
Tannic acid . . .		Heavy, flocculent, yellowish-white precipitate.
Lead acetate . . .		" " "
Copper acetate . .		" " "

The platinochloride is obtained by precipitation as a light, flesh-colored, granular precipitate. It is readily soluble in water, from which it can be reprecipitated by addition of absolute alcohol. From aqueous solution, when allowed to evaporate slowly, it crystallizes in long, thick needles.

The mercurochloride is thrown down from solutions of the hydrochloride in absolute alcohol, by alcoholic mercuric chloride, as a heavy, white, granular precipitate. This readily dissolves on the addition of a small quantity of water, and can be perfectly reprecipitated by addition of absolute alcohol. On treatment with hydrogen sulphide it is readily decomposed, yielding the pure hydrochloride.

The aurochloride is very soluble in water and alcohol. From the alcoholic solution it may be partially precipitated by ether as a light-yellow, oily precipitate, which is adherent to the sides and bottom of the tube.

Physiological experiments.—By a series of preliminary experiments made with sterilized culture-fluid on animals, it was shown that a relatively large amount was necessary to cause fatal results in rats. Thus, 50 c. c. of the culture-fluid of the hog-cholera bacillus were sterilized by heating one hour at 60°, then acidulated with hydrochloric acid, and concentrated at a low temperature on a water-bath to 6 c. c. Of this, 3 c. c., representing 25 c. c. of the original culture-fluid, were neutralized and injected subcutaneously into a young white rat. At first the animal was quite uneasy and jumped about, and the respiration became rapid; but it soon became quiet, the head most of the time resting, and the eyes closed. In about half an hour the gait became staggering, and a sleepy condition, with unwillingness to move, prevailed. About four hours later the animal became comatose, lying with the head horizontal, the respirations were slow and deep, and it finally died in this position. Post-mortem examination showed some bloody infiltration under the skin; a jelly-like mass at the seat of inoculation; the heart in diastole; lungs bright-red; some exudate in the pleural cavity; liver soft, but otherwise normal in color and size; kidneys and spleen normal.

The general course of the symptoms thus observed corresponded exactly to those obtained by inoculating rats with unsterilized cultures, except that in the latter case, where the disease lasted several days, a thick secretion formed between the eyelids and the animal passed abundant soft fæces.

In another experiment the clear culture-fluid, after being sterilized by heating to 60° for one hour, was evaporated on a water-bath, without neutralization with an acid, to dryness. The residue was taken up in a little water, and a portion of this solution, corresponding to 15 c. c. of the original culture-fluid, was injected subcutaneously into a young rat. The animal remained in a perfectly quiet condition for some hours, with, perhaps, slightly increased respiration. Its hind legs soon appeared to be affected, for the animal sat upright with difficulty, and showed a tendency to topple over; the eyes were closed; ears pale. About four hours later it recovered somewhat, and was able to crawl about, though it had but partial control over its hind legs. Eight hours after the inoculation the animal seemed to have recovered, but the next morning was found in a very depressed condition, lying perfectly quiet, with the eyelids closed, and conjunctivæ filled with a thick secretion. It remained in this condition during the entire morning, but about 1 P. M. toppled over on its side, and was unable to rise, though kicking vigorously. Finally, after some time, it regained an upright position, remained thus all the afternoon, and died during the evening. The post-mortem examination corresponded to that described above.

This experiment showed that the sterilized culture-fluid retained its toxicity, when evaporated, without neutralization, to dryness. When smaller quantities of the liquid were employed for injection the animals survived. The equivalent of at least 15 c. c. had to be injected in order to produce fatal results.

To test the physiological action of the syrupy hydrochloride, the following experiments were made: About 100 mg., dissolved in a little water, were injected subcutaneously into a young rat. The animal was at first quiet, apparently unwilling to move. After some ineffectual attempts at jumping it settled down in a recumbent position, and when placed on its side was unable to rise. Respiration was at first retarded, later increased, but toward the end was again very slow. Convulsive tremors shook the body at frequent intervals. The animal kicked vigorously. Reflexes were present almost to the end. As death approached, the red eyes whitened and took on a glazed, opaque appearance. Death resulted in one and a half hours. The animal was on its side, the feet extended. Post-mortem examination showed the heart arrested in diastole, lungs rather pale, stomach contracted, serum in thoracic cavity, subcuta pale and œdematous.

A second animal was given half of the preceding dose. It appeared very much affected in the course of the following hour, moving with difficulty; the next morning it was found with eyes closed, in a sleepy condition, and very unwilling to move. Forty-eight hours later this animal was given a second dose, the same in quantity as the first. This injection was borne without any apparent manifestation. Accordingly, the idea to make a third inoculation suggested itself, this time with the virulent pure culture of the bacillus, in order to see what degree of immunity, if any, had been secured. The animal was, therefore, inoculated subcutaneously with 1.5 c. c. of the bouillon-culture of the bacillus. As a control, two animals, from the same litter as the preceding, were selected, and were given by injection 1 and 2 c. c. of the same culture, respectively. Both controls died the next day, whereas the test-animal did not show any signs of indisposition for more than twenty-four hours after the death of the controls. On the third day a moist secretion appeared about the eyes, and the animal became unwilling to move, but ate well. This condition continued during the fourth day, and the animal finally died on the morning of the fifth day, more than three days after the death of the control-animals.

This experiment would, indeed, seem to indicate that a partial immunity had been conferred upon the animal by the injection of a pure ptomaïne. It would have been very desirable to repeat it upon a series of animals; but, unfortunately, the material was not abundant, and it was thought best to reserve the remainder for purpose of analysis. Whatever may be the significance of this last experiment, it is evident that the new base is decidedly toxic in action.

Toxalbumins of hog-cholera.—The researches of Brieger and Fränkel, Baginski, Stadthagen, Hankin, and Christmas, already referred to, suggested the desirability of examining cultures of the hog-cholera bacillus, with reference to the presence or absence of these new toxic substances.

For this purpose some pork-bouillon which had been inoculated with the bacillus of hog-cholera, was kept at 35-37° for a period of five and a half weeks. About 600 c. c. of the clear, filtered liquid were concentrated in vacuo at 36° to less than one-fourth its volume. The concentrated aqueous solution thus obtained was added, drop by drop, with constant stirring, to six or eight times its volume of absolute alcohol. The flocculent precipitate which formed was allowed to subside, then received upon a filter, and well washed with absolute alcohol. The filter was then spread open, and allowed to dry at the temperature of the room. There was thus obtained a light, dry, whitish, crumbling powder, which is readily soluble in water, yielding a slightly opalescent solution.

To test its action upon the lower animals, 100, 50, and 25 mg., respectively, were injected into three young rats, from one litter. The animal which received 100 mg. shortly afterward began to crawl vigorously around the side of the cage, on its belly, unable to rise. The eyes were soon flooded with a thick secretion, and its toes became red. Finally, it became quiet, lying on its belly, with the feet extended. The respiration became deeper, and a coma-like condition set in. The animal died, without struggles or convulsions, in about three hours. The animal which received 50 mg. went through the same course of symptoms, though to a less degree. It died under exactly the same conditions four hours after the injection. The animal that received 25 mg. became very sick, but finally recovered. The eyes were covered with a thick secretion, the toes were red, and the animal showed no disposition to eat or move. It passed a large quantity of soft fæces. This condition lasted about two days, and on the third it disappeared.

As a control to the preceding experiments, as well as to test the virulence of the liquid which had been concentrated in vacuo, a young rat, belonging to the same litter as the preceding, was given 3 c. c. of the concentrated liquid. The animal passed through exactly the same symptoms as those observed in the rat which had been given 25 mg., and finally died two days later.

One week later the rat which survived the injection of 25 mg. was given a second dose of 30 mg., with scarcely any effect following. Inasmuch as this indicated the establishment of a tolerance for the poison, it was decided to continue the injections at intervals with successively increasing quantities, and then, if the animal survived the maximum dose of the poison, to inoculate finally with a culture of the virulent germ, and thus obtain immunity to the disease. This expectation was realized. The animal was given, subcutaneously, at intervals of five, three, five, two, and four days, respectively, 40, 50, 75, 100, and 125 mg., without any effects. Control-animals inoculated with 100 and 125 mg. invariably died in from three to six hours. Three days after the last injection of 125 mg. the experimental animal was inoculated with 1 c. c. of a bouillon-culture of the highly-virulent germ. Only a slight temporary effect was observed during the first day, after which the animal recovered its former activity and appetite, and has remained in good condition ever since. A control-animal, which was given the same quantity of the same culture, sickened on the next day, refused to eat or drink, rested most of the time in a perfectly motionless condition, and finally died one week later.

From this experiment it will be seen that complete immunity can be produced in rats against the action of the bacillus of hog-cholera by previously introducing into the animal successively increasing doses of the toxalbumin generated by this microörganism.

A further study of this interesting toxic proteid is now being made, and the results obtained will be published in due time. It may be stated now, however, that the toxic properties of the substance are not destroyed when the dry powder is heated for one hour at 72°, but are effectually destroyed by heating for the same length of time at 100°.

To summarize the results which have been obtained from the study of the chemical products of the bacillus of hog-cholera, we may say that when grown in proper nutrient material it forms:

1st. A basic toxic substance, or ptomaine—*susotoxine*.

2d. A toxic proteid substance, or toxalbumin.

3d. That this toxalbumin is capable of producing immunity in rats against the action of virulent bacillus.

In conclusion, I desire to express my thanks to my friend Mr. Charles J. Greenstreet, who kindly executed the elementary analysis in this work.

REFERENCES.

Löffler.—Experimentelle Untersuchungen über den Schweinerothlauf. Arbeiten aus dem kaiserl. Gesundheitsamt. Bd. i. S. 46, 1885 ; Berlin.

Schütz.—Ueber den Rothlauf der Schweine und die Impfung mit demselben. Arbeiten a. d. kaiserl. Gesundheitsamt. Bd. i. S. 56. Ueber die Schweinesenche

Arbeiten Bd. i. S. 376, 1886. Die Schweinepest in Dänemark.

Lydtin und Schottelius.—Der Rothlauf der Schweine, seine Entstehung und Verhütung, Wiesbaden, 1885.

First and Second Annual Reports of the Bureau of Animal Industry. Washington, 1884, 1885.

Investigations of Swine Disease : Department of Agriculture, 1886, p. 603.

Hog-cholera : Its History, Nature, and Treatment. Department of Agriculture, Washington, 1889.

L. Brieger und C. Fränkel.—Untersuchungen über Bakteriengifte. Berliner klin. Wochenschrift, March 17, p. 241 ; March 24, p. 268, 1890.

A. Baginski und M. Stadthagen.—Ueber giftige Producte saprogener Darmbakterien. Berliner klin. Wochenschrift, March 31, p. 294, 1890.

Hankury Hankin.—British Medical Journal, 1889, p. 810.

Christmas.—Annales de l'Institut Pasteur, 1888, p. 469.

HYGIENIC LABORATORY, UNIVERSITY OF MICHIGAN.

A PRELIMINARY STUDY OF THE PTOMAINES FROM THE CULTURE-LIQUIDS OF THE HOG-CHOLERA GERM.[1]

BY E. A. v. SCHWEINITZ, PH.D.,
CHEMICAL LABORATORY, BUREAU OF ANIMAL INDUSTRY, WASHINGTON, D. C.

DRS. SALMON and SMITH, of the Bureau of Animal Industry, U. S. Department of Agriculture, were the first to demonstrate that the substances produced by bacteria in their growth in culture-media could be used for purposes of preventive inoculation. This they proved by a number of experiments upon pigeons, in 1887. They succeeded in producing immunity from hog-cholera by inoculating pigeons with sterilized culture-liquids of the hog-cholera germ. With a view to learn more of the products of these and other disease-germs, a chemical laboratory was recently attached to the Bureau of Animal Industry, and for a short time I have been engaged in studying the products in the culture-liquids of the hog-cholera germ. The bacteriological work was done by Dr. Moore, of the Bureau of Animal Industry. The advice of Drs. Salmon and Smith has also been very valuable, and it was at their suggestion that the work was undertaken. Although the experiments are not complete, we think it best to make now a preliminary statement in regard to some of the results obtained, reserving for the near future a more extended account of the work.

The researches of Brieger, Baginsky, Salkowski, Selmi, and others, have shown that the multiplication of a number of different bacilli produces basic substances of an alkaloidal character. called *Ptomaïnes*. Some of these bodies are very poisonous. and a number of them have been shown to be

[1] Read before the Chemical Section of the American Association for the Advancement of Science. August, 1890.

identical with certain of the artificially prepared amines. In general, the best results have been obtained by allowing the germs to multiply in beef-bouillon, and after a number of experiments we have found an acid bouillon containing 2 per cent. of peptone to be the most satisfactory medium for the growth of the hog-cholera germ. Erlenmeyer flasks of 500 c. c. capacity were used, the mouths of the sterilized flasks being closed with a cotton plug. After inoculating the liquid with the germ the flasks were allowed to stand in the incubator for from two to three weeks, at a temperature of about 37° C. At the end of this time the liquid had become cloudy, and considerable precipitate, due to the growth of the germ, was found at the bottom of the flask and in suspension. The fluid had a decidedly alkaline reaction. Careful examination showed that the culture-liquid had not become contaminated with foreign germs.

In endeavoring to isolate the chemical products from these liquids, the methods, with some slight modifications, by which Brieger obtained such brilliant results, were followed.

The culture-liquid, after being acidified with dilute HCl, was evaporated on the water-bath. The residue was then extracted with 98-per-cent. alcohol, and the filtered solution treated with mercuric chloride. A heavy crystalline precipitate was formed which increased upon standing. After filtration this precipitate was treated with water, and decomposed with sulphuretted hydrogen, and the mercury sulphide removed by filtration. From the filtrate, after removal of the excess of H_2S and concentration, I was able to isolate cadaverine, and a primary amine which I have not yet identified. The filtrate from the mercuric chloride precipitate was freed from excess of mercury by sulphuretted hydrogen, and the mercury sulphide filtered off. The residue, after concentrating this filtrate, was extracted with absolute alcohol, the solution thus obtained showing the presence of a salt of an alkaloidal character. The reactions were as follows:

With phosphomolybdic acid—light-yellow precipitate.

With bismuth-potassium iodide—red needles.

With phosphotungstic acid—a white precipitate.

With potassium iodide and iodine—brown-red precipitate.

With platinum chloride—yellow crystalline precipitate.

With gold chloride—yellow-red crystalline precipitate.

The double salt obtained with Pt Cl_4 was submitted, after crystallization from 96-per-cent. alcohol, to a preliminary analysis, giving results which correspond to the formula $C_{14}H_{34}N_2Pt\,Cl_6$.

The free base I have not yet succeeded in obtain-

ing in a pure form, and will not be ready to give this ptomaïne a name until more is learned of its constitution. The hydrochloride of this base is soluble in absolute alcohol, but I have obtained the salt only as a thick syrup, which so far will not crystallize over sulphuric acid in vacuo.

By treating the original culture-liquids of the hog-cholera germ with a large excess of absolute alcohol a white flocculent precipitate was obtained, a portion of which was soluble in water, and could again be precipitated by alcohol. By repeated treatment in this manner with water and alcohol a small quantity of an albuminoid body containing C, H, N, O, and S was finally obtained. This substance, which we will call albumose, when dried over sulphuric acid in vacuo, crystallized in white translucent plates. After drying, it was still soluble in water, though it dissolved with more difficulty. The water solution gave with $PtCl_4$ an almost insoluble precipitate, appearing under the microscope as needle-like crystals.

The toxic effects of this albuminoid body and of the ptomaïne were tested by subcutaneous inoculation of guinea-pigs. At the point of the inoculation with the albumose there was swelling and the formation of a hard lump, which disappeared after four or five days. There was also a rise in the temperature of the animal for a few days, but in other respects it seemed to suffer no inconvenience.

After subcutaneous injection of a small quantity (½ c. c. or about 0.005 gramme) of the neutral solution of the hydrochloride of the new base before referred to, a rise of temperature in the animals was noted for a few days, and also necrosis and slight ulceration at the point of inoculation, otherwise the animals appeared well. The salt of this base, as well as the albumose, are, therefore, not virulent poisons. It may be added that special attention was given to keeping the solutions sterile, by means of a Pasteur filter, and that the absence of germs was determined by making plate-cultures.

According to an article in the *Berliner klinische Wochenschrift*, March, 1890, Brieger and Fränkel have succeeded in isolating from culture-liquids (containing 10 per cent. of blood-serum) of the diphtheria, typhoid fever, and cholera-infantum germs, albuminoid bodies which they call tox-albumose, and which are very poisonous in small doses.

From culture-liquids of beef infusion with peptone and 2 per cent. of blood-serum, we have also obtained with the hog-cholera germ an albumose, having chemical properties similar to those described by Brieger, but not virulently poisonous to guinea-pigs when given subcutaneously, though there was considerable ulceration at the point of inoculation.

The detailed results of the experiments in preventive inoculation which have been conducted are not quite ready for publication. The statement may be made in advance, however, that by inoculating guinea-pigs with certain chemical compounds which I have prepared, the animals have been rendered immune from hog-cholera.

Having, therefore, made considerable progress in the study of the culture-liquids of this hog-cholera germ, and also in preventive inoculation with chemical compounds, the results of this line of work are reserved for the present, and until more detailed results of the experiments can be given, which are promised for the near future.

COCAINE AND ANTIPYRINE COMBINED IN THE TREATMENT OF OBSTINATE VOMITING, AND AS A LOCAL ANÆSTHETIC FOR MINOR SURGICAL OPERATIONS.

BY E. STUVER, M.S., M.D.,
OF RAWLINS, WYOMING.

SEVERAL years ago, while treating a case of fever complicated by obstinate vomiting, the stomach rejecting everything taken into it, even small quantities of iced water, I first resorted to the use of cocaine muriate for the relief of this condition. One-eighth grain of the drug, in aqueous solution, administered about twenty minutes, or long enough to obtain its anæsthetic effect, before giving food or medicines, entirely relieved the vomiting, which did not recur during the illness. Since that time I have used cocaine in quite a large number of cases of various diseases for the relief of this aggravating, and at times serious, symptom. In a large proportion of the cases so treated the relief was prompt and satisfactory, but in others it was only transitory or entirely absent. In thinking over the subject it seemed logically conclusive to me that if cocaine could be combined with some remedy possessing analgesic and sedative effects, a more pronounced and persistent result would be obtained. Antipyrine, from its well-known influence in subduing pain, appeared to offer the greatest number of advantages for this purpose. Accordingly, for more than a year, I have treated cases of obstinate vomiting, whether due to central or to peripheral causes—vomiting caused by acute infectious or contagious diseases, as scarlatina, rubeola, etc., that due to acute indigestion, and other forms of gastric irritation, also the vomiting of pregnancy—by a combination of these two remedies, and have obtained better general results than by any other treatment; indeed, success often followed when our old, tried, and trustworthy remedies failed to afford relief. I trust, however, that no one will impute to me the claim of specificity for these remedies. They, like every-

thing else, will fail at times, and this fact, in connection with their well-known potency, may render a caution against their indiscriminate use advisable, and impress the importance of carefully selecting cases in which the well-known physiological and therapeutic properties of the drugs are most clearly indicated.

The following cases will serve as examples of the effects produced:

CASE I.—On May 9, 1890, I was asked to prescribe for a woman suffering from obstinate vomiting of pregnancy. She had used all ordinary remedies without avail, and had become so weak that she could scarcely move about. She could not retain even a swallow of cold water. I gave the following:

R.—Cocaine muriate (P. D. & Co.'s) 12 grains.
  Antipyrine . . 1 drachm.
  Water . . . 6 ounces.

One teaspoonful to be taken every half-hour until vomiting was relieved.

This acted promptly and effectively, and she was much elated over the result.

CASE II.—S. B., aged seven years. In this patient every systemic disturbance causes irritability of stomach, nausea and vomiting. In April, 1890, while passing through an attack of parotitis the vomiting was very severe, and the stomach would retain nothing. I prescribed:

R.—Cocaine muriate (P. D. & Co.'s) 2 grains.
  Antipyrine . . 16 "
  Water . . . 2 ounces.

Of this she was directed to take half a teaspoonful every hour until vomiting ceased. A few doses produced the desired effect and she had no further trouble during the attack.

This child had a severe attack of measles about June 1st, attended during the pre-eruptive stage by obstinate nausea and vomiting, which were promptly relieved by a few doses of the same mixture.

CASE III.—On June 27, 1890, D. S., aged fourteen months, was suddenly taken with a severe attack of acute indigestion, attended by free emesis. Though the vomiting removed all, or the greater part, of the offending material, marked gastric irritability persisted and everything swallowed was promptly ejected. There was considerable fever (pulse 150), and intense thirst, which was aggravated by the inability to retain even small quantities of nearly ice-cold water. I gave $\frac{1}{24}$ grain cocaine and $\frac{3}{4}$ grain antipyrine in aqueous solution and repeated the dose in an hour. Fifteen minutes after taking the first dose the child drank water freely and suffered only slightly from nausea; a little later he nursed, and vomiting caused no further trouble. Two grains of calomel given in the evening produced free catharsis the following morning. This, together with the treatment above indicated, and careful regulation of the diet, were the only therapeutic measures employed, and resulted in a prompt and satisfactory recovery.

While the size of the dose and the frequency of administration have been varied to meet the exigencies of particular cases, I have obtained the best results from small, frequently repeated doses. My standard for an adult has been: cocaine ⅛ grain, antipyrine 1 grain, in aqueous solution every half-hour or hour as required.

While not pertinent to the subject just considered, I will take this opportunity to state that I have found concentrated solutions composed of five per cent. and fifteen per cent. each of cocaine and antipyrine, far superior as a local anæsthetic, to cocaine alone. The effect is more decided and much more persistent. I have used this solution with highly satisfactory results in minor surgical operations, also for obtunding the sensibility of the gums before extracting teeth. If, before the latter operation, this solution be thoroughly applied to the gums for about fifteen minutes, and the region of the external auditory meatus (a method first suggested, I believe, by a French physician) be well sprayed with ether, the extraction of teeth is attended by very slight pain.

For an external operation, where a more decided anæsthesia than can be obtained by simple application to the surface is desired, the effect can be greatly enhanced by applying the solution to the part to be operated on by means of a galvanic current strong enough to produce a decided impression. For this purpose a galvanic battery should be used, as it is needless to say the ordinary faradic battery or electro magnetic machine has but slight effect.

MEDICAL PROGRESS.

The Extraction of Unripe Cataract.—In the Berlin Medical Society, July 2, 1890, PROFESSOR SCHWEIGGER read a paper on this subject, discussing at some length the vague and varying views as to what constituted "ripeness," and claiming that the term and its practical outcomes are now largely obsolete. The importance of the matter, as is well known, lies in the question whether the lens can be wholly removed in the operation; for not only will portions of the unripe lens-substance cling to the capsule, and by their later opacity annul the benefits of the operation, but the presence of these swelling masses will often give rise to serious or destructive inflammations. The usual criterion, that the lens is opaque to the periphery, and that no shadow is cast by the iris in oblique illumination, he holds to be erroneous; since much time may be needlessly lost and the patient kept waiting in blindness for this stage, long after the eye is ready for the operation. He regards the age of the patient as the sole basis for judgment. In that period of life when the accommodation is annulled by the physiological changes in the lens, that is, toward the close of the fifth decade, and quite surely after the sixtieth year, we can extract any cataract as soon as defective vision makes the operation desirable, even if the greater part of the lens is still unclouded. In this case it is necessary to combine iridectomy with the extraction, and the old classical flap-operation with the retention of the normal pupil, to which Schweigger returned some years ago, finds here a valuable field. At earlier periods the question is more difficult, and the old criterion has weight. Total opacity is important, and here artificial ripening has its place: v. Graefe's discission, carried deep into the lens, being better before the fortieth year, but after that age Förster's trituration of the lens-cortex is preferable. Neither procedure needs iridectomy; and the extraction can generally be done from four to five days after the discission, or from one to two weeks after the trituration.

In the discussion, Professor Hirschberg, while concurring in most points, was still more radical. After the fortieth year any cataract is hard, or at least the nucleus is, and through an ample section any lens can be cleanly extracted whether the cortex is ripe, immature, or hypermature.—*Centralblatt f. prakt. Augenheilkunde*, july, 1890.

Ulcerative Stomatitis.—DR. NIL J. SOKOLOFF (*Vratch*) describes an epidemic of ulcerative stomatitis in which he saw thirteen cases, all adults. In nearly all, the tonsils and posterior wall of the pharynx were simultaneously affected. The disease usually commenced with intense malaise, vomiting, diarrhœa, and fever. In severe cases the fever lasted during the whole course of the affection, its type on the whole resembling enteric fever, while in mild cases the temperature returned to the normal about the end of the first week. In some patients abscesses under the tongue, or in the organ itself, were observed; in two, an erythematous confluent rash occurred; in two, albuminuria was present. The liver and spleen remained normal in all cases. The duration of the affection varied between fourteen and fifty-six days. In one case direct infection was noticed —a patient who was recovering from some grave disease contracted ulcerative stomatitis from his neighbor. Bacterial examination revealed the presence of ordinary streptococci, but no specific microbes.

PROFESSOR SIMANOVSKY also describes eight cases of the disease. In two of the cases the ulcerative process was confined to the mouth, while in the remaining six the fauces or the pharynx was involved. The faucial lesions were usually limited to one side, the ulcer being either on the tonsils or half-arches. In one of three cases in which the urine was examined, albumin was discovered. Search for bacteria gave negative results. The treatment consisted in gargling and painting with a solution of potassium chlorate (1 drachm to 4 ounces), a two-per-cent. solution of boric acid, or a solution of salol made by adding two teaspoonfuls of a six-per-cent. alcoholic solution to a glass of water.—*Journal of Laryngology and Rhinology*, August, 1890.

The Proper Time to Administer Quinine.—In the *Annales de Thérapeutique Médico-Chirurgicales*, July, 1890, CHARPENTIER gives the following directions as to the administration of quinine:

1. The action of quinine is chiefly felt about six hours after its ingestion, and for this reason it should be given, not at the time of an expected malarial paroxysm, but six hours before.

2. In the case of quotidian fever the quinine should not be given six hours before the chill, but eight hours before, so that the full effect may be present two hours before the chill, for though the chill is the apparent onset, the real onset is still earlier.

3. When the fever is tertian, Charpentier thinks that the quinine should be used twelve hours before, and where it is quartan, eighteen hours before the attack is expected.

The drug should be given in massive doses, not in fractional doses, for the reason that it is rapidly eliminated by the urine, and in small amounts would have no effect; although when the stomach is too irritable to stand heroic amounts, fractional doses should be given every three-quarters of an hour.

Treatment for Ozæna.—COZZOLINI recommends the following powder for the treatment of this troublesome affection:

R.—Salol . . . . 2 drachms.
Boric acid . . . 1 drachm.
Salicylic acid . . . 12 grains.
Thymol . . . . 5 "
Powdered talc . . . 3 "
Use as an insufflation.
—*Provincial Medical Journal*, August, 1890.

Theobromine as a Diuretic.—GRAM, in the *Annali di Chimica e di Farmacologie*, xi., 1890, sums up his opinions of this drug as a diuretic in heart and renal disease as follows:

1. Theobromine when *pure is absorbed with difficulty, but its absorption is followed by pronounced diuresis. It is without action on the heart and provokes diuresis by a direct action on the kidneys.

2. If salicylate of sodium is combined with theobromine it facilitates the absorption of liquids and increases their elimination. The effects of theobromine are not disagreeable and the author noticed only one instance in a weak subject in which vertigo occurred.

The ordinary daily dose is 1½ drachms of the salt divided into 15-grain doses.

Retinol in the Treatment of Vaginitis.—BALZER, in the *Revue Obstétricale et Gynécologie*, July, 1890, writes of retinol, which is extracted from colophony by distillation. It is a hydrocarbon which presents itself in the form of a liquid of the consistency of linseed oil, and of the color of tan—dark-brown, or sometimes golden-yellow, according to its mode of preparation. Its reaction is acid and it evaporates slowly at ordinary temperatures. It is balsamic in nature, and possesses antiseptic powers. It has been used in America in gonorrhœa and metritis and similar diseases. When used in vaginitis it may be applied to the mucous membrane by means of an applicator and speculum, or on a tampon, and is particularly useful where vegetations are growing or recur after removal. When used on a tampon an excess acts very severely, and it is often best used by making it into a paste with boric acid and introducing a ball of this into the vagina or against the diseased spot. As the paste is very diffusible it may in some cases produce a good deal of pain and even intense inflammation.

So far, Balzer has not employed retinol sufficiently to recommend its use, but he expects to prove that it is valuable as an antiseptic, and as a cauterant and local application in certain cases of diseased mucous membranes.

Bromidrosis of Feet.—SCOTT recommends the following:

R.—Biborate of sodium } of each 2 drachms.
Salicylic acid }
Boric acid . . 30 grains.
Glycerin at 86° F. } of each 1 ounce.
Alcohol }
Mix, and use as a wash three times a day.

This application is particularly useful in those cases where much maceration of the skin is present, and where remedies of other kinds have failed.

Amylene Hydrate in Epilepsy.—NACHE agrees with Wildermuth as to the value of amylene hydrate in epilepsy, even where bromides have failed, and where the attacks are, not only very frequent but severe. He uses a 10-per-cent. solution of the drug, and gives from one to two tablespoonfuls a day (from 30 to 90 grains). Nache also believes that *petit mal* and nocturnal epilepsy are benefited by the drug.

Operative Treatment of Bubo.—PÖLCHEN, of Königsberg, gives the following directions for the treatment of bubo produced either by gonorrhœa or chancre:

After all antiseptic precautions are taken the bubo is to be incised in a line parallel to the longitudinal axis of the body, and not parallel to Poupart's ligament. The length of the incision should be about that of the swelling. After the gland is exposed, it is to be carefully dissected away from the surrounding tissues, care being taken to avoid the great vessels, and every portion of diseased tissue removed. The space surrounding the gland is now to be packed with iodoform-gauze while search is made for other diseased parts. At this time the hæmorrhage should be almost nothing. For the total destruction of the disease-process we may cauterize all the affected glands with caustic potash, using antiseptic gauze to protect the healthy parts, instead of scraping the glands. The advantages of the latter plan consist in the ease of the operation and its freedom from danger, while it is asserted that the dangers from general infection are much decreased by the action of the caustic and that the cure is completed in the majority of cases without fever. It is true, on the other hand, that healing is postponed a little longer than after the simple use of the knife. This inconvenience, is however, counter-balanced by the fact that the patient can return to his usual occupations almost at once, and the secretion from the wound amounts to almost nothing.

Treatment of Syphilis by Rectal Injections of Iodides.—According to the *Revue Générale de Clinique et de Thérapeutique*, the following formula may be used by the anus, whenever the stomach is disordered:

R.—Iodide of potassium . . 15 grains.
Extract of belladonna . ¼ grain.
Water . . . . 4 ounces.—M.

The solution must be warm, and is said to be well borne and effective.

Treatment of Metrorrhagia by Ergotine Injections.—When ergotine is badly tolerated by the stomach, it is recommended that it be used in the following manner in metrorrhagia:

The bowel having been first evacuated of fæcal matter and the rectum washed out, a teaspoonful of the following is to be mixed with two tablespoonfuls of hot water and injected:

R.—Ergotine . . . 150 grains.
Distilled water . . 2½ ounces.
Glycerin . . . 6 drachms.
Salicylic acid . . 6 grains.

—*Revue Gén. de Clin. et de Thérapeutique*, Aug. 6, 1890.

Treatment of Acne.— In the *Revue Thérapeutique Médico-Chirurgicale*, ISAACS recommends the following for acne:

R.—Camphor ⎫
Vaseline ⎬ of each . 150grains.
Beta-naphthol ⎭
Precipitated sulphur . . 1½ ounces.
Green soap . . . ½ ounce.-M.

Apply to the affected part for from three to fifteen minutes, according to its susceptibility. After using this lotion, use in its place, after thoroughly drying the skin:

R.—Resorcin ⎫ of each . . 7 to 15 grains.
Salicylic acid ⎭
Oxide of zinc . . . 30 grains.
Vaseline . . . . 6 drachms.—M.

This is to be allowed to remain on all night, or a less time if it is too stimulating, and is itself to be followed by an emollient, such as cold cream or chalk powder.

Prescription for Flatulent Dyspepsia.—DR. PAUL CHÉRON prescribes the following powder to cases of flatulent dyspepsia:

R.—Magnesia ⎫
Calcium phosphate ⎬ equal parts.
Powdered charcoal ⎪
Sulphur ⎭

A teaspoonful to be taken in water when necessary.—*Provincial Medical Journal.*

Hypodermic Injection for Delirium Tremens.—In *La Semaine Médicale*, July 30, 1890, the following formula is given:

R.—Methylal . . . . 75 grains.
Distilled water . . . 5 ounces.
Mix, and use for hypodermic injections.

This mixture is to be injected, hypodermically, in three or four doses during twenty-four hours, and its use continned for four or five days. It produces less evil effects under these circumstances than most of the drugs devoted to the treatment of delirium tremens. Fischer states that these injections are never followed by abscess, and may be employed when an attack of *mania-a-potu* is imminent, as a prophylactic measure.

Tests for Arsenic in Wall-paper.—The *British Medical Journal* describes the following simple tests for arsenic in wall-papers: Turn down an ordinary gas-jet until the flame is wholly blue. Then a strip of the suspected paper, about one-sixteenth of an inch wide, is brought in contact with the outer edge of the flame. If arsenic is present, a gray coloration will be seen in the flame, and, if the paper is burned a little more, a garlic-like odor can be detected in the fumes. If, on removing the paper from the flame, the charred portion is of a reddish color, copper is present (arsenic used for this purpose is usually in the form of arsenite of copper). On again placing the charred paper in the flame a green coloration, due to the copper, is seen.—*The Sanitarian*, July, 1890.

Treatment of Acute Vaginitis.—In the *Revue Générale de Clinique et de Thérapeutique*, July 2, 1890, ELOY gives the following treatment for vaginitis: He divides the disease into the initial or primary stage, and terminal or final stage.

For the primary condition he advises the employment of hot injections of liquid vaseline and cocoa-butter, combined with 300 grains of boric acid to each pint of this mixture, the injections to be made every few hours. This is to soothe the irritated parts.

In the terminal stages, when acute inflammation has passed, one of the following injections is useful:

Sulphate of iron . . . 300 grains.
Distilled water . . . . 1 pint.
Or,
Chloral . . . . . 300 grains.
Distilled water . . . 1 pint.
Or,
Permanganate of potassium . 2½ grains.
Distilled water . . . . 1 pint.

After several days, if the discharge persists, the vagina should be packed with cotton tampons saturated with glycerole of tannin made as follows:

Tannic acid ⎫ of each . . 2 drachms.
Glycerin ⎭

After each removal of these, the mucous membrane should be touched with a strong solution of silver nitrate.

Nylander's Test for Glycosuria. — DR. BRANDRETH SYMONDS advocates the use of Nylander's solution in testing for sugar in the urine (*New York Medical Journal*, July 12, 1890). The solution consists of bismuth subnitrate, 31 grains (2 grammes); Rochelle salt, 62 grains (4 grammes), dissolved in 3⅓ ounces (100 c. c.) of a 10-per-cent. solution of sodium hydrate. On boiling this with glucose a dark-brown or black precipitate of bismuth suboxide and metallic bismuth is produced. The most delicate mode of applying the test is to half-fill a test-tube with urine, then add about one-third of the solution. Boil the upper layers, watching for any reduction.

Though less delicate than Fehling's test, detecting only a tenth of one per cent., it has the advantages of not changing, even when kept for a long time, and of not giving a reaction with chloral, pyrocatechin, or glycosuric acid. Dr. Symonds thinks the test sufficiently delicate for ordinary clinical work, and is the one which he usually applies.

THE MEDICAL NEWS.

A WEEKLY JOURNAL
OF MEDICAL SCIENCE.

COMMUNICATIONS are invited from all parts of the world. Original articles contributed exclusively to THE MEDICAL NEWS will be liberally paid for upon publication. When necessary to elucidate the text, illustrations will be furnished without cost to the author.

Address the Editor: H. A. HARE, M.D.,
1004 WALNUT STREET,
PHILADELPHIA.

Subscription Price, including Postage.

PER ANNUM, IN ADVANCE . . . . $4.00.
SINGLE COPIES . . . . 10 CENTS.

Subscriptions may begin at any date. The safest mode of remittance is by bank check or postal money order, drawn to the order of the undersigned. When neither is accessible, remittances may be made, at the risk of the publishers, by forwarding in *registered* letters.

Address, LEA BROTHERS & CO.,
NOS. 706 & 708 SANSOM STREET,
PHILADELPHIA.

SATURDAY, SEPTEMBER 6, 1890.

PURULENT CAPILLARY BRONCHITIS IN THE PHTHISICAL, DUE TO THE PNEUMOCOCCUS.

EVERY physician of large clinical experience with the phthisical must have observed many cases in which the more or less sudden termination has seemed to be due to something above and beyond the mere tuberculous condition. That is to say, either physical examination fails to show—and autopsy to reveal—an extent of pulmonary infiltration or destruction sufficient to necessitate a fatal issue at that time, or even to account for the severity of the constitutional symptoms; or, on the other hand, while conditions of great pulmonary destruction have long been recognized, yet the final breaking-down of vital powers in general, is of a suddenness not to have been expected from the slow progress of the chronic disease. The most plausible explanations hitherto offered for the phenomena are sudden, generalized infection from penetration of bacilli into the circulation, or lethal intoxication with ptomaïnes.

An investigation recently undertaken by MM. DUFLOCQ and MENETRIER (*Archives Générales de Médecine*, June and July, 1890) throws a certain amount of new light upon the subject. In the course of their researches into the pathogenetic activities of the pneumococcus, other than as the cause of pneumonia, they have observed clinically, and ex-amined post-mortem, a number of cases of phthisis, upon which an acute capillary bronchitis had supervened, apparently from secondary infection, which they attribute to the pneumococcus.

At the autopsy they have invariably found the lesions of the tuberculous and bronchitic infections coëxisting, but not coëxtensive; the anatomical relations being such as to leave no doubt of the priority of the tuberculous process. While the lesions of tuberculosis were found principally in the upper lobes, the capillary bronchitis involved the middle and inferior portions of the lung; that is to say, regions relatively free from bacillary localization. The bacillus was always wanting in the pus of the bronchioles, while the pneumococcus was encountered only exceptionally and in very small number, in the liquid contents of cavities. Having determined beyond doubt, by culture and by inoculation, that they were dealing with the veritable pneumococcus, the authors ask, Why is it that this microbe gave rise in the cases under consideration, not to pneumonia, but to capillary bronchitis? The answer they give is, in brief, that while ordinarily the pneumococcus must act in conjunction with other pathogenetic parasites—as, for example, the streptococcus or the pneumo-bacillus of Friedländer, or some more common pyogenetic germ—yet in these particular cases it was the sole agent in the infection; the irritation produced by the presence of the tubercle bacillus and the passage of tuberculous fluids over the bronchial mucous membrane having rendered the tissues vulnerable without other intervention.

If these observations are correct, it will readily be seen how a comparatively limited and quiescent pulmonary tuberculosis can be suddenly converted by this additional infection into a very grave and dangerous condition. Such additional infection will explain the heightened fever, the renewed symptoms of septic toxæmia, and the physical signs of obstructed respiration and impaired circulation disproportionate to the extent of the existing tuberculous lesion.

In these remarks, as in the researches quoted, the well-known liability of the subjects of slow, chronic phthisis to sudden and frequently fatal pneumonia has not been under consideration.

STOMACH-WASHING IN CHILDREN.

STOMACH-WASHING in the treatment of the gastric disorders of childhood has been practised chiefly by

Epstein, and in this country, to a limited extent, by Seibert and a few others. Recently DR. WILLIAM D. BOOKER (*Johns Hopkins Hospital Bulletin*, July, 1890) has used the method in the treatment of nearly two hundred cases of gastro-intestinal disturbances in children, all the cases occurring in hospital or dispensary practice. Although, as Booker himself writes, it is too early to estimate the exact position of the procedure in the therapeutics of childhood, it is undoubtedly of great value in the treatment of certain conditions.

Booker's observations seem to show that stomach-washing is of especial value for the relief of vomiting due to indigestion. In many of his cases relief was immediate, and in only one case was it necessary to stop giving milk. The vomiting of dysentery was less markedly influenced, though in some cases it was checked. In the summer diarrhœas benefit often followed the washing, and was evidently due to the fact that undigested food was prevented from entering the intestines. In some of the latter cases, however, the curative influence was very slight. A few cases of constipation due to gastro-intestinal catarrh were also improved by systematic stomach-washing.

The apparatus used by Booker was a Nélaton catheter, No. 8, 9, or 10, attached by a rubber tube two feet long to a two-ounce glass funnel. To perform the operation properly the child should be held in a sitting position on the nurse's lap, with the head slightly inclined forward and the hands confined by the nurse's left arm. The tube, moistened with water, is then steadily passed back to the pharynx and downward into the stomach. Gagging may be produced when the end of the catheter reaches the pharynx, but usually ceases when it reaches the stomach. One or two ounces of water are then poured into the funnel, held above the child's head, and the moment the funnel becomes empty it is lowered and the contents of the stomach siphoned out. This should be repeated until the water returns clear.

Booker also made some interesting observations upon the contents of the stomach in normal and in disordered digestion, but it is to the therapeutical aspects of the subject that we wish to direct attention, and to advise washing out the stomach in the treatment of gastro-intestinal diseases in children, *after* careful regulation of the diet and other measures have failed. We do not believe that it will, or should, supplant other methods of treatment, but that it is a valuable addition to our resources in the management of serious and often obstinate diseases.

THE NEW SURGEON-GENERAL.

DR. JEDEDIAH H. BAXTER, formerly Chief Medical Purveyor of the United States Army, has just been appointed its Surgeon-General, and we congratulate the President upon his wisdom in making such an appointment. While it has been claimed by certain opponents of Dr. Baxter that he has never seen much active frontier service, it nevertheless remains a fact that such service is not the training necessary to make a good surgeon-general, who needs executive ability and experience in matters closely connected with what Dr. Baxter has been accustomed to attend to since the war. Further than this, his prolonged residence in Washington has given him complete information as to the central management of the service, and his executive ability must soon make itself felt now that he has succeeded Surgeon-General Moore, and has at last reached a rank where he may use his powers. Promotion according to rank is a custom too often disregarded, and we are glad that in this instance at least the regular line of promotion was followed out. Dr. Baxter has before him a period of many years before the retiring age arrives, and we are confident that these years will be used for the good of the service.

SPECIAL CORRESPONDENCE.

THE POLICY OF SURGEON-GENERAL BAXTER.

To the Editor of THE MEDICAL NEWS,

SIR: On the 28th ult. the Senate wisely confirmed the appointment of Colonel Jedediah H. Baxter to the Surgeon-Generalship of the United States Army, vice Surgeon-General John Wood, retired. General Baxter's service of over thirty years in the Army, twenty-five of which were in the administrative department, his sequence in line of promotion, and his well-known ability amply warrant the appointment.

The long period during which Dr. Baxter will fill the highest office within the medical department of the Army renders the lines upon which the service will be conducted a matter of interest beyond the circle of army surgeons. Your correspondent, therefore, is happy to be able to assert authoritatively, that increased effort will be made to improve the efficiency of this arm of the service.

To this end, examinations for admission to the service will aim to test more thoroughly than heretofore the practical ability of the applicant, rather than his fund of theoretical knowledge, and in all cases a sound general education will be an essential for appointment. Previous hospital experience will rate more highly than heretofore in an applicant's qualifications, and will be esteemed in accordance with its length and the standing of the institution. The physical condition of the applicant will be inquired into as strictly as is the case in other arms of the service. The necessity of this measure has been evinced by the proportion of appointees who, after a few months of active service, become physically disqualified.

Another plan that cannot fail of excellent effect is, that assistant surgeons after a reasonable term of service at isolated posts shall be given leave of absence for the purpose of " brushing up " their medical knowledge by attendance at post-graduate and hospital courses in the larger cities.

Rapid promotion and the consequent increased pay will render the position of army surgeon more attractive and induce an increased number of applicants. With this object in view, it is Surgeon-General Baxter's intention to secure the adoption of measures that will enable disabled surgeons to enter upon the retired list without the vexatious delays now experienced, and thus reduce the number of contract-surgeons employed. When the latter are required, a much more strict preliminary examination will be enforced than has been the custom in the past.

These are but a few of the many plans Dr. Baxter entertains for the benefit of the department of which he is the head. Many others concern minor matters of detail of little general interest, others are not yet sufficiently developed to entitle them to publication ; but that all will prove for the benefit of the service and for the welfare of its officers, the long experience and tried ability of Dr. Baxter are ample guarantee.

WASHINGTON, D. C., August 30, 1890.

BRIGADIER-GENERAL J. H. BAXTER was born in Strafford, Vermont, May 11, 1837. He is the son of the late Hon. Portus Baxter, who represented the Third District of Vermont in Congress during the War of the Rebellion.

General Baxter was graduated from the University of Vermont, receiving the degree of A.B. in 1859, and that of M.D. in 1860. He is also a graduate of the Law Department of the Columbian University of the District of Columbia.

Dr. Baxter entered the army at the outbreak of the war, as surgeon of the 12th Massachusetts Regiment of volunteers, and was mustered into the United States service June 26, 1861. He has been in continuous service in the volunteer and regular army from that time.

He was promoted to be Brigade Surgeon, U. S. Volunteers, April 4, 1862, and served in the Peninsular campaign with the Army of the Potomac, on the staffs of Generals Banks and McClellan. He was taken ill with fever while on duty in the field and ordered to Washington.

Having partially recovered, he was assigned to the charge of Campbell Hospital, Washington, D. C., one of the largest United States General Hospitals during the war. He organized the hospital, which contained about 1500 beds, and was in full charge until January, 1864, when he was called by the order of the Secretary of War Stanton to take charge of the medical department of the Provost Marshal General's Bureau, at the request of General James B. Fry, the Provost Marshal General.

On the reorganization of the regular army on a peace-footing, after the close of the war, the services of volunteer officers who had achieved distinction during active service were recognized in filling original vacancies created by Congress in the several staff departments, which had been increased commensurate with the growth of the standing army.

Surgeon Baxter was appointed Assistant Medical Purveyor, with the rank of Lieutenant-Colonel, July 20, 1867, and March 12, 1872, was appointed Chief Medical Purveyor with the rank of Lieutenant-Colonel ; and Chief Medical Purveyor with the rank of Colonel, June 23, 1874.

He has been the senior officer in the Medical Department, next to the Surgeon-General, for many years, and on the retirement of Surgeon-General Moore, August 16, 1890, the President, on the same day, sent to the Senate the name of Colonel Baxter to fill the vacancy. He was unanimously confirmed by the Senate, August 27th.

SOCIETY PROCEEDINGS.

THE GYNECOLOGICAL SOCIETY OF CHICAGO.

Stated Meeting, April 18, 1890.

THE PRESIDENT, JAMES H. ETHERIDGE, M.D.,
IN THE CHAIR.

DR. FRANKLIN H. MARTIN exhibited a cancerous uterus that he had removed by vaginal hysterectomy. The cervix was first thoroughly scraped away to as near the healthy tissue as possible. In about three weeks the disease returned. When it began to involve the vagina, Dr. Martin advised the operation of vaginal hysterectomy, which was done, January 15, 1890. The bases of the broad ligaments were ligated with silk, and for the remaining portion of each broad ligament clamp-forceps (Byford's pattern) were used. The operation was performed without difficulty or complications, and the patient was discharged in about four weeks. On April 16th, there was still no recurrence.

DR. HENRY T. BYFORD then showed a suppurating kidney. The patient was thirty-one years old ; married for five years, and had had no children. She had been subject to periodic attacks of septic fever for more than a year. The temperature would reach 103° to 104° F. during the attack, with great tenderness in the right side of abdomen. After a discharge of pus and granular material with the urine, the symptoms would subside for a time. The organ was felt to be enlarged at each examination.

The kidney was removed through an incision made in the linea semilunaris, through which the other kidney was first palpated and found to be healthy. The tissues about the diseased one were healthy, but the uterine appendages were extensively diseased. He completed the operation by establishing drainage with iodoform-gauze through a small opening in the lumbar region, and closed the abdominal incision completely. The ureter was ligated with fine silk at about one and one-half inches from the kidney, and placed so that any suppuration that might arise from it would find its way out through the lumbar opening. The temperature remained between 99° and 100° F. for a few days, and then became normal.

Dr. Byford also showed a specimen of probable sarcoma of the uterus and one of fibroma of the uterus. The patient with the sarcoma was at about the period of the menopause. The tumor was growing rapidly and causing pain, and the bloodvessels about the uterus were exceedingly large. He based his diagnosis upon the appearance of the tumor, the excessive vascularity, the absence of a capsule, and the manner in which it was attached to the bladder. Microscopical examination had not yet been made.

In the case of the fibroma, the diagnosis was obscure. Ten years previously the condition had been diagnosed and treated as pelvic inflammation and pyosalpinx. The abdomen, when the patient was seen by Dr. Byford, was so tympanitic that it was impossible to make a satisfactory bimanual examination. The patient was taking liquor and opiates, was very nervous, and was losing ground. This was the sixth case that Dr. Byford had operated upon by the following method:

The broad ligaments are tied off, the uterus amputated below the tumor, and the stump sewed up somewhat after Schröder's method, but with catgut and silkworm-gut. The bladder is separated, and an opening made into the vagina through the anterior fornix at the junction with the cervix. The silkworm-gut sutures are used for traction, and the cervix is drawn down and forward into the vagina and a clamp put on through the vagina. He usually holds the stump loosely with clamps, so that the apposed surfaces may heal up, as after trachelorrhaphy. As in all his earlier cases but the second the edges sloughed, he now prefers ligating rapidly with silk, and clamping firmly with a hollow clamp, so that the slough will separate early and come off in the clamp. The clamp prevents the contact of the slough with the patient's tissues, and avoids septic trouble.

After the stump is turned down he sews the peritoneum from behind the bladder to the posterior wall of the cervix. There is no raw surface left for extensive adhesive inflammation in the pelvis, with its consequent peritonitis and obstruction of the bowels. He has used drainage in all of the cases but one, because he does not usually operate on simple fibroids, there being generally some disease in the broad ligament and an oozing surface left. When he puts on the clamp from below he inserts a finger from above in the cul-de-sac of Douglas behind the cervix and a thumb in front of it, then pushes a pair of hæmostatic forceps up from the vagina through the anterior fornix between his thumb and the cervix, and enlarges the rent by scissors-snipping and stretching.

In discussion, DR. PARKES said that he regarded the specimen of kidney as very interesting and unusual in the length of time that it had existed without following the usual disposition of such diseases toward external suppuration. The only explanation of this is the peculiar enlargement of the ureter, which enabled it to carry the accumulated matter in the pelvis of the kidney into the

bladder. Usually in suppurating kidney almost the first manifestation is the formation of a tumor and the development of a perinephritic abscess which opens externally. Surgeons have always found difficulty in the removal of such kidneys, on account of the surrounding cicatricial tissue. It is almost a rule, he said, that suppurating kidneys should not be removed, and this rule is sustained by the results in many cases. But this case was very exceptional in that there were no surrounding complications; all the trouble was inside the kidney and could be attacked without the usual difficulties. He had always dreaded to remove them, on account of the complications arising from the presence of adhesions and the danger of septic poisoning, and has adopted the plan of laying them widely open, which is not very satisfactory, as the patient often apparently recovers, but the disease returns, owing to the many pockets in which pus accumulates. The idea of continuous irrigation has suggested itself to him in these cases.

DR. MARTIN said that he had had the pleasure of witnessing two of these operations by Dr. Byford with his method of treating the stump. The only objection that could be offered to the operation is that, for a nervous, rapid operator, the procedure is altogether too long. Dr. Byford spends from two and a half to three hours in performing this operation, and the abdominal cavity is perfect after the stump is secured.

In the discussion which followed a paper by DR. T. J. WATKINS on the

AFTER-TREATMENT OF ABDOMINAL SECTION,

DR. JAGGARD said that he was particularly interested in the allusion to ether as a renal irritant, and the reader's reference to two cases in which ether was responsible for fatal nephritis. Dr. Jaggard thought that this was one of Emmet's ideas and that the evidence that ether was a renal irritant had never been proven. Dr. Weir, of New York, has published a very interesting paper on the effect of ether upon the kidneys, and the results show that ether employed as an anæsthetic is not a renal irritant. In not one case has Dr. Weir been able to establish the fact that ether produces more irritation of the kidney than does any other extremely volatile substance. It would be interesting, he said, if Dr. Watkins would give the evidence upon which he based his conclusion that ether was responsible for two cases of fatal nephritis. Can he exclude septic infection? Dr. Jaggard also said that he had used ether in a number of cases of puerperal convulsions, contrary to the teaching of Emmet, and that he had never seen bad effects. He considers ether given hypodermically a valuable diffusible stimulant in chloroform-narcosis, and has never seen local irritation when the hypodermic needle was sterilized.

In regard to the length of time that a woman should remain in bed after an abdominal section, he described two cases. In one woman, two weeks after the operation left her bed, travelled five miles in a carriage, and, a week later, died of peritonitis. In the other case the woman went home by railway, eighteen days after the operation. On the journey the incision opened and the intestines protruded. The incision was closed again by her family physician, and she recovered.

DR. PARKES referred to the fact that after abdominal section the temperature might rise even to 104°, from no other cause than constipation. In such conditions he does not believe that the administration of antipyretics is proper, though, if there are general symptoms such as malaise and headache, he advised cold sponging.

DR. DUDLEY spoke of the management of abdominal section in the Woman's Hospital of New York, when he was an interne in the institution, fifteen years ago. At that time patients were kept on a restricted diet during the week preceding the operation. They were also given large doses of quinine, and, to prepare the system for the shock of the operation, large doses of opium. These drugs were continued after the section. The percentage of deaths was enormous, though, of course, many died from the absence of asepsis.

Dr. Dudley also said that he had adopted the enema— a half-ounce each of glycerin, sulphate of magnesium, and water—recommended by Dr. Watkins for the treatment of tympany, and that it had proven very satisfactory.

DR. BYFORD said that he had frequently noticed that a patient who had been long under ether—two or three hours—was less likely to vomit than a patient who had taken comparatively little ether. He did not consider it a good rule to take out the drainage-tube in twenty-four hours, nor did he think that the stitches should be removed in six days.

In closing the discussion, DR. WATKINS said that he still adhered to the belief that the drainage-tubes should be removed early, for, if fluid remains in the abdominal cavity, it will well up through the track of the tube.

He was unable to see any reason for the opinion expressed that etherization does not produce nephritic congestion. No one doubts that ether is eliminated by the kidneys, and that when given in small amounts it has an active diuretic effect. It is, moreover, a therapeutic fact that all active diuretics, when given in excess, produce nephritic congestion. Scanty secretion of urine, pain in the region of the kidneys, nausea, and cephalalgia not infrequently follow etherization, and these symptoms are usually relieved by increasing the functional activity of the kidneys.

In regard to the method of etherizing, he said that, though the Clover inhaler is theoretically bad, practically it works well. When properly used, not more than two ounces of ether are necessary for the first hour, and frequently one ounce suffices for an operation. The liability to vomit is much lessened when little ether is used, and congestion of the kidneys and air-passages is necessarily much less frequent.

CORRESPONDENCE.

LONDON.

The Annual Meeting of the British Medical Association. The Address of the President. Mr. Lawson Tait's Address. Professor Hamilton on Acid Dyspepsia.

To the Editor of THE MEDICAL NEWS,

SIR: The annual meeting of the British Medical Association has, of course, been overshadowed by the International Congress at Berlin; but, nevertheless, the gathering at Birmingham was one of considerable im-

portance, and deserves some recognition. In the first place, it was evident that the ill-feeling in a certain quarter last year against the Association, which led to the resignation of some seventy members, had not had any permanent damaging effect on the Association. Dr. Wade, one of the oldest practitioners, and certainly the most distinguished physician in Birmingham, was elected President and worthily upheld the dignity and traditions of the office. His address dealt almost entirely with medical education, the important medico-political problem of the day. The General Medical Council has, in its wisdom, decreed that at no very distant date the medical curriculum shall be at least five years, instead of four, as at present, and has proposed a scheme by which the first year shall be entirely devoted to physics, chemistry, biology, etc. Dr. Wade is not quite satisfied with this arrangement, and would like to see two years devoted to the study of the preliminary sciences, as we may call them. He thinks that the study of these subjects should be commenced at the age of fifteen, as by that time a boy has had ample opportunity for a sufficient general education. One difficulty with this plan is that the majority of boys at the age of fifteen have not decided what profession to follow. In cases where they have arrived at this decision, there can be no question that it is greatly to their advantage to begin the study of the sciences at an early age.

As to the main question of what is to be done during the additional year, I am in hopes that the time will be added to the end and not to the beginning of the curriculum, for I am quite sure that our students are much more in need of additional clinical work than of preliminary study, and I would make the extra year count only from the time of passing the final examination. So long as students have an examination before them the majority will make no attempt to learn anything but what is necessary to enable them to scrape through the examination; and it is my firm conviction that the addition of a year at the commencement of the medical curriculum will not make them one whit better practitioners than they are under the present *régime*.

Mr. Lawson Tait, who delivered the Address in Surgery, which, it goes without saying, was both vigorous and practical, denounced very strongly the unpractical character of the teaching of the present day and the enormous amount of time wasted upon the biological training of the modern student. He would like to return to the old system of apprenticeship; but, although many of our leading practitioners of the present time were educated under that *régime*, and are never weary of advocating it, I do not anticipate that it will ever be reintroduced. If a system of apprenticeship at the end of the curriculum could be established, it would, I believe, be of great service.

One of the most important papers read at the meeting was that of Professor Hamilton, of Aberdeen, on "Acid Dyspepsia." His main point was that the disturbance was, in the first instance, one affecting mainly the quantity or the quality of the gastric juice. Variations in the quantity of the hydrochloric acid in the gastric juice are exceedingly common, and it is chiefly on these variations that the symptoms of dyspepsia depend. The second cause arises from a deficiency in the quantity of hydrochloric acid and the formation of lactic acid in excess. Normally, lactic acid is formed in only very minute quantities. So that acid dyspepsia may be the natural consequence of a too abundant formation of hydrochloric acid in the stomach, or of a deficient formation of it; and the recognition of these two forms is, of course, all important in treatment, as it is obvious that they will require different measures.

An active discussion followed Sir Dyce Duckworth's paper on "Functional Disorders of the Heart."

Of course, the social festivities and entertainments were not neglected at this meeting, and the hospitalities of the Mayor and other local celebrities cannot have failed to leave a pleasant recollection on the minds of the twelve hundred members who received them. This is the fourth time that Birmingham has been the meeting-place of the Association; and since its last meeting there, seventeen years ago, the Association has trebled its membership, now including in its roll more than half the practitioners in the United Kingdom.

NEW INVENTIONS.

A NEW SET OF REFRACTION LENSES.

BY H. F. HANSELL, M.D.

I HAVE recently had made a set of test-lenses adapted to the needs of medical men who do not practise ophthalmology as a specialty. It contains comparatively few lenses (50—Natchez 212), yet so arranged that, either singly or in combination, all practical strengths of sphericals and cylinders may be obtained, and all remediable errors of refraction corrected. The advantages are low cost, light weight, and small size; the single disadvantage is the slightly greater expenditure of time necessary in adjusting the lenses, as compared with the larger cases.

The plus and minus spherical lenses are pairs of 0.25 and 0.50, singles of 0.75, 1, 1.50, 2, 3, 4, 8, 13; cylinders, singles of 0.25, 0.50, 0.75, 1, 1.50, 2, 3, 4; prisms, 1°, 2°, 4°, 8°, 20°. The box contains a Natchez frame so modified that it will hold in position four lenses on each side at the same time. The case is made and sold by Borsch & Rommel, 1324 Walnut St., Philadelphia.

NEWS ITEMS.

Examinations for Appointment in the Medical Corps of the United States Army.—An army medical board will be in session in New York City during October, 1890, for the examination of candidates for appointment in the Medical Corps of the United States Army, to fill existing vacancies.

Persons desiring to present themselves for examination by the board will make application to the Secretary of War, before October 1, 1890, for the necessary invitation, stating the date and place of birth, the place and State of permanent residence, the fact of American citizenship, the name of the medical college from whence they were graduated, and a record of service in hospital, if any, from the authorities thereof. The application should be accompanied by certificates based on personal knowledge, from at least two physicians of repute, as to professional standing, character, and moral

habits. The candidate must be between twenty-one and twenty-eight years of age, and a graduate from a regular medical college; as evidence of which, his diploma must be submitted to the board.

Further information regarding the examinations may be obtained by addressing Surgeon-General J. H. Baxter, U. S. Army, Washington, D. C.

Foreign Students in France.—The *Gazette Médicale de Paris* gives the following figures in regard to this question: The foreign students registered in the faculties of medicine for the scholastic year of 1889-90 numbered 908. Of these Paris has 822, made up as follows: 6 Germans, 51 English, 7 Austrians, 7 Belgians, 8 Bulgarians, 34 Spanish, 34 Greeks, 6 Dutch, 12 Italians, 1 Norwegian, 18 Portugese, 85 Roumanians, 261 Russians, 25 Swiss, 71 Turks, 159 Americans, 13 Egyptians, 1 Persian, 1 Australian.

Bordeaux has 17 foreign students, of whom 2 are English, 2 Belgians, 1 American, 1 Egyptian, 5 from Mauritius, 5 from Argentine Republic, and 1 from Cuba.

Lille has 3 foreigners: 1 English and 2 Russians.

Lyons has 8 foreigners, namely, 1 Russian, 2 Swiss, 3 Turks, 2 Egyptian.

Montpelier has 53 foreigners: 2 English, 14 Bulgarians, 3 Spaniards, 7 Greeks, 1 Italian, 2 Roumanians, 4 Russians, 16 Turks, 4 Egyptians.

Nancy has 4 foreigners, namely, 3 German and 1 American.

In *résumé* we have 907 foreign students, as follows: 9 Germans, 56 English, 7 Austrians, 9 Belgians, 22 Bulgarians, 37 Spaniards, 41 Greeks, 6 Dutch, 13 Italians, 1 Norwegian, 18 Portugese, 87 Roumanians, 268 Russians, 27 Swiss, 90 Turks, 161 Americans, 19 Egyptians, 5 Mauritians, 1 Persian, 1 Australian, 5 Argentine Republicans, and 1 Cuban.

American Rhinological Association.—The American Rhinological Association will hold its eighth annual session at Louisville, Ky., October 6, 7, and 8, 1890.

Many subjects relating to nasal and naso-pharyngeal diseases will be opened for discussion by Fellows of the Association. The medical profession is cordially invited to attend.

The Secretary, Dr. S. Knode, Omaha, Nebraska, will furnish any information to physicians desiring to become members.

Dr. John K. Mitchell has returned to Philadelphia after a long absence made necessary by an attack of typhoid fever last autumn, and has moved into a new office at No. 211 South Seventeenth Street.

OFFICIAL LIST OF CHANGES IN THE STATIONS AND DUTIES OF THE MEDICAL CORPS OF THE U. S. NAVY FOR THE WEEK ENDING AUGUST 30, 1890.

HOEHLING, A. A., *Medical Inspector.*—In addition to present duties, ordered as President of Medical Examining Board at Philadelphia, convened by Department Order, June 9, 1890.

KENNEDY, R. M., *Assistant Surgeon.*—In addition to present duty, ordered as member of the above Board.

OGDEN. F. N., *Passed Assistant Surgeon.*—In addition to present duty, ordered as member of the above Board.

MCCLURG, WALTER A., *Surgeon.*—Granted a month's leave of absence from September 1st.

KERSHNER, EDWARD, *Surgeon.*—Granted two weeks' leave of absence from September 1, 1890.

THE MEDICAL NEWS.

A WEEKLY JOURNAL OF MEDICAL SCIENCE.

Vol. LVII.   Saturday, September 13, 1890.   No. 11.

ORIGINAL LECTURES.

REMOVAL OF AN INTRA-LIGAMENTARY CYST.

A Clinical Lecture,
delivered at the Hospital of the University of Pennsylvania.

BY WILLIAM GOODELL, M.D.,
PROFESSOR OF GYNECOLOGY.

[Reported by LEWIS H. ADLER, JR., M.D.,
RESIDENT PHYSICIAN OF THE EPISCOPAL HOSPITAL; LATE RESIDENT
PHYSICIAN OF THE UNIVERSITY HOSPITAL.]

GENTLEMEN: The woman I bring before you this morning is thirty-seven years old. She has been married thirteen years, but has been sterile, and she has a tumor which developed eighteen months ago. Examination shows what seems to be a multiple fibroma of the uterus, together with another abdominal tumor, the nature of which I have not yet determined. The fact that she has uterine fibroids suggests that the growth is fibro-cystic; but, as this is rare, and as the tumors are separated from each other, I am more inclined to think that it is an ovarian growth. If it is fibro-cystic, it is more serious. The strongest reason against its being a fibro-cystic tumor is that there is no increase in the amount of the monthly bleeding. Whatever it is, I propose to cut into the abdominal cavity, in order to see what can be done in the way of removal. The amount of fat in the abdominal walls is small, and this circumstance renders the operation easy.

Just here, whilst the patient is being etherized, allow me to say a few words about the preparation of a patient for an abdominal section.

In the first place, all the emunctories of the body should be active. If the patient has travelled a long distance, rest in bed and tonics are indicated; if the patient is strong, moderate exercise will do no harm. In all these cases a good, substantial, easily-digested diet is required. On the day previous to the operation I order a full dose of castor oil, compound liquorice powder, or Epsom salt, given early in the morning. During the afternoon of the same day, after the patient has had a soap-and-water bath, the abdomen is thoroughly scrubbed, clean clothes are put on, and she goes to bed. In the evening, should there be sleeplessness, some hypnotic should be given, but not opium, as this drug checks both secretion and excretion and tends to nauseate. The morning of the operation the patient is given an enema of soap and water, followed by another bath, and a vaginal douche of bichloride of mercury, 1 to 2000. A carbolized towel is then placed over the abdomen, covered with waxed paper, and retained by a binder.

Our patient now being ready, we will begin the operation. I make the incision in the median line, cutting through skin and fat, with the intention of reaching the linea alba beneath—not always an easy matter, especially when the walls of the belly are not distended. An excellent way to find the linea alba is to pass a grooved director across each rectus muscle, as you see me do here, to the right, and then to the left, and the point of arrest indicates the line. Carefully dissecting through this line, I come to the peritoneum, which lies behind the recti muscles, separated by a cellulo-adipose tissue.

Before opening the peritoneum, hæmorrhage is checked with catch-forceps. I now pick up, with a pair of forceps, the peritoneum, and gently cut through it, taking care not to wound any stray loop of intestine. By inserting two fingers in the opening made, I am enabled, by means of a pair of blunt-pointed scissors, to enlarge the wound to the required extent. I am now in the abdominal cavity and have exposed the wall of the tumor. It is not an ovarian cyst, because it is not nacreous-hued, and besides, it has too great a number of muscular fibres in its walls. It may, however, be an intraligamentary cyst. There is also present some ascitic fluid which must be removed. I think I shall find this to be a tumor covered with the broad ligament.

There are many adhesions, and as I am afraid to break them at once, I shall make the abdominal incision larger so that I may the more readily get at them. These adhesions are upon the transverse colon. None are free, and therefore I must work with extreme care, lest I wound the intestine. There are also other numerous and strong adhesions below, which I try to wipe away with a sponge, but without success.

Now, after working for some time, and with very careful dissection, I have succeeded in enucleating the tumor from the broad ligament. It is an intraligamentary cyst—a variety of tumor that is most difficult to remove. The vessels are now clamped so far as is thought necessary. Other large and most formidable adhesions, extending to—I cannot tell where—make it necessary for me to wash out the cavity of the peritoneum after the operation, because of the escape of clotted blood into the cavity. The tumor is really fastened down by adhesions to the bones of the pelvis behind. As you notice, the patient is greatly emaciated and she has been growing more and more so each day; therefore, without the operation she would have lived but a short time. I do not know yet, as I now take out this tumor, whether it is a uterine or an ovarian tumor. If by any means I open the aorta or vena cava, the patient is done for. Yet I have to run that risk, as I am compelled to work blindly. I am getting along, but it is slow and dangerous work and my heart is in my mouth. I believe now that this is primarily a fibro-cystic tumor, growing from the womb; but the adhesions arising from the posterior bones of the pelvis make its removal especially difficult. It is impossible to break up these adhesions without using force that in this instance would be attended with the greatest danger. At length I have the pedicle separated so that it can be tied. I am very much afraid that this growth is malignant, and, that therefore, the prognosis is not very good—although I have seen patients quite similar to this, recover without a bad symptom, after just such an operation.

The nerve-strain on me in this operation has been fearful. The fear was that I should wound the intestine or a large bloodvessel. I have lost but one patient on the table, though another died fifteen minutes after the operation.

The particulars of the former case were as follows: I had to go to a town a short distance from Philadelphia, and while there was asked to see a school-mistress who was suffering with vomiting and constipation. She had also two abdominal tumors, and investigation showed that there was a stricture of the rectum. I left directions for the stricture to be dilated, and when I returned, the patient having in the meantime been placed upon tonics and nutrient food, I operated. Unfortunately the etherizer became too much engrossed in my part of the work, as this was the first operation of the kind that he had seen. Both tumors were removed; but the patient died on the table from sheer exhaustion; and, as no one of the other physicians was willing to tell the family of this, it became my sad duty to do so. One of the assisting physicians had diabetes mellitus; the shock to his nervous system was so great that he never fully recovered from it. Every precaution was taken, but without avail. Finally, he tried a change of climate, but this too was a failure, and he died a few months later. This was the sequel to the case. But to return to the accident. The news of it spread through the town like wildfire and everybody wanted to have the minutiæ of it explained to them. I was exceedingly anxious to get home as soon as possible, but found to my horror that there was no regular train until the next day. Fortunately there was an express that passed there in the afternoon, and by telegraphing to headquarters, I got permission to stop this train. I was exceedingly thankful to get away, but, to my discomfiture, when I got on the cars I found that two of the townsmen got on with me, that they knew of the circumstance, and that I had to entertain them with a rehearsal of the details on the way to Philadelphia.

Now to return to the present tumor. There is either a piece left on the sigmoid flexure of the colon, or there is upon that viscus an independent tumor which it is impossible to remove, as it completely encircles the intestine. There is some deep-seated bleeding; and though, as a rule, I would rather tie the vessels than use Paquelin's cautery, I have to use the cautery here. I do not hesitate to touch the bleeding points on the intestines and on the back of the womb. I remove the left ovary and tube also, and the fact of their being separate from the other tumor proves the growth to be fibro-cystic. I now carefully smell the abdominal cavity to learn whether there is any fæcal odor. There is none. If fæcal odor were present, of course it would indicate that there had been an intestinal wound with extravasation. This would necessitate the discovery and closure of the opening. There is still some bleeding going on within the abdominal cavity, and I will attempt to control it by what I am pleased to call the "toilet of the peritoneum," for which purpose I use a clean Davidson's syringe and hot carbolized water. When the water returns perfectly clear I know that the peritoneal cavity is

free from blood and clean. Thoroughly draining the abdomen of all fluid, I close the incision; but before doing this I place a clean sponge in Douglas's pouch, another in the sulcus between the bladder and the womb, and a third (large, broad and flat) over the intestines under the wound to catch the blood that may ooze from the cut surfaces.

The sutures have a needle upon each end—which allows them to be passed from within outward. Each needle is inserted about a quarter of an inch away from the edge of the wound, and it is well to include in the sutures all the layers of the parietes—cutaneous, muscular, aponeurotic, and peritoneal. I would lay especial stress on including the muscular layer, although many ovariotomists think that by so doing abscesses in the recti muscles are apt to follow in the suture-tracks. But it seems to me that it is better to run the risk of a stitch-abscess than the more serious and grave one of ventral hernia.

Having inserted all the sutures, I remove the sponges from the abdomen, and am rejoiced to find that there is scarcely any blood on them. This tells me that there is but little bleeding from the sutures or from the abdominal cavity itself. I now count my instruments and sponges, and find the number correct, and then close the incision without having to use a drainage-tube.

My method for closing the wound is by grasping in one hand all the sutures on my side, while my assistant does the same upon the opposite side; thus the edges of the wound are brought firmly together, and at the same time all air is expelled from the abdominal cavity. Each suture is then tied with the surgeon's knot. The entire wound being closed, the ends of the sutures are gathered together and cut off several inches from the knots. The wound is dressed with the usual antiseptic precautions: First, it is thoroughly cleansed and dried; next iodoform is freely sprinkled over the surface of the abdomen, and particularly into the umbilicus; then several layers of carbolized gauze are placed over the wound, and over the gauze adhesive strips of rubber plaster are fastened; last of all comes a wad of cotton-wool which has been thoroughly baked in order to destroy all germs. This is held in place by a flannel binder.

I shall now give the patient a suppository of opium, not only to soothe the pain, but especially as a nerve stimulant; because her peritoneal cavity was open for more than an hour and there were numerous adhesions, perhaps later she may require another suppository.

The after-treatment will consist in keeping the patient on her back, and without food for twenty-four hours. Hot cans will be applied to the body, care being taken that they do not come in too close contact with the skin, as the burns which they make are unusually severe. She will be allowed to see no one but the physicians and the nurse for several days, as absolute quietness must be observed.

Should obstinate vomiting occur, ice will be given or sinapisms applied to the epigastrium. If there is much flatulence, it will be relieved by inserting a flexible catheter high up into the rectum, or by enemata of turpentine, soap and water.

As a rule, it is necessary to catheterize for a day or so after the operation, but it should be avoided if possible, as the too frequent use of the instrument is likely to cause an irritable bladder that is slow to respond to treatment.

On the second day we will give half an ounce of milk every two hours, gradually increasing the quantity as her condition demands it.

If her temperature should reach 101° or over, ice will be applied to the head, the body sponged, a saline cathartic given, or some antipyretic administered.

On the fourth or the fifth day the bowels will be freely opened with castor oil, or compound licorice powder. If these fail to act, they will be supplemented by an enema.

In from seven to nine days the dressing will be ready to be removed and the stitches will be taken out.

ORIGINAL ARTICLES.

PROGNOSIS IN PULMONARY TUBERCULOSIS.

Based upon an Analysis of Five Hundred and Fifteen Cases.[1]

BY KARL VON RUCK, B.S., M.D.,
DIRECTOR OF THE SANITARIUM FOR DISEASES OF THE LUNGS AND
THROAT, ASHEVILLE, S. C.; MEMBER OF THE AMERICAN CLIMA-
TOLOGICAL ASSOCIATION, THE AMERICAN MEDICAL
ASSOCIATION, ETC.

IF I should state that of 515 cases of pulmonary tuberculosis 59 recovered and 65 showed material and lasting improvement, and that the percentage of recoveries was eleven and a fraction, such statement would aid but little in the prognosis of a given case, and also would be unreliable as to the necessary mortality of cases, unless all of them came under treatment and observation at the same stage of the disease and remained under the same conditions until the outcome was determined. Should I endeavor to base a prognosis upon the first 181 cases of my series, in which there were but 3 recoveries, I might well doubt my diagnoses, and take it for granted that in these 3 cases my senses deceived me, and that the disease was always fatal.

Statistics based upon the diagnosis of tuberculosis previously to 1883, or upon cases in which bacilli were not invariably demonstrated, would, in all probability, include some cases of non-bacillary disease. My deductions are based upon cases in which the microscopical diagnosis was clear, which have been under my own observation, and of which I have not only the histories and records while under my care, but have also been able to ascertain the course of the disease up to the date of my inquiry, by direct and indirect communications with patients and their friends, or their physicians. I take this opportunity to express my thanks to the physicians to whom I frequently appealed for careful replies, without which the number of cases available for classification would be much smaller. I hope that the vast

[1] Read before the Buncombe County Medical Society, Asheville, N. C., July 7, 1890.

amount of labor involved in correspondence and detailed inquiries may be justified by a more ready appreciation of the various points which bear upon prognosis directly or indirectly, and perhaps by the adoption of means, or avoidance of influences, which appear to affect the course of the disease.

It may be well to explain here my meaning when speaking of *improved* or *recovered* cases. Under the former I include all patients in whom general and local improvement lasted for a number of months, the temperature, as a rule, not exceeding 100° F. ; who gained in flesh and strength and were able to resume their vocations ; in whom cough and expectoration were materially diminished, but still present at the time of their discharge, and who, as far as ascertainable, still show tubercle bacilli in the sputum. (In some of these cases sputum examinations have not been made for several years; some sent me specimens by mail ; others had examinations made at home.)

As *recovered* cases, I report those in which all local and general symptoms have disappeared, no active symptoms having been present for six months or more ; cough and expectoration having nearly or quite ceased, with continued absence of bacilli in the sputum, if slight expectoration still exist. A number of the improved cases could have been included among the recovered were it not for the bacilli which still appear in the slight expectoration.

The following table shows the influence of age and the general mortality of my cases. Among the fatal cases I have also included patients who are still alive, but who are growing worse, and in whom the termination will probably be fatal :

Age.	Total number of cases.	Number that have died or are growing worse.	Per cent.	Improved and are still doing well.	Per cent.	Recovered.	Per cent.
5 to 15	5	5	100	0		0	
15 " 20	24	22	91.6	1	4.2	1	4.2
20 " 30	186	153	82.2	16	8.6	17	10.5
30 " 40	216	152	70.4	39	18.0	25	12.0[1]
40 " 50	67	46	68.6	7	10.4	14	20.8
50 " 60	16	12	75.0	2	12.5	2	12.5[1]
60 " 70	1	1	100	0		0	
Total,	515	391	76	65	12.5	59	11.5

The influence of age.—Of the 391 cases who died or have become hopelessly advanced in the disease, there are 223, or 57 per cent., who, at one time, while under my care, showed somewhat encouraging improvement ; 67 of these to such an extent that permanent arrest seemed probable. In these 67 cases (38 per cent.) the relapses were, with few exceptions, due to preventable causes—as a rule, to

[1] One of the recovered cases that died of other disease.

the too early abandonment of climatic and general treatment, obstinately continued over-exertion, or to imprudent exposures. In 8 cases the relapse was clearly referable to epidemic influenza. The latter disease also caused serious relapses in several cases in which the disease was nearly arrested. Four cases that I had considered as cured I have excluded from my report of recovered cases, as I am unable to determine the exact nature of the lung disease which accompanied the influenza, and which continned until death, the patient not being under my care at the time, and microscopical examinations of the sputum not having been made by the attending physicians.

The apparent influence of age upon prognosis is shown by the table to be favorable in proportion to the number of years up to fifty, after which the effects of advancing age seem to influence the prognosis somewhat adversely. The number below twenty years and above fifty is, however, so small that no conclusions are really justifiable.

The influence of sex.—Of the 515 cases, 290 were males, of whom 212, or 73.2 per cent., died or have grown worse ; 38, or 13 per cent., improved ; and 40, or 13.8 per cent., recovered. Of females, there were 225, of whom 179, or 79.6 per cent., died or have grown worse ; 27, or 12 per cent., improved ; and 19, or 8.5 per cent., recovered. If, however, of female patients we include only those between the ages of fifteen and forty years, we find that the dead and hopeless cases amount to 85.3 per cent., with improvement in 9 per cent., and recovery in 6 per cent. Furthermore, I find that the climacteric period furnished a proportionally larger number of female patients, as compared with men of the same age. Of the 67 patients, between the ages of forty and fifty years, the number of females was 41, or 61 per cent., whereas male patients predominate during every other period, except that between ten and twenty years, where females again are in the proportion of 18 to 12, or 68 per cent. This may be coincidence, especially with some cases that were treated at my institution, or at a distance from their home, yet it seems reasonable that the two great epochs, puberty and the climacteric, especially if complications incident to these periods exist, may lead to nutritive disturbances, such as chlorosis and anæmia, and thereby predispose the individual more strongly to infection.

Whereas all the female patients between the ages of ten and twenty years, died or became hopeless cases, the 41 cases, between forty and fifty years, furnish the largest percentage of recoveries, being 10 recoveries, or 25 per cent., against 4 recoveries, or 15.4 per cent., in males of the same age. In 33 of these 41 female patients, menstruation had permanently ceased when they came under my care.

I have frequently noticed that female patients are apt to lose ground during the menstrual week, and this often in the absence of any special disturbance of their menstrual function. Fever if absent is apt to return, and if fever has been present it is several degrees higher, for a day or two, immediately preceding the menstrual flow. If the period is entirely missed or is delayed the increased temperature has often been observed to continue throughout the time corresponding to the menstrual week. In addition, increased cough, diminished appetite, and digestive disturbances, are frequent, and a loss of several pounds in weight has been noticed in a number of such cases who had been gaining. When such disturbances are repeated monthly they interfere, sometimes quite seriously, with the favorable progress of a case, and must to some extent influence the prognosis.

The occurrence of pregnancy, during any stage of pulmonary tuberculosis, renders the prognosis serious, even in an otherwise favorable case. Of my 225 cases, 13 became pregnant during the earlier stage of the disease ; all went to term and were delivered of apparently healthy children ; in all active symptoms returned or increased within nine weeks after delivery ; in 4 marked temporary improvement again occurred, 12 died, and 1, otherwise a very favorable case, recovered.

It would, therefore, appear that in the female the prognosis is less favorable if her menstrual function be accompanied by the disturbances that are mentioned above, and more favorable if the climacteric period has been passed.

The influence of heredity.—There are few practising physicians who will be convinced by the laboratory student that hereditary influences have nothing to do with the etiology of tuberculosis and that the acquirement of the disease is accidental. I not only feel absolutely convinced that heredity is an indirect factor in the acquirement of tubercular disease, but it appears also from my records that *the prognosis in such cases is much less favorable.*

No one to-day maintains that heredity means the transmission of the morbific agent which causes the disease. Those who believe that heredity is a factor claim, on clinical grounds, that the subjects of such heredity furnish a larger proportion of cases of pulmonary tuberculosis than those with no inherited tendency, and that had heredity no influence in causing the disease, the number of cases should be the same in those who have and those who have not a consumptive family history.

Among 100 interrogations from patients with phthisis (casually made as I had opportunity and in a locality where phthisis is prevalent) I received 88 negative answers, as to the disease having been present in their respective families. Granting, however, that such a history could be shown in 18 per cent. of the entire population, why is it that more than twice this percentage of tubercular patients show such a history? It is generally accepted that parents transmit physical and often mental peculiarities to their children, why not believe that diseased, weakly and constitutionally depraved individuals should produce weak offspring? We require no predisposition of tissues, only a generally depressed and weak constitution, which causes the organism to be deficient in its nutritive processes, in its force-producing, injury-resisting, and repairing powers, as compared with individuals who have no such heritage.

Observing physicians believe that such people have little power to resist, and readily become victims to tubercular infection. This would be still more probable if such persons also inherited, or acquired by faulty development, a phthisical thorax, a small heart, a tendency to glandular enlargement, etc., all of which would lead to nutritive disturbances in general and of the lungs in particular. The non-resistance of such persons is only relative. In the cases of acute miliary tuberculosis, or acute phthisis, in which, at least after infection has taken place, non-resistance to the progress of the disease is apparent. In other people the resisting power may be more or less, according to their individuality; all being influenced for the time being by the various conditions of general health, and the intactness of the part in which the infecting germs lodge. I do not believe that any human being possesses an absolute immunity from infection and I have no doubt that if enough of the tubercle bacilli find entrance into the organism, no matter by what avenue, infection will result. The behavior of the infected organism toward the progress of the disease, and in repairing the damage done, may, however, be very different in the constitutionally strong than in those who are predisposed in the sense that I have explained. Speaking for myself as a strong believer in hereditary predisposition, and in a larger sense than the term is generally applied, I would be most unwilling to inhale even the smallest number of tubercle bacilli, although I am in no sense predisposed to infection.

According to my understanding, the predisposition by heredity need not be the result of phthisical disease of the ancestors, which I have termed *direct hereditary predisposition.* Want of resisting power in the offspring may be the result of a variety of conditions, under which the parents produced a child that easily succumbs to various causes : but if it lives long enough and if circumstances are favorable, it falls a victim to tubercular infection. This I have termed *indirect hereditary predisposition.*

In my 515 cases the question of heredity was

11*

fully answered and recorded 501 times—in 14 cases the patients knew so little of their family history that they could not be satisfactorily classified.

Direct hereditary predisposition (phthisical family history) was shown to have existed 202 times as follows :

From the father's side alone in . . 51 cases.
From the mother's side alone in . 80 "
From both parents in . . . 11 "
From father and grandfather alone in 12 "
From mother and grandmother alone in 20
From both parents and both grandparents in . . . . . 3 "
From grandfather alone (skipped one generation) in . . . . 8 "
From grandmother alone (skipped one generation) in . . . . . 17 "

Total, 202 cases, or 39.2 per cent. of all.

As may be seen, the mother and grandmother seemed to transmit a predisposition most frequently. The possibility of this was present in 131 and is evident in 117 cases, whereas on the part of father and grandfather it was possible in 85 and evident in only 71 cases.

Indirect hereditary predisposition could be shown in 217 cases, or 42.3 per cent., as follows:

(*a*) Ninety-two cases were children, the sixth or later in large families, often born in rapid succession, none of the older children having acquired the disease ; but in 26 cases younger brothers or sisters were also suffering from or had died of phthisis. The history of these patients was almost without exception that they had been less strong and robust than the older children, or had been sick from various causes a great part of their lives.

(*b*) Twenty-two cases were either one of twins, or the mother had given birth within a year previously to another child. In these cases again, the tubercular patient had nearly always been the weaker one, and delicate from childhood. In two instances the other twin had already died of phthisis.

(*c*) In 59 cases one or both parents were suffering from impaired general health at the time of conception or during pregnancy—chronic diarrhœa, chronic dyspepsia, cancer, syphilis, disease of the genito-urinary organs, uterine disease, etc. There were also histories of sickness or death of brothers or sisters from meningitis (tubercular?), chronic disease of joints, rickets, spinal disease, scrofula, etc. In 14 cases death in the family from measles and whooping-cough was stated to have occurred, and 28 patients gave a history of scrofula in childhood. In 19 cases brothers or sisters were suffering from or had died of phthisis.

(*d*) Forty-four cases gave as part of their histories, that one or both parents were suffering from severe nervous disease previously to the birth of the patient, including insanity, paralysis, locomotor ataxia, and epilepsy. In 9 instances brothers or sisters were or had been suffering from epilepsy or from chorea; in 8, brothers or sisters were suffering or had died from phthisis.

In 78 of these 217 cases the so-called phthisical habitus was noted, although no phthisical history was present, against 136 in the 202 cases in which direct hereditary predisposition was shown.

Considering, now, these 217 cases, their percentage and the circumstances under which the patients were born, is it surprising that such persons have acquired a depraved constitution, or a predisposition to fall more readily victims to disease?

Is it not reasonable to suppose that the minimum amount of infecting material which in such cases would produce phthisis, would be resisted and overcome by stronger persons coming of a better stock?

There remain now 96 cases in which the family history was good, both as to direct and to indirect predisposition, and in which the health was, as a rule, good from infancy. In these we can believe that either they received a sufficiently large dose of infecting material, that such infecting material was of unusual virulency, to which their relative good resisting-power was inadequate, or that they had become temporarily predisposed. In 56 cases the health was said to be good to the time of the development of phthisis; in 4 the disease followed typhoid fever; in 3 croupous pneumonia; in 8 catarrhal pneumonia; in 5 childbirth; in 1 puerperal fever; in 3 peritonitis; in 1 acute pleurisy; and in 1 measles. The others, as most tubercular patients do, ascribed as a cause "catching cold," by which, perhaps, we should understand "catching tubercular infection."

To show the influence on prognosis of direct, indirect, or no hereditary predisposition, we find from an analysis of my cases that the prognosis does not materially differ, whether direct or indirect predisposition existed. But I was much surprised to find that when hereditary predisposition was absent, six times as many recovered. I have gone over these cases again and again to prove that no error is present; each time with the same result. I then divided the cases into groups according to the years of their occurrence, again with practically the same result.

Table showing the Influence of Heredity upon Prognosis.

	Grouped under.	Number of Cases.	Recoveries.	Per Cent.
I. Direct hereditary predisposition (family history of phthisis),		202	9	4.5
II. Indirect hereditary predisposition,	a	92	6	6.5
" " "	b	22	1	4.5
" " "	c	59	3	5
" " "	d	44	3	7
III. No hereditary predisposition,		96	37	37.6

In view of this extraordinary showing, it is very desirable that other observers consult their records, or make proper inquiry hereafter, and publish their results. This will show whether my results are correct or incorrect. For such inquiries a systematically arranged series of questions is absolutely necessary. It is essential that the patient should understand that a full statement of the facts, even if it is necessary to make inquiry of friends, has a most important bearing on their individual case.

The influence of the stage of the disease.—Of course the earlier a case, which is susceptible of improvement, comes under proper treatment and management, the better will be the outlook, and no statistical evidence is required to prove this self-evident proposition. Of the 515 cases, 81 were classed as in an early stage and 434 in an advanced stage. Of the 81 early cases, 11 remained under treatment for so short a time that no material change could be expected; 34, or 55.5 per cent., showed improvement and then relapsed, as a rule from causes within their control —all these have since grown hopeless or died; 17 cases, or 21 per cent., are improved, and 20 cases, or 24 per cent., have recovered. Of the 434 advanced cases the disease progressed without material improvement in 125, or 29 per cent.; improvement more or less temporary occurred in 189, or 43.5 per cent.—all relapsed, many from preventable causes, and have grown worse or have died. Marked improvement with prospective arrest of the disease occurred in 33, or 7½ per cent.; all these have relapsed, often from causes within their control, and have grown worse or died; 48, or 11 per cent., of the cases still remain much improved, and 39, or 9 per cent., have recovered. From a scrutiny of these results it is apparent that had an ideal course been pursued in all cases, many more recoveries would have resulted. The fact is, that such a course was pursued only exceptionally. Taking the improved and recovered cases together we have in the early stage 45 per cent. and in the advanced stages 20 per cent. Of the 515 cases there were three females and one male in whom, although they came under observation early, the disease followed a rapidly fatal course—all deaths occurred within four months. Every effort seemed unavailing to cause even a temporary halt. Aside from the slower course of these cases they differed clinically from acute miliary tuberculosis, in that pulmonary symptoms were more prominent, and the stage of breaking-down and excavation was reached. Physical examination showed the evidence of diffused bronchitis, with many small areas where the respiratory murmur resembled the bronchial. Very little change in the percussion-note was manifest.

In one case the infection could be traced to a cut upon the finger of the left hand, which became inflamed, as did the lymphatics of the arm, and was soon followed by a glandular swelling in the axilla. The general health began to fail after this and before any attention was attracted to the lungs. The patient and her friends, I was told, had obstinately refused to have the swelling incised, though the tubercular character of this was not suspected. The case came to me with this history and a cough, supposed to be bronchitis, which had existed for three months. The slightly-fluctuating, enlarged gland was still noticeable. The patient died ten days later.

Although I could find no source for infection through the blood in the other three cases, I cannot but believe that it must have existed. They all pursued almost an identical course, and the diffused tubercular deposits with numerous broncho-pneumonic centres throughout both lungs were characteristic of all.

The extent of lung tissue involved in any stage necessarily influences prognosis. Under proper management further involvement of the healthy tissue of other lobes, and especially of the opposite lung, as long as general infection has not occurred, can, as a rule, be prevented. The bacilli having no independent motion must probably be first expectorated to reach with the inspired air healthy parts of the lung, though further infection may also occur by the gravitation of the secretions. For this reason it is important that an already infected case does not inhale more bacilli, and one of the first conditions of proper management is so to take care of the excretions, and especially of the expectoration, that the danger from this source may be reduced to a minimum. The tendency to extensive destructive processes without connective-tissue repair, which determines the formation of cavities, and with the latter an increased liability to severe arterial hæmorrhages, and to long-continued suppuration from the walls, with the attending danger of septic absorption and amyloid degeneration of other organs, influences the prognosis very much. But the mere fact that a cavity exists does not necessarily cloud the prognosis, if the cavity is of moderate size and located favorably. It is then of more importance to determine the presence of still active disease and its extent, and whether the cavity is secreting and enlarging, or is dry with a tendency to cicatrize and to become obliterated or lined with smooth, fibrous wall. If there is cicatrization the patient has passed through the critical period of softening and suppuration, and he may continue upon a course of uninterrupted improvement. Large cavities in the lower portions of the upper lobe, and those in the lower lobes, or those that for any reason have an imperfect outlet, are apt to remain inflamed, to secrete profusely, and to discharge irregularly. Such cavities frequently continue to enlarge by progressive breaking-down of

their walls and to cause exhaustion, particularly if there is much fever.

The influence of the digestive organs.—As long as a fair degree of digestive power and of assimilation of food can be maintained, and if the disease is not hopelessly advanced, we should not despair. On the other hand, it matters little how how many encouraging signs we may see in a case ; unless we can keep up the nutrition our efforts must ultimately prove fruitless. Many cases acquire gastric and intestinal disturbances by the injudicious use of alcoholics and improper food, and by the use of drugs and patent medicines, especially those which contain opiates. There is also a tendency to sympathetic functional disturbances, especially of the stomach. All such disturbances can, as a rule, be controlled by a proper regimen. If, however, structural disease of the digestive organs exists, be it due to the abuse of alcohol, or to long-continued gastric catarrh from other causes ; if we have reason to suspect amyloid disease of the vessels of the intestines, of the liver or of the spleen ; if we have fatty liver, or tubercular disease of the biliary passages or of the intestine, we cannot hope to nourish our patient thoroughly. In several cases in which I had the opportunity of seeing the results of autopsies upon patients who had followed the so-called "whiskey cure," I was not surprised at my failure to improve the nutrition. There was atrophy of the gastric glands in one case, with dilatation of the pylorus. In another case the stomach was in a state of severe catarrhal inflammation.

Of functional disturbances none has resisted efforts for permanent relief so obstinately as gastric and intestinal accumulations of gas. In mild cases I have succeeded well enough with diet and the administration of salol ; but I have had a number of cases in which all measures failed, and the distress occasioned, as well as the interference with the absorption of food, seemed to hasten materially the downward course of the patients. I could not believe that the gas was due to fermentation, but rather attributed it to non-absorption by the intestinal mucous membrane. Occasional watery stools were also present and some slight fullness of the right side of the heart, with variable increase in the size of the liver. The distress was least after maintaining the recumbent position for a number of hours, causing me to suspect that the abdominal viscera were in a state of passive congestion, which interfered with absorption. In neither of these cases was there any improvement.

Purely functional disturbances of the digestive organs frequently accompany the initial stage of the disease, and simulating dyspepsia they divert the attention from the real cause. Much time may be lost by treating the dyspepsia alone, and harm may be done by restricting the diet, frequently to artificial food-products, which are poor substitutes at all times. Such conditions if improperly managed cause rapid advance of the lung affection, and require forced feeding with milk, eggs, light meats, and especially with vegetables, in small quantities frequently repeated, to be increased by fats after some improvement has been made. Among medicinal agents creasote, bitter tonics, and wines have seemed beneficial.

There are cases that seem to have no disturbance of their digestive organs and have a good appetite, and yet gain nothing in weight or even continue to lose. Upon inquiry it is found that these cases have daily two to three large evacuations. In such cases if the nutrition is not improved by giving less food and by administering it in frequently repeated, small quantities, the prognosis is unfavorable.

Slight peptonuria, demonstrated by Ehrlich's method, has been noted in a number of cases of recent date, no tests having been made in my earlier cases; profuse and continued peptonuria was found only in rapidly progressing and ultimately fatal cases.

Absolute increase in the amount of urates and uric acid I have frequently seen. It is probably due to diminished oxygenation by obstruction and increased venous tension, diminished respiratory surface, and diminution of red corpuscles. Such patients for the time lost flesh. If this condition could not be relieved by inhalations of oxygen in large quantities, and if it persisted, it affected the prognosis unfavorably.

The influence of fever, cough, and expectoration.— Fever, cough, and expectoration are common to all cases of pulmonary tuberculosis. It is their intensity and persistency rather than their presence which influence prognosis. In considering them we should also consider the stage of the disease, the previous management, and the deportment of the patient. The fever, in a case under proper management, and when indiscretions of the patient are excluded, pretty clearly reflects by its amount, the activity and extent of pathological processes at the seat of the disease, and reaches, as a rule, its maximum during the stage of softening, absorption, and excavation. If during that period it is moderate, if areas of softening are small and circumscribed, and if we have one lung or a considerable portion of both lungs unaffected, we need not despair. It is a nice question of judgment to estimate the probable duration of this stage. If the patient's nutrition is still fairly good, and if we succeed in preventing serious loss of flesh, or, better still, if he should show a slight gain, we have good reason to believe that the process will remain circumscribed, that tissue-repair will probably take place, or that the cavities will be small

and speedily made, and that the patient will pass safely through this stage. After this, improvement will follow. Such has been my experience with the cases I am considering. When large areas are involved, when the temperature rises very high and becomes several degrees subnormal, once, and occasionally twice in twenty-four hours, and if the rise is accompanied with a distinct chill, it is not often that the patient's nutrition can be kept up, and, as a rule, the stage is indefinitely prolonged, and leads to a fatal result. Afebrile periods usually correspond to periods of improvement.

The cough bears a certain relation to the fever, and unless due to non-specific bronchitis is not often troublesome in cases in which the temperature is below 100° F., if over-exertion and fatigue are avoided.

The cases in which the bronchial mucous membrane was extensively involved—the so-called broncho-pneumonias—usually ran their course with higher temperatures, and in these the cough was most severe and exhausting, yielding to nothing short of opiates. The intensity of the cough, its interference with rest, and the effects of opiates on the patient, certainly influenced the prognosis, which appeared, however, always less favorable in the broncho-pneumonic form of the disease. Cough due to catarrhal states of the upper air-passages, or to the symptomatic catarrhal bronchitis, yielded, as a rule, to proper local treatment by inhalations, etc., and did not affect the prognosis.

The quantity and quality of expectoration stand in intimate relation to the stage of the disease. Bloody sputa in the early stage betoken inflammatory changes and extensions; later the sputum comes from ulcerated, inflamed, or congested cavities, especially when the patient has over-exerted himself. The color of the expectorated blood depends upon the time it remained upon the respiratory surfaces; it is, therefore, an aid to diagnosis, but only indirectly of prognostic significance. Purely purulent sputa is rare in phthisis, and belongs to abscess or empyema. A muco-purulent character is the rule, and it is greatest in quantity during the stage of softening and excavation. Cheesy particles in the sputum come from recent cavities; sand-like or calcareous concretions from old inspissated, purulent, or cheesy deposits, or degenerated bronchial glands. They have no special prognostic significance, except that their presence in the lung is likely to cause suppuration until the particles are expelled.

It has been thought that the number and form of the tubercle bacilli in the expectoration could be made a basis for estimating the intensity of the pathological process and for prognosis. I, too, have endeavored to draw some inferences, but offer my conclusions with some diffidence, and shall be glad to be corrected if I am wrong. It has seemed to me that I am not mistaken. I realize, of course, that the number of bacilli varies greatly, as we select for examination a cheesy particle or one of only muco-pus. To avoid this source of error I have used various expedients which I need not mention in detail, the object being to get a uniform specimen, and I find that I can obtain a pretty equal distribution of the bacilli upon the prepared cover-glasses. If now, repeated examinations showed a steady decrease in the number of the bacilli until finally but a few and occasionally none were found, and especially if the bacilli were very small and thin, and if the peculiar effect in staining, believed to be due to the presence of spores, was absent or but rarely noted, the specimen came from a case that was improving in general health, and in the local conditions, in every instance. In cases running an unfavorable or indifferent course no such results were observed.

The influence of the pulse.—Many of my predisposed cases, in fact almost all of them, showed a much increased pulse-rate, as is common in phthisis, even in the absence of fever, and when the latter was present the frequency of the pulse was usually out of proportion to the temperature. A congenitally small heart, which was frequently associated, does not show compensatory hypertrophy when obstruction exists in the lesser circulation, if fever and other nutritive disturbances are present. Even a heart of normal size soon shows the results of such injurious conditions by a less perfectly filled radial artery and a more frequent pulse-rate. The auspicious cases had a comparatively slow pulse, and when fever was absent the pulse-rate approached the normal. This was observed in all my greatly improved and recovered cases.

The influence of concomitant tubercular disease in the upper air-passages.—In 81 cases, in the early stage of phthisis, tubercular laryngitis was present in 5 only. In the 434 advanced cases it was noted 111 times. I propose to make these cases a special study in the future, especially with a view to show the effects of various modes of treatment according to the extent, location, and stage of the lung affection when the disease of the larynx made its appearance. I may say here that in the majority of cases no results were obtainable from treatment as long as the lung disease was progressive, but in 2 cases in an early stage, and in 10 in an advanced stage, complete cicatrization occurred. These 12 cases still belong to the improved or recovered cases. No case recovered in which the ulcerative and destructive processes were extensive. The epiglottis was seriously involved in 19 cases, none of which recovered. The painful deglutition seriously interfered with nutrition, and the severe paroxysms of cough, too, tended to exhaust the patients, who were nearly all in the last stages. In only 1 case was the pharynx the seat of tubercular disease, and this case also had a small tubercular ulcer of the tongue, with, however, but slight pulmonary deposit; the patient did not improve, but is still alive.

The influence of pulmonary hæmorrhage.—I notice a material difference between the frequency of pulmonary hæmorrhage in my patients in private practice and in those treated in my institution. In the former it occurred in about one-third of all cases; in the latter, in less than one per cent. Besides the anatomical changes which make hæmorrhage possible, over-exertion nearly always preceded it in the cases in private practice and in every case in my institution. In the early stages the hæmorrhage is moderate, results from inflammatory changes, and is simply a diapedesis. In the latter stages moderate hæmorrhage comes from granulating cavities; when severe, it is arterial, and due to the rupture of sacculated or degenerated and still pervious vessels in the cavities. In estimating the effect upon the future course of the disease we must consider the presence or absence of the various other factors which enter into the prognosis. Even a slight hæmorrhage is at least a temporary hindrance to favorable progress, excluding the exceptional cases in which cough and other symptoms are relieved by the local bleeding of a congested area. But tubercular patients can ill afford the loss of blood even in small quantities. The necessary confinement and the loss of blood itself must certainly, for the time being, check further improvement. If treated by all sorts of mineral and vegetable astringents, ergot, etc., given by the mouth, and if the patient is kept on a diet of ice pills and, perhaps, a few spoonfuls of milk or broth, the loss in nutrition is a further hindrance. Profuse hæmorrhage, especially if repeated, leads to rapid exhaustion, and may terminate a case abruptly by suffocation.

The effect of pleurisy.—Pleurisy, if dry and circumscribed, did not influence the prognosis. Indeed, pleurisy may be conservative by causing thickening and adhesive inflammation over cavities which might otherwise perforate and lead to pneumothorax, a complication which is the beginning of the end. Simple pleurisy, with serous effusion occurred in 5 of my cases, and did not seem to exert any material influence upon the subsequent course of the disease, except that the patients lost flesh and strength during their confinement. Tubercular pleurisy, as a complication, has been recovered from in but 2 of my cases; in these the effusion subsequently became purulent, and required resection of a rib. For a time after the operation the patients improved remarkably, but were then lost from observation, and have since died.

The influence of nasal stenosis. — In 483, or 90 per cent. of cases, catarrhal affections of the nose and throat were present, and there was evidence that they had preceded the lung disease in the great majority of cases. In 221 cases the catarrh was associated with nasal obstruction from turbinated hypertrophies, polypoid growths, septal thickenings, deviations and excrescences that markedly interfered with free respiration through the nose, especially at night; but often during the day also, the patients were obliged to breathe with the mouth open when taking exercise. To what extent these conditions may have favored the deep inhalation of infecting bacilli I cannot here consider, but I am sure that nasal stenosis frequently interfered with improvement, which in many cases occurred only after the obstruction had been removed by proper treatment.

The influence of rectal fistula and peri-rectal abscesses. — Rectal fistula was noted in 27 cases. In 3 cases in the early stage I operated successfully, and 2 of these finally recovered; 24 cases were in an advanced stage of the disease; 1 of these recovered and was subsequently operated on at home. In neither of the other cases was an operation attempted, nor did the fistulæ seem to exert any influence on the disease, though they were an annoyance, frequently became inflamed, and discharged continuously. Small peri-rectal abscesses I have observed more frequently, but have not always kept a record of their occurrence. In all but 4 cases they were immediately incised when discovered, and healed kindly. In the 4 cases in which incision was delayed by the patient neglecting to call attention to the swelling, fistula resulted. In several of such cases tubercle bacilli were found in the pus.

In conclusion, the personal hygiene and the healthful environments of patients; their steadfastness of purpose and determination; their own proper estimation of the importance of early measures and of implicit compliance with advice; their willingness to make necessary sacrifices, and also the painstaking management of the physician in charge, and his ability to prevent even slight complications, all exert influences which are none the less real or important because their effects are an unknown quantity.

SELECTED SURGICAL CASES.[1]

BY DONALD MACLEAN, M.D.,
OF DETROIT, MICH.

THE following cases have been selected for presentation in the hope that, whether regarded from a theoretical or a practical standpoint, they may be deemed worthy of consideration. They will be de-

[1] Read before the Surgical Section of the Michigan State Medical Society, at Grand Rapids, June 19, 1890.

tailed with as much brevity as is consistent with intelligibility.

I desire to call attention here to the value of subcutaneous section of the anterior annular ligament of the wrist, and to a similar operation in the neighborhood of the ankle-joint, especially for the relief of the condition known as compound ganglion. In a communication presented to the American Surgical Association in 1885, I invited attention to this subject, and reported a number of characteristic cases occurring in my own experience. Since that paper was published I have had numerous opportunities to test the value of this method; moreover, I have come to believe that this simple procedure is of great value in other conditions besides the one referred to.

In rapid and violent inflammations involving the tissues of the palm, or those of the dorsum of the foot, whether from a poisoned wound or other cause, the subcutaneous division of the anterior annular ligament will not only afford immediate relief to the patient's suffering, but will do much toward giving the constricted and inflamed tissues an opportunity to recover their normal equilibrium; somewhat in the same way, and on the same principle, that iridectomy affords relief and benefit in certain diseases of the eye.

From a number of characteristic cases I have chosen the two following for the purpose of illustrating this subject:

CASE I. — On November 20, 1887, I was called by telegram to Springport, Jackson County, Michigan, for the purpose of amputating the right hand of Mrs. W., aged thirty-five years. I found the patient suffering intensely from extensive suppuration of all the tissues of the right palm, and with corresponding constitutional irritation and alarming depression.

She was tired of suffering, and willing to submit to anything for relief. On inquiry I found that for at least eight years she had been troubled with a large compound ganglion of the palm. Various methods of treatment had been tried without effect, and a few weeks previously to my visit a seton had been used. Suppuration supervened, and when I saw her the condition was in every respect most critical.

I determined to try one more expedient before sacrificing the hand. Accordingly, chloroform having been administered, I made a thorough division of the anterior annular ligament, from which on recovering consciousness the patient declared herself materially relieved. I did not see this patient afterward, but her medical attendant, Dr. Winslow, informed me that the relief proved permanent, and that, notwithstanding a severe continued fever, with which she was attacked a few weeks after my visit, she made a good recovery, with a perfect, or nearly perfect hand.

CASE II. — This case will serve to demonstrate the

value of the operation in a different and, no doubt, more common class of cases:

Mr. A. H., Mount Pleasant, Michigan, aged forty-two years, married, was admitted to the Hospital of the University of Michigan November 14, 1888.

While at work in a saw-mill, November 3d, he bruised the fingers of his right hand in the machinery. The little finger was the only one much injured, and that not so seriously as to stop his work. But he thinks that, on November 7th, he sprained the right hand and wrist. It immediately began to swell, and to give him great pain. The swelling and intense pain continued up to the time of his admission. His family physician used poultices and other applications, but with no relief. When admitted, the right hand and forearm were enormously swollen, and the patient was suffering intensely. Dr. Abbott immediately opened the hand and fingers by free incisions, and evacuated a large amount of pus and dark, decomposing blood. The hand and arm were then placed in hot water, and the patient experienced some relief. On November 15th, he presented himself at the clinic. The good effects of Dr. Abbott's highly judicious treatment had disappeared, and the patient was again in great agony.

Here was a case in which a slight bruise of the fingers had led to the involvement of the entire hand and forearm in a severe inflammatory process, and it was very apparent that unless arrested this process would soon lead to destruction of the parts by gangrene.

Without using an anæsthetic the anterior ligament was at once divided with a fine, sharp-pointed tenotome. Slight hæmorrhage followed the operation, and the patient experienced immediate relief.

November 16. The hand was dressed in bichloride gauze, and a firm bandage applied.

20th. Bandage has been applied, wet, every day, and the patient is improving rapidly. Temperature normal now, while it has been up to 105° during most of the past week.

22d. Glycerin and iodine were painted over the hand and arm to promote absorption. No fever.

24th. Swelling greatly reduced, and pain almost gone. Movement returning gradually. Discharged.

December 20. A letter just received from the patient states that he has resumed work with complete use of his hand. There is slight stiffness of the fingers, which is rapidly disappearing.

REMARKS.—The first hint of this practice undoubtedly came from Syme, the author and source of many advances in practical surgery. Syme, however, operated by free incision, and I trust that I am not presumptuous in claiming, in this instance, an improvement upon his practice by substituting the subcutaneous for the more heroic and certainly more dangerous open method.

The following case of neuroma of the median nerve has seemed to me to possess more than one point of interest:

CASE III.—Mrs. C., aged thirty-one years. Introduced to me by my friend and former pupil, Dr. Frazer, of Sarnia, Ontario.

Patient had had a tumor in her right forearm nearly all her life. Ten years ago it became very painful, and led her to seek medical advice. Removal was suggested, but this she declined and came to Michigan, preferring to place her case in the hands of a quack, who undertook to eradicate the growth by the application of caustic plasters. This treatment resulted in her confinement to bed for a period of eight months, during which her sufferings were very severe, and at the end of that time her tumor was somewhat larger, and a great deal more painful.

On May 8, 1890, I saw the patient and examined the tumor, which was situated about four inches above the wrist, on the right forearm, and was evidently connected with the median nerve. It was impossible to manipulate it much owing to its extreme tenderness. Nevertheless, I was able to determine the important diagnostic fact that it permitted moderately free movement laterally, but in no other direction, a characteristic feature of nerve-tumors.

In short, every fact in the case pointed toward that diagnosis, and as the patient was almost exhansted by her sufferings she readily assented to my proposition to excise the growth. This was done under chloroform without difficulty or delay, although it is only right to record the fact that the patient came nearer to dying from the anæsthetic than any case I have ever seen during the thirty years that I have used chloroform.

Artificial respiration, energetically and persistently applied, proved ultimately successful, and she made a good recovery. In this emergency Dr. Frazer proved a cool and efficient assistant.

REMARKS.—In reference to this case Dr. Frazer recently wrote that the parts supplied by the median nerve were somewhat numb, but that there was a moderate amount of sensation and good motor power. She still occasionally complains of pain in the course of the nerve, but the severe lancinating pains are entirely gone, and the patient looks and feels better than she has done for many years. This case serves to impress the principle that nerve-tumors, if amenable to treatment at all, should be excised. It might also be used to teach the people of Michigan that there are worse things than nerve-tumors, and that of all the ills that human flesh is heir to, the cruelest and most cold-blooded is the quack.

CASE IV. *Tumor of forehead.*—E. S., aged twenty-nine years, a resident of Marshall, Mich., came to my clinic at Ann Harbor, April 8, 1889. Two months previously the patient had received a slight bruise over the middle of his forehead, which was rapidly followed by the growth of a cystic tumor. For this he consulted Dr. Smiley, who tapped the cyst, and on its refilling repeated the operation and injected iodine. Still it did not disappear, but rather grew worse.

On admission the patient was in good health, but much alarmed about the tumor, which being about the size of a small orange, caused serious disfigurement as well as a good deal of pain.

Pulsation was a marked feature of the growth. Profiting by Dr. Smiley's experience I determined upon radical measures, and at once proposed excision, to which the patient promptly assented. Chloroform having been administered, I made a crucial incision of a sufficient extent to afford free access to the tumor, which I then dissected out from its intimate attachments to the tissues. It was necessary to execute the latter steps of the operation with great care, as the tumor had caused absorption of both tables of the skull, and was intimately attached to the dura.

Its removal was safely accomplished, and the wound carefully dressed antiseptically, and with every facility for free drainage. In three weeks the wound had healed, and the patient was dismissed cured, and, so far as I know, he has continued well.

REMARKS.—It seems very strange that so slight an injury should have resulted in the development of a thick-walled, rapidly-growing, cystic tumor, and that complete absorption of the bones of the forehead should have followed in so short a time. It is also rather remarkable that no further trouble has developed at the seat of operation. It is only reasonable to suppose that in this case a small, unobserved cystic tumor had previously existed, and that the injury caused its rapid development.

CASE V. *Complicated injury of the shoulder-joint.* —H. B. M., aged forty-two years, of Alepna, Mich., had always enjoyed good health until the receipt of the injury to be described.

On December 12, 1889, while employed at his trade of a millwright, the patient received a blow by the falling of a beam fifty feet long and ten by twelve inches thick. The blow was received on his right shoulder and arm. He was knocked first against another timber and from there precipitated to the hard, frozen ground fifteen feet below. A comrade working with him was so severely injured by the falling beam that he died soon afterward.

Investigation ultimately demonstrated that Mr. M.'s injuries consisted of :

1. Fractures of several of the upper ribs near the sternum.

2. Similar fractures near the articulation of the ribs with the spine.

3. A fracture of the anatomical neck of the scapula ; that is to say, the glenoid cavity was broken off, and, with the head of the humerus, was carried downward and inward so as to rest upon the thoracic wall below the clavicle.

4. A fracture of the body of the scapula, so that the axillary margin of the bone was completely detached, and driven into the axilla, where it was afterward found lying parallel with the shaft of the humerus.

5. A fracture of both bones of the forearm.

As might reasonably be expected in so complicated a case, some of these lesions were overlooked by the medical men who first examined him.

Within a few days, however, an effort was made to restore the head of the humerus to its proper position, and this effort was repeated several times, but proved unsuccessful.

Five weeks after the injury the patient called on me at Detroit, and on examination I found that while the fractured ribs and forearm had united, the entire right arm was in a position that rendered it a useless and distressing burden. Throughout its entire extent it was greatly swollen and œdematous ; voluntary power was absolutely lost, although a slight degree of passive movement could be made at the upper end where the head of the humerus rested on the ribs. The elbow, wrist, and fingers were immovable. Excessive deposits of callus had taken place at the different points of fracture. It would hardly be possible to imagine a more uninviting or unpromising case for treatment.

On careful consideration two courses seemed open in the way of operative interference, viz. :

1. Amputation at the shoulder-joint, which would give the patient—a young, strong man—a good prospect of rapid recovery, though with the loss of his right arm.

2. Something in the nature of a resection of the upper end of the bone, by which a more or less useful arm might be preserved. It was only too plain that unless something very decided could be done to relieve the mechanical obstruction in the axilla, and to improve the general condition of things in that region, amputation would be desirable, as the arm was neither useful nor ornamental to the patient. Of course, without operation, any chance of material improvement or relief was out of the question.

February 18. I operated, having previously obtained the patient's full consent. The operation was undertaken for the purpose of discovering the precise condition of things in the neighborhood of the shoulder, and with the determination to rectify these, if possible ; but it was also distinctly understood that, if necessary, the arm should be amputated.

I began by making a long, straight incision down to the humerus, exposing the head and upper part of the shaft, which were deeply imbedded in inflammatory deposit. The head was lodged in and firmly articulated to a well-formed glenoid cavity, which, from its depth and capaciousness, looked more like the cotyloid cavity of the hip-joint.

Careful examination at this stage of the operation conclusively demonstrated that without removing the upper end of the humerus further progress was out of the question. Consequently this was done, with much difficulty, by means of the chain-saw. Serious obstacles to the return of the upper end of the humerus to anything like its original position still existed, and it also appeared that a large, dense mass was in the axilla, in close relation to the upper end of the shaft of the humerus. To this I naturally attributed the compression and strangulation of the extremity as a whole, and I determined to investigate still further, and, if possible, to remove the mass. With extreme difficulty, and in the face of a great dread of inflicting injury upon the axillary nerve and vascular trunks, I at length succeeded in dissecting out and removing a fragment of bone. This fragment was the inferior costa of the scapula deprived of its glenoid cavity, which latter had been broken off and carried inward with the head of the humerus.

When the removal of this fragment had been safely accomplished everything assumed a much more favorable appearance. The arm was easily restored to a comparatively natural position, and the wound was dressed as after an ordinary resection of the shoulder-joint, a counter-opening having been made so that the fluids could find ready escape from the large and deep cavity left by the operation.

No important vessels were wounded, but the operation was a long one, and a considerable amount of blood was lost. Still, the patient rested well, and, although pretty extensive suppuration occurred, he made a good recovery. The most, if not the only, unsatisfactory part of his condition is the persistent stiffness and swelling of the hand and fingers, for which, in my opinion, the fracture of the radius and ulna is chiefly to blame. But even this will, I hope, in time be relieved.

In the performance of the operation here described, as well as of many others, I was ably assisted by Drs. W. G. Henry, F. W. Mann, and Abbott.

CASE VI. *Suppuration, with destruction of the entire left lung, treated by resection of ribs and drainage.*—E. B., aged eight years, was first brought to me at my clinic at Ann Arbor, in June, 1889, when I diagnosed an abscess of the lung, and recommended an operation for the evacuation of its contents and drainage, but I was not afforded an opportunity to carry this into execution. Before long, however, an opening was made by another doctor, who simply punctured the cavity through an intercostal space, and at its upper part. Great aggravation of all his symptoms followed this procedure, and some weeks later he was brought to me in Detroit. By this time the little fellow was in a deplorable condition of weakness and emaciation from excessive discharge of the most fœtid pus, and, of course, with septicæmia.

I now lost no time in making an effort to save his life, although it seemed almost too late. The cavity was tapped, and thoroughly drained by excision of a portion of two ribs, the ninth and tenth, at the lowest point of the abscess-cavity. Through this opening an enormous quantity of horribly offensive pus was evacuated; the cavity was thoroughly douched with hot water, and a large drainage-tube was inserted. through which daily ablutions with boric acid solution and other medicaments were easily and painlessly effected. The quantity of the discharge rapidly diminished, and its quality improved. In a few days the tube was dispensed with, but the ablutions were continued for several weeks. The child's health gradually improved. the discharge entirely ceased, and he is now in perfect health.

CASE VII. *Osteo-sarcoma of the scapula.*—William W., aged twenty-six years. married, a resident of

Grand Haven, Michigan, was admitted to the Hospital of the University of Michigan, May 10, 1889, suffering from a large and rapidly-growing tumor of the scapula. Patient was tall, slim, and apparently very delicate. He stated that he had been in his usual health until seven weeks previously to admission. At that time he first observed the growth in his shoulder. It had given him no pain until during the past two weeks, when he received a severe wrench of the arm and shoulder, and from that time on he suffered severe pain, and the tumor grew more rapidly. It had been diagnosed as abscess, and incision recommended.

I at once suspected osteo-sarcoma limited to the scapula, and advised the operation of immediate excision of that bone. The patient's anæmic and emaciated condition, however, made me hesitate, and I placed him on tonic treatment and determined to wait for some improvement in his health. This took place, so that on May 28th, I performed excision of the entire scapula. Chloroform having been administered, I made an incision from the point of the acromion process backward, along the superior margin of the scapula, to the median line of the back, and from the middle of that incision a vertical one downward, to a point at least two inches below the lower angle of the bone. With these free external incisions I was sure to have plenty of room for the subsequent steps of the operation. The hæmorrhage from these preliminary incisions was very severe, and it seemed that the only chance of safety consisted in a rapid completion of the operation. I first freed the posterior margin and the lower angle by rapid sweeps of the knife. I then disarticulated the shoulder-joint, and finally separated the deep attachments of the bone in front and above. The suprascapular artery, much enlarged, was divided and instantly secured. The subscapular was also much enlarged, and was divided and ligated half an inch from its origin from the main trunk. Numerous smaller branches were also ligated. Although the patient was in the amphitheatre only twelve minutes in all, and although every precaution was taken to limit the flow of blood, still a good deal was lost, and he suffered very seriously from the shock. for which stimulants were freely administered. In about twelve hours reaction was fully established.

The subsequent progress of the case was extremely satisfactory. One week from the date of operation the patient walked into the amphitheatre to have his wound dressed, when it was demonstrated that the whole extent of that vast wound had healed by first intention. In three weeks he was dismissed in good condition, and with every prospect of complete restoration to health. Before leaving the hospital he had recovered good movement of and control over the arm.[1]

The tumor was examined by Dr. Gibbes. who pronounced it osteo-sarcoma. The specimen is now in the University Museum.

REMARKS.—Before leaving this case I desire to refer very briefly to the history of the operation of exci-

---

[1] Since the above was written I have heard with regret of the death of this patient from causes unconnected with the operation.

sion of the entire scapula, and to recall some practical deductions in relation to it. Professor Syme performed this operation in 1856, with at least temporary success, and he believed that no one had preceded him. In a brief preface to his paper, entitled, "Excision of the Entire Scapula," he says: "In the present advanced state of surgery any real addition to its resources must be regarded as a subject of interest. I, therefore, venture to hope that the following account of an entirely new operation will be deemed worthy of separate publication."

Syme's first case was performed in the Royal Infirmary of Edinburgh, October 1, 1856. He was, however, mistaken in believing that no one had preceded him, for Langenbeck had done it successfully a few months previously. This fact, however, does not in the least detract from the merits of Syme's work, which was certainly original and independent. Not only so, but he has left behind him a description of the *modus operandi*, as well as a summary of the principles involved, which, bearing as it does the unmistakable stamp of his surgical genius, will stand for all time as the most authoritative utterance on the subject.

From his first case he deduced the following doctrines:

1. "That the entire scapula may be disarticulated from the shoulder-joint without loss of blood to any great extent.

2. "That the wound resulting from this operation does not necessarily occasion an excessive amount of discharge.

3. "That the arm which remains is not a useless appendage, but a serviceable limb."

So far as I have been able to learn, the tumor removed in my case is by far the largest on record, as it weighed about eight pounds.

In my operation every effort to secure asepsis was used, and certainly the union by the first intention of so extensive a wound might justly be quoted as a testimonial to our modern methods, of which my celebrated preceptor, in 1856, had never even dreamed. But let me quote his own words, immediately following the description of his operation:

"Everything went on favorably after the operation, and a great part of the wound healed by the first intention."

According to the *International Encyclopædia of Surgery*, forty-two cases of excision of the entire scapula have been recorded. Of that number, eight were by American surgeons, and of the whole number exactly 20 per cent. died.

72 LAFAYETTE AVENUE.

The Death of Dr. Frederich Arnold.—The death is announced of Dr. Frederich Arnold, emeritus professor of anatomy in the University of Heidelberg. Dr. Arnold was nearly ninety years of age.

COCOANUT-WATER AS A CULTURE-FLUID.

BY GEORGE M. STERNBERG, M.D.,

MAJOR AND SURGEON, U. S. ARMY.

THE fluid contained in unripe cocoanuts is known in the West Indies as *agua coco*, or cocoanut-water. Unlike the fluid contained in the ripe nut, which has a milky appearance, it is perfectly transparent.

In countries where the cocoanut is indigenous this *agua coco* is very popular as a refreshing drink, and by some is thought to possess valuable diuretic properties. At railway stations in the country, and at places of refreshment in towns, piles of the unripe nuts are to be seen, and at a moment's notice one may obtain a tumblerful of the fluid at very small expense.

At the time of my first visit to Cuba, in 1879, the idea occurred to me that this fluid might be a useful culture-medium for bacteria, and upon making the experiment I found that various species grew in it most luxuriantly.

As it is contained in a germ-proof receptacle no sterilization of the fluid is required when it is transferred with proper precautions to sterilized test-tubes, or is drawn directly from the nut into the little flask with a long and slender neck, which I am in the habit of using for fluid cultures. In these it may be preserved indefinitely, remaining perfectly transparent and ready for use. Heating the fluid causes a slight precipitate.

In the investigations which I have made in Havana during the past two years I used this fluid very extensively and found it a great convenience to have a sterile culture-fluid always at hand ready for use at a moment's notice. Moreover, it has certain special advantages for the study of the physiological characters of various bacteria and for the differentiation of species. It contains in solution about four per cent. of glucose in addition to vegetable albumin and salts, which alone would make it a useful nutrient medium.

Certain microörganisms multiply in it without appropriating the glucose, while others split this up, producing an abundant evolution of carbonic acid, and giving to the fluid a very acid reaction. As obtained from the nut it has a slightly acid reaction, which makes it unsuitable as a culture-medium for certain pathogenic bacteria, but when desired it is a simple matter to neutralize it. For a large number of species of bacteria and for the saccharomycetes it constitutes a very favorable medium. Since my return from Cuba I have obtained an analysis of this fluid through the kindness of Professor Remsen, of Johns Hopkins University. Six unripe cocoanuts sent to me by my friend, Dr. Daniel Burgess, of Havana, were placed by Professor Remsen in the hands of Mr. L. L. Van Slyke,

Ph. D., for chemical examination. I have received from Dr. Van Slyke the following report of the results of his analyses:

1. Weight of fluid obtained from each nut varies from 230.5 grammes to 383.7 grammes, the average being 339.1 grammes.

2. The specific gravity (at 15.5° C.) varies from 1.0215 to 1.0246, the average being 1.02285.

3. The amount of water in the fluid from each nut varies from 94.37 per cent. to 96.43 per cent., the average being 95 per cent.

4. The amount of ash or inorganic matter in each varies from 0.575 per cent. to 0.675 per cent., the average being 0.618 per cent.

5. The sugar is mainly in the form of glucose, with traces of cane-sugar. The amount of glucose varies from 3.45 per cent. to 4.58 per cent., the average being 3.97 per cent.

6. The fat varies from 0.084 per cent. to 0.145 per cent., the average being 0.119 per cent.

7. The amount of albuminoids in each varies from 0.095 per cent. to 0.205 per cent., the average being 0.133 per cent.

HYSTERICAL APHONIA.

With Especial Reference to a Plan of Treatment, and with the Report of Cases.[1]

BY J. A. BACH, M.D.,
OF MILWAUKEE, WIS.

ONE of the many manifestations of hysteria is the so-called hysterical paralysis of the muscles of the vocal cords, resulting in aphonia, a condition that is most interesting and instructive, inasmuch as it can be so readily observed from its full development to perfect cure. The lack of proper central stimulation is well illustrated here. Examination with the laryngeal mirror shows the cords to be of nearly a normal color. If a strong effort at intonation be made by the patient, the cords quickly approximate but as quickly recede, so that voice is not produced, although apparently the effort of the patient is continued. The central nerve-stimulus is lost and 'the muscles of phonation are practically paralyzed. This condition is often accompanied with paresis of the muscles of the tongue and pharynx.

It is well established that the impediment to conduction is not situated in the peripheral motor nerves, for the electrical reaction remains normal. It would further seem, from the results of treatment in the following cases, that there is no impediment at all to conduction, but only a lack of the production and correct application of a central stimulus.

The etiology of hysterical aphonia is similar to

---

that of other hysterical conditions. It is less a local trouble than a general one manifesting itself locally. In many cases no cause is apparent, and the voice may disappear either suddenly or gradually. The affection is limited to the period between puberty and the menopause.

Treatment.—The various modes of treatment practised and advocated have met with success in probably the majority of cases, but the results have often been only temporary or incomplete. This has been the result with the various methods of electrical treatment, whether centrally or locally directed ; also, with the administration of the different nerve tonics and sedatives, as well as with other medicinal means. Furthermore, the time consumed in securing definite results has, in many cases, been considerable.

The plan of treatment to which I wish to draw special attention proposes to do away with all such means, and teaches the patient inductively to regain control of the larynx, to innervate properly the muscles of the cords, and to produce voice as a beginner on the cornet would learn to produce his first tones.

The greatest difficulty with the hysterical patient is the production of the first tone, as such patients are generally unable, through their own efforts, to produce any sound whatsoever. This initial difficulty, however, can always be overcome in a few moments by the assistance of reflex action. For this purpose a strong irritant, whether mechanical or chemical, may be applied to the larynx so as to excite cough. This, of course, requires no effort on the part of the patient. Having excited this cough once or twice the patient will be able to reproduce it independent of the irritant. The cough is short and of an explosive character.

After repeating the cough five or six times the patient will have gained sufficient control of central stimulation to produce a cough. It now becomes a simple matter to continue this cough and to pronounce, more or less distinctly, the vowel "*a*" at each effort, and after a few efforts to substitute the vowel "*e*," and so on, until all the vowels have been coughed. After this is repeated several times, the element of cough can easily be eliminated from the vocalization, when we have left the pure vowel-sound, which, without effort on the part of the patient, can be combined with consonants, as, for instance, with "*d*" — "*ad*," "*ed*," "*id*," "*od*," "*ud*," first placing the vowel before the consonant and then reversing this. It would not be advisable to attempt the articulation of words at this stage, but better to combine the vowels with single consonants, gradually increasing the duration of the sound. The patient is thus led to speak words without resisting, wilfully or uninten-

[1] Read before the Milwaukee Clinical Society, June 10, 1890.

tionally. The time occupied in this procedure need not be more than half an hour, although it is advisable to give several treatments, in order to place the patient beyond the possibility of relapse by impressing her with the fact that she produced the sound by her own efforts, and that it is due to a lack of effort if the voice is again lost. Show her how, by coughing if necessary, she can go through the same process as before.

A report of the following cases will illustrate results obtained in apparently unfavorable subjects.

CASE I.—Miss B., aged twenty-eight years, poorly nourished. anæmic, and of a neurotic type, came under my care for treatment in June, 1889. For about seven years she had been unable to speak or whisper, and she carried with her a tablet upon which all communications were written. She was very despondent, and had but little hope of relief, as she had had nearly continuous treatment of various kinds for more than three years.

Upon examining the larynx I found a very characteristic picture of hysterical paralysis of the vocal cords, and, in addition, an infiltration of the ventricular bands, yet not sufficient to prevent the proper action of the cords. Although the paralysis had existed so long the resulting atrophy was not very marked. One peculiarity of the case was her imagined inability to whisper. As her breathing power was fair there was no good reason for this complication. The patient was of a fairly intelligent class and I explained to her the condition as well as I could, assuring her that with her coöperation it would be perfectly possible to effect a cure in a short time. After having shown her the folly of not being able to whisper, and that whispering is not a function of the vocal cords or larynx, and is produced by the modifying influences upon the breath by organs above the larynx, she gained confidence, and I had at least a whisper to begin with. It now remained again to direct properly central innervation of the vocal muscles, which, according to the plan proposed, was accomplished as readily and in as short a time as if she had been aphonic for only a week. The other pathological conditions of the larynx were treated for some time before the patient was discharged.

CASE II.— Mrs. J. H., a Jewess, aged forty-three years, married. This lady was well nourished and in perfect general health, but for about ten weeks had been unable to speak, for which difficulty she had been treated without result. The laryngeal picture was one of hysterical aphonia, with considerable congestion ; no other changes were found. Patient asserted that she had contracted the trouble through a severe cold, but I elicited the additional fact that a quarrel in the family about the time of contracting the cold played a rather more important factor than the cold itself.

Treatment was applied as in the preceding case, and at the second visit the patient was discharged, perfectly cured.

CASE III.—Miss W. B., a teacher, aged thirty years ; well nourished, and of a neurotic type, had,

seven months previously, lost her voice. In consequence of this she was obliged to give up her occupation as teacher.

During this time she had been under various modes of treatment by different physicians. One doctor told her that her throat and larynx were "swollen shut."

Here again the laryngeal image was characteristic. The condition was uncomplicated, and my prognosis was favorable. The treatment resulted in a cure in fifteen minutes, although she made a second visit before I discharged her.

The results in these cases were so satisfactory and so direct that all other means of treatment would seem superfluous.

It has occurred to me that, could other hysterical conditions be brought under such direct control and treated upon a similar plan, we would not so frequently hear of Christian science and faith-cures after so-called medical science has failed.

CLINICAL MEMORANDA.

SURGICAL.

A Case of Malignant Disease of the Kidney.—February 14, 1890, I was called to see J. J. P., male, aged forty-three years, a farmer by occupation. His pulse was 100, and his temperature 99.2°. He complained chiefly of a lame back and pain in the lumbar region, extending down the thighs to the knees, and occasionally to the ankles, on attempting to move. The pain was more marked on the left side than on the right. He was able to move about on crutches, and was more comfortable while sitting up than when lying down. Just before my visit he had had several paroxysms of severe pain in the region of the stomach, accompanied with dyspnœa.

Upon examination I found a tumor in the left lumbar region, extending from the last rib to the crest of the ilium and the same distance transversely, with its centre about at the external border of the erector spinæ muscle. With a hypodermic syringe I drew out, from about one inch below the surface, a sero-sanguinolent fluid, which was odorless. Upon inquiry I found that his previous health had been good, as was also his family history.

His account of his present illness was as follows : About june 1, 1889, he began to be troubled with pain and lameness which interfered with his work. He also could feel what he described as the sensation of a lump in his abdomen. As time passed on, the original sensation of a tumor was replaced by pain. He was seen on November 23d, and again December 23d, by a reputable practitioner, who treated him for rheumatism. From December 23d, he was confined to his home.

In January he was seen by another practitioner and the first diagnosis was confirmed, although the tumor was at that time quite prominent. As the other symptoms increased the patient began to be troubled with constipation, which was evidently due to pressure on the descending colon. At no time was there much pain in the tumor itself.

I did not examine the urine microscopically, but chemically I could detect nothing abnormal except an excess of urates.

I could get no history of anything that threw light on the case, except a sprain of the back, in April, 1889.

My diagnosis was nephritic or perinephritic abscess, and I advised an operation.

February 21st, Dr. G. L. Pritchett, of Fairbury, Neb., saw the patient with me, confirmed my diagnosis and also advised operation. He thereupon proceeded, with my assistance, to open the cavity by a free incision about midway between the last rib and the crest of the ilium, extending in the direction of the fibres of the external oblique muscle. About a pint of sero-sanguinolent fluid and broken-down tissue, apparently kidney tissue, escaped. All parts within reach of the finger seemed to be normal except the kidney, which was so disorganized to be unrecognizable. The wound was irrigated with bichloride solution, a drainage-tube inserted to a depth of three inches, the cavity packed with iodoform-gauze, and dressed externally with iodoform-gauze and bichloride cotton.

There was considerable discharge at first; later it grew less but never stopped.

The results of the operation were the disappearance of pain and great relief to the patient. On March 15th he walked from his chair to his bed without crutches for the first time for two months. His temperature had gradually fallen to normal. He sat up from one to four hours a day after March 10th. Until March 15th he improved so much that his ultimate recovery seemed certain. On March 7th I dressed the wound with bichloride-gauze and stopped using iodoform, after which there was more pus. Between March 29th and April 14th, I opened three small cavities, containing pus, near the original opening; one in the cicatrix formed by the partial healing of the first operation. In each I inserted a tube to a depth of from two to four inches.

On April 20th, Dr. G. L. Pritchett, assisted by Dr. Eaton, of Fairbury, Neb., and myself, again opened the cavity, removed much broken-down tissue and packed the wound with bichloride-gauze. The patient's general health did not fail much until June, but the wound was more unhealthy after about March 15th. It did not heal after the second operation, but grew deeper and small cavities occasionally opened into the main one. The swelling increased until it was about ten inches in diameter. It also seemed to increase internally and to press on the nerves—causing a return of the original pain though to a less severe degree.

From April 1st, the temperature varied irregularly from the normal up to 104°, and there was an occasional chill. After the first operation he had attacks of vomiting, but during most of the time his appetite was good. About June 15th, he became unable to sit up, and the discharge increased and was very foetid. From then until his death, June 26th, the discharge was so great that it was necessary to place an oilcloth under the sheet, and to change the bedclothes several times a day. The odor became very offensive. Gangrene appeared about two days before his death, that is, in the parts exposed to view. judging from the odor I am sure that internally it commenced earlier.

For about a week before death the urine was much diminished in quantity. It contained no albumin. Further examination was omitted for want of instruments.

Death occurred by asthenia. My opinion is that the abscess was caused by a malignant growth, although no autopsy was held.   A. C. AMES, M. D.
REYNOLDS, NEBRASKA.

Abscess of the Prostate Cured by Perineal Section.—Abscess of the prostate of idiopathic origin is sufficiently rare and serious to warrant the report of the following case:

Mr. C., aged seventy-two years, a prominent agriculturist and legislator, was attacked quite suddenly with pain in the perineum and anus. He had suffered for several months from constipation, and thought the "straining at stool brought on piles," as he expressed it. His family physician gave him some soothing ointment, but it afforded him no relief. The parts about the anus became greatly swollen, evacuation of the bowels was very painful and the urine was voided with great difficulty. He had fever, lost appetite, and had remitting pain of a throbbing character.

I saw him in consultation after he had been sick a week. He was delirious, had chills every few hours and profuse sweats. Anodynes and quinine were being used freely. The parts about the anus were so œdematous that a digital examination *per rectum* could be made only with difficulty. However, a smooth oval tumor was felt in the region of the prostate. It encroached upon the rectum and appeared to push the bladder upward and backward, elongating the urethra. There was no history of previous urethral or vesical disease, and a sound met little obstruction on the way to the bladder.

I diagnosed an abscess and felt an indistinct sense of fluctuation on placing my finger in the rectum behind the tumor and pushing it forward toward the perineum, where I made counter-pressure with the finger of my other hand. Without an anæsthetic a sound was passed into the bladder and given to an assistant to hold, as in the operation for perineal lithotomy—the patient being in the lithotomy position. Then I pushed or pulled the tumor down against the perineum with a finger of my left hand in the rectum, and introduced the point of a straight bistoury through the integument in the median line of the perineum about one inch in front of the anus, and pushed the blade straight back into the tumor, while the urethra was held up out of the way of incision by my assistant with the sound. As the pus began to flow the incision was carried toward the anus until it was free enough to empty the abscess thoroughly, which contained about two ounces of pus.

The subsequent treatment was washing the abscess cavity daily with a fifty-per-cent. solution of peroxide of hydrogen and the internal use of bitter tonics. The patient's recovery was perfect and uninterrupted.

HAL C. WYMAN, M.S., M.D.,
Professor of Surgery in the Michigan College
of Medicine and Surgery, Detroit.

OBSTETRICAL.

Double Cephalhæmatoma.—A cephalhæmatoma on either parietal bone in a newly-born infant is quite common.

There is probably not a general practitioner of any experience in obstetrics who has not become familiar with it. At least ten have been seen by the writer in hospital and private practice. A double hæmatoma, on the contrary, is very rare and gives the infant's head a much more deformed appearance. Curiously enough, two cases have occurred in the writer's service in the Maternity Hospital within eighteen months. The first was bilateral, on each parietal bone, and unusually large; it was reported in the *University Medical Magazine*, with an illustration. The second has been under observation for more than three months. The blood-tumors were situated on the right parietal bone and on the right side of the occipital bone. Each was as large as though a small crab-apple had been inserted under the scalp, and the two together gave the head a very curious appearance. They appeared three days after birth. The mother was a primipara, and the labor lasted in its three stages respectively six hours, two hours, and ten minutes. The labor was easy, the position of the vertex was right occipito-anterior. Nothing was done for the tumors and they slowly subsided; but still, three months from their appearance, there are decided lumps on the infant's head. If the blood-tumor is large, and if the child cannot be kept under observation a long time, it is a question whether it would not be better to aspirate antiseptically about a week or ten days after the formation of the tumor, as at this time there would be little likelihood of a fresh subcranial effusion.

BARTON COOKE HIRST, M.D.,
Professor of Obstetrics in the University of
Pennsylvania.

MEDICAL PROGRESS.

The Uselessness of Quinine in Non-malarial Diseases.—We use the term "malarial" to define a certain group of symptoms, but more frequently to hide our ignorance of the true nature of diseases, especially of those that are attended with febrile phenomena. Hence the common use of quinine in many varieties of diseases.

The observations of Roux, Laveran, Collin, and others, have almost established the fact that malaria is a disease of the country, and that large cities seem gradually to create for themselves an immunity against paludal disorders.

DR. JOAQUIN L. DUEÑAS (*Crónica Médico-Quirúrgica de la Habana*, Havana, July, 1890, No. 7) publishes an able article on the use of quinine in a variety of diseases, and his results corroborate the experience of Laveran, Maillot, Dutrenlean, Jaccoud, and others, with regard to the use of the drug in the treatment of disease.

Dr. Dueñas's observations were made in Havana. He asserts that this city, contrary to what might be expected, is particularly free from malarial infection, and that it is only in a few sections of the town, where the pavement is imperfect, and where there is much decomposing organic matter, that cases of true malarial fever are met. Thus, of 3961 patients treated by him in the course of nine consecutive years the death-rate was only $7\frac{7}{8}$ per cent. Of this large number of persons, 1694 suffered from apyretic disorders, while 2267 presented febrile symptoms. Of these fever cases, 774 were

of an infectious character, and of the latter only 70 could be classed as malarial, thus: intermittent fever 42; remittent fever 18; pernicious fever 6; malarial cachexia 4. Of the 8 deaths from paludal poisoning, among the 70 cases, 6 were due to pernicious fever and 2 to remittent fever. The remaining 704 pyretic affections comprised typhoid fever, yellow fever, smallpox, varicella, measles, scarlatina, miliary tuberculosis, erysipelas, and septicæmia.

With regard to the employment of quinine in this large number of cases, Dr. Dueñas used it extensively in the 70 malarial cases, and in the non-malarial diseases, only in a certain number of cases of typhoid fever and erysipelas.

In the 1694 cases of a non-febrile character the remedy was employed more especially as a cardiac and vascular tonic and as a nerve stimulant. Of these cases, 1435 completely recovered, 83 died, and the results in 173 could not be ascertained, giving a mortality of 5.65 per cent. The diseases most commonly met with were the catarrhal affections of a rheumatic origin, neuroses, chlorotic neuralgias, and scrofula.

Quinine was found of great service in certain congestive conditions, in hæmorrhages, non-febrile rheumatism, idiopathic and constitutional neuralgias, migraine, asthma, cardiac weakness, whooping-cough, and in other diseases, which, although not dependent upon malaria, frequently assume the intermittent type. Of all these latter diseases, neuralgia was found to be the most frequent, and it yielded easily to the use of quinine. Of 228 cases treated successfully by the drug only two were due to a distinct malarial poisoning.

But the most important part of Dr. Dueñas's experience is with reference to the employment of the drug in febrile disorders not dependent upon malaria. Of the 2267 cases of this nature treated, 993 were catarrhal affections and diseases of the mucous membranes; 774 infectious pyrexias; 272 organic and other inflammations; 124 tubercular and rheumatic diseases, and the remainder were such specific diseases as diphtheria, dysentery and tetanus, and ephemeral or continued fevers.

Although possessing excellent antiphlogistic and antiperiodic properties, quinine was often harmful in certain catarrhal affections of the respiratory apparatus, such as laryngitis, bronchitis, and acute broncho-pneumonia. In these diseases a marked reduction of temperature after the administration of quinine was never observed.

The same results were observed in the treatment of catarrhal affections of the digestive organs. In cases of mucous and hepatic disease, in febrile stomatitis, and in acute gastritis, the temperature could be lowered only by means of ipecacuanha, and the resolution of the disease was hastened by the application of local emollients, rest, diet, and hygienic measures. It was noticed that in such cases quinine prolonged the febrile stage and the duration of the disease. Cases of acute enteritis, enterocolitis, cystitis, endometritis, and other local diseases of the mucous membranes, were successfully treated without the aid of quinine. In many of the cases the drug exercised an injurious influence, even when the disease was malarial. The drug was also found harmful, and even hastened death, in cases of infantile broncho-pneumonia.

In the infectious febrile disorders, Dr. Dueñas used the remedy only to reduce high fever and as a cardiac and vascular tonic, except in cases with malarial symptoms. He employed it in moderate amounts in. some septicæmic diseases, in erysipelas, in typhoid fever, and in miliary tuberculosis; but never in smallpox, measles, scarlatina, or yellow fever. After a short experience the drug was discontinued in the treatment of typhoid fever and septicæmias.

It was found useless in malarial disorders of an adynamic type. In the few cases of pernicious fever in which quinine was used as the chief remedy, death was invariably the result. But whether death was due to the medicine or to the disease cannot be determined.

In malarial remittent fever, quinine produced excellent results; but in those forms of disease known as typho-malarial, in which the most prominent symptoms are typhoid, the uselessness of quinine was most remarkable. Here the drug, owing to its local action, prolonged the irritation of the gastro-intestinal mucous membrane: besides, it seemed to weaken the system, to diminish organic resistance, and to predispose the patients to attacks of syncope, in which the degeneration of the cardiac fibre was a frequent cause of death.

The remedy was found useful in erysipelas and in the treatment of acute articular rheumatism, but useless in dysentery, diphtheria, and all forms of septicæmia, especially that occurring in the puerperal state.

In localized cerebral congestions dependent upon tubercular disease, quinine often did good when given in moderate doses. In the hyperæmia of the meninges, so frequent during the period of dentition, and in other infantile disorders, the alkaloid produced most brilliant results in doses of from 3 to 4 grains, according to the age of the patient. On the contrary, in meningeal irritation due to anæmia, the remedy was not only useless, but dangerous.

Dr. Dueñas found quinine useless in the fever of syphilitic, chlorotic, and hysterical subjects, and in the fever of dentition.

Treatment of Pediculi Pubis.—

R.—Vinegar . . . . 5000 parts.
　　Corrosive sublimate . . 1 part.—M.

This is said to be recommended by BROCQ.—*Revue Thérapeutique Médico-Chirurgicale.*

Treatment of Paroxysmal Tachycardia.—HUCHARD, in a

clinical lecture delivered at the Hospital Bichat, gives the following directions as to the treatment of this severe affection; dividing the treatment into first that devoted to the care of the patient during the attack, and second, to his care between the paroxysms.

If the man is standing, he must be made to lie down on the right side in as nearly a horizontal position as possible, and every measure taken to relieve him of mental or physical disturbance. Compression may be applied over the right carotid artery, while in some cases a deep inspiration may give relief. In either case the remedial result is due to the effect on the vagus nerve. While these measures are useful in some cases, Huchard himself employs others, such as the application of a bichloride of methyl spray to the præcordium, the back of the neck, or the chest. Sometimes active vesication

over the præcordium is useful. He also gives at the time of the onset of the attack, digitalis by the mouth, if possible, or, if the stomach is irritable, by rectal injection, and finds that in moderate doses it does great good. When the attack is prolonged and threatens life, and when cardiac dilatation is imminent, venesection may be resorted to, or, in a plethoric person, local bloodletting from the præcordium be carried out. When cardiac weakness is very marked and syncope is a pressing symptom, hypodermic injections of ether or caffeine may be used, and nitroglycerin given or nitrite of amyl inhaled. These last remedies are absolutely contraindicated in those instances in which low arterial tension already exists.

The stage of intermission is to be treated by dieting and the proper use of drugs. The patient must take neither coffee, tea, nor alcoholic drink, nor must he use tobacco. All stimulating foods must be forbidden, and everything done which will tend to efface any tendencies to subsequent attacks. In each case we must seek for a cause and overcome it. Huchard uses arsenic as a general systemic tonic, and as an alterative particularly affecting the nervous centres. In those instances in which the arterial tension is below normal, he recommends pills of sulphate of quinine and ergot, as follows:

R.—Sulphate of quinine　　}
　　Aqueous extract of ergot } of each 1 drachm.
　　Extract of nux vomica . . . 1½ grains.

Make into 40 pills, and give 2 or 3 pills two or three times a day for six weeks or two months, and accompany them with 1 to 2 drops of Fowler's solution. Digitalis may be given in constant but small doses for a long period if cardiac weakness is present. In some cases prolonged avoidance of mental or physical exertion is absolutely necessary if a cure is to be arrived at.

Treatment of Chilblain.—BOELZ, of Tokio, states that

the treatment of chilblain should consist, first in washing with hot water, and second in applying to the surface the following mixture:

R.—Caustic potash . . . ¼ grain.
　　Glycerin　　　　}
　　Rectified spirit } of each 6 drachms.
　　Distilled water . . . 2 ounces.—M.

This preparation is generally not too irritating, and produces a cure in the space of two to three days.—*Rev. Gén. de Clin. et de Thérapeutique.*

Syrup for Infantile Constipation.—

R.—Podophyllin . . . 1 grain.
　　Alcohol . . . 1¼ drachm.
　　Syrup of red raspberry . 3 ounces.—M.

Dose: from a teaspoonful to a dessertspoonful every morning, according to the obstinacy of the constipation.—*L'Union Médicale,* August 5, 1890.

Treatment of Sycosis.—ROSENTHAL applies the following in this condition:

R.—Tannic acid . . . 15 grains.
　　Milk of sulphur . . . 30 "
　　Vaseline . . . . 5 ounces.—M.

During the day no applications are used, but at night the ointment is thoroughly applied. The following, recommended by Hebra, may also be resorted to:

R.—Tannic acid . . . 75 grains.
   Milk of sulphur . . . 150   "
   Oxide of zinc } of each . 9 drachms.
   Starch   }
   Vaseline . . . . 1½ ounces.—M.

After the ointment is applied, it is covered with iodoform-gauze.—*Rev. Gén. de Clin. et de Thérapeutique.*

Ointment for Syphilitic Alopecia.—According to *L' Union Médicale,* july 31, 1890, MAURIAC recommends the following application for the relief of syphilitic alopecia:

R.—Sulphate of quinine } of each 7½ grains.
   Turpeth mineral   }
   Suet . . . . . 1 ounce.—M.

Make this into a pomade, and apply night and morning. Every second day use the following wash:

R.—Carbonate of sodium } of each 15 grains.
   Boric acid   }
   Distilled water . . . 8 ounces.

If the disease persists, a lotion of mercuric chloride of the strength of 1 to 500 or 1 to 1000 may be used, or in other instances yellow precipitate ointment will be more efficacious.

A Simple Ointment for Pruritus.—BALFOUR reports that he has almost never failed to obtain prompt relief, in cases of pruritus of the anus and vulva, from an ointment containing eighty grains of calomel to the ounce of vaseline or other unguent.

A Death from Chloroform.—M. SOTTAS (*Arch. Génér. de Méd,* July, 1890) reports a case of death under chloroform in a patient who had previously been chloroformed on several occasions, the last time but one month prior to the fatal anæsthetization. The chloroform used was mixed with one-fourth of ethylic alcohol. The patient had been operated upon several times for tubercular disease of the bones, but was coughing very little and presented no signs of advanced pulmonary tuberculosis.

He bore the early administration well; the conjunctival reflex, the pulse, and breathing being carefully watched. The patient was turned upon his side, in order to reach the dorsal region, where a cold abscess was situated, the opening of which was the object of the operation. At this moment a general muscular contraction of the trunk took place, and he suddenly and without warning ceased to breathe. The eyelids opened, the pupils dilated, the conjunctival reflex disappeared, the face and chest became dark-colored, and, in spite of prolonged artificial respiration, electrical stimulation, oxygen inhalations, and ether injections, he gave no sign of life except a few attempts at spontaneous respiration. Two huge pockets containing pus were found at the autopsy, the one in front of the dorsal spine pushing the heart forward and displacing the aorta to the left, the other posterior to the spinal column in the lumbar region, and reaching down to the sacrum. A fistulous communication existed between the two pockets. The heart was normal in size, and filled with dark blood. The lungs were adherent to the pleura, much congested, and the aorta was slightly atheromatous.

The Effects of Salol on the Kidneys.—HESSELBACH (*Practitioner,* August, 1890) has made a valuable study of the effects of carbolic acid and salol on the kidneys. He finds that carbolic acid continuously administered to rabbits produces anæmia and fatty degeneration of the renal cortex, with disintegration and destruction of the epithelium. Salicylic acid given in the same manner produces hyperæmia of the cortex with extravasations into the interstitial tissue and the tubules. Salol given continuously produced pathological changes almost identical with those caused by carbolic acid, showing that the latter constituent and not the salicylic acid gives to salol its toxic properties.

Hesselbach deduces the following practical conclusions from his observations:

1. The large proportion of carbolic acid contained in salol renders it so toxic a substance that its unrestricted therapeutic use is fraught with danger.

2. In renal disease, acute or chronic, salol is contraindicated.

Cystitis in Diabetes.—SCHMITZ (*Berliner klinische Wochenschrift,* No. 23, 1890) draws attention to the occasional occurrence of cystitis in the course of diabetes. It is caused, he thinks, by fermentation of the saccharine urine. Schmitz distinguishes three stages of the chronic form—acute cystitis in diabetes being unusual. The first is mild with no subjective symptoms; the urine is somewhat turbid, faintly acid, and contains numerous mucous corpuscles and a few pus-cells. From this the second develops, when the urine becomes more turbid, has an unpleasant smell, and contains bacteria, phosphates, and more pus. In the third stage the fermentation may cause the evolution of gas which is passed through the urethra, and the subjective symptoms of cystitis are marked.

To cure this condition the bladder should be frequently washed out with a solution of salicylate of sodium, to prevent decomposition of the urine; the diabetes, of course, being carefully treated by the usual methods.—*Practitioner,* August, 1890.

Lactic Acid in the Treatment of Diarrhœa.—HAYEM (*L'Médecine Moderne,* July 5, 1890) calls attention to the value of lactic acid in the treatment of the diarrhœas of adults as well as in those of children. He thinks that in small doses it increases the power of gastric digestion; that in moderate quantities it is probably absorbed and changed in the blood; but that after large doses—more than 2½ drachms daily—it appears in the urine and fæces. The large doses, however, do not cause any disagreeable symptoms, and Hayem has given as much as 2½ drachms daily for several weeks. He prescribes the acid as follows:

R.—Lactic acid . . . 2½ to 3 drachms.
   Syrup . . . . 6 ounces.
   Water . . . . 7 ounces.—M.

Half a tumblerful to be taken between each meal.—*London Medical Recorder,* August, 1890.

THE MEDICAL NEWS.

A WEEKLY JOURNAL
OF MEDICAL SCIENCE.

COMMUNICATIONS are invited from all parts of the world. Original articles contributed exclusively to THE MEDICAL NEWS will be liberally paid for upon publication. When necessary to elucidate the text, illustrations will be furnished without cost to the author.

Address the Editor: H. A. HARE, M.D.,
1004 WALNUT STREET,
PHILADELPHIA.

Subscription Price, including Postage.
PER ANNUM, IN ADVANCE . . . . $4.00.
SINGLE COPIES . . . . 10 CENTS.

Subscriptions may begin at any date. The safest mode of remittance is by bank check or postal money order, drawn to the order of the undersigned. When neither is accessible, remittances may be made, at the risk of the publishers, by forwarding in *registered* letters.

Address,　　LEA BROTHERS & CO.,
Nos. 706 & 708 SANSOM STREET,
PHILADELPHIA.

SATURDAY, SEPTEMBER 13, 1890.

GASTRIC NEUROSES.

WITHIN recent years considerable progress has been made toward a clearer understanding of the various morbid conditions which have long been classified under the rather vague and ill-defined heading of "dyspepsia," with, perhaps, the occasional addition of an adjective, like "functional" or "nervous," which added but little to our knowledge. The readers of THE MEDICAL NEWS have been kept fully informed of current researches, not only by comments in the editorial columns, but by original communications—notably a paper read by DR. FREDERICK P. HENRY before the Philadelphia County Medical Society—and by abstracts of the more important communications to other journals, American and foreign.

The highly elaborate classifications proposed by many authors might, however, be much simplified without loss to our comprehension of the subject-matter—the more so as the association of morbid states is usually complex, derangement of secretory function being usually an accompaniment of disturbance of motor function, and *vice versa;* and, as just exemplified, no matter how elaborate our subdivision of morbid conditions, we are still unable to escape from the use of such general terms as "disturbance," "derangement," etc.

To a purely palliative treatment it may, of course,

make considerable difference whether the gastric juice contains an excess of acid to be neutralized by the administration of alkali or whether it is deficient in acidity, requiring artificial aid for digestion by acids medicinally ingested. And so with the other refinements as to excess or lack of secretion. The careful physician will seek to inform himself as accurately as possible of the existing conditions in each individual case. When, however, more radical treatment is considered, the question is not as to what particular aberration of secretion or motion may be present, but whether that aberration has a local or a central cause. For not only may either a local or central cause apparently give rise to similar conditions, but the same cause, whether local or central, may give rise in different individuals to dissimilar conditions.

The circumstances modifying the causative action, so that what brings about supersecretion in one case, in another brings about superacidity, and in a third, perhaps, a diminution of secretion or qualitative lack of acid, are probably transient and unimportant. They are like the currents of wind determining the fall of an apple upon this or that particular spot; while the determining cause of aberration, independent of its direction, is some imperative action, like the gravitation which makes the apple fall, whether here or there.

REMOND (*Archives Générales de Médecine,* June, 1890) publishes a contribution to the study of "Mixed Neuroses of the Stomach," which contains the history of several instructive cases. In one the predominant phenomenon was excessive secretion, which occurred with any excitation or even independent of excitation. In such a case we have, evidently, an instability of the nervous apparatus controlling secretion, an excessive catabolic action, leading, eventually, to a failure of compensatory anabolic action, when the phenomena presented would be those of deficient secretion—a want of catabolic action for lack of material. But an original nervous disturbance might have taken the reverse direction, so that what appears in the case referred to as a secondary condition is, no doubt, in many cases primary. Thus, Remond, in the article cited, collates a considerable number of cases of disturbance in the secretory function of the stomach presenting very diverse phenomena, occurring principally in hysterical patients and in ataxics. Finally, he traces by the following path the connection between supersecretion and that

condition of atony to which Meyer has given the
name *phthisis ventriculi.*

The stomach, from some morbid state of its nervous apparatus, secretes an abnormal gastric juice.
The patient has pyrosis; the stomach at each meal
responds with undue activity to the stimulation of
food, and finally vomiting occurs to relieve the viscus from the excess of acid. The vomiting, on the
one hand, increases the irritability of the nervous
apparatus of the stomach, and, on the other, depresses the patient's spirits, thus adding to the
original trouble. The morbid activity of the
glands is increased until, finally, exhaustion occurs,
and they fail to respond to any stimulus, dilatation
and wasting being the final results. Remond does
not agree with Rossbach, Riegel, and others, who
attribute dilatation to spasm of the pylorus from irritation by too acid a secretion. The long duration
of his first case, without dilatation, negatives this, to
his mind. He believes that histological alterations
are produced in the secretory structures—a sclerosis,
in fact, which may either seal up the orifices of the
glands, producing retention-cysts, if of superficial
origin ; or destroy their secretory cells, if of deeper
location. As to the underlying cause, Rosenthal
suggests a degeneration of the sympathetic ganglia,
citing, in support of this theory, the results of
autopsies by Köhler, Demange, Landouzy, and
Dejerine. Jürgens, in a case of grave secretory
trouble of the stomach, found extensive degeneration of the plexus of Meissner and of Auerbach.
Blaschko and Sasaki found similar lesions in cases
of gastro-intestinal glandular atrophy.

From all that is known of the subject it is evident
that, in any case, the gastric clinical phenomena
are of less importance than the information to be
derived from a careful study of the general condition of the patient, in order to determine the nature
of the underlying neurosis—whether it is structural
or functional, ataxic or neurasthenic. Lavage, and
other local measures, to relieve the irritation present, may succeed in diminishing morbid reaction
and in preventing some of the unfortunate sequelæ,
but it is the neurosis which demands treatment, if
cure is to be effected.

Marine-Hospital Service.—The present status of this
service as a branch of the Treasury Department's work
may be changed. It is stated that a movement is on
foot to make the Marine-Hospital Service a department
of the medical service of the navy.

REVIEWS.

THE THROAT AND NOSE, AND THEIR DISEASES. By
LENNOX BROWNE, F.R.C.S.E. Third edition, re-
vised and enlarged. 8vo., pp. 716. Philadelphia:
Lea Brothers & Co., 1890.

MR. BROWNE's work on diseases of the nose and throat
is to-day, probably, more widely used as a text- and
reference-book than any other work on the same subject,
and deservedly so, for it is the result of enormous experience and a critical observation of the practice of other
laryngologists, and is almost absolutely free from dogmatism.

The chief change noticed in the third edition is that
the chapters upon intra-nasal diseases are much fuller,
one hundred pages being devoted to diseases of the nose
and accessory cavities, beginning with an excellent
chapter upon etiology. Mr. Browne attributes great importance to the cilia lining the respiratory tract of the
nose in maintaining a healthy condition of the mucous
membrane, and believes that destruction or injury of the
cilia by smoke, irritating vapors, etc , is often the starting-
point of a chronic catarrh.

In reviewing the causes of ozæna the author suggests
that, in some cases at least, the condition is due to a congenitally imperfect development of the lining membrane
of the nose, and that in such the tissues have at no time
been able to perform their proper functions.

The entire subject of reflex diseases of nasal origin is
very thoroughly discussed, and in a perfectly unbiassed
spirit. The evidence is so logically stated that the most
sceptical, after reading the pages devoted to this, cannot
fail to be convinced that many diseases, and often those
in which such a connection would not be expected, arise
from some nasal abnormality, and can be cured in no
other way than by intra-nasal treatment.

As to the etiology of chronic hypertrophic rhinitis, our
author is fully in accord with the views of Dr. J. N. Mackenzie, namely, that the disease is the result of recurring
attacks of acute and subacute catarrh ; and he cannot
agree with Bosworth, that septal spurs or deviations are
factors, although admitting that their removal constitutes
an important part of the treatment. In the treatment of
hypertrophic rhinitis he thinks that sprays and douches
are of little use, and that surgical measures must be
chiefly relied upon. In cases uncomplicated by septal
deformities the galvano-cautery will usually accomplish
all that is desired ; but in those which are not relieved
by such measures, he has had encouraging results from
the use of gelatin bougies formed on a rigid wire nucleus
and medicated with iodol, chloride of zinc, etc. He thinks
that paresis of the alæ nasi not infrequently prevents
complete cure, and for the relief of this he advises the use
of stimulating smelling-salts, menthol inhalations, and
"gymnastic exercise of the nasal dilator muscles." In
a few instances he has resorted to faradism. Unfortunately, he does not tell us why inhalations should relieve
the paresis, nor how "alar gymnastics" can be performed.

Septal diseases—perforation, deviations, and hyperostosis—are thoroughly discussed, and clear directions
given upon the operations indicated, and the proper
methods of performing them. Mr. Browne is opposed

to Adam's operation of refracturing the septum for traumatic deviation, and believes that rectification can be secured by removing the obstruction by means of a saw or trephine. He writes enthusiastically of Curtis's nasal trephine, and considers it the most useful instrument devised for the relief of hard obstructions.

The least satisfactory portion of the work is that upon aural diseases, though even here there is much sound advice, and Mr. Browne shows that he is more familiar with otological work than are most laryngologists.

In the second edition of this book Mr. Browne was very distinctly opposed to the operation of intubation in laryngeal diphtheria. Now, however, he confesses that his former objections have been almost entirely dissipated, chiefly by observing the results of the operation in America.

In this brief sketch we have purposely confined ourselves to the points in which the third edition of the work differs from the second, and have necessarily passed by much that is valuable, but with which all laryngologists and many general practitioners are already familiar. In general appearance the treatise differs but little from the preceding editions, and, indeed, it could not well be improved in this particular. The binding is substantial, the type clear, and the illustrations—many of which are reproductions of Mr. Browne's drawings—are numerous and above criticism.

CORRESPONDENCE.

ORIENTAL MEDICINE.

To the Editor of THE MEDICAL NEWS,

SIR: Oriental medicine in the post-mediæval period has received so little attention in the study of the history of medicine, and the materials for research are so scanty, that I venture to think the recipes below may be of interest. They are written on the fly-leaves of the *Williams Codex*, the property of Mr. Robert S. Williams, of Utica, N. Y., and are the subject of an elaborate prolegomena by Dr. Isaac H. Hall, published by the johns Hopkins University, in 1886, with *fac-similes* of the Syrian Antilegomena epistles which it contains. The translations of the prescriptions given below are, however, by Dr. Van Dyke, of Beirut, Syria. The extracts date, in all probability, from about 1471, the MSS. being dated july 4, 1471, and the prescriptions, in Arabic, being written at about the same time, and in Mesopotamia, probably near Husn Keifa. I dare say, most European physicians at the time would have deemed them useful, as they antedate Paracelsus and are contemporary with Campegius. "Steeped water of fresh glass" is, of course, a periphrasis for distilled water, and the day is still, I believe, in the future when the necessity for this precaution will be both accepted and acted upon by all our own apothecaries.   TALCOTT WILLIAMS.

Recipe for the Philosopher's Electuary—they also call it "The Matter of Life." "It is useful in excess of phlegm, and strengthens the soul, and rejoices, and digests, and eructates, and appetizes, and increases the capacity to commit to memory and to remember, and acuteness of intellect, and loosens the tongue, and re-moves indigestions, and stops 'stillicidium urinæ,' and quiets flatulencies, and increases the seminal fluid, and strengthens the penis, and makes firm the teeth, and removes pains in the joints and back. It is made of pepper and long pepper, and myrobolans and Myrobolans Bellerica, and Amyros Zeilanica, and Aristolochia (roots), rolled, and male orchis, and twigs of chamomile, and heart of pine seeds (and) citron. To be pounded and sifted and moistened like other electuaries. The dose of it is about the size of a walnut, and God is the healer of all pains."

A trial of dentifrice composed of fennel (?). (Reading doubtful. The lines apparently not perfect.)

Electuary of assafœtida (benefits) from all stings of insects and quartan fever, and from . . . assafœtida, pepper, rue . . . to be pounded and sifted and mixed (" fiat massa "). The dose . . . removes . . . (Much effaced, and words where . . . appears are obliterated.)

The dose of myrrh is half a drachm.

Talikûn. [No such word known in Arabic—probably a Mesopotamian corruption of Talcûn—Talc]: This vitriol (or alum) its scar will not granulate nor heal, and if with tweezers made of this vitriol (or alum) the hair be extracted, it will not grow at all, ever; and if a small hook be made of it, there will be caught a large fish; it debilitates it and makes it drunk; and if there be made of it a probe (*i. e.,* anything used for touching the eyes with stibium), and a sore eye be touched with it, it cures it; and it has, beside these virtues, high properties. It is made (thus): to be taken, zinc (calamine) prepared with hot water and steeped in the urine of cattle a long time, then taken out and dried, and to be taken some red coral and ground fine and steeped water of fresh glass next ten days, then taken out and dried, then all pulverized together. Then melt purified copper, and when melted in the crucible, inoculate it with the (above) medicine a times until it becomes cleansed. To every ten (parts) add two of the medicine.

To catch . . . take berries of solanum nigrum . . . bruise the leaves . . . and hang it . . . Another like it: take tartar and drug, and flour of barley and blood . . . equal parts; pound the whole . . . the place in which is . . . to it from every place, and if it is made . . . linen and let down to . . . the fish they can be caught with the hand. . . . Another, from Said el Hammam: Take horse beans and cook them with sulphur . . . and seeds of hyoscyamus niger, any bird . . . to the earth and does not (sit) high . . . take it by the hand, and if you wish pour oil . . . into its mouth.

NEWS ITEMS.

The American Association of Gynecologists and Obstetricians.—The American Association of Gynecologists and Obstetricians will hold its next annual meeting in Philadelphia, on Tuesday, Wednesday, and Thursday, September 16, 17, and 18, 1890, in the hall of the College of Physicians, corner Thirteenth and Locust Streets. All physicians interested are invited to attend the several sessions.   E. E. MONTGOMERY, M.D., *President.*
          W. WARREN POTTER, M.D., *Secretary.*

American Dermatological Association.—The fourteenth annual meeting of the American Dermatological Association was held at Richfield Springs, New York, September 2, 3, and 4, 1890. After a brief business meeting the President, Dr. Prince A. Morrow, delivered his address. Papers were read by Drs. R. W. Taylor, L. A. Duhring, R. B. Morrison, J. N. Hyde, J. C. White, H. W. Stelwagon, and others.

The American Orthopœdic Association.—The fourth annual meeting of the American Orthopædic Association will be held at the College of Physicians, Philadelphia, September 16, 17, and 18, 1890. A large number of papers will be read, and the meeting promises to be an interesting one.

Mississippi Valley Medical Association.—The medical profession is cordially invited to attend the sixteenth annual meeting of the Mississippi Valley Medical Association, to be held at Louisville, Ky., October 8, 9, and 10, 1890. The President of the Association is Dr. Joseph Mathews, Louisville; Secretary, Dr. E. S. McKee, Cincinnati; Chairman of the Committee of Arrangements, Dr. I. N. Bloom, Louisville. Elaborate preparations will be made for the entertainment of visitors. Papers from the East are promised by Drs. Frank Woodbury and H. A. Hare, Philadelphia; Dr. John A. Wyeth, New York; Dr. William C. Wile, Danbury, Conn.; and Drs. Sutton, Daly, Wood, and Murdoch, Pittsburg. Papers are also promised by many other prominent men in the profession.

This Association is an outgrowth of the old Tri-State Medical Society, which comprised members from Indiana, Illinois, and Kentucky, and now includes all the territory in the valley of the Mississippi.

The interest of the occasion will be further increased by the annual meeting of the American Rhinological Association, which will be held in Louisville October 6 7, and 8.

The Reported Case of Cholera in London.—Regarding the case reported as one of cholera, in London, a note in *The Lancet* says that though the clinical symptoms point to Asiatic cholera, there would appear to be nothing incompatible with the diagnosis of severe so-called English cholera, or cholera nostras, cases of which are by no means uncommon in England during the summer months. Every possible precaution has, however, been taken in the interests of the public health. The vessel from which the patient came has been fumigated, and her water-tanks emptied and cleansed. The conveyances by which he travelled have been disinfected, while the house, clothing, etc., have been thoroughly fumigated and cleansed. The improbability of the case being one of Asiatic cholera rests on the facts that no other cases of a like nature have occurred on the voyage or since, although all clothing and effects in the possession of the patient had been used by him during the voyage; and, further, that he was in his ordinary health on arrival. A possible source of infection has been suggested in the wearing of a suit purchased in a Calcutta bazaar. It has, however, been proved that the suit was bought in London after his arrival. The patient is rapidly recovering.

Stramonium Poisoning.—Two children were poisoned in Philadelphia, September 5th, by eating the seeds of Datura Stramonium. One, a girl three years old, died in a few hours; the other, a boy of the same age, recovered.

Dr. Gray's Treatise on Nervous Diseases.—The many friends of Dr. Landon Carter Gray will learn with pleasure that the literary labor on his forthcoming work on *Diseases of the Nervous System* is drawing toward completion. Throughout it has been Dr. Gray's aim not simply to record that which is already known of this obscure class of troubles, but to add the increment of his personal experience and give to his work the impress of personal individuality that must add largely to its value.

OFFICIAL LIST OF CHANGES IN THE STATIONS AND DUTIES OF OFFICERS SERVING IN THE MEDICAL DEPARTMENT, U. S. ARMY, FROM SEPTEMBER 2 TO SEPTEMBER 8, 1890.

WOODHULL, A. A., *Major and Surgeon*—Is granted leave of absence for one month, on surgeon's certificate of disability, with permission to go beyond the limits of the Department.—Par. 1, S. O. 122, *Headquarters Department of the Missouri, St. Louis, Mo.*, September 5. 1890.

WOOD, LEONARD, *First Lieutenant and Assistant Surgeon.*—Is hereby granted leave of absence for one month, to take effect on or about October 20, 1890, with permission to apply for an extension of one month.—Par. 1, S. O. 74. *Department of California, San Francisco, Cal.*, August 30, 1890.

DE WITT, THEODORE F., *First Lieutenant and Assistant Surgeon.*—Is granted leave of absence for one month, to take effect September 15, 1890.—S. O. 76, *Headquarters Department of Texas, San Antonio, Texas*, September 1, 1890.

APPOINTMENT.

BAXTER, JEDEDIAH H., *Colonel and Chief Medical Purveyor.*—To be Surgeon-General, with the rank of Brigadier-General, August 16, 1890, vice Surgeon-General Moore, retired from active service.—*Headquarters of the Army, A. G. O., Washington*, September 1, 1890.

OFFICIAL LIST OF CHANGES IN THE STATIONS AND DUTIES OF THE MEDICAL CORPS OF THE U. S. NAVY FOR THE WEEK ENDING SEPTEMBER 6, 1890.

WISE, J. C., *Surgeon.*—Detached from Torpedo Station, and ordered to the U. S. S. "Alliance."

FITZSIMMONS, PAUL, *Surgeon.*—Ordered to the Torpedo Station, Newport, R. I.

BRIGHT, GEORGE A., *Surgeon.*—Detached from the U. S. S. "Constellation," and ordered to the Naval Academy.

OLCOTT, F. W., *Assistant Surgeon.*—Promoted to be Passed Assistant Surgeon.

WENTWORTH, A. R., *Passed Assistant Surgeon.*—Requests to withdraw resignation; granted.

CRAWFORD, M. H., *Passed Assistant Surgeon.*—Detached from the U. S. S. "Monongahela," and granted two months' leave of absence.

KEENEY, JAMES F., *Assistant Surgeon.*—Detached from the U. S. S. "Richmond," and granted two months' leave of absence.

LOWNDES, CHARLES H. T., *Assistant Surgeon.*—Detached from the Naval Academy, and ordered to the U. S. S. "Richmond."

THE MEDICAL NEWS *will be pleased to receive early intelligence of local events of general medical interest, or of matters which it is desirable to bring to the notice of the profession.*

Local papers containing reports or news items should be marked. Letters, whether written for publication or private information, must be authenticated by the names and addresses of their writers—of course not necessarily for publication.

All communications relating to the editorial department of the NEWS *should be addressed to No. 1004 Walnut Street, Philadelphia.*

THE MEDICAL NEWS.

A WEEKLY JOURNAL OF MEDICAL SCIENCE.

VOL. LVII.　　　　SATURDAY, SEPTEMBER 20, 1890.　　　　No. 12.

ORIGINAL LECTURES.

HISTORY OF THE ADMISSION OF LIGHT IN THE AFTER-TREATMENT OF CATARACT OPERATIONS.

A Clinical Lecture,
delivered at the Charleston City Hospital, July 28, 1890.

<blockquote>

BY MIDDLETON MICHEL, M.D.,
PROFESSOR OF PHYSIOLOGY AND MEDICAL JURISPRUDENCE IN THE MEDICAL COLLEGE OF THE STATE OF SOUTH CAROLINA, AND ONE OF THE SURGEONS OF THE CITY HOSPITAL OF CHARLESTON, S. C.
</blockquote>

GENTLEMEN: We shall select for our clinical remarks this morning the cataract operation performed several weeks ago upon this woman, sixty years old. After rendering the eye, instruments, and hands aseptic, and using a four-per-cent. solution of cocaine, the linear method was adopted, performing an iridectomy, removing the lens, then closing the eye with isinglass-plaster alone—a plan of dressing the eye which we have exhibited to our classes for several years. The patient was allowed to sit up in the open ward after the operation and to take her ordinary food, though she was not permitted to go into a bright light nor to smoke her pipe, both of which my assistant, Dr. T. S. Bratton, informs me she did in a few days.

I bring this case before you as one which might be termed a perfect result, for the conjunctiva and cornea are clear; there is a well-formed coloboma with no imprisonment of the iris; the pupil is clear; the linear cicatrix is of no great extent, and vision is good for objects at a distance. Out of this window she sees the lawn, and says that she sees some object crossing over the grass. With a two-inch cataract-glass she could doubtless thread a needle. When, however, the eye has undergone so severe a mutilation of its dioptric media, you should watch it with jealous care for weeks, before subjecting it to tests with proper glasses that will prove whether, indeed, you have met with perfect success.

An eye is necessarily hypermetropic after losing its lens, the removal of which destroys its power of accommodation also; if the dioptric apparatus, thus absolutely impaired even when the operation appears successful, is to be of any ultimate use to the patient beyond mere light-perception, it must first be rendered emmetropic for clear vision at a distance; and, secondly, must be rendered myopic for clear vision at 20 or 40 cm. from the eye. To ascertain what has been the result of your surgery, visual acuity must be tested with at least a 10 D. for the one purpose, and with about a 14 D. for the other. This must not be done on a feeble and injured eye for some weeks after your surgical intervention; therefore I desire to guard you against rushing with prurient haste into statements of statistical results until you are certain of the ultimate condition of this sensitive organ. During my service in the hospital last year, three patients entered whose eyes had been operated upon for the removal of cataract a few months previously. One of these eyes was in such a condition as to endanger its healthy fellow, and I was soon obliged to enucleate the ball. Another of the patients suffered from an irido-cyclitis of some months' duration and lost the sight completely, while the third patient went through iritic complications which, I doubt not, by this time have destroyed the sight.

Entanglement of the iris, after a cataract operation, may exist for some time before giving rise to iritis; a pupil perfectly clear on inspection may, after a short time, reveal a delicate floating fragment of wrinkled anterior capsule, so transparent as to be scarcely discerned, yet quite enough to interfere permanently with vision; and plastic lymph may be organizing into indestructible adhesions which, sooner or later, will surely ruin the results of the operation. Remember, that the size, direction, and health of your incision, whether this be corneal, scleral, or corneo-scleral, almost always determine the subsequent result of your operation. The incision either avoids or leads to the production of cyclitis with the resultant contraction of the cicatrix and adjacent tissues; or perhaps yet more frequently to incarceration of the iris, which, if it do not involve the eye in panophthalmitis, may, even under the most favorable circumstances, cause chronic cyclo-iritis. An awkward incision is often succeeded by a flattened cornea, produced by a cicatrix that contracts, distorts, and occludes the pupil, dragging it toward the scleral border; and when defervescence of inflammation occurs, such an eye may retain a certain amount of vision for a while, but blindness eventually supervenes from the intra-ocular pressure caused by an abortive iridectomy, a detached retina, and a shrunken vitreous. Postpone judgment, then, respecting your supposed success until the patient uses glasses and can *see* with them.

I will not detail the steps of the operation which you witnessed the other day. I shall not inflict you, nor waste your time with the platitudes that are too frequently spread out in printed pages of redundant and battologized instructions—how to cleanse the eye, to hold the knife, to make the section, and to extract the lens. These things, by this time, you have seen so often, and concerning which you have read so much, that, with your present knowledge as graduates, you will only be the more ready to criticise severely should you discover me to be a delinquent respecting any of them. Nor shall I indulge in complacent dogmatism respecting any particular method that you should adopt in every case. With the knowledge and judgment which I presume you to possess, you will of course modify your methods according to the particular case. When you take up your keratome, "take no trenchant blade in hand" with dictatorial asseverations against iridectomy. At least let the names of de Wecker, Knapp, and others hold your Delphic utterances in abeyance. Perform iridectomy when it is obviously indicated; occasionally leave the iris with its perfect pupil when this brilliant result can be effected; while in the aged, in whom the suspensory ligament is feeble or relaxed, extract the lens in its capsule, as you saw me do in this woman, so as to avoid the possibility of a secondary pupillary membrane. Indeed, gentlemen, eclecticism in surgery is a lesson which experience is sure to teach.

My object, however, on this occasion is to speak to you of the after-treatment of cataract operations without excluding light. I can give no offence to the historian of our professional literature in dwelling exegetically upon the open method of dressing the eye after the extraction of cataract, as I thereby will furnish you with such information respecting our varied methods of treatment that you shall not suppose that what you and others have seen me do is an innovation of my own.

Toward the end of the last century Daviel, a Frenchman, first taught us that a cataractous lens could be extracted through a large corneal flap; a most difficult and extremely delicate operation, attempted for many years after by only a few expert surgeons, for the eye became practically opened in half its corneal extent, and was therefore often evacuated—vitreous, lens, and all its contents—by sudden contractions of the recti muscles. After such a corneal section it was found absolutely necessary to place the eye in a specially secured condition against anything like spasmodic contractions, or even movements associated with those of the muscles of the opposite eye. It became requisite then to put the eye up in splints, so to speak; while it was on physiological principles equally important to prevent the other eye from roaming about, so as to check what we know constitutes the associated movements of the recti muscles of these organs. Therefore was it that both eyes were bandaged; and for the careful adjustment of compresses that could exert the minimum of pressure with the maximum of resistance to accidental, spasmodic, or associated movements of the eyes, every variety of appliances and bandages were invented from Daviel's to the popular bandage known as Liebreich's.

Again, the painful ingress of light which, of course, very naturally followed upon the first exposure of these organs for simple inspection after the operation, was found to be so distressing, oftentimes so intolerable, and even dangerous through sympathetic retinal excitation, that a darkened room, or bed inclosed by curtains, came to be resorted to; not that light itself was thought to be injurious, but its sudden entrance through preternaturally dilated pupils and impingement upon the now sensitive retina, excited reflex sympathetic trouble in the eye that had been operated upon.

It is very significant that as soon as Beer invented the well-known and well-devised knife that facilitated a safer and easier performance of the corneal-flap operation without escape of the aqueous, and that secured a more frequent cicatrization of the wound, that he himself became the first to advocate the introduction of light into the patient's apartment, and urged others to follow his example; but it was not until von Gräfe introduced his peripheral linear incision through the upper segment of the cornea, of such inconspicuous extent as to heal

readily in a few hours or days, that so much danger was obviated, and so much more confidence felt in its performance even by the most inexpert, that the idea of disencumbering the eyes of heavy dressings, and of no longer enforcing precautionary measures against improbable accidents suggested itself.

It is a valuable thing to be possessed of an idea that rests upon a rational scientific basis; and that is carried out with patient, earnest, persevering conviction of its ultimate usefulness and success. The thought becomes so affiliated with one's nature, that the expectant results in their minutest details present themselves ever and anon to the mind until its accomplishment is theoretically and practically fulfilled. Such a predominant idea evidently occupied the mind of Walton while adopting his aftertreatment of cataract. In his published record we find the method announced with the fulness of a completed achievement, and with every argument that justifies the method. So important are Walton's precise yet epitomized directions that I shall read them to you word for word from the *Medical Times and Gazette*, December 3, 1870. He says:

". . . . The first thing is to close the eyelids with a couple of strips of court-plaster about an inch and a half long and a quarter of an inch wide . . . . this insures adaptation and supports the corneal flap. . . . Such closure accomplishes all that can be done for the wound without disadvantage. . . . . The tears and the aqueous readily escape because some portions of the eyelids are uncovered. Bandages and compresses of all kinds are injurious. They are hurtful in proportion to their action. All pressure, beyond that which is naturally produced from closing the eyelids, must tend to be prejudicial, and at times to be positively damaging. Whatever keeps the eye hot must be bad—whatever soaks up the secretions is objectionable. I am well aware that some surgeons pack the eye with cotton-wool or charpie and subsequently apply a bandage. This system is like the French method of treating a stump after an amputation. I believe it to be important that the patient be well fed, and, therefore, I allow him a full diet. It is a mistake to prescribe liquid food under the idea that chewing is hurtful to the eye, for in man the muscles of mastication cannot in any way influence the eyeball. It is different in most of the lower carnivora."

Now, this was Walton's treatment in 1868–69, concerning which he goes on to say:

"I believe its simplicity is the chief reason why this— my practice—is not more generally followed. It leaves nothing for meddlesome fingers to do."

But Beer, as I have already said, opposed bandages and was in the habit of closing the lids by "*strips of sticking-plaster*," which he carried, however, down over the cheek. Beer was followed, as we could show, by many German operators; and all this was in 1801.

Lawrence, in his celebrated lectures delivered at the London Ophthalmic Infirmary, and published afterward in the *Lancet*, October, 1825, p. 145, objects to bandaging the eyes, and writes:

"The application of a bandage to the eye is not to be regarded as an essential point of treatment; it is rather employed to keep the eye quiet and to guard it from any slight accident. On this account gentle confinement during the night is expedient; but the part may be left uncovered, or with a damp rag over it, while the patient is awake."

Lawrence states, also, that:

"Mr. Tyrrell has suggested that when the patient has the advantage of a good attendant, he might remain for a few hours on a couch or easy chair; so that he will be less likely to fall asleep than in bed, and thus have a better chance of sleeping at night."

The most liberal praise must, however, be awarded to Walton, whose practical injunctions on this subject more particularly arrested the attention of oculists, though receiving, perhaps, scarcely deserved prominence until Wilde, of Dublin, confirmed these teachings and practice. It was from Wilde that our own lamented friend, the late Dr. C. R. Agnew, obtained his knowledge respecting this treatment, and adopted the same in his own practice. Writing to me in July, 1885, in the letter which you here see, Dr. Agnew refers thus to this important matter:

"In the proceedings of the American Ophthalmological Society for 1869 you may find a paper by your humble servant, with the title 'A method of dressing eyes after cataract extraction and other ophthalmic operations requiring rest by exclusion of light.' In that paper I take ground against shutting patients in the dark. In founding the Brooklyn Eye and Ear Hospital, in 1868, provision was made to provide light in the wards. The same was true and continues to be so in the case of the Manhattan Eye and Ear Hospital, opened in 1869. Both these hospitals are as light as any other hospital that I have seen. I have taught in the College of Physicians and Surgeons for more than twenty years against incarcerating eye patients in the dark."

The merits and advantages of so beneficent a release offered to cataract patients were not long withheld from American surgeons who keep abreast with the progress of their science. So we find that in Philadelphia Drs. Levis and Roberts at once acknowledged the importance of such a course, and for years have followed no other in the Pennsylvania and in the Wills Eye Hospital. Since the establishment of an Ophthalmological Department in the Jefferson Medical College Hospital, in 1877, Dr. Thomson also has banished the proscriptive measures usually enforced under such circumstances. The American editors of the fourth edition of Stellwag's *Diseases of the Eye*, 1873, on page 641, say:

"The discussion in this country of the subject of cataract and its treatment being an almost everyday occurrence, American surgeons have been led to modify materially the after-treatment. The patients are not confined to their beds so long as formerly, and surgeons are not so particular in excluding every ray of light. A few turns of a flannel roller-bandage, or even a piece of black silk placed over the eyes and retained in position by strips of adhesive plaster, is all that is ever used, and then the room is moderately darkened for several days."

The same course has been adopted for years by many oculists; thus we are informed that Dr. Charles E. Michel, of St. Louis, has for eighteen years pursued a like plan, and has published his reasons in its favor. Dr. Joseph A. White, of Richmond, Va., in his annual report of the work done at the Eye, Ear, Throat, and Nose Infirmary, refers to the success of dressing with goldbeaters' skin, after Dr. Michel's plan, in favorable cases and in docile patients. Impressed with the results of Dr. Michel's practice, Dr. Chisolm, of Baltimore, has been recently induced to give the method a trial.

I could furnish exhaustive proof by an unbroken web of evidence of the value of this method of after-treatment did time permit; but enough has surely been said to rectify any misapprehensions as to the source whence we have derived our knowledge of this simple, soothing, beneficent, and defensible method; and it only remains to recommend it highly to your attention, not only for its intrinsic value in almost every case, but for the avowed popularity it has attained both in Europe and America. Isinglass and rubber strips, undarkened apartments, and freedom from restraint in the management of cataract and iridectomy operations, are not now under trial for the first time among ophthalmologists; the names of Walton, Wilde, Lawrence, Tyrrell, and Agnew will assuredly permit you to take their counsels in this matter safely "on trust;" in resorting to it, then, in your future practice you will not be treading upon doubtful ground, and will not have to watch with anxious solicitude lest some untoward accident should befall your patient.

ORIGINAL ARTICLES.

SURGERY OF THE LATERAL VENTRICLES OF THE BRAIN.

Résumé of Paper read before the Surgical Section of the Tenth International Medical Congress, Berlin, August, 1890.

BY W. W. KEEN, M.D.,

PROFESSOR OF SURGERY IN THE JEFFERSON MEDICAL COLLEGE, PHILADELPHIA, PA.

AFTER alluding to the fact that puncture of the brain for the relief of hydrocephalus dates back to the case of Dean Swift in 1744, Dr. Keen pointed out that the early operations were done through the anterior fontanelle, and not by trephining. In 1881 Wernicke first proposed to trephine and puncture the lateral ventricles. This proposal was adopted by Zenner, of Cincinnati, in 1886.

On November 7, 1888, Dr. Keen read a paper before the College of Physicians of Philadelphia,[1] in which, in ignorance of these earlier propositions, he proposed to trephine, puncture, and drain the lateral ventricles. The idea was suggested to him by a case of exploratory trephining for supposed abscess in the temporo-sphenoidal lobe. The post-mortem examination showed that there was distention of the lateral ventricle in consequence of tubercular meningitis, and that the drainage-tube had reached to within a quarter of an inch of the ventricle without producing inflammation. He pointed out the fact that the brain would not bear pressure nearly as well as the other viscera, and hence the need for early trephining. He then reported the following three cases of his own.

CASE I.—A boy, four years old, was threatened with blindness from acute hydrocephalus. This

---

[1] THE MEDICAL NEWS, December 1, 1888.

condition was thought to be due probably to tumor of the cerebellum, though on which side was doubtful. Dr. Strawbridge had examined the eyes and had found that there were choked disks with retinal hæmorrhages and swelling. The swelling of the disk measured 2.30 mm. in each eye, and in view of the rapidly-increasing blindness he brought the child to Dr. Keen for operation. This was done at the Woman's Hospital, Philadelphia, January 11, 1889.

A puncture was made at a point one inch and a quarter behind the left meatus and the same distance above "Reid's base-line." A half-inch button of bone was removed and the brain punctured by a hollow needle (No. 5 French catheter scale), which was directed toward a point two and a half inches vertically above the opposite meatus. At a depth of about an inch and three-quarters the resistance suddenly ceased, and the cerebro-spinal fluid began to escape. Three stout doubled horsehairs were then passed into the ventricle. No peculiar phenomena occurred during the operation. The highest subsequent temperature was 101¾° for a brief interval, but most of the time it was normal. In two days the swelling of the optic nerves had fallen to 1.57 and 1.63 mm. in the right and left eye respectively, and by the sixth day to 1.09 mm. in both eyes. By the seventh day the swelling of the optic nerve had increased, and the drainage was not very free. The tumor was sought for by probing through the drainage-opening into the occipital lobe, almost to the occipital bone. No tumor being found by this procedure, an opening a quarter of an inch in diameter was gouged in the occipital bone below and to the left of the inion. The cerebellum was explored by a probe to the depth of two and one-quarter inches in the direction of the left lobe, and again obliquely across into the right lobe, but no tumor was found. This wound healed by first intention without any fever.

On the fourteenth day the horsehairs were removed and a small rubber drainage-tube was inserted into the ventricle in order to give free vent to the fluid. This was attended by no pain or discomfort. By the twenty-eighth day the child had become somewhat restless, and the swelling of the disks, which had fallen to 0.83 mm., had again increased to 1.33 mm. in each eye. Accordingly, the right side of the skull was trephined at the corresponding point above and behind the ear, and the occipital lobe was punctured to the tentorium, but no tumor was found. A drainage-tube was then passed directly into the right ventricle, being inserted without the prior puncture by a hollow needle.

On the thirty-second day, by a fountain-syringe, the bag of which was raised about six inches above the head, the ventricles were irrigated from side to side with warm boric acid solution—4 grains to the ounce. While the connection was being made with the tube the child was a little restless, but so soon as the warm water began to flow into the brain he became quiet and said that "it felt good." The fluid slowly escaped from the opposite side. The bag of the syringe was then elevated until the escape

became quite free, but not a continuous stream. It was estimated that about eight ounces passed into the ventricles, of which about two ounces escaped from the opening on the opposite side, consequently about six ounces were retained. No phenomena whatever were apparent during the process described except the comfort shown by the child.

On the thirty-fourth day the ventricles were again irrigated from side to side with plain boiled water, which gave less relief than the boric acid solution, but produced no ill effects. A few days later the child was evidently not so well, and he died on the forty-fifth day, the first drainage-tube having been in place nearly continuously after the operation.

At the autopsy the cerebro-spinal fluid was found perfectly clear, more so than that obtained at the first tapping, which was slightly turbid. The ventricles were greatly distended with fluid. In the left lobe of the cerebellum a sarcoma was found, which had compressed, as had been suspected, the straight sinus and the veins of Galen, and had encroached upon the fourth ventricle. The sinuses through which the rubber tubes passed were not surrounded by an inflammatory zone. There was no injury of the opposite wall of the ventricle, and no trace remained of the punctures in the cerebrum or cerebellum. The oblique puncture made in the latter had gone through the tumor, which, however, was too soft to be perceived at the time.

CASE II.—A boy, aged three and a half years. Hydrocephalus set in four or five months after birth. His mental condition was extremely weak.

On March 5, 1889, the left ventricle was tapped in the same manner as in Case I. At a depth of an inch and a quarter the resistance suddenly ceased, and the cerebro-spinal fluid immediately escaped. As in the first case, the fluid was slightly turbid. Drainage by horsehairs was in this case also not very effective. The highest temperature after the operation was 100¾°, and there was marked increase in the use of the right arm, which had been paretic. The drainage being insufficient, on the fourth day the ventricle on the opposite side was opened, and a small drainage-tube inserted in each ventricle. These were stopped by disinfected plugs of wood, with a V-shaped slot cut in each, so as to permit the escape of the fluid at the rate of about thirty-five drops a minute. As this seemed to be too free, after four and a half hours other disinfected plugs were inserted with smaller slots. Convulsions began the next day, and when Dr. Keen reached the patient he found the convulsions constant. He then decided to replace the fluid that had been drained away, and having no time for the preparation of an artificial cerebro-spinal fluid, he used plain boiled water for this purpose. This was siphoned from a height of about eight inches. When the warm water began to flow into the ventricles the spasms ceased. The flow was then immediately stopped by squeezing the tube, and in a few minutes the convulsions returned. They were immediately arrested again by allowing the water to flow. Eight times the convulsions returned and each time they were arrested by a siphonage of from half an ounce to one ounce of fluid. Dr. Keen estimated that the amount of fluid injected was nearly a pint. No further spasms occurred, but the child gradually failed, and died in the afternoon. The post-mortem showed great hydrocephalic distention, but no injury from the operation.

CASE III.—This was a case of tubercular meningitis, with unilateral acute internal hydrocephalus of the left ventricle. The foramen of Monro, as determined at the autopsy, was closed. This closure was attended by unilateral distention, and produced right hemiplegia. In this respect the case is probably unique. The left ventricle was tapped through the arm-centre. The child was almost *in extremis* when the operation was performed, and died about four hours later. At this operation also it was easy to determine when the ventricle was reached.

Dr. Keen next referred to the case reported by von Bergmann in his *Surgical Treatment of Brain Lesions*, as the first case ever operated upon, though not published until after the reader's paper and a note upon his first case. Von Bergmann's case was operated on, July 15, 1887, by the anterior route, and proved fatal on the fifth day. Dr. Keen then described two cases reported to him by letter by Mr. Mayo Robson, of Leeds, as follows:

A girl ten years old, without preceding illness, began to have pain in the left ear, and was feverish, December 19, 1888. In three days a discharge followed, which gradually lessened, but was still present a month later when admitted to the hospital. There had been also rigidity of the neck and twitching of the right angle of the mouth. No vomiting; slight mental disturbance. On admission, January 19, 1889, her temperature was 105°; she complained of pain in the left side of the head; there was paresis of the right arm and leg which gradually developed into complete hemiplegia and aphasia. Optic disks inflamed.

Operation, February 7, 1889: Trephining was done over the arm-centre; the dura was found healthy. On exposing the brain it did not pulsate, and seemed to be compressed. An exploring-needle was passed deeply in various directions in the hope of reaching pus, but failing to find any the needle was pushed into the lateral ventricle and a half-ounce of clear fluid was drawn off. After this, pulsation returned in the brain. The wound was closed as usual, no drainage being employed.

On the next day there was slight power in the arm, soon after in the leg, and on the third day she could answer simple questions. Within a month the hemiplegia was gone, and six months later she was perfectly well.

Even a half-ounce of fluid seems to have imperilled life by pressure, and the operation undoubtedly saved the patient's life—a most important and encouraging lesson for the future.

· Mr. Robson's second case was one of an infant who was trephined for rapidly-increasing hydrocephalus, following treatment of spina bifida by Morton's injection. The skin was trephined an inch in front of the Rolandic fissure over the second frontal convolution. The dura was opened and the needle of an exploring-syringe inserted into the

12*

ventricle, which was reached an inch from the cerebral surface. By means of Lister's sinus-forceps a rubber drain was inserted, following the needle as a guide. The drainage was so free that it wet the dressings and ran on the floor, and after this the patient seemed much relieved. The drainage soon became less free, and on the third day the child died in convulsions. The post-mortem showed that the brain had shrunk so much that the end of the tube was lying between the dura and the brain.

Dr. Keen then referred to the case of Ayers and Hersman, in which, on December 4, 1888, puncture was made over the coronal suture an inch and a half from the middle line. The operation was repeated on April 28, 1889, by Dr. Hersman. The first operation was followed by the escape of from four to eight ounces of cerebro-spinal fluid, which caused evident improvement. At the second operation no fluid was found in the ventricle, and the child was very much improved.

Of the 7 cases thus far reported, 2 have recovered and 4 died—a mortality of 71 per cent., which, for a new operation, and for so extremely a dangerous condition, is far from discouraging.

Dr. Keen then entered into the question of the technique of the operation, and pointed out that it was not difficult or dangerous, and that the rules that he had laid down in his former paper[1] had proved to be correct, and that in his judgment the lateral route is the best, except in special instances. From his experience in these three cases he urges that the puncture be made by a canula (No. 13 French catheter scale), and that the drainage shall not be secured by a tube, but by a sufficiently large bundle of horsehairs, and that too much haste shall not be used in draining off the fluid, as such haste may cost the life of the patient, as in Case II.

The speaker then took up the question of hæmorrhage into the ventricles, and referred to the following case, reported to him personally by Professor Frederic S. Dennis, of New York. It is the first case in which a clot has been removed from the lateral ventricle.

A man, aged thirty-six years, was struck on the right side of the head by a falling ladder, but was not rendered unconscious by the blow. An hour after admission to the hospital his left arm became paralyzed, and later, the face and leg also. A diagnosis of cerebral hæmorrhage was made, and six hours after the accident he was operated upon.

A linear fracture without depression was discovered, and trephining was done over the arm-centre. No epidural and no subdural clot was found, nor was any clot discovered when the brain tissue was incised. Accordingly, an incision was made directly into the ventricle, and when the retractors were slightly separated a blood-clot about the size of a pullet's egg shot out of the ventricles with enough force to fall several feet from the patient's head.

---

[1] Loc. cit.

Gentle irrigation and drainage were used, and the wound was dressed in the ordinary manner. The patient never recovered from the paralysis, became delirious, and in three days died comatose.

The autopsy confirmed the diagnosis, and also showed that there had been great laceration of the cerebral substance, to which fact death was due. There was no meningitis and no suppuration.

The author then narrated four cases of abscess bursting into the lateral ventricle, beginning with the historic case of Detmold, in 1849, and adding three cases ; one of Pancoast's, one of Morehouse's, and one of Morton's. All of the cases died, a result that would be expected after so serious an accident.

The next class of cases mentioned was that due to rupture of the ventricles by compound fracture. Two cases were referred to, one of Massa's, the other of Hewitt's, in each of which the lateral ventricles were primarily torn and there was free discharge of cerebro-spinal fluid. Both of these cases recovered.

Of secondary opening of the ventricles he mentioned seven cases, reported by Bouchacourt, Berenger de Carpi, Erichsen; Rodenstein, Cheever, and himself. Strange to say, four of these seven cases recovered.

Five cases of rupture of the lateral ventricles, from simple fracture of the skull, were also referred to, one each described by Thompson, Haywood, and Erichsen, and two by Lucas. All of these cases were in young children, five years of age or less, and all showed secondary soft swelling under the scalp. The cerebro-spinal fluid was removed, either by tapping, or, as in one case, by rupture. Of the five cases three recovered.

After consideration of the entire subject the following conclusions were reached :

1. Injuries involving the ventricles, the result of compound fracture or of trephining, and involving great disturbance of the cerebral substance, are not necessarily fatal, for ten of the twenty-six cases here reported have recovered. In these few cases compound fractures and extensive injuries, unless primarily fatal, seem to be less dangerous than rupture of the ventricle from simple fracture. They should be treated antiseptically by drainage and the usual treatment of wounds in other regions. If pus follows, or if the cerebro-spinal fluid becomes dammed back, causing symptoms of pressure, incision and free drainage should be resorted to.

2. In cases of simple fracture involving the ventricles, experience would seem to indicate that it would be wise not to attempt any operative procedure unless threatening symptoms supervene. If necessary to interfere, the cyst containing cerebrospinal fluid should be continuously and slowly drained by a small bundle of horsehairs, rather than by freer evacuation. In the majority of cases constant pressure, and but little active treatment, may be all that is necessary.

3. Abscess of the brain bursting into the lateral ventricle has been thus far uniformly fatal, and demands the promptest treatment possible. The suggestion made for immediate bilateral trephining and irrigation of the ventricles can, at least, do no harm, although the possibility of its doing good is but slight in so serious a condition.

4. Hydrocephalus, whether acute or chronic, is usually a fatal disease. Surgical procedures for tapping the ventricles for its relief are easy, and certainly do not *per se* involve great danger. Whether they will cure the disease is, as yet, not determined.

5. In acute effusions, tapping, with or without drainage, as may be thought best, will certainly save some lives otherwise doomed to be lost ; and, in the chronic form, long-continued slow drainage at an early period is at least worthy of a trial, with a reasonable hope of success in a few cases.

6. The methods here described for performing the operation, especially by the lateral route, are at least worthy of a trial, with a view to determine the value of such surgical procedures.

7. After trephining and tapping the ventricles, irrigation of the ventricular cavities from side to side is not only possible, but it does no harm. In abscess involving the ventricle, and possibly in other conditions, it may possibly do good. The fluid used for such irrigation should not contain anything which, if retained and absorbed, might do harm. An artificial cerebro-spinal fluid, or a simple boric acid solution, would seem to be the best for such use.

8. Convulsions, due to too rapid withdrawal of the cerebro-spinal fluid, may be checked by injecting an artificial cerebro-spinal fluid, or such other innocuous fluid that is available.

9. In either irrigating or injecting the ventricles it is probably desirable that the air should not enter, but such entrance of air does not seem to be productive of mischief.

10. In hæmorrhage into the lateral ventricle, at least of traumatic origin, immediate trephining and evacuation of the clots should be done, which in a few cases will probably be followed by a cure, unless the injury of the cerebral tissue is so great as to be incompatible with life.

THE SO-CALLED MOUNTAIN-FEVER OF COLORADO AND ADJACENT REGIONS, ITS DESCRIPTION AND TREATMENT.

BY L. HUBER, M.D,.
OF ROCKY FORD, COLORADO.

IN Colorado it is very common to hear the term, mountain-fever, both from the laity and from physicians. The term is not confined, however, to this

State, but is used more or less throughout the whole Rocky Mountain region. It will be interesting to know just what type of fever is meant by this, and its probable etiology, symptoms, and successful treatment.

Types of fever vary with diversities of climate, soil, altitude, etc. I am quite certain that I first observed cases of the so-called mountain-fever in the Arkansas River valley, in western Kansas. There it was not known by the above appellation; nevertheless, several years' experience with the disease convinces me of its identity with mountain-fever. In 1884 and 1885 there was rapid occupation and settlement of new lands in the vicinity of Kinsley, Kansas, where the writer was then in active practice. During these years there was an exceptionally heavy rainfall. Farmers were encouraged, vast tracts of prairie were converted into farms, and cities and towns were built. In this rush after homes and business little attention was paid to the source and quality of the drinking-water, a pool, or stream, or shallow well supplying it. The result was that many communities were fever-stricken. After the first extensive outbreak isolated cases continued to appear, and may occasionally be found at the present time.

In 1887 I removed to Rocky Ford, Colorado, a small town, 4100 feet above sea-level. Here, too, under the development of the irrigation system of agriculture, a rich valley was being rapidly converted into a farming country. The Arkansas River, the only stream or body of water in the vicinity, flows in a well-defined channel, and with a strong current. The current is also strong in the several irrigating canals, and there is no stagnant water from which effluvia would be expected to arise. Water was freely distributed over the newly-cultivated soil. The supply of drinking-water was drawn from the open ditches, filtered more or less thoroughly, and stored in cisterns. When carefully filtered and kept in clean reservoirs the water is clear and tasteless, and develops no odor for many months, if at all. It is, however, "hard," and is called *alkali* water.

Even in the mountain districts the same system of irrigation and water-supply exists, and the same types of fever prevail. The soil of the valley is a sandy loam, very rich and productive. The natural grasses of the valley are rather sparse, and the timber-belt is confined to narrow limits along the Arkansas.

With our previously conceived notions of the origin of malarial poison, it is difficult to believe that the fever in question is of malarial origin. A dry, almost rainless climate; a dry soil, sparsely covered with vegetation before the introduction of agriculture; an elevation of 4100 feet above sea-level, no marsh lands; and no stagnant waters—the very opposite to countries where we usually find the mala-

rial poison. Yet, some eminent authorities recognize that the agent producing malarial fever is found under these circumstances. Professor Bartholow, in his *Practice of Medicine*, in defining the limits of malaria, says: "One important factor is elevation, malaria not breeding higher than 5000 feet above the sea, which seems to be its maximum limit. The apparent exceptions to this, afforded by the so-called 'mountain-fever' of Colorado will be alluded to hereafter." The same writer also observes: "That malarial poison is soluble in water, and is contained in the surface-water of infected districts, seems now to be well established. The author found the surface-water of Kansas to produce malarial fevers and cholera." Yet, withal, it is not difficult to find physicians of large experience who will deny the malarial origin of mountain-fever. As for myself, I have seen well-defined ague in persons who have not been away from the vicinity of Rocky Ford for a number of years. These cases were certainly contracted there. I have also met with typical remittent fever. These are not classed with the form of fever usually known as mountain-fever.

The description of several cases taken from the writer's note-book will prepare the way for a correct description of the disease, and perhaps furnish a true picture of it:

CASE I.—Walter B., aged twenty-one years; usually strong and healthy. He had been complaining for a few days, when, on April 9th, was taken with a chill, followed by high fever, headache, pain in right groin and in back and limbs. He was much depressed, and quite weak. I saw him on April 10th, and found the above symptoms persisting. Temperature 102°; pulse 100, and rather feeble. He had had several large watery stools. Tongue was rather heavily coated, but the tip was bare and red. I ordered the following:

R.—Aromatic sulphuric acid . . 2 drachms.
　　Infusion of digitalis . . 2 ounces.
One teaspoonful every three hours.

Also:

R.—Sulphate of cinchonidine . . ½ drachm.
　　Extract of cascara sagrada . 6 grains.—M.
Divided in six capsules, of which one was taken every three hours.

I also directed a milk diet to be employed.

April 10. Morning temperature 103.5°; pulse 105; no nausea; no delirium; skin moist; bowels moved once during the day. Treatment continued.

11th. Morning temperature 101.5°; pulse 90, and strong. In the evening the temperature and pulse were unchanged. Patient has taken three pints of milk, and without discomfort. Treatment continued.

12th. Morning and evening temperature 99°; pulse 85. Headache and pains entirely gone. Tongue cleaning; patient feels stronger.

From this time he continued to convalesce: but

from the time required it was evident that the disease, even in its short course, had made quite a profound impression on his system.

CASE II.—J. H. G., adult; strong, and of a full habit; had been working on an irrigating canal for several days, and drank water therefrom. He had had slight diarrhœa, and felt weak. In the night he was taken with chills and diarrhœa; severe headache and pains in back and limbs. The stools, he says, were fœtid and ochre-colored.

On examination I found the temperature 102°; pulse 83. There was perceptible enlargement of spleen, and some tenderness over the abdomen. Patient's face was congested, and the eyes quite injected. I ordered the following:

R.—Sulphate of quinine   .   .   .   5 grains.
      Sanguinarine   .   .   .   .   ¼ grain.—M.
To be taken at night.

Also:

R.—Dilute hydrochloric acid, } of each 2 drachms.
      Glycerin,   }
      Water sufficient to make .   . 2 ounces.
A teaspoonful every three hours.

A milk diet was ordered.

On the evening of the following day I found my patient quite comfortable; tongue cleaning; pulse and temperature normal. I ordered a dessertspoonful of elixir calisaya after meals, and dismissed the case.

CASE III.—Richard D., aged seven years; taken on the night of April 5th with a chill, and severe pain in the gastric region. I found him with a temperature of 104°; pulse 120, and small; tongue coated, with the papillæ prominent; tip red and strawberry-like. The child was in great pain.

I directed warmth to be applied to his feet and limbs, and gave him two-drop doses of fluid extract of gelsemium every hour until the skin became moist, and the pain somewhat relieved.

April 6. At 7 A. M. patient much the same; temperature 104.5°; pulse 128; some delirium; headache; pain in spine and in back of neck; nausea and vomiting. Can discover no tenderness over the spine. The coldness of the extremities has disappeared; bowels are confined. I ordered the gelsemium to be continued in two-drop doses every two hours, and also one grain of calomel every two hours until five doses were taken. For the thirst I allowed an effervescing draught. Tepid compresses were employed to reduce the high temperature.

7th. Patient passed a restless night, the fever at times rising above 105°; pulse 130; is nervous, and tosses about in bed; headache still present, and uneasy sensations along the spine are complained of. Vomiting has ceased, and the patient retains milk. No tenderness along the spine. During the day the temperature fell more than a degree. No evacuation from the bowels. Pupils contracted. The gelsemium and the tepid-water compresses were continued. I ordered 5 grains of sulphate of quinine by the rectum every three hours.

8th. Temperature 104° at 6 A. M.; pulse 120; patient lies with arms flexed and rigid; stupor;

pupils dilated. The bowels acted freely during the night; some tenderness along the spine, especially over the upper vertebræ; movement of the limbs causes pain; no vomiting; thirst considerably abated. Mild counter-irritation along the spine was ordered; quinine discontinued.

9th. Temperature 103°; pulse 114; patient sleeps naturally at intervals, and wakens less delirious; coughs considerably at times; takes milk freely at regular intervals; bowels have acted twice; tongue moist, and coated toward the tip; raised in flakes. Treatment continued.

10th. Temperature 103°; pulse 105; patient comfortable and rational, and takes milk freely. Expression good; changes his position readily. At 3 P. M. his pulse fell to 101.2°; pulse 96, and compressible; still coughs considerably. At 6 P. M. he was sweating freely, and passed a large quantity of urine. Later, his temperature became normal, and he slept well.

From this date there was slow convalescence, though on alternate days, for some time, mild fever appeared. With the administration of the following mixture, to which I am very partial under certain circumstances, the patient recovered:

R.—Dilute nitric acid   .   .   .   1 drachm.
      Sanguinarine   .   .   .   .   1 grain.
      Glycerin   .   .   .   .   .   3 drachms.
      Water, sufficient to make   . 2 ounces.—M.
One teaspoonful three times a day.

This case is rather typical of the disease in children, and my note-book could furnish other very similar examples. They all show the profound impression made upon the spinal cord and brain.

Symptomatology.—From these and similar cases the history of the disease may be sketched as follows: The premonitory symptoms are usually a chill, or chilly sensations, followed by fever more or less marked and persistent. The temperature ranges from 102° to 105° at the onset, but usually falls several degrees during the first week. There are no uniform or marked remissions, but, often, intermissions will follow the onset, and continue for a week, if the case is untreated, when the fever will return and assume a continued type, lasting from two to four weeks. There are often localized pains, and especially in children there is severe distress in the gastric region. The head, back, and limbs usually ache. These symptoms often very closely simulate those of spinal meningitis, as the above reported cases show. In adults the tongue is coated, except ing the tip, and sometimes the edges. A clean tip is always seen in cases that ultimately assume the typhoid type. In children the enlarged papillæ project through the coating, and the tip of the tongue is strawberry-like. The pulse and temperature usually preserve the normal ratio; if not, the former is rather slow. There are often nausea and vomiting, though these do not generally persist. The bowels may be loose or confined. In children they are often stubbornly constipated, and difficult to regulate with medicines. The liver and spleen are frequently perceptibly enlarged. As a rule, there is no tenderness in the right iliac region, though this and a tympanitic condition sometimes arise.

The headache is often excruciating. Delirium is not usual, but when it exists it is low and muttering. The spinal symptoms are often marked, and consist in shooting pains passing up and down the spine and into the extremities. There may be tremor. Sometimes the patient loses the power of motion.

In not a small percentage of cases cough and bronchial irritation are present.

The eyes are usually suffused, and show slight signs of jaundice. In children the pupils are widely dilated. The skin is generally dry, sweating occurring only as the fever abates. Often the disease breaks up with a copious sweat and several free evacuations from the bladder and bowels.

Convalescence is slow and accompanied with a strong tendency to the development of a mild but obstinate intermittent fever, quotidian in type. Relapses are apt to follow at the septenary periods, unless the case is closely watched and carefully treated.

Treatment.—Having already specified the measures and remedies available in this disease, it would seem that little more need be said regarding the treatment. However, with a riper experience and wider observation I am constrained to speak in very positive terms on this subject.

The first proposition is that this so-called mountain-fever tends, under favorable circumstances, to pursue a benign course, but this does not signify that treatment is useless. By proper nursing, dieting, and medication, the disease can be shortened, and the suffering of the patient greatly mitigated. Baths are very useful, and should be systematically given. The temperature rarely rises to the danger-point, yet, for the harsh, dry skin, sponging with tepid water is effective. In children, when the temperature reaches the highest point, I direct tepid-water compresses to be applied over the abdomen and thighs. These often abstract enough heat to cause a perceptible fall in the temperature. For the hot, throbbing temples cold applications often add greatly to the patient's comfort.

The diet is not to be overlooked. I almost invariably order several ounces of milk to be given every three hours. It is not often that this regimen disagrees. When I find some contra-indication or some obstacle to its use, I order broth or some good beef-extract. The reason that I insist upon a fluid diet is that the bowels are already loaded, and slow to respond to medicines. When diarrhœa exists absorption is so interfered with that only the most assimilable foods enter the system.

The patient having no appetite, it will not do to consult his preferences and leave him without sustenance, or allow hurtful articles to be given. A due allowance of cold drink contributes greatly to the patient's comfort and welfare.

As to medicines, there are several that do positive good. Gelsemium, in from two- to five-drop doses of the fluid extract every three hours, will frequently control the fever, mitigate the spinal pains, and break up the disease. I have tried it alone in many cases, and with very uniform results. Even after quinine had been employed without satisfactory results gelsemium produced good effects.

The mineral acids, nitric or hydrochloric, or a combination of the two, are also useful. It is usual with me to employ a combination of the acids and gelsemium.

As to the use of quinine and its congeners, for some reason they are not satisfactory. They will check the disease, but they are slow in producing their effect, and in the high altitudes where this fever is found they cause an untoward impression on the whole nervous system. Usually there is more or less pulmonary congestion, and the quinine increases this. It requires large doses of the remedy to produce any early result.

After convalescence is established the septenary periods must be watched. It is always well to continue some mild antiperiodic for two or three weeks.

For isolated symptoms and complications the usual measures employed in other fevers are admissible. It is useless to try heroic measures to regulate the fever. In some regions it is customary to attack it with ponderous doses of mercurials and quinine, but the complications that then arise in the nervous system become serious. As hitherto remarked, the fever tends to self-limitation, but when thrown out of its course seems to take a firmer hold upon the patient, and to be more grave. On general principles it may be said that medication should be directed primarily to the maintenance of open emunctories and the elimination of the *materies morbi* through them.

THE SURGERY OF THE THYROID GLAND [1]

BY A. H. LEVINGS, M.D.,
OF APPLETON, WISCONSIN.

THE thyroid gland, like the spleen and the thymus and suprarenal glands, has no duct. Its function is not well understood.

In its normal condition it is described as consisting of two lobes situated on the sides of the trachea, and connected by an isthmus which overlies the second and third rings of the trachea.

In its histological structure (Schenk) it is com-

---

[1] Read before the Wisconsin State Medical Society, June, 1890.

posed of connective and elastic tissue so interwoven as to form numerous meshes in which are found closed vesicles. These vesicles consist of a homogeneous membrane, lined with cylindrical epithelia and filled with a clear albuminous fluid. The cylindrical epithelia are often found detached and floating in the albuminous fluid, or forming small aggregations in different parts of the vesicles. A fine meshwork of blood- and lymph-vessels surrounds each vesicle. The nerves supplying the thyroid are derived principally from the sympathetic, but also to some extent from the pneumogastric.

Although the thyroid in its normal condition has but two, or at most three lobes, one on each side of the trachea, and the third, the pyramid, connected to the isthmus, in its pathological state, associated, connected or disconnected lobules are sometimes found. These associated lobules are in form and consistence not unlike the lymph-glands. They are situated, according to Wölfler, in the space bounded below by the arch of the aorta, on the sides by the carotids; and above by the hyoid bone. Gruber divides the accessory thyroid glands into superior, inferior, and posterior. The first two groups he further divides into median and lateral. The superior are those lobules found between the upper edge of the thyroid isthmus and the hyoid bone. The lateral glands or lobules are those found between the hyoid bone and the clavicle, generally situated near or associated with the lateral lobes. Of especial interest are the posterior accessory glands, found beneath the thyroid, between the trachea and œsophagus or below the œsophagus.

The enlargement of the thyroid gland, producing what is usually called goitre, occurs sometimes before birth, frequently during childhood, more often at the age of puberty, and occasionally in later life. It may be confined to one lobe or to some part of it, or may affect the entire gland. It may be temporary, from congestion caused by valvular heart-disease, during the period of menstruation, at the time of confinement, or it may be permanent. The permanent cases are either benign or malignant. In the benign enlargement there is an increase of tissue of one or more of the component parts of the gland, but it retains the gland-structure. In the malignant enlargement the growth of tissue does not conform to the structure of the gland. It is an adventitious tissue, usually carcinoma or sarcoma, and occurs most frequently where goitre is endemic or epidemic.

In the formation of goitres three principal varieties may be considered, namely, the follicular, the fibrous, and the vascular. In the follicular variety the first step is an increase of the cylindrical epithelia lining the vesicles. This leads to a growth of the vesicle itself which finally divides, forming two. Thus, in this variety, there is not only an increase in size of the vesicles, but also an increase in number. The vesicular goitre is soft and semi-fluctuating. Cysts are formed by the pressure of these vesicles producing absorption of the adjacent walls, thus converting many vesicles into one cyst. The fibrous form is produced by an increase of the connective tissue forming the framework of the gland, and which surrounds the vesicles. It may be increased to such an extent that the vesicles are almost entirely obliterated, and the gland feels hard and resistant.

In describing the vascular form it must be remembered that the thyroid gland is supplied by four, sometimes by five arteries; two superior thyroids from the external carotid, two inferior from the subclavian, and occasionally a middle thyroid from the innominate artery. These arteries enter the gland, divide and subdivide in the connective tissue, and finally form a network around each vesicle. The blood is returned by six veins. The two superior open into the internal jugular. The two middle make a connection with the thyroid circuit and open into the internal jugular. The two inferior open into the right and left innominate veins. In the vascular form of goitre the arteries may be especially enlarged—those on the surface as well as the branches which penetrate the gland-substance—giving it a strong pulsation which is often very noticeable on inspection. The veins are enlarged much oftener than the arteries—the so-called *struma varicosa*. The small veins in the glands become varicose, tortuous, and greatly enlarged. The veins on the surface are often enlarged into wide channels.

The cysts which are found in goitre, instead of containing the clear albuminous fluid natural to the vesicles, are often filled with a colloid substance, colorless, yellowish, or of a greenish color. It is thick and sticky, and contains "kernels" and epithelia, and, according to Virchow, is probably produced by a chemical change of the normal albuminous contents of the vesicles. The cysts may also be filled with blood, due to the rupture of a bloodvessel in the cyst-wall, generally caused by amyloid degeneration rendering the arteries inelastic and brittle.

Etiology.—Among the predisposing causes of goitre are age, and especially the period of puberty. The menstrual period and pregnancy are apt to lead to a swelling of the gland, which is at first only vascular, but which often results in an increase of connective tissue which is permanent. An increase of the circulation from nerve-irritation is also a cause, as seen in Basedow's disease. The blowing of wind-instruments, ascending mountains, lifting heavy weights, an imperfect return of the venous blood as in heart-disease (right side), may each be causative. It may be congenital. Some countries are almost entirely free, while in others, especially in valleys lying between high mountains, as in parts of Styria, Tyrol, and Switzerland, goitre is endemic and often epidemic. In some valleys nearly every inhabitant is affected. Not only those who have always lived there, but also those who for a considerable time make their residence there. The disease often attacks whole garrisons of soldiers and schools. In these regions where goitre is so constant, idiots, mutes, and cretins form a large portion of the population. Individuals suffering from idiocy or cretinism generally have goitre.

In Styria the government has established a large hospital for cretins, which is full to overflowing, and yet only a small part of the cretins of the country are accommodated.

The cause of goitre in these countries has long and diligently been sought. The social relations, the air, the water, the telluric conditions have each and all been most persistently examined. The air influenced by the surrounding mountains and by moisture has been thought, at different times and by different observers, to have much to do with the production of goitre. The water, usually strongly impregnated with lime and magnesia, has had its adherents as a causative condition. The state of the soil, often saturated with moisture and impregnated with deposits from the overflowing mountain streams, has also had many adherents. Dr. Theodore Kocher, in 1883–84, in the Canton Berne, had the surroundings of 76,606 children between the ages of seven and sixteen years examined, with a view to determine, if possible, the cause of goitre. There was a most minute and searching examination made of the soil and water, and it was found that in regions where goitre was most frequent the soil was richest in organic material; that the inhabitants drank surface-water impregnated with organic matter and rich with microörganisms; that there were some families entirely free from goitre, and that these used water from meadow springs, nearly free from both organic matter and microörganisms. From these investigations his conclusions were that in these regions the cause of goitre was the organic matter of the drinking-water.

The actual cause of goitre in these regions is yet in doubt, but the theories advanced by Lücke, Klebs, and Bircher, that goitre is caused by a microörganism, have many followers. Thus far, however, their theories have not been substantiated.

Symptoms.—The growth of goitre is usually slow, and ordinarily produces no marked symptoms until it has attained a large size, when it may seriously impede respiration from pressure on the larynx or trachea. Lobules situated beneath the sternum, on the trachea, or between the trachea and œsophagus, are very apt to produce injurious pressure; or when

one lobe or part of a lobe is considerably enlarged, harm is produced by pressure on the side of the trachea.

Where the gland is much enlarged and the sternohyoid and thyroid muscles are rigid, they press the gland down tightly and thereby cause stenosis of the trachea. It is also held that by considerable and long-continued pressure on the larynx or trachea fatty degeneration is produced, making them pliable, and that by a sudden twisting of the gland a kink in the trachea may be produced, resulting in death from asphyxia. Pressure of the gland may produce paralysis of the vagus or of the recurrent laryngeal nerves with a fatal result. Billroth states that such deaths, resulting from goitre, are much more frequent than is generally supposed. Death may be produced not only by paralysis, but also by irritation of the nerves, causing spasm of the muscles of the larynx.

Stenosis of the œsophagus with difficult deglutition may also occur when a portion of the gland has grown between the œsophagus and trachea.

Pressure on the carotids may occur, producing anæmia of the brain, and on the jugular veins, causing a stasis of blood in the head.

Treatment.—The approved methods of treatment practised at the present time may be considered under five heads:

1. The use of iodine.
2. Electrolysis.
3. The treatment of cysts.
4. Ligation of the thyroid arteries.
5. Extirpation.

The treatment of goitre by iodine, externally, usually in the form of a salve, and internally by the administration of potassium iodide, has long been practised, and often with good results, especially in cases which have not attained a large size, and are not of long duration. Its action consists chiefly in causing absorption of the connective tissue, and its external use may also produce, in the superficial parts, inflammation, matting together, and consequent shrinkage.

The parenchymatous injection of tincture of iodine is followed by much better results. This was first recommended by Lücke, in 1867. It is especially applicable in cases of goitres which are soft and which involve only a part of the gland.

In advanced age a goitre usually undergoes degeneration, becomes hard from the deposit of lime salts; or large cysts with rigid walls are formed. In these cases injections are useless. Practised with strict anatomical and antiseptic precautions injections are attended with but little danger. Still there have been cases with great difficulty of respiration, and even death following the procedure. Bruns ascribes death, in some cases, to paralysis of the vagus. In other cases suppuration has followed, and in still others the injection has entered one of the large veins, producing thrombus.

Dr. Heymann has collected the records of sixteen deaths from parenchymatous injection, but these unfortunate results are so very rare that they may almost be disregarded. In making the injections the strictest antiseptic precautions should be observed—the syringe carefully cleansed either by heat or by carbolized solution, and the patient's neck well washed with a carbolized solution. Avoiding any large veins that may be on the surface of the gland, the needle is thrust directly into some enlarged portion, care being taken first to fix the part with the thumb and finger, then one-third or one-half of a syringeful is slowly thrown in. The injections are practised usually twice a week, but the frequency and the amount of iodine injected are governed by the degree of reaction. Generally after one or two injections an entire syringeful can be used, selecting a new point where the gland is soft. Before the injection is finished, or immediately afterward, the patient complains of severe pain in the teeth, eye, ear, or in the maxillary articulation, always on the side on which the injection has been made. If the injection has been made low down near the sternum, the patient will complain of severe pain in the chest, and there may be for a time difficult breathing. In over-sensitive girls this pain may continue for several hours. The injections produce an inflammation in the substance of the gland, matting the tissues into a hard lump which causes shrinkage at that point. Its specific alterative effect is also considerable.

CASE I.—Annie H., aged eighteen years; enlargement of both lobes of thyroid, which had been noticeable for two or three years. A neck-chain that she formerly wore, would not clasp by an inch; the gland was soft. Four injections were made, two on each side, at intervals of three days. This reduced the gland to two hard nodules, and she could again wear the neck-chain.

CASE II.—Annie R., aged twelve years; enlargement of both lobes of thyroid, but especially of the right. Enlargement was very marked and produced a feeling of suffocation. Eight injections were made, when the visible swelling had almost entirely disappeared and only some hard nodules could be felt.

The foregoing was substantially the result in a large number of cases in which the injections have been used, and in no case have unpleasant results followed any of the injections. It would seem that in this part of the country, where goitre is sporadic, few if any cases would attain considerable size if timely injections were practised. Substances other than iodine have been used, such as diluted alcohol, solutions of ergotin and of arsenious acid, and iodoform emulsion, but none of them has been found

to produce such uniformly good results as iodine, while the injection of some has led to the production of suppuration.

Electrolysis.—Mr. John Duncan[1] gives the results of treatment of this method in fourteen cases of goitre. Six were entirely cured, and the others more or less benefited. Weimbaum reports two cases cured by electrolysis. This method of treatment promises well, and is practised by using a galvanic current of from six to eight cells. The electrodes are needles, which are thrust into the gland and moved about in its substance. The sitting is maintained for from ten to fifteen minutes.

In long-standing goitre cysts may occur. In some cases there will be but one cyst, in other cases many. They are formed by the enlargement and coalescence of the original vesicles. As the vesicles' enlarge they are closely pressed together, their adjacent walls become absorbed, and a large cyst may be formed from many small ones. In old cases the walls of these cysts are often thick, rigid, and infiltrated with lime salts.

There are three methods of treating the cysts usually recommended :

1st. Puncture and the injection of iodine.

2d. Incision.

3d. Enucleation.

Puncturing a cyst with a canula, and injecting iodine, is the simplest method, and can be practised with success in single cysts, with thin walls. Where the cyst-walls are firm, or where several are in close conjunction, incision offers better results.

Incision should be done under strict antiseptic precautions, cutting down to the cyst-wall, which is stitched to the skin before opening (Kœnig). The cyst is then incised to the full extent of the external wound, irrigated with a carbolic acid solution, and drained. If there is much bleeding from the cyst-wall the cavity should be packed with iodoform-gauze. Healing is not so certain as after the old method of leaving an open, suppurating, granulating wound, but it is far less dangerous.

In cysts with thick, rigid walls, or containing much solid matter, enucleation is to be preferred. This is performed by making an incision down to the wall, and then shelling out the cyst with the fingers, with closed scissors or with dressing-forceps. The cavity is then irrigated and drained, and an antiseptic dressing applied.

CASE III.—Mrs. H., aged thirty-four years; sought relief from a cyst of the right lobe of the thyroid, near the median line. There had been a gradual enlargement for several years, which at the time of the consultation was the size of a small apple. Its walls were thin, and the cyst superficial. After thoroughly cleansing the region, a small trocar was

1 British Medical Journal, November 3, 1888.

thrust into the cyst, its contents, a thin albuminous fluid, were allowed to drain off, and half a drachm of tincture of iodine thrown in through the canula and allowed to remain. The reaction was slight, and complete obliteration of the cyst followed.

CASE IV.—Maggie H., aged twenty-four years; consulted me on account of a cyst of the thyroid, directly over the trachea. The cyst had been growing for four or five years, and was the size of a small hen's egg. The patient was anæsthetized, the parts carefully cleansed, and an incision made directly over the cyst and down to its wall, when it was easily shelled out. The pedicle containing the bloodvessels was ligated with antiseptic silk and an antiseptic dressing applied. Healing occurred by first intention.

In order to avoid the misfortunes and dangers which have sometimes attended or followed extirpations of goitre, Wölfler, during the last few years, has revived the operation of ligating the thyroid arteries. In his monograph, published in 1887, on the history of goitre operations, he gives Walther (1814) the credit of first ligating the superior thyroid arteries for the purpose of producing atrophy of the gland, and to Porta (1850) the credit of first ligating the four thyroids for the same purpose, with successful results. The number of cases to which the operation is applicable seems limited. Billroth[1] states that the operation should be performed only in cases of goitre that are well nourished. In cases in which degenerative processes or large extravasations of blood have taken place, in which the goitre is largely cystic with thick, firm walls, or in which there is a deposit of lime salts in the tissues, the operation is contra-indicated. The operation is applicable to much the same class of cases as are the parenchymatous injections. Performed under strict antiseptic precautions the operation should be practically free from danger, though often difficult, and in well-selected cases it seems probable that it may take the place of the more radical and dangerous operation of extirpation.

The superior thyroid arteries are the first branches given off from the external carotids. In tying them, an incision two inches long is made at the anterior border of the sterno-cleido-mastoid muscle, with the middle of the incision over the space between the thyroid cartilage and hyoid bone. The integument, superficial fascia, and platysma myoides are divided, the deep fascia torn through with dissecting-forceps, or divided on a grooved director. When the operator reaches the artery, it should be ligated in two places with imbedded aseptic silk sutures.

In tying the inferior thyroid Billroth recommends an incision at the posterior border of the sterno-mastoid muscle, the incision terminating an inch above the superior border of the clavicle. The skin and platysma are cut through, tying any veins, with

two ligatures, that may be in the line of the incision, before cutting them. When the deep fascia is incised one comes directly upon the scalenus anticus muscle with the phrenic nerve coursing down its centre. This is the deep landmark of the region. Then, by raising the border of the sterno-mastoid muscle and separating the connective tissue, the inferior thyroid artery is reached.

In this incision the operator does not see the origin of the artery, and in order to be sure that the vessel is the one desired it should be traced upward, when it will be seen to curve under the common carotid artery. For greater security the artery should be ligated in two places and incised.

CASE V.—Mrs. D., aged twenty-seven years. At the age of nineteen she first noticed a slight fulness and pulsation in the neck. The increase in size was gradual until she became pregnant, four years after first noticing the enlargement. During this and a subsequent pregnancy the increase was rapid ; there was much difficulty in respiration, which was noticeable at all times, especially at night, when it was necessary for her to be propped up in bed. She was also almost constantly troubled with a hoarse, croupy cough. The gland pulsated strongly in every part. Her neck measured above the gland 34 centimetres, and over the greatest enlargement 48 centimetres.

August 22, 1889. The four thyroid arteries, excepting the right inferior thyroid, were tied at one sitting in the usual manner. In the region of the right inferior thyroid the gland extended so far beneath and beyond the external border of the sterno-mastoid muscle that it was feared great difficulty might be experienced in reaching the artery ; consequently an incision was made one inch above and parallel with the clavicle, incising integument, platysma, and deep fascia. The anterior border of the sterno-mastoid being forcibly raised with the index-finger and the deep connective tissue torn open, I easily came upon the first portion of the subclavian artery, doubly ligating and dividing the middle thyroid vein which crossed the deep part of the wound. The thyroid artery was then exposed and doubly ligated. The artery was very large—the size of a large goose-quill. All pulsation in the gland had now ceased ; it felt like a sponge saturated with water and could be easily emptied. The wounds were irrigated with bichloride solution, drained and united with a continuous silk suture. A very heavy antiseptic dressing was applied, extending well down on the chest, the bandage encasing not only the neck, but the head and chest as well, in order that the muscles of the neck would be at rest. The dressing was changed on the seventh day. the tubes and sutures removed. and complete union found. The cough and difficult breathing were completely relieved. and thus far there has been no return. The gland decreased to about one-half of its original size, when it remained stationary.

Extirpation.—Perhaps no operation in surgery has had a more varied experience than extirpation

[1] Wiener klinische Wochenschrift. No. 1, 1888.

of the thyroid—at times recommended by some of the best surgeons and strenuously opposed by others equally good.

In 1791 Desault made the first successful extirpation of one-half of a goitre, and in 1800 Hedenus made two total extirpations, both successful (Wölfler). Still, the operation was, perhaps, justly condemned, and it was not practised to any extent until the advent of antiseptic surgery. In 1875 Küster made the first extirpation with strict antiseptic methods.

In 1877 both Albert and Billroth extirpated goitre under antiseptic precautions. From this time the operation became more popular. The favor with which it was now held was not entirely due to the antiseptic precautions, but perhaps quite as much to a better technique.

As illustrating the disfavor in which the operation was formerly held I quote the following from Gross's *Surgery* :[1]

" But no sensible man will, on slight considerations, attempt to extirpate a goitrous thyroid gland. If a surgeon should be so adventurous or foolhardy as to undertake the enterprise I shall not envy him his feelings while engaged in the performance of it, or after he has completed it, should he be so fortunate as to do this. Every step he takes will be environed with difficulties, every stroke of his knife will, if he is not perfectly self-possessed and most cautious, be followed by a torrent of blood, and lucky will it be for him if his victim live long enough to enable him to finish his dissection."

This would perhaps be as true now as then, were it not for better methods of operating. There were formerly two great dangers attending extirpation, namely, hæmorrhage and suppuration. These two sources of danger are now happily almost wholly under control.

In the experience of surgeons who have had most to do with this operation other difficulties also have followed, namely, tetany and cachexia strumipriva. If tetany occurs it is usually on the day following the operation. There are at first pains in the extremities, which are soon followed by muscular spasms in the legs. The upper extremities are also soon affected, as well as the muscles of the face. These tonic muscular contractions may be of short duration, the patient quickly recovering, or they may continue for an indefinite period, reducing the patient very much or even leading to death. In Billroth's first seventy cases of extirpation, tetany occurred seven times (Wölfler). The cause of tetany in these cases is not well understood, but it is thought to have some connection with impoverished blood, and perhaps it is excited by irritation of the recurrent laryngeal nerve. Dr. James Stewart[2] affirms that tetany never occurs unless the entire gland has been removed.

[1] Edition of 1872, page 431.
[2] American journal of the Medical Sciences, November, 1889.

What is of far more serious import is cachexia strumipriva. This condition has been especially observed in Switzerland (Reverdin and Kocher). It generally occurs during the first month after the operation. There is general disturbance of nutrition, loss of flesh, and muscular weakness. The mind is benumbed, the lips and tongue and eyelids swollen, and difficulty of speaking occurs. This condition is one of cretinism and is lasting, but occurs only when the entire gland has been removed, and more especially in young persons. So uniformly has this been the case, that it has become a rule never to extirpate the entire gland before puberty. If even a small portion of the gland is left the cachexia does not occur. In persons past the age of puberty the condition is not apt to occur even after complete extirpation.

Schiff has advanced the opinion that the thyroid gland has a regulating function on the circulation in the brain, and that after complete removal the marasmus is produced by chronic anæmia of the brain.

The most approved method of operating at the present time is that of Kocher and Billroth. According to Wölfler, these two surgeons have removed more goitres than any other two men in the world. An incision is made in the median line, from near the sternum to the hyoid bone, and if necessary it may be extended on either side, or on both sides, in the form of the letter Y, to the sterno-cleido-mastoid muscles. The anterior jugular vein, and perhaps the external jugular, may be under the line of the incision ; if so, they should be doubly ligated and incised. In separating the tissues it will be found necessary to touch the sterno-hyoid and omo-hyoid muscles if the gland is large. When the capsule of the gland has been reached the knife should be laid aside and all tissue doubly ligated *en masse* before being cut. The dissection is made with dissecting-forceps and with the fingers, the gland being shelled out first at the superior border of one side. Reaching the superior thyroid vessels, artery and vein, they are doubly ligated and incised ; the dissection is carried down the same side until the inferior thyroid vessels are reached, which are also doubly ligated and cut. The greatest care should be exercised in this region not to injure the recurrent laryngeal nerve. The dissection is now carried below, tying the middle thyroid vein and artery, if the latter exists, separating the gland from the trachea, and ligating any vessels that may be found. The goitre is then lifted from its bed and the vessels on the opposite side ligated. The wound is irrigated and drained, united with a continuous silk suture, and a large antiseptic dressing applied.

In this operation one of the most important considerations is the prevention of hæmorrhage, and the advice of Billroth on this subject should never be forgotten; namely, that when the capsule of the gland has been reached, lay the knife aside and doubly ligate all tissues before cutting them.

CASE VI.—G. D., aged twenty-four years, first noticed the neck enlarging five years ago. Numerous attempts were made to check the growth by the external application of iodine, but with no effect. The increase in size was continuous. In August, 1889, both lobes were found very much enlarged. Some difficulty in respiration was experienced and great inconvenience felt on account of the increased size of the neck in wearing a collar. The gland felt firm and hard to the touch. August 13th, extirpation was performed. Great difficulty was experienced in separating the overlying tissues from the gland, as they were matted together in consequence of the iodine applications; and in making the separation a cyst the size of a large crab-apple was broken into. After the gland was freed from the overlying tissues, little difficulty was experienced in shelling it out. The vessels were ligated as they appeared, the wound was irrigated, drained, and united with a continuous silk suture, and a heavy antiseptic dressing was applied. On the eighth day the dressings were changed and the wound found united throughout. Patient has remained perfectly well up to date.

AN ANALYSIS OF THE OCULAR SYMPTOMS FOUND IN THE THIRD STAGE OF GENERAL PARALYSIS OF THE INSANE.[1]

BY CHARLES A. OLIVER, M.D.,
OF PHILADELPHIA.

THESE observations and their deductions, which form a part of, and in fact conclude those which were presented to the American Ophthalmological Society at its last annual meeting, are here given in hope of offering a few more facts to the ocular symptomatology of general paralysis.

Care was taken that each subject was seemingly free from any gross extraneous disease or local disorder, and discretion was exercised that competent and authoritative medical opinion had been given as to the type and stage of the general complaint; also, for reasons given in the previous paper, the study has been limited to the male sex.

In a disease of such complex symptomatology, where doubtless quite a number of pathological peculiarities exist at one time, accurate pathognomonic changes cannot be expected in each case, and for this reason a great number of seemingly similar cases have been studied in the effort to obtain an idiocratic picture of a few of the oculo-motor and retinal changes to be found in this disorder. However, as the disease seems, as shown by the microscope, to expend its greatest force upon both the

[1] Paper read before the American Ophthalmological Society, july 17, 1890.

motor and sensory regions of the cerebral cortex, with involvement of the related higher mental areas, the symptoms which are improperly described as paretic only, assume types of both motor and sensory derangement, with associated mental peculiarities of a distinctive character. As a part of these, the ocular apparatus, with its six channels on each side to the cortex of the brain, becomes not only a useful situation from which to study these changes, but is really invaluable as an exponent of the intracranial changes.

Observations.[1]—1. Direct vision for form was reduced in every instance where obtainable to any degree of certainty.

2. Direct vision for color was subnormal in the few instances in which it could be properly studied, showing itself more particularly for green and red.

3. Accommodative action: though impossible to obtain any reliable results by various subjective methods, yet by objective means (retinoscopy) this was seemingly lessened in every unequivocal case tried.[2]

4. Visual fields: no determinate answers could be obtained.

5. Pupils, as a rule, were somewhat larger than normal.

6. Pupils were ofttimes unequal in size, and, in some instances, had a difference of one or two millimetres in their longer diameters.

7. Pupils were frequently oval and ovoid in shape; their long axes being opposed to one another at placed at equivalent angles.[3]

8. The pupillary border of the iris in several instances was quite irregular in outline, without any evidences of localized inflammatory change.

9. Changeability of pupillary form still persistent in one case in which it had been so noted in the second stage of the disease.

10. Irides were devoid of any gross peculiarities in comparative tint.

11. Irides, as a rule, were either extremely slow in response or absolutely immobile to the strongest light-stimulus, though fairly responsive to efforts for convergence and accommodation.

12. The iris of the larger pupil, in some instances, was not so responsive to light-stimulus as its fellow, this inequality of action seeming to bear no relation to the degree and character of refraction-error, and, in some cases, seemingly free from the apparent amount of optic-nerve change.

[1] A portion of these observations will form a part of the Fifth Annual Report of the Ophthalmological Department of the State Hospital for the Insane at Norristown, Pa.

[2] Curiously, one case upon several occasions gave distinct ophthalmoscopic evidence of spasm of accommodation.

[3] It must not be forgotten that the pupils of many of the mentally healthy present similar characteristics, especially in cases of astigmatism, where asthenopia is complained of.

13. The secondary movements of the iris were almost, if not entirely, lost in all instances in which light-stimulus produced a reflex act.

14. Irides, in quite a number of cases, were very feebly responsive to efforts for accommodation and convergence only; the want of this character of action being very changeable and unequal at the same time upon the two sides.

15. Irregular and incomplete dilatation of the pupil followed the employment of strong solutions of atropine—sufficient to give full mydriasis in ordinary subjects—the comparative positions of the greatest amounts of pupillary enlargements being unequally situated at fifteen and thirty degrees differences, although several cases yielded peculiar and fantastic forms.

16. Insufficiency of the interni was noted in several cases, though on account of the mental condition of the subject nothing could be positively determined.

17. Ataxic nystagmic motions of the extra-ocular muscles were present at times in a few cases, especially noticeable with the third and sixth nerve distributions, either in separated or conjoined action.

18. The optic disks, in many instances, were decidedly and unequally semi-atrophic, the degeneration being especially pronounced in the deepest layers and on the temporal side of the nerve.

19. The capillarity of nerve-substance was materially lessened, the greatest amount of blood-supply being recognized in a rather narrow crescentic area on the nasal side of the disk.

20. The disk, in a few cases, was of a suffused and gelatinous appearance, its edges being plainly seen, and the surrounding retina somewhat œdematous.

21. A series of minute venous and arterial loops in the retinal vessels on the disk were seen in one well-marked case.[1]

22. The scleral ring was sharply cut all around and quite broad; this, as a rule, being more noticeable on the temporal side of the disk.

23. Blackish crescents of pigment, broken and somewhat absorbed beyond the scleral ring, at the outer edge of the optic-nerve head, were frequent.

24. Pigment-lines of different widths and varying degrees of absorption were seen beyond the scleral ring at the inner edge of the optic-nerve head.

25. The pigment-layer of the retina was, as a rule, diminished in thickness, the greater amount of striation being seen at the superior and inferior borders of the optic disk.

26. Retinal striation, in a few instances, was very pronounced, rendering the disk-edges quite hazy.

27. Retinal arteries were reduced in size and sometimes slightly tortuous.

28. Retinal veins were somewhat undersized and quite tortuous in a number of cases.

29. Blood-currents of the retinal vessels were apparently normal in tint.

30. Very few lymph-reflexes were seen, these being generally situated in the walls of the main retinal stems.

31. Fine pin-point opacities in the retina between the disk and the macula were seen in two cases; no other gross changes in the retina.

32. The choroid was granular and disturbed in the majority of cases.

33. Refraction was generally hypermetropic, with a marked degree of astigmatism.[1]

Summary and Conclusions.—1. The oculo-motor symptoms of the third stage of general paralysis of the insane, which consist in varying, though marked degrees of loss and enfeeblement of iris-response to light-stimulus, accommodative effort and converging power; lessening of ciliary muscle tone and action; weakening and inefficiency of extra-ocular muscle motion—all show paretic and paralytic disturbances connected with the oculo-motor apparatus itself, of greater amount and more serious consequence than those seen in the same apparatus during the second stage of the disease.

2. The sensory changes of the third stage of general paralysis of the insane, which, though similar to those found in the second stage of the disorder, are so pronounced as to show a semi-atrophic condition of the optic-nerve head and marked reduction in the amount of both optic-nerve and retinal circulation, with consequent lowering of centric and excentric vision for both form and color—all indicate a degenerate condition of the sensory portion of the ocular apparatus, with impairment of sensory nerve action.

3. The peculiar local changes seen in these cases, which consist in conditions of the choroid and retina indicative of local disturbance and irritation of these tunics, more pronounced than those seen during the second stage of the disease—all represent the results of greater wear and tear given to a more delicate and a more weakened organ.

4. Both the motor symptoms and the sensory changes of the ocular apparatus, as thus described in the advanced or third stage of general paralysis of the insane, furnish not only evidences of a local disturbance of a more pronounced type than those shown in the second stage of the disorder, but plainly show themselves as one of the many peripheral expressions of fast-approaching degeneration and dissolution of nerve-elements most probably connected with related cortex-disintegration and death.

---

[1] Acquired syphilis was suspected in this case.

[1] Thanks are due to Drs. Henry Sidebottom and Henry C. Cattell for their kind assistance during the study of these cases.

CLINICAL MEMORANDA.

SURGICAL.

Abscess of the Liver. Operation: Recovery.—T. R., aged twenty-seven years, laborer, entered the Philadelphia Hospital, August 16, 1889, suffering from fever and severe pain in the side. He stated that he had always enjoyed good health, with the exception of an attack of jaundice from which he suffered for six weeks when in his sixteenth year. During May last, while much exposed, he contracted dysentery. This became severe in type and confined him to his bed for two weeks. He resumed work before recovery was complete, suffering from occasional bloody stools for nearly two months. About the first of August he experienced considerable pain over the right iliac crest. The bowels were at this time costive. Shortly afterward he noticed a tumor in the region of the liver. At no time were there chilly sensations. His symptoms steadily grew more pronounced until he entered the hospital.

On admission the temperature was 103°, the pulse 100, the respiration 30. The liver-dulness extended three inches below the ribs in the liver-line, forming a distinct tumor visible on inspection and tender on palpation, but showing no signs of fluctuation or superficial œdema. Auscultation failed to detect friction-sounds. Rectal examination showed the absence of any accessible ulcerating foci. The following day the temperature reached 104°, and the general condition of the patient had markedly altered for the worse. An operation for the evacuation of pus was at once performed. An incision three inches in length was made over the most prominent part of the tumor. The abdominal muscles were divided to the full extent of the wound down to the peritoneum, and the cavity of the latter was opened just below the tumor. The tumor at its most prominent part was found to be firmly adherent to the peritoneum. The opening into the general cavity was protected by a sponge and the point of the knife was thrust through the adhesions into a liver-abscess the size of a large orange. By means of the finger passed into this cavity, the walls of two other abscesses were broken through and about a pint of thick, bile-stained pus was evacuated. Two large drainage-tubes were carried to the deepest parts of the suppurating cavities, the wound was washed out with sterile normal saline solution (0.7 per cent. sodium chloride) and the wound was closed. The patient was under ether for thirty minutes. On the following day the temperature dropped to normal, and the subsequent course of the case was one of uninterrupted recovery, with the exception of a small stitch-abscess which developed on the fifth day and sent the temperature up to 101°. In two weeks the drainage-tubes were removed, the discharge having entirely ceased, and in three weeks the patient was sitting up. His subsequent history shows that he has enjoyed robust health and has never suffered from any trace of his liver trouble.

It is interesting to note in this case that, although the suppurative trouble was immediately due to septic emboli carried from ulcers of the lower bowel; the operation was successful in evacuating all abscess-cavities of the liver. A study of many autopsies shows that such abscesses are generally multiple, the liver frequently being completely riddled and destroyed. Indeed this is so frequently the picture that many pathologists advise against operation in these cases, maintaining that the trouble is so disseminated as to be beyond the help of the surgeon's knife. Though the abscesses were multiple in the case reported, they were separated from each other by such thin walls that the latter were readily broken down. Even had this latter procedure not been deemed advisable, it is more than probable that in one or two days the most these remaining collections of pus would have ruptured in the direction of least resistance, thus spontaneously evacuating their contents.

A month after operation a blood-count was made to see whether such extensive destruction of liver-tissue had any effect upon the number of corpuscles. The latter seemed normal in color, and as a result of repeated observation gave an average number of 4,000,000 to the c.mm., a percentage not lower than could be reasonably expected after a month's stay in a crowded hospital-ward.

EDWARD MARTIN, M.D.,
Assistant Surgeon to the
Hospital of the University of Pennsylvania.

RHINOLOGICAL.

Anosmia from Tobacco-poisoning.—Tobacco-amblyopia is now a well-recognized disease, and is daily becoming a more familiar example, and an alarming evidence, of the growing abuse of tobacco-smoking.

A recent case leads us to believe that the nerve of smell as well as, though less frequently than, the nerve of sight, is sometimes injured by excessive smoking. Reference has been made to many of the standard works on the subject of anosmia, and various are the causes which are said to produce it. In the order of their frequency syphilis, traumatism, catarrh, obstruction of the nares, strong fumes, and malaria are enumerated, but we are unable to find that tobacco is held responsible for the loss of smell. This fact leads us to bring to the attention of the profession what we believe to be a case of tobacco-anosmia.

In March, 1890, Mr. A. S. F. applied for treatment, and stated that about a year ago he began to suffer from dryness of the post-nasal region and a disposition to clear his throat. Then he noticed a feeling of fulness or stuffing in his nose and a slight difficulty in nasal respiration, sometimes in one nostril, and, again, in the other. Lately he had observed that he had lost the sense of smell.

There was no specific history. He was, however, an inveterate smoker, and was in the habit of blowing the smoke through his nostrils.

Examination showed pharyngitis and an atrophic rhinitis. His sight was also slightly impaired, and this led us to suppose that tobacco was the cause of the condition.

This diagnosis subsequently proved correct, as was conclusively proven by the cure of the disease by removing the cause.

The treatment consisted mainly in total abstinence from tobacco-smoking, the administration of one-thirtieth grain of strychnine three times a day, and in the application of electricity to the nasal mucous membrane by means of a pledget of wet cotton on the end of an electrode. In about a month the power of smell began to improve, and when last seen and tested he could recognize almost any moderately strong odor.

The effect of tobacco on the eye is known to be an atrophic condition of the optic nerve resulting in amblyopia ; hence it is an organic disease.

Now the sense of smell, though primarily dependent on the olfactory nerve, is secondarily dependent on several conditions, the most important of which are moisture and an unobstructed nasal passage.

Hence, anosmia may be either organic or functional, and tobacco-poisoning is, in our opinion, capable of producing either, or both. The anosmia is functional, when we have an interference with the secondary conditions necessary for the sense of smell ; organic, when we have the nerve-sensibility destroyed by atrophic changes.

From personal experience and from actual observation and inquiry, we are convinced that smoking is especially injurious to the nasal and post-nasal fossæ, and that by it the sense of smell is apt to be impaired, and may be destroyed.

EDWARD F. PARKER, M.D.
CHARLESTON, S. C.

MEDICAL PROGRESS.

Aristol in the Treatment of Skin Diseases.—In a letter to the *Journal of Cutaneous and Genito-urinary Diseases*, September, 1890, DR. L. BROCQ, of Paris, communicates some of his results with aristol in the treatment of cutaneons diseases. In his experience the drug acts only as a cicatrizant. In chancroid its use does not seem to exert a favorable influence on the virulence of the disease. In tertiary syphilitic ulcerations it apparently hastens cicatrization, provided that appropriate general treatment with mercury and potassium iodide is also used. Cicatrization in tuberculous diseases of the skin is also hastened by applications of aristol. Applied to non-ulcerated lupus vulgaris or erythematous lupus, it exercises no useful influence. In tuberculous ulcerations of mucous membranes it is useful, and by means of it Dr. Brocq was able to secure cicatrization of an extensive tuberculous ulcer of the arch of the palate. In superficial epithelioma aristol does not seem to exert any destructive influence on the pathological cells ; but, if the growth has been destroyed by caustics, by curetting, or by the hot iron, the drug hastens cicatrization. The author's method of treating this disease is to curette the base thoroughly, and if he believes that the diseased tissue is completely removed, to dress with aristol. If the disease is apparently not completely removed, he applies potassium chlorate, either in powder or solution, for a few days, and then uses aristol.

In the treatment of psoriasis, aristol has given the author scarcely appreciable results. To test its value thoroughly in this disease, he has treated all his cases with aristol on one side of the body, and with the ordinary applications on the other.

In no instance has Dr. Brocq seen aristol produce toxic symptoms.

Incision and Drainage in the Treatment of Hydrocephalus. — POTT (*Der Kinder-Arzt*, August, 1890) reports the case of a child, four weeks old, with marked hydrocephalus, in which he punctured the skull and drew off ten ounces of fluid. The psychical symptoms immediately improved, though for only a short time, and in twenty-four hours the fluid had re-accumulated, distending the skull to its former size. The author then made an incision through the lower third of the right fronto-parietal suture, inserted a drainage-tube, and applied a compressing bandage to the head. The child at first improved, but died on the twelfth day after the operation. At the autopsy both lateral ventricles were found full of fluid, and, as there was no communication between them, the evacuation of one had not reduced the fluid in the other.

Methods of Disinfecting the Hands.—GEPPERT (*Central-blatt für die medicinische Wissenschaften*, july 26, 1890) advises the following method of disinfecting the hands previous to operating: Cover the hands with a paste made by mixing 100 parts of powdered chloride of lime with 45 parts of water. Then dip them for a few moments in a three-per-cent. watery solution of hydrochloric acid. Or, in place of this, the hands may be alternately dipped into a chloride of lime solution and three-per-cent. hydrochloric acid solution.

MIKULICZ (*Der Frauenärzt*, August, 1890) disinfects his hands by first cleaning the nails, then scrubbing the hands for three minutes with potash soap and water, soaking them for half a minute in a three-per-cent. carbolic acid solution, and finally washing them off with a 1-to-200 sublimate solution.

Prognosis in Extravasation of Urine.—According to DR. J. BLAKE WHITE (*Journal of Cutaneous and Genito-urinary Diseases*, September, 1890), the prognosis of operations in cases of urinary extravasation can be estimated as follows:

1. Should the infiltration not have extended beyond the perineal structures before operation, the prospects of recovery are favorable.

2. Should the infiltration have involved the scrotum and the perineal structures, the operation, though affording the best chances of recovery, is not without hazard.

3. Should the infiltration extend into the perineum and scrotum, and involve also the ileo-abdominal region, the danger to the patient is greatly increased.

4. Should the infiltration descend to the ischio-rectal space, the prospects are exceedingly gloomy, since it threatens deep-seated sloughing, and, in consequence, profound shock.

Large Doses of Potassium Iodide in Tertiary Syphilis.— WOLF (*Revue de Thérapeutique*) administers potassium iodide in doses of from 450 to 750 grains daily to obstinate cases of tertiary syphilis. The drug is dissolved in a decoction of rice in order to prevent iodism, any free iodine formed in the stomach being immediately converted into iodide of starch.—*London Medical Recorder*, August, 1890.

The Diazo-reaction in Diagnosis.—DR. L. RÜTIMEYER, who has made between two and three thousand trials of the so-called diazo-reaction in the urine from 260 patients, believes that it is a very useful guide, both in diagnosis and prognosis, being especially valuable in phthisis and typhoid fever. In phthisis he regards it as denoting the absorption of caseous matter, and, when it is persistent, as implying rapid mischief and an early and fatal termination. In cases of general miliary tuberculosis it was always obtained. A large number of typhoid cases were examined and the presence of the reaction was very constant, and could generally be obtained early. It does not seem to be present in pyrexial intestinal catarrh.

In the diagnosis of typhoid fever, if the reaction is not obtained during the first or second week, the case, if typhoid at all, must be a very slight one. It cannot, however, be affirmed that a well-marked and constant diazo-reaction is a sign of a fatal termination, as with phthisis.

The reaction is never given by the urine of healthy persons, and was not observed in hysteria, hepatitis, diabetes, cystitis, pyelo-nephritis, gastro-abdominal catarrh with fever, or in a number of surgical diseases. It was occasionally present in cancer of the stomach and œsophagus, chronic nephritis, caries of bone, pyæmia, scarlatina, pleurisy with serous effusion, tubercular meningitis, and heart disease. It was more frequently obtained in croupous pneumonia.

The method of testing is very simple, two special solutions only being required, namely, a concentrated solution of sulphanilic acid in water, and a solution of nitrite of sodium of the strength of 1 to 200. The actual test-solution is prepared immediately before use, by mixing 200 parts of the sulphanilic acid solution with 10 of pure hydrochloric acid and 6 of the nitrite of sodium solution. This mixture is added to an equal volume of the urine, and sufficient ammonia added to render the whole alkaline. A bright or carmine-red coloration denotes the diazo-reaction. After from twelve to thirty-six hours a deposit occurs, the upper part of which is green or black.—*Lancet*, August 23, 1890.

Local Anæsthesia by Means of Carbonic Acid.—According to VOITURIEZ, the anæsthetic effects of carbonic acid, described by Brown-Séquard, can be obtained in an extremely simple manner by means of the ordinary siphons containing mineral water charged with the gas. The anæsthesia is secured by projecting from a distance the contents of two or three siphons of seltzer water, limiting the application to the part to be operated upon. The insensibility to pain lasts about five minutes and then slowly disappears. The method is chiefly applicable to the limbs, as about the head and trunk the irrigation is somewhat inconvenient.—*London Medical Recorder*, August, 1890.

Gargle for Tonsillitis.—The following prescription for the treatment of tonsillitis is quoted by the *Canada Medical Record* :

℞.—Ammoniated tinct. of guaiac } of each 4 drachms.
Compound tinct. of cinchona }
Potassium chlorate　.　.　.　.　2　"
Honey　.　.　.　.　.　.　4　"
Powdered acacia　.　.　.　.　q. s.
Water　.　.　sufficient to make　4 ounces.—M.

Use from one-half to one teaspoonful as a gargle every two hours.

Mixture for Irritable Bladder.—DR. W. P. CHUNN uses the following mixture in the treatment of vesical irritation when due to excess of phosphates in the urine :

℞.—Benzoic acid　.　.　.　.　2 drachms.
Borax　.　.　.　.　.　3　"
Water　.　.　.　.　.　12 ounces.—M.

Dose : One teaspoonful three times daily.—*Canada Medical Record.*

Eczema.—According to *L'Union Médicale*, LUSTGARTEN recommends the following application for eczema :

℞.—Oleate of cocaine　.　.　.　10 to 15 grains.
Lanoline　.　.　.　.　3 drachms.
Olive oil　.　.　.　.　½ drachm.

This is to be made into an ointment, and will be found particularly useful in eczema of the anus and genital organs. Two applications a day are to be made, and followed by dusting the parts with dry absorbent powders. If there is much secretion, with the formation of scabs, warm baths may be used and the foreign materials removed by either mild or strong soaps, as the case may require. In cases of pruritus of the anus, Lustgarten recommends suppositories of the oleate of cocaine.

Formula for Pulmonary Phthisis.—GILBERT recommends the following :

℞.—Creasote　.　.　.　.　30 to 45 minims.
Arseniate of sodium　.　.　½ grain.
Quinine wine　.　.　.　1 pint.

Two small wineglassfuls should be taken directly after each meal.

Treatment of Herpes of the Genitals.—FEULARD, in *L'Union Médicale*, states that where the eruption of herpes of the genitals is widespread but not severe, lotions with pure water, vinegar and water, or aromatic wine are useful, and that the small ulcers may be covered with powdered bismuth, talc, or starch. If the ulcers be severe, he recommends that they be touched with a feeble solution of nitrate of silver of the strength of from 4 to 10 grains to each 6 drachms of water ; or, in place of this, the same quantity of the silver salt in the same amount of vaseline. In those cases in which there is a tendency to recurrence, it is necessary to place about the glands or under the prepuce a small piece of absorbent cotton, or similar substance, laden with tonic astringent applications.

Where the herpes is idiopathic and depends upon digestive disturbance, he recommends the use of an emetic, the employment of non-exciting foods, abstinence from alcohol, and the use of alkaline waters.

The Analgesic Action of Methylene-blue.—According to EHRLICH and LEPPMANN, in painful effections of the nerve-trunks methylene-blue possesses marked analgesic properties. The action is usually manifested about two hours after the administration of the remedy, and, if given in sufficient amounts, increases in intensity until the analgesia is absolute. The dose required to produce complete anæsthesia is 1 grain hypodermically or 2 to 4 grains if given by the mouth. In some cases as much as 15 grains in gelatin capsules was given daily without causing any toxic symptoms or disagreeable effects. For hypodermic administration they employed a two-per-cent. solution, which occasioned no pain and no local reaction other than a slight tumefaction which disappeared within a few days.

The authors have not discovered that the drug has any effect upon inflammatory swellings, nor were its effects very evident in the osteocopic pains of syphilis or the pain of gastric ulcer. — *Therapeutic Gazette*, August, 1890.

Hypnotism as a Therapeutic Agent.—At the recent meeting of the British Medical Association at Birmingham, papers upon hypnotism were read by DR. NORMAN KERR and DR. G. C. KINGSBURY, which excited an interesting discussion.

Dr. Kerr said that he accepted practically all the alleged hypnotic phenomena as facts, but that in hypnosis he could see only a disordered cerebral state with exaltation of receptivity. In order to decide whether hypnotism is a desirable remedy, he said that certain facts should be taken into consideration, namely:

1. That only a certain number of persons can be hypnotized.

2. That the after-effects are a disturbance of mental balance and nerve-exhaustion, and that frequent repetition tends to cause intellectual decadence and moral perversion.

3. That hypnosis is a departure from health, a true neurosis embracing the lethargic, cataleptic, and somnambulistic states.

4. That, although suffering may be assuaged by hypnosis, the underlying disease is not necessarily cured.

5. The dangers of hypnotism are great ; each *séance* may bring the patient more under the control of the hypnotist, and may result in the complete submission of the former to the will of the latter.

The greatest success of hypnotism is said to be in the treatment of nervous diseases, but these are the very ailments that Dr. Kerr has seen intensified. In inebriety or narcomania no physician of repute has found hypnorism of any value.

He strongly deprecated public mesmerism as degrading, and hoped that Great Britain would follow the example of Holland and Switzerland, and prohibit such entertainments.

Dr. Kingsbury differed from Dr. Kerr in many respects. He denied that only a few people were susceptible. He thought that the unfortunate association of hypnotism with charlatanism should not prejudice us against it or prevent us from giving it a fair trial.

DR. HACK TUKE thought that, up to the present time, the field of hypnotism in therapeutics has been very limited, but that there are sufficient grounds to warrant a further and unprejudiced trial.

DR. C. L. TUCKEY believed that hypnotism, if skilfully practised, is absolutely harmless, and, in support of that opinion, gave his own experience with 500 cases.— *British Medical Journal*, August 23, 1890.

Indications for the Use of Glycerin Enemata.—The observation of the effects of glycerin enemata and suppositories in a large number of cases has led DR. COLUBINSKI

(*Deutsche medizinal Zeitung*) to the following conclusions :

Glycerin irritates the mucous membrane of the rectum, as shown by the burning sensation produced and by a local rise in temperature. The increased temperature and the desire to defecate are of short duration, and the latter can often be voluntarily overcome by the patient.

The irritation of the mucous membrane does not excite secretion, since the fæces evacuated after a glycerin enema are covered with glycerin only. The best results are obtained when the rectum and sigmoid flexure are filled with scybala ; if fæces are in the upper part of the intestine only, glycerin is useless. According to the author, then, the cases in which glycerin enemata and suppositories are indicated are :

1. Those in which the fæcal masses are already in the rectum.

2. Cases in which the fæces are immediately above the rectum—a frequent condition in the lying-in period.

3. Those in which there is mechanical obstruction of the rectum or sigmoid, as by pelvic new-formations, pregnancy, etc.

4. Scrofulous children.

5. Persons in whom, although they have a daily evacuation from the bowels, the act of defecation is accompanied with difficulty and pain, and in whom the fæces are excessively compact.— *Therapeutic Gazette*, August, 1890.

Antifebrin and Camphor in the Treatment of Pneumonia.— DR. SHESHMIUTZEFF (*Novosti Terapii*) writes that he has had excellent results in the treatment of pneumonia by the administration of antifebrin combined with camphor. To an adult he gives about five grains of the former and two and one-half grains of the latter every four hours.

According to this author, the camphor prevents the depressing effects of the antifebrin, and the temperature falls without rigors or collapse—*St. Louis Medical and Surgical Journal*, September, 1890.

The Treatment of Gonorrhœal Rheumatism.—According to the *Wiener klinische Wochenschrift*, August 28, 1890, RUBENSTEIN has found potassium iodide a rapidly-effective remedy in the treatment of gonorrhœal rheumatism. He gives small doses, usually ordering one drachm of the iodide in five ounces of water, of which he directs the patient to take one or two tablespoonfuls in the morning, and four or five tablespoonfuls in the afternoon. In some cases he gives a still weaker solution, the patient taking one tablespoonful every hour. After a very few hours, in most cases, the pain is markedly lessened, swelling subsides, and a cure is brought about in two or three days.

As to local treatment, the author usually envelops the joint in cloths saturated with a one-per-cent. carbolic acid solution. In some cases he uses a dressing of blue ointment, in others cold, moist cloths, and in still others a solution of common salt. When the pain has disappeared he applies an elastic bandage, and if there is effusion he aspirates. Rubenstein has treated in this manner fifteen cases, some of which were acute, others chronic, and all were cured.

THE MEDICAL NEWS.

A WEEKLY JOURNAL
OF MEDICAL SCIENCE.

COMMUNICATIONS are invited from all parts of the world. Original articles contributed exclusively to THE MEDICAL NEWS will be liberally paid for upon publication. When necessary to elucidate the text, illustrations will be furnished without cost to the author.

Address the Editor: H. A. HARE, M.D.,
1004 WALNUT STREET,
PHILADELPHIA.

Subscription Price, including Postage.

PER ANNUM, IN ADVANCE . . . . $4.00.
SINGLE COPIES . . . . 10 CENTS.

Subscriptions may begin at any date. The safest mode of remittance is by bank check or postal money order, drawn to the order of the undersigned. When neither is accessible, remittances may be made, at the risk of the publishers, by forwarding in *registered* letters.

Address, LEA BROTHERS & CO.,
NOS. 706 & 708 SANSOM STREET,
PHILADELPHIA.

SATURDAY, SEPTEMBER 20, 1890.

THE PART PLAYED BY DOMESTIC ANIMALS IN THE TRANSMISSION OF DISEASE.

FROM time to time the daily papers or medical journals contain some small note detailing an instance where a contagious malady has been conveyed from place to place by means of pet cats and dogs, or, equally commonly, instances are given in which some domestic animal has itself suffered from a contagious disease capable of afflicting man, and so caused an isolated case or an epidemic. One of the most prominent instances where such transmission occurred was that known as the Hendon outbreak in England, in which it was supposed by some that the milk of a herd of cows affected by a disease resembling scarlet fever produced an epidemic among the children who took the milk. It has also been asserted that the fur of cats and the hair of dogs are ready carriers of contagium, and it is not at all unlikely that the cat may itself suffer from diphtheria, and that many instances of untraceable exposure to disease may have their explanation in these facts. Our attention has been called very forcibly to this subject by the report of several cases of diphtheria, due to the presence of this disease in a pigeon, by BILHAUT in the *Journal de Médecine de Paris* of July 13, 1890. A man who was very fond of keeping these birds noticed that one of them was ill and showed evidences of severe sickness, which he could not explain, although it was evident that the respiratory passages were involved. The pigeon died, and the veterinary surgeon found post-mortem that the creature had succumbed to diphtheria. From this case the father, daughter, and a child were infected, and all suffered from diphtheria of the fauces and tonsils, with swelling of these glands and all the evidences of a typical attack of the disease. The possibility of the development of diseases in animals which generally affect the human being, is overlooked chiefly because very few of these diseases are supposed to be capable of existence in blood possessing so high a temperature as that of most of the domestic animals, and particularly that of the pigeon, whose normal temperature is so very high. That a cat in its daily wanderings may play in the room of a sick child and then return to that of a well child is so possible that it is curious we do not see more instances in which such an accident occurs. Perhaps contagion is frequently so carried, though we fail to recognize the fact.

THE VALUE OF SALOL.

WHEN a new drug comes before the profession for trial it goes through two stages of existence, in the first of which it is generally praised by authors because they are attracted by its novelty or they wish to have their names connected with the recommendation of a new medicament. In the second stage the "bears" of the medical stock-market find an opportunity for attracting attention to themselves by decrying that which others have lauded to the skies, and thereby giving the editorial shears a second opportunity of cutting out the names of those who have written and are writing about the remedy in question.

Those of the profession who gave an instant's thought before using it, to the chemical composition of the drug which is now under consideration, realized at once that it must surpass salicylic acid in its power of producing aberrant and dangerous symptoms even when given in very small doses to the ordinary individual, or when administered to a patient having idiosyncrasy to either one of its parts, namely, salicylic and carbolic acids.

In the numbers of the *London Practitioner* for July and August, 1890, is a very interesting and able paper by Dr. Hesselbach, of Halle, in which this author considers the action of salol upon the kidneys in relation to its effects when given in poisonous doses, and he has also recorded a case of a young man who took by mistake two drachms of salol, thereby producing death.

His conclusions, after quite a prolonged physiological and toxicological study, are as follows:

1. The large proportion of phenol contained in salol renders it so toxic a substance that its unrestricted therapeutic use is fraught with danger.

2. In renal disease, acute or chronic, salol is contra-indicated.

It should be remembered that when we administer salol that with every one hundred grains of the drug given we give no less than forty grains of carbolic acid, so that if this amount is used during the day an extremely large dose of a very lethal and irritating agent is ingested.

REVIEWS.

SAUNDERS' QUESTION COMPENDS: ESSENTIALS OF THE DISEASES OF THE EYE, NOSE, AND THROAT. By EDWARD JACKSON, A.M., M.D., and E. BALDWIN GLEASON, S.B., M.D. With 118 illustrations. Philadelphia: W. B. Saunders, 1890.

THIS book is the fourteenth of its series, and we understand that still others are to follow it, namely, one on Diagnosis, by Dr. D. D. Stewart, one on Practice, by Dr. Henry Morris, and one on the Diseases of Children, by Dr. Wm. M. Powell. Like its predecessors we can highly recommend this compend to students who desire such an aid, as we believe it is the best short epitome of the subjects of which it treats that we have. We are sorry that in the section on the eye so little is told us about correcting errors of vision by means of glasses, but the omission is excusable in so limited a space, and in a book arranged in this manner.

Dr. Gleason's part of the book is very well done, but we wish that the proof-reading had been more careful in all parts, although this book is better than some of its predecessors in this respect. Thus, on page 139, in the second paragraph, the word "failure" is used where the word feature is evidently intended, and in the endeavor to be concise clearness has sometimes been sacrificed to brevity, chiefly by the omission of "a" and "the." So many short books on the eye and throat are now on the market that no great sale can be expected for any of them, but if any succeed this one should do so.

RAILWAY SURGERY. By C. B. STEMEN, A.M., M.D., LL.D. Illustrated. St. Louis: J. B. Chambers, 1890.

THIS book is an interesting evidence of the growth of railway surgery in importance. While it is a valuable contribution in this respect, it contains very little that cannot be found in general surgical text-books, and is disappointingly imperfect in some of its parts. The chapter on anæsthetics is wofully behind the times, particularly in view of the great prominence of this subject at the present day; and the advice given as to the treat-

ment of shock possesses no particular advantages over any other treatment that we are familiar with, and is not as good as it should be. Finally, the book bears unmistakable evidence of having been dictated instead of written, and in consequence shows the ineffaceable evidences of hurry or carelessness, and lack of easy diction. Much of the work is copied *ad libitum* from other writers on the subject treated of, and while due credit is given in each instance, this causes a lack of originality.

CORRESPONDENCE.

CHICAGO.

To the Editor of THE MEDICAL NEWS,

SIR: At a recent meeting of the Chicago Pathological Society, Dr. Homer M. Thomas read a paper on "Nasal Catarrh." After dealing with the physiology of the nasal passages and the etiology of the affection, he dwelt upon the symptomatology and referred to the presence of ocular symptoms in nasal disease as an interesting feature. A certain group of eye-symptoms, such as lachrymation, photophobia, conjunctival hyperæmia, are observed in a number of patients who go to rhinologists, and yet an examination of their eyes reveals no anomaly; the vision is normal, there is no eyestrain, the conjunctivæ are healthy, and the tear-ducts are open. In such cases relief of the coexisting rhinal affection usually results in the cure of the eye-symptoms. An interesting case was reported. A woman was troubled with severe hypertrophic rhinitis, and stated that she had been unable to use her eyes longer than five minutes at a time for several years. The turbinated bones were well cauterized, after which the patient was referred to an oculist. She returned in two weeks, and stated that she had not been to the oculist, for the reason that after her hypertrophies were cauterized she was able to read at night without eye-symptoms.

Dr. Thomas said that the basis of the successful treatment of nasal catarrh is a thorough application of the principles of antisepsis. Given a case in which it is possible to medicate efficiently the anterior and posterior openings of the nasal passages as often as necessary, a cure can usually be produced. The nasal passages should permit the free entrance and exit of air during inspiration and expiration, and anything that interferes with this normal function is the starting-point of nasal catarrh.

Conditions may exist in the nasal passages which require surgical treatment, such as the straightening of a deflected septum, or the removal of portions of the superior turbinated bones. If there is an obstruction that interferes with free nasal respiration, there can be no successful treatment until the obstruction is removed. It has been estimated that out of six hundred people there are not more than ten who have perfectly straight and smooth passages; hence internal deviations of the passages are not a cause of disease, unless they interfere with perfect nasal respiration. Dr. Thomas believes that a great deal of unnecessary surgery is done upon the nasal passages, and that a large proportion of cases do not require any surgical procedures.

The remedies he advocates are strong astringents, strong solutions of nitrate of silver applied with a post-nasal syringe, sprays of the tincture of chloride of iron, tannic acid, etc.

At the outset the nasal cavities are sprayed with Dobell's solution, or with listerine. Seiler's antiseptic tablets are also very effective; and albolene, too, is an excellent medicament. A powder which has been found very satisfactory in its action on the mucous membranes of the nasal organs, consists of one grain each of borate and bicarbonate of sodium, three grains of the carbonate of magnesium, four grains of cocaine, and a sufficient quantity of sugar of milk to make one hundred grains. This combination allays acute inflammatory attacks, and also temporarily relieves hypertrophies of the turbinated bones. Dr. Thomas uses it by insufflation, both anteriorly and posteriorly. The action of the powder seems to be due to its stimulation of the vasomotor nerves, causing contraction of the vessels of the terminal bulbs of the peripheral nerves and diminishing their blood-supply.

The Railway Brotherhood Hospital Association was chartered at Springfield a day or two since. Its object is to establish ultimately hospitals for the sole benefit of railroad men at convenient points between New York and San Francisco. It is expected that all the railroad brotherhoods will eventually come in and give the scheme their financial and moral support. A hospital in this city has already been secured. It is the old Bennett Hospital, on the corner of Ada and Fulton Streets.

Dr. John B. Chaffee, who has been a practising physician in Chicago for nearly a quarter of a century, and at one time one of the best-known practitioners in the southern part of this city, died at his home, September 7th. He came from New York State, and graduated at the McDowell Medical College in 1861. During the war he served as surgeon under General Sheridan, and was wounded on several occasions. His wounds resulted in lameness of his left side, which lasted until his death. The cause of death was brain and spinal disease, from which he had been suffering about two weeks.

Thomas Kelly, M.D., C.M., M.R.C.S., has been elected Professor of Medical Chemistry in the College of Physicians and Surgeons, and Dr. Frank B. Earle Assistant to the Chair of Practice.

Dr. James B. Herrick has been appointed Lecturer on Materia Medica and Therapeutics in the Woman's Medical College, and Dr. Edwin M. Smith Professor of Anatomy.

The Chair of Professor of the Principles and Practice of Medicine, in Rush Medical College, will be filled hereafter by Dr. Henry M. Lyman, in the place of the late deceased Dr. James Adams Allen; and the Chair of Professor of Physiology, by Dr. Harold N. Moyer.

Dr. Elbert Wing has received the appointment of Lecturer on Nervous and Mental Diseases and Medical jurisprudence in the Chicago Medical College, Dr. Walter Hay, it is understood, having resigned the professorship of this chair at the close of the last lecture term.

The new medical society, recently chartered, and known as the Chicago Academy of Medicine, will, we are informed, soon begin its strictly scientific work. Among the incorporators are Drs. J. G. Kiernan, Harold N. Moyer, and S. V. Clevenger.

Professor I. N. Danforth recently returned from a trip to Berlin, where he attended the International Medical Congress. His remarks before the September meeting of the Chicago Pathological Society, relative to the social affairs and scientific work done by the Congress, were very instructive and entertaining.

According to our city medical directory, recently issued by Mr. J. Newton McDonald, there are in Chicago, 1621 physicians (including homœopaths, regulars, and eclectics), 27 chemists, 18 microscopists, 574 druggists, 147 nurses, 352 dentists, 18 pharmaceutical, medical, and dental publications, 5 dental colleges, 8 medical colleges (1 eclectic, 2 homœopathic, 4 regular, and 1 physio-medical), 3 polyclinics, 2 colleges of pharmacy, 3 colleges of midwifery, 23 charity and benevolent institutions, 19 dispensaries, 34 hospitals, and 9 training-schools for nurses.

NEWS ITEMS.

Medical Achievement in China.—It is said of Dr. Kerr, a medical missionary at Canton, that he has, in the past thirty-six years, treated over 520,000 patients, and has prepared twenty-seven medical and surgical books. He has trained one hundred medical assistants, chiefly Chinese. China now possesses one hundred and four hospitals and dispensaries, at which, in 1889, more than 348,000 patients received treatment.

Dangerous Public Baths.—The New York City public baths are located at points along the North and East rivers in close proximity to the outlets of sewers. As a consequence, many of the boys who patronize these baths have been reported as under treatment for ophthalmia due to the irritating effects of the polluted water. A preliminary report to the Board of Health tended to confirm the fact of this origin of the trouble, although further investigations show that the number of cases was greatly exaggerated.

La Grippe and Witchcraft.—The prevalence of influenza in Alaska last winter was the cause of many deaths among the natives. Witchcraft and superstition had full sway among them, and in one of the tribes a little boy, aged seven, the nephew of the chief of that tribe, was for some reason supposed to be responsible for the epidemic. It is alleged that after torture the child was about to be burned to death, but was rescued by a courageous white miner.

Typhoid Fever at Princeton, N. J.—The town authorities at Princeton and the College trustees have entered into an agreement to construct a system of sewerage. The College will bear one-half the expense of the original plant. Typhoid fever prevailed to a moderate extent during July, and by the townspeople it was feared that the disease might become epidemic, but on August 1st, the number of cases was known not to exceed seven, all of which were recovering, and that no new cases had developed within several weeks. Analyses of water and milk, suspected causes of the disease, were made, but with negative results. In the case of one suspicious dairy it was found that the cows were allowed to drink from a brook into which fæcal sewage found its way, but the milk from that dairy, after analysis, was declared pure. Although the sanitary status of the College is believed to be above suspicion, the introduction of a modern plant of sewers has been deferred until this outbreak indicated that a longer delay would be dangerous.

Law for the Prevention of Blindness.—The legislature of New York has adopted a law, the substance of which is given below, for the prevention of that element of the causation of blindness which follows ophthalmia neonatorum. The statistics of our institutions for the blind show that not far from one-fifth of all their cases arise from that disease, and the sufferers belong largely to a class of our population that is attended by midwives and untrained nurses. The New York law, which went into effect on September 1st, is as follows:

"Section 1. Should any midwife or nurse having charge of an infant in this State notice that one or both eyes of such infant are inflamed or reddened at any time within two weeks after its birth, it shall be the duty of such midwife or nurse so having charge of such infant, to report the fact in writing within six hours to the nearest health officer or some legally qualified practitioner of medicine of the city, town, or district in which the parents of the infant reside.

"Section 2. Any failure to comply with the provisions of this Act shall be punishable by a fine not to exceed one hundred dollars, or imprisonment not to exceed six months, or both."

Obituary.—The death of DR. JAMES MATTHEWS DUNCAN has been announced by cable as having occurred at Baden, on the 3d instant. He was the distinguished professor of midwifery at the St. Bartholomew's Hospital School, and a valued authority in the departments of gynecology and pediatrics. He was born in Aberdeen, in 1826, and the schools of Edinburgh were the scene of his labors and eloquent lectures during the first twenty-five years of his professional life. In 1877 he went to London, and became eminent as a professor, author, and consultant, although his name and fame were world-wide long before he left the Scotch capital.

—— SIR WILLIAM CARTER HOFFMEISTER, M.D., of Cowes, Isle of Wight, died July 29th, aged seventy-three years. He was for many years the attending physician of the Queen, the Prince of Wales, and of many of their relatives and descendants, not a few of whom were ushered into the world under the ministration of this eminent obstetrician and physician. He obtained the honor of knighthood in 1884, in recognition of these services.

—— DR. ROBERT W. JONES, Professor of Therapeutics in the College of Physicians and Surgeons of Chicago, died suddenly on September 12th.

OFFICIAL LIST OF CHANGES IN THE STATIONS AND DUTIES OF OFFICERS SERVING IN THE MEDICAL DEPARTMENT, U. S. ARMY, FROM SEPTEMBER 9 TO SEPTEMBER 15, 1890.

By direction of the Acting Secretary of War, a Board of Medical Officers, to consist of EDWARD P. VOLLUM, *Colonel and Surgeon;* GEORGE M. STERNBERG, *Major and Surgeon;* ALBERT HARTSUFF, *Major and Surgeon;* and WILLIAM E. HOPKINS, *Captain and Assistant Surgeon,* is constituted to meet in New York City, on October 15, 1890, or as soon thereafter as practicable, for the examination of candidates for admission to the Medical Corps of the Army.—Par. 8, *S. O. 213, A. G. O., Washington, D. C.,* September 11. 1890.

By direction of the Acting Secretary of War, JOSEPH K. CORSON, *Major and Surgeon,* is relieved from duty at Fort Sherman, Idaho, and will report in person to the commanding officer Washington Barracks, District of Columbia, for duty at that station.—Par. 4. *S. O. 212, A. G. O.,* September 10. 1890.

By direction of the Acting Secretary of War, the following changes in the stations and duties of officers of the Medical Department are ordered: HEIZMANN, CHARLES L., *Major and Surgeon,* is relieved from duty at San Antonio, Texas, and will report in person to the commanding officer at Fort Clark, Texas, for duty at that station, to relieve Edward P. Moseley, Captain and Assistant Surgeon, who, upon being relieved by Major Heizmann, will report in person to the commanding officer at San Antonio, Texas, for duty at that station.—Par. 23, *S. O. 211, A. G. O., Washington, D. C.,* September 9. 1890.

CARTER, EDWARD C., *Captain and Assistant Surgeon.*—Is granted leave of absence for one month.—Par. 2, *S. O. 108, Headquarters Department of the Columbia,* September 6, 1890.

By direction of the Acting Secretary of War, NATHAN S. JARVIS, *First Lieutenant and Assistant Surgeon,* is relieved from duty at Fort Verde, Arizona Territory, and will report in person to the commanding officer San Carlos, Arizona Territory, for duty at that station.—Par. 2, *S. O. 208, A. G. O., Washington, D. C.,* September 5. 1890.

OFFICIAL LIST OF CHANGES IN THE STATIONS AND DUTIES OF THE MEDICAL CORPS OF THE U. S. NAVY FOR THE WEEK ENDING SEPTEMBER 13, 1890.

WOOLVERTON, THEORON, *Medical Director.*—Ordered to the U. S. S. "Philadelphia," September 15th.

PENROSE, THOMAS N., *Medical Inspector.*—Detached from the U. S. S. "Richmond." .

GARDNER, J. E., *Passed Assistant Surgeon.*—Detached from the U. S. Fish-culture Steamer "Albatross."

DRAKE, N. H., *Passed Assistant Surgeon.*—Detached from the U. S. Coast-survey Steamer "McArthur," and ordered to the U. S. Fish-culture Steamer "Albatross."

BERRYHILL, T. A., *Passed Assistant Surgeon.*—Detached from the Hospital, Mare Island, Cal., and ordered to the U. S. Coast-survey Steamer "McArthur."

HEFFINGER, A. C , *Passed Assistant Surgeon.*—Ordered before Retiring Board, October 1, 1890.

OFFICIAL LIST OF CHANGES OF STATIONS AND DUTIES OF MEDICAL OFFICERS OF THE U. S. MARINE-HOSPITAL SERVICE, FROM AUGUST 12 TO SEPTEMBER 6, 1890.

VANSANT, JOHN, *Surgeon.*—Granted leave of absence for thirty days, to take effect upon return to duty of Assistant Surgeon J. C. Perry, September 5, 1890.

WYMAN, WALTER, *Surgeon.*—To proceed to Cape Charles Quarantine Station, on special duty, August 25, 1890.

STONER, GEORGE W., *Surgeon.*—Granted leave of absence for four days, August 19, 1890.

CARMICHAEL, D. A., *Passed Assistant Surgeon.*—Leave of absence extended fifteen days, August 26, 1890.

AMES. R. P. M., *Passed Assistant Surgeon.*—To proceed to Memphis. Tenn., on temporary duty.

DEVAN, S. G., *Passed Assistant Surgeon.*—Leave extended five days, on account of sickness, August 12, 1890.

WILLIAMS. L. L., *Passed Assistant Surgeon.*—Granted leave of absence for thirty days, September 5, 1890.

GOODWIN, H. F., *Assistant Surgeon.*—Granted leave of absence for thirty days, August 21, 1890.

COBB, J. O., *Assistant Surgeon.*—To proceed to Marine Hospital, Detroit, Mich., for duty, August 16, 1890.

HUSSEY, S. H., *Assistant Surgeon.*—Granted leave of absence for thirty days, August 19, 1890.

PERRY, J. C., *Assistant Surgeon.*—Granted leave of absence for twenty days, to take effect when relieved, September 3, 1890.

YOUNG, G. B., *Assistant Surgeon.*—To rejoin his station, at St. Louis, Mo., when relieved, September 3. 1890.

APPOINTMENT.

ROSENAU, MILTON J., *Assistant Surgeon.*—Commissioned as an Assistant Surgeon by the President, August 25, 1890. Ordered to Chicago, Ill., for temporary duty, August 27, 1890.

THE MEDICAL NEWS.

A WEEKLY JOURNAL OF MEDICAL SCIENCE.

VOL. LVII.   SATURDAY, SEPTEMBER 27, 1890.   No. 13.

ORIGINAL LECTURES.

MACEWEN'S OPERATION FOR CONGENITAL INGUINAL HERNIA.

A Clinical Lecture.

BY D. A. K. STEELE, M.D.,

PROFESSOR OF THE PRINCIPLES AND PRACTICE OF SURGERY AND CLINICAL SURGERY IN THE COLLEGE OF PHYSICIANS AND SURGEONS, CHICAGO.

GENTLEMEN: The patient we present to-day is this little child, with the following history: He is now eighteen months old. His mother states that soon after his birth she noticed a swelling in the lower part of the abdomen, appearing simultaneously over each inguinal canal. When the child was about three weeks old, it was seen that the swelling extended lower down; the mother noticed that the swelling increased along the course of the inguinal canal when the child made any violent effort, such as coughing, crying, straining, or any exertion that brought into play the diaphragm or abdominal muscles. Some weeks later she took the child to a dispensary, where a truss was adjusted, but the instrument, did not prevent the reappearance of the swelling in the scrotum. During the past year a number of trusses have been applied, but none of them prevented the recurrence of the hernial swelling.

Now, when an infant is brought to us suffering from a tumor of the scrotum, it may be one of a variety of diseases, and it is well to make a diagnosis by exclusion. Let us enumerate some of the various tumors that may occupy the scrotal pouch. We may have either a hernia, hydrocele, epididymitis, hæmatocele, varicocele, œdema, or an orchitis, or a complication of two or more of these affections. How shall we differentiate these varied conditions? What will aid us in a correct diagnosis in a given case? For diagnostic or clinical purposes tumors of the scrotum may be divided into two general classes, namely: reducible and irreducible. The reducible tumors include all varieties of hernia (except strangulated), varicocele, and congenital hydrocele. Irreducible tumors include those connected with the testicles, all hydroceles (except congenital), and strangulated hernia. Tumors of the tegumentary surface of the scrotum, such as inflammatory œdema, elephantiasis, and epithelioma, are usually so characteristic in their history as to offer no special impediments to a correct diagnosis.

Scrotal hernia may be mistaken for (1) hydrocele of tunica vaginalis, or cord, or for encysted hydrocele; (2) sarcocele of the testicle, either simple, tuberculous, cystic, or malignant; (3) varicocele; (4) hæmatocele; (5) bubo or an undescended testis.

In scrotal hernia, as a rule, the tumor is soft and doughy to the touch, light in weight, smooth and regular, and painless, unless inflamed or strangulated. Its advent is sudden, and from above downward; it is resonant on percussion; fills the inguinal canal; has an impulse on coughing; and is of normal opaque color, and gurgles on pressure. It may exist on either side; the spermatic cord is concealed; the tumor does not fluctuate; aspiration gives negative results, and the bowels may be embarrassed. It can be reduced, unless the hernia is strangulated or incarcerated.

In hydrocele of the testicle the tumor is ovoid or pyriform; develops slowly from below upward; is firm, tense, and elastic; is translucent, fluctuating and dull on percussion, and is reducible. The spermatic cord is neither concealed nor displaced; the inguinal canal is empty; the bowels are unaffected, and aspiration reveals fluid.

In congenital hydrocele the fluid completely disappears within the peritoneal cavity if the tumor is compressed for a short time.

In sarcocele of the testicle the tumor is usually hard and resistant; heavy; often nodular and irregular; painful; grows slowly, and is dull or flat on percussion. The inguinal canal is empty; there is no impulse on coughing; the bowels are unaffected; the tumor is irreducible, and there are no auscultatory sounds. Simple sarcocele is a chronic orchitis, both the epididymis and body of the gland being affected, and the cord is usually thickened. Abscess of the organ may occur, and is usually caused by an injury followed by inflammatory deposits. Tubercular sarcocele is met with most frequently in early manhood, and may occur in any variety of constitution—in the strong and robust, as well as the weak and cachectic—and although often associated with tuberculosis of other organs, it is not uncommon to find the tuberculous nidus in the epididymis, not as a sequence of gonorrhœal inflammation or some slight injury followed by inflammatory infiltration, as was formerly believed, but as a coincident. The progress is slow and insidious. The gland at first moderately enlarges, with little or no pain, the hypertrophy being especially marked in the globus major. Presently the outline of the tumor becomes nodulated, and it extends around the testicle from behind forward. After several months, the adventitious tissue exceeds in size the testicle proper, and then it begins to soften, and one or more abscesses burst and discharge a thin, shreddy pus. The vas deferens is greatly enlarged.

In syphilitic sarcocele, or gumma, the history of the patient guides us in the diagnosis. We also find that the body of the gland is usually the seat of the infiltration which takes place in the connective tissue between the tubuli seminiferi, the epididymis undergoing little, if any enlargement. The cord and vas deferens are unaffected. There is little or no tenderness, and the peculiar sensation elicited by squeezing a healthy testicle is absent. The tunica albuginea is very greatly thickened. Hydrocele is a frequent complication, and tapping is often required to establish a diagnosis.

Cystic tumors of the testis closely resemble hydrocele, and differ chiefly in being opaque instead of translucent. Aspiration should be practised before pronouncing positively upon their character.

Cancer of the testicle primarily invades the body of the gland, and almost invariably assumes the encephaloid form. Most observers doubt the existence of other varieties of malignant disease in this organ. The development of the disease is rapid. The patient has a sensation of weight, pain, and dragging in the testis; the scrotum becomes distended, and reddish or purplish, and the superficial veins are enlarged. The skin adheres to the gland, ulceration occurs, fungous growths protrude, the inguinal glands are secondarily involved, and the patient by this time presents the characteristic cancerous cachexia.

In varicocele the tumor develops gradually; is knotty and irregular, like a bag of worms; is bluish in color, and is most frequent upon the left side. It increases in size upon the application of heat; is dull on percussion; fluctuation is doubtful, and the spermatic cord is not affected, nor is the inguinal canal involved. There is no cough-impulse. The tumor disappears when the patient assumes any position that favors increased venous return, but immediately returns when he stands up, notwithstanding pressure at the ring. There is a sensation of weight and dragging in the scrotum.

In hæmatocele the advent is sudden, and usually follows traumatism. The tumor grows from below upward, if it arises spontaneously; at first it is soft and fluctuating, but when coagulation occurs it becomes hard. It is pyriform in shape; ecchymotic, irreducible, heavy, and dull on percussion. The spermatic cord is unaffected, and the inguinal canal empty. There are often pallor and prostration from loss of blood. The bowels are unaffected.

Bubo is seldom mistaken for a scrotal tumor, and it is unnecessary to name the differential points.

An undescended testicle is painful, and pressure upon it causes a peculiar, sickening pain. The scrotum is imperfectly developed upon the same side, and, of course, does not contain the testicle. It is sometimes mistaken for bubonocele.

Now, gentlemen, I trust that this minute enumeration of diagnostic points may not be considered tedious or unnecessary, and that a remembrance of them will aid you in making a correct diagnosis.

Let us return to the patient before us. We have here a soft, elastic, compressible, reducible swelling, occupying both sides of the scrotal pouch; cough-impulse is present, and gurgling is plainly felt. Upon flexing the thighs, elevating the hips, grasping the scrotum gently, and making moderate compression, the tumor disappears within the abdominal cavity. Inversion of the bottom of the scrotum by the little finger enables us to follow readily the receding mass through the dilated inguinal canal and distended inguinal ring into the abdominal cavity. With the history presented, and with the result of this physical examination, we are enabled to make a diagnosis of *double congenital oblique inguinal hernia.*

Now, inasmuch as persistent efforts during the past year have been made by able surgeons to retain this hernia *in situ* by various trusses, without success, what plan of treatment shall we adopt? The treatment of the affection, as you know, may be divided into *palliative* and *radical*, or *curative*. Palliative treatment consists in the use of such apparatus, instruments, or trusses, fitting over the inguinal ring, as will prevent the extrusion of the hernial tumor. They must be fitted with sufficient nicety to the contour of the parts to inflict the minimum amount of pain, and yet with sufficient firmness to resist the intra-abdominal and intra-thoracic pressure produced by coughing, crying, straining during urination or defæcation, or any exercise of the voluntary muscles that causes downward pressure upon the abdominal viscera. In a large proportion of cases a properly adjusted truss, continuously worn during the first few months or year or two of infantile life, will effect a permanent occlusion of the distended inguinal ring; but occasionally we meet with cases, such as the one we have just examined, where cure by means of a truss is impossible.

If it is impossible to retain the hernia within the abdomen, then it becomes necessary to resort to more radical measures—to closure of the enlarged canal by means of a surgical operation. One of the best operations for this purpose is that devised by Macewen, of Glasgow.

Macewen's operation consists, first, in a thorough cleansing of the field of operation with soap and water, and removing by means of turpentine all animal oil from the surface. The parts are then covered with lint saturated with a bichloride solution. In the case of an adult, the hair of the pubes and neighboring parts is closely shaven. The patient is then anæsthetized, and the limb on the side of the swelling is flexed at the knee and retained in that position by a pillow placed beneath. After having reduced the bowel, the operator makes an incision sufficiently large to expose the external abdominal ring. An exploration of the sac and its contents is then made, and the finger introduced through the canal examines the abdominal aspects of the internal ring, and determines the position of the epigastric artery. The following steps of the operation may then be divided into two parts—the one relating to the establishment of a pad on the abdominal aspects of the internal ring; the other to the closure of the inguinal canal. The details are as follows:

The surgeon frees and elevates the distal extremity of the sac, preserving any adipose tissue that may be adherent to it. When that is done, he pulls upon the sac, and, while maintaining the tension, introduces the index-finger into the inguinal canal, separating the sac from the cord, and from the parietes of the canal; he then inserts the index-finger outside of the sac until it reaches the internal ring, and there he separates the peritoneum for about half an inch around the abdominal aspects of the ring. Next, a suture is firmly secured to the distal extremity of the sac, and the free end is passed in a proximal direction several times through the sac, so that when pulled upon the sac becomes folded upon itself like a curtain. The free end of this stitch, threaded on a hernia-needle, is made to traverse the canal and to penetrate the anterior abdominal wall about an inch above the internal ring, the wound in the skin being pulled upward so as to allow the point of the needle to project through the abdominal muscles without penetrating the skin. The needles that Macewen uses are corkscrew-shaped, with an eye in the point, and are made rights and lefts. The thread is relieved from the extremity of the needle, when the latter is withdrawn, and is pulled through the abdominal wall; and when traction is made the sac is thrown into a series of folds, its distal extremity being drawn backward and upward. An assistant maintains traction upon this stitch until the introduction of the sutures into the inguinal canal, and when this is completed the end of the first suture is secured by passing its free extremity several times through the superficial layers of the external oblique muscle. The pad of peritoneum is then placed upon the abdominal side of the internal opening, where, owing to the abdominal aspect of the circumference of the internal ring having been freshened, new adhesions may form. The sac having been returned into the abdomen and secured to the abdominal circumference of the ring, the inguinal canal is closed outside of it in the following manner: The finger is introduced into the canal between the inner and lower borders of the internal ring; the threaded hernia-needle is then introduced, and, guided by the index-finger, is made to penetrate the conjoined tendon—first, from without inward, near the lower border of the conjoined tendon; second, from within outward as high as possible on the inner aspects of the canal. This double penetration of the conjoined tendon is accomplished by a single screw-like turn of the needle, when a single thread is withdrawn from the point of the needle by the index-finger; after which the needle, with the other extremity of the thread, is removed. The inner side of the conjoined tendon is therefore penetrated twice by the thread, and a loop is left on its abdominal aspect. The other hernia-needle, threaded with that portion of the stitch which comes from the lower border of the conjoined tendon, is guided by the index-finger into the inguinal canal, and introduced from within outward through Poupart's ligament and the aponeurotic structures of the internal and external oblique muscles. It penetrates these structures at a point on a level with the lower stitch in the conjoined tendon. The needle is then completely freed from the thread and withdrawn. The needle is now threaded with the suture, which protrudes from the upper border of the conjoined tendon, and is introduced from within outward through the internal and external oblique muscles on a level corresponding with the upper stitch in the conjoined tendon. It is then freed from the thread and withdrawn. There are now two thread-ends on the outer surface of the external oblique muscle, and these are connected with a loop on the abdominal aspect of the conjoined tendon. To complete the suture, the two thread-ends are drawn together and tied in a reef-knot; thus firmly uniting the internal ring. The same stitch may be repeated lower down the canal, if thought desirable. In adults it is well to do so. The pillars of the external ring are likewise brought together, and, in order to avoid compression of the cord, it should be examined before tightening each stitch. It is advisable to introduce all the sutures before tightening any of them. When this is done, they all may be drawn tight, and maintained so, while the operator's finger is introduced into the canal to ascertain the result. If satisfactory, they are then tied, beginning with the one at the internal ring, and taking up the others in order.

During the operation the skin is retracted from side to side to bring the parts into view and to enable the stitches to be fixed subcutaneously. When the retraction is relieved the skin falls into its normal position, the wound being opposite the external ring. The operation is, therefore, partly subcutaneous. When the canal has been brought together, a decalcified bone drainage-tube is placed with its one extremity next to the external ring, the other projecting beyond the lower border of the external wound. A few chromicized gut sutures are then introduced along the line of the incision in the skin. Iodoform is dusted over the wound, a small portion of sublimated gauze is applied, and over this a sublimated pad, held in position by an aseptic bandage. When the patient is laid in bed, a pillow is placed under his knees, while his shoulders are slightly raised, so as to relax the tissues about the canal. The temperature is taken night and morning, and the dressings are left undisturbed for from fourteen to twenty-one days, unless they are stained or the temperature is elevated.

From four to six weeks after the operation the patient is allowed to rise from the bed, but is not permitted to work until the end of the eighth week, and is further advised not to lift heavy weights until the end of the third month. Adults engaged in laborious occupations are advised to wear a bandage and pad as a precautionary measure, but in the majority of children the closure is so complete and firm that further treatment by a pad is unnecessary.

In the case of this little child, who is now under the influence of an anæsthetic, we will modify this operation, inasmuch as we have to deal with a congenital hernia in which the loop of bowel and the testicle occupy a common sac—there is no tunica vaginalis. After the preliminary incision, I will separate the sac from its connections; then open it transversely about an inch and a half above its distal extremity, and form the lower part into a tunica vaginalis by closing it with fine continuous catgut suture. The upper part of the sac is now pulled down as far as possible, split longitudinally behind, a portion of it closed around the cord, which is carefully preserved, and that part which is left is now dealt with as the sac of an acquired hernia; passing a stitch through its distal portion a number of times, so that it becomes folded up as a curtain. Then with the finger I separate the attachments around the circumference of the abdominal ring. I then pass a needle through the abdominal wall an inch above the ring, bringing the thread out, where it is held by an assistant. Traction upon this cord forms the intra-abdominal pad or boss —a firm buttress that resists the intra-abdominal pressure.

I now proceed to close the internal ring in the manner described, passing two or three sutures along the course of the canal, drawing them snugly together, yet not tight enough to strangulate the cord. A drainage-tube is now passed from the upper angle of the wound and brought down through a slit in the bottom of the scrotum, so as to afford perfect drainage. The parts are now irrigated with a 1-to-3000 solution of bichloride, the wound closed with interrupted catgut sutures, dusted with iodoform, and hermetically sealed with cotton and collodion, so as to prevent infection from the urine, which is liable to occur in the case of infants or young children. In closing the wound in this way we reduce the risk of infection to a minimum. A heavy antiseptic dressing will now be applied, and covered with a starch bandage. The child will be kept as quiet as possible, small doses of camphorated tincture of opium will be administered from time to time, and the dressing will probably have to be changed every second day. The mother will be directed to keep the child lying on the left side as much as possible, so as to avoid soiling the dressing during urination. The operation on the left side will be deferred until permanent healing of the right has taken place—probably for two or three weeks.

[NOTE.—A week later the child was presented to the class, and showed primary closure of the wound, except at the upper angle and the scrotal button-hole through which the drainage-tube emerged. Slight suppuration had taken place along the course of the drainage-tube. The highest temperature was 100.5°, on the day following the operation; the second day it dropped to 98.5°, and remained normal, the child showing no symptoms or evidences of having undergone a serious or dangerous operation, the result so far being in every way emiuently satisfactory.]

ORIGINAL ARTICLES.

CONTINUOUS DRAINAGE IN THE TREATMENT OF ASCITES—ABDOMINAL SECTION FOR INTESTINAL OBSTRUCTION.[1]

BY T. A. HARRIS, M.D.,
OF PARKERSBURG, W. VA.

I HAVE been prompted by certain articles on the "Benefits of Successive Tapping in Ascites" to report my success with continuous drainage in similar cases. It seemed to me that the continuous drainage of serous effusion would prove beneficial in cases with no organic disease of either the liver, kidneys, or heart.

CASE I.—In August, 1888, I was requested by a country friend to see Mrs. B., with him. The history of the case was that the patient had been delivered by my friend after a tedious labor, some five or six months before; that the placenta had been retained, and that he had introduced his hand into the uterus and delivered it. The patient had a slow "getting up," and had not been well since. Some three months after her delivery the abdomen began to enlarge. The enlargement was evidently ascitic. She suffered with soreness and tenderness over the abdomen. The secretion of urine was very scanty, but normal in character. When I saw her the abdomen was about as large as that of a woman at term. She was somewhat emaciated, but complained of nothing except the inconvenience and discomfort of the abdominal enlargement. Upon examination I could find no disease either of the heart, liver, or kidneys. She had had four children. She said that while carrying the last child she had had some soreness in the region of the right ovary; that when the doctor removed the afterbirth with his hand, it caused pain

[1] Read before the West Virginia Medical Society, June 13, 1890.

in the same region, and that afterward she was very sore over her entire abdomen.

I tapped her and drew off a large amount of ascitic fluid, a peculiarity of which was that it contained quite an amount of whitish flocculent matter. She was greatly relieved by the operation; the action of the kidneys was restored and she passed urine freely. But the dropsical effusion gradually returned, with the former symptoms, and in a month she was as large as before. I visited her again and found her in about the same condition as when I had first seen her. I then determined to make the second operation, if possible, more effective than the first. I had come prepared to introduce a drainage-tube, and to leave it in place. This I did, with the necessary antiseptic precautions. After introducing the trocar and canula I withdrew the trocar, and at once passed a drainage-tube through the canula. I then withdrew the canula and allowed the fluid to flow through the drainage-tube. About as much fluid escaped as after the first tapping. In order to prevent the drainage-tube from slipping in or out, I stitched it to a piece of adhesive plaster placed over the abdomen, and through which the end of the tube projected. Here I made my mistake, for in three days there was so much inflammation about the tube that it was necessary to remove it. Under simple treatment all the irritation quickly subsided, but there was again a return of the former trouble, so that in three weeks she was nearly as large as before. At the third tapping I determined that nothing should be lacking, and I left the tube in place with most careful antiseptic precautions. Three weeks from the date of the operation she travelled fifteen miles on the railroad to see me; the drainage-tube still in place. She said that the discharge for the first week had been quite free, but during the last two weeks much less. As there was still some discharge when she was in the recumbent position I did not think it best to remove the tube, and asked her to see me again in another week. She did not return until the expiration of two weeks, when she said that there had been no discharge for more than a week. I then withdrew the tube.

This was more than a year ago, and I have seen the patient several times since, once within the past month. She is well and has had no return of the trouble.

I know that "one swallow does not make a summer," and that one case does not establish a principle, but I have recently had a very similar case (October, 1889):

CASE II.—I was again asked by a brother-practitioner to see a patient, and was given the general statement that the case was one of dropsy following confinement. On making the visit, I found an apparently healthy woman with an ascitic enlargement equal to that of the seventh month of pregnancy. She had been confined about four months before, and easily delivered of her fourth child. She was attended only by a neighboring woman. There was nothing unusual during her convalescence, but a few weeks later she noticed that her abdomen was enlarging. This did not at first cause her any uneasiness, as she said that she had noticed a similar, though slight, condition after the birth of her previous children. There was no discoverable disease of any of the viscera, and this fact, in connection with her statement as to enlargement after previous confinements led me to regard the effusion as due to some peritoneal irritation, if not to inflammation of a mild type; and I decided to try the effect of continuous drainage. With the usual precautions the drainage-tube was introduced through the canula and held in position by a strip of adhesive plaster, through which it passed and to which it was stitched. The case was left in the hands of my friend, who has since informed me by letter that the day after the operation he was summoned in haste to see the patient, and that he found her with a temperature of 102°, and a pulse of 110, and complaining of much pain over the region of the right kidney. The drainage-tube was all right and there was no abdominal pain. With warm fomentations over the region of the kidney and the use of an anodyne and antipyretic, the pain, the temperature, and the pulse were reduced by the next day, and from this time the course of the case was uneventful. There was some discharge from the tube for a few days, but by the end of a week there was none. The tube was retained for two weeks and then removed. There has been no return of the ascites; the patient is up and attending to the duties of a country housewife.

CASE III.—In July, 1888, I was asked to see a patient in an adjoining State, said to be suffering from dropsy. I found a woman whom I had seen several years before, on account of a uterine fibroid, and who was at that time in fair health, and suffering in no way from the tumor. I had advised against any operation for its removal, and told her that no medicine would be of any special advantage to her. Not satisfied with this advice, she had gone to a quack in a neighboring town, who promised to relieve her by medical treatment. She suffered much at his hands, from purgatives and diuretics, all to no purpose. She then fell into the hands of a homœopath, whose promises were about as futile as those of the quack.

When I saw her the second time she was so distended that respiration was seriously interfered with. I tapped, and drew off a large amount of ascitic fluid. The uterine fibroid was in its former place. The woman was in an extremely exhausted condition. I expressed the opinion that the fluid would again accumulate, and promised that if it did I would remove it, and make provision against its further return. In about a month I was recalled to the case, and found things about as at first, except that the patient's general condition was worse. I again tapped, introduced a drainage-tube, and left it in place. I did not see her again, but learned that the tube was effective in preventing any re-accumulation of fluid, but that there was some slight discharge until the time of her death, more than a month after the tube had been inserted.

CASE IV. *Abdominal section.*—I was sent for on March 9, 1890, to consult with Dr. William Kurn, of Lubeck, upon a case of obstruction of the bowels, in a boy of about fourteen years. The obstruction was of five days' duration, and there had been stercoraceous vomiting during the day. All reasonable and proper efforts had been made to produce a movement of the bowels.

I found a decided lump in the right iliac region, which was quite tender on pressure. There was a moderate amount of tympany. Under the circumstances I decided that there was but one thing to do, namely, to open the abdomen and find the cause of the obstruction. With the consent of the family this we did, at midnight, by the light of two small lamps, and in a log-cabin, from which we had to expel a crowd of people, several dogs, and a coop of chickens. The abdomen was opened with antiseptic precautions, by an incision over the lump in the right iliac region. The first thing that presented was the distended small intestine, which was healthy in appearance. Passing my finger in, I drew into sight the empty and flaccid ascending colon, and then the cæcum. Replacing these, I drew out the small intestine, working my way down toward the ileo-cæcal valve, when, after a little resistance, I drew out six or eight inches of deeply congested intestine. This was evidently the portion which had passed into the ileo-cæcal valve. Its withdrawal was attended with a gurgling sound, due to the rush of the contents into the cæcum. The obstruction was relieved. I then reversed my mode of procedure, and worked my way up the intestine as high as possible, and tried to force down with my fingers the contents of the distended small intestine into the colon. I found it easy to press onward the liquid contents, but the gas slipped through my fingers, leaving the small intestine about as much distended as at the beginning. I closed the wound with deep sutures of silver and superficial of silk, dressed it antiseptically, and put the boy to bed. He rallied well. I saw him again on March 13th, when I opened the dressing, and found the wound in good condition, excepting a superficial abscess just above the upper end of the wound. I cut the upper silk stitch, and let out about a teaspoonful of pus. After this the course of the case was uneventful. The bowels moved twenty-four hours after the operation, and continued open. Six weeks from the date of the operation, the boy rode six miles in a wagon to my office. He said that he was "well, and wanted to go to work."

I have reported this case in order to encourage early operations in cases of intestinal obstruction. I have seen a number of such cases, and this is the first that did not die. The operation was performed under very unfavorable circumstances as to time. place, and assistance, and yet was entirely successful. Why, then, shall we hesitate under more favorable circumstances, when the dire alternative of death stares us in the face?

In a case of intestinal obstruction I think that milder measures, such as purgatives, enemata, and massage, should be persisted in, *only* until the occurrence of stercoraceous vomiting. or of some other critical condition ; then an exploratory incision should be made, without reference to the obscurity of the diagnosis, for whatever condition the obstruction is dependent upon, there is little chance of recovery by other than operative treatment. Nor do I think the surgeon should stay his hand, let the condition of the patient be ever so desperate. Desperate conditions require desperate remedies, and in the average surgical mind I think that the operation is regarded as more desperate and dangerous than the facts warrant, when it is done with the precautions demanded by modern surgical teachings.

HYPNOTISM IN A RELIGIOUS MEETING.

BY THEODORE DILLER. M.D.,

CLINICAL ASSISTANT TO THE CHAIR OF PSYCHIATRY AND NEUROLOGY, MARION-SIMS MEDICAL COLLEGE, ST. LOUIS.

IN a large tent in St. Louis, capable of holding 3000 or 4000 people, most extraordinary "religious meetings" have recently been held. These so-called "revival meetings" were led by one Maria B. Woodworth, who is, in my opinion, a paranoiac of a strongly religious type.

The writer's attention was called to the subject by several of my patients, who averred that Mrs. Woodworth was a prophetess sent directly from Heaven, and that people were so impressed with her preaching that they were prostrated to the ground, and that while in this condition many had visions of heaven, angels, etc.

Together with Dr. Wellington Adams, I attended some of the meetings and found the statement to be correct that "people were prostrated to the ground," and I doubt not many had visions such as they describe. The meetings, for a time, increased in size, while the number hypnotized each evening increased proportionately. One evening the crowd in the tent was estimated at 5000 (many standing) while, it is said, nearly an equal number were turned away for want of room.

The beginning of the meeting is principally ocenpied by Mrs. Woodworth, who speaks to the audience. The address, for the most part, is an incoherent, unintelligible jargon, but occasionally a few sentences can be understood. The latter usually have to do with the supernatural occurrences related in the Bible, such as the Transfiguration, the descent of the Holy Spirit on the Apostles, or the miracles. Perhaps her favorite themes are the visions, especially those related in the Book of Revelations. She frequently interrupted herself (if such a discourse can be said to be interrupted) to tell of visions which she herself has had, or to describe one of the very many "cures" of physical ailments which have been effected by the "power" manifested in her meetings. Her address is usually very long and I noted that she never became excited nor

did she have any tendency to "shout," or unduly elevate her voice, as is so common in the ordinary revival meeting. On the contrary, there was a quiet confidence expressed in her manner which was very suggestive of the delusional, self-conceited paranoic, strong in her own beliefs.

Toward the end of her discourse she begins to exhort her hearers to "Look up to the Lord"— "Hold up your hands "—" Have faith." Her followers obey her injunctions literally ; they fix their eyes steadfastly on the electric lights high above them, or on the intricate mass of converging tent-ropes beyond. In this position a few of the more susceptible of her believers succumb. They go into the first or cataleptic stage of hypnotism while the exhorter is relating from the Bible or from her own experience the visions of heaven. A hymn then follows which is of a peculiar, monotonous character and well adapted to assist in promoting the hypnotic condition in many who are slightly or not at all influenced by the visual impressions alone. The hymn is usually repeated a number of times. During the singing, Mrs. Woodworth and her assistants (of which there are several) walk up and down the long platform encouraging those who are nervous, uneasy, or in any way visibly affected, to "hold up their hands, look up, and think of the Lord." The greatest number succumb during the singing.

As may be expected, more women than men are affected. At one large meeting the number more or less hypnotized must have been fully one hundred. Some were typical cases, exhibiting the three stages of hypnosis, namely, catalepsy, lethargy, and artificial somnambulism. When laid upon their backs on the platform, where the subjects were brought as rapidly as they became affected, those representing the typical condition lay with the eyes wide open, pupils dilated, and with a vacant or fixed stare ; the arms unsupported extended upward and outward. One young woman whom I watched closely did not wink or move her eyeballs during the ten or fifteen minutes that I observed her. I attempted to place my finger upon her eyeball but was, in sharp terms, forbidden to do so by the attendant at her side. Many were more or less affected while on their feet ; others while observing the directions of the leaders entirely failed in the consummation of their purpose.

A particularly shocking feature of the meetings was the hypnosis of children, of whom several were usually affected.

The force of example must have a strong influence with many. In Charcot's clinic the subjects for hypnosis are several times shown others in the hypnotic condition before any attempt is made to hypnotize them. This preparation causes a mental impression which makes the subsequent actual attempts at hypnosis more generally successful and with fewer trials. Now most of Mrs. Woodworth's subjects have precisely this preparation ; *i. e.*, they attend a number of meetings, become mentally impressed, and at subsequent meetings succumb with ease.

The question as to whether Mrs. Woodworth is an impostor or a case of religious insanity naturally arises. Judging from the meetings, from her autobiography, and more especially from an interview that I had with her, I am strongly of the latter opinion.

She states that she was born in 1845, in a small town in Ohio, but soon removed to Salem, in the same state. She denies inherited mental taint, but says that her husband was mentally unsound at one time. Four out of five of her offsprings died in childhood—one of "scrofula," another of some lingering malady.

She states that she never knew what the "power" was—never witnessed it until she had been engaged in evangelistic work for two years. When a child of thirteen she knew that the Lord had ordained her to go out and preach the gospel, and she became converted, but she fought against God. One day while sitting alone in her room she saw the vision of the Bible on the wall. The letters were raised and the book shone as brightly as the sun. This call to preach was an audible call, heard with her ears just as she hears anyone's voice now. After this she had many visions. At first the voice of God frightened her very much, but in time she became accustomed to it. The idea of going out to preach was so repugnant to her—because a woman—that she seriously contemplated suicide. A vision of the devil, who came and tempted her, also exerted a depressing effect upon her. Her lack of education, she also felt, was a serious obstacle. During this time of struggle and indecision the Lord came and persuaded her to go. She saw a bright light, too, and angels flying all around her.

She married at an early age. After marriage the struggle continued, and the devil came to tempt her, but the Lord told her that she must go out and preach or lose her soul. In this particular vision the Saviour was on the cross ; his face was so bright that she could not see it distinctly. There was a crown of thorns at His feet. This vision occurred when she was at the age of thirty-four. She told the Lord of the difficulties which she felt were in her way—lack of education, etc., when the Lord gave her power to preach just as he had given it to the Galilean fisherman. She then began her work. During the first few years of her preaching no one was stricken down in the meetings, and she was frightened when she first saw the people fall down. In this extremity the Lord came to her again and said:

13*

"Sister, don't you remember the vision of the grain?" This vision she had beheld some time before, and was as follows: One day angels came into her room—"a whole flock of them." They carried her up and into the West, miles and miles away, over prairies and forests, and lakes and rivers. Then they stopped, resting in the air on their wings, and she saw a long, wide field of waving grain. She then began to preach, and saw the grain fall into sheaves. This she compares to Ezekiel's vision. Christ then came to her and said : "Be not afraid, that is the way you'll do when you preach to real people."

At present she seldom has visions except when "under the power," but frequently hears voices while sitting in her room, or while in bed, and she often converses aloud with the Deity. Her assistant or attendant states that she frequently finds Mrs. Woodworth standing in her room with fixed gaze and wholly immobile.

One evening during the progress of the meeting, Mrs. Woodworth herself became apparently unconscious, the condition coming on very gradually. But the phenomena in her case presented a marked contrast to those of her hypnotized followers. Instead of the expressionless, cataleptoid state common in them, the leader's appearance was that of great exhilaration—ecstasy. The face assumed a peculiar, radiant expression ; the eyes became fixed, while the body remained immobile in a dramatic position. Her condition at that time was described as pure ecstasy. Her appearance was so striking, so supernatural that it would have impressed anyone. It is not a matter of surprise that the more susceptible of her followers are able to see at such times an actual halo of light about their leader's head. She may possibly at other times have attacks of catalepsy or hystero-epilepsy, but this I was unable to determine. Mills[1] states that the three conditions are commonly associated in the same individual.

The woman, I believe, is a case of *religious monomania* (paranoia). Her early struggles ; her visions of hell and heaven ; her strong temptation at one time to commit suicide ; the nature, character, and evolution of her delusions, transforming the ignorant country girl into the undaunted, direct agent of the Deity—all confirm this theory. The two prominent characteristics of paranoia, namely, personal egotism and a feeling of persecution, are prominent features in the character of Maria B. Woodworth.

History is full of examples of religious characters such as hers. Spitzka[2] says:

"More than one insane fanatic of the middle ages has been responsible for the fierce campaigns waged against dissenters and alleged infidels, and not one of the least remarkable incidents of this period of history is the fact

---

[1] Pepper's System of Medicine. vol. V. p. 339.
[2] Manual of Insanity. p. 318.

that for two centuries Europe poured out its best strength in the Crusades, under the influence of the prayers, sermons, and visions of a Peter the Hermit, who undoubtedly suffered from this form of monomania."

Mills[1] describes a number of historical characters who, at times, would pass into the condition of ecstasy. Both Elizabeth of Hungary and Joan of Arc were cataleptics and ecstatics.

Gibbon's[2] description of the state of ecstasy as it occurred in the monks of the Oriental Church is classical.

The visions of Swedenborg and John Englebrecht were conceived during the ecstatic trance.

A notable case is that of Bernadette Soubirons, who, near a mountain stream of the Pyrenees, saw in the niche of a rock a female figure of great splendor, with an aureola about her head ; her body also being very bright. She saw this vision a number of times, and believed it to be the Virgin Mary. The place has been made a shrine, and is visited by persons of all nationalities.

Cataleptic, ecstatic, hysterical, and allied manifestations in religious gatherings might be recounted at great length, but a few notable historical occurrences must suffice. The Buddhist fasts to render his body weak. He then fixes his eyes and thoughts intently on a single object, when he easily brings himself into the trance condition.

Often wonderful visions appear to subjects in the cataleptic state, and these are described to others.

The "dancing mania" occurred in 1374, principally in France and Germany. It is said that persons affected were unconscious, and insensible to pain, and that many beheld celestial visions. This epidemic was very widespread, the presence of one affected person being sufficient to excite the disease in a large crowd.

In the famous Kentucky revival of 1810 scores were prostrated at a single meeting. Some became cataleptic ; others became possessed of a sort of "dancing mania" or "jerks." This latter manifestation was most remarkable. The body would sway violently forward and backward, the arms and hands striking out in any or all directions. The slave and his master, the delicate woman and the rugged backwoodsman, the preacher and his hearer, were alike affected.

The "jerks" appeared in Ireland about the year 1859, during the progress of a very remarkable religious movement. The manifestations were very similar to those of the famous Kentucky revival. Visions of various kinds were common, and thousands of persons were affected. An interesting feature noticed in many of the subjects was the appearance of stigmata on the hands or feet. For a

description of those curious phenomena the reader is referred to the admirable articles of Hammond,[1] Clymer, and Mills.[2]

The reader of history—secular, medical, and religious—will find many more examples similar to those briefly referred to here.

These movements, or "jerks," of course, chiefly affect the neuropathic and hysterical or those predisposed to such conditions. Becoming more extensive the epidemic affects persons who are healthy, or at least who have enough mental and nervous stability to carry them through life, under ordinary circumstances, without abnormal manifestations of the nervous system.

Working upon religious feeling—the strongest in the human mind—is it to be wondered at that enthusiasts and religious monomaniacs have with their pseudo-religious fervor wrought such woful harm in the past ? Who can estimate ultimate results in the way of hereditary transmission of nervous instability ?

Laws governing the practice of hypnotism are now in force in Belgium, France, and Russia, and the writer hopes that efficient laws will soon be enacted in this country. An attempt on the part of Dr. Wellington Adams and myself to abolish the Woodworth meetings in St. Louis was futile, as there is no law by which that end could be attained. The cry may be raised by the unsophisticated and the ignorant that to forbid the Woodworth meetings would be a menace to religious liberty. To those we can answer that the law would not or should not permit the habitual use in religious exercises of agents, such as ether, chloroform, or opium, which will cause a person to lose consciousness. Neither should the use of a more subtle agent, such as hypnotism, be permitted. All these are universally recognized by physicians as exceedingly harmful in their effects when used habitually and indiscriminately, and by ignorant and unauthorized persons.

It should always be remembered that it is a serious matter to cause any person to lose his very *Ego*—through whatever agency.

The enlightenment of our age, and the scientific basis upon which hypnotism is beginning to rest, lead us to hope and believe that hypnotism as a factor in the hands of religious fanatics can never in the future do as much harm as it has done in the past.

Resignation.—Dr. George Strawbridge has resigned from the Chair of Otology in the University of Pennsylvania.

---

[1] Pepper's System, vol. v. p. 340.
[2] Decline and Fall of the Roman Empire, vol. vii. p. 64.

[1] On Certain Conditions of Nervous Derangement. New York, 1881.
[2] Pepper's System, vol. v. p. 348.

SUPPURATION OF THE TYMPANIC ATTIC AND PERFORATION IN SHRAPNELL'S MEMBRANE.

BY B. ALEX. RANDALL, A.M., M.D.,

PROFESSOR OF DISEASES OF THE EAR IN THE PHILADELPHIA POLYCLINIC; OPHTHALMIC AND AURAL SURGEON TO THE EPISCOPAL AND CHILDREN'S HOSPITALS, PHILADELPHIA.

THE human drum-membrane is inserted into a grooved bony ring—the annulus or tympanic bone of the infant—which is incomplete above, where the auditory plate of the squamosa fills the gap between its anterior and posterior extremities or spines. This notch varies considerably in size and shape, giving considerable diversity to the appearance of the entire drum-head, but especially to the thin membrane which occupies it. This upper segment was first well studied by Shrapnell,[1] who described its "flaccid" character, and clearly differentiated it from the "membrana tensa" below, and it is now quite generally known by his name.

Rivinus had described, in 1689, an opening in this region (previously noted by Marchetti and others), and not a little controversy has raged as to the presence of a "foramen" at this point, Bochdalek and others claiming that it is a constant feature, although sometimes hard to discern; while some have almost denied its existence and insisted that it is rare and accidental. Hence the association of the name of Rivinus with this region, and the edge of the squamosa is often known as the "Rivinian margin" and an opening here as a "foramen Rivini." The embryological views of Huschke explained this opening as a colobomatous gap left by the incomplete formation of the drum-membrane across the bottom of the auditory canal; but modern studies have shown that no such formation takes place, since a complete septum between the external canal and the tympano-tubal fissure is present at all stages. While it is conceivable, therefore, that the foramen may in rare instances be congenital, since its bilateral presence has been associated with cleft palate and similar defects of growth, it is usually inexplicable on any such ground.

Within and above the flaccid membrane lies that portion of the tympanic cavity which lodges the larger upper portions of the malleus and incus. Leidy has brought into clear view the separate and variable character of this "recessus epitympanicus," and has most conveniently named it the "attic" in distinction from the other parts of the tympanum, the lower "atrium," and the posterior "antrum;" and Blake and others have shown the great variations in the bands within it, forming septa about the ossicles, as Politzer and Prussak had demonstrated the bands constituting the "pouches" in front of the neck of the malleus.

[1] London Medical Gazette, x. p. 120, 1832.

Crystallizing about this convenient name, "attic," much study has of late been given to the diseased conditions met in this locality; and the advocacy of the excision of the drumhead and ossicles in suppurative affections of the attic, has called for full investigation of the matter in all its aspects.

Moos seems to have been the first of modern otologists to describe (in 1864) suppurative perforation in Shrapnell's membrane, and a number of cases were figured by Hinton in his atlas (1874); but the studies of J. Orne Green (1874), Blake, Buck, Burnett, and Miller, in America, and of Politzer, Morpurgo, and Hessler, abroad, placed the subject in full view and left little for later students to add. Yet there are several points on which investigators are not in accord, and further study seems urgently called for; and as I have been directing attention to several of these of late, I beg leave to offer here the results thus far obtained.

The successful treatment of these cases is of course the special end of their study, and the questions of the origin, frequency, and seriousness of the lesions are of fundamental importance. If suppuration of the tympanic attic were rare, unimportant, or easily treated, much of the attention which has been given to it would seem misplaced; but there is evidence to show that it is by no means rare in aural practice, and I have elsewhere[1] given reasons for believing that aural affections constitute two per cent. or more of medical work. If not an element of much size in the practice of the physician, it makes up for it by its serious importance. It is not without cause that suppurations of the ear are bars to life insurance; and more often in these than in any others do we have caries just where the meninges are nearest.

The upper pole of the drum-membrane is often difficult to study owing to the narrowness of the canal or the configuration of its walls; and in any case the view is easily obstructed by flakes of epidermis, cerumen or inspissated discharge. Careful cleansing is often essential to the investigation of the Shrapnell membrane, and delicate and skilful manipulation of the probe and forceps is called for in order to clear the way. A considerable number of cases will then be found to present a depression of the membrana flaccida, with a clearly visible opening at its centre or a less certainly discernible foramen at the extreme upper margin. This is the so-called "foramen of Rivinus," and is met in about one out of five to ten cases. Its lack of physiological explanation has been already noted; while its persistence as a pathological perforation is readily comprehensible. Its symmetry and the lack of suppurative history may in some cases be cited in support

[1] Address in Otology, Transactions of the Pennsylvania State Medical Society. 1888.

of its congenital character; but any one who has seen much of ear-disease knows that the most interesting findings are often in the ear which the patient insists is not, and never has been, affected in any way, and will be a little sceptical as to the negative history. Most children have cried during an entire night with ear-ache, and timely study frequently shows in such a case a bulging or a perforation of the flaccid membrane. Cure is gained without sensible discharge, for only a single drop may have needed to be exuded in order to give immediate relief; so an otorrhœa is of course denied, as it sometimes is even when profuse. It seems a point worthy of note that I have rarely met these dry foramina in very young children; and I believe investigation would show them to be several times as frequent in adult life.

A further and more important point is clearly brought out by a routine study of the flaccid membrane. There is often a brownish scale covering the region and removable only with difficulty; and study will at once show that it is not cerumen, as may have been expected (the ceruminous glands do not extend thus far in), but a leathery crust similar to those formed in the nose. The exposed surface of the upper pole will be found red, perforated, and with a trace of moisture in the opening, barely enough to be wiped away, yet sufficient to renew the crust in a few hours. Opinions may differ as to whether these are to be regarded as cases of suppuration of the attic, since the scanty flow is of mucus rather than pus and some secretion is of course merely physiological; yet any extended observation will dash the hopes of anyone who expects these cases to remain quiet and innocuous. Sooner or later, upon slight occasion or without any really appreciable reason, an exacerbation will almost always take place that is unmistakably a suppuration of the attic. It is further noteworthy that the probe will detect bare surfaces of bone even in some of the dormant cases, the rough areas being usually either on the neck of the malleus or on the Rivinian margin. In not a few instances the loss of substance is not confined to the membrane, and a considerable opening will be found, due to loss of the bony margin, which exposes the head of the malleus if this be present, and opens the attic to view. Polyps, granulations or pearly masses of epithelium may fill the opening, and pus of a sickening odor be present in an ear that gave to the casual examination no evidence of disease.

So much for the external appearances in these cases. Within the tympanum important conditions are often present. If by any means the drum-cavity is inflated, there may be evident action upon the membrana tensa, and yet no perforation-whistle or other sign of exit of air through the opening at the upper pole. The intra-tympanic syringe may be vigorously used without carrying a drop of fluid to the pharynx through the Eustachian tube, although this may promptly result from injection into a lower opening in the same case. Morpurgo found that the air passed freely out through the normal flaccid membrane when incised; but could not be passed again until the engorgement due to the little operation had passed away. The reason for these things, as also for the limitation of disease to this small portion of the tympanum, has been well given by Blake and others who have minutely investigated the anatomical relations of these parts. Besides the ligaments of the ossicles, so well described by Helmholtz, numerous variable folds of mucous membrane are present, especially in this part of the cavity, which form septa dividing the area into more or less isolated compartments. From these the drainage is limited, yet usually sufficient; but it needs only a slight congestive thickening of these septa to close the avenues of escape for any retained secretion. Such a pouch was long since well described by Prussak as fairly constant between the flaccid membrane and the malleus neck. Politzer showed a series of such cavities in some of his preparations, while Kretschmann has shown that the form varies greatly, yet regards as most usual a pouch larger than that described by Prussak, and bounded within by the incus and its articulation with the malleus, as well as by the neck of that ossicle.

These isolated portions of the tympanum share in any inflammatory process, however caused, but they not infrequently fail to share in the resolution which may promptly take place below. The congestive occlusion of the Eustachian tube may be but transient, and the atrium recover its normal drainage before retained secretion has forced its way through the drum-membrane; but the attic, or a portion of it, be left congested and distended. Resorption or caseation of the secretion may follow; but resolution is apt to be imperfect, and a focus of future trouble formed.

The peculiar character of tympanic inflammations must not be lost sight of. The drum-cavity is lined with a delicate mucous membrane, readily involved by continuity in the catarrhal affections of the pharynx and nares, yet its inflammation is not a simple catarrh. It constitutes the periosteum of the ossicles and bony walls, and all except the superficial inflammations have some of the nature of a periostitis. Hence the ease with which caries can result from affections primarily catarrhal, for ulceration of the mucous membrane means denuding of the subjacent area of bone. The presence of a cheesy mass of retained secretion in contact with the neck of the malleus can hardly fail to be detrimental to the bone, and it is not surprising that lesions at this point are not rare.

Another fact in the anatomy explains the peculiar vulnerability of the Rivinian margin. The external part of the attic overhangs the auditory canal and is separated from it by only a thin wedge of bone dependent for its nutrition upon the mucous lining within and the delicate cutaneous covering without. These are the direct continuations of the flaccid membrane, are generally involved in its inflammations, and are all too ready to leave unnourished this thin *scute* to undergo caries or necrosis. Further, the suppurative process within the attic can gain partial exit at this point and burrow out sub-periosteally along the auditory canal, to form abscesses behind, before, or above the ear, sometimes involving most of the side of the head. The mastoid may be wholly uninvolved in these cases, although the abscess be on its outer surface; and a delicate probe may show that the fistulous track leads directly to the Rivinian region.

Inflammation of the tympanic attic probably occurs in almost all cases of otitis media, and in the larger number of cases shares the fortune of the general condition. Yet in a considerable group, conditioned doubtless by the anatomical variations above noted, the affection runs an independent course in the upper cavity. Shut off by the swelling of its lining from its usual communication, its pent-up secretion finds an exit through the thin, flaccid membrane, sometimes bagging it down into a long, polyp-like sac before rupturing it. Whether perforation of the membrana tensa, or even its total destruction, has previously taken place, matters little; the obstacle to drainage is above it, and even the total removal of the drum-membrane and malleus may not afford the requisite freedom of outlet. Drainage is usually bad, so that the ossicles and bony walls are extremely likely to suffer in the chronic cases. Treatment is difficult because access is imperfect; and the location of the process immediately below the meninges does not add to the comfort of the surgeon having such a patient in charge. Serious results are not uncommon; and without that, the exasperating obstinacy of many of these cases and their tendency to recurrence give them a most unwelcome reputation among aurists.

Part of this notoriety is hardly deserved. The bad cases are very bad; but there are many of less intense perversity and malign character, which are often earlier stages of the same condition, but much more amenable to treatment if promptly recognized and combated. Here lies almost all of what the writer can add to the previous contributions upon the subject. These attic inflammations with perforation in the Shrapnell membrane are not rare. Walb noted twenty cases among the 1231 patients of one year at the Bonn clinic; and Bezold, in Munich, eighty-eight among the 8227 patients seen in six years. In like manner at least fifty cases have been met by the writer among somewhat less than 2000 new patients treated during the past twenty months, although this record is probably incomplete. Numerous instances of dry perforations in this location, and of suppurations, suspected but not definitely proved to belong to this category, could be cited; but it is safer to accept the minimum figures, as they are sufficient to prove the frequency of the lesion. In point of fact, fifteen cases were met among the 500 seen in the first half of 1889, twenty-three among some 600 in the similar period of 1890, and seven among 100 patients in August, 1890, the periods during which strict records were kept. Only five were *noted as such* in my records for the latter half of 1889, although it is almost certain that more were seen; so I was prepared to admit that the earlier half of the year might show more cases, at least of the recent lesion. But this August experience would hardly bear out such a view.

The detailed histories of the cases seen in the first half of 1889, with five, previously noted and sketched, were presented at the meeting of the American Otological Society of that year; and the additional cases met up to July, 1890, were brought forward in the same place this year. Repetition of them here is quite needless. It may be well, however, to cite some recent details of a recent instance of the affection, in order to make clear some of their varying clinical features.

The certain recognition of the condition in question was made in this latest case only as these lines were being written.

Mr. H. P. was sent to me by Dr. Charles K. Mills, on August 26th, suffering with pain that for several nights had prevented sleep, accompanied by slight discharge from the left ear. Suppuration had been occasionally noted for several years, but the absence of any severe symptoms had led to neglect, since the hearing was little impaired except when the canal was clogged with discharge. A large polypoid mass was found growing from the upper wall of the canal about half way out and preventing any view of the fundus. Its removal was painful and had to be divided between several sittings, as the patient's endurance had been much reduced by his sleeplessness and sufferings; and the sinus around which, as usual, the mass had grown has not yet been followed to the uncovered bone which without doubt lies beyond it. The hearing was almost normal when the canal was cleansed, but the character of the lesion was suspicious, and the imperfect glimpses obtained of the Rivinian region increased the suspicion.

On September 5th the obstruction was so far removed that study became possible, and a considerable opening above the short process of the malleus was distinctly seen and the probe discovered carious bone within the attic. Intra-tympanic syringing with peroxide of hydrogen gave pain enough to

SUPPURATION OF THE TYMPANIC ATTIC.

limit its employment somewhat, yet brought away much pus and cheesy secretion from the opening. The lower membrana tensa is thickened, somewhat opaque and macerated by the pus which has bathed it, but the hearing remains nearly normal, a fact which, however curious, is by no means unusual, although some authorities state the contrary. The patient has been quite comfortable since the first treatment, except for several hours after a deep cauterization with chromic acid, and has been able to attend to his work. He is satisfied with his condition, as well as with his progress, and is likely to demur decidedly if the caries of the malleus proves so considerable as to call for the excision which is becoming rather fashionable.

It seems here in place to comment upon the operation of excision of the malleus and drum-membrane, in cases such as these, of which Dr. Sexton is the most ardent American advocate. It rests upon the rational idea of removing carious bone and endeavoring to establish free drainage from the attic. The operation, though delicate, is not very difficult; but may be tedious from obstruction by bleeding. The tendon of the tensor tympani is first cut by a needle curved on the flat introduced close behind the short process and pressed upward until the slight snap of the tenotomy is felt and the malleus handle is found to move more freely outward. The drum-membrane is then divided around the periphery with a suitable knife, and the malleus extracted by means of a snare loop around the handle. This last may prove difficult, as the placing of the loop is apt to be obscured by the bleeding, and the traction must be made inward as well as downward, lest the ossicle be broken through the neck. Probably the incus should be extracted before the malleus, as it is wholly useless in the absence of the first ossicle, and may, like it, be carious. Its disarticulation from the stapes must be delicately done, since dislocation of this last ossicle seriously imperils the hearing. As renewal in some fashion of the drum-membrane generally takes place, it is wise to carry the excision to the extreme periphery up and back, in the endeavor to prevent closure here by removing a part of the tendinous annulus. A portion of the chorda tympani is usually resected in such a case; but healing quickly follows, and the loss of taste on that side of the tongue is often unnoted by the patient during its brief duration. Little reaction is to be expected if proper cleanliness is observed— as an antiseptic the peroxide of hydrogen may be used in conjunction with styptic injections of hot water.

Such is the operation long in use by Schwartze and others, and of late most enthusiastically advocated, by Sexton especially. Its minor details are varied to meet individual preferences. It would seem to have given, in many instances, practical fulfilment

of its theoretical value, but has yet to gain any wide acceptance among aurists. In the three cases of suppuration in which I have practised it the value was almost nothing, since the caries involved the Rivinian segment as well as the ossicles. Drainage seemed not appreciably improved, and in one case a new sinus formed above, while the suppuration continued freely from the lower opening.

In the less severe cases the process may often be brought to a halt by less radical measures; and while this cessation had best be esteemed as merely a hollow truce, it has been found to persist for two years or more in some cases, which is as much as can often be claimed for the operation at its best. The danger of these conditions naturally seems small to a patient who has had a suppuration for years that gives him little inconvenience; and, as before stated, the hearing may be practically normal and more likely to lose than gain by the operation. Consent to surgical interference may be wholly refused, and is apt to be accorded only in the worst cases. In these the results are not likely to prove brilliant; and while I expect to offer the interference to some of my patients, and even to urge it upon a few, it will be with no expectation of striking results or rapid cures. The cases in which these are at all possible, are those in which caries is limited to the ossicles and can be eradicated with them; and unless the diagnosis of such limitation can be made with much more certainty than is usually possible, the prognosis had better be a guarded one. Where the hearing is much affected and the presence of caries of the ossicles has been established, the chances of improved hearing and greater accessibility to the diseased structures speak in favor of the operation, since it is attended with little danger.

For the majority of cases the most thorough possible cleansing constitutes the best treatment. This will require painstaking care and some little skill, as the opening is apt to be too small to admit fluid except when the syringe-tip is carried directly into it. Enlargement of the perforation should be made when much difficulty of this kind is met, any granulations should be snipped off with the snare or forceps, and rough, bare surfaces of bone should be rubbed with the cotton-tipped probe in order to detach spicules and excite reparative inflammation. A long-nozzled syringe must be used in order to secure the needed penetration of the fluid—that of Blake serving admirably, although I use by preference a large lachrymal syringe with the hollow probe known as de Wecker's canula. The canula commended by Schwartze and Hartmann is generally too clumsily made and the curve at its extremity is oftener a danger than an aid. The delicate glass canula of Buck can be made by anyone at all skilled in working glass, and used with the fountain-syringe or a bulb-syringe worked by the patient, will do excellent service. It need hardly be reiterated that full illumination by the forehead mirror is essential to these manœuvres, which require a full view of the affected region, and generally the use of both hands.

In this connection it may be remarked that the construction of most forehead mirrors is very faulty in giving too limited a range of movement, and that one with a *double* ball-and-socket joint is far superior to that with the single, and enables the surgeon to get good illumination under the most difficult circumstances. The mirror may be brought very close to the eye, and looking through a large sight-hole, the advantages of central illumination may be combined with entire freedom from interference with binocular vision. The left hand may be used to make traction upon the auricle, draw forward the tragus and at the same time furnish a rest for the syringe—a very important item in the use of a piston-syringe.

The peroxide of hydrogen is probably the best fluid for intra-tympanic use, the twelve-volume solution being diluted with three to six volumes of hot water. Dizziness is but little more common under these measures than in the simple syringing of the canal, and can generally be avoided by gentleness and a proper temperature. The great value of the peroxide lies in its power to oxidize rapidly any purulent matter with which it comes in contact, and the resulting evolution of gas distends the cavity, forces the fluid into its remotest recesses and also aids in its evacuation. As this frothing, if active, may be disagreeable to the patient, the dilution is advisable, which also secures the desired warmth of the fluid. The delicate cotton-carrier will do good service in clearing the way before and after the syringing, and delicate forceps often are useful in removing detached flakes of epithelium, etc. The air-douche has but limited value in these cases, as before noted; yet it should generally be employed as a possible aid to the cleansing—due attention being paid, of course, to the naso-pharyngeal condition.

Numerous fluids have been employed topically in these attic suppurations with doubtful benefit. The nitrate of silver has undoubted value, but its employment is not free from risk except in weak solution, as is also the case with the mineral acids, which are credited with power to hasten the removal of dead bone. Boric acid in powder may be dusted into the opening or injected as a saturated solution, serving probably as well as any of the antiseptics accredited with more potency to keep the cavity sweet in the intervals of the cleansing.

Good results may be expected from this treatment in all the recent cases, and even among the chronic and carious affections gratifying improvement is common. Apparent cures may be quickly gained, yet relapses must be looked for in most of them, and the prognosis in the intractable cases is grave. In one of the patients reported in 1889 the attic affection remained in abeyance for some ten months, and started up only after a cold-taking which caused acute inflammation of both tympana. The caries of the malleus-neck and the growth of granulations from the Rivinian margin recommenced, and were slow in yielding to treatment, as they had also been slow to renewed activity.

The point to be especially insisted on in these, as in most aural suppurations, is the necessity of most painstaking cleansing at all times, in order that first the exact condition of matters may be recognized as promptly and clearly as possible, and second that the treatment may be applied, not to the exfoliated products of the inflammation, but to the affected tissues themselves. Thus only can we learn what we are dealing with, make sure that we are actually utilizing the measures undertaken for its relief and fairly compare the effects of various applications. It can be confidently predicted that the instances of attic suppuration with perforation in the flaccid membrane will be not infrequently met, under these circumstances, and that the shortcomings of the conservative treatment, properly applied, will not be found as great as the advocates of excision are inclined to claim. The serious, intractable cases will be found rather in the minority, since they will be attacked in the earlier stages; and the operative interference, confined to the instances which really require it, will be able to show its actual value in the cases not amenable to less radical measures.

Study of my fifty cases shows that all ages, from three to sixty-nine years, were represented, and that ten of the patients were less than ten years of age, while twenty-one were in the second decade. The perforation was in Shrapnell's membrane alone (as in Fig. 1) in twenty-three instances, being supplemented by a second opening or a cicatrix (Fig. 2) in the lower portion of the drumhead in a little more than one-half the cases. Polyps of notable size were present in almost a half, and caries was discovered in nearly as many. Destruction of the Rivinian margin (as in Figs. 6 and 8) had occurred in five cases, and loss of the malleus, and probably of the incus, in the same number. In one, the latter ossicle alone seemed to have been lost, and through the thin cicatrix which promptly formed in the posterior opening, the stapes and stapedius tendon could be plainly seen (Fig. 7). The perforation was usually in the central part of the flaccid membrane, above and before the short process, as in Figs. 2, 4, 5 and 7, less often involving the posterior part, as in Fig. 3 and to a less extent in Fig. 1.

FIG. 1.   FIG. 2.   FIG. 3.   FIG. 4.

FIG. 5.   FIG. 6.   FIG. 7.   FIG. 8.

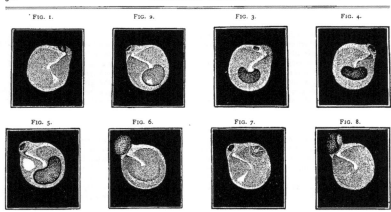

The results of treatment cannot be fully and accurately stated. In fifteen of the patients the suppuration was brought sooner or later to a stop; and this apparent cure is known to persist after periods varying from two to twenty months, sometimes in spite of conditions which have set up suppuration of the other ear. For these it is fair to claim cure, with little reserve. In seven cases, on the contrary, the condition is known to be as bad as when first seen—in two of them, in spite of excision of the drum-membrane and ossicles. For the remainder, including the recent cases which are still under care, moderate success can be claimed. Many of them passed out of view apparently cured, but the maintenance of this condition cannot be asserted. Others were more or less improved, but uncured, when they ceased attendance. It can at least be urged, then, in favor of the less radical treatment that it rarely fails to bring about marked and often permanent improvement; and although recurrence of the trouble is common and always to be anticipated, that it may be rare and slight and with long intervals of immunity and apparent health.

MALIGNANT ŒDEMA.

(Gangrenous Emphysema; French, "Gangrene Gazeuse.")

BY K. HOEGH, M.D.,
OF MINNEAPOLIS, MINN.

A GIRL, eleven years old, was brought to me late on the night of June 28, 1890, with the history that, on June 25th, she had stepped barefooted on a nail in a barn, the floor of which was covered by manure and stable-soil. The nail caused a punctured wound of the right foot, about two inches behind the head of the second metatarsal bone. She complained of severe pain; there was very little bleeding, but the pain steadily increased, so that her sleep was disturbed. On the next morning the foot was considerably swollen, and there was marked redness of the dorsum and toes. During the second night her sleep was much more disturbed, and the pain increased to such an extent that she was in misery the whole day. The night of the 27th there was no sleep, and at three o'clock in the morning, about sixty-five hours after the injury, her mother noticed that the toes were "white as lard," cold, and insensible. Later in the day they were black. After a railroad journey of nearly one hundred and fifty miles, the child was brought to me, about eighty hours after the receipt of the injury. The foot was then black and gangrenous up to the tarsal bones. There was no suppuration, but small gas-bubbles were present; there was considerable œdema and a purplish discoloration up to the ankle, and above that streaks, as of lymphangitis, along the inner side of the leg, and some mottled redness in spots over the lower part of the leg. The original wound could not be seen. Her pulse was 120; temperature 101°. There was great pain; her mind was not quite clear, and she was in a condition suggesting collapse. As it was late, and I was not quite sure of the nature of the case and of the proper treatment, she was put to bed in St. Barnabas Hospital, with no other local treatment than elevation of the leg and permanent irrigation with an antiseptic fluid; whiskey was given, and also a hypodermic of morphine.

She passed a miserable night, and on the morning of the 29th her temperature was 103°; pulse very rapid. The gangrene had extended as high as the malleoli, and the œdema had reached to about two inches below the knee. In the presence of Drs. H. E. Holmes and E. Wood, house-surgeons to the hospital, and with their kind assistance I amputated the leg at the lower third of the femur, about four days and four hours after the receipt of the injury. Careful antisepsis was observed, and the wound was drained with iodoform-tampons.

The amputated limb was carefully examined; the foot was black, as that of a cadaver that had been for a long time in water, and the epidermis came off like a glove. The corium was moist. Upon incising the foot no pus was found, but gas escaped. There was crackling, as of lung-tissue, when the soft parts were cut into. The track of the punctured wound was found; it was filled with a black coagulum. The œdema above the gangrene was very firm. Large quantities of greenish serum escaped after cutting into the leg. Here and there, over the gangrenous parts and the neighborhood, were large bullæ filled with a limpid fluid.

Two rabbits were inoculated with the serum and the contents of the bullæ, but, as their subsequent history proved, with no effect upon their health.

The night after the operation there was still some pain, but the patient was perfectly conscious. Her lips, as well as the skin generally, had a peculiar dusky appearance, which the mother declared was not the patient's natural color. She improved during the day; toward evening her temperature was 100°, pulse 90, pain less. From the next day recovery was uninterrupted. In about three weeks the patient went home well, and with a healed stump.

This case was diagnosed as one of malignant œdema or gangrenous emphysema (*gangrène gazeuse*), a disease of not very common occurrence. The characteristic signs and symptoms of this disease are a rapidly spreading gangrene, with the development of gases in the soft tissues, with no putrid smell, at least in the beginning, before contamination with putrefactive germs, and no formation of pus, but with marked constitutional intoxication manifested by fever and great depression of the nervous system. The local process goes on with rapidity and the constitutional symptoms increase *pari passu.* A case formerly observed by me terminated fatally on the sixth day. In the case described above the constitutional symptoms promptly disappeared after removing the infected limb.

The disease depends upon the presence of a specific bacillus, the bacillus of malignant œdema, which is described in Baumgarten's *Lehrbuch der pathologischen Mykologie,* 1890, from which the following notes are largely extracted.

In 1877 Pasteur described the bacillus under the name of *vibrione septique,* but the first complete and accurate description was given by Koch in 1881. The bacillus is, morphologically, very similar to the anthrax bacillus, with which it seems that Pasteur confounded it, but it has very distinct characteristics. It is more slender, the ends are rounded, and the bacilli are joined together in a somewhat different manner. It is further distinguished from the anthrax bacillus by having a spontaneous motility, a quality not belonging to the anthrax bacillus, as is well known. There are also differences in the spore-formation and in the behavior of these two bacilli in culture-media. The bacillus of malignant œdema is strictly anaërobic, and cannot live in the presence of oxygen. Biologically and pathologically, it is nearly allied to the tetanus bacillus, and like the latter its natural habitat is in the soil, especially in rich soil. It is very widely distributed, but it is questionable if it is found in uncultivated soil. It is found in the upper strata, but not on the surface, because it does not thrive in the presence of light and air.

Garden-soil seems to be particularly rich in these bacilli, just as it is in tetanus bacilli. Accidentally, they are taken into the animal organism, but do not produce spores during the life of the animal. After the death of the animal they multiply in the body. Like the tetanus bacillus the œdema bacillus not uncommonly invades horses, usually with fatal effects. Pure cultures of this bacillus, when inoculated in animals, produce an extensive œdema, but do not produce gaseous gangrene. Inoculation with garden-soil, however, produces gaseous gangrene, probably owing to the simultaneous inoculation of the "pseudo œdema-bacillus." Nearly all domestic animals, mice, guinea-pigs, and rabbits are susceptible to these inoculations; only the cow seems to be exempt. To produce the disease the inoculations must be subcutaneous, as surface-wounds cannot be infected, and the quantity used must not be small. Injections into the bloodvessels give negative results.

After inoculation the œdema is apt to spread to the deeper parts, and unlike the anthrax œdema, is sanguinolent, not gelatinous. Inoculated animals occasionally survive, and the inoculation produces a decidedly less malignant infection than that caused by the anthrax bacillus. If an animal is killed and examined immediately, the bacilli are found only in the œdema of the superficial parts, never in the blood; thus resembling also in this the tetanus bacillus, and differing from the anthrax bacillus. A further similarity to the tetanus bacillus is the fact that one attack of the disease does not produce immunity against new infection.

If animals are inoculated with garden-soil malignant œdema and tetanus are common results, but the longer the earth has been dried the less is the probability that it will cause malignant œdema. The tetanus bacillus, however, or its spores, will retain their virulence in dry earth for almost an unlimited period.[1]

The so-called "pseudo œdema-bacillus" is commonly found accompanying the œdema bacillus, both in soil and in infected animals. These bacilli are, morphologically and biologically, easily distin-

----

[1] Faber on Tetanus. Copenhagen. 1890.

guished from each other ; the pseudo œdema-bacillus is anaërobic, and produces a gas, owing to its strong fermentative qualities. It seems probable that, biologically, these two bacilli may be to some extent dependent upon each other ; for instance, by creating products of mutual benefit. Their strongly anaërobic qualities seem to make such an assumption possible.

Experiments in regard to the resistance of these bacilli and their spores, to our usual chemical antiseptics may have been made, but, if so, their results are not generally known. The experiments of Faber[1] prove that the tetanus bacillus is not destroyed by five-per-cent. carbolic acid solution nor by a 1-to-1000 sublimate solution, but only by heat.

Thus we have an explanation of the fact that punctured wounds have always been considered dangerous ; we know now why such wounds, if they are infected by earth or by dust from the soil may be followed by tetanus and malignant œdema. Sufficient disinfection is not only difficult, owing to the narrowness and depth of the wound, but also to the fact that at least one of the bacilli which lurk in the soil is unusually resistant to chemical antiseptics. Hence, it becomes our duty to treat each punctured wound, which may be thus contaminated, in the most radical manner. After producing artificial anæmia by means of Esmarch's apparatus, the wound should be laid freely open, when it can then be seen and examined to the bottom. After removing foreign bodies, thorough cauterization with a galvano-cautery or hot iron is recommended, then ordinary antiseptic dressings. If tetanus develops experience has proved the inutility of amputation ; but in a case of malignant œdema we should not hesitate to sacrifice a limb, as amputation may save the life of the patient.

MEDICAL PROGRESS.

The Treatment of Phthisis with Boric Acid.—For five years DR. GAUCHER has been studying the action of boric acid on pulmonary tuberculosis. He at first determined by means of experiments on animals the toxic limits of the drug, which he found to be in the ratio of about fifteen grains to each two and one-half pounds of the bodyweight. He also found that it was eliminated rapidly by the kidneys, and that there is little danger of its accumulating. It is also eliminated by the lungs, and can be found in considerable amounts in the sputum of patients who are taking the drug.

Some of his experiments are interesting, and should encourage a careful trial of boric acid in the treatment of phthisis. For example, he injected with a hypodermic needle a few drops of a pure culture of tubercle bacilli into the lungs of several rabbits. In this way he set up a local tuberculosis, which soon became caseous, but

not generalized. Some of the animals died from pulmonary tuberculosis, others were killed, and in all pulmonary phthisis was found at the autopsy. He then repeated the inoculations on healthy rabbits, but fed them on bran mixed with boric acid. After a time these animals also were killed, but in all the lungs, as well as the other organs, were quite free from tuberculosis.

As to clinical results, treatment with boric acid caused a notable diminution in the expectoration, which became more fluid and less purulent. Considerable time is, of course, necessary before the final results can be determined, but in the cases under observation it may be said that they improved in every way, while the tubercular disease in the lungs seemed to be at a standstill. The amount administered in these cases was fifteen grains, in divided doses, in twenty-four hours. As a rule, it will be found not to disorder the stomach, and in some of Dr. Gaucher's cases it seemed to check diarrhœa. As it has no disagreeable taste it is easily taken.—*Lancet*, August 16, 1890.

Antiseptic Treatment of Scarlatina.—According to the Paris correspondent of the *Archives of Pædiatrics*, PROFESSOR HUTINEL has endeavored to determine the cause of the various complications of scarlet fever. His studies lead him to believe that these complications are due to secondary infection, and that the causative germs enter through the pharynx. If these hypotheses are true, the first indication in treatment is disinfection of the pharynx, and on this principle Dr. Hutinel has treated a number of cases with good results. As children cannot gargle, he uses irrigation by means of a large enema-syringe, through which a three-per-cent. boric acid solution is injected into the pharynx several times daily. He is careful to use a separate canula for each patient.

In addition to this, the throat is cleansed by mopping with a cotton tampon saturated with borated glycerin, and a few drops of borated vaseline-oil are dropped into the nostrils several times each day. The diet is confined to milk alone.

In 35 cases of scarlatina treated in this way there was 1 death. As to complications, 6 of the cases had albuminuria, 1 had rheumatism, 1 pleurisy, 1 otitis, and 1 diphtheria, but all the complications were promptly cured.

Creolin as an External Application in Inflammation.—STAFF SURGEON v. KOBYLECKI (*Wiener medizinische Presse,* August 17, 1890) writes enthusiastically of creolin as an external application in inflammation from various causes. In a case of fracture at the ankle, which, when it came under his observation some hours after the injury, was ecchymotic, and very much swollen, applications of creolin in water reduced the swelling in four days. Since then he has used creolin-water in all cases of inflammation of the joints resulting from contusion or sprain, saturating the dressings every two hours or oftener, and always with good results.

In orchitis and epididymitis the applications are also of great benefit, and diminish the duration of the disease. In these affections the patient should remain in bed with the scrotum elevated, and should paint the latter once daily with pure creolin until recovery ensues. No other

---

[1] Loc. cit.

treatment is necessary, and, unless the application is made too often, no irritation is produced.

Hypodermic Injection of Bichloride of Methylene in Typhoid Fever. Hypodermic Injection of Chloroform in Strychnine-poisoning. — In *L'Union Médicale*, August 19, 1890, MARTINEZ reports from Zapateca, in the Republic of Colombia, the following interesting cases. In the first, tetanic contractions came on during the course of typhoid fever, and were cured by the hypodermic injection of bichloride of methylene; and, in the second, poisoning by strychnine was relieved by the hypodermic injection of chloroform.

A man, aged twenty-two years, of a strong, robust constitution and sanguine temperament, was attacked with a low form of typhoid fever complicated by well-marked tetanic spasms associated with trismus, the contractures affecting the upper and lower limbs and the muscles of the body, and being accompanied with constipation and retention of urine. The attacks came on at frequent intervals and lasted about five minutes. Dr. Martinez had recourse at this time to hypodermic injections of bichloride of methylene, giving from twenty to thirty minims. After the first injection there was appreciable improvement. The use of the bath to control the temperature, and the application of affusions to the nape of the neck to diminish congestion and relieve pain in the head, were also followed by favorable symptoms. The patient was given, in addition, bromides and chloral to allay pain and nervousness. He took his nourishment well, and passed a comfortable night. Soon afterward he had a copious movement from the bowels, and passed urine freely. Rapid convalescence set in and the cure of the entire attack ultimately resulted, the chief cause of relief being, in the author's mind, the use of the hypodermic injections, without which the convulsions would have killed the patient.

In the second case, one of strychnine-poisoning, a man, about twenty-eight years of age, married, but separated from his wife, for various reasons became desperate and resolved to attempt suicide by the use of strychnine. A quarter of an hour afterward he confessed to having taken the poison, and was immediately put to bed. The convulsive movements became severe. The treatment consisted in the hypodermic injection of fifteen minims of chloroform, followed by washing out of the stomach. Recovery ultimately took place, and, although at one time bromide · of potassium and chloral were freely used, the reporter believes that the chloroform was the principal agent in producing a cure.

Chloroform Liniment.—

℞.—Chloroform . . . . 4 ounces.
Camphor . . . . . 1 ounce.
Fluid vaseline, sufficient to make 8 ounces.

· Dissolve the camphor in the chloroform and then add the fluid vaseline. Of course, the amount of vaseline may be varied according to the strength of the liniment desired. It is said that this makes a much more useful application than chloroform liniment made with olive oil.

Gunshot Wounds of the Stomach and Intestines.—SENN (*Journal of the American Medical Association*, Sep-

tember 6 and 13, 1890), in a valuable paper on gunshot wounds of the abdomen, draws a number of conclusions, of which the following are the most important :

1. In gunshot wounds of the abdomen, in the absence of fæcal extravasation or prolapse of the omentum, it is absolutely necessary to determine whether penetration has taken place, by enlarging the wound.

2. Absence of visceral lesions requiring abdominal section is most frequently met with in perforating gunshot wounds of the abdomen if the wound of entrance is at or above the level of the umbilicus, and if its course is antero-posterior.

3. In transverse and oblique gunshot wounds at a point below the level of the umbilicus, multiple perforations of the intestines are extremely probable.

4. The general and local symptoms, with the exception of external fæcal extravasation, are absolutely of no value in the differential diagnosis between simple penetrating gunshot wounds of the abdomen and those complicated by visceral lesions.

5. Dangerous internal hæmorrhage caused by perforating wounds can be recognized by the symptoms of acute anæmia and by the physical signs of fluid in the peritoneal cavity, and such symptoms and signs are positive indications for abdominal section.

6. After opening the peritoneal cavity for the treatment of hæmorrhage, temporary hæmostasis should be secured by digital compression of the aorta, or by packing with sponges, until the bleeding points can be found.

7. Wounds of the stomach and intestines large enough to permit the escape of the contents of these organs can be infallibly demonstrated by the hydrogen test before the abdomen is opened.

8. Direct distention of the stomach through an elastic tube is preferable to rectal insufflation, when it is probable that the stomach is wounded.

9. Thorough insufflation, without evidences of free tympanites or escape of gas through the external wound, proves either the absence of perforations, or that, if present, they are too small for leakage to take place, and is a strong argument in favor of non-interference.

10. The hydrogen test should invariably be used in searching for perforations after the abdomen is opened, as this test makes extensive eventration unnecessary, and never fails to reveal every perforation.

11. After the lowest perforation has been discovered by rectal insufflation, the succeeding tests should be made through the perforations, and the external wound should never be closed until the entire gastro-intestinal canal has been tested.

12. The hydrogen test ordinarily does not cause fæcal extravasation.

13. By following the indications furnished by the test the surgeon relieves himself of all medico-legal responsibility in the operative treatment of gunshot wounds of the abdomen.

14. The closure of bullet wounds of the stomach and intestine is accomplished most speedily, and with a sufficient degree of safety, by one row of interrupted sero-muscular sutures of fine aseptic silk. The operation should be undertaken as early as possible.

15. If enterectomy is unavoidable, the continuity of the intestinal canal should be restored by making lateral

anastomosis between the closed ends by means of decalcified, perforated, moist bone-plates.

16. Flushing of the abdominal cavity is to be reserved for cases in which the peritoneum has been contaminated by the escape of the contents of the stomach or intestines.

17. Drainage is necessary if the peritoneum has become infected, and in wounds of the kidney, spleen, or pancreas not treated by partial or complete extirpation. Also in wounds of the liver.

18. The necessary diagnostic skill and manual dexterity in the operative treatment of gunshot wounds of the stomach and intestines can be acquired only by experiments upon the lower animals.

Intravenous Injections of Quinine in Malaria.—BACCELLI publishes (*Berliner klinische Wochenschrift,* June 2, 1890) an interesting communication on the intravenous injection of quinine in malaria. Believing that if the specific medicament was brought into direct contact with the blood-cells the destruction of the parasite would be accomplished more quickly and more permanently, he undertook a series of investigations to determine the following points :

1. The minimum dose which is required for complete and permanent cure.

2. The proper moment for the use of the medicament to prevent the paroxysm, to restrict it as much as possible, or to prevent a return.

3. The histological modifications brought about in the blood, already altered by the infection, through contact with the medicament.

In medical literature he found no example of injection of quinine into the vessels for therapeutic—that is to say, for antimalarial—purposes, although many physiologists had practised this expedient for purposes of investigation. The latter had, however, used acid solutions, and the author's investigations upon animals led him to believe that such solutions are extremely dangerous. Under these circumstances he employed a neutral solution of quinine hydrochlorate in distilled water with the addition of sodium chloride, to obviate the destructive action of the water upon the red blood-cells. The formula is as follows :

Quinine hydrochlorate   1.00 gramme (15 grains).
Sodium chloride   .   0.75   "   (11½ ").
Distilled water   .   . 10.00 grammes (2½ drachms).

This solution is perfectly clear if employed lukewarm.

Having ascertained from repeated experiments that doses of five and ten centigrammes were perfectly harmless to guinea-pigs, the author employed the same doses upon man. After the veins of the forearm had become turgid, as the result of compression with a circular bandage above the elbow, he injected the solution with a Pravaz needle, inserted from below upward into the interior of one of the smallest veins, and immediately removed the bandage. The most rigorous antisepsis was observed, the solution being filtered and again boiled. The injection was made slowly, in order to observe that no swelling of the subcutaneous tissue took place, and, therefore, to be sure that the needle was in

the interior of the vessel. The point of puncture was closed with collodion.

With the exception of one case, in which a number of abscesses developed, no injurious local effect resulted in any of the experiments. In two cases, in which the needle was not properly inserted into the interior of the vessel, and in which the solution was therefore partially injected into the subcutaneous tissue, there was œdema of the arm, but no other evil consequences. With doses of from ten to thirty centigrammes, no noteworthy physiological effects were observed. After the employment of from thirty centigrammes to one gramme, in three cases some of the characteristic symptoms of quinine intoxication immediately developed, namely, bitter taste, vertigo, loss of consciousness ; at first a small and infrequent, afterward a fuller and slower, pulse-beat; and coldness of the skin. In general this condition disappeared in from fifteen to twenty minutes. In but a single case was cardiac weakness prolonged for several hours, so that the employment of cardiac stimulants became necessary. The usual dose of the quinine solution was from forty to sixty centigrammes. The results were good in so far as that, in many cases, the fever was at once brought to an end; and, if this were not done, there was always produced a diminution of the temperature succeeding the injection, frequently as much as 2° C. With doses of one gramme, in none of his patients was there a genuine recurrence of the attack under eight days. The author believes that when there is no idiosyncrasy against quinine, as much as three grammes of the solution can be injected into the veins without danger.

The great value of the method is in pernicious fever, for in other cases of malarial fever the ordinary methods of administration of quinine are usually efficient. In pernicious fever, one gramme of the solution should be the tentative dose. Of this form, 5 cases were treated by Baccelli with good results. Of these, 3 were of the somnolent variety, 1 was associated with hemiplegia, and 1 with bulbar symptoms. In addition to the quinine injections, analeptic and cardiac remedies were administered, especially repeated injections of ether, in large doses—five to ten grammes in twenty-four hours. The effect of the specific treatment in these cases was shown rather by the disappearance of the dangerous symptoms than by reduction of temperature, for in such cases temperature is frequently moderate, or even remains normal (*larval malaria*). In general, the following results were noted : The injections did not prevent or modify the fever paroxysm, if made at the acme, at the beginning, or even as many as three hours previous to the access. If made at the end or during the decline of the paroxysm, the succeeding paroxysm was either entirely prevented or much reduced in intensity. In the sub-continued forms of fever, which are usually rebellious to medication, it was found useful to make the injection during the period of remission, the effect being to transform the type into that of an intermittent, usually with an accelerated crisis.

We would especially call the attention of practitioners in the Western and Southern States of the Union to this important research, which seems to furnish them with a better method of combating the pernicious forms of malarial infection than has yet been at command.

THE MEDICAL NEWS.

A WEEKLY JOURNAL
OF MEDICAL SCIENCE.

COMMUNICATIONS are invited from all parts of the world. Original articles contributed exclusively to THE MEDICAL NEWS will be liberally paid for upon publication. When necessary to elucidate the text, illustrations will be furnished without cost to the author.

Address the Editor:　H. A. HARE, M.D.,
1004 WALNUT STREET,
PHILADELPHIA.

Subscription Price, including Postage.

PER ANNUM, IN ADVANCE . . . . $4.00.
SINGLE COPIES . . . . 10 CENTS.

Subscriptions may begin at any date. The safest mode of remittance is by bank check or postal money order, drawn to the order of the undersigned. When neither is accessible, remittances may be made, at the risk of the publishers, by forwarding in *registered* letters.

Address,　　LEA BROTHERS & CO.,
NOS 706 & 708 SANSOM STREET,
PHILADELPHIA.

SATURDAY, SEPTEMBER 27, 1890.

EXOPHTHALMIC GOITRE.

WHEN the classical triad of symptoms—rapid heart, protruding eyeballs, and enlarged thyroid gland—is present, nothing is easier than the diagnosis of the affection to which English authors attach the name of Graves, and German writers that of Basedow. Quite different is it, however, if one or more of these signs should be absent or so slight as to escape notice unless searched for. The writer of this article remembers very well a case in his early practice which he mistook for phthisis on account of the repeated occurrence of hæmoptysis; and he has now under his care a case also attacked by pulmonary hæmorrhages, which had been variously diagnosed as phthisis, ·nervous dyspepsia, and hypertrophy of the heart. These two cases further agreed in the absence of exophthalmos, and in the fact that the thyroid enlargement was not perceptible upon casual observation, being hidden by the clothing of the patient, and very slight withal.

The early recognition of the affection, however, is a matter very often of prime importance; for it may be stated that, as a rule, the favorableness of the prognosis as to cure varies inversely with the duration of the disease. The difficulty of diagnosis is sometimes as great when the goitre presents itself as a prominent symptom, as when the goitre must be sought for; the most important of the three symp-toms being the disturbed condition of the heart. In any case of overacting heart, especially in a neurotic subject, and more especially when associated with other phenomena of vasomotor ataxia, Graves's disease should be taken into consideration in the diagnosis and should not be lightly excluded. Even in the absence of demonstrable goitre, a thrill felt within, or in the immediate neighborhood of, the suprasternal notch, associated with a soft systolic blowing murmur, though not pathognomonic, is significant. When this symptom· is found, careful observation will often bring to light the existence of a condition of intermittent ,enlargement of the thyroid gland, which would render the diagnosis certain.

SEELIGMUELLER (*Deutsche medicinische Wochenschrift*, May 29, 1890) has collated the most recent observations upon the symptomatology, pathogenesis, and therapy of the disease. According to this author, tremor, to which attention was first directed by Charcot in 1883, has assumed considerable importance as an initial symptom; thus Lewin observed it in thirteen out of twenty-seven cases as the first manifestation of the disease. One of his patients, a boy of nine years, after a severe fright suddenly exhibited muscular trembling and stuttering speech, while the full clinical picture of exophthalmic goitre did not present itself until the patient reached his seventeenth year. In the case of an hysterical girl, seventeen years old, who came under the writer's care at the medical clinic of the Jefferson Medical College Hospital, nystagmus had existed since childhood; goitre and cardiac disturbance suddenly developing after a fright consequent upon a fall from a step ladder. In this case exophthalmos developed under observation.

Diminution of electrical resistance of the skin, first observed by Vigouroux and confirmed by Charcot, Eulenberg, von Martius, and Kahler, while not pathognomonic is an important symptom. It is plausibly attributed to increase of moisture the result of insensible perspiration. Irregular temperature is another indication of vasomotor instability which may be an aid in the diagnosis. Complications with epilepsy, tabes, ophthalmoplegia externa, irregular bulbar paralysis, polio-encephalitis, paralysis of the limbs, diabetes, polyuria, hysterical paralysis, etc., are reported. The importance of hysterical symptoms in diagnosis has long been known.

Of the more recent theories of pathogenesis, only

two demand attention : that which places the origin of the affection in the medulla, and that which seeks it in the thyroid gland. Durdufi has repeated Filehne's experiment upon animals and has succeeded in producing protrusion of the eyeball by section of the medulla at the level of the auditory nucleus, though he was not able, as Filehne was, to produce goitre and cardiac disturbance.

Hale White has reported the results of an autopsy on a patient who died from pneumonia, after having for years suffered with exophthalmic goitre, in which he found in the floor of the fourth ventricle a number of small hæmorrhagic infarcts. These he attributed to the influence of the circulatory sequelæ of the pulmonary inflammation, upon a place of lowered resistance.

Paul Moebius first put forth the idea that disturbance of thyroid function is the primary stage in the general clinical features of the affection, thus making the disease correlated with myxœdema and cachexia strumipriva. Gautier upholds this theory by citing cases in which surgical operations upon the goitre have caused the disappearance of all symptoms. The study of early cases, however, must negative this view—at least in the eyes of the clinician.

In the matter of therapy, recent contributions do not help us much ; although instances of recovery under various methods of treatment continue to be reported. In our own experience, picrotoxin, as recommended by Bartholow, has proved of service.

SOCIETY PROCEEDINGS.

AMERICAN DERMATOLOGICAL ASSOCIATION.

Fourteenth Annual Meeting, held at Richfield Springs, New York, September 2, 3, and 4, 1890.

THE President, DR. PRINCE A. MORROW, of New York, called the meeting to order and delivered

THE PRESIDENT'S ADDRESS,

in which he said that those engaged in the practice of dermatology had abundant cause for congratulation. Only a few years ago dermatology had but little standing in America, as shown by the fact that until 1876 only twelve medical schools gave special instruction in diseases of the skin. To-day, as he had learned by the answers to circular letters sent to one hundred colleges, dermatology was a part of the curriculum in eighty-six. But, he said, there is reason to believe that there are many and grave defects in the existing system of instruction, and that the capacity of some of the teachers in our medical schools is doubtful, while the clinical

material in the majority of cases is inadequate. Even in large cities the clinical material is too much dispersed. In New York, for instance, instead of having a central hospital for all dermatological cases, as in Paris, the clinical material is scattered in various dispensaries and hospitals.

In the matter of nomenclature, Dr. Morrow said that new names are being introduced into dermatology which are not destined to retain a permanent position, and that while an essentially new disease requires a new name, yet he protested against the present neological craze.

DR. R. W. TAYLOR, of New York, then read a paper entitled

OBSERVATIONS ON PRURIGO, CLINICAL AND PATHO-LOGICAL.

The author said that new interest in this disease had been excited by Dr. Zeisler's paper, read at the last meeting of the Association, in which twelve cases were described which had been seen by Dr. Zeisler in Chicago. The combined experience of all present at that meeting included only eighteen cases. Dr. Taylor thought that the disease is more common in America than is generally supposed. It is probable that many cases escape recognition and are classed as eczema, scabies, pediculosis, ecthyma, impetigo, and even ichthyosis.

Dr. Taylor then described a case that he had recently seen, and also alluded to the casual concomitants and modifying conditions during the course of the disease. The patient was a healthy girl, nine years old, of healthy American parents in good circumstances, and with healthful surroundings. When four years old she began to scratch, and little red pimples appeared on the face, forearms, and legs, which the parents thought were mosquito-bites. The disease has recurred every year. When first seen by Dr. Taylor, january, 1890, the expression of the child's face was rather dull and her color was the typical white, somewhat ashy hue of prurigo. Over the forehead, temporal region, and cheek was a copious eruption of small conical papules, some whiter than the skin, others of a yellowish hue, and some well capped with a blood-crust the result of scratching. They were not upon the site of sebaceous glands. There was no marked dryness or want of vitality in the hair, although there was slight mealy desquamation in the scalp, such as Hebra describes. The eruption did not appear on the neck and nucha, but began where the shoulder merged into the neck. The principal eruption was on the back of the hand and forearm and on the external and anterior surface of the legs, where the papules were as large as a split pea. There were also some on the arms, buttocks, and thighs. They were scattered and without a semblance of grouping.

DR. W. T. CORLETT, of Cleveland, Ohio, followed with

A CLINICAL STUDY OF PRURITUS HYEMALIS—WINTER-ITCH, FROST-ITCH.

This affection, he said, was first pointed out as a disease by Dr. Duhring, and at about the same time by Mr. Jonathan Hutchinson. In one case in Dr. Corlett's practice it had recurred during the cold season for more than twenty-two years. In another case the eruption had at times the appearance of urticarious patches two or three inches in diameter, confined to the extremities, subsiding in about ten minutes, and leaving for a short time a dark yellowish spot. A third case was in a negro, showing that that race is not exempt.

The author's experience showed that the state of the general health had no appreciable effect on the pruritus; that the local irritation of the clothing, although capable of aggravating the malady, is not by itself able to produce it; and that meteorological conditions seem to be the main etiological factor. The disease is most common when the temperature and humidity are low, with a wind blowing from the northwest. Under these conditions evaporation is rapid, and the low temperature reduces the glandular activity of the skin to the minimum. As a consequence the skin becomes harsh, the peripheral nerves are irritated, and the disease results. He did not think the primary irritation could be central, else in time it would give rise to a more permanent disease.

The treatment is largely palliative. Internal medication seemed to have little effect in Dr. Corlett's cases, but he had used with advantage an application of ichthyol and resorcin.

DR. E. B. BRONSON, of New York, read a paper on

PRURITUS.

and was followed by DR. J. T. BOWEN, of Boston, who reported a series of cases of

CUTANEOUS TUBERCULOSIS,

and gave the results of his histological studies.

DR. L. A. DUHRING, of Philadelphia, spoke on the

TREATMENT OF DERMATITIS HERPETIFORMIS.

He said that as the several papers published by him on dermatitis herpetiformis contained no reference to treatment, it seemed appropriate to speak now of the treatment of this exceedingly rebellious disease. Each group of cases based on the etiological factors at work require special handling. A speedy cure cannot be expected. It must be remembered that the disease, as a rule, is multiform in character, and that the several varieties require different applications. His experience has been that milder remedies are called for in the erythematous than in the vesicular and bullous forms. A difficulty to contend with is the tendency of the disease to repeat itself, a new crop coming out before the old one disappears. Almost all his cases were chronic, and had previously undergone all manner of treatment.

He has reached the conclusion that the most benefit is derived from stimulating applications, especially those which act as revulsives, such as tar, carbolic acid, sulphur, thymol, ichthyol, resorcin, etc. That which in his hands has proved of the greatest value is sulphur ointment—two drachms of sulphur to the ounce of ointment, applied by thorough and long rubbing, so as to make a positive impression upon the skin, causing, as it were, local shock. Dr. Duhring especially emphasized the manner of making the application. Internal remedies had proven of little avail in most cases.

DR. F. J. SHEPHERD, of Montreal, reported a case of

ATROPHIA MACULOSA ET STRIATA, FOLLOWING
TYPHOID FEVER,

and showed photographs of the patient, a boy fifteen years old, who was admitted to the hospital with typhoid fever. During the course of the fever he was delirious, and had epileptic attacks. Macular lines formed, extending across the patellæ and around the anterior aspect of the thighs to near the middle, some being several inches long. They were at first of a reddish color, but became paler, were not distinctly shiny, and were grooved. The interesting point in the case was the occurrence of the atrophic lines in a boy during acute fever.

DR. J. C. WHITE, of Boston, followed with a paper upon

IMMIGRANT DERMATOSES,

in which he said that on a ship the conditions tending to induce skin affections are: homesickness, seasickness, filth, foul air, constipation, inability to take exercise, and contact with others having contagious disease. It is not uncommon for young persons to be attacked, a week or ten days after landing, with an urticarial, bullous, or eczematous eruption. Of imported affections the most common is scabies. The rare affection, melanosis lenticularis progressiva, which Dr. White thought is not seen in native American stock, also occurs. Prurigo also might be regarded as an imported disease, and is scarcely seen elsewhere than in cities with a large foreign population.

The prevalence of vegetable parasitic affections among us is likely to be largely increased by immigration. Tinea favosa, tinea trichophytina, and tinea versicolor are more common in countries from which we receive many immigrants than they are here. The same is true of tubercular affections of the skin, and he is disposed to regard lupus, scrofuloderma, scrofulous gummata, tuberculosis verrucosa, etc., as closely-allied affections, inoculable and auto-inoculable.

In conclusion, the author suggested the propriety of addressing a memorial to the national government with regard to carrying out the following measures: (1) To remove all animal parasites from immigrants on landing, by cleansing the person and clothing. (2) To retain in quarantine all immigrants with contagious skin diseases, including venereal affections. (3) To return to their homes all persons affected with the contagious diseases that cannot be treated in quarantine, such as leprosy, tuberculosis, and advanced syphilis. (4) To provide efficient medical inspection at foreign ports of immigration, with the power to prevent the importation of dangerous diseases to this country.[1]

DR. R. W. TAYLOR then described

A CASE OF SECOND INFECTION WITH SYPHILIS, AND A
CASE OF SYPHILITIC INFECTION IN A PERSON
HEREDITARILY SYPHILITIC.

The first case was that of a sickly-looking woman, aged thirty-eight years, who entered the Charity Hospital in January, 1890. Eleven years ago she had syphilis, accompanied with a hard swelling of the external genitals, enlargement of the glands, and an eruption entirely over the body. The second year she had rheumatoid pains and mucous patches; the third year, serpiginous syphilides, etc.

---

[1] Later the Council was given power to carry out this suggestion in a modified form, and to send a memorial to the United States and Canadian governments upon the propriety of these measures.

She married and gave birth to two weak children, which soon died. Her husband dying, she again became a prostitute, and entered the hospital broken-down in health. There were typical miliary syphilides scattered over nearly the entire surface of the skin; all the ganglia were markedly enlarged; there were mucous patches of the tongue and mouth, and evidences of alopecia, and pain in the joints which was worse at night. The second attack was much more severe than the first. She is improving under mercurial treatment.

The second case was one of acquired syphilis in a person hereditarily syphilitic. The woman came to Dr. Taylor in 1879, when she was nineteen years old. At that time he treated her for a destructive syphilitic sore on the face, due to hereditary syphilis, a clear history of which was afterward given by her mother, who acquired syphilis three months before the child's birth. The child had a rash, condylomata cuta, sniffles, etc. In 1885, five years after the patient's first visit, she returned, and then had a roseola, scaling syphilides over the entire body, condylomata of the genitals, mucous patches of the pharynx, etc. The infection began in the right labium, and was contracted from her husband. All the glands were enlarged, and there was alopecia. She has since been cured.

DR. G. T. JACKSON, of New York, then read a paper on

ELECTROLYSIS IN THE TREATMENT OF LUPUS VULGARIS,

in which he said that the advantages of electrolysis, in the treatment of lupus vulgaris, over other and older methods are as follows:

1. It is comparatively painless, and does not require the administration of an anæsthetic.

2. There is not the slightest loss of blood, and thus there is no dread of a surgical operation.

3. The patient is not kept a moment from his occupation, there is no deformity caused by the treatment, and no disfiguring applications are required. He is also spared the discomfort of a swollen face, the ordinary attendant of the arsenical or pyrogallic acid treatment.

4. The treatment goes to the root of the disease with far more exactness and less damage to the surrounding skin than any other caustic or surgical method, and the scar left is smooth and not unsightly.

5. The result obtained is as good as, if not better, than that of any other method of treatment.

DR. H. W. STELWAGON, of Philadelphia, then showed photographs of

A CASE OF PLICA

which he had seen a few months ago, although he was not sure that plica is the right name for the disease. The woman came to be treated for acne, and called his attention to a lock of hair as thick as one's thumb springing from the middle of the occipital region, closely matted together and falling as low as the ankles, terminating in a brush-like end. It had begun to grow four years before, from no apparent cause; it was not sticky. The rest of the hair fell over the shoulders, and was not matted.

DR. C. W. ALLEN, of New York, followed with a paper on

THE TREATMENT OF ERYSIPELAS,

based upon the results of treatment, during the past two years, of 419 cases in the hospitals on Blackwell's Island, not under his care, and 47 cases in his own practice during the same time. Of the former, 21 died; of the latter, 4. Various forms of treatment were employed, and consisted chiefly in applications of different kinds. Dr. Allen thought that, although tending to pursue a definite and usually favorable course, the disease can be checked by treatment. Among the applications used were boric acid, iodine, resorcin, bicarbonate of sodium, ichthyol, collodion, aristol, scarification with the knife, and plaster strips. He is disposed to think favorably of scarification and adhesive plaster, separately or combined, but has tried them in only two cases.

DR. H. G. KLOTZ read a paper entitled

NOTES ON PILOCARPINE IN DERMATOLOGY,

in which he reviewed the history of pilocarpine in dermatology, and said that it had not met with the acceptance which one would have expected if its therapeutic virtues were at all proportionate to its diaphoretic qualities. The author has employed the remedy in a few cases, including eczema, pruritus of the anus, and affections with dryness and irritation as symptoms. The results were such as to encourage him to give it a further trial. It can be given internally, or by hypodermic injection, in small doses and continued for a long time. A tenth of a grain is probably sufficient to keep the skin moist.

DR. C. W. ALLEN then related his experience with

ARISTOL,

which, he concluded, possesses excellent cicatrizing, granulating, and stimulating qualities, is free from the objectionable odor of iodoform, and seems valuable in certain dermatological cases.

DR. C. C. RANSOM, of Richfield Springs, then reported, by invitation, the

RESULTS OF TREATMENT OF DERMATOLOGICAL CASES BY SULPHUR WATER AT RICHFIELD SPRINGS.

He said that since the new bathing establishment had been completed, 22 cases had been treated, including 9 of eczema, 1 of psoriasis, 4 of seborrhœa, 1 of pruritus, and 2 of urticaria. In nearly all of these cases there was marked improvement, and in some a cure. The temperature of the baths was usually from 95° to 106° F., and they lasted from seven to fifteen minutes. A longer stay in the sulphur bath has a depressing effect which continues for some hours.

The officers elected for the ensuing year are Dr. Greenough, of Boston, President; Dr. F. N. Denslow, of St. Paul, Vice-President; and Dr. G. T. Jackson, of New York, Secretary and Treasurer.

AMERICAN ORTHOPÆDIC ASSOCIATION.

Fourth Annual Meeting, held in Philadelphia, September 16, 17, and 18, 1890.

FIRST DAY—MORNING SESSION.

THE Association met in the Hall of the College of Physicians, and was called to order by the President, DR. DE FOREST WILLARD, of Philadelphia, at 10 A. M.

After a short business meeting, the President delivered his

ANNUAL ADDRESS.

In a few well-chosen words he welcomed the members of the Association as a Philadelphian, and extended to them the hospitalities of the city.

Referring to orthopædic surgery in Europe, Dr. Willard said that during his trip across the water he had found it in a far less advanced state than he had anticipated. In America it stands farther ahead in its surgical aspect, and in the ingenuity of its mechanical contrivances, than it does across the ocean. Such men, however, as Macewen, Edmund Owen, and Howard Marsh are doing excellent work. He was pleased with Macewen's clear-headed, strong and earnest advocacy of laminectomy and other operations which promise to give relief and assistance in a certain number of cases of caries of the spine with pressure-paralysis.

Following Dr. Willard DR. E. H. BRADFORD, of Boston, read a paper entitled

TREATMENT OF DEFORMITIES OF SPASTIC PARALYSIS,

in which he said that orthopædic surgeons have not done full justice to the surgical treatment of this affection, because the disease has been but little understood, although it is one which occasions distortion and difficulty in locomotion. Light, however, has been thrown upon the subject recently by neurologists, and it is now recognized and studied. The author has not been able to gain permanently satisfactory results by the use of appliances, although in infantile paralysis—sometimes confounded with spastic or cerebral paralysis—appliances are of great assistance. He has not derived any benefit from the use of electricity, and but very little from massage in these cases. Where the lower extremities are affected by this disorder, he has had satisfactory results from tenotomy and myotomy of the resistant muscles,—*i. e.*, the tendo-Achillis, hamstring muscles, and the adductor muscles. After the operation a light appliance should be worn to aid locomotion for a month or so. Permanent benefit may be expected in children free from mental deficiency. His experience included fourteen cases, with ages ranging from four to sixteen years. He had had no experience in operating upon adults suffering from this affection.

DR. ARTHUR J. GILLETTE, of St. Paul, Minnesota, contributed a paper on

TENOTOMY FOR RELIEF OF DEFORMITY IN SPASTIC PARALYSIS,

and reported a case.

The patient was eleven and one-half years of age. The deformity consisted in the flexion of the right forearm upon the arm. Whenever the patient became excited the muscles of the arm became rigid, as did the fingers of the hand of the same arm. The right foot was in the position of talipes equinus, and when the patient attempted to walk so that weight was thrown upon the foot, it was brought into the position of talipes equino-varus.

Dr. Gillette divided the tendo-Achillis, which permitted the foot to come into good position. It also relieved the flexion at the knee. He then placed the foot in plaster-of-Paris and allowed it to remain in this dressing a few weeks, the child playing and walking as much as she desired. When he removed the plaster he applied an ordinary ankle-brace with a "stop-joint" to prevent the foot from returning to its former position. It is now eight months since the operation was done, and the child has not yet had the slightest spasm of any of the muscles of the foot. The ankle-joint will permit of almost all the normal movements, and the patient walks with but a slight limp.

DR. AP MORGAN VANCE, of Louisville, read a paper entitled

AMPUTATION AS AN ORTHOPÆDIC MEASURE.

He said that the introduction of amputation as an orthopædic measure was something out of the recognized lines, but as orthopædists are expected to relieve patients of deformity it is obvious that if amputation in some cases is the best and often the only way this can be done, the operation may be performed by the orthopædic surgeon. In the past ten years quite a number of cases had come under his observation and care in which there was no doubt in his mind that amputation performed for convenience' sake would have been better than any other treatment. Among those in which the knee can be saved will be found a few cases of old infantile paralysis (talipes), and adult cases of congenital talipes, where painful bursæ have developed and life is often unendurable from the pain caused by walking. On the other hand, old subluxated knees with ankylosed patellæ, with flail joints and great shortening, are not uncommon. Some of these cases can be converted from hopeless cripples into useful members of society by a proper amputation and adjustment of a good artificial limb.

Dr. Vance then reported four cases illustrative of the good done by amputation performed for orthopædic purposes.

AFTERNOON SESSION.

DR. HENRY LING TAYLOR, of New York, described

A READY METHOD OF COUNTER-TRACTION AT THE KNEE.

He said experience had shown the obstinate and serious nature of many cases of synovitis and arthritis of the knee, and the frequency of grave sequelæ, unless treated with the utmost care and precision. Properly applied counter-extension with fixation and recumbency usually affords prompt and often marvellous relief to the intense suffering in the active stage of the trouble, and at the same time provides conditions favorable to the proper nutrition of the joint and the subsidence of the inflammatory process. Fixation alone, or simple traction by means of the weight and pulley, however useful in an emergency, give by no means the same results. Dr. Taylor is convinced that the early application of some form of counter-extension is of extreme importance in surgical inflammations of the knee-joint.

DR. F. H. MILLIKEN, of Philadelphia, contributed a paper on the

TREATMENT OF INFANTILE CLUB FOOT PRELIMINARY TO OPERATION.

He offered some suggestions regarding the treatment to be used in cases of club-foot before proceeding with the operations of tenotomy and osteotomy. Not infrequently we hear of tenotomy, and even of osteotomy, as having been performed on the feet of infants not more than two or three months old. This he considers premature practice.

In private practice and among people possessing a fair amount of intelligence, the traction principle is by far the preferable method of treating infantile club-foot ; but in dispensary practice the surgeon meets with a different class.

The directions are not faithfully attended to, and cases show little improvement. For this reason the fixed dressing is preferable for the class of cases that apply for treatment at the dispensary clinic. But neither the fixed dressing nor any other can be depended upon to correct a case of severe club-foot or effect a permanent cure without a final resort to the use of the knife.

DR. BENJAMIN LEE, of Philadelphia, in a paper entitled

SACRO–ILIAC DISEASE,

reported two cases, and from them deduced the following corollaries :

1. Disease of the sacro-iliac symphysis induces a characteristic deformity of the spine, of which the features are a lateral displacement of the entire trunk in a direction away from the affected side, a single curve comprising the entire length of the spine, and the almost complete absence of rotation.

2. It also induces a peculiar rolling or waddling gait.

3. It is often the cause of inveterate and excruciating sciatica.

4. It is useless to attempt to remedy the spinal distortion so long as its cause remains unrelieved.

5. The existence of chronic pain in the sciatic nerve, not yielding in a reasonable space of time to medication, should always lead the practitioner to make a careful examination of the spine and of the region of the sacro-iliac juncture.

6. This affection is met with more frequently in adult than in child-life.

7. Its appropriate treatment consists in splinting the pelvis and thus preventing motion between the opposing surfaces of the symphysis, motion not being its natural function.

8. For the same reason extension cannot be expected to produce the favorable results in this affection that we obtain from it in arthrodial joints.

9. The disease is often of extremely slow development.

10. Its first symptom is often abdominal pain, whence it may readily be mistaken for peritonitis, ovaritis, cystitis, and the like.

11. This pain is principally referred to the side on which the lesion exists.

12. The existence of severe unilateral abdominal pain, accompanied by little or no febrile action, should lead to the suspicion of the existence of this affection.

13. An instrument-maker may, by a happy chance, give temporary relief to a patient suffering from this disease, but as he is entirely ignorant of its seat and nature, he is not perhaps the safest person to refer the patient.

DR. ROYAL WHITMAN, of New York, read, by invitation, a paper on

THE TREATMENT OF PERSISTENT ABDUCTION OF THE FOOT,

in which he said that the successful treatment of any chronic affection demands a personal, persistent attention to details on the part of the surgeon.

The two principal objects in the treatment of this affection are : (1) to overcome the contraction and spasm of the abductors ; (2) to straighten the adductors. This is best accomplished as follows :

The patient being etherized, the affected foot is forcibly extended and adducted—that is, both the heel and toes are turned inward so that the inner border of the foot is bent like a bow ; it is then forced inward under the leg to a position of extreme equino-varus, the operation being attended with audible cracking of adhesions in all of the diseased articulations. In this position a well-fitting plaster bandage is applied with the object of persistently overstretching the shortened ligaments and contracted muscles and holding the foot firmly in its new position. The bandage may remain on a variable length of time according to the subsequent pain and the difficulty that has been experienced in the reposition. From one to three weeks is the average time for it to remain, after which it may be removed.

(*To be continued.*)

CORRESPONDENCE.

THE MEDICAL EXAMINING BOARD OF VIRGINIA.

To the Editor of THE MEDICAL NEWS,

SIR : In connection with a letter appearing in your issue of August 16, 1890, from a correspondent in Seattle, Washington, concerning " Medical Law in the State of Washington," it may be interesting to compare the medical examination as recently held by the State Medical Board of Virginia.

The Virginia Board is composed of thirty-two regular physicians and five homœopathists, and in its *personnel*, in the grade of the questions asked, and in the result of its labors, is excelled by none and equalled by but few, if any, other State boards in the country.

The thirty-seven members composing the board are divided into committees to preside over the examinations upon the following branches : chemistry, anatomy, hygiene, and medical jurisprudence ; physiology, materia medica and therapeutics ; obstetrics and gynecology ; practice of medicine, and lastly, surgery. Six questions are asked upon chemistry, eight upon anatomy, six upon hygiene and medical jurisprudence, eight upon physiology, twelve upon materia medica and therapeutics, twelve upon obstetrics and gynecology, twenty upon practice of medicine, and twenty upon surgery.

The examinations are entirely written, and each applicant is known by a number which is placed opposite his name by the secretary of the board, he being the only member possessing this information. Thus all possibility of prejudice or favoritism influencing the decision of an examination is obviated.

The standard required is a general average of 75 per cent., but a grade of less than 33⅓ per cent. on any one of the subjects examined upon calls for the rejection of the applicant receiving it.

Before the board at its last meeting, on the 3d and 4th of September, 1890, twenty-four applicants for licence to practise in Virginia presented themselves for examination. Of this number, thirteen received the required average, and eleven fell below it, and were, therefore, refused certificates.

The examinations occupied two days, beginning on the morning of each day at nine o'clock and terminating in the evening at eleven o'clock; three hours were devoted to each branch examined upon, and one hour each for dinner and supper was allowed. It will thus be seen that, aside from the mental task, the time required to answer the questions imposed no small physical exertion. The length of time devoted to each branch also conveys some idea of the severity of the examinations.

Your correspondent, who was one of the applicants before the board at its last meeting, went to the examination with the impression that the board was prejudiced against outsiders and against those who are graduates of colleges not situated in Virginia. This impression was received from various sources and your correspondent believes it to be the one generally held in Philadelphia. Never was an impression more falsely founded, and it gives him pleasure to be able to bear testimony to the universal courtesy and fair treatment received from every member of the board before whom he appeared. That so many men, graduates and residents outside of Virginia, have been rejected by this board is due solely to the fact that the applicants have not been fitted to pass an examination before such a body of men as compose the Virginia State Board.

That nearly all the men who are graduates of the Virginia colleges pass these examinations is not on account of any favoritism shown them, but because they are well prepared, in theory at least, to stand the examination. For instance, the University of Virginia requires at its final examination a general average of 83⅓ per cent., a grade certainly not demanded by any college in Philadelphia. The examinations are both written and oral, and your correspondent was assured by a graduate of that institution that its examinations are fair in every particular, and that no cheating is indulged in by the student, a fact of considerable importance in judging of the relative merits of men from different colleges, in some of which, it must unfortunately be admitted, the evil exists to a considerable degree. Of course, such a training as is given its men by the University of Virginia, theoretical though it be, must have its effect in an examination which is in itself necessarily theoretical.

That the Medical Board of Virginia is doing a good work in keeping out of the State men of improper qualifications may be judged by the number of men it yearly rejects, and one cannot but believe that these rejections are just when one hears some of the answers to the questions asked. At the recent examination one of the applicants, who was of course rejected, to the question, "Describe an operation for the radical cure of inguinal hernia," replied that he did not know what hernia was; that it was "one of those new-fangled ideas that had recently cropped up," and that he had not yet heard of it. Another man, a graduate of a Northern college, received a grade of but twenty on chemistry, and one but little higher on anatomy. At the examinations held last year, to the question, "What is a cell, and describe its physiological functions," a brilliant follower of the healing art replied: "A cell is a place of confinement." This answer proved him to be deficient himself in cells—at least of the cerebral gray matter.

Of course this class of men has not been allowed to practise in Virginia, and these facts prove in an unanswerable manner the benefit the Virginia Medical Board is bestowing upon the profession of that State. It also clearly demonstrates the folly and negligence of those States that have not organized examining boards to judge of the qualifications of men desiring to practise medicine within their boundaries. If such poorly equipped men appear before the Virginia State Board, knowing that they will be obliged to stand a rigid examination, what must be the extent of the medical knowledge of some of the men who flock to those States where no State examination is required!

PHILADELPHIA, September, 1890.

ST. LOUIS.

To the Editor of THE MEDICAL NEWS,

SIR: The year 1890 will be a somewhat notable one in the history of medical colleges in St. Louis. Never in this city have there been erected in one year so many buildings expressly for purposes of medical instruction.

I have already mentioned in a previous letter the burning of the Beaumont Medical College building at Clark Ave. and Sixteenth St., and the subsequent purchase of a lot at Jefferson Ave. and Vine St. On this lot the faculty have so far completed the erection of a building that they feel warranted in announcing that the lectures of the regular term will commence there next month, while those of the preliminary course are being delivered in a hall near the college building. The building is an imposing one in external appearance, and it is well adapted to the special uses for which it is designed.

More ornate and showy architecture is seen in the new building of the Marion Sims Medical College on Grand Ave. and Caroline St., an elevated point in the western part of the city commanding an extensive view in all directions, and affording a fine opportunity for the display of architectural effect which has been utilized to the fullest extent. Whether that elegant residence neighborhood will afford material for extensive clinics, which seem so important an adjunct to college-work, remains to be seen.

Another large and stately building is being erected on the corner of Gamble St. and Jefferson Ave. for the College of Physicians and Surgeons. This is, I think, a much more desirable site than the old one at North Market and Eleventh St.

In addition to these three large and handsome buildings nearly or quite prepared for use this fall, it seems probable that the old St. Louis Medical College is about to join the procession and move westward, for it is stated in the daily papers that the faculty have sold for $75,000 their property on Clark Ave. and Seventh St., which has become very valuable for warehouse purposes on account of its proximity to the railroad and depots, and undesirable as a site for medical college in every respect except for the vast amount of clinical material which is gathered from the densely populated district surrounding it. Where the College will secure a new location is yet to be decided.

The several medical societies have resumed their stated meetings. The Medico-Chirurgical Society, in accordance with a vote taken last winter, will hold weekly meetings instead of bi-weekly as formerly.

An important practical question for early consideration by this society will be that of location. For the past four years the society has rented a hall in the building of the Post-Graduate School of Medicine, which is centrally located, commodious, accessible, and convenient both as an assembly room and as a library and reading-room. Now that the Post-Graduate School has been absorbed by the Missouri College, it is thought by many that the best interests of the society will not be conserved by having the meetings in the college building, and probably a change of location will be deemed advisable. It would be a consummation devoutly to be wished if the different societies would combine their forces and rent a suitable building, or better yet, erect one, which could be occupied by all, as no two hold their meetings on the same evening. By some such combination of resources it would be practicable to render the libraries of the several societies of much greater practical value to the members, as it would then be entirely feasible to have a paid librarian in constant attendance in the reading-room who could issue books to those desiring to read them at home, and preserve the files of journals.

One reason why comparatively few papers from St. Louis physicians find their way into the medical journals of other cities is that the policy of the St. Louis medical societies has been to make a contract with some home journal by which that journal shall publish all papers and discussions presented or occurring at society meetings. At present the *St. Louis Courier of Medicine* has secured the right to publish papers read before the St. Louis Medical Society, the Medico-Chirurgical Society, and the St. Louis Obstetrical and Gynecological Society.

DOUBLE CEPHALHÆMATOMA.

To the Editor of THE MEDICAL NEWS,

SIR : The great interest I felt in the cases reported by Dr. Barton C. Hirst of this rare affection in the newly-born infant, has encouraged me to add two cases from my own practice, which are almost fac-similes of those reported by him.

Last April, I was called to attend Mrs. T., primipara, twenty-two years old. Labor was normal, lasting in its three stages, respectively, nine hours, two hours, and twenty minutes. The child was a male, weighing ten pounds. The head was large, and there was extensive overlapping of the flat bones.

Three days later my attention was called to a small swelling on the left parietal bone. On the following day I noticed a similar swelling on the right parietal bone. In a few days these blood-tumors had reached the size of a hen's egg, the left somewhat larger than the right. Elasticity and fluctuation were distinct, but there was no tenderness on pressure.

I did nothing for these tumors, and when I discontinued my visits to the mother at the end of three weeks they had diminished in size considerably.

Two weeks later, however, I received a note from the mother, asking me to call, as "something was wrong with the bones of the child's head." The tumors had entirely disappeared ; but the borders of the parietal bones were rough and raised one-half inch above, and overlapped the occipital bone. I could lay my finger between the bones. Near the posterior fontanelle, from the left parietal projected a piece of bone one-fourth of an inch long, so that the head presented a unique and marked deformity.

As the child was well, I did nothing. He was kept under observation, however, for about three months. At the end of that time his head assumed its normal shape.

In the second case the tumors were on the left parietal bone and on the left side of the occipital bone. Both were small. They subsided in three weeks, without treatment, leaving no deformity.

FRANCES HATCHETTE, M.D.

PHILADELPHIA.

THREE PROPOSITIONS TO DR. ERNST.

To the Editor of THE MEDICAL NEWS,

SIR : In volume V. of the *Annual of the Universal Medical Sciences*, 1889, Dr. Ernst states that Novy and I, in our little volume on *Ptomaïnes and Leucomaïnes*, make the suggestion that "bacteria may be the products of these alkaloids." In your issue of July 6, 1890, I asked Dr. Ernst to be kind enough to inform me on what page of the volume I could find the " suggestion." Dr. Ernst replied by quoting a part of a sentence, which by being isolated is made to appear to have a wholly different meaning from that which it has in the text, and which has no relation whatever to the question at issue.

Now the difference between Dr. Ernst and myself is easily stated. In the work on ptomaïnes and leucomaïnes, on the first page of the first chapter, I make the following statement concerning the relation between bacteria and ptomaïnes : "Since all putrefaction is due to the action of bacteria, it follows that all ptomaïnes result from the growth of these microörganisms." Dr. Ernst persists in stating that I teach the very opposite doctrine, *i. e.*, that bacteria are produced by ptomaïnes. I have these propositions to make to Dr. Ernst : I will submit the work on ptomaïnes, the article of his in the *Annual*, and our correspondence in THE MEDICAL NEWS, to any three teachers of bacteriology in America whom he may mention, and ask them to report over their own signatures whether or not "the suggestion that bacteria may be the products of ptomaïnes " can be found in the little volume written by Novy and myself.

My second proposition is to submit to the same men the question whether or not, in our correspondence in THE MEDICAL NEWS of July 5th, Dr. Ernst has fairly and honestly answered the questions which I ask.

My third proposition is to submit to any three scientific men in America, whom Dr. Ernst may select, and ask them to report their answer to THE MEDICAL NEWS over their own signatures, the following question : Is it fair and honorable to take from the sentence, " Indeed, so long as the investigation goes no further than this, we are justified in saying that the microörganism may be an accompaniment or consequence of the disease," the clause "we are justified in saying that the microörganism may be an accompaniment or a consequence of the disease," and print it as an independent sentence, and give it as the meaning of the writer of the complete sentence?

I will ask you, Mr. Editor, to submit this letter to Dr. Ernst, and to inform him that I await his reply.

Respectfully,

V. C. VAUGHAN, M.D.

ANN ARBOR, September 16, 1890

NEWS ITEMS.

A Quack Libel Suit.—Suit has been entered by William Radam, manufacturer of Radam's Microbe-killer, against the *Druggists' Circular*, of New York, for $200,000 damages, the largest amount, so far as heard from, that was ever asked for in a libel suit of this kind. The pleadings show that the action is brought to recover damages claimed to have been done the business of the plaintiff by an article published in the *Druggists' Circular* for September, 1889. This article gave the result of an analysis of the Microbe-killer made by Dr. R. G. Eccles, a prominent chemist of Brooklyn, who stated that an identical preparation could be made by the following formula:

Oil of vitriol (impure) .	. .	4 drachms.
Muriatic acid (impure)	. .	1 drachm.
Red wine, about .	. . .	1 ounce.
Well or spring water	. . .	1 gallon.

This mixture, it was alleged, could be made at a cost of less than five cents per gallon, for which Radam charged three dollars.

It was further alleged that while, when properly used, sulphuric acid, the principal constituent of the Microbe-killer, was a valuable medicine, it was, when taken without due caution or advice, a slow but certain cumulative poison; and the theories advanced by Radam, as to the causes of diseases and the proper method of treatment, were alleged to be totally erroneous. Col. Robert G. Ingersoll, the famous lecturer, is the counsel for the plaintiff.

The *Druggists' Circular*, which is published at 72 William Street, New York, expresses a desire to hear of any case in which unfavorable results have followed the administration of the Microbe-killer, or of any other fact that would be interesting under the circumstances. They claim to have published this analysis without malice and with the sole intention of protecting the public from the loss of their health and money by the use of a dangerous nostrum.

Honors of a Female Medical Student.—Miss Ann Frances Piercy, a student at the London School of Medicine for Women, has gained triple examination honors and two gold medals. In materia medica she held first place, with a medal; in anatomy, second place, with a medal; and in physiology and histology she was first-class.

The Aseptic Hand of the Surgeon.—An aphoristic saying of von Bergmann, on the importance of cleanliness of the hands of the surgeon, has been almost universally quoted by the German journals, as follows: "Infection by contact with the practitioner's hands plays no inconsiderable part in the etiology of the diseases of wounds, and the much-prized skilled hand of the surgeon may bring the greatest harm with the tenderest touch."

An Association of Medical Legislators.—The medical members of the French parliament have united to form an association for the purpose of taking concerted action upon proposed laws regulating the medical profession and the sale of medicines. The profession is more largely represented than before, in recent years, upward of eighty being physicians.

Accidental Poisoning in Bellevue Hospital.—In the case of a typhoid-fever patient who recently died from an overdose of carbolic acid in Bellevue Hospital, New York, the coroner's jury censured the nurse for his carelessness in administering strong acid when dilute acid had been ordered. The jury further found that the "said negligence was, in part, attributable to the authorities of Bellevue Hospital, who neglected to label properly the medicine prescribed by the regular physician, and who allowed made-up prescriptions for internal use to be mingled in the same chest with poisons of a violent nature, intended for external use only, and the whole to be placed in the control and custody of inexperienced nurse pupils, and in this case of one below the average intelligence."

Rhinoplasty in India.—A notable literary and scientific production, from the native press of Junagadh, India, is a description of one hundred cases of rhinoplasty, by Surgeon Trilovandas Motichand Shah, chief medical officer at the Junagadh Hospital. The author has collected the cases within four years, under peculiar circumstances. The deformities for which this procedure was required were not the results of disease, but of wilful mutilation committed either in revenge or as a causeless outrage on innocent persons, by a class of miscreants known in that country as the Makrani outlaws. The book is illustrated by photographs, which clearly show the extent to which the facial mutilation is carried by these criminals, as well as the signal improvement effected by surgical treatment. The author, who has worked upon his subject with much zeal and success, strongly advocates the old operation, in which the flap is taken from the forehead. It requires less time than the cheek-flap operation, and the subsequent disfigurement is much less, the forehead scar being readily concealed by the turban almost universally worn by the people of the province where these mutilations chiefly occur.

An Epidemic of Beri-beri.—A whaling bark has arrived at New Bedford, Massachusetts, after a cruise of five years. While off the coast of Patagonia several months ago the seamen were attacked with what is believed was beri-beri. Thirty-four of the crew of thirty-seven were ill with the disease at one time, and nine cases proved fatal.

Burns from Chlorate of Potassium.—According to the *St. Louis Medical and Surgical Journal*, workers in chlorate of potassium manufactories have their clothes so completely saturated with the salt that recently one of them was severely burned by striking a match on his trousers. His clothes were at once a mass of flames, and, although immediately plunged into a pool of water, it is probable that the burns will be fatal.

Medical Work in the Cholera Districts.—It is stated that the physicians at work in the cholera-infected districts of Spain continue to be ill-used by the peasants, who are opposed to the enforcement of precautionary measures. Notwithstanding that the physicians are provided with a military escort, three have been killed by the peasantry.

Leprosy in Surinam.—The Bishop of Dutch Guiana, who was recently in Baltimore, made an appeal for the lepers in his diocese. The disease has been unchecked by any sanitary precautions of the government, and has spread to a serious extent in Surinam. Three priests who came in contact with the diseased have become leprous, and one of them is now paralytic and helpless. This heroic priest, like the late Father Damien, of Malakao, left his home to spend his life among the neglected lepers of a foreign land. He first noticed the signs of the disease in himself in 1880.

A Prelate's Charity.—Cardinal Manning, not long since, was presented by his friends with an illuminated address and a purse of $37,000, in token of the silver anniversary of his episcopacy, and he soon afterward made public his intention to devote a large portion of the money-gift to the *endowment* of a bed in the accident ward of the London Hospital, for the use, *in perpetuo*, of humble workingmen who may be injured on or along the River Thames.

The Montreal General Hospital.—This conservative and venerable institution has turned over a new leaf, and, according to the *Montreal Medical Journal*, has never before been in so good a condition, The house staff are uniformed in white patrol-jackets, while the trained nurses are dressed in pink and white, with caps and badges. The wards look fresher and more business-like. The out-patient department has been enlarged, and fitted for the accommodation of the specialists. Clinical instruction will be better provided for than in the past. "The venerable institution has merely been drowsy; and is not yet moribund."

Obituary.—DR. PHANUEL EUCLID BISHOP, of Pawtucket, R. I., died of Bright's disease, September 21st, at the age of forty-six years. The deceased entered Brown University in 1862, but at the end of one year enlisted in the Union army. Soon rising to the rank of Second Lieutenant he was sent to New Orleans, and was for a time stationed at Fort Jackson. He was subsequently made Captain, was detailed as judge-advocate on court-martials, and was provost-marshal of St. Mary's parish in New Orleans. After the war he went West and graduated from a business college in Chicago, was superintendent of schools in a city of Iowa, and travelled considerably. Returning to Pawtucket, he was connected with the public schools for some time as teacher, and then as superintendent. At this time the degree of Master of Arts was conferred upon him by Brown University. Meanwhile he had found time to study medicine and attend lectures at Bowdoin and Dartmouth medical schools. He practised successfully in Paw-

tucket for seventeen years. He was a Fellow of the Rhode Island Medical Society, a Mason, an Odd Fellow, and a Forester. Two children and an only sister survive him.

—— DR. JOSEF VON JELENFFY, an eminent laryngologist of Hungary, did not return home alive from the Berlin Congress. He was able to attend the meetings of one day only, when he was prostrated by cardiac disease and was taken to the Catholic Hospital. He died soon after. At his funeral, which was attended by all the members of the laryngological section then remaining at Berlin, Dr. B. Fränkel, president of that section, delivered an address commemorative of the life and services of the deceased, speaking of him in most sympathetic terms.

OFFICIAL LIST OF CHANGES IN THE STATIONS AND DUTIES OF OFFICERS SERVING IN THE MEDICAL DEPARTMENT, U. S. ARMY, FROM SEPTEMBER 15 TO SEPTEMBER 22, 1890.

MIDDLETON, JOHNSON V. D., *Major and Surgeon.*—Is relieved from duty at David's Island, N. Y., and will report in person to the commanding officer Fort Columbus, New York City, for duty at that station, relieving Joseph Gibson. Major and Surgeon, and reporting by letter to the commanding general Division of the Atlantic. Major Gibson, on being relieved by Major Middleton, will report in person to the commanding officer David's Island, N. Y., for duty at that station, and by letter to the Superintendent of the Recruiting Service.—Par. 1, *S. O. 219, A. G. O., Washington,* September 18, 1890.

By direction of the Acting Secretary of War, the following changes in the stations and duties of officers of the Medical Department are ordered:

SPENCER, WILLIAM G., *Captain and Assistant Surgeon,* will, upon the abandonment of Fort Bridger, Wyoming (his present station), report in person to the commanding officer of Fort Omaha, Nebraska, for duty at that station, relieving Alfred E. Bradley, First Lieutenant and Assistant Surgeon. Lieutenant Bradley, on being relieved by Captain Spencer, will report in person to the commanding general Department of the Platte, for duty as Attending Surgeon at the Headquarters of that Department.—Par. 16, *S. O. 214, A. G. O., Washington, D. C.,* September 12, 1890.

By direction of the Acting Secretary of War, leave of absence granted WILLIAM N. SUTER, *First Lieutenant and Assistant Surgeon,* in Special Orders No. 149, June 26, 1890, from this office, is extended fourteen days.—Par. 6, *S. O. 214, A. G. O., Washington, D. C.,* September 12, 1890.

By direction of the Acting Secretary of War, the leave of absence for seven days, heretofore granted HENRY McELDERRY, *Major and Surgeon,* by the Superintendent of the U. S. Military Academy, is extended to November 10, 1890, on account of sickness.—Par. 5, *S. O. 214, A. G. O., Washington, D. C.,* September 12, 1890.

By direction of the Acting Secretary of War, JOHN J. COCHRAN, *Captain and Assistant Surgeon,* now on duty at Fort Adams, R. I., will proceed to Mount Vernon Barracks, Ala., and report in person to the commanding officer of that post for temporary duty, and, on completion of the duty contemplated, he will return to his proper station.—Par. 2, *S. O. 214, A. G. O., Washington, D. C.,* September 12, 1890.

By direction of the Acting Secretary of War, leave of absence for three months, commencing about October 1, 1890 is granted FRANK J. IVES, *Captain and Assistant Surgeon,* provided one of the Assistant Surgeons serving in the Department of the Missouri can be assigned to duty in his stead at Fort Sill, Oklahoma Territory, during that time.—Par. 26, *S. O. 213, A. G. O., Washington, D. C.,* September 11, 1890.

OFFICIAL LIST OF CHANGES IN THE STATIONS AND DUTIES OF THE MEDICAL CORPS OF THE U. S. NAVY FOR THE WEEK ENDING SEPTEMBER 20, 1890.

OLCOTT, F. W., *Passed Assistant Surgeon.*—Ordered to the U. S. S. "Alert."

THE MEDICAL NEWS.
A WEEKLY JOURNAL OF MEDICAL SCIENCE.

| Vol. LVII. | Saturday, October 4, 1890. | No. 14. |

ORIGINAL ARTICLES.

THREE TYPES OF CEREBRAL SYPHILIS PRODUCING MENTAL DISEASE.

By C. M. HAY, M.D.,
ASSISTANT PHYSICIAN AND PATHOLOGIST TO THE STATE ASYLUM
FOR THE INSANE, MORRIS PLAINS, NEW JERSEY.

THE effects of the syphilitic poison upon the brain are so variously expressed that it is important to remember that mental disease is, at times, produced by syphilis without any physical symptoms being present to aid us in diagnosis. This is now a too well-authenticated fact to need particular emphasis. That syphilis is frequently overlooked, however, in cases of beginning insanity there is much reason to believe, and I will cite a case in which only the accidental discovery of the fact that the man had previously contracted syphilis led to correct therapensis. In certain rare cases of simple mental disorder following syphilis there is no local pain, convulsions, or significant cranial-nerve spasms or paralyses to indicate the presence of a gross lesion, and a clear specific history or the therapeutic test alone will indicate the real cause.

Commonly, however, the proofs of the existence of organic lesions of the brain or its membranes are not wanting, and a cranial-nerve palsy or spasm, a convulsive seizure, a sudden or gradual attack of hemiplegia, or violent local head-pain, with, perhaps, other neuralgic symptoms, will make us suspect that syphilis is the true cause of the patient's mental disorder. It is generally said that any form of mental disease may be the result of syphilis, and yet the *rôle* that the latter plays, particularly in the production of general paralysis of the insane, has been, and is to-day, still wholly unsettled, some authors rating it as a very prominent, and others as a comparatively insignificant, cause of that affection. That syphilis can produce a form of general paralysis which is curable is admitted by many. In connection with this, Professor H. C. Wood[1] writes:

"In conclusion, I may state that it must be recognized as at present proved that syphilis may produce a disorder the symptoms and lesions of which do not differ from those of general paralysis; that true general paralysis is very frequent in the syphilitic; that the only constant difference between the two diseases is as to curability; that the curable sclerosis may change into or be followed by the incurable form of the disease."

[1] Nervous Diseases and their Diagnosis, p. 463.

This view is also held by Griesenger, Mendel, Foville, Esmarch, Legardelle, Lamet, Rollet, and many other prominent clinicians. Another school maintains that the encephalopathies produced by syphilis are distinguishable from true general paralysis.

Therefore, although the question cannot be considered to be settled, still, in reading over the literature of this subject, it would seem that the burden of proof rests with those who, with Professor Wood, consider the syphilitic form indistinguishable from true general paralysis. Assuming this to be the case, the recognition of the presence of syphilis is, in all incipient cases of general paralysis of the insane, very important, and in all doubtful cases specific treatment should be adopted as the therapeutic test between the two forms of the disease.

Syphilis is, however, so constantly thought of in connection with general paresis that probably it very rarely escapes recognition, and I believe it is in the case of less marked psychoses that it is more likely to be overlooked as an etiological factor. The frequent inability to get a true history of the case and the remote period at which symptoms may occur are additional reasons for very careful exclusion of the syphilitic diathesis in all cases of obscure origin. In some cases that I have seen during the past two years the recognition of syphilis as the true cause of the mental disease has resulted in a complete cure of the patients, who, otherwise, were undoubtedly doomed to hopeless dementia; and the impressions received from the observation of those cases form the subject of this paper. It would seem, therefore, that the point cannot be too strongly insisted upon that, when rather atypical mental symptoms appear in a subject over twenty-five years of age, the presence or absence of syphilis should, if possible, be determined, especially when other apparent causes are wholly wanting, and that the therapeutic test should be applied, if syphilis cannot be otherwise excluded. No harm can be done to the patient by its careful application, and, if syphilis should be present, there will be, in the majority of cases, the most gratifying amelioration of all the symptoms, and perfect cures are by no means rare.

In the cases of syphilitic brain-disease that have come under observation in the New Jersey State Asylum a comparatively large proportion have exhibited a progressive dementia. In two cases this was very marked, and closely resembled an attack of that rare mental disease, primary dementia. There did not appear to be anything in the condition of these two cases to distinguish them from primary dementia. So that while differential points may be entirely wanting between certain cases of syphilitic psychosis and acute primary dementia, in the former there will usually be the history of syphilitic infection and the absence of any obvious exciting cause, such as sudden grief, fright, remorse, or exhausting illness. The different periods of life in which these two affections occur will also guide us; for, while primary dementia usually occurs before the age of twenty-five years, syphilitic mental disease is far more common after that age. Sex, also, should be considered, males being more subject to syphilis, while sex exerts little influence in the causation of primary dementia. These distinctions are by no means fixed, and the diagnosis between the two conditions must at times be difficult. Still, the above considerations usually furnish valuable hints as to the probable diagnosis, and combined with the therapeutic test they furnish a fairly adequate line of reasoning.

The following cases are taken almost at random from my notes, but they may serve to illustrate some types of syphilitic mental disease, other than general paralysis of the insane, which I have reason to believe, are of quite frequent occurrence:

CASE I.—Mr. R., aged forty years; married; native of New Jersey. Admitted, April 15, 1890. No hereditary predisposition to nervous or mental disease. No history of syphilis could be obtained on admission. His attack had commenced two months before with melancholia and a "numb feeling" in the head.

At the time of his admission his physical condition was good, and no local disease could be discovered. His mental condition was one of listless apathy; he would sit for hours with a perfectly expressionless face; he answered questions slowly and aimlessly, and appeared to take very little interest in his surroundings. He failed to comprehend conversation well, his replies being at times irrelevant and meaningless. After being aroused by a question he would immediately relapse into silence, with the same dull, vacant stare, and the eyes looking straight forward. It was learned that he had had an attack of "grippe" some time previously, and that at two periods—six and two years ago, respectively—he had had slight attacks of melancholia, which were attributed to some domestic trouble.[1]

For two months succeeding his admission he grew worse, dementia became more marked, and the probable diagnosis of primary dementia was made, when by accident it was discovered that the man

[1] Since the recovery of the patient he has informed me that those attacks were due to the knowledge that he was the victim of syphilis contracted eight years before his admission here.

had acquired syphilis. He was at once given potassium iodide, commencing with 30 grains three times daily and rapidly increasing the dose until 1 drachm three times daily was taken. He was kept upon these doses for a time, but at present he is taking 15 grains three times daily. The effects of this treatment were marked, and the improvement in the mental condition could be noted from day to day. Memory came back slowly, but surely; the face took on expression, and reasoning and judgment returned. He began to converse freely and intelligently, and the "slightly dead or numb feeling" in the head coincidently disappeared. To-day he considers himself in about his usual health, but he will continue to take the iodide for some time to come. In this case the mental disease corresponded exactly to some cases of primary dementia which have occurred here.

The next case exemplifies a more frequent type. In the preceding case a peculiar, drowsy dementia, with slight "numb feeling" in the head, were the only symptoms; but the class of patients of which the following is an example give a history of sudden or gradual hemiplegia, with or without aphasia, and if not preceded, usually followed, by convulsive phenomena. To what extent the mental symptoms are due to direct irritation from gross lesions, or, on the other hand, to a direct action of the syphilitic virus on the brain cortex, can only be conjectured, and it is of no practical importance to determine, for, with our present knowledge of the subject, there can be but one rational treatment for such cases.

CASE II.—Mr. S., aged thirty-one years; married; has no children; native of New Jersey; fairly educated, and a clerk by occupation.

Admitted, April 15, 1889, with the following letter from his physician: "Patient underwent treatment for primary syphilis about four years ago. One year ago he had a stroke of paralysis during the night, after a hard day's work, and since then has shown, at times, signs of mental derangement. The power of speech has not been good since then, and there is a tendency to cry and to be forgetful, and, of late, mental confusion and an inclination to wander away from home. He has also threatened suicide."

Examination on admission showed the following conditions: Medium-sized man, of light complexion, with pale, relaxed features and soft, flabby muscles. The left pupil was slightly smaller than the right. Field of vision, ocular movements, accommodation, and color-sense good. There was difficulty in speech, the pronunciation being jerky, uncertain, and irregular. The tongue protruded nearly straight, but was tremulous and clumsy in movement. There was inability to select proper words quickly, but if time were given the patient he could usually complete his thought. The right arm and leg showed marked incoördination of movement and a slight paresis of this side when compared with the left side of the body. A pin was picked from the floor awkwardly, and his writing was almost illegible, but the spelling was correct. The patellar-reflex was highly increased on the right side and slightly so on the left side. The sensations of pain, heat, and cold seemed normal.

The mental condition was one of melancholia mingled with a considerable degree of dementia. Memory was lost for recent events and much impaired for remote ones. He seemed to be in a hopeless, dazed, emotional state, with, at times, mental hebetude approaching complete dementia. He could, however, be readily roused into conversation, which he would, sometimes, carry on in a fairly intelligent manner. For several months prior to admission he had been wholly unfit for business, and frequently wandered off to distant cities, where he would be found, unable to explain his curious conduct. He had no delusions.

He was immediately given 30 grains of potassium iodide with $\frac{1}{24}$ grain of bichloride of mercury three times daily. During the first two months of treatment he showed little improvement, and had four convulsive seizures, affecting the right side of the body. After these seizures the aphasia and the incoördination and paresis of muscles were decidedly worse. The convulsions were ordinary epileptiform attacks, and were attended by no further eye-symptoms than those already noted. After this period the convulsions did not recur, and rapid improvement began. The mind cleared, speech became easy and natural, and the incoördination and paresis almost wholly disappeared from the right arm and leg. He remained under treatment three months after he considered himself fit for business, and was discharged, practically cured, December 14, 1889. I have since frequently heard from him, and he is still well and attending to business, having had no return of his mental or physical troubles. At his discharge he weighed thirty pounds more than on admission, his muscles were hard and complexion ruddy, notwithstanding the large doses of the iodide. The mercurial was omitted from the treatment after four months, when decided improvement had begun, and the potassium iodide was increased until, at one time, he was taking 200 grains daily. Regular out-door exercise constituted an important element in treatment while the patient's mind was returning to its normal condition. At no time did symptoms of salivation or iodism appear.

The case just detailed is instructive in showing the good effects of long-continued large doses of anti-syphilitic remedies in such cases. Had the treatment been abandoned as useless after the first two months, during which time convulsions and no perceptible improvement gave a hopeless aspect to the case, it is only fair to presume that the patient would have gone rapidly downward, and that a long terminal dementia, or death from exhaustion or in a fit, would have been the end. Hence, persistent treatment should be adhered to for months, even if improvement does not occur.

The last case that I will describe is one of a class having very definite symptoms of organic lesions, which usually appear gradually, and may be preceded, accompanied, or followed by mental disease. The case also illustrates the remarkable improvement which will sometimes follow huge doses of specific remedies under apparently desperate circumstances. Another important lesson taught by this case is that death is frequently due to neglect of treatment. which, in the present instance, afforded us an autopsy. There is no doubt that a final recovery would have occurred in this case also, had his medicine been continued for a sufficient length of time. The failure to carry out treatment is a frequent cause of relapse in such cases, and patients cannot be too emphatically told of the risks they run in neglecting to follow a long course of treatment after all active symptoms have passed away.

CASE III.—Mr. C. Y., aged thirty-nine years; native of New Jersey; a plumber by occupation, and with no trace of mental or nervous disease in his family history. His previous diseases were only those incident to childhood and youth. He contracted syphilis at about the age of thirty-four years.

Thirteen months before admission he began to show mental symptoms consisting of causeless melancholy, unstable temper, with emotional periods. when he would cry over some imagined woe. He became restless, roamed about the town, and worked only fitfully at his trade. He was utterly disheartened, especially in the mornings. With these symptoms, memory rapidly failed, and at his admission to the asylum, November 5, 1888, it was almost entirely gone. He also lost in weight. On June 7, 1888, he had a slight stroke of paralysis, affecting the right side, and after this, mental deterioration was more rapid. He imagined that his mother was dead, and various other delusions also occurred at this time.

For the following notes of his condition, shortly after his admission, I am indebted to my friend, Dr. L. L. Mial, under whose care the patient was, until December 1, 1888, when I first saw the case. Dr. Mial informs me that, beginning with violent pain in the left frontal region, there was progressive paralysis, occurring as follows: Partial ptosis of left eyelid, gradually becoming complete, accompanied with external strabismus and, later, with dilatation of the pupil of the same eye; then paresis, deepening into paralysis, of the left arm, and after the arm, the left leg became similarly affected. Sight remained good. Sensation was normal. The face and tongue were unaffected. His speech-memory was absent. Dr. Mial placed the patient on the mixed treatment, and by the time he came under my care, December 1, 1888, he had nearly recovered from his paralysis, and intellection was fairly good. The treatment was continued, and two months later he passed from observation, nearly cured mentally and physically.

Through neglect he did not continue to take the remedies prescribed, and he returned, March 1. 1889, with extensive paralysis, which had commenced a few days previously. First, the left arm became "numb," and memory completely failed; on the following day the left arm was completely paralyzed, and the left leg was "very cold," while, at the same time, the right arm showed decided weakness. On the third day the bladder was paralyzed and the right arm was flaccid, and the day following the development of these symptoms the right leg was paretic. On March 7, 1889, the man was almost completely paralyzed, the only exceptions being the face and tongue, and the right leg, which could be very feebly moved. Elsewhere the paralysis was perfect and complete. Rapid emaciation had occurred prior to the paralysis, and on admission he was in a very feeble condition. He was placed upon general tonics, with stimulants and potassium iodide 40 grains, with biniodide of mercury $\frac{1}{16}$ grain, three times daily.

March 11. Right hand can be feebly extended. Urine drawn. Iodide increased to 50 grains three times daily. Areas of anæsthesia were noted over chest and abdomen and left extremities.

16th. Moves right arm, hand, and leg slightly, and slight voluntary movements of left hand can be performed. Left leg still completely paralyzed. Pupils nearly equal in size, but the right is slightly more dilated than the left; both react to light. Temperature, 99°–102½°. Pulse weak, 100, and occasionally drops a beat. Urine acid; specific gravity 1020; no albumin or casts; contains excess of phosphates.

19th. Power in right side increased. Left arm can be raised from the bed, but movements of the wrist or fingers are not performed. Mental condition is one of stupor, from which he can be easily roused and made to answer questions intelligently. Memory totally gone; cannot remember my name longer than two or three seconds. Biniodide of mercury omitted from treatment. Tongue, heavily coated, is protruded well, and does not deviate. Fever continues. Sight remains unaffected.

31st. The same amount of fever and paralysis.

April 4. Muscular power is fairly good on right side, and there has been decided gain in left arm. Wrist- and finger-movements are now feebly performed. Pupils equal and of about the normal size. Bedsores forming.

18th. No change in paralysis. Abscess of right thigh evacuated of about a pint of apparently gummatous pus. Extensive bedsores. Patient failing.

25th. Patient died to-day, from exhaustion.

Autopsy: Calvarium very thin and brittle, diploë diminished. Dura abnormally adherent to the bone. A slight excess of cerebro-spinal fluid. No marked atrophy of brain, and no gross lesion of the cortex. Weight of brain, 41 ounces. In the left hemisphere, and involving the anterior third of the optic thalamus, was an area of bright reddish-yellow pigmentation surrounding a dark centre, the whole being nearly the size of a silver dollar. The dark centre, the size of a five cent piece, was situated in the anterior end of the optic thalamus, and consisted of broken-down brain-substance infiltrated with blood, and, under the microscope, disorganized brain-tissue, blood-coloring matter in masses, and

the products of fatty metamorphosis were seen. In the left crus, just above and including the point of exit of the third nerve, was a patch of similar color, but without any broken-down area, the deep pigmentation being the only macroscopic appearance. Microscopically, abundance of pigment-granules, with numerous round-cells infiltrating the area, were seen. The nerve-fibres appeared to be separated in places by aggregations of these cells. No notable destruction of the fibres was detected.

In the right hemisphere, just beneath the floor of the lateral ventricle and between the optic thalamus and the caudate nucleus, was an abscess, three-quarters of an inch antero-posteriorly and half an inch in width. This involved the anterior extremity of the optic thalamus only to the extent of a line, and was thus situated somewhat more anteriorly than the lesion on the left side. It involved the fibres of the anterior segment of the internal capsule from the knee forward for a distance of three-quarters of an inch. The abscess was about three-eighths of an inch deep. Surrounding it was an area of red softening about three lines wide, and outside of this zone was another of bright reddish-yellow pigmentation exactly similar to the condition found in the left hemisphere. Microscopically, the contents of the abscess were found to consist of compound granule-cells, broken-down nerve-tissue, pigment-granules, and granular débris, with cells resembling ordinary pus-corpuscles.

With the exception of increased adherence to the bones of the skull and a little thickening along the vertex, the dura was normal.

The arachnoid was generally slightly opaque. The pia was not adherent to the brain-substance anywhere and presented only increased vascularity. The brain-substance, and particularly the cortex,[1] were congested. No other gross lesions were discovered in the brain-substance.

The vessels showed marked thickening of the internal coat, and the left, middle, and anterior cerebral arteries were especially affected. In places the calibre of the vessels was notably diminished.

The post-mortem changes found in this case would seem to explain fully the paralytic symptoms that existed during life. The remains of the lesion of the left crus, revealed at the autopsy only by deep pigmentation and the results of what apparently had been an inflammatory condition, probably originated from the extensive disease of the vessels— syphilitic endarteritis. The three lesions found seemed exactly similar in nature and differed only in degree. The one in the right hemisphere was the most destructive, producing an abscess; the one in the left hemisphere was of less serious consequence to the brain-substance, a small necrotic area in the anterior part of the optic thalamus being its result, while the appearances around both of these lesions were identical and corresponded exactly to

---

[1] Microscopical examination of the cortex has not yet been completed, but will probably appear in the next annual Pathological Report of the New Jersey State Asylum for the Insane.

the area of the left crus which has been described. Whatever the process of formation of these lesions— and the appearances certainly strongly indicate the presence of at least a reactive inflammatory process —there can be little doubt that the attack of ocular paralysis on the left side, with left brachial monoplegia, was due to the lesion in the crus, with, of course, the possibility that at the same time the lesion in the right hemisphere also participated in the causation of the left-arm paralysis. The prompt treatment which the patient underwent at that time apparently had the effect of so modifying the crus-lesion that nerve-conduction was restored, as was shown by the disappearance of the paralytic symptoms and the patient's recovery at that time. The nearly symmetrically situated lesions of the hemispheres sufficiently explain his last and fatal attack and the bilateral paralysis. While the left arm regained a little motion, the left leg remained completely paralyzed until death; this is interesting in view of the more extensive lesion of the right internal capsule, half the diameter of which must have been included in the abscess-cavity. That the right side recovered power is only what would be expected in looking at the lesion of the left side, which scarcely interfered with the internal capsule, except by a zone of pigmentation.

The local severe frontal pain, complained of during his first attack, in November, 1888, is not explained by the post-mortem examination. Reasoning from the appearance of the lesion in the right hemisphere, and from the crus-lesion, which was evidently older, I am inclined to the belief that the latter was mainly responsible for the symptoms occurring in November, 1888, and that the two other lesions were coincidently developed, the right one being more extensive and serious in its effects upon the brain. Taking into consideration the extensive arterial lesions present, it does not seem unlikely that the primary pathological process was thrombosis, with secondary reactive inflammation and softening. This view is somewhat supported by the symmetry of the lesions.

These three cases, I think, are pretty fairly illustrative of the types of syphilitic brain-disease combined with mental disease to which I have referred. Other syphilitic manifestations, of course, occur in conjunction with insanity, and I have selected these three types only because common ones, and also because they illustrate the good effects of early and persistent anti-syphilitic treatment. The class of cases illustrated by Case I., and, to a less degree, by Case II., would seem the most important from the standpoint of diagnosis, for early treatment is all-important as regards the cure of the patient. In many cases sudden hemiplegia is the first symptom noticed by the patient, and when this occurs in a comparatively young man there is reason for suspicion.

The practical conclusions suggested by the observation of these cases are as follows :

1. That primary mental disorder following syphilis can often be completely relieved by energetic anti-syphilitic treatment.

2. That it is of vital importance that the patient continue under treatment for not less than one year after active symptoms have ceased.

3. That in some cases of bilateral paralysis the cause is bilateral syphilitic lesions of the internal capsules.

INCREASE OF HYPEROPIC ASTIGMATISM.

BY EDWARD JACKSON, M.D.,
PROFESSOR OF DISEASES OF THE EYE IN THE PHILADELPHIA POLYCLINIC.

THERE is little reason to doubt that, as is commonly believed, in the great majority of eyes the amount of astigmatism remains the same throughout life. That in progressive myopia, changes in the shape of the eyeball should to some extent involve the cornea, and so cause changes in the amount or direction of the astigmatism, was rather to be expected, and the expectation has been justified by reported cases. At one of the early meetings of the American Ophthalmological Society Dr. O. D. Pomeroy described the case of an artist who seemed to have acquired a myopic astigmatism from straining his eyes at portrait-painting.

Increase of hyperopic astigmatism is, however, a different matter. Here we are not led to expect the changes in the shape of the globe that attend the increase of myopia; although cases reported by Risley and Norris show that diminishing hyperopia may be essentially the same morbid process as increasing myopia.

In 1885 Dr. S. Theobald reported to the Ophthalmological Society three cases of astigmatism markedly increased after intervals of some years, of which one was hyperopic. And although the latter case was that of a young man whose eyes had not been submitted to the influence of a mydriatic at each examination, it is probably a case of the kind now under consideration. Two years ago Dr. J. B. Emerson reported to the Society a very striking case of this kind; and at the recent meeting of the American Medical Association Dr. O. B. Frothingham reported a similar ease.

My attention was drawn to the subject by the increase of three-fourths of a dioptre in my own compound hyperopic astigmatism. I have since noted seventeen cases which are elsewhere detailed, being all the cases that I have met with in private practice in which the change of astigmatism in either eye

[1] The substance of a paper read before the American Ophthalmological Society. July 17. 1890.

amounted to 0.5 D. or over, the refraction having in each instance been carefully and repeatedly measured under full mydriasis.

In all of these cases the balance and strength of the ocular muscles were carefully and repeatedly tested. In several of them no tendency toward deviation of the visual axes was discovered ; in most of the others apparent tendencies of this kind disappeared under the constant wearing of correcting lenses for the anomaly of refraction. In only one was there a marked, persistent tendency of this kind —esophoria. My observations, therefore, do not indicate any special relation between defects of the extra-ocular muscles and increase of astigmatism.

It would be very interesting to know something of the frequency of these cases relatively to the whole population, but my series of seventeen cases throws no positive light on the subject. One cannot estimate what proportion of his patients would return to him should there be a recurrence of their asthenopia, or other symptoms, after the lapse of four and a half years, the average interval in these cases. I have on my records a large number of cases that came to me from competent colleagues with glasses that did not correct the hyperopic astigmatism that their eyes presented. And, doubtless, my colleagues have on their books cases coming from me in a similar condition. Then there are, probably, many in whom the change of 0.5 D. in the astigmatism of one or even of both eyes has not led to a recurrence of asthenopia or other annoyance, for there are many in the community who do not have trouble from that amount of original error of refraction.

Should I hazard a guess at the frequency of these cases of progressive hyperopic astigmatism, it would be that they constitute about two per cent. of all cases seeking relief on account of anomalies of refraction. The cases in which, after the lapse of an equal length of time, the use of a mydriatic has shown me no change in the amount of astigmatism, outnumber them very decidedly ; and cases of mixed and myopic astigmatism are relatively, not absolutely, more frequently progressive.

It is of interest to note that no case of regressive astigmatism was encountered, none in which the astigmatism diminished so much as half a dioptre. But it is not improbable that such cases do occur.

It seems probable that progression of astigmatism is determined in some cases by the chronic congestive and inflammatory conditions allied to those of progressive myopia ; but acting rather on the anterior segment of the eyeball, and determining a change in the shape of the cornea. But, while the change in the shape of the cornea may thus be caused by distention, the normal gradual increase of hyperopia, which Priestley Smith has shown to be due to the gradual increase in the size of the crys-

talline lens, would cause the change in refraction to be, chiefly, in the direction of increased hyperopia in all meridians, as was observed in most of my cases.

In many of the cases there is a clear history of renewed symptoms of congestion or chronic inflammation, coincident with the change in the amount of astigmatism, quite similar to those which occur in progressive myopia ; and in six of the cases there was actual diminution of the hyperopia in one principal meridian of one or both eyes. The condition of impaired nutrition in the ocular coats might be part of some general impairment of nutrition, though none of the cases is noted as giving a clear history of such general ill-health (a history very frequently obtainable in conical cornea) ; or it may arise from eye-strain due to unusual exertion of the eyes, of which there was a clear history in several cases, or from uncorrected hyperopia due to the normal increase of the lens.

On the other hand, it is likely that in some of these cases the increase in astigmatism is directly due to an unsymmetrical increase in the bulk of the lens, causing more rapid increase of the hyperopia in some meridians than in others. The binocular symmetry of the increase, in certain cases, points toward an individual developmental tendency ; while the blood-relationship between some of the patients seems to indicate a family tendency in others. Thus, two of the patients were brothers, two were sisters, and two were first cousins, and in each pair of relatives the astigmatism was progressive at about the same period of life, and in about the same meridians.

From this series of cases we must conclude that liability to change in the amount of astigmatism is not confined to any particular period of life, though such changes are more frequent in early life. My study of the subject leads me to these conclusions :

1. Astigmatism is by no means constant in degree, though decided changes are exceptional.

2. Changes in its amount, and slight changes in the direction of its principal meridians must be looked for. These changes are not due to muscular defects nor confined to any particular period of life.

3. When a patient comes with lenses prescribed some time previously by a colleague, and which do not now correct the ametropia, we must not jump at the conclusion that these lenses were inappropriate at the time they were ordered.

A CASE OF EXTRA-UTERINE PREGNANCY. WITH SPONTANEOUS RECOVERY.

By LESLIE DEWEES, M.D.,
OF SHELBYVILLE, MO.

On May 11, 1887, I was called to see Mrs. K., thirty-four years of age. She was tall and slender, weighing 130 pounds before her illness. She had been married twice, and was a multipara. Her health previous to April 15th was good, though her menses sometimes appeared at intervals of a fortnight. About April 15th, slight pain and soreness were felt in the right ovarian region. The pain at first was only occasional, but soon became constant and severe. The menses, expected at this time, did not appear, and the pain and soreness steadily increased for two weeks before medical aid was sought.

About two weeks after what should have been the menstrual period—the time at which the pain and soreness were first noticed—the patient discovered a small tumor at the seat of pain. The alarm caused by this discovery induced her to send for a physician, who, after examination, concluded that the menstrual flow was obstructed, a condition that he endeavored to relieve by the use of tents, probes, etc. Several efforts were made with this object in view. The physician at this juncture failing in the regularity of his attendance, the writer was called until the former should resume charge of the case.

My first call was made on May 11, 1887, when I found the patient with a pulse of 120, temperature 102° F., and respiration 28. Anorexia, headache, and pain in the back were prominent symptoms. Pain and formication in the right hip and lower extremity were also complained of. Frequent micturition with a burning sensation, and constipation seemed also to cause considerable annoyance.

Palpation revealed the existence of a tumor the size of an orange, situated to the right of and posterior to the uterus. There was cellulitis, which was circumscribed, or at least chiefly to the right of the median line. The constipation was only partly relieved at this time by the use of enemata.

Her physician now returned, and I did not see the case again until May 26th, when I saw her in a consultation with Dr. A., and learned that on the previous day Drs. M. and O. had seen the patient, and decided that nothing could be done for her more than to administer palliatives. At the time of this visit the patient was excited, and had a high temperature, quick, wiry pulse, rapid respiration, and seemed fearful that an operation of some kind was contemplated. She was decidedly emaciated. The tumor seemed almost centrally located, as large as a small cocoanut, but flattened upon and attached to the uterus, so that no line of separation could be felt between the tumor and that organ.

Complete occlusion of the bowel had existed for several days, and this condition was relieved with the greatest difficulty by means of a soft rubber catheter attached by a piece of tubing to the nozzle of a hand-ball syringe. By means of a long, flexible probe the catheter was passed beyond the tumor. Through this apparatus a half-pint each of sweet oil and soapsuds were injected, and within half an hour a large quantity of liquid fæces was passed, greatly to the relief of the patient.

The speculum revealed an open os, with the lips everted and patulous. A sanguino-purulent discharge came from the cavity of the womb. Much irritation was present from the former use of tents. The uterus was somewhat enlarged, and the fundus 14*

was displaced forward and toward the left side. The cavity of the uterus was increased in proportion to the size of the organ, and was markedly convex on the side next to the tumor.

An operation appeared out of the question, unless the inflammatory condition should subside and the patient greatly improve. Attention was, therefore, given to the cellulitis and the general condition, with the hope of operating subsequently. However, consent was never obtained for the performance of an operation.

But little change took place from the date of the above-mentioned visit until near the middle of July, except that the patient became weaker, and perhaps the tumor grew a little larger.

The cellulitis, which, up to this time, was diffuse and severe, began to grow less, and the temperature was lower. Profuse sweats, with an occasional chill, occurred during the latter part of July. The bowels were relieved by the use of enemata when necessary. Micturition was frequent. The urine was scanty, and contained some pus. Operation was still declined by the patient. On August 1st, after having taken an enema, and during an effort to evacuate the bowels, there was a sudden gush of about two quarts of pus and liquid fæces, which materially reduced the size of the tumor. In the pus were found numerous epiphyses, about the size of tomato-seeds, for which they were mistaken by the patient. I was at once notified of this occurrence, but did not see the patient. None of the larger fœtal bones were discharged, except two or three ribs. The tumor refilled, and in about three weeks again discharged through the rectum, but the amount of pus was less, and there were fewer epiphyses.

After this, pus continued to flow from the bowel till about October 1st, when it ceased, and the tumor began to enlarge. For a time, but rather more slowly than before. About December 25th, the tumor showed signs of pointing in the vagina to the right of the cervix, and a few days later it opened spontaneously, discharging a large amount of pus, and several fœtal ribs, about 1¼ inches long, an ulna, and portions of other bones.

I saw the patient again, January 1, 1888, when one of the parietal bones was arrested in the vaginal opening of the pus-cavity, and by its sharp edge was producing much pain. Under an anæsthetic I succeeded in removing this bone, with several others. Owing to the patient's condition all the bones within the sac could not be removed at this time. For a month after this, bones continued to be discharged. The patient's general condition now began to improve, and when I saw her again, on April 22d, she was able to sit up for an hour daily. The appetite was good, the action of the bowels free and regular.

Micturition, however, was still frequent, perhaps due to the contractions of the tissues about the bladder. The tumor had now nearly disappeared, though a hard cicatrix could be felt in its former place. The larger bones, which had been carefully saved, were counted at this time, and all but two or three were found, and it is probable that these had been lost.

The opening from the sac into the vagina had closed, and aside from the possible continuance of the frequent micturition, together with a tendency to the opium-habit, recovery seemed probable.

On May 12, 1888, I again saw the patient, who could then walk without fatigue, but could not stand erect, which she said was due to a "drawing" sensation in the lower part of the abdomen. She weighed about as much as before her illness.

March 4, 1889. The patient had been complaining of a cutting, or stinging, sensation near the median line and half way between the umbilicus and symphysis pubis, and which she thought was caused by another bone, but which on careful examination I found was caused by a tense condition of the tissues. This tension was probably due to cicatricial contraction, and was distinct only when the spinal column was straightened, or bent backward. On flexing the thighs upon the abdomen the cicatrix could be felt, and was not sensitive to pressure.

The uterus was displaced upward so far that it could not be felt with the finger, and could be seen only by dilating the vagina with a pair of forceps passed beyond a Cusco's speculum. The vagina was also much narrowed by the upward traction of the cicatricial tissue.

It was, of course, impossible to determine in this case at what part of the tube the ovum lodged, and there was nothing which indicated the time that the rupture occurred. The latter fact might suggest that the pregnancy was abdominal, or extratubal, but from the previous active habits of the patient, together with the location of the tumor when first noticed, I deem this quite improbable.

It would be difficult to determine with any degree of accuracy the length of time that the fœtus lived, but the history and the size of the bones indicate that it died at about the end of the third month.

Doubtless, this case, like many others, might have been cured by an early abdominal section, but after the development of the inflammation there seemed to be no time at which an operation could be safely undertaken.

THE PRODUCTION OF IMMUNITY WITH THE CHEMICAL SUBSTANCES FORMED DURING THE GROWTH OF THE BACILLUS OF HOG-CHOLERA.

BY E. A. v. SCHWEINITZ, PH.D.,
CHEMICAL LABORATORY, BUREAU OF ANIMAL INDUSTRY, DEPARTMENT OF AGRICULTURE, WASHINGTON, D. C.

As a continuation of the preliminary paper on the ptomaïnes from the hog-cholera germ, presented by us to the Chemical Section of the American Association for the Advancement of Science, in August, and published in THE MEDICAL NEWS, September 6, 1890, we present now a somewhat detailed account of the successful experiments in the production of immunity in guinea-pigs which have been made up to date. The work from this standpoint again is of course a practical continuation of the experiments of Drs. Salmon and Smith, made upon pigeons in 1887, in which sterilized culture-media were used for preventive inoculation. We refer further to the bulletin of the Bureau on "Hog-cholera," published in 1889, in which are recorded a number of experiments upon hogs, sterilized culture-media being used for the purpose of producing immunity.

This work of Drs. Salmon and Smith was the pioneer work in preventive inoculation with other than some form of the germ of the disease itself, and the work now recorded was of course under the advice and direction of Dr. Salmon as head of the Bureau of Animal Industry. Without the careful bacteriological study of hog-cholera which has been made by the Bureau of Animal Industry, our work would have been impossible. For our laboratory experiments guinea-pigs were used, as being convenient to handle and susceptible to hog-cholera. They have proved very satisfactory. The material used for inoculation was prepared in the chemical laboratory by modifications of methods already described, and by other methods which will be explained in more detail at some future date. The testing of the materials used, to determine that they were free from germs, and the greater part of the preventive inoculations, were made by Dr. Moore, with such quantities of substance and at such times as we thought best. The autopsies were also made by Dr. Moore, and the work thereby greatly facilitated.

As to the name which should be given to the ptomaïnes and albumins from the hog-cholera culture-liquids, until their chemical constitution is more thoroughly studied, it would seem best, as there are several distinct swine-diseases, to call the ptomaïnes from the hog-cholera germs, as a class, *Sucholotoxins*, and the ptomaïne which appears to be the principal factor *Sucholotoxin* (from the Greek Σῦς, a hog, Χολέρα, cholera, from Χολή, bile, and *toxus*, poison). *Sucholo-albumin* would seem to be sufficiently distinctive for the albumin of these culture-liquids. As Hankin [1] shows, the name *toxalbumin* is hardly the correct one to apply to these substances. We shall, therefore, refer to the ptomaïnes and albumin by the names given above.

The first of our experiments that we will record were made with sucholotoxin.

EXPERIMENTS I.—Two guinea-pigs, each weighing about three-fourths of a pound, were treated with a solution of about 0.05 gramme of sucholotoxin each. The solution was introduced under the skin of the inner side of the left thigh. Immediately after the operation the animal appeared uncomfort-

[1] British Medical Journal, 1889, p. 810.

able, but was not made ill. For a few days there was a rise in temperature and also a slight swelling at the point of inoculation, which, however, disappeared in about five days, and the animal was then well.

Two more guinea-pigs were now selected as checks, approximately of the same size and weight as those which had been treated, and the four animals were then inoculated with 0.1 c.c. of hog-cholera virus each (0.1 c.c. beef-infusion and peptone culture one day old, plus 0.2 of sterile, normal salt solution). This is the dose which previous experiments made in the Bureau had shown to be the proper quantity to kill a guinea-pig in from eight to ten days. The inoculations with the virus were also made subcutaneously in the thigh. The checks died in eight and nine days. Post-mortem examination showed a large swelling at the point of inoculation, infiltration of a purulent, grayish substance into the connective tissue, and necrosis of the superficial layer of the muscles of the thigh. Enlargement and reddening of inguinal glands. Peyer's patches enlarged and pigmented; liver pale and covered with a number of necrotic foci; spleen very much enlarged, dark-colored, and friable. Cover-glass preparations from the spleen and liver showed hog-cholera germs. This was the characteristic appearance of all the check guinea-pigs upon post-mortem examination, and it will not be necessary to repeat these details.

Of the animals which had been first treated with the substance mentioned, and afterward inoculated, one died two days after the last check. Autopsy revealed the following: At the point of inoculation in the left thigh the subcutaneous tissue was infiltrated with a grayish-white substance, and the superficial layer of muscles over the inner side of thigh, and 4 square centimetres of the abdominal wall were necrosed. Liver pale. Spleen much enlarged, dark-colored, and friable. Cover-glass preparations from the spleen showed a large number of hog-cholera germs. Both ventricular walls of the heart were light-grayish and very brittle (necrosed). The other guinea-pig of this set was quite ill for ten days, with a large swelling at the point of inoculation. This finally opened and healed and the animal was quite well within three weeks after the inoculation, and has continued so to date—five months.

EXPERIMENTS II.—The next series of experiments were made with sucholo-albumin from beef-infusion and peptone culture-media.

Two guinea-pigs were again selected and treated with about 0.008 gramme each of sucholo-albumin. There was a slight rise of temperature in the animals and the formation of a small, hard lump at the point of injection. This disappeared by the eighth day, and the animals were quite well. Two more guinea-pigs were now taken as checks, and all four animals

were inoculated with 0.10 c.c. of hog-cholera culture. The checks died within seven days. The post-mortem appearances were practically the same as those noted in the first series. The two guinea-pigs which had been treated with the sucholo-albumin died *ten* days after the checks. This indicates considerable resistance to the disease. Autopsy showed, at the point of injection with the albumin, the subcutaneous tissue thick and reddened. The animals were considerably emaciated. At the point of inoculation a cyst the size of a walnut, and composed of a grayish, purulent substance, was also found. The muscular wall surrounding this was sprinkled with punctiform hæmorrhages. Peyer's patches swollen and pigmented; mucous membrane of small intestine covered with a dry, yellowish, firm layer of mucus; stomach contained a considerable quantity of liquid; liver pale, and showed fatty degeneration; spleen slightly enlarged and dark. Cover-glass preparations showed no germs, but a culture made from the spleen showed hog-cholera germs. Beneath the peritoneum in the region of the spinal column, and in the mesentery was a considerable number of small grayish tubercles. Several other experiments were made by treating guinea-pigs with the albumin in varying quantities, all showing resistance, and subsequently immunity.

EXPERIMENTS III.—Three guinea-pigs were treated with sucholo-albumin, 0.1 gramme being given to each, subcutaneously in the thigh. The albumin for two of the animals was derived from cultures containing blood-serum, the albumose given to the third was from ordinary beef-infusion peptone culture. Ugly ulcers formed at the point of inoculation, which healed, however, in from ten to fourteen days, and the animals with the exception of a slight rise of temperature were well.

Two checks were again selected and the five animals were inoculated with 0.1 c.c. hog-cholera virus. The checks died respectively in eight and ten days from hog-cholera. The animals which had received the preventive treatment were slightly ill for a few days with swelling at the point of inoculation, which finally opened and then healed nicely, and within a week the guinea-pigs were well.

Three weeks after the inoculation, one of these animals was chloroformed and examined post mortem. Not the slightest scar could be discovered, all the organs appeared perfectly normal, and no germs were found.

EXPERIMENTS IV.—Four guinea-pigs were treated, two with a mixture of sucholotoxins, two with sucholotoxin and albumin. The injections were made as before, subcutaneously in the thighs, and at intervals extending over a period of four weeks. The sore caused by each injection was allowed to heal before the next one was made. After the animals had recovered from the last treatment two checks were selected, and the six were each inoculated with $\frac{1}{110}$ c.c. hog-cholera virus. The checks died, one in eight and the other in ten days, the post-mortem examination showing characteristic hog-cholera lesions. The animals having the preventive treatment were ill for about four days, those that received only the sucholotoxins being more dull than the others. There was also slight swelling at the point of inoculation with the germ, which subsided in ten days, after which the animals were perfectly well, and have remained so—four months.

EXPERIMENTS V.—Six guinea-pigs were inoculated for this experiment, two with solution of the sucholotoxin and four with a solution of the mixed sucholotoxins. The sucholotoxin solution produced only slight local lesions, while the mixed toxins caused ulceration at the point of injection which did not heal for two weeks. The treatment in this case again extended over a period of from three to four weeks. The animals having by this time recovered, the test-experiment with hog-cholera virus was tried. Four of the animals mentioned above were taken—two from each set—and also two checks, and the six were inoculated. The checks died in eight and nine days, the autopsies showing the characteristic conditions of death from hog-cholera. Those that had the preventive treatment were ill and dull for from four to six days after the inoculation. At the point of inoculation there was also some swelling and infiltration, very slight, however, compared with the similar swelling on the checks. In the treated animals the swelling sloughed and healed, and within ten days after the inoculation they were perfectly well. To test the resistance of the animals that had been treated by this method, to ordinary exposure the following experiments were conducted.

EXPERIMENTS VI.—Two guinea-pigs that had received the preventive treatment, two blanks—*i. e.*, animals that had received no treatment—and two check animals that were inoculated with hog-cholera virus were placed in one large cage. The checks became ill and died in eight or nine days from hog-cholera. During this time the cage was cleaned only three times, so as to give full and free opportunity for contagion. One week after the checks had died one of the blanks became ill, and died within ten days. The autopsy showed hog-cholera lesions. The second blank became ill a few days after the first blank succumbed, and died within thirty days. The animals which had the preventive treatment are now and have been quite well, though continually exposed for five weeks to every opportunity for contagion.

EXPERIMENTS VII.—These experiments are a step in advance of those already recorded, and although not quite so conclusive, indicate that the proper methods have been adopted.

A pure chemical compound prepared synthetically in the laboratory, was used for treating the guinea-pigs. Three animals were taken, and this compound was administered to them by the method already used. There was a slight rise in temperature of the animals and swelling and soreness at the point of injection. After this had healed these animals and two checks were inoculated with $\frac{1}{10}$ c.c. of hog-cholera culture. The checks died in eight and nine days. The animals which had been previously treated became ill, two dying five and six days after the checks. The third entirely recovered.

Post-mortem examination of the two that died showed the following: At the point of inoculation the skin had sloughed away over an area of 1 sq. cm. The superficial muscular layer was necrosed over an area of about 3 sq. cm. and to a depth of 1 mm., lymphatics in the fold of the knee much enlarged; Peyer's patches enlarged and pigmented; spleen *very slightly enlarged and not discolored;* kidneys reddened; lungs normal. Cover-glass preparation from the spleen showed a few hog-cholera germs. On both sides of the spinal column were several grayish tubercles, from $\frac{1}{4}$ to 2 mm. in diameter, lying just beneath the peritoneum. This material is being more fully tested, and experiments which promise to be successful are also being made upon hogs. Autopsies made from the animals of Experiments VI., three or four weeks after their recovery, showed that the parts were perfectly normal, not even a scar being left upon the skin, and the immunity produced was therefore *perfect.*

It is important to add that in all the experiments great care was taken that the solutions used were free from germs, cultures always being made. In cases in which the albumin is used this is particularly important. A single precipitation with absolute alcohol does not suffice to destroy the germs, and it is necessary to free the solution from germs by means of a Pasteur filter, or in some other suitable way. Therefore experiments made with material which has not been tested for germs are practically of no value. As to the poisonous character of the ptomaïnes, a single large dose is sufficient to kill a guinea-pig in from one hour to two days. The autopsy of a case of this kind is as follows: Liver, pale and fatty; subcutaneous tissue over abdomen, necrosed and infiltrated; muscle, soft and friable. Other organs apparently normal.

The experiments here recorded show:

1. That in guinea-pigs *complete immunity* from hog-cholera can be produced by *chemical inoculation.*

2. The sucholotoxins and sucholo-albumin are equally effective in this respect, and a mixture of

these two products gives greater immunity than either used by itself. The effect of the albumin in producing immunity from anthrax has already been pointed out by Hankin, his experiments being very successful.

3. The sucholotoxins given in large doses produce death. To produce immunity it is necessary that they should be administered in small quantities at a time and at frequent intervals, the system being in this way accustomed to the poison and enabled to resist it.

Further study in this interesting line of work is in progress.

The tabulated results of the foregoing experiments are appended :

They, with eight or ten companions, found a truck, used for moving stone, standing by the roadside. They got hold of it, some pulling and others pushing, and dragged it up a steep hill. Reaching the summit, they turned it around, got aboard, and let it go down. What the ultimate fate of all the adventurers was after they started on their journey down the hill we are unable to record, but a police officer, hearing the noise of the truck and the screams of the children, hurried into the field, to find the truck capsized near the foot of the hill, and two boys lying about midway down the declivity, both being unconscious, and one apparently dead. The Harlem Hospital ambulance was sent for, and, on its arrival, Dr. F. P. Hammond, the ambulance-surgeon, found W. P., the older boy, apparently moribund. He breathed only in gasps, at long

TABULATED RESULTS OF EXPERIMENTS IN PRODUCING IMMUNITY FROM HOG-CHOLERA IN GUINEA-PIGS.

Number of experiment.	Material used for treatment.	Hog-cholera Virus used for each animal	Number of animals used.	Number of checks.	Number of days between inoculation with Virus and death of checks.	Result in treated animals.
I.	Sucholotoxin . . .	0.10 c.c.	2	2	8 and 9	1 died in 11 days; 1 recovered.
II.	Sucholo albumin . .	do	2	2	7	Died in 17 days; great resistance.
III.	Sucholo-albumin . .	do.	3	2	8 and 10	Recovered; immunity.
IV.	1. Sucholotoxins . . .	do.	2			Recovered; immunity.
	2. Sucholotoxin and albumin	do.	2	2	8 and 10	
V.	1. Sucholotoxin . . .	do.	2			
	2. Sucholotoxins . . .	do.	2	2	8 and 9	Recovered; immunity.
VI.	Sucholotoxins . . .	do.	2	2 blanks	8 and 9	Blanks died in 18 and 30 days.
				2 checks		Others not affected; immunity.
VII.	Pure chemical . . .	do.	3	2	8 and 9	Two died in 13 and 14 days. Third recovered; immunity.

TWO CASES OF FRACTURED SKULL.

Recovery in One; Death from Chloroform in the Other.

BY THOMAS MANLEY, M.D.,
VISITING SURGEON TO THE HARLEM HOSPITAL, NEW YORK.

ALTHOUGH traumatic lesions of the cranial shell, in large cities, are of frequent occurrence, those of the kind here described are rarely seen. Both cases are singularly interesting in causation, age of the patients, location and similarity of the lesions, clinical history, pathological conditions, and in the state of the nerve-centres when the patients came under observation.

Now, that cerebral localization is being investigated with great care and minuteness, it is interesting to note how far experiments on the lower animals can be utilized for clinical purposes in man. And further, since the two Hyderabad Commissions have given their, rather conflicting, but, nevertheless, very full and exhaustive, reports on the lethal action of chloroform, it is timely to note precisely the phenomena which attend the mortal action of this drug on man.

The two boys who are the subject of this history were injured on the afternoon of June 11, 1890.

intervals; the pulse was absent in one wrist, and in the other only a feeble flicker could be detected. Respiration was stertorous; blood mingled with saliva was oozing from the mouth and nose, and there was a bloody fluid flowing from the left ear. Dr. Hammond vigorously stimulated the patient by hypodermic injections, sponged out the mouth, and douched the face with cold water. The little fellow gradually reacted, and in half an hour was in the ambulance.

The other boy, B J., lay on his back, bleeding freely from a wound of the head, and was also insensible. His general condition was not bad, and before he reached the hospital he regained consciousness.

In each case antiseptic dressings were immediately applied with as much care as possible.

I saw the cases three hours after they were admitted to the hospital. They were then perfectly conscious, but could not give a clear account of the accident. The older boy was still suffering from shock. His pulse was slow, 60 beats to the minute, and the pupils were markedly contracted. The outline of the features was regular, and the nose, ears, and lips of an ashy pallor. The extremities were cool, with marked, though not total, abolition of the reflexes. There were areas on the inner side of the thighs in which sensation was wholly lost, and others on the palmar surface of the hands where, though sensation was intact, mobility was lost. When asked to move a limb he did so slightly, but with great effort, and on one side only. He was somewhat deaf. Immediately behind the right ear there was a scalp-wound exposing the bone. There was free hæmorrhage from the nose, mouth, and left ear, and from the latter the blood was somewhat serous and straw-colored in character.

His condition indicated fracture of the base of the skull, probably with free hæmorrhage into one of the great cavities of the body.

He was brought into the operating-room, and, as a preliminary to the examination of the wound, we adopted the recommendation of Dr. F. S. Dennis, and shaved the entire scalp, in order that antisepsis might be more rigorously carried out. At the seat of injury we found a fracture which was almost circular, with its greatest diameter from before backward. The large disk of bone was driven into the brain, being wholly detached at its circumference. The position of the fracture was on a line with, and immediately behind, the concha of the ear. The skull surrounding the fracture was fissured in a radiating manner, the fissures extending backward and toward the base being the deepest and most widely separated. Considering the cranio-cerebral topography of the lesion, it was evident that the left lateral sinus was nearly in the centre of this depressed plate of bone, which was evidently a part of both the parietal and occipital bones.

The safest course to pursue was now a question which did not permit much deliberation. Whether, bearing in mind the close proximity of the large venous channel, it might not be safer to cleanse the parts thoroughly, and let the fracture alone—as, independent of the eyes, we had no distinctive indication of cerebral pressure—or whether it would not be better to trephine at once, were the questions which had to be decided. We all know that hæmorrhage from vessels within the skull is sometimes difficult or absolutely impossible to check. We know, too, that an aseptic blood-clot—if not large or within the brain—often undergoes disintegration, organization, or absorption, without causing serious harm. We know further—though, unfortunately, operators are loath to report such cases—that an operation to remove depressed bone, or large blood-clots, may in itself be fatal. I have had, in about one hundred and fifty fractured skulls which I have treated, two such cases.

In one we were removing a large fragment of bone driven into the brain, almost at the confluence of the cranial sinuses. The spicula of bone came out quite readily, but it was followed by a deluge of blood which could not be controlled. In the other case, I trephined above the ear, over the temporo-parietal articulation, for symptoms of compression following an injury. We came at once, upon a very large intradural coagulum. After I had gnawed away, with the rongeur, sufficient bone to remove the clot, I commenced to crush it gently with the fingers, working cautiously until I believed it was nearly displaced, when a jet of dark, tarry blood welled up from the bottom of the space

left by the clot. It came in torrents, and our compresses and hæmostatic forceps were useless. We had re-opened a large trunk which the clot had plugged, and it was fatal. I may add, that I have heard of similar disasters, in the hands of others, but they have not been published.

To return to the present case. I decided to try to elevate, as the fragment was driven in so far that I was able, by chipping off enough bone from the overlapping margin, to get my elevator between the dura and the skull, using the edge as a fulcrum. Happily, I was able to raise quite easily the fragment to its normal position. Very little blood was lost, and the wound, with the entire cranium, the neck, and the eyes, were enveloped in soft antiseptic gauze.

During the night, following the operation, the patient moaned, groaned, cried, and vomited. He had two or three sinking spells and became cold; but Dr. Guest, the house-surgeon, used heat and stimulants energetically, and the boy reacted.

I saw him at 10 A.M., June 17th. At this time it seemed that he could not recover. His pulse was 186, and his temperature subnormal, and he had the heaving respiration which Bell[1] has so well described, as a sure precursor of death. But by noon he commenced to rally and he has made a good recovery; although both pupils are dilated, and he has double convergent squint. Hearing has been perfectly regained and there is no trace of paralysis.

It is interesting to note that in this case we had almost unequivocal evidence of fracture through the base of the skull, and yet the patient made a good recovery, the only organic disturbance at this date being confined to the organs of vision.

Dr. Ferrier in his recent Croonian lectures on "Cerebral Localization," tells us that "the occipto-anterior region is the visual area of the cortex." It seems that this conclusion has been reached, mainly by experiments on monkeys and clinical observations on man. Considering the location of the lesion, in the case just described, and the marked disturbance of the visual organs, at the time of the injury and since, I think that the patient's condition is strong evidence in favor of the correctness and accuracy of the statement made by Dr. Ferrier.

There can be no doubt that considerable blood escaped into, and through the cerebral substance, and that, following the line of fracture, it ultimately lodged in close contact with the base of the pons Varolii and the corpus pyramidale, where, by pressure, it interfered with the nutrition and functions of the ocular nerves, notably and persistently with the abducens.

With the ultimate reduction and absorption of the effused blood, I expect perfect restoration of accommodation.

[1] Sir Charles Bell: Nervous System, second edition, p. 203.

The younger of the two boys, B. J., when I saw him, had a large hæmatoma directly behind the right ear, in precisely the same situation as the wound in the preceding case, except that the tumor extended slightly downward into the cellular tissue of the neck. The house-surgeon had made a diagnosis of fracture of the skull. The patient had almost no constitutional disturbance, but there had been nasal hæmorrhage. He did not complain of pain, and moved about in bed without difficulty. He was slightly pale, however, and vomited twice after entering the hospital.

The contour of the hæmatoma, with its firm, bevelled border and depressed centre—characters common to all cranial hæmatomata—and the total absence of any cerebral symptoms, led me to believe that there was no fracture.

The scalp over the swelling was shaved and cleansed, after which I made an incision into the tumor and evacuated it, when I found well-marked linear fractures; one running antero-posteriorly, intersected by another passing toward the base. The greatest extent of fracture was in the occipital bone, extending but two or three lines into the parietal. There was very slight depression of the upper boundary of the divided plate. Under strict antisepsis, I closed the incision with a continuous suture, and applied the usual dressing.

The following morning the patient was in excellent condition, and speedy recovery seemed probable. At noon of this day he vomited. At 2 P.M. the temperature was 102°. Internal squint of the left eye, varying in degree, was noticed, and the pupil was slightly dilated. He was able to urinate and had no paralysis of the extremities.

On June 17th it was noted that he had passed a restless night. At 8 A.M., temperature was 103½°, and at 10.40 A.M. was the same; at 12.30 P.M. temperature was 103¾°. At 1.20 A.M., June 19th, temperature was 103¾°; at 2 P.M. temperature was 104⅕°.

I saw him at 3 P.M. on this date. He now had well-marked symptoms of compression with meningitis. His pulse was very rapid, the temperature high, and he was incessantly moving about in the bed. Marked congestion of the conjunctival vessels clearly indicated cerebral hyperæmia.

His mental condition at this stage presented many features of interest. He would have intervals of repose, in which he would lie on his back, with his eyeballs immovably set and the lids widely opened, muttering incoherently to himself. Every few minutes he would arouse from this condition for a short time. When asked how he felt, he would look up, answer intelligently and complain of great pain throughout his head. Then he would immediately lapse into a semi-conscious condition with his eyes open.

It was only too apparent that serious mischief had resulted from the injury, but whether from local conditions, as the pressure of a shattered internal table, or of a clot, was difficult to determine. It was too early for pus to have formed.

I had recently seen two cases of traumatic meningitis in boys: one from fracture of the skull, the other from an infected scalp-wound. In both there were well-defined cortical lesions, with all the typical symptoms. On trephining these cases, however, nothing was found but a general meningitis, a diagnosis confirmed by autopsy.

In the present case, it seemed to me that there were no symptoms which could be relied upon as an indication to operate. Besides, in refraining from operating I followed the opinion of the veteran French surgeon Verneuil, who says : "Qu'on fasse dans le laboratoire toutes les expériences, qu'on vondra ; mais qu'on se garde les transportes au lit du malade."[1] This entirely harmonizes with my own experience.

I was anxious to ascertain the condition of the wound, and, if I found indications of incipient ostitis, to trephine, as recommended by Bryant.[2] My intention was to remove one or two sutures, inspect the line of incision, and reclose the wound without using an anæsthetic. But I found the tissues behind the ear puffed, œdematous, and discolored. On freeing two or three of the sutures I saw that the whole wound was in a bad condition. The edges were covered with a dirty grayish exudate, and were slightly everted, and the whole had an appearance indicative of disease beneath the bone.

As I saw that our operative procedures would be somewhat tedious, and as the patient was keenly sensitive to pain, and, excepting his temperature, in a good general condition, I decided to give him a few whiffs of chloroform, presuming that this would be taken with less resistance and more rapidly than ether, and that it would not congest the vessels of the brain.

Dr. F. P. Hammond, third assistant-surgeon of the hospital, an extremely cautious and painstaking man, administered the chloroform by sprinkling a few drops on lint placed in a tumbler. I had denuded the skull, and removed a piece of bone with a small trephine and rongeur, when I noticed, in an instant, several terrible changes. The patient ceased to breathe ; his features were black and bloated ; he foamed at the mouth ; the eyes bulged, and plainly he was asphyxiated. Feeling for the radial pulse, I was amazed to find it full, slow, and regular—about 60 to the minute. We had before us a genuine case of chloroform-poisoning, with all the symptoms which have been described by other authors and investigators.

The *respiratory centres yielded first.* This was clear and unmistakable. All our resources were immediately applied, namely, artificial respiration, inversion, inhalation of nitrite of amyl, hypodermic injection of atropine, drawing the tongue forward, douching of the face, and friction of the body. After an interval of what seemed five, though in reality not more than two, minutes, the patient gasped several times. A little later he breathed again, but very irregularly, and would cease unless artificial respiration were continued. Respiration seemed quite fairly reëstablished at one time. It was interesting

---

[1] Mercredi Médical. May 27, 1890.
[2] Surgery, third edition.

to note the condition of the brain in the meantime. With dyspnœa and apnœa the brain-tissue crowded into the gap made by the rongeur. The vessels were enormously distended, and of a deep black color. With partial return of respiration the brain gradually receded, and the vessels collapsed to their usual calibre and assumed their normal tint. I had noticed, however, before the symptoms of asphyxia developed, that the cerebral vessels were greatly distended.

No more chloroform was given after the first lethal symptoms were manifest.

Although respiration was partially restored, the deep cyanosis remained, the breathing continued stertorous, and frothy mucus, tinged with blood, oozed from the mouth. In about five minutes, or possibly a little longer, there was another break in the rhythm of the breathing. This time all our efforts were futile. As in the first instance, the pulse continued to beat fully two minutes after the patient was apparently dead, or rather had ceased to breathe.

Although I have witnessed the administration of ether and chloroform a great many times, this is the first case in which I have seen death immediately and directly attributable to the anæsthetic.

This case so clearly and absolutely proves that the lethal action of chloroform begins by benumbing the respiratory centres, that no one can question it. The condition is a veritable asphyxia. The phenomena, to the eye, are precisely the same as those seen in cases of spasm or stenosis of the larynx ; in persons who have been submerged in water, and in those struggling through an epileptic fit, when the laryngeal muscles are temporarily convulsed.

It was in the *initial* stages of anæsthesia that the respirations ceased, and after very little chloroform had been given. The vaso-motor nerves and the cardiac centres were affected *consecutively*. The blood, surcharged with carbonic acid, soon destroyed the vitality and irritability of the pneumogastric and sympathetic nerves.

Clearly perceiving, then, how the action of the drug manifests itself, we are in a position to deal with it intelligently. We should act with two objects in view : first, to unload the vascular system, and the brain ; and, second, to keep up respiration. It may be said that when breathing ceases the respiratory centres are paralyzed, and all efforts at resuscitation are useless.

But we see many cases which prove that this is not always true. A case of tracheotomy, for instance, reported by me in the *New England Medical Monthly,* January, 1890, is an illustration. In this case, after the trachea was opened, the patient inspired blood. He ceased to breathe, but the pulse continued to beat for some time. With the body limp and apparently lifeless, we worked fully five minutes with artificial respiration, when the patient gasped, and shortly revived, ultimately making a good recovery.

A surgeon related to me, how in a case of croup, he called in a consultant, who advised tracheotomy. Some blood was drawn into the windpipe, the infant had a terrible convulsion, and turned over apparently dead. The consultant, quite shocked at the result, and fearing the maledictions of the parents, immediately left. But the attending physician remained at his post, wiped out the bleeding opening, and with his own lips blew into the child's trachea. In a few moments—fully ten, he thinks—the child commenced to breathe, and finally made a good recovery.

In the case reported above, had we worked more diligently at renewing the air in the lungs, and given less attention to the incision, the result might have been different. But we were too confident ; besides, I had to search for and ligate a small meningeal vessel which commenced to spurt freely. When respiratory paralysis occurred for the second time, had we done a tracheotomy and used the invaluable apparatus of Dr. Joseph Fell, of Buffalo, for forced respiration, I am confident our patient might have been saved.

The unfortunate termination of this case has more strongly than ever convinced me of the imperative need of an experienced and trained anæsthetizer—one who will give his whole attention to administering anæsthetics ; a man of good judgment and who is solely concerned with the patient's general condition. He should be specially licensed, and the administration of an anæsthetic, other than in an emergency, by anyone not professionally and legally qualified should be regarded as a misdemeanor. The present custom is dangerous, and little short of being positively criminal. Usually the anæsthetic is committed to the junior assistant, who is almost wholly ignorant of practical work. He is often more interested in the operation than in giving the anæsthetic, so that when he finally looks into his patient's face, and feels the pulse, perchance the patient is dead. Let us hope that a reform in this matter will soon be accomplished.

The physical characteristics of the two fractures demand only brief mention. From a medico-legal point of view, they are full of interest, and also to those who may be called on, in a court of justice, to testify as to the quality and direction of force brought to bear in traumatic lesions of the skull.

It will be noted that the children were found alone and unconscious, in an open field. No one has been found who saw the accident, or at least who will admit that he saw it.

In each case, so similar were the osseous lesions in extent and direction, that it would certainly seem that they were inflicted with precision and deliberation. The violence must have been great and concentrated. Its point of impact was very limited, and chiefly in the direction of the base. There were no rocks in the place where the boys were injured. It is hard to conceive how these boys, of light weight, precipitated from a stone-truck, about two feet from the ground, to soft, elastic turf, could receive such injuries. Did the wheels pass over their necks or heads? There were no abrasions or contusions except those immediately over the wounds, and if the wheel had passed over their heads the wounds would have been larger.

Had not the boys regained consciousness, or had they been found dead, so that no history could have been obtained from themselves, the state of the integument, the shape, direction, and extent of the fractures would have thrown no light on the injury.

These cases would seem to prove that there are serious bone-lesions in which we are absolutely unable, from the condition of the parts, to say what was the nature of the force, or in what direction it was applied; hence the importance of the surgeon proceeding with great caution when giving testimony, on which great consequences or even a human life may depend, when such testimony is merely presumption or hypothetical premises.

REPORT OF A CASE OF SPONTANEOUS RECESSION OF A LARYNGEAL PAPILLOMA AFTER TRACHEOTOMY.

BY WARWICK M. COWGILL, PH. B., M.D.,
OF PADUCAH, KENTUCKY;
FORMERLY CLINICAL ASSISTANT AT THE NEW YORK OPHTHALMIC AND AURAL INSTITUTE.

MR. LENNOX BROWNE, in his work on *Diseases of the Throat*, under the heading of "Treatment of Benign Growths of the Larynx," warns against harsh methods in attempting their removal. He says:

"The number of persons to whom the advice to wait and watch is given, must be very small, but, without doubt, there is a very large proportion of cases which never require treatment, and, if left to themselves, never assume a serious aspect. There is no reason to doubt that while many of these formations remain thus stagnant a large proportion would, on no less authority than that of Virchow, if untreated, frequently disappear spontaneously, being subject, as they are, to slow atrophy and resorption."

Dr. G. Hunter Mackenzie,[1] of Edinburgh, has reported a case of spontaneous disappearance of laryngeal growths after tracheotomy.

"The case was that of a boy aged five years, who, in 1883, underwent tracheotomy for laryngeal stenosis from warty growths. The growths disappeared after the canula had been worn for a year. The canula was then removed and complete recovery ensued, and without the development of sequelæ."

I wish to add the following:
In the latter part of April, 1885, I was called in

---

[1] Lancet, April 6, 1889. Abstracted in the Journal of Laryngology and Rhinology, June, 1890.

consultation by Dr. John G. Brooks, of Paducah, to see Minnie B. I found a delicate, pale, little girl, six years of age, laboring for breath, inspiration being somewhat more difficult than expiration. I at once made a laryngoscopic examination. The child was making the fullest exertion in its power to inhale sufficient air to support life, and was naturally averse to any additional interference with respiration, so that it was impossible for me to get a good view of the larynx. But I was able to recognize an obstruction in the upper portion of the larynx. The nature of the obstruction I did not then attempt to determine, though I believed that it was a neoplasm. The history of the case was, briefly, that difficult breathing had been first noticed four years previously to this time—that is, when the child was but two years old—and that the difficulty had slowly increased up to the time of my examination. I advised tracheotomy to relieve the urgent dyspnœa, and as a preliminary step toward removing the obstruction.

On May 5th, a few days after I had first seen the child, I performed laryngo-tracheotomy, which gave instant relief to the obstructed respiration, and in a few moments the pale, bluish face and the blue lips were red with the now well-oxygenized blood. Not a bad symptom followed, and on the eighth day after the operation the child was allowed to return home, about five miles into the country.

As soon as she was sufficiently strong I had her brought to my office for further examination. At this time, with the aid of cocaine, I obtained an excellent view of the larynx. In the lumen of the larynx, above the vocal bands, was a pale-red, mulberry-like growth, about the size of a large filbert, and almost filling the cavity. From its appearance, slow growth, and the age of the patient, we arrived at the conclusion that the neoplasm was a benign papilloma. At this time, and afterward, I made repeated attempts to remove the growth with forceps, but the patient being so young, and much frightened by the instruments, I did not succeed in my attempts. After the ineffectual attempts to remove the growth *per vias naturales*, I suggested thyrotomy, but the parents strongly objected to any further cutting operation, as the patient seemed to be doing so well.

The child grew stronger and suffered but little inconvenience from wearing the tracheotomy tube. I, of course, admonished the parents as to the danger of the child breathing unwarmed air through the tube, and she was well protected from exposure to sudden atmospheric changes.

The condition of the case changed little, if at all, for about two years. At the end of this time, however, the mother believed that the child could talk a little more distinctly, and on examination, I thought I detected some diminution in the size of the growth. From this time on we waited and watched. The growth gradually receded until, in December, 1888, three years and eight months after the tracheotomy, the only remaining sign was a small papilla, about one line in length, projecting from the posterior wall of the larynx. The canula was then finally discarded, and the artificial opening was closed. Up to the present writing there is no sign of any return of the growth.

In concluding, I wish to call attention to the term *spontaneous*, as used in this report. Strictly speaking, it can hardly be said that the growth disappeared spontaneously, for if irritation of the mucous membrane is one of the most active causes in the production of papillomata of this structure, then the absence of irritation upon a papillomatous growth—or, in other words, rest, as was secured in this case, by tracheotomy—must have been an active agent in producing its recession.

MEDICAL PROGRESS.

Extra-uterine Pregnancy.—The following case, reported by BOISLIEUX, of Paris, in the *Nouvelles Archives d'Obstétrique et de Gynécologie* of August 25, 1890, was one of extra-uterine pregnancy at the third month, terminating spontaneously with the expulsion of the decidual membranes. The patient had been previously subject to pelvic peritonitis, and had been treated for this disease. Six years before the occurrence of extra-uterine pregnancy she was delivered of a living child after a normal labor. At the end of the third month in the extra-uterine pregnancy a few drops of blood were lost, and ergot was given to control the hæmorrhage, which, however, shortly returned, requiring a second administration of ergot and opium by injection twice a day. Some days later the patient appeared exsanguinous, the pulse was small—120 beats a minute, and there was great pain in the right groin ; the uterus was anteflexed, and the fundus was bound down and immovable, being incarcerated below the promontory of the sacrum. On palpation a distinct swelling could be found on the right side pressing down into Douglas's pouch.

The diagnosis made was that abortion was imminent, and, as a consequence, the ergot was stopped and the opiates continued; the vagina was also packed with iodoform-gauze. After this the pain in the uterus ceased, but persisted in the right groin. There was no trace of lymphangitis or œdema.

Several days later, after persistent pain for six hours, there was expulsion of the fœtus and membranes.

Microscopical examination of the membranes which were expelled showed that they were, beyond all doubt, derived from tubal pregnancy. The swelling in the groin rapidly decreased in size, and the woman ultimately entirely recovered.

Flushing the Bladder without a Catheter.—STAFF-SURGEON ROTTER, of Munich, recommends the following process of flushing the male bladder, which obviates the introduction of a catheter, and makes it impossible to introduce septic matter into the bladder. An irrigator, filled with a quart of some disinfecting, and perhaps slightly astringent, liquid, at a temperature of from about 82.5° to 86° F., having a tube six feet or more in length, with a perforated and somewhat pointed end—which, according to the size of the meatus, is covered with more or less gauze previously saturated

with the disinfecting fluid and greased with antiseptic vaseline—is used. For patients with a very small meatus a thin, gutta-percha drainage-tube a few inches in length is attached to the end of the tube, which is exhausted, and then completely filled with the warm fluid. The patient is told to micturate, if possible, and then to lie on his back, with his legs a little drawn up and his pelvis supported. The end of the tube is then introduced into the urethra to the depth of about an inch, and there held by the physician, who continually presses the glans against the tube. The irrigator is then raised, first three feet high, and then six feet, and in from half a minute to two minutes, or, in patients with a very strong sphincter, in three or three and a half minutes, the liquid begins to flow into the bladder. The amount used is easily determined if the irrigator is made of glass ; or, if not, by the vibration that is communicated to the corpora cavernosa. If it is intended to fill the bladder completely, percussion, the appearance of the bladder above the symphysis, and, in many cases, the patient's sudden desire to micturate, will give the necessary information.—*Lancet,* August 30, 1890.

Condurango.—In a paper published in the *Bulletin Général de Thérapeutique,* of August 30, 1890, GUYENOT, after a careful study of this drug, reaches the following conclusions :

1. In the form of a powder it is very efficient in the treatment of painful affections of the stomach, and particularly when they are due to ulceration or irritation of the mucous membrane of this organ.

2. In cases of cancer of the stomach, which have been reported as cured by condurango there has certainly been an error in the diagnosis, the real condition present being in all probability that of gastric ulcer.

3. The active principle of condurango has a curious and interesting action, for it produces a true experimental locomotor ataxia.

Guyenot recommends this drug in the following forms :

In powder it may be given in the dose of from a half to one drachm in capsules, or the tincture may be given in the following manner :

R.—Tincture of condurango   .   3 drachms
    Syrup of bitter orange peel . 2 ounces.—M.

Sig. A teaspoonful to a dessertspoonful three times a day ; or the bark may be made into an infusion by adding half an ounce to three teacupfuls of water and taking one teacupful morning and night ; or, a third method of administration consists in taking a half ounce of powdered bark, and adding thereto fifteen drops of hydrochloric acid, and adding to this five ounces of syrup of bitter orange. Of this last mixture a teaspoonful may be taken every two hours.

Use of Iodides in Infantile Scrofulosis. — Tincture of iodine may be administered to very young infants in the dose of a drop a day diluted with a small quantity of barley-water or milk. BESNIER uses iodoform in minute doses for the same purpose in infants.

Remedy for Dyspnœa.—HUCHARD states that aspidospermine, the active principle of *aspidosperma quebra-*

cho, is a useful remedy in the treatment of dyspnœa. When powdered it may be prescribed in the dose of one-half to one and one-half grains a day, or it may be injected hypodermically provided that the hydrochlorate is employed, the solution being made by adding seven grains of the drug to every two and a half drachms of distilled water.

Snuff for Coryza.—In the *Journal de Médecine de Paris*, ASCHMANN recommends the following powder in coryza:

R.—Finely-powdered naphthalin   6 drachms.
"   "   boric acid   6   "
Powdered camphor   .   .   15 grains.
Extract of violets   .   .   15   "
Essence of rose   .   .   10 drops.

To be used as a snuff in coryza.

The Human Body Forty Years under Water.—A very interesting report has just been issued by DR. KÖNIG, "Gerichtsarzt" (judicial physician) of Hermannstadt, on the state in which the human subject, after forty years' immersion in water, may be found by the physiologist. In the revolutionary upheaval of 1849, a company of Honvéds, as the Hungarian militia are called, having fallen in the vicissitudes of war, were consigned to the waters of the Echoschacht, a pool of considerable depth not far from Hermannstadt. Their bodies have recently been brought up to the light of day, and subjected to a careful and minute investigation from the physiologist's point of view. Dr. König found them in perfect preservation, without a single trace of any decomposing process. Externally, they had the appearance of having been kept in spirit. The epidermis was of a whitish-gray color; the muscles rose-red, feeling to the touch like freshly-slaughtered butcher's meat. The lungs, heart, liver, spleen, kidneys, bladder, stomach, and alimentary canal were of the consistence of those in a newly-deceased corpse; while the brain was hard and of a dirty gray color, as if preserved in spirit. Structurally, the organs retained their outline perfectly, and were so easily recognizable in tissue as well as configuration that, according to Dr. König, they might have been exhibited for "demonstration" in an anatomical lecture-room. After forty-one years under water these are indeed remarkable phenomena. The large intestine contained fæces of a yellowish-brown color, quite unaltered and inodorous; while the bladder was partially filled with straw-colored urine. But perhaps the most significant feature disclosed by these corpses is the following: In their interior a large amount of chloride of sodium, crystallized in cubes, had been deposited and fixed on the several tissues and organs, and this salt had not penetrated, mechanically, into the dead bodies from without. In the completely closed and perfectly unimpaired pericardium, and also on the outer surface of the heart itself, crystals of the same kind were found. This, according to Dr. König, clearly shows that, in the water, particles held in solution may pass through the skin and the muscles, and find their way into the most deeply-seated organs. Herein, he adds, we have confirmatory proof, if such were needed, that the specific virtues of mineral baths exercise in this way their salutary effect on the internal economy of the bather. There is a notable difference, however, between the time spent in the bath by an ordinary bather at a "Curort" and the forty-one years during which the Honvéds remained under water. The phenomenal quietness of the Echoschacht may also have been a material factor in this impregnation of the corpses with chloride of sodium. But, with every allowance for such considerations, Dr. König has furnished a striking illustration of the permeability of the immersed human subject to salts in solution, and we hope his painstaking researches will lead to others in the same important direction.—*The Lancet*, August 9, 1890.

On the Assimilation of Natural and Artificial Butter and Tallow in Healthy Persons.—In order to throw some light on this matter, DR. NIKOLAI F. FLORIN, of St. Petersburg, has carried out (*St. Petersburg Inaugural Dissertation*, 1890, No. 24, pp. 50) a series of elaborate and most careful comparative experiments on nine men (including himself) aged from 21 to 35 years, and a lady (the author's wife) aged 27 years. In each case the experiment lasted ten days, being divided into two periods of equal duration. In seven of the ten experiments, during one of the periods, artificial butter (obtained from a local manufactory and prepared after somewhat modified methods of Mége-Mouriès and Mott) and during the other period genuine butter was given. The remaining three persons were similarly taking artificial butter and tallow. Besides the fats, the dietary consisted of cooked meat, fatless beef-tea, thick gruel (*Kasha*), wheat or rye bread, the whites of eggs, tea, sugar and salt. The essential outcome of the researches may be given as follows: First. The assimilation of natural butter oscillates between 94.74 and 97.81 per cent. (of the fat ingested), averaging 95.89; that of an artificial butter, between 92 and 95.25, averaging 94.82; that of tallow, between 92.55 and 93.07, averaging 92.75. Second. Therefore artificial butter is not assimilated by healthy adults as well as a genuine one (the difference amounting to 2 per cent.), but better than tallow (at the rate of 1.91 per cent.). Third. Artificial butter is tolerated by healthy people quite well (if it is prepared of the best materials and under the strictest precautions in regard to cleanliness, etc.). Fourth. Nevertheless there is no necessity whatever for artificial butters—at least so far as Russia is concerned. Hence, the government should prevent the establishing any new butter factories, while exercising the strictest sanitary supervision of those already in existence.—*St. Louis Medical and Surgical Journal*, September, 1890.

Ointment for Pigment Spots of Pregnancy.—The following prescription for the treatment of cloasma of pregnancy is quoted by the *Revue de Thérapeutique*:

R.— Zinc oxide   .   .   .   .   1 drachm
White precipitate .   .   .   1½ grains.
Castor oil   .   .   .   .   2 drachms.
Essence of rose   .   .   .   10 drops.
Cocoa butter   .   .   .   2 drachms.—M.

Apply morning and evening.

The Relations between Quinine and Malaria.—The close association of malaria and hæmoglobinuria is undoubted, and in a series of attacks of tertian ague the earlier ones may be simple, and the later complicated with hæmoglobinuria. To the Italian physicians it is an important question whether the large doses of quinine that they are in the habit of giving do not induce hæmoglobinuria. TIRABOSCHI discusses the question and describes cases in which hæmoglobinuria began with the administration of 10 grains of quinine three times a day, and others in which the symptom disappeared under the same circumstances. He can find no cases of malarial disease in which quinine alone, without the factor of paroxysmal fever, produced hæmoglobinuria. Consequently he is inclined to attribute little or no influence to the drug in the causation of the symptom. He can trace no clear analogy between any action of quinine and what he considers the two chief sources of hæmoglobinuria, namely syphilis and cold.—*Practitioner*, September, 1890.

Induction of Premature Labor in Contracted Pelvis.—DR.

E. AHLFELD (*Centralblatt für Gynäkologie*, July 26, 1890) reviews his results of the induction of premature labor in 111 cases of contracted pelvis, and concludes:

1. That the induction of premature labor is a better procedure than Cæsarean section in cases of contracted pelvis, if the conjugate is not less than 7 cm. This is proven by the fact that of the author's 111 cases, only one mother died, and of the 101 children born alive, 61 lived.

2. That Krause's method—the introduction of a flexible bougie—is the best method, and can be performed in a private house as well as in a hospital.

3. The operation should be delayed as long as possible.

4. Under ordinary circumstances induced premature labor should be conducted in the same manner as normal labor.

5. If the life of the mother only is considered the labor should be terminated quickly by rupturing the membranes and evacuating the uterus, but otherwise the membranes should be preserved intact.

Pills for Dysentery.— BOUDIN, in *L' Union Médical*, September 2, 1890, recommends the following pills for the treatment of dysentery:

R.—Ipecacuanha . . . 5 grains.
Calomel . . . 1½ "
Extract of opium . . . 1 grain.

To be made into three pills and one given every hour and used either for dysentery or diarrhœa dependent upon exposure to heat.

Ointment for Tinea Tonsurans.—

R.—Caustic potash . . . 30 grains.
Carbolic acid . . . 15 "
Lanolin and cocoa butter each 1½ ounces.
Essence of lavender a sufficient quantity to perfume the mass.

These materials are to be made into an ointment and well applied at night to the affected part, limiting its application to the diseased tissues or a little beyond them. There is generally an improvement after ten days, but in very marked cases relief may not be obtained for as long a period of three months.

Formula for Scrofulosis.—In *L' Union Médical*, August 26, 1890, the following prescription of GUÉPIN for scrofulosis is given:

R.—Iodide of potassium . . 75 grains.
Chloride of ammonium . 30 "
Simple syrup . . . 1½ ounces.
Distilled water . . . 4 "

A teaspoonful of this is to be taken night and morning and may be accompanied by cod-liver oil. The patient, if possible, should stay for as long a time as possible at the seashore.

Syrup for Rheumatism.—The following prescription, recommended by AUDHOURI, is given for rheumatism:

R.—Iodide of potassium . . 75 grains.
Salicylate of sodium . . 5 drachms.
Syrup of bitter orange peel . 10 ounces.

Of this syrup two to four dessertspoonfuls are to be given each day to an adult for the purpose of relieving the pain and quieting the patient, or if the patient is a child, a coffeespoonful three times a day will generally be sufficient. It is always best to give at the same time that this mixture is administered a small dose of morphine to relieve any pain which may be present.

Treatment of Gonorrhœal Arthritis.—

R.—Camphor . . . . 100 grains.
Extract of opium . . 75 "
Alcohol . . . . 1 drachm.
Extract of belladonna . 75 grains.

This is to be made into a cataplasm and applied over the part from ten to twelve hours, the joint being made immobile by proper dressings.

Insanity and Bright's Disease.—DR. ALICE BENNETT has made a thorough study of the relations between Bright's disease and insanity, and in an exhaustive paper read before the Pennsylvania State Medical Society draws the following conclusions:

1. That, contrary to the generally received opinion, affections of the kidney are very common among the insane.

2. That "uræmic poisoning" is one of the most frequent causes of insanity.

3. That while the mental manifestations may be as varied as there are different centres subjected to irritation by these unknown poisons, the most prominent and constant symptom is some form of *mental pain*, which may range from simple depression, through all degrees and varieties of delusions of persecution, self-condemnation and apprehension, with or without hallucinations, up to a condition characterized by a frenzy of fear, with extraordinary motor excitement, and rapid physical prostration—the "grave delirium" or "typho-mania" of some authors.

4. That the motor centres are specially liable to be affected, as evidenced by the restlessness and incessant activity of many cases, less frequently by convulsions and convulsive twitchings; occasionally by choreic movements; occasionally by cataleptoidal states.

Dr. Bennett cites a large number of cases in support of her deductions.

THE MEDICAL NEWS.

A WEEKLY JOURNAL
OF MEDICAL SCIENCE.

COMMUNICATIONS are invited from all parts of the world. Original articles contributed exclusively to THE MEDICAL NEWS will be liberally paid for upon publication. When necessary to elucidate the text, illustrations will be furnished without cost to the author.

Address the Editor: H. A. HARE, M.D.,
1004 WALNUT STREET,
PHILADELPHIA.

Subscription Price, including Postage.

PER ANNUM, IN ADVANCE . . . . $4.00.
SINGLE COPIES . . . . 10 CENTS.

Subscriptions may begin at any date. The safest mode of remittance is by bank check or postal money order, drawn to the order of the undersigned. When neither is accessible, remittances may be made, at the risk of the publishers, by forwarding in *registered* letters.

Address,   LEA BROTHERS & CO.,
Nos. 706 & 708 SANSOM STREET,
PHILADELPHIA.

SATURDAY, OCTOBER 4, 1890.

THE TREATMENT OF TUBERCULOSIS OF THE LARYNX.

TUBERCULOUS disease of the larynx is so distressing a complication of a most distressing malady that every observation upon its treatment is deserving of attention. While this condition does occur as a primary localization—a fact long disputed, but finally settled by the studies of J. Solis-Cohen, published in 1881—it is most frequently associated with pulmonary tuberculosis. The special therapeutic problem to be solved, then, is not so much how to bring about the absolute recovery of the patient—for this is bound up with the larger question of the treatment of internal tuberculosis in general, and pulmonary tuberculosis in particular—but how we may bring about healing of the local lesions, or how we may mitigate the sufferings to which those lesions give rise.

It has long been held by competent authorities that in a certain small proportion of cases tuberculous ulceration of the larynx will heal under measures of cleanliness and antisepsis, such as washing with detergent sprays and the insufflation of iodoform—proper attention, of course, being given to general measures of nutrition. Of the truth of this view we can recall a most remarkable instance, that of a patient who came under our observation in 1883,

and is still living, apparently well. This man, a commercial traveller, learned how to insufflate iodoform into his own larynx, and for more than a year practised this expedient thrice daily while on his journeys.

It must be admitted, however, that the proportion of such cases is small, and hence, since the discovery of the tubercle bacillus has led to general acquiescence in the theory of the local origin of the morbid processes, renewed efforts have been directed toward discovering feasible methods for radical extirpation of the diseased tissues. Instances from pre-bacillary times were not wanting, in which good results had followed such measures, instituted on the general principles of good surgery. Thus, J. Solis-Cohen, in 1870, excised the epiglottis of a woman with phthisis, on account of limited tuberculous ulceration, and the patient was reported alive and well twelve years later.

The great difficulty in the majority of cases, however, lies in the comparative inaccessibility of the lesions. Tuberculous lymph-glands of the neck, tuberculous joints, and the like, are readily amenable to direct surgical procedures. Manipulations within the larynx are not easy under the most favorable circumstances, and are extremely difficult in the tortured and enfeebled subjects of tuberculous disease. Thyrotomy for better access is not likely to be successful, for the chances are that infection of the wound will prevent healing, and lead to a more rapidly fatal issue. It would be an exceptional, almost unimaginable case, that would justify laryngectomy.

Krause, of Berlin, encouraged by the success of von Mosetig-Moorhof in the use of lactic acid in the treatment of epitheliomata, employed that agent to destroy laryngeal tissues infiltrated with tubercle, and the reports of his good results have encouraged specialists throughout the world to resort to the same procedure.

The larynx being thoroughly cocainized, ulcerated parts are curetted and harshly rubbed with a sponge or cotton wad, saturated with a solution of lactic acid. The strength of the solution varies from 30 to 40 per cent. at first, to from 50 to 80 per cent. finally, according to the severity of the reaction. Chromic acid, the electric cautery, and superficial electrolysis, according to Voltolini's bipolar method, have also been resorted to.

Krause has likewise vigorously applied lactic acid without preliminary curetting, to reduce the infiltration of non-ulcerated structures, and he claims excellent results; a claim which has been confirmed by other good observers.

In a communication to the Berlin Congress upon the curability of laryngeal tuberculosis by surgical treatment, Luc (*Archives de Laryngologie*, August, 1890) reviews the various procedures instituted with this object. Many specialists, he says, have not succeeded in obtaining results as brilliant as those reported by Krause, Hering, and others, from curettage and lactic acid, and have, therefore, despairingly fallen back upon purely palliative measures. To illustrate the possibilities of success in radical treatment of accessible lesions, he reports the case of a man, thirty-five years old, affected with tuberculosis of the naso-pharyngeal mucous membrane, in whom Krause's local treatment, combined with superalimentation and other appropriate general measures produced a perfect cure. He also reports a case of limited laryngeal tuberculosis, in which energetic curetting and lactic acid applications had apparently brought about recovery. The patient, however, returned some two months later, after a sojourn in the country, much improved in general health, but with a new local lesion. This latter case, he believes, emphasizes the importance of continuous local treatment; the combination of proper topical applications, with the most approved measures to promote general nutrition, being absolutely necessary in every case.

From a large number of observations the author concludes that the method of Krause is capable of producing good results in well-selected cases; but he deprecates its indiscriminate employment. On account of the pain and distress to which the patient is put, he considers that it is the part of humanity not to resort to this expedient when the condition of the lungs or other organs is such as to render the case absolutely hopeless, or when the laryngeal lesions are so situated that thorough treatment is not possible. On the whole, this is sound advice; though, in certain cases, even with advanced pulmonary lesions, it may be advisable to perform tracheotomy, and then actively curette, and apply lactic acid to the larynx, in the endeavor to avert the difficulty of nutrition, which arises in late stages from the exquisite pain in swallowing, due to the passage of food over ulcerated surfaces. The truth is, that in no disease is more discretion required of the physician in applying general rules to individual cases.

REVIEWS.

TRANSACTIONS OF THE AMERICAN ORTHOPÆDIC ASSOCIATION. Vol. II. Published by the Association. Philadelphia, 1890.

THE development of the various departments of surgery has been so rapid that it is practically impossible for the general practitioner of medicine to follow the advances in the year's work; and although the papers read before the American Orthopædic Association have, in the main, appeared elsewhere, their collection in one volume is most serviceable, since in an hour's reading the subscriber is able to appreciate the best thought and best methods of the most progressive orthopædists.

As would be expected, hip-joint disease is discussed at length, and it is a satisfaction to perceive that the tendency of the present day is not toward conservative treatment.

Dr. W. R. Townsend contributes a paper upon "Acute Arthritis of Infants," tabulating a long series of cases. In the treatment he has nothing new to offer, beyond meeting the well-known indications of suppurative processes.

Dr. DeForest Willard contributes two papers—one upon " Rest and Fixation in Joint Disease," the other upon "The Operative Treatment of Hip Disease." Both of these are characterized by sound common-sense, always noticeable in the writings of this distinguished surgeon.

It is interesting to note that the general drift of all the papers is toward greater attention to what may be called the minor details of treatment; new splints, new applications of old methods are advanced. There is no indication of any radical change of treatment, of any great advance, but in this volume will be found hints and suggestions of the greatest possible value.

ELECTRICITY IN THE DISEASES OF WOMEN, WITH SPECIAL REFERENCE TO THE APPLICATION OF STRONG CURRENTS. By G. BETTON MASSEY, M.D. Second Edition, revised and enlarged. Philadelphia and London : F. A. Davis, 1890.

THIS little volume and the methods which it advocates have been subject to much adverse criticism—criticisms, for the most part, on the part of those ignorant of the principles here set down; but such of his critics as are severe and unjust Dr. Massey can well silence by pointing to the second edition of his work so quickly following the first. Indeed, the popularity of this work is, to a certain extent, a guarantee of its value, or at least an assurance that it is not without value; and of the sincerity of its author none who reads its pages can doubt. The list of cases and of reported cures would be conclusive, were such reports from one man ever conclusive. It will not be until we have the experience of many observers, and of those not primarily in favor of electricity, that a decision as to the true value of this agent as applied to the diseases of women can be reached.

The first few chapters of this work are rightly devoted to a description and explanation of apparatus. Chapter XI. is upon the subject of the electrical treatment of fibroid tumors of the uterus. The author has certainly made out a strong case for his side of the question.

The electrical treatment of uterine hæmorrhage, of subinvolution, of metritis and endometritis, of inflammatory diseases of the uterine appendages, of pelvic pain, of uterine displacements, of extra-uterine pregnancy, and of miscellaneous conditions, are next considered.

It will be a surprise to those opposed to electricity to learn that Dr. Massey has devoted his twentieth chapter to the "Contra-indications and Limitations to the Use of Strong Currents," for according to their statements, it would seem that, in the mind of the electrician, there are neither contra-indications nor limitations. This, however, is unjust and untrue; and, considering the strength of his belief in his methods, Dr. Massey is singularly fair in his conclusions.

SOCIETY PROCEEDINGS.

AMERICAN ORTHOPÆDIC ASSOCIATION.

Fourth Annual Meeting, held at Philadelphia, September 16, 17, and 18, 1890.

(Continued from p. 310)

SECOND DAY—MORNING SESSION.

This day was devoted to the subject of

ROTARY LATERAL CURVATURE OF THE SPINE.

DR. BENJAMIN LEE, of Philadelphia, read a paper on

THE NERVOUS AND MUSCULAR ELEMENTS IN THE CAUSATION OF IDIOPATHIC CURVATURE,

in which he remarked that the maintenance of equilibrium is the first necessity, and that a very small lumbar curve will necessitate a large dorsal compensating curve. It is not strange that the comparatively trifling lumbar curve often goes unnoticed and that the large dorsal curve is the first to attract the attention of the mother or the dressmaker. In fact, in the large majority of cases, the mother does not detect the former even when it has become aggravated, until the surgeon points it out to her. Under ordinary circumstances it is not conceivable that the use of the muscles which move the upper extremity should draw the spine toward the extremity. The extremity must of necessity be drawn toward the spine. We cannot attribute the dorsal curve to direct traction by those muscles, however excessively they may be developed.

DR. CHARLES L. SCUDDER, of Boston, contributed a paper on

THE MUSCULAR ELEMENT IN THE ETIOLOGY OF ROTARY CURVATURE,

which was a preliminary report of an investigation to establish an index of muscular strength in growing girls for each year from the tenth to the nineteenth year of age. The report was based on an examination of the backs of 1041 of the schoolgirls of Boston. The examinations were conducted by means of a chair especially constructed for the purpose, the strength of the back-muscles as a group being measured by a self-registering dynamometer. The results of the investigation show a gradual increase in the strength of the back-muscles of the growing child. The importance of this investigation, as establishing a firm scientific basis for a further study of the muscular element in the etiology, was shown, as well as its bearing upon the treatment, the prognosis, and the recording of lateral curvature cases.

DR. R. W. LOVETT, of Boston, contributed a paper on the

ETIOLOGY OF LATERAL CURVATURE,

and DR. A. B. JUDSON, of New York, one upon the

MECHANISM OF ROTATION IN LATERAL CURVATURE.

Dr. Judson said that rotation is a necessary accompaniment of curvature of the spine in disease and also in health. It may be seen in a thin person when the trunk takes a strong curve to the right or left, and is readily observed in a gymnasium. It is one of the normal functions of the spinal column and adds a sinuous grace to the movements of the trunk. Its cause is found in the fact that when the spine curves laterally, the bodies, forming the anterior part of the vertebral structure, are free to move laterally in the cavities of the chest and abdomen, while the processes forming the posterior part of the column are prevented from the same degree of lateral displacement by being entangled in the parietes, composed of ribs, muscles, and fasciæ.

An important effect of rotation in the deformity produced by lateral curvature is that the curve is greater in the anterior part of the column than in the posterior. A slight curve in the process means a considerable curve in the bodies, and an early diagnosis may be made by looking for rotation rather than for curvature. Rotation may be recognized in a case of incipient lateral curvature by detecting scapular obliquity and a prominence of the transverse processes on the side of the convexity. Its effect on the ribs is to produce an inequality in the diagonal diameters of the chest. In the absence of positive knowledge of the etiology he assumed that lateral curvature is an expression of inability (very likely of nervous origin) on the part of the muscles to hold the spine erect.

He disapproves of the use of braces applied for the forcible arrest or reduction of curvature, as he believes that the mechanical difficulties are too great. A knee can be straightened by applying pressure from before backward in the neighborhood of the joint and counter-pressure from behind forward at points remote from the joint on the long bony levers which compose this joint, but he would not try to straighten by pressure an upright column composed of many short bones thrown into a double or triple curvature with the added complication of rotation at two or three points in opposite directions. He would advise the patient to avoid fatigue from whatever cause, and to assume for as many hours in the twenty-four as is practicable those attitudes in which there is the nearest approach to symmetry. The patient should sleep supine with lordosis produced by an air pillow. The same position should be assumed a portion of every day. Suspension should also be practised up to, but not beyond, the point of fatigue.

AFTERNOON SESSION.

Papers on the *Treatment of Lateral Curvature* were read by Drs. E. H. Bradford, of Boston, and Henry Ling Taylor, of New York.

THIRD DAY—MORNING SESSION.

DR. JOHN RIDLON, of New York, read a paper entitled

A REPORT OF SIXTY-TWO CASES OF HIP-DISEASE OBSERVED IN THE PRACTICE OF HUGH OWEN THOMAS.

He presented for consideration further facts regarding the use of the Thomas hip-splint. Conclusions could not be drawn from his study of the cases, but he ventured the following suggestions:

Very many of the cases had had the short splint applied before muscular spasm and pain had subsided and before deformity had been reduced, and they had been allowed to walk about without high patten and crutches. Those whose joints had been only partially immobilized, without being protected from the pressure, superincumbent weight, and the concussion of walking, presented a slight degree of adduction, absence of motion, and in a few cases slight flexion, and in one instance in-knee. On the other hand, those cases that had worn a long splint until cured, that remained in the horizontal position till all pain and muscular spasm had subsided and had then used the high patten and crutches, and had had the benefit of intelligent care and nursing, have been cured without flexion or other deformity than a shortening due to actual erosion of bone and arrested growth; a very large proportion have shown motion, and in not a few has there been normal motion.

The average duration of limp before treatment was commenced was, in the 62 cases, a little over ten months. Average duration of treatment was not computed, as only a few cases were cured, and many had been under treatment but a short time. Of the 58 cases that had been under treatment for a longer or shorter time, 24 had shortening, 24 had adduction, 5 had abduction, 3 had inward rotation, and 2 had outward rotation. In the cases where abduction coëxisted with the shortening, it was an advantage, as it compensated in a measure for the shortening.

DR. JAMES K. YOUNG, of Philadelphia, followed with a paper on

DISEASES OF THE EYE ASSOCIATED WITH CARIES OF THE SPINE.

He said that the diseases of the eye associated with caries of the spine are, from necessity, of the same pathological nature—strumous or tubercular.

Scrofulosis may be considered the constitutional predisposition to caseation; tuberculosis the same condition infected with bacilli of tuberculosis. Both the lesions of the eye and the caries of the vertebræ yield more readily to constitutional and local treatment combined.

Referring to the relation between scrofula and tubercle, Treves has given the following conclusions:

"1. The manifestations of scrofula are commonly associated with the appearance of tubercle; or, if any fully-formed tubercle be met with, a condition of tissue obtains that is recognized as being preliminary to tubercle. Anatomically, therefore, scrofula may be regarded as a tuberculous or tubercle-forming process.

"2. The form of tubercle met with in scrofulous diseases is usually of an elementary and often of an immature character; whereas in diseases called tuberculous in a strict clinical sense, a more perfect form of tubercle is met with in the form of gray granulation or adult tubercle.

"3. Scrofula, therefore, indicates a milder form or stage of tuberculosis, and the two processes are simply separated from each other by degree."

DR. SAMUEL KETCH, of New York, read a paper on

POSTERIOR RACHITIC CURVATURE OF THE SPINE.

He said that of the deformities of the spine whose underlying cause is found in the condition known as rachitis, those most commonly seen in practice are the lateral and posterior.

The etiology and pathology of posterior rachitic curvature of the spine are essentially those of rickets in general, the deformity being simply one of the local manifestations of a general diathesis. Dr. Ketch believes that the causation is largely mechanical, and furthered by such movements as tend to throw the weight of the body on the weakened vertebræ and their appendages. Rachitis of the vertebræ evinces itself, as does rachitis usually, at a very early period of life, by an irregularity in the process of ossification, by cartilaginous enlargements, and by marked diminution of the harder substances entering into the formation of bone, notably the lime-salts. In consequence of this unstable condition of the rachitic vertebræ we find in the long axis of the spinal column many soft places, in some cases including the upper and lower surfaces of all of the vertebræ, in others localized to a few.

A large number of cases show a limitation of the curve to the dorso-lumbar spine, a favorite position for the occurrence of Pott's disease. In addition to the deformity we may have more or less pain, spinal rigidity, pseudo-paralysis, or any of the distinctive symptoms relating to the area of the disease.

In the treatment of young children from one to two years old, he never advises the use of mechanical supports, the tissues being so unstable that any pressure is apt to be badly tolerated. In such cases the constant recumbent position, with fresh air and sun-baths, together with internal treatment and close attention to the diet, is usually sufficient.

AFTERNOON SESSION.

The following papers were read and discussed:

Relief of Paraplegia, by Dr. A. J. Steele, of St. Louis; Lateral Deviation of the Spinal Column in Pott's Disease, Dr. R. W. Lovett, of Boston; Prognosis of Pressure Paralysis, by Dr. T. Halsted Myers, of New York.

DR. A. B. JUDSON exhibited an apparatus by which it was demonstrated that the strain falling on the tendo-Achillis when a person stands on tiptoe on one foot greatly exceeds the weight of the body. The foot was shown to be a lever, its long arm being the distance from the ankle to the toe, and the short arm extending from the ankle to the heel. In the apparatus shown, the four pounds representing the weight of the body appeared as twelve pounds on the spring-balance which represented the tendo-Achillis. To estimate the tension of the tendon, the weight of the body is to be multiplied by the number of times the distance from the ankle to the heel is exceeded by the distance from the ankle to the toe. If the former is one-third of the latter, in a man weighing two hundred pounds, the tension of the tendo-Achillis is six hundred pounds.

OFFICERS FOR 1891 :

President.—Dr. A. B. Judson, of New York.

First Vice-President.—Dr. Ap Morgan Vance, Louisville, Ky.

Second Vice-President.—Dr. George W. Ryan, Cincinnati, O.

Secretary.—Dr. John Ridlon, New York.

Place of meeting, Washington, D. C., 1891, in connection with the Congress of American Physicians and Surgeons.

MEDICAL SOCIETY OF VIRGINIA.

Twenty-first Annual Meeting, held at Rockbridge Alum Springs, Virginia, September 2, 3, and 4, 1890.

THE twenty-first annual session of the Medical Society of Virginia convened at Rockbridge Alum Springs, Virginia, Tuesday evening, September 2, 1890, and adjourned Thursday evening, September 4th, to partake of a banquet tendered by the managers of the Springs to the Society and its guests.

The session was called to order by the President, Dr. Oscar Wiley, of Salem, Va. There were also on the stand the Secretary of the Society, Dr. Landon B. Edwards, of Richmond, Va.; the several ex-Presidents of the Society, and the following invited guests: Dr. Landon Carter Gray, of New York City; Drs. Joseph Price and Joseph Hoffman, of Philadelphia; Dr. E. S. Ricketts, of Cincinnati; and Dr. George Herndon, of the U. S. Navy. Among other distinguished visitors at the Springs to whom the same compliment was extended, was General Joseph E. Johnston.

After prayer by the Rev. E. F. Garrison, of Philadelphia, and the cordial address of welcome on the part of the Rockbridge Springs Company, by the resident physician, Dr. J. Edgar Chancellor, of the University of Virginia, DR. JOHN S. APPERSON, of Marion, Va., delivered the

ANNUAL ADDRESS TO THE PUBLIC AND PROFESSION,

in which he dwelt upon the value to the public of regular medical societies.

Following this address, the committee appointed to examine the essays which had been presented for the Hunter McGuire prize of one hundred dollars for the best original essay on the *Diagnosis, Pathology, and Treatment of Chronic Cystitis in the Male,* after having carefully examined each of the seven papers presented, decided that the essay signed "*Causa cessante, cessat effectus,*" possessed the greatest merit. On opening the envelope corresponding to this motto, the author was found to be Dr. R. M. Slaughter, of Theological Seminary, Virginia. This essay will soon be published in full in the *Transactions* of the Society, and in the *Virginia Medical Monthly,* and probably in other journals.

Dr. Hunter McGuire, who was present, after awarding the prize by mail (the author not being at the meeting), authorized the announcement that he would award another prize of one hundred dollars at the next annual session of the Society to the practitioner residing in West Virginia, Virginia, or North Carolina presenting the best original essay on some subject that will soon be announced by the Secretary. All essays offered in competition must become the property of the Society, and will be disposed of by it or its Publication Committee.

During the session about one hundred and fifty physicians were in attendance, the total membership being about eight hundred. Nearly fifty new members joined during the meeting. A large number of non-professional men and women were present during the session of the first night, and throughout the several daily meetings Mrs. Mary Young Ridenbaugh, the granddaughter of Dr. Ephraim McDowell, was present as an interested spectator and listener, and received the compliment of being formally introduced to the Society by the President.

SECOND DAY.

At 11 A.M., the President, DR. OSCAR WILEY, delivered his

ANNUAL ADDRESS,

which was retrospective, suggestive, and prospective, as to the profession of Virginia in particular, and was extremely interesting.

THE TREATMENT OF THE SUMMER DIARRHŒAS OF CHILDREN

was the subject selected for a general discussion which occupied several hours. While the discussion was interesting, and some practical points were brought out, nothing was said that indicated a marked advance in our knowledge of the nature and treatment of these diseases.

The appointed leader in the discussion was Dr. C. T. Lewis, of Clifton Forge, Va., who opened the discussion by reading a paper on the subject. Dr. J. N. Upshur, of Richmond, also read a paper.

Extempore remarks were made by Drs. Thomas J. Moore, J. S. Wellford, W. W. Parker, Thomas J. Riddell, and Jacob Michaux, of Richmond; Dr. J. Edgar Chancellor, of the University of Virginia; Dr. T. James Taylor, of Brunswick County; Dr. J. E. Copeland, of Rectortown; Dr. E. T. Brady, of Marion; and Dr. Jacob Simmons, of Obenshain.

During the afternoon the election of officers for the ensuing year took place. The following were elected :

President.—Dr. William W. Parker, of Richmond.

Vice-Presidents.—Drs. J. W. Dillard, of Lynchburg; Jacob Michaux, of Richmond; and H. M. Patterson, of Staunton.

Recording Secretary.—Dr. Landon B. Edwards, of Richmond.

Corresponding Secretary.—Dr. J. F. Winn, of Richmond.

Treasurer.—Dr. Richard T. Styll, of Hollins.

The committees remain about as they were, except that ex-President Hunter McGuire, of Richmond, was made Chairman of the Executive Committee, in place of Dr. Parker, elected President.

Dr. Charles M. Blackford, of Lynchburg, was appointed to deliver the Address to the Public and Profession, in 1891.

Acute Dysentery was selected as the subject for general discussion, which will be opened by Dr. P. B. Green, of Wytheville.

Dr. A. C. Palmer, of Norfolk, was nominated to the Governor of Virginia to fill a vacancy occasioned by the resignation of a member of the State Medical Examining Board.

On nomination by Dr. Blackford, of Staunton, Lynchburg was chosen as the place for the next annual session; the time of meeting, October, 1891; the day to be fixed by the Executive Committee.

EVENING SESSION.

The evening session was devoted to the section on Ophthalmology, Otology, and Laryngology.

DR. ROBERT L. RANDOLPH, of Baltimore, the reporter on the progress of Ophthalmology, spoke of the new treatment of detached retina by injection of tincture of iodine, and of the value of fluorescein as an aid in the diagnosis of corneal lesions. He also narrated some experiments of his own and of Kolinski's, with reference to the production of cataract in the lower animals by feeding them on naphthalin.

DR. WILLIAM F. MERCER, of Richmond, the reporter on the progress of Otology and Laryngology, spoke of investigations as to the transformation of benign laryngeal growths into malignant growths due to intra-laryngeal operations; the early treatment of naso-pharyngeal and throat affections in young children as a cure or preventive of certain nervous troubles; of nasal intubation as an easy and ready cure of hypertrophy of the soft intra-nasal tissues and deviations of nasal septa; and of the easy diagnosis of abscess of the antrum by illumination of the maxillary bones by an electric lamp introduced into the mouth. He also spoke of the importance of early recognition and treatment of acute suppurative otitis media following scarlatina.

DR. JOSEPH A. WHITE, of Richmond, Va., read an interesting and valuable paper on the

IMPORTANCE OF NASAL SURGERY AND NASAL THERAPEUTICS IN THE TREATMENT OF AURAL CATARRH.

He also presented a paper by title on the

RELATIONS OF REFRACTIVE ERRORS AND MUSCULAR DEFECTS IN ASTHENOPIA, OCULAR HEADACHES, ETC.

DR. CHARLES M. SHIELDS, of Richmond, read a paper entitled

WHEN SHALL WE OPERATE FOR CATARACT AND STRABISMUS?

He said that a large proportion of cases of cataract in children are zonular, and that an operation is too often postponed until the retina has lost its functional activity. He referred to five cases in his practice, in three of which operation was deferred till the patients were between ten and thirteen years old, but with unsatisfactory results; whereas in two cases—one three years and the other six months old—the results were very satisfactory. As to the age for alternating-strabismus operations, six or seven years is proper; but in the unilateral form of strabismus the earlier the operation the better.

DR. ALEXANDER DUANE, of Norfolk, read a paper on the

MODERN TREATMENT OF STRABISMUS,

contrasting the old methods with the precision of modern operations. Carefully and repeatedly test, he said, the static and dynamic condition of the eyes before operating. In spastic, in periodic accommodative, and in some cases of paralytic squint, treatment of the cause is required; in concomitant and in other cases of paralytic squint an operation is called for. In concomitant strabismus he made a sharp distinction between cases with tendon-tension and those with tendon-relaxation—in the latter advancement, in the former tenotomy being required. He described a remarkable instance of tendon-relaxation in which an apparently divergent squint was immediately benefited by advancement of the external rectus. In paralytic squint he has employed, whenever possible, tenotomy of the antagnostic muscle as recommended by v. Graefe, and, in paralysis of the superior and inferior rectus, advancement of the affected muscle.

DR. JOHN HERBERT CLAIBORNE, JR., of New York City, forwarded a paper on

BOILS IN THE EAR,

of which the following is a summary: (1) Furunculosis of the external canal is a local disease. (2) The cause is infection by pyogenic microbes. (3) Treatment should consist in local antisepsis, such as applications of solutions of boric and carbolic acids, moist heat, and incisions of the furuncles when they point.

DR. LAURENCE TURNBULL, of Philadelphia, forwarded a paper entitled

CATARRHAL OTITIS MEDIA,

in which he condemned most of the so-called hearing-restorers or artificial drums. The only form of artificial covering suited to diseased perforations of the drum-membrane is, he said, delicate gauze or rubber, charged with an antiseptic solution to protect the ear from floating microbes and from temperature-changes. As to the treatment of chronic aural catarrh, in addition to the means mentioned in his book, he suggested, in suitable cases, massage of the ears, valerianate of strychnine, and residence in an elevated region.

DR. CHARLES M. BLACKFORD, of Lynchburg, then described a

NEW METHOD OF LIFTING THE EPIGLOTTIS,

which was devised by Dr. Samuel P. Preston, of Lynchburg. He uses an ordinary silver laryngeal probe, which is bent at a right angle half an inch from the end. Through rings soldered to the shaft the third and fourth fingers of the left hand are passed. Let the bent portion of the probe press down on the glosso-epiglottidean ligaments, so as to tighten them, and this tightening will elevate the epiglottis. The pressure should be gentle.

DR. ALFRED C. PALMER, of Norfolk, described in a short paper a new method of treating deformities of the eyelids, which he termed

PALPO-TRACTION.

He claimed that many distortions of the eyelids might be permanently improved by this conservative plan, but said that it must be applied in infancy when the tissues are pliable and easily moulded by manipulation. He asked obstetricians to pay strict attention to the formation of the lids of newborn infants, and in all forms of entropion, ptosis, and contracted palpebral fissures, to begin at once to shape the lids and retract them to their proper forms and positions.

THIRD DAY.

The Section on Obstetrics and Diseases of Women and Children being called to order, DR. I. S. STONE, of Lincoln, read a brief paper on the

DIAGNOSIS OF PELVIC DISEASE, AND WHEN TO OPERATE.

He said that the profession is united in advising operation for pelvic and abdominal tumors, extra-uterine pregnancy, pyosalpinx, etc., and that electricity in such conditions is hazardous. Salpingitis in country practice is a common result of puerperal diseases, but its symptoms so closely resemble those of pelvic peritonitis and cellulitis as to render the diagnosis impossible. Conorrhœa is rare in the country, and, therefore, pyosalpinx is not as frequent as in cities. The impossibility of determining the extent of pelvic diseases, and the complications, are the real dangers of operations. He spoke of tubercular salpingitis, and remarked that the cause of each case of pelvic disease should be investigated before deciding to operate. Many cases are aggravated by marriage.

In discussing the paper, DR. GEORGE TUCKER HARRISON, of New York, said that Dr. Stone treated puerperal malarial fever as too trivial a disease. It is a common complication or sequel of labor, although it is not always easy to determine the cause. It may occur even after a perfectly aseptic delivery, lasts for weeks or months, and is often followed by rheumatism. As to the removal of the uterine appendages, operations are often undertaken without a diagnosis having been made. No radical operation should be undertaken until every other means of relief has been tried, unless, of course, it is plain that the organs are structurally diseased. As to extra-uterine pregnancy, the operation should be performed early. Tait confounds hæmatocele and hæmatoma with extra-uterine pregnancy in his writings on the diagnosis of the condition.

DR. JOSEPH PRICE, of Philadelphia, wished to emphasize Dr. Harrison's remarks as to operations upon the female pelvis. They should be undertaken only for an objective disease. Pelvic surgery has also suffered because many operations have been imperfectly done. The mortality from abdominal section for ovarian, tubal, and uterine diseases has been reduced to about two per cent., and the results of McGuire's suprapubic cystotomies conclusively show that simply opening the abdomen should not prove fatal. Dr. Coe, he said, had made some drawings of pus-tubes which are influencing professional opinion and action, but the drawings are unfortunately not true to nature. Dr. Price said that if the presence of pus in the tubes or pelvic cavity can be determined, it should be evacuated, as from any other part of the body. He advises that all forms of fibroids, even if small, be extirpated. Battey's operation, so far as it implies " normal ovariotomy," he said, should be consigned to oblivion. Dr. Price also condemns tampering with so-called intra-uterine medication by curettes, caustics, electricity, and sounds, and said that Emmet has not passed a sound for fifteen or twenty years. The palliative treatment of all intra-uterine diseases should be conducted on the most conservative principles. More prominence should be given to the ravages of gonorrhœa in unsuspecting wives as a cause

of disease. He then spoke of extra-uterine pregnancy, advising operation as soon as the condition is recognized. He has found rupture of the pregnant tube to occur almost invariably near one of the fimbriated extremities.

DR. HUNTER McGUIRE corrected a statement of Dr. Harrison's. It was not Dr. Barker, but the late Dr. Otis F. Manson, of Richmond, who first described puerperal malarial fever.

With reference to the use of the uterine sound, Dr. McGuire said that he has never had the slightest reason to think that he has done harm by its use; on the contrary, he is sure he has often done good. As to Battey's operation, he believed that it would soon become obsolete. To take out a normal ovary for a neurotic trouble, hereafter, he thinks should be considered a crime. But when there are pathological changes in the organ, and when all other remedies have failed, then an operation to remove the ovaries or appendages, or anything in the female pelvis that is causing ill-health, is justifiable. He did not agree with Dr. Price that all fibroids should be removed.

DR. JOSEPH HOFFMAN, of Philadelphia, said that it is a mistake to suppose that more than about one per cent. of diseases of women are essentially cellulitis. Tubal pus-cavities are like links of sausage; hence, to open one does not open all.

DR. EDWIN RICKETTS, of Cincinnati, spoke of the history of abdominal sections, remarking that McDowell was born in Rockbridge County, Va., within a few miles of where the Society was assembled.

The tendency now, he said, is toward too much pelvic surgery, and it should never be forgotten that discredit comes upon surgery when the surgeon fails to make his diagnosis clear, and hence fails to give that benefit which the patient seeks.

DR. ISAIAH H. WHITE, of Richmond, spoke especially of the importance of an early diagnosis of extra-uterine pregnancy, in order that an operation may be performed in time to avert the dangers ahead. But some cases pass through the stage of rupture and collapse, and the products of conception remain in a quiescent state until some additional cause of inflammatory or ulcerative action takes place, as, for instance, the occurrence of pregnancy. There are many cases in which extra-uterine pregnancy is first discovered years after impregnation, by reason of the escape of fœtal bones. Such cases suggest the propriety of the treatment recommended by some, viz., to kill the fœtus by electricity as soon as the diagnosis is clear, allowing the mass to become encapsulated and remain in the abdomen. What are known as the " remnants " of an extra-uterine pregnancy—excluding, of course, the fœtus itself—are most probably only the products of the inflammation excited by the passage of the fœtus through the tube into the peritoneal cavity. The appearance of the tube in cases of pyosalpinx, which reminds one of sausages, is due to the adhesive bands formed around the tube. Dr. McGuire was undoubtedly correct in deploring the so-called normal ovariotomy.

DR. LANDON CARTER GRAY, of New York, in response to requests for remarks, condemned Battey's operation for the cure of nervous diseases, just as he did Baker Brown's clitoridectomies, Sayre's wholesale circumcisions, and Stevens's general cutting of eye-muscles. In nearly all the cases in which such mutilations have been resorted to for the cure of nervous diseases, the relief that has followed in some cases has been of too short duration to justify the operations. These operations do good only upon the theory of mental impression. Esquirol recorded his tests as long ago as 1828, and why they are ignored now by men high in the profession Dr. Gray could not understand. Esquirol divided his epileptic patients into groups. To one group he gave one class of remedies, with the strong adjuvant of mental impression as to the benefit that would result; to a second group he gave another class of drugs, with the same adjuvant of mental encouragement; while to a third group he gave colored water, but with the same encouragements. Each group of cases did about equally well for a time; but relapses soon began to occur, and all the cases finally relapsed to their former condition. If an operation is to be performed simply to get the benefit of mental impression, let that operation be as slight as possible.

DR. WILLIAM W. PARKER, of Richmond, could not lay aside the education of a large experience which taught him that intra-uterine injections are perfectly safe if proper precautions are observed.

DR. HARRISON did not wish to put himself on record as wholly opposed to Battey's operation; for there are serious nervous troubles in which, although the ovaries are apparently only moderately diseased, the patient is permanently relieved, if not cured, by the operation. Dr. Battey's original error—which, however, has long since been corrected—consisted in naming his operation "*normal* ovariotomy."

DR. STONE, in closing the disussion, said that, in his opinion, the so-called Barker's, but more properly, Manson's, puerperal malarial fever is usually only an evidence of pus in the Fallopian tube, although he would not deny the existence of a pure type of the disease, such as Dr. Manson, and, later, Dr. Barker, have described as puerperal malarial fever. As to Battey's operation, he has undertaken it but once, and the results were very unsatisfactory in what he thought was a well-selected case.

In the section on Practice of Medicine papers by Drs. William H. Bramlett, of Pulaski City; William R. Cushing, of Dublin; P. B. Green, of Wytheville; William W. Parker, of Richmond, and others were read by title.

DR. LANDON CARTER GRAY read a paper on

VERTIGO,

in which, after detailing the various forms of vertigo from organic disease of the nervous system, he spoke at length of the vertigo to which Murchison gave the name of lith-æmic. He stated that he has reached the conclusion that this is due to imperfect digestion of the nitrogenized or farinaceous articles of diet, and that it should be treated principally by aiding the digestion and by hepatic stimulants.

Dr. Joseph T. Logan, of Atlanta, Ga., was then elected an Honorary Fellow of the Society, and the elected officers were installed.

AFTERNOON SESSION.

DR. GEORGE B. JOHNSTON, of Richmond, described a method of securing

PERMANENT DRAINAGE OF THE MALE BLADDER BY A RETAINED CATHETER INTRODUCED ABOVE THE PUBES.

He adds to Van Buren's trocar and canula a steel guide twice the length of the trocar, over which the outer canula may be easily withdrawn from the bladder and replaced.

DR. JOSEPH PRICE, of Philadelphia, followed with a paper on

THE PRESENT STATUS OF ABDOMINAL SURGERY.

He insisted that it was the duty of the surgeon to prepare himself for the unexpected when he undertakes abdominal operations. Vaginal punctures, he said, are more dangerous than incisions through the abdominal wall. As to ectopic pregnancy an operation should be performed as soon as the condition is discovered. The placenta should be removed, if possible; if not, it should be emptied of blood and the cord tied, after which it may be digested by the peritoneum. Flushing the abdomen with hot water in abdominal section is beneficial if there is a tendency to shock. He does not use antiseptics but depends upon cleanliness. As to treatment after such operations he allows neither food nor drink until the stomach becomes quiet; then gives small quantities of liquid diet—butter-milk being excellent. The patient should be kept in bed at least three weeks after an abdominal section.

DR. EDWIN RICKETTS, of Cincinnati, then read a paper entitled

EARLY EXPLORATORY INCISION AS AN AID TO THE DIAGNOSIS OF SOME SURGICAL DISEASES OF THE ABDOMINAL CAVITY,

in which he said that he had found it difficult in many cases to make a diagnosis previously to incision. To open the abdomen is easy enough, but afterward to do the best thing, and that promptly, bearing in mind that half-completed surgical procedures are rarely excusable, is often difficult. He then briefly reported eleven cases that had come under his observation, in which the diagnosis could not be made without an exploratory incision.

DR. HUNTER MCGUIRE, of Richmond, then reported a number of cases of

DISEASES OF THE BRAIN AND SPINAL CORD FOLLOWING URETHRAL STRICTURE.

He believes that long-existing urethral strictures are often followed by painful and dangerous neuroses.

DR. JOSEPH HOFFMAN, of Philadelphia, then read a paper entitled

THE SALIENT POINTS IN APPENDICITIS—ITS DIAGNOSIS AND TREATMENT.

He pointed out that a purely physiological rotation of the cæcum may excite congestion without the presence of any irritating matter whatever. As to treatment, those surgeons who operate between attacks represent the progressive surgery of the day. In women, it is usually best to cut through the median line, for the chances are that in them the disease will not be found in the vermiform appendix, and through the median incision any other abdominal operation may be performed. He condemned exploratory incisions. In man, the presence of an indurated mass in the right iliac fossa, with pain and fulness in the region detected by rectal examination, is important. The right leg is also often drawn up.

DR. M. D. HOGE, JR., of Richmond, then read a paper on the

MODERN TREATMENT OF EPILEPSY.

DR. E. M. MAGRUDER, of Charlottesville, reported a

CASE OF REMOVAL OF A LARGE VESICAL CALCULUS (ABOUT 2 × 3 INCHES) THROUGH THE VAGINAL WALL.

EVENING SESSION.   •

DR. GEORGE TUCKER HARRISON, of New York, read a paper entitled

REMARKS UPON ANTEFLEXION OF THE UTERUS.

After describing normal changes in the shape and position of the uterus, he stated that pathological anteflexion is simply the stability of the flexion. When metritis attacks an anteflexed uterus the angle of which had been variable up to that time, it becomes fixed. The usual symptoms of anteflexion are dysmenorrhœa and sterility—the dysmenorrhœa being due to associated metritis ; and the sterility to the endometritis. If these inflammations be removed before they have caused permanent pathological changes, conception may take place. As to treatment, the peri- and para-metric inflammations should be removed. If the uterus becomes sensitive it should be scarified just before menstruation, and the dysmenorrhœa will be moderated. For the persistent uterine catarrh, after dilating the uterine cavity with aseptic laminaria tents and then by steel dilators, the uterine cavity should be washed out with a solution of carbolic acid. Lately, he has been much pleased with ichthyol, incorporated with lanolin, and applied around the portio vaginalis, as an aid in clearing up old peri- and para-metric adhesions.

Following this paper, Dr. L. Ashton, who is about to remove to Dallas, Texas, was elected an Honorary Fellow. Dr. Ashton has been an influential working member of the Society for many years, a Vice-President, a member of the Medical Examining Board of Virginia, and has contributed a number of papers during his many years of Fellowship. The retiring President, Dr. Oscar Wiley, of Salem, was also elected an Honorary Fellow.

CORRESPONDENCE.

CEPHALHÆMATOMA.

To the Editor of THE MEDICAL NEWS,

SIR : In THE MEDICAL NEWS of September 6, 1890, Dr. H. A. Kelly, writing of cephalhæmatoma, says : "Few men outside of the ranks of the pure specialists are aware that such a disease as cephalhæmatoma exists. Cases which occur in the practice of the general practitioner are diagnosed and treated by him upon ' general principles.' The information which he possesses upon this subject is fairly comparable to that of a physician practising early in the last century." In THE NEWS of September 13th, Dr. Barton C. Hirst says : "A cephalhæmatoma on either parietal bone in a newly-born infant is quite common. There is probably not a general practitioner of any experience in obstetrics who has not become familiar with it."

Now, each of these gentlemen is a teacher in a leading medical college, and an authority in the obstetric art. A general practitioner who has seen and diagnosed cephalhæmatoma from specific knowledge of the condition asks, Which one is more nearly correct? Is the general practitioner of this day as ignorant as the opinion of Dr. Kelly indicates?

In Condie's work on *Diseases of Children*, a well-known text-book of twenty-five years ago, is a full account of this condition, he devoting some six pages to its consideration. In the latest American work on diseases of children — *Keating's Cyclopædia* — Professor Parvin evidently considers one page sufficient.

It is true, however, that in most of the text-books on obstetrics there is little or no mention of the subject.

In Volume III. of *Holmes's Surgery*, Mr. Holmes, writing of sub-aponeurotic extravasations of the scalp, shows the difference between them and cephalhæmatoma, and further says " that the same ridge bounding a small circumscribed collection of fluid is also familiar to surgeons as a frequent symptom in blows on the head, and a frequent cause of mistake to inexperienced observers, who confound these appearances with those of depressed fracture." So even the surgeons seem to be familiar with cephalhæmatoma.

Respectfully,

W. H. SHARP, M.D.

PARKERSBURG, W. VA.

NEWS ITEMS.

Fire in a Texas Insane Asylum. — On the night of September 18th the Insane Asylum at Austin, Texas, was partly burned. No lives were lost, but the inmates of one of the female wards were asleep at the time, and were with difficulty rescued before the building was destroyed. A laundry was attached to the ward, and it was there that the fire originated.

The Chair of Chemistry in the Chicago College of Physicians and Surgeons.—James A. Lydston, M.D., Ph. G., late chief of the Eye and Ear Department, Pension Bureau, Washington, D. C., has been elected to the Chair of Chemistry of the Chicago College of Physicians and Surgeons.

Honor to Sir Joseph Lister.—The Cameron prize in therapeutics of the Edinburgh University has been awarded to Sir Joseph Lister for his development of the antiseptic system of surgery. Mr. Lister will deliver an address before the University during the approaching session, in which he will sum up the results of his labors in recent years.

Influenza in Germany.—It is said that influenza has broken out again in parts of Germany, and that pneumonia is a very frequent complication.

Experiments on an Executed Criminal.—According to the *Lancet*, some interesting observations were recently made in Paris on the body of a criminal who had been guillotined. The heart continued to beat for more than six minutes, and experiments were performed to determine the independence of ventricular and auricular contractions. A study of the reaction of the contents of the gastro-intestinal tract was also made.

Hypnotism in Russia.—The medical department of the Russian Ministry of the. Interior has decreed that, "considering the evils resulting from a public display of hypnotism, public *séances* of hypnotism and 'magnetism' are forbidden," and that the "application of the method for therapeutic purposes is to be permitted only in the presence of several physicians."

First Meeting of the Board of Medical Examiners of New Jersey.—The State Board of Medical Examiners of New Jersey will meet in the Senate Chamber of the Capitol, at Trenton, Thursday, October 9th, at 9 A. M., for the purpose of examining candidates presenting themselves for a licence to practise medicine in New Jersey.

Prizes for Essays on Vivisection.—The American Humane Society offers two prizes, each of $250, for the best essays on the question whether vivisection should be permitted in the interests of humanity, and, if so, with what restrictions. Essays should be sent to George T. Angell, No. 19 Milk Street, Boston, before January 1st.

A Song from the International Congress.—The following was sung at the banquet of the Rhino-laryngological Section of the Tenth International Medical Congress, Berlin, August 6, 1890:[1]

RHINOLOGY.

BY MICHAEL, OF HAMBURG.

For all the ills we now endure
  With calm philosophy,
There's only one sure, certain cure—
  It's Rhinochirurgy.

Chorus.—The nose must straightway be burned out;
  'Twill always cure beyond a doubt.
  Tiralalalalalala tiralalalalala.

Whoever through his nose doth speak,
  Whosoever's nose is clogged,
Whose breath's asthmatic all the week,
  Whose sleep is much befogged;

His nose must straightway be burned out,
  'Twill cure him sure. beyond a doubt, etc.

And he who suffers from migraine,
  Whose head is dull alway,
Who feels somewhere some little pain,
  Or fev'rish gets from hay,

His nose must straightway be burned out, etc.

The maiden, too, with goitre dread,
  Whose heart beats pit-a-pat,
Whose eyes seem starting from her head—
  Basedow described all that—

Her nose must straightway be burned out, etc.

Then, when acid chloracetic
  Fails, as fails aristol,
Pyoktanin energetic,
  Or useless iodol,

The nose must straightway be burned out, etc.

[1] International Centralblatt f. Laryngologie und Rhinologie, September, 1890. (Translated by a Philadelphian.)

Whoever holds his nose too high,
  Or pokes it where he shouldn't,
Or gets it twisted all awry,
  And pointing where it wouldn't,

His nose must straightway be burned out, etc.

If bent, or straight, or small, or big,
  Or short, or long, or lame,
Or dirty, or of famous rig—
  It's all and one the same—

That nose must straightway be burned out, etc.

To woman, now, a thund'ring cheer,
  ' Let ev'ry man ring out!
Who don't join in, or doth appear
  Unwillingly to shout,

Let his nose straightway be burned out;
  'Twill cure him, sure, without a doubt.
  Tiralalalalalala tiralalalalala.

OFFICIAL LIST OF CHANGES IN THE STATIONS AND DUTIES OF OFFICERS SERVING IN THE MEDICAL DEPARTMENT, U. S. ARMY, FROM SEPTEMBER 23 TO SEPTEMBER 29, 1890.

TESSON, LOUIS N., *Captain and Assistant Surgeon* (Fort Sidney, Nebraska).—Is granted leave of absence for twenty days, to take effect when his services can be spared by his post commander.—*S. O. 72, Department of the Platte, Omaha, Nebraska,* September 25, 1890.
  In view of the abandonment of Fort Crawford, Colorado, to which post he is at present assigned for station, J. S. PHILLIPS, *Captain and Assistant Surgeon*, is relieved from duty at that post, and will, upon the expiration of his present leave of absence, proceed to Fort Logan, Colorado, and report to the commanding officer for duty.—Par. 1. *S. O. 135, Department of the Missouri, St. Louis, Mo.,* September 27, 1890.
  In view of the abandonment of Fort Gibson, Indian Territory, to which post he is at present assigned for station, W. O. OWED, JR., *Captain and Assistant Surgeon,* is relieved from duty at that post, and will, upon the expiration of his present leave of absence, proceed to Fort Sill, Indian Territory, and report to the commanding officer for duty.—*S. O. 135, Department of the Missouri, St. Louis, Mo.,* September 27, 1890.
  In view of the early abandonment of Fort Elliott, Texas, to which post he is at present assigned for station, J. P. KIMBALL, *Major and Surgeon,* is relieved from duty at that post, and will, upon the expiration of his present sick-leave of absence, proceed to Fort Supply, Indian Territory, and report to the commanding officer for duty.—Par. 2, *S. O. 131, Department of the Missouri,* September 24, 1890.
  Under the provisions of General Orders No. 43, *c. s.,* Headquarters of the Army, Adjutant-General's Office, the post of Little Rock Barracks, Arkansas, will be abandoned, to take effect not later than October 1, 1890. PAUL R. BROWN, *Captain and Assistant Surgeon,* will accompany Company " E " to Fort Supply, Indian Territory, and there take station until further orders.—*G. O. 15, Headquarters Department of the Missouri, St. Louis, Mo.,* August 11, 1890.
  EWING, C. B., *Captain and Assistant Surgeon.*—Is granted leave of absence for one month, to take effect the 1st proximo.—Par. 5. *S. O. 131, Headquarters Department of the Missouri,* September 22, 1890.
  APPEL, AARON H., *Captain and Assistant Surgeon.*—The leave of absence for seven days, granted by the commanding officer Fort D. A. Russell, Wyoming, is extended twenty-three days.—Par. 3. *S. O. 70, Department of the Platte,* September 17, 1890.

THE MEDICAL NEWS *will be pleased to receive early intelligence of local events of general medical interest, or of matters which it is desirable to bring to the notice of the profession.*

Local papers containing reports or news items should be marked. Letters, whether written for publication or private information, must be authenticated by the names and addresses of their writers—of course not necessarily for publication.

- All communications relating to the editorial department of the NEWS *should be addressed to No. 1004 Walnut Street, Philadelphia.*

THE MEDICAL NEWS.

A WEEKLY JOURNAL OF MEDICAL SCIENCE.

VOL. LVII. SATURDAY, OCTOBER 11, 1890. No. 15.

ORIGINAL ARTICLES.

THE PREVENTION OF SHOCK DURING AND AFTER OPERATIONS.

BY STEPHEN SMITH, M.D.,
PROFESSOR OF CLINICAL SURGERY IN THE UNIVERSITY OF THE CITY OF NEW YORK.

AT the meeting of the American Surgical Association at Washington, in 1888, one of the subjects of discussion was the prevention of shock during and after operations. It appears that, notwithstanding the great improvements in the treatment of wounds, the mortality from operations, due to primary and secondary shock, has not diminished, if, indeed, it has not increased. Failure of operations, due to shock, was attributed to prolonged procedures, nausea from the anæsthetics, and to the chilling dressings now applied. In a word, it was stated that pain and bleeding are less frequent; that slow cutting, nausea, exposure, and low temperature are more frequent; that primary shock has diminished, but that secondary shock has increased.

The truth of these statements is a matter of every-day observation. Rapidity of operation was a cardinal feature of the reputation of operators before the days of anæsthetics. The chief concern of the operator was to lessen the period of pain. Every detail of the procedure was carefully arranged with a view to celerity of execution. But it is evident that precision was then sacrificed to rapidity, and many operations failed to attain their ultimate objects owing to imperfections in the management of details. When, however, anæsthetics removed pain as an element in operations, the attention of surgeons was directed to precision in details, and with very happy results. Not only were the immediate and ultimate results of operations greatly improved, but the range of operations was immensely increased. These advantages were gained, however, only at the expense of prolonged anæsthesia, necessitated by the more complicated procedures and by the greater attention to all the steps of the operation. It follows that, notwithstanding the vast improvements in the details of operations, we are still confronted with shock as an even more fatal complication than formerly.

The preventive measures proposed in the discussion at Washington were simply such as every prudent surgeon adopts, viz., wait for reaction; calm the patient by a cheerful word; give stimulants before the anæsthetic; make anæsthesia short; operate as rapidly as practicable; dress quickly; avoid chilling the patient. After the operation apply dry heat; give liquid nourishment, with stimulants and laudanum, by the rectum; inject brandy subcutaneously; by the mouth give aromatic spirit of ammonia, and also black coffee and brandy; secure quiet, a horizontal position, and sleep; assure the patient that all is over and doing well. But in spite of all of these precautions it was alleged that secondary shock is very liable to occur and prove fatal.

Long since, impressed with the dangers of shock in many modern operations, owing to the long continuance of the anæsthesia, the liability to chilling and to depression from the loss of blood, I have been accustomed, where time will permit, to prepare patients for operations by stimulation to the extent of semi-intoxication. The results have been most happy, especially with feeble patients whose condition has rendered the propriety of an operation very doubtful. The course which I pursue is to give the stimulant in hot milk, beginning from *eight to ten* hours before the operation. Such quantities are given, and so frequently, as to secure a state of happy indifference to the operation on the part of the patient. If the operation is to be at three o'clock in the afternoon, I give directions to commence at six or eight o'clock in the morning. I prefer whiskey to brandy, owing to its slow and persistent operation over a much longer period.

If the patient is not accustomed to the habitual use of stimulants I order an ounce of whiskey every two hours in half a pint of hot milk. If at twelve o'clock, or even at ten, sufficient progress has not been made to render it quite certain that semi-intoxication will be secured at the appointed time, I give an ounce of whiskey in milk every hour during the remaining time. When the requisite effect has been obtained the stimulation should be discontinued. In the case of habitual drinkers I have given two ounces every hour. It is important to give the stimulant in hot milk, which will furnish a large supply of easily-digested and readily-assimilated food, in a form most useful to sustain the vital energies during the critical period of a severe operation, or during a necessarily-protracted operation.

The patient thus prepared has suffused eyes, a flushed skin, a slow full pulse, and complete indifference to the operation, though perhaps previously extremely timid. Frequently he jests and sings when taken to the operating-table. He is warmly covered except on the part to be exposed for the operation. The assistant who administers the anæsthetic is directed to suspend it as frequently as possible. It will be a matter of surprise to anyone who first administers an anæsthetic to a person partially, or quite, intoxicated by the foregoing means, to observe how quickly, and without a struggle, the patient comes fully under its influence, and how small the quantity required. The pulse remains at its normal standard throughout the operation, the breathing is quiet and regular, the skin continues warm and red, and without unusual perspiration.

During the twenty-four to forty-eight hours subsequent to the operation the condition of the patient remains good. The pulse continues full, the skin natural. the respiration undisturbed, and the mental state is that of indifference, or hopefulness. Neither primary nor secondary shock occurs under such circumstances.

To prevent chilling, the patient should not only be protected by warm clothing, but the wound should be douched with hot water containing the disinfectant. The exact temperature of the water is a matter of much importance, as the term "hot" is indefinite and misleading. In the haste of an operation the hand is often employed to determine the temperature of the water. This test varies somewhat with different individuals, as one person will shrink from placing his hand in water at a temperature which another may bear with little inconvenience. I have frequently tested the temperature of water in which an assistant could thrust his hand, though compelled to withdraw it instantly. This temperature does not exceed 150° F., but more often is 145° F. The hand I regard as a sufficiently good test for a temperature of 145° F. to 150° F. Nor should I care to apply water at a higher temperature than 150° F. to the wound. The late Dr. Varick, of Jersey City, who urged the use of hot water, advocated using water "slightly" below the boiling-point on operation wounds. Water at that temperature would, however, be destructive to tissues, for in my experience water at a temperature of 150° F. will destroy living tissues if it is allowed to remain in contact with them. It can be used at this temperature as a douche only—that is, it must be dashed on the wound. When applied to a fresh wound the surface should be rendered of a dull-gray color. The patient is usually instantly aroused by the heat. The best method of applying the water is by pouring from a pitcher; but not continuously; it should rather be dashed into the wound so that it will penetrate every recess. The effect of the hot water is also seen in the arrest of all oozing of blood from the wound, and this arrest of hæmorrhage is permanent, and prevents secondary bleed-

ing. The application of the dressings immediately follows, and as these consist of materials retentive of heat, there can be no chilling of the patient by the dressings.

During the past ten years I have pursued the above method of preventing shock, and in no instance has that complication occurred.

FEMORAL PHLEBITIS IN TYPHOID FEVER

BY S. C. CHEW, M.D.,
PROFESSOR OF THE PRACTICE OF MEDICINE IN THE UNIVERSITY OF MARYLAND, BALTIMORE.

IN the following report of cases of femoral phlebitis complicating typhoid fever, the term phlebitis is used in a clinical rather than in a strictly pathological sense. Cruveilhier and other pathologists of his time, as well as later pathologists, regarded the presence of coagula in veins as proof of the existence of phlebitis; but the investigations of Virchow conclusively showed that arterial and venous obstruction may be brought about by embolism and thrombosis independently of inflammatory change in the vessels. In fact, the changes in the walls of the vessels wrought by inflammation, such as roughening and thickening, which were thought to be especially causative of coagula, may, it is known, exist to a very great extent without producing any such obstructions. It is, for example, not uncommon to find the intima of the aorta and other vessels excessively roughened even by extensive calcification, without the occurrence of clotting.

Into the minute pathology of this subject, which is still under discussion and needs much elucidation, I do not now propose to enter. My object is to call attention to a particular form of venous obstruction that occurs as a complication of typhoid fever, and which cannot be regarded as very uncommon, and yet relatively to many other complications of this disease is perhaps infrequent. The seat of the obstruction in the cases referred to is the femoral vein. The thrombus occasioning it is termed *marantic* or *marasmatic*, and in accordance with the meaning of this term it is believed by some to be due to feebleness of the circulation resulting from heart-weakness and consequent retardation of the blood-current. Whether such slowing and enfeebling of the circulation are of themselves sufficient to produce the thrombus, is, I think, at least open to question. What share the accumulation of blood-plaques or hæmatoblasts may have in its production, as they have been shown to have in the case of other thrombi, has not yet been clearly shown.

In THE MEDICAL NEWS of September 7, 1889, three cases of femoral phlebitis complicating typhoid fever are reported as occurring in the clinic of Professor J. M. DaCosta. All of the cases were in men between twenty and thirty years of age. In all of them the phlebitis was first observed in the third week of the disease; in all the affection was in the left leg and thigh; and in all recovery took place. In this report it is mentioned as a curious fact, of which no accurate explanation has yet been given, that as a rule the left leg is the one involved in the trouble. It is further remarked that as nearly all cases recover, the pathology is difficult to get at. But the result is not always as favorable as in Dr. DaCosta's three cases; for Dr. Austin Flint, Sr., mentions a case in which sudden death occurred in typhoid fever from an embolus being detached from the thrombus and occluding the pulmonary artery,[1] and of course the possibility of such a result exists in every case. Liebermeister reports thirty-one cases of this complication with two deaths; and Murchison seventeen cases with three deaths, which, however, he thinks were not attributable to the complicating phlebitis alone.

The course of typhoid fever is indeed traversed by so many "downward slopes to death;" its fatal termination may occur in so many ways—as cardiac failure from high temperature; cardiac failure from muscular degeneration or exhausting diarrhœa; intestinal hæmorrhage; perforation; hypostatic pneumonia; or brain-lesion—that a person may readily die *with* femoral obstruction, and yet not *from* it.

I have said that this complication is absolutely not very uncommon. In addition to the writers already referred to, it is mentioned by Christison, who states that several examples of it occurred in Edinburgh between 1817 and 1820.[2] He remarks that it resembles the phlegmasia dolens of puerperal women, and says that it was first described by Dr. Tweedie, in 1828, as an occasional sequel of continued fever in the London Fever Hospital.

Strümpel speaks of swelling of one of the lower limbs, caused by venous thrombosis due to cardiac weakness, as sometimes occurring during convalescence from typhoid fever, but as happening in other cases too early to be attributable to weakness of the heart, and therefore due to some local specific cause.[3]

Hutchinson refers to it as resulting from heart-weakness, and states that he has seen both femoral veins obstructed at the same time.[4] None of these writers, however, except Professor DaCosta, as above quoted, refers to its special occurrence on the left side.

On the other hand, I have said that in comparison with many other complications of the disease, this one may be regarded as infrequent, and this statement is borne out by the fact that there is no mention of its occurrence in that storehouse of pathological facts, Cruveilhier's *Pathological Anatomy;* in Harley's very elaborate and learned article on typhoid fever in *Reynolds's System of Medicine;* in the lectures of Sir Thomas Watson; in Professor Loomis's *Text-book of Practical Medicine;* in Professor Bartholow's *Treatise on Practice;* nor in the writings of the late Professor George B. Wood.

In a considerable experience with typhoid fever derived from a practice of many years, I have never chanced to meet this complication among the cases which I have attended primarily, but I have witnessed it in four cases which I was called to see in consultation with professional friends, and the case occurring in the practice of each of these individual physicians was, I believe, the only one that he had ever encountered.

CASE I.—The first instance of this affection that I saw occurred in a married man about twenty-eight years of age, whom I was asked to visit in consultation by Dr. Charles H. Riley, in December, 1883. This patient, during the second and third weeks of his attack of typhoid fever, had been as near to death from cardiac exhaustion as I have ever known one to be who ultimately recovered. After convalescence was fairly established he was suddenly attacked with pain in his left thigh along the course of the femoral vessels and running down to the leg, which rapidly reached the degree of intense agony. The vein could be felt as a hard, corded line, and the whole limb became swollen and presented the tense and shining appearance that is seen in phlegmasia dolens. As the temperature of the limb, especially in its distal part, was somewhat lowered, it was kept enveloped in cotton-batting, and the pain was controlled as far as possible by hypodermic injections of morphine. In the course of a few days this pain subsided so that the morphine could be omitted. The swelling of the limb gradually lessened, and the case terminated in perfect recovery.

CASE II.—This occurred in September, 1884, in the practice of Dr. James Bosley, who requested me to see the patient. The patient was a married man about thirty-five years old, and was in the third week of typhoid fever, when he developed a condition of the left thigh and leg resembling that in Case I., except that the pain, while severe, was of less agonizing intensity. The œdema and the corded condition along the limb were as marked as in Case I. The treatment was the same, and the patient slowly recovered.

CASE III.—This case I saw in June, 1888, in Bel Air, Maryland, in consultation with Dr. B. H. Richardson. There were four cases of typhoid fever in the family, three out of the four being of great severity, and one nearly proving fatal from excessive intestinal hæmorrhage. Another one of the three, a girl seventeen years of age, showed very grave symptoms from an early period of the disease. In the fourth week the left thigh and leg became swollen and painful. The pain was much increased by pressure, but was not severe enough to demand

[1] Practice of Medicine, sixth edition, p. 963.
[2] Library of Practical Medicine, vol. i. p. 198.
[3] Text-book, p. 15, American edition.
[4] Pepper's System of Medicine, vol. i. p. 294.

morphine. The cord-like hardness along the femoral vessels was especially marked. The symptoms gradually abated and recovery ultimately took place.

CASE IV.—In August, 1888, I saw a fourth case of this kind in consultation with Dr. Tall, of Baltimore. The patient was a young married woman who had nearly passed through a well-marked, but not very severe, attack of typhoid fever, and had entered upon convalescence, when the same symptoms as those described in the preceding cases occurred in the left thigh and leg. The pain in this case was not violent, but the swelling of the limb and the hardness along the course of the vessels were very great. The subsidence of the symptoms was, however, rapid, no treatment being used except enveloping the limb in cotton-batting.

Four cases of this somewhat unusual complication of typhoid fever have now been described, two being male and two female subjects, so that as far as this number of cases indicates, no sexual proclivity is shown. In all, the left lower limb was affected, and all ended in recovery.

Whether there is any special anatomical explanation of the selection of the left limb I am unable to say. The left common iliac vein is, it is true, somewhat longer and more oblique in its course than the right, but the difference is hardly sufficient to account for the fact that the left femoral vein is so much more frequently affected by a condition from which its fellow altogether escapes.

Again, our Anatomies teach us that in some cases the left common iliac vein, instead of joining the right one in the usual position between the fourth and fifth lumbar vertebræ, ascends on the left side of the aorta as high as the kidney, where, after receiving the left renal vein, it crosses the aorta to join the right iliac. Whether this unusual length and tortuous course of a vessel having no valves may account for the occurrence of the obstruction in conditions of great weakness of the circulation, such as exists in typhoid fever, is a conjecture that may be hazarded ; but the explanation could be established only by finding the unusual course in a post-mortem examination of a case in which the complication had occurred. Opportunities for such examinations are seldom presented, and I know of no record of any having been made. Some more probable reason for the complication may exist, but at present I can only look upon it as, as Professor Da Costa does, as a curious fact of which no accurate explanation has been given.

EMPYÆMA, WITH REPORTS OF CASES, INCLUDING A CASE OF DOUBLE EMPYÆMA.

BY W. A. BATCHELOR, M.D.,
OF MILWAUKEE, WIS.

THE following brief histories of a few cases of empyæma are presented not as examples of any new plan of treatment, but simply as additional experience with what are now probably regarded as the best methods of treating a condition which is interesting alike to the physician and to the surgeon.

The subject is one upon which much has been written, and the attention thus called to it has, no doubt, stimulated a greater accuracy of observation, whereby fewer cases of the disease than formerly are overlooked. The discussions and recorded experience of the last few years have, I believe, also done much to improve the methods of treatment. The changes and improvements which have thus been made are epitomized in the two ideas of simplicity and cleanliness.

At the present time I think it may be laid down as an axiom that the presence of pus in the pleural cavity, be it in child or adult, is an indication for incision and free drainage. Cases undoubtedly do recover without operation by spontaneous absorption, by absorption after one or many aspirations, by rupture into the lung and discharge through a bronchus, or by rupture externally through an intercostal space. But the recovery under these circumstances is slow.; the patient becomes emaciated, anæmic, and weak, pleural adhesions may render subsequent expansion of the lung difficult or impossible, or the occasional residual products of spontaneous absorption may form a focus for a renewal of suppuration.

The subject of diagnosis may be briefly referred to. The physical signs of a pleural effusion are well known, and if the effusion is large the signs are unequivocal—absolute dulness with displacement of the mediastinum, a sensation of resistance to the percussing finger, a short, wooden percussion-note, and fulness or bulging of the intercostal spaces. The differential diagnosis between purulent and serous effusions is well stated by Money in his book on children's diseases, as follows: "The signs that tell for empyæma as against serous effusion are emaciation, anæmia, long duration, with sweating, fever, clubbing of the fingers, œdema of the affected side, with extra heat of the skin there and enlargement of the veins." An early diagnosis, however, and a *positive* diagnosis at any time, is best made by means of a hypodermic syringe with a large needle, though even the evidence thus obtained is not always absolutely unimpeachable. In a doubtful case I should advise repeated punctures, and, in children that are not easily controlled, puncture under the influence of an anæsthetic. In this sort of exploration let it not be forgotten that skin, needle, syringe, and hands should be *absolutely* clean.

CASE I.—Otto O., aged four and one-half years, operated on, June 4, 1888. He had been in my care for the four weeks immediately preceding this, for what I considered as left-sided catarrhal pneumonia. He had passed through the acuter stages of the trouble, the fever had abated, and there were signs of improvement. My visits and examinations had become less frequent. The improvement, however, was slow, some fever, poor appetite, etc., persisting. In the latter part of this period of four weeks, examinations of the chest were not made so frequently as they should have been, and pleurisy had not been thought of. Finally an examination showed that the chest was enlarged, distended, and dull almost to the clavicle. An exploration with a hypodermic needle made the presence of pus positive, and a quart was withdrawn by aspiration. Two days later a pint was drawn off in the same manner. Two days after this an incision was made between the sixth and seventh ribs in the axillary line, two rubber drainage-tubes were inserted, one long, the other short, and the cavity was freely washed with Thiersch's solution. The chest was washed out at each of the five or six subsequent dressings, at intervals of from two to four days. The dressing consisted of a mass of aseptic gauze, rubber tissue, cotton, and bandage. The long tube was gradually shortened. One tube was removed on the nineteenth day after operation, the remaining tube on the twenty-fifth day, after which the wound quickly and completely healed. The patient is now well and has been since the cicatrization of the wound.

CASE II.—Mamie S., aged seven years. First seen, May 27, 1889. Diagnosis, pleurisy of left side with circumscribed pneumonia. On June 8th, puncture with a hypodermic needle revealed pus.

Operation, June 11th: Free incision and drainage as in Case I., irrigation of the pleura with iodine water. No irrigation at subsequent dressings. Tube finally removed, July 3d. Recovery was prompt and the patient is now in good health. In this case a diagnosis was made early, and the early operation prevented the accumulation of any large amount of pus. About four ounces were removed at the time of the incision.

CASE III.—Mrs. S., aged thirty-six years, was operated upon in November, 1888. Two years before this the patient began to poultice the lower part of the left thorax, on account of pain which had existed in a greater or less degree since an attack of pneumonia some four or five months previously. Very soon a fistula formed, and continued to discharge pus. During this time the patient had been in poor health, and at the time of my first examination, November, 1888, was in a most unfavorable condition; fever constant, though not excessive, 101° to 103° being about the limit; pulse 120 to 135. She was anæmic, and the urine was albuminous. The left thorax was dull to the clavicle, the apex of the heart was at the right of the sternum. The patient had not menstruated for five months, and for some time previous to that menstruation had been irregular and scanty. Digital examination of the womb revealed no marked enlargement or displacement.

The operation was done November 22, 1888, the intention being to remove portions of four or five ribs. After removing sections of two ribs the condition of the patient was such that it was deemed advisable to complete the operation as quickly as possible, and to defer further excision for a secondary operation. Digital examination through the opening thus made revealed a cavity bounded below and anteriorly by the diaphragm and pericardium. The upper boundary could not be reached by the examining finger. A large quantity of pus and thickened masses of fibrin were removed through the opening. The cavity was well irrigated with iodine water, and the operation hastily completed. This case remained under my care for more than a year, the last drainage-tube being removed December 23, 1889, and the wound permanently closing soon after. The condition of the patient remains most excellent up to the date of writing. During all this time the wound was dressed at intervals of from one to three or four days.

An interesting and important event in the history of this case was the discovery, a month or more after the operation, of a tumor in the abdomen. Reviewing her menstrual history, it was feared that an ovarian tumor had appeared to complicate matters. No positive opinion was given, however, and it was soon evident that the patient was pregnant. Seven and a half months after the operation she was delivered, apparently at full term, of a healthy, large male child. The pregnancy was, no doubt, an important factor in the closing of the empyæmic cavity.

After the thorough drainage there was a considerable but slow expansion of the lung. The excision of two ribs permitted some depression of the chest-wall, and the upward pressure of the diaphragm by the pregnant uterus was an element quite as important as the other two in the obliteration of the cavity. The child, her fourth, is now over a year old, and is strong and healthy. The first child was stillborn, the second lived three days, and the third three months.

CASE IV.—Erna T., aged ten years, was first seen June 8, 1889. A diagnosis was soon and satisfactorily made of catarrhal bronchitis and left-sided pleurisy. After ten or twelve days an accumulation of fluid was evident. Later, the fever and sweating, and the slight œdema over the left side, suggested pus. An exploratory puncture under chloroform, with permission to operate, if necessary, was advised, but was at first declined. No improvement following, permission was given. On July 3d, the left thoracic cavity was aspirated, and three or four ounces of thick pus were withdrawn. On the following day the cavity was incised and drained. Between the time of the aspiration and the time of operating there seems from the history of the case to have been a rupture through the lung into a bronchus, for there was increased cough and expectoration of what was said to resemble pus. Some pus, I think, was swallowed, for after the incision the flow of pus, though free, was not so great as I had been led from previous physical examination to expect. The opening into a bronchus was proved by the distinct odor of chloroform at the incision. The pleura was not washed out. On

July 24th, one drainage-tube was removed. On July 31st, the remaining tube was found to have been accidentally pushed or drawn out of the wound, and the opening was practically closed. No attempt was made to reopen the wound. On August 1st and 2d there was a marked rise of temperature. On August 3d the temperature was normal, and a good recovery was soon established.

CASE V.—This case was one of double empyæma, and is worthy of note chiefly on account of the rarity of this condition, the operation and treatment being similar to those detailed in the cases already described.

Alban P., aged five years, was taken sick on March 21, 1890. He had an ordinary bronchitis, with considerable pain referred to the left side. Effusion was soon manifest on this side, and after puncture with a hypodermic needle the operation of incision with drainage was made, April 14th. At this time examination of the right side revealed slight dulness low down posteriorly, but the respiratory murmur was transmitted, though faintly, through the dull area. This dulness increased in intensity and extent, and the right side was incised, April 29th. No irrigation was used in this case. The fact that thicker pus and fibrous masses were obtained from the right side would seem to indicate that the trouble began in both sides at the same time. The patient made a most excellent recovery, the first opening being closed on May 16th, and the second four days later.

These are all the cases that have been under my own care. Another may be mentioned as a further illustration of the same simple mode of treatment. The patient was a youth, aged eighteen years, with empyæma of the right side, and was seen by me with Dr. C. H. Lewis. Incision and drainage, as above described, were followed by a satisfactory recovery.

Two other cases are also perhaps worthy of mention. One was that of a child about a year old. There were cough, emaciation, and fever, with dulness over the lower half of the right pulmonary area. An unsatisfactory puncture with a hypodermic needle was made, and two drops of yellowish serum, which may or may not have contained pus, were found in the needle. Puncture under chloroform, and an operation, if then found to be indicated, were advised and declined. The child improved somewhat while taking cod-liver oil, but died suddenly about six weeks later. The other was the case of a little girl, aged about seven years. The symptoms were somewhat obscure, except that pain was prominent. On about the ninth day there was dulness over the lower part of the left chest, somewhat more marked anteriorly. There was doubt as to the cause of the dulness, and the request to settle it by exploration with a hypodermic needle resulted in a change of doctors. The child died about a week later.

TREPHINING AND OPENING THE DURA MATER AS A DIAGNOSTIC MEASURE IN DISEASES OF THE BRAIN—WITH THE REPORT OF A CASE.[1]

By MILES F. PORTER, A.M., M.D.,
PROFESSOR OF SURGICAL ANATOMY AND CLINICAL SURGERY IN THE FORT WAYNE COLLEGE OF MEDICINE.

THE patient was a boy twelve years old. His family history was unimportant. He was active and healthy, except for the usual diseases of children, until May, 1888, when he had a convulsion, followed in twenty-four hours by an attack of mumps. He recovered from this, and had no further trouble until the following September, when he had a second convulsion. He was now placed in my care, and with the use of bromides he averaged about one fit weekly until July, 1889. From this time until the following September he had none. In October of the same year he had two in one day, and after that two each month until January, 1890. From the latter date until March, 1890, they were more frequent. The patient was then taken to another physician, under whose treatment he improved, and from the first week in March until the last of April he had no fits, when, notwithstanding the continuation of the treatment, he grew worse, and was brought again to me on May 1st, when he was having from twenty-five to fifty convulsions every twenty-four hours. I now learned that he had had *la grippe* in April, and that before he had entirely recovered he fell into the water and remained outdoors in his wet clothes for some time. When he reached his home his neck was stiff and the head drawn to the right side. Until May 1st, his attacks were those of ordinary epilepsy, with an aura on the outer side of the right leg and thigh, except that they usually commenced in and were most marked on the right side, and that sometimes when he felt a fit coming on "he would get up and run about for a minute or two, belch considerably," and thus prevent a major attack.

After May 1st, he did not lose consciousness during the attacks, which would commence by flexion of the fingers of the right hand, quickly followed first by tonic then clonic spasm of the right upper and lower extremity, and right side of the face, in the order named.

Paralysis commenced May 1st, involving first the thigh and leg, then the arm, and lastly the face on the right side; motor aphasia developed with the facial paralysis. The paretic symptoms increased until July 2d (the date of operation), at which time he was unable to walk, could not raise his hand to his mouth, sat with his head falling forward and to either the right or left, and with a decided lack of expression in the right side of the face. He spoke with great hesitation and difficulty. There was no ptosis. Though his slowness in replying to questions and lack of facial expression made it appear that his mental faculties were failing, yet I feel certain, from frequent examinations, that they were as active as

---

[1] Read before the Fort Wayne Academy of Medicine. August 12, 1890.

ever, or nearly so. So far as I could determine, none of the muscles were completely paralyzed, but only in a condition of marked paresis. There was no loss of sensation, and the patellar reflexes were normal. He was given 90 grains daily of bromides, in different combinations, from May 1st until the operation. For the three weeks preceding the operation he also took from 75 to 120 grains of potassium iodide daily.

I should state that in 1884 the boy fell and received a scalp-wound in the left occipital region, but there were not then, nor are there now, any signs of fracture of the skull, nor is there any tenderness in the region of the scar.

The patient was sent to Dr. K. K. Wheelock for an examination of the eyes, but absolutely nothing abnormal was found. During last June his temperature was found on several occasions to be from one to two degrees above normal.

There was no tenderness upon percussion, but there was slight headache, referred to both temporal regions. On three occasions only was any peculiarity of the pupil noticed—dilatation of the right. Having presented the patient to the Fort Wayne Academy of Medicine, and being unable with the aid of the Fellows to arrive at a diagnosis, and in view of the fact that the patient was steadily growing worse, I proposed an exploratory trephining, to which the parents and the patient gladly assented, each remarking that death was preferable to existence in the present condition. It was understood that whatever was revealed by the exploration should be dealt with in whatever manner seemed best. It was explained to the parents that we might find no visible lesion, and that in that case there would yet be a *faint hope* that the operation would be beneficial.

Operation.—The operation was performed, July 2d, in the City Hospital in the presence of Drs. Jelleff and Boyers, of Decatur, and Drs. Dills, Mary Wheery, H. S. Myers, C. Proegler, and Greenawalt. Dr. W. P. Wheery administered the chloroform, while Drs. A. P. Buchman and H. McCullough assisted.

The left Rolandic fissure was located according to the method of Championnière, as described in *Wyeth's Surgery*, the lines on the scalp being marked in ink and a fine bone-drill used to mark the skull after the flap was turned down. A long horseshoe-shaped incision was made, the flap turned down, and two buttons of bone were removed with a seven-eighth-inch trephine, the second being a little below and in front of the first. The intervening bone was removed with a rongeur, thus exposing the dura overlying the ascending parietal and frontal convolutions and a portion of the foot of the third frontal. Nothing abnormal appearing, the dura was divided by a curved incision to the length of the opening in the bone and turned aside. Examination of the areas supposed to be involved, by inspection, palpation, and by the use of a probe and exploring-needle, revealing nothing, the dura was stitched, the flaps were united and dusted with iodoform, and the parts covered with carbolized gauze and a bandage. Silk was used for all the
15*

stitches. Strict asepsis was observed and nothing but boiled and strained water was used in cleansing the wound. The dressing was changed at the end of twenty-four hours, as the outer bandage was stained by the oozing. It was not removed again until the seventh day, when the stitches were removed and complete primary union found to have taken place. From the 5th to the 14th of July the patient was under Dr. H. McCullough's care, during my absence from the city, and for his kindness I desire here to offer my thanks.

There was nothing of importance in the convalescence so far as concerns the operation *per se*. The highest temperature—100½°, with a pulse of 140—was found on the day following the operation. Contrary to Dr. McCullough's wishes, the patient left the hospital on the tenth day after operation, and since that time has not been confined to bed.

The convulsions steadily decreased up to the sixth day, when the patient had only four; they then increased until the ninth day, when he had eleven; while on the tenth and last day in the hospital he had seven. After he went home they continued to decrease, so that between July 25th and 31st he had but one.[1] With the decrease in number there has also been a decrease in severity, while there is a very marked improvement in his speech, and he walks unassisted, and is able to throw objects to a distance of 100 feet with his previously paralyzed arm and to feed himself with it. His facial expression is likewise improved, he is cheerful, sings, plays, and, in short, enjoys life once more.

REMARKS.—I do not wish to be understood as reporting this case as one of epilepsy permanently benefited by operation, nor as one which promises complete recovery. Time alone can decide as to the ultimate results.

Before the operation I was inclined to look upon the case as one of epileptoid convulsions due to organic disease of the cortex or subcortical substance about the Rolandic fissure, and I am still inclined to that opinion. The number and character of the convulsions, of late, and the paresis exclude, it seems to me, the diagnosis of functional epilepsy. Acquired syphilis is out of the question, while the family history and the treatment by the iodides set aside the idea of inherited syphilis. The paresis of only certain groups of muscles, together with the absence of sensory paralysis and eye-symptoms, is against a diagnosis of basal disease. Certainly the clinical history of the case since May 1, 1890, clearly points to the diagnosis of Jacksonian epilepsy due to a lesion of the Rolandic zone, commencing probably in the upper and extending thence to the lower portion. And in view of the normal appearance of the cortex and the absence of tenderness on percussion we may conclude that the sub-

---

[1] The patient walked to my office, a distance of more than a mile, to say that he had had no convulsions for eight days. His paresis also continues to improve.

cortical substance is the seat of the trouble. In the absence of paralysis we would be less warranted in thus localizing the trouble, for then we might reasonably conclude that the irritation originated at some distance from the seat of explosion.

"But if following these limited spasms paralysis of motion should occur in the parts formerly convulsed . . . . and still more so if a succession of monoplegia should result in a general hemiplegia, then we may with certainty diagnose organic disease of the Rolandic zone of the opposite cerebral hemisphere."[1]

But what shall we say of the attacks prior to May 1st, when, as I have said, they resembled ordinary attacks of *grand mal,* except that the convulsions usually commenced, and were worse, on the right side.

It must also be remembered that while at first the attacks began in the outer side of the knee and thigh, that after May 1st they began with flexion of the fingers. This raises the question as to whether we may not have in this patient a functional epilepsy followed by organic changes, such changes being the result of the epileptic attacks or a complicating disease. I was not able to see the patient in one of the attacks prior to May 1st, but had the symptoms been noted by a trained observer my opinion is that, taken with the history since that time, we would have a well-defined clinical picture of Jacksonian epilepsy.

The most important point connected with this, as well as with all similar cases, has not yet been touched upon. I have concluded—and for the sake of argument will assume that the reader agrees with me— that the trouble is organic and involves the subcortical substance in the Rolandic zone ; but, what is the exact nature of the disease ?—is it a tumor ? and if so, is it fluid or solid ? and if solid, is it encapsulated ? To decide these and similar questions exploratory trephining is not only warrantable but demanded in many cases, and it is to add my mite to the statistics of this question and to excite a discussion by the Fellows of the Academy that I report this case so soon after the operation. Ferrier, as quoted by Gray in the article previously referred to, says: "In the absence of definite indications as to the character of the tumor . . . . trephining is, in my opinion, justifiable as a diagnostic measure."

I desire to state as my opinion that it is advisable as a diagnostic measure in cases other than those of tumor ; for while it may not, as in my case, clear up the diagnosis, it is *per se* an operation attended by very trivial danger considering the gravity of the cases in which it should be resorted to.[2] If the dis-

ease proves amenable to operation, we avert death, which is otherwise inevitable ; if it cannot be removed by operation, or nothing is found, we have done our duty. Besides, the operation will occasionally, albeit rarely, cure, though nothing further than trephining and exploration be done. How the cure is brought about in such cases no one knows, any more than we know why or how exploratory laparotomy cures tubercular peritonitis, or removal of spinous processes and lamina of vertebra cures spinal paralysis, or dilatation of the cervix uteri cures the vomiting of pregnancy. To my mind the most satisfactory answer to this question is that given by Dercum and White,[1] who say :

"It would seem as though the local shock had been promptly followed by a corresponding reaction, in which the vitality of the tissues had been raised sufficiently high to determine a return to the normal state."

Several other points of interest suggest themselves in connection with this case, but these I will leave until a future time, when I shall report the further progress of the patient. I will conclude with the statement that it is my firm conviction that exploratory operations should occupy the same relation to brain surgery that they do to abdominal surgery.

100 FAIRFIELD AVENUE.

THE TREATMENT OF HÆMORRHOIDS BY EXCISION.[2]

BY CHARLES B. PENROSE, M.D., PH.D.,
SURGEON TO THE GYNECEAN HOSPITAL AND TO THE OUT-PATIENT
DEPARTMENT OF THE PENNSYLVANIA HOSPITAL.

MY object in presenting this paper is to urge the more general use of Whitehead's operation of excision in the treatment of certain cases of hæmorrhoids.

In 1887, Mr. Whitehead, of Manchester, reported[3] three hundred consecutive cases of hæmorrhoids which had been successfully treated by the method of excision and suture. His operation is performed in the following manner :

1. The patient is placed on a table in the lithotomy position, with the hips well elevated.

2. The anal sphincters are then thoroughly paralyzed by digital stretching.

3. The mucous membrane of the rectum is divided at its junction with the skin around the entire circumference of the bowel.

4. The mucous membrane, with the attached hæmorrhoids, is dissected from the submucous tissue, and the cuff or cylinder thus formed is dragged below the margin of the skin.

5. The mucous membrane above the hæmorrhoids is then divided transversely, thus removing

1 Ferrier, quoted by Gray in the Annual of the Universal Medical Sciences, vol. ii. p. 2, 1890.
2 I mean, of course, when performed with thorough antiseptic precautions.

1 Annals of Surgery, July, 1890.
2 Read before the Philadelphia County Medical Society, September 10, 1890.
3 British Medical Journal, February 6, 1887.

the pile-bearing area, and the operation is completed by suturing the upper margin of the severed membrane to the free margin of the skin.

The advantages claimed by Whitehead for this method of treatment are based on pathological and on surgical reasons. He considers that the internal hæmorrhoids, which are generally regarded as localized distinct tumors, amenable to individual treatment, are, as a matter of fact, component parts of a diseased condition of the entire plexus of veins surrounding the lower rectum, each venous radicle being similarly, if not equally, affected by an initial cause, constitutional or mechanical.

The operation of excision is the only one which removes this whole diseased area. It is, therefore, demanded for this pathological reason. It is in addition surgically more perfect than any other method of treatment, because it provides for the readjustment of healthy tissues with the object of securing primary union and rapid convalescence. It does not leave the sluggish ulcer of the cautery, nor is it attended with the pain and slow convalescence of the ligature.

My experience with this operation is limited to ten selected cases. Only those cases were selected in which there existed a complete circle of hæmorrhoidal tumors surrounding the lower margin of the rectum, since for such cases Whitehead's method of excision seems to be particularly adapted.

The details of the operation are simple and easy to execute. In dividing the mucous membrane from the skin it is best to begin at the posterior margin of the anus in order to prevent the blood from obscuring the field of operation. No skin should be sacrificed, even though there appear to be redundant tags around the margin of the anus. The skin always retracts somewhat and the tags shrivel and disappear before firm union has taken place. Failure to observe this rule may result in subsequent serious trouble. Kelsey[1] reports the case of a woman who had been subjected to a so-called Whitehead operation and who presented herself to him with a complete circle of excoriated mucous membrane extending for one inch outside the anus. It is probable that in this case the operator had sacrificed too much skin.

On the other hand, the upper section of the mucous membrane should be made in the same horizontal plane throughout, in order to prevent subsequent ectropion ani.

The dissection of the mucous membrane from the underlying tissue is exceedingly easy except in some cases of long-standing piles. The attachment of the submucous tissue is very loose, and separation can be effected with the finger or with the handle

---

[1] New York Medical Journal, October 5. 1889.

of the scalpel. It is not always possible to dissect the piles completely from the underlying structures, as they may involve not only the mucous but the submucous tissues, and in such cases it is necessary to cut partly through the piles until the healthy mucous membrane above is reached. Repeated attacks of inflammation of course render closer the adhesion of the pile-area to the underlying structures. In one of my own cases in which the piles had existed for forty years, and had frequently been inflamed, the adhesions to the two sphincters were so close that a few muscular fibres were cut away during the removal.

The amount of blood lost during the operation is surprisingly small. Whitehead states that he has often operated on severe cases and not found it necessary to twist a single vessel. In five of my cases no hæmostasis was necessary. Bleeding is avoided by adhering closely to the mucous membrane in the dissection, as the larger arterioles lie beneath the submucous tissue. Arterial bleeding occurs in those cases of old piles which have been subjected to previous operation or to attacks of inflammation, and in which dilatation of the rectal and anal arteries has taken place secondary to dilatation of the hæmorrhoidal veins. The bleeding from the upper divided edge of the mucous membrane can be reduced to a minimum by following Whitehead's method of inserting the sutures as each portion is divided, or by adopting Marcy's plan of introducing a circle of shoemaker-stitches of catgut around the mucous membrane above the piles before cutting the mass away.

Whitehead's advice is to remove in all cases the complete cylinder of mucous membrane, whether or not the whole of this area appears to be diseased. He gives this advice for the reason which I have already stated, that he considers the individual piles as but part of a general pathological condition, involving all the lower hæmorrhoidal veins of the rectum.

Whether we accept this pathological view or not, it is best to follow his plan, and to make a complete circular division of the mucous membrane, as by this method the most perfect surgical results are obtained, and ectropion ani prevented. I have seen a case in which only one-half of the circumference of the mucous membrane of the rectum was removed, and a few hours after the operation an œdematous swelling formed in the other half, which has now resulted in a hæmorrhoidal tumor almost as annoying as the one for which the operation was performed.

In attaching the mucous membrane to the skin Whitehead uses interrupted silk sutures. He never removes the sutures. but allows them to ulcerate through—a process which is very easily accomplished. In my own cases I have used the continuous catgut suture.

The treatment of these cases after operation is very simple. It is rarely necessary to use opium or the catheter. An opium and belladonna suppository introduced immediately after the operation is in most cases all that is required. The bowels can be moved in from twenty-four hours to four days, and with very little pain. Absence of pain after Whitehead's operation is due to the thorough paralysis of the sphincters, and to the fact that no source of irritation is left beyond that of a clean linear incision, united without tension and without strangulation of tissue.

A glance at the histories of my own cases shows that they were all cases of aggravated hæmorrhoids, in which the piles covered the whole circumference of the lower part of the rectum. In all the cases the disease had existed for many years, and two had been previously subjected to operation by the ligature.

In only one case was there anything like free bleeding during the operation.

In all the cases a suppository of ½ grain of extract of opium and ½ grain of extract of belladonna was introduced immediately after the operation, and this was all the opium required except in three cases, in which ⅙ grain of morphine was subsequently administered.

The catheter was used in only three cases, and in these for a period not longer than twenty-four hours. The length of time that the case is confined to bed depends to a great degree upon the social standing and the disposition of the patient. In my cases it varied from two to ten days. Every case should be able to sit up in four or five days, and to resume work in ten days or two weeks.

The bowels were opened without pain in from twenty-four hours to four days after operation.

No complications of any kind followed these operations. Union takes place quickly, and generally one dressing, taken off when the bowels are moved, is all that is necessary. In no case was there incontinence from paralysis of the sphincters, or any tendency to stricture from contraction of the scar.

Since the publication of Whitehead's paper his method of operating has been tested by many surgeons. The operation cannot be criticised on surgical grounds, as it is certainly the most perfect plan of treatment, surgically speaking, which has been proposed.

The immediate removal of the tumors, the coaptation of healthy tissues, and primary union, are substituted for slow strangulation by the ligature, or removal by the cautery and healing by granulation.

The applicability, or the necessity, of this operation in all cases of hæmorrhoids, is, however, open to criticism. If we accept Whitehead's views in regard to the pathology of piles, and believe that the whole venous plexus surrounding the anus and the lower end of the rectum is in a pathological condition in every case of hæmorrhoids, even though there may be present only one or two isolated tumors, then, of course, the complete removal of this area is indicated.

But that this view is not true is proved by the thousands of cases which have been permanently cured by the ligature and the clamp. The method, however, is indicated in all cases of aggravated hæmorrhoids in which the vascular tumors cover the whole or the greater part of the circumference of the bowel. In such cases the operation presents no great difficulties. Statistics show that it is at least as safe as operation by the ligature or the clamp, and it is certainly followed by a more rapid convalescence, and much less pain and discomfort.

PERNICIOUS ANÆMIA, WITH A REPORT OF FIVE CASES.

BY A. McPHEDRAN, M.B.,
LECTURER ON CLINICAL MEDICINE IN THE UNIVERSITY OF TORONTO, ETC.

EACH of the following cases possesses features sufficiently interesting for publication. My experience leads me to believe that pernicious anæmia is much more common than is generally supposed, and that, as in other diseases of an obscure nature, a diagnosis is seldom, if ever, made until the case has lasted some time. This has been true in all my own cases, and I have seen nothing in the reports of cases which would lead me to believe that my experience differs from that of others. It would be very interesting to know the effects of treatment begun in the early stage.

CASE I.—B. T. P., aged forty-nine years, a physician practising in the northern part of Canada, came under the joint observation of Dr. Byron Field, of Toronto, and myself, on May 1, 1889. His family history contained nothing of moment. He had been subject to "bilious" attacks occasionally for several years; his health was otherwise good until three or four years ago, when he noticed that he was less vigorous, and that his "bilious" attacks were more frequent. He gradually became anæmic, but this did not attract particular attention till the autumn of 1888, when anæmia was quite decided. He continued to attend to his laborious practice, though with increasing difficulty. Toward the end of the winter of 1888–89 he found it almost impossible to continue his work, but he persevered until he was compelled to give it up—about April 15th. He had been under treatment for some time for anæmia, taking iron and digitalis freely but without benefit.

After giving up work he grew rapidly worse, and on the evening of May 1, 1889, when first seen by

Dr. John Ferguson, Dr. Field, and myself, he was in a state of marked delirium, from which he could be recalled to only a semi-conscious condition. He had just passed through an extremely severe chill; his temperature was 104° F., pulse 120, small and weak. The body was well nourished, but there was extreme pallor with a decided lemon color. Vomiting troublesome; the stomach was distended with gas, much being belched up; and there were frequent loose motions with considerable flatus and colicky pains. The heart and lungs presented nothing abnormal; the liver and spleen did not seem to be enlarged.

On the next day the blood was examined; it had a venous tinge and appeared diluted. The corpuscles showed no tendency to form rouleaux; they varied greatly in size and shape, measuring from three to twelve μ. Of the large ones the greater number were irregular in shape, being oval, pear-shaped, balloon-shaped, and pointed. Some seemed to be budding, the bud being from one-fifth to one-third the size of the corpuscle. All the corpuscles were pale, but some were decidedly paler than others. There was also some granular débris, rather dark in color. In estimating the number of corpuscles Gowers's hæmacytometer was used. There were 745,000 per c.mm.—an average of 100 squares. No increase in the number of white corpuscles. Not having the appliances the percentage of hæmoglobin was not estimated, but it was very low, though probably relatively higher than the corpuscles. The patient was given champagne at short intervals until the stomach became quiet; then a pill of arsenious acid, $\frac{1}{15}$ grain, every three hours, the interval to be shortened to two hours after a few doses. Diet: milk, raw or peptonized, matzoon, beef peptonoids, etc.

May 3. Another chill; temperature 104°; enemata of milk and whiskey given.

4th. He was more rational; had a slight hæmorrhage from the mucous membrane of the mouth and spat a few clots. He retained medicines and nourishment, but was extremely restless and obtained only short periods of sleep; diarrhœa troublesome. The urine had to be drawn by a catheter. It was high-colored, specific gravity 1010, acid, no albumin. Not examined with the microscope. The arsenic was given every two hours, except during sleep. He received ten doses (⅔ grain) in twenty-four hours.

6th and 7th. Polyuria—about 100 ounces of urine being passed daily, which was acid, and darker than such dilute urine should be; specific gravity 1005. Great thirst and restlessness.

8th. A severe chill lasting fifty minutes at 1 A. M. Temperature during chill 104°. Very restless and delirious. Often refused food. Temperature had fallen to normal at 5 A. M.

10th. His appearance was better. Dr. R. A. Reeve examined the eyes and found the fundus very pallid and containing many small hæmorrhages. There was a large hæmorrhage into the conjunctiva of the right eye. The blood on being drawn looked like cherry-juice. Corpuscles were more regular in shape and seemed higher colored; less débris; 731,746 per c.mm. Some tendency to form rou-

leaux. Bowels regular. Urine paler and in considerable excess.

20th. Progress slow; greatly troubled with flatulence. Consciousness gradually returned. Has taken increasing amounts of nourishment, and with relish. A hasty examination of the blood showed about 1,000,000 red corpuscles per c.mm.; corpuscles much more regular in shape; no débris; fewer microcytes. Arsenious acid, ¼ grain daily.

25th. Greatly improved in appearance; a decidedly pink tinge to lips and finger-nails. A few days before this the veins on the back of the hands were of a peculiar magenta color. His appetite was good and had to be restrained. As more convenient, the arsenic was given every three hours, and liquor arsenicalis substituted for arsenious acid, from thirty to forty minims being taken daily without any gastric disturbance being caused. Some sores in the mouth healed rapidly after applications of nitrate of silver.

30th. Able to take a full diet. Corpuscles showed more tendency to form rouleaux, and were more regular in shape, but still varied in size; 1,676,687 per c.mm., the average of 80 squares.

June 7. Color greatly improved; able to sit but not to walk. Corpuscles 2,300,000 per c.mm., quite regular and scarcely distinguishable from normal.

11th. The fundus oculi still pallid, arteries small but otherwise normal.

18th. Corpuscles 2,500,000 per c.mm.

July 1. Corpuscles 3,217,000 per c.mm.; rouleaux fairly formed; a few irregular corpuscles found; diameter varied from 6.6 to 10 μ. Felt well; appetite and digestion good; bowels regular. He slept well, and was able to walk a mile. Still taking 30 minims of liquor arsenicalis daily. A few days after this he went home.

About July 15th, a copious purpuric rash appeared on the feet, legs, and body, with severe pain and some swelling of the feet, which were relieved by rest and elevation. He said that he had had wandering pains in various parts of the body for four or five weeks before this acute attack. He stopped taking the arsenic and these symptoms soon improved. The rash lasted ten days, but the pains disappeared slowly, and even now pain in the feet troubles him somewhat. It is possible that the rash was due to the arsenic, as a few cases are on record of such a rash from the medicinal use of the drug.[1] The pain and tenderness of the feet may have been due to neuritis caused by the arsenic, but this is very improbable, as such a result is all but unknown. More probably the pains were rheumatic.

July 27. Corpuscles 4,500,000 per c.mm.. normal in size and shape; rouleaux well formed.

November 6. Looked and felt well. Able to attend to a fair amount of professional work without becoming tired. General health better than it had been for three or four years. Some disagreeable numbness in feet and a little in hands. Urine normal. Corpuscles 4,100,000 per c.mm., by a hasty estimate.

Since then he has continued well and is attending

---

[1] Duhring. Diseases of the Skin.

to his practice as usual. He writes me that he feels in better health than he has for several years.

CASE II.—The notes of this case are from my hospital case-book, and were taken by Dr. R. W. Palmer, my clinical clerk.

W. J. H., aged thirty-nine years; born in the United States; family history good; a piano-tuner. A small man, not robust, and with a fastidious appetite. Temperate in the use of alcohol, but smoked excessively for some years. His health was fair until 1885, when he had troublesome diarrhœa for some months, and he has not been very well since then. In the winter of 1888, he said, he had pleurisy and pneumonia, and while recuperating from this in the following June, his attention was first called to his extremely anæmic appearance. His complexion had been high-colored. He was in the Toronto General Hospital during most of the winter without improving. He went out in February and returned in May, 1889, after which he was unable to leave his bed. He was extremely anæmic, with a decided greenish-yellow or lemon tint. Conjunctivæ pearly. He was of spare habit but not emaciated. The skin was moist. Temperature, A. M. 99°; P. M. 99.8° F.; pulse 100, fairly full but soft. Heart and lungs normal; soft murmurs at base of the neck. Liver normal; spleen slightly enlarged. Bowels irregular and diarrhœa frequent. Urine high-colored, normal in quantity, acid, specific gravity 1017. No albumin or sugar, but some uric acid crystals. Night-sweats troublesome. Blood-corpuscles 606,000 per c.mm., the average of sixty squares of Gowers's hæmacytometer. No rouleaux formed, many corpuscles were oval, tailed, budding, and pointed. Their size varied from three to eleven μ. Liquor arsenicalis was given, at first 3 minims three times a day, and later 5 minims every three hours. But he soon complained of epigastric pain and diarrhœa, and the abdomen became distended so that the arsenic had to be withdrawn until these symptoms abated. It was then given again, but in three or four days the pain returned and the arsenic was again intermitted. Fearing that he magnified his suffering, an arsenical pill ($\frac{1}{30}$ grain) was ordered under the name of "pil. anæmiæ," that he might not know he was taking arsenic. The pills were given three times a day at first, increasing to six daily, by which time the pain became unbearable. The pills were omitted until the symptoms abated, when they were again taken, to be omitted when the pain became troublesome.

In this manner the treatment was kept up until he left the hospital for the Convalescent Home. At the same time the most nourishing food he could take was given to him, reliance being placed chiefly on milk and nitrogenous foods. The blood was examined from time to time and found to improve gradually, the improvement in the character of the corpuscles being much more rapid than the increase in their number. The temperature remained about normal, occasionally rising to 100°; at such times his urine was darker and he was feeling worse.

June 1. Corpuscles 606,000 per c.mm.

July 3. Corpuscles 1,043,000 per c.mm.

18th. Corpuscles 1,560,000 per c.mm.

August 9. Corpuscles 1,810,000 per c.mm.

16th. Corpuscles 1,620,000 per c.mm.

25th. Corpuscles 1,950,000 per c.mm.

September 4. Corpuscles 2,180,000 per c.mm.; much more nearly normal in shape; tendency to form rouleaux.

16th. Corpuscles 2,520,000 per c.mm.

October 8. Corpuscles. 2,600,000 per c.mm.; only an occasional irregular corpuscle; a few microcytes; rouleaux better formed.

He was then removed to the Convalescent Home, a supply of medicine being given him, with directions to omit it when the pains became troublesome and to resume it again when they disappeared. The matron of the Home was so much alarmed at the pain produced that she refused to allow him to remain if he continued to take the medicine. He called to tell me this on October 19th. He was then apparently greatly improved. Corpuscles 2,780,000 per c.mm.; very little irregularity; rouleaux well formed; the color of the corpuscles uniform and not so dark as in June. He was directed to omit all medicines.

November 6. Corpuscles 3,250,000 per c.mm.; no abnormal ones seen. Looked and felt well. Walked a great deal.

December 24. Corpuscles 4,560,000 per c.mm.; normal. Did not remember having ever felt so well, looked perfectly healthy, and weighed 130 pounds—five pounds more than his ordinary weight. Had taken no medicine since leaving the hospital in October.

When last seen, this summer, he was in excellent health and without any trace of his illness. There has not been an opportunity since December to examine the blood.

CASE III.—This case I had the privilege of seeing with Dr. George Acheson, of Toronto.

Mrs. M., young, of healthy parentage, gave birth to her second child in January, 1889. She passed through the puerperal period satisfactorily, except that she was rather pale and did not regain her strength readily. Lactation was well established. The pallor progressively increased, and there were recurrent attacks of diarrhœa. She was given iron in various forms without benefit. Some febrile movement was discovered in February and sepsis was feared, but nothing could be found to account for the fever which was not marked or constant. The increase in the anæmic condition was gradual, and pernicious anæmia was not thought of as a possibility until March 1st, by which time a lemon tint of the skin had developed—this tint never became very marked. The urine had been high-colored, of normal volume, and low specific gravity. The blood was found to contain only 1,781,000 red corpuscles per c.mm.; their size varying up to 13 μ. No rouleaux were formed, and there was decided irregularity in the shape of the corpuscles. There was also a considerable number of Eichhorst's corpuscles present. The eyes were examined by Dr. R. A. Reeve, and two hæmorrhagic patches found in one eye and three in the other.

Calomel was given to empty the bowels of any offending matter, and naphthalin to keep them disinfected as far as possible. Liquor arsenicalis, from 10 to 20 minims daily, was given as the stomach would bear it. At the same time the patient was allowed to drink freely of a chalybeate water and red wine.

There was but little improvement in the condition of the blood during March. The temperature gradually fell to normal. She then began to improve slowly, with occasional slight relapses, and by the end of five or six months she had regained her usual health.

The condition of the house not being above suspicion, an examination was made. Under the cellar floor the ground was found covered with stable manure, placed there by the workmen while building. This was decomposing and giving out a very unpleasant odor. There is little doubt that this had much to do with the patient's illness, as other persons in the house became more or less indisposed also. The conditions following parturition rendered her more susceptible, and caused the poison to affect her in the manner described. Whatever the explanation may be, she presented all the phenomena of a decided case of pernicious anæmia, and we must consider it as such until fuller knowledge of the pathology of that disease enables us to exclude everything not belonging to it, no matter how close the resemblance. Should the now rather prevalent opinion that pernicious anæmia is due to a special poison gaining access to the system through an unhealthy gastro-intestinal tract prove correct, then it will be easy to see the connection between that unsanitary cellar and Mrs. M.'s illness.

CASE IV.—Dr. A. T. C., a highly-esteemed physician of Toronto. His history is briefly as follows: He had an attack of *la grippe* in January, 1890, and was confined to his house for three weeks. Though far from well, he attended to his professional duties during February. He had a second attack of *la grippe*, in March, and has been quite ill since then. Marked anæmia followed this second attack. At one time malignant disease was suspected, as vomiting, almost at once after food was taken, was a prominent symptom. There were some evidences of Bright's disease, and still are. In April he went to Long Island for the change of climate. He returned in June slightly improved, and since then has been sometimes better, sometimes worse. His temperature is often slightly elevated, at times 101° F. His color occasionally has a decided lemon tint, but usually only slightly so. Though he has lost flesh he is not emaciated. He is subject to attacks of diarrhœa at short intervals, and irregular vomiting.

The blood was examined in June by Dr. John Carden, who found about 1,800,000 corpuscles per c.mm, with very marked poikilocytosis. On July 31st I found the number of corpuscles to be 1,750,-000 per c.mm, very irregular, no rouleaux, size from 3 to 13 µ. No increase of white corpuscles. Some reddish-yellow granular débris. The urine was dark, and required dilution by about an equal volume of water to reduce it to normal color ; specific gravity 1017 ; decidedly acid in reaction, and contained about one-sixth volume of albumin. Numerous granular casts, some large and irregular,

and most of them containing a large amount of dark granular pigment. Few renal cells, much granular débris of yellowish color.

August 12. Corpuscles, 1,780,000 per c.mm. They appeared less irregular and of better color. The patient felt and looked much better, his appetite improved, bowels were regular, urine much paler, specific gravity 1018. A trace of albumin and a few casts were found, but no yellowish pigment. He always feels worse when he has diarrhœa, and the urine becomes of a higher color. The mouth becomes sore, and the excoriations of the anus—always present—increase. He has been taking no arsenic for some time.

15th. Has had what he calls a "bilious attack"—vomiting and diarrhœa—since yesterday. Took a podophyllin pill, ¼ grain, last night. Ordinarily this would just move the bowels. Urine darker, specific gravity 1018, some pigment-granules and casts ; becomes cloudy on heating. He had tried arsenic in solution and pill-form, and found that it always caused disturbance of the stomach and bowels in a few days, with a metallic taste and soreness of the mouth, and increase of the anal affection. It is very doubtful if the arsenic was entirely responsible for these attacks, for he had precisely similar ones such as the attack above described, without arsenic having been taken for days. So much was I impressed with this opinion that I strongly advised him to persevere with the arsenic, notwithstanding the discomfort caused, omitting it when these attacks showed their first symptoms, and returning to it again as soon as they passed off. The ultimate success after long perseverance in Case II. amply justified such advice. He was also advised to try minute doses of corrosive sublimate at short intervals for its antiseptic and tonic effect. He has been at the seaside for a month and has now begun to improve.

CASE V.—Elizabeth H., aged twenty-eight years. Married. Family history unimportant. She has not enjoyed very good health since she began to menstruate, at the age of twelve years. She entered the Toronto General Hospital, September 1, 1890, and gives the following history of her present illness:

Two years ago she first noticed a slight greenish-yellow hue to the complexion ; she was then in indifferent health. From January until April, 1889, she was quite ill, suffering as she is now, the jaundiced hue being then marked. Bowels irregular, urine at times very dark, appetite poor, and occasional vomiting. During the summer she regained fair health and was able to do her own work, her complexion becoming much more natural. This state of health continued until last winter, when she had an attack of *la grippe*, and since then has been in poor health, with a return of the jaundiced complexion. She gave birth to a child, her fourth, July 25th. She was very well for three days after labor, when her appetite failed. She got up on the tenth day, but had to return to bed and has not been able to be up since. She has had irregular diarrhœa all summer, alternating with constipation lasting for a few days. She usually vomited every morning. Appetite various, at times craving, and at others no desire for food. She is a spare woman, but not emaciated, very pallid, and with well-marked lemon tint; conjunctivæ pearly.

Physical examination revealed nothing except a slightly enlarged spleen. Heart normal; pulse 100, and very small. Temperature has varied from 100° to normal since her entrance into the hospital, showing no regular gradations. No chills. Urine high-colored, specific gravity 1020 to 1025, some flocculent deposit; no casts or granular matter; no albumin or sugar, reaction acid. About 1,200,000 red corpuscles per c.mm, not very irregular in shape. They varied in size from about 4 to 13½ μ. No increase in white corpuscles.

The treatment consisted in the administration of beta-naphthol, 5 grains three times a day, to disinfect the bowels as far as possible, and liquor arsenicalis 30 minims daily in divided doses every three hours. The diet was milk, yolks of eggs, etc.

The results in the first three of these cases are eminently satisfactory. All the cases present to a greater or less degree the typical features of pernicious anæmia, namely, the marked pallor with the lemon tint and without emaciation; the febrile disturbance; the high-colored, acid urine of low specific gravity, but not increased in amount; the disturbance of the digestive tract as shown by the occasional vomiting and irregular diarrhœa; and lastly, the typical blood-changes.

In all, the pallor was very marked, as was also the lemon tint, except in Case III., in which it was only slight.

Except during the attack of polyuria in Case I., the urine in all the cases was characterized by a high color and low specific gravity, especially during the paroxysms in Cases I., II., and IV. In Case IV. the only one except Case V. in which a microscopical examination of the urine was made, renal casts infiltrated with many granules, were found, and after an exacerbation of symptoms, when the urine was much darker in color, many spherical yellow granules, usually in masses, were found in every specimen. When the exacerbation passed off and the patient improved, the urine became more nearly normal in color, and the granules were not present. Hunter, Mott, and others attach great importance to the presence of these signs in the urine, and think that the phenomena are sufficient of themselves to establish the diagnosis of pernicious anæmia.[1] They indicate a great destruction of red blood-corpuscles with liberation of hæmoglobin, and that the blood-destruction occurs in the portal circulation, as shown by the condition of the liver and the absence of hæmoglobinuria.

These cases agree also in the constancy with which they present disturbances of the digestive tract, the intestine being more severely affected than the stomach. The recovery of the first three cases proves the absence of any serious organic disease—

the symptoms point rather to a mild catarrhal condition of the mucous membranes.

Another feature worthy of note is that commencing improvement was characterized by a better shape and color of the red corpuscles rather than an increase in their number. This was true at least in Cases I. and II.; in Case III. no note was made on this point, and in Case IV., in the few observations made, the corpuscles were found more regular in shape during the period of improvement than during the exacerbation. It would seem that the corpuscles damaged during the exacerbation had been completely destroyed, and that the new corpuscles were affected to a less degree by the destructive agent which is probably thrown into the blood during the exacerbation. The absence of marked irregularity of the corpuscles in Case V. is to be noted. It is not exceptional to meet with cases of pernicious anæmia in which, though the corpuscles are very large, the poikilocytosis is not marked.

Pernicious anæmia is characterized by no constant anatomical lesions, though lesions are, however, exceedingly numerous and of great variety. The most constant are those of the digestive tract, and so frequent are these that they have been considered by some as the essential lesions of the disease. In the gastro-intestinal tract have been found malignant disease, atrophy of the peptic glands, inflammatory thickening of the interstitial tissue of the gastric mucosa, and degeneration of the nervous structures of the intestinal walls. In a few, intestinal worms —ankylostoma duodenale and bothriocephalus latus —or a foreign body, as a nail, have been present and their removal followed by recovery. None of these, however important they may be in individual cases, can be regarded as the essential cause of the disease. They exist in many cases without the development of any of the phenomena of pernicious anæmia, while they are absent in other cases of the disease.

Of the anatomical changes resulting from pernicious anæmia, the most important, next to those occurring in the blood itself, indicating as they do the nature of the disease, are found in the liver and kidneys. The hepatic cells in the periphery of the lobules are deeply infiltrated with granules of free iron. Similar granules are found in the epithelium of the convoluted tubules of the kidney. Mott found an abundance of this iron pigment in the small branches of the hepatic vein also, but none in either the intestinal or hepatic branches of the portal vein.[1]

These changes in the liver and kidneys, together with the brownish-yellow "droplets" of hæmoglobin occurring in the high-colored urine, indicate that pernicious anæmia is characterized by excessive

---

[1] The Practitioner, December, 1889.

[1] The Practitioner, August, 1890.

destruction of blood, which is more or less paroxysmal, and occurs in the portal circulation, with
the liberation of hæmoglobin. The hæmoglobin is
carried to the liver, where it is decomposed into
bile-pigment and free iron, the latter being deposited
in the hepatic cells, and, when too abundant for the
liver to dispose of, in the renal epithelium, the former
being largely excreted as normal or pathological
urinary pigments.[1]

The question now arises, What is the morbific
agent that causes this blood-destruction in the portal
system? In a recent paper[2] Dr. William Hunter,
of Cambridge, than whom probably none has done
more to elucidate the pathology of this obscure
disease, as the result of a careful investigation of a
case ending fatally, has, he believes, shown that
there were greatly increased putrefactive changes
occurring in the intestinal tract, as proved by the
increased excretion of aromatic sulphates in the
urine. He also succeeded in isolating a ptomaïne
that he had not hitherto found in connection with
ordinary putrefaction. As ptomaïnes are formed
from proteids by the agency of bacteria, and not
from ordinary tissue-metabolism, he thinks that this
ptomaïne may signify the presence in the intestinal
canal of a specific microörganism. In the light
of his studies he ventures the following conclusion:

"The special factor required to initiate the symptoms
peculiar to pernicious anæmia is the presence, under
certain favorable conditions, ·of organisms of specific
nature within the gastro-intestinal tract.

"These conditions may be either local and permanent
—malignant disease, various forms and degrees of gastritis, with atrophy of gastric glands; or general and
removable—a specially unhealthy condition of the
mucous membrane of the stomach and intestine, induced by the presence of intestinal parasites, or by prolonged bad nourishment."[3]

This is a very fascinating theory, and one cannot
but wish that it would stand the test of future investigation, but as yet it is "not proven."

Delépine, as the result of a careful study, shows
that the liver has, what he suggests might be called
a "*ferrogenic*" function, by which he means that it
"separates iron from effete iron-containing pigment, stores it in the form of a loose compound,
and gradually elaborates it into a more stable albuminous compound, analogous, if not identical, with
hæmoglobin, ready for assimilation by the young
red blood-corpuscles."[4]

Mott,[5] as the result of a study of three cases of
pernicious anæmia, and in the light of the observations of Delépine, suggests that the disease is an
exaggeration of a normal physiological process, due
to the presence of some abnormal product. Pep-

tone, he says, if not changed, has a marked influence upon the blood, and might lead to such disturbance of this "ferrogenic" function of the liver
as to cause increased hæmolysis. In connection
with Hunter's theory of a chemical product of the
growth of some microörganism, Mott observes that
he did not *always* find a relation between the pyrexia,
the diminution of the corpuscles, and the color of
the urine. In my own cases, as far as my observations extended, this relationship was very marked,
and especially so in Case IV.

From all these observations it seems safe to conclude that pernicious anæmia consists in an excessive hæmolytic process in the portal system,
remittent and often progressive in character. As to
the active agent in this destructive process there is
not so much certainty, but at present it seems probable that a variety of poisons may be capable of
producing it. In one case it may be a ptomaïne, in
another one of the multitude of albumoses, or both a
ptomaïne and an albumose may be present. It is
possible that such a variety of poisons may explain
the varying results obtained from treatment.

Medicinal Treatment.—With an increasing knowledge of the disease the treatment should become
more rational. Since gastro-intestinal derangement
is so often associated with the disease, our first
efforts should be directed to correcting these disorders as far as possible. In the majority of cases
an occasional calomel purge seems to be beneficial.
Something should be expected of intestinal antiseptics, of which, probably, the best are thymol, beta-
naphthol, naphthalin, and similar compounds.
Thymol is, probably, the most powerful, but many
patients find it the most difficult to take on account
of disturbance of the stomach produced, often with
vomiting. Beta-naphthol is more easily borne.
Naphthalin, it is said, may cause choroidal hæmorrhages, which may possibly simulate retinal hæmorrhages,[1] so that the eyes should be examined before
beginning its administration. Small doses of the
perchloride of mercury might prove useful both as
an antiseptic and as a tonic.

Arsenic still stands preëminent as the remedy
for pernicious anæmia. It has effected a cure in a
large number of cases, and when it has failed seldom
has recovery been attained. It is characteristic of
the majority of cases that they bear large quantities
of arsenic without any signs of disturbance. Case I.
took a fourth of a grain daily for weeks. Some,
however, bear it badly, and others not at all. This,
as already pointed out, may be due to the degree of
gastric catarrh present. Various theories to explain
its action have been advanced. By some its effects
have been attributed to local antiseptic properties,
a very improbable explanation in view of the small

[1] Lancet, 1888, vol. ii. Practitioner, 1889.   Guy's Hospital
Reports, 1889.
[2] British Medical Journal, 1890, vol. ii.   [3] Ibid.
[4] The Practitioner, August, 1890.   [5] Ibid.

[1] Kolinski: Arch. de Physiologie, April, 1890.

quantity that suffices for the cure of some cases, unless there is a special poison present over which arsenic has peculiar powers; and if this were true, it should always succeed. Others have attributed good effects to stimulation of blood-formation and metabolism. This would not account for the arrest of the excessive hæmolysis that is going on. A third view is that it affects the blood-corpuscle, enabling hæmoglobin to resist the tendency to be dissolved in the blood-serum—in other words, that it increases the resistive powers of the blood to the morbific agent, if there is such an agent. This view is certainly more in accord with the probable pathology of the disease.

Judging from my own limited experience, I think that the greatest amount of benefit will result from the administration of arsenic in frequently repeated small doses, the maximum quantity that the patient will bear being given. If it cannot be taken for more than a few days it should be intermitted until the symptoms of irritation abate. Some patients bear minute doses, a drop or half a drop of the liquor arsenicalis every hour or two, when larger doses disagree. Its administration should be persevered with, if possible, until there is decided benefit, when it may be intermitted probably without disadvantage. Case II. indicates that in some cases at least arsenic is not necessary after convalescence is well established, and that then nothing more but good food and proper care are needed to complete the cure.

In those cases in which arsenic fails, or is not well borne, iron in some form should be tried, as in a few it has succeeded after arsenic had failed. It is a matter of surprise that iron has proved of so little use in this disease. If Hunter's opinion as to the increased putrefactive processes going on in the intestinal tract be true, iron in large quantities is indicated. It has been well established, especially by Bunge,[1] that the good effects of iron in anæmia are due to its powers of neutralizing the alkaline sulphides resulting from putrefaction in the intestines, converting them into stable iron sulphide, thus preventing the sulphides from destroying the iron in the hæmatogen of the food, from which only, and not in the least from the iron of medicines, the blood derives its iron for the hæmoglobin.

Hydrochloric acid, also, should prove of benefit, as in all these cases there must be a deficiency in the digestive fluids, and the more perfect the digestion the more rapid the absorption and the less the putrefaction. Hydrochloric acid alone is, for this reason, sufficient to cure many cases of ordinary anæmia.

Diet.—Our natural impulse, in view of the pro-

found poverty of the blood, is to give those foods which contain an abundance of nutriment for the blood-corpuscle, such as milk, yolks of eggs, meat, and such vegetable substances as the cereals. Until some other course is definitely proven to be better, it would appear best to follow our natural impulses in this matter. Food should be given in small quantities, and often, so that digestion may be rapid, thus giving less time for decomposition.

As the result of a short experience in his last case Hunter advises a trial of a more or less exclusively farinaceous diet, believing that it may be attended with less blood-destruction.[1] In health a nitrogenous diet causes a much greater destruction of blood than a farinaceous or fatty one. While this should be of very little moment in a disease in which the blood is destroyed by a special poison, yet the improvement resulting from the change of diet leads him to believe a trial of the nitrogenous foods desirable. This would certainly seem worth bearing in mind in the treatment of cases that are not doing well on ordinary diet.

In view of the decided benefit usually resulting from the use of arsenic in this disease, and of the fact that nearly all anæmias are benefited by the administration of the remedy, it seems highly desirable to resort to its use in all persistent anæmic conditions of doubtful character without waiting for a positive diagnosis. If this were done much valuable time would be saved in many cases, and possibly we would have fewer failures to record in the treatment of even pernicious anæmia.

ULCERS OF THE LOWER EXTREMITIES.[2]

BY J. A. MACK. M.D.,
OF MADISON. WIS.

WITHOUT attempting to discuss the pathology of ulcers, it may be said that whether resulting from occupation or any other non-specific cause, the venous circulation surrounding them will always be found faulty. The veins before ulceration are overloaded, distended, and tortuous; their valves give way and partial stagnation occurs, with transudation of serum, loaded with excrementitious matter, into the surrounding tissue; swelling results, beginning at the most dependent parts and gradually ascending, accompanied with constant irritation of the skin caused by the attempt to eliminate the effete material with which the serum is surcharged. Then if a rupture of a venous radicle, or if the slightest injury of the integument occurs, an ulcer results; or to relieve the intense itching and burning (both being worse at night), scratching is indulged in

---

[1] Lehrbücher Phys. und Path. Chemie, Leipzig, 1889, p. 84-95.

[1] British Medical Journal. vol. ii., 1890.
[2] Read before the Central Wisconsin Medical Society, June, 1890.

until finally a small sore results, which gradually enlarges, growing painful as it increases in size.

The arbitrary varieties of leg-ulcers described in the text-books are somewhat misleading. For instance, it is said that an ulcer may become chronic from the age of the patient, improper treatment, or the character of the tissue involved; and that an ulcer may be indolent and irritable from like causes. Yet the fact is, that they all are both chronic and irritable, and so much depends upon the situation, the treatment, the avocation of the patient, and last but not least, upon the patient's susceptibility to pain, that classification is of little moment. As a rule, these cases are not seen until all home remedies have been indiscriminately tried, consequently there is much nerve-irritation in addition to a constantly-growing sore.

The foul, dirty, at times gangrenous, ill-smelling ulcer, covered with some rancid dressing and a bandage saturated with the discharge, may well be called indolent, and speaks forcibly of its owner's habits. To this class a lecture on personal hygiene never comes amiss, but unless the patient is watched the directions are never carried out.

Another class of ulcers are those with a glazed, hardened base, with thick and sometimes everted edges, that are deep, quite extensive, and accompanied with great swelling of the limb and with some eczema. Patients with these suffer greatly, both mentally and physically, and have usually been under the care of many physicians.

Sex is a factor in the symptomatology, for it matters not where situated, or whether indolent or chronic, these sores in the female can always be classed as irritable.

Having had a large experience with these cases (numbering about two hundred) during the past twelve years, and without a failure in treatment, I have arrived at the following conclusions:

1. That the average leg-ulcer is usually treated too harshly.

2. That the surface of the ulcer is a non-absorbing one.

3. That absolute rest is unnecessary.

4. That the age of the ulcer is of no importance.

5. That if the bodily functions are well performed, and if the patient is in fair health, without specific taint, internal medication is uncalled for.

Of all forms of treatment so far proposed, the rubber bandage and absolute rest are best known. My objections to these are, that where eczema exists it is aggravated; that if not present it is likely to be induced, especially in warm weather; that it is impossible to know just how much pressure each turn of the bandage will make, owing to its natural retraction; and that absolute rest is a hardship, especially if the patient's existence depends on his daily labor.

In my practice the following method has been pursued, and with such good results that I am not likely to change:

Gently douche the ulcer with either warm or cold water, dry the limb by enveloping it in a towel and dress with the following ointment: White-lead in linseed oil (common white paint) and vaseline, equal parts; carmine, a sufficient amount to color slightly. Spread thickly on lint, and apply to the ulcer, being careful that the margins are well covered. Immediately over the ulcer, and upon the dressings place a pad of absorbent cotton; now bandage carefully from the toes to the knee, applying the bandage with moderately firm, even pressure. The bandage that answers the requirements best is made from unstarched bleached muslin, and is two inches wide and from eight to ten yards long. If well applied, it is unnecessary to renew it oftener than every second day. A loose bandage or soaked dressing should be immediately changed. A good rule to follow is to renew the dressings often enough to sustain pressure and to keep the limb comfortable.

Additions may be made to the ointment to meet indications; thus, if the ulcer is sluggish or gangrenous, the addition, for a few days, of ten grains of iodide of lead to each ounce of ointment, acts as a mild stimulant, without escharotic action, and also as a disinfectant.

In applying the bandage let the patient sit on a chair with the limb straight, and the heel supported on another chair.

After healing has taken place a well-fitting elastic stocking should be worn.

MASTOIDITIS INTERNA PURULENTA FOLLOWING ERYSIPELAS.[1]

BY J. A. LIPPINCOTT, M.D.,
OF PITTSBURG, PA.

THE following case, especially interesting from an etiological standpoint, presents some additional features which help to make it worthy of being placed on record:

E. S., twenty-eight years old, had always enjoyed excellent health, and had never suffered from any aural affection, his hearing on both sides having been, indeed, exceptionally acute.

He was attacked on March 27, 1890, with erysipelas of the face and scalp, which produced great tumefaction. Ten days later two large abscesses, one below the left eye, and the other above the occiput, were evacuated with a bistoury. The swelling and the discharge of pus gradually subsided during the next four weeks.

One week after the beginning of the attack, without previous pain or special local swelling, and

1 Read before the American Otological Society, july, 1890.

without any symptoms in the throat or nose, pus began to flow from the right ear. His medical attendant, Dr. McCormick, of Greensburgh, an intelligent physician, states that at this time the walls of the external auditory canal were normal, and that the pus obviously came from the middle ear through an opening in the drum-head. About May 15th (the otorrhœa in the meantime continuing) the neighborhood of the ear became swollen, and extremely painful. Under hot poulticing these symptoms yielded in about a week. On June 22d the pain and swelling recurred, and continued until I saw the patient June 29th, when the condition was as follows :

Decided swelling and tenderness over whole mastoid region on the right side. Doubtful fluctuation in upper mastoid region. External auditory canal filled with pus, on removing which, at a point about two-thirds of the length of the canal from the external meatus, was seen a furuncular-looking mass with its base attached to the posterior wall, and large enough to render a view of the tympanic membrane impossible. Pus was seen coming from behind this mass, but apparently very little came from the mass itself. A watch of forty inches hearing-distance was heard when lightly pressed against the ear. Examination of the throat and nares negative. The patient complained of deep-seated pain behind the ear, and he was considerably emaciated.

I advised an operation on the mastoid as the quickest way of securing thorough drainage and consequent relief.

Two days later the patient returned and went to the hospital, where an anæsthetic was administered and the mastoid perforated in the usual way. A small collection of pus was found under the perlosteum, at a point about three-fourths of an inch above the meatus externus ; but neither there nor at any other place could any trace be found of an opening into the mastoid cells.

On perforating the external wall, which was thin, the cells were found extensively broken down, the cavity thus formed being filled with a greenish, unhealthy-looking pus, which reminded me strongly of the appearance of the pus removed some years ago from an orbital abscess following erysipelas. A warm solution of boric acid, thrown into the opening by means of a syringe, escaped through the auditory canal. The syringe was subsequently used daily, but no pus afterward issued either from the mastoid opening or from the meatus.

All the unpleasant symptoms were promptly terminated by the operation. On the fourth day the protrusion from the posterior wall of the canal had almost disappeared, and the tympanic membrane could be easily examined. A perforation in the centre of the latter, about three mm. in diameter, was seen, from which, by means of the 'cotton probe, a very minute trace of pus was removed. The hearing on the fifth day had improved so that the watch could be heard at two inches. Patient went home in a week with the suggestion to Dr. McCormick to continue the irrigation, and to keep the wound open as long as might seem necessary.

Erysipelas as a cause of mastoiditis interna must be rare. In the limited period which has elapsed since I saw the case above described, I have not been able to find a report of any other case arising in this way.

The sequence of the pathological phenomena is not without interest, nor, it may be added, without uncertainty. The mastoid disease may have been metastatic in character, and so, in a sense, primary. The history of the case before I saw it, however, perhaps tends to show that the first link in the chain was a painless abscess in the middle ear. Then followed invasion of the mastoid cells, accompanied with violent symptoms, and finally rupture through the posterior wall of the auditory canal, which gave temporary relief. The recurrence of the pain and swelling probably arose from blocking up of the opening in the auditory canal.

CLINICAL MEMORANDUM.

OBSTETRICAL.

Eclampsia Fifteen Days after Labor. Death.—J. H., aged thirty-six years ; nervous temperament ; had been married for four years when she first became pregnant. In the latter part of gestation she had a mild but persistent diarrhœa, and also œdema of the vulva and lower extremities. The œdema of the vulva was excessive and troublesome, but was relieved by treatment. Labor was normal, with but little hæmorrhage and without nervous manifestation. The patient was anæmic, but improved at once with the use of iron and arsenic. One week after confinement there was some irritation of the stomach, but this was readily controlled. She also complained of headache, which her husband stated she had been subject to for some years. Aphasia manifested itself, and when asked how she felt, she would answer, "I feel—I don't know what." The attendants stated that she occasionally had brief "nervous spells," but these attracted no attention. Temperature slightly elevated ; pulse 120.

On the fourteenth day after labor damp clothes were put on her, and a few hours later she complained of severe pain below the knee extending upward to the hip and to the abdomen. Morphine and hot applications gave relief. On the next morning her pulse was 130, temperature nearly normal, appetite fair. At 2 P. M. convulsions began, four or five paroxysms following at short intervals. Inhalation of a small quantity of chloroform and the administration of chloral controlled them. Vaginal irrigation with carbolized water had been used for some days, but thinking the trouble might possibly be caused by reflex irritation from the uterus, I now used an intra-uterine douche. The os was somewhat patulous and discharged a slightly-stained mucus which was not offensive. Rapid respiration and coma followed, with death thirty-six hours after the first convulsion.

C. V. MOORE, M.D.

FAIRMOUNT, IND.

MEDICAL PROGRESS.

Euphorine.—Under the name of euphorine, SANSONI (*Therapeutische Monatshefte*, September, 1890) describes the physical and therapeutical properties of a new compound which, chemically, is phenylurethan. It is a white crystalline powder, with a faint aromatic odor and a slight taste suggesting that of cloves. It is sparingly soluble in cold water, readily dissolves in alcohol, and is best administered in white wine, in which it is easily dissolved.

Given to healthy men, in doses of from 1½ to 3 grains, euphorine has no apparent effect upon the pulse, the respiration, or the temperature; and in dogs large doses do not lower the blood-pressure, as determined by the manometer. Still more important is the fact that it causes no changes in the blood—in animals the blood remaining normal even after toxic doses have been given.

Clinically, Sansoni finds that euphorine possesses valuable antipyretic, antiseptic, antirheumatic, and, in some cases, analgesic effects. As an antipyretic, he has employed the drug in fever from various causes, such as typhoid fever, croupous pneumonia, phthisis, acute rheumatism, pleurisy, orchitis, influenza, etc., administering it either as a powder or dissolved in wine. The fall of temperature begins within an hour after the administration, reaches its maximum usually in about three hours, and continues, as a rule, for from five to seven hours. In some cases the fall is more brief, and in a few it continues for fourteen hours. The subsequent rise of temperature is usually sudden and accompanied with a chill, the duration and severity of which are proportionate to the intensity of the disease. During the period of apyrexia the patient has a feeling of well-being. Cyanosis is seldom observed, and the pulse and respiration are regular. The antipyretic effect varies in different persons, and it is best to begin with a small dose (1½ grains), increasing until the proper amount is determined. To most adults, from 15 to 22 grains can be given daily without producing harmful effects, its antithermic power being about twice that of antipyrine.

In rheumatism, both acute and chronic, the doses of euphorine should be larger than those given to reduce temperature. From 22 to 30 grains, or even more, should be given daily. In acute rheumatism the good effects appear very soon after the drug has been administered; the temperature falls, and the pain, whether due to inflammation or to the pressure of the swelling, disappears.

As an analgesic, euphorine is very useful in orchitis, less so in sciatica, lightning pains of tabes and trigeminal neuralgia, and is almost useless in intercostal neuralgia and migraine.

The observation that carbolic acid is formed when euphorine is brought in contact with an alkali, led Sansoni to test its antiseptic powers, which, in the case of an obstinate ulcer and one of chronic ophthalmia, he found were excellent.

The Relations of the Cœliac Plexus to Diabetes.—LUSTIG, in a series of experiments on animals to determine the function of the cœliac plexus, found that extirpation of the plexus, electrical excitation, and irritation by acetic acid produced similar symptoms, namely: glycosuria, usually temporary, but occasionally permanent; acetonuria, which, when of long duration, led to severe symptoms; and subnormal temperature. Further, to determine whether the cœliac plexus is a necessary organ in the production of diabetes, Lustig punctured the diabetic area in the medulla in dogs from which the plexus had been removed. Diabetes resulted from the puncture, showing that the cœliac plexus is not always concerned in the production of the disease.—*Centralblatt f. klinische Medicin*, September 6, 1890.

Pill for the Treatment of Chronic Constipation.—In the treatment of chronic constipation NOTHNAGEL advises the use of the following, when a laxative is necessary:

R.—Podophyllin . . . . 4½ grains.
Extract of aloe }
Extract of rhubarb } of each . 45 "
Extract of taraxacum, a sufficient quantity.

Mix and divide into forty pills, of which one, two, or three may be taken at bedtime.—*Therapeutische Monatshefte*, September, 1890.

Removal of a Portion of the Liver by an Elastic Ligature.—TERRILLON reports a case in which a portion of the liver was removed by means of an elastic ligature. The patient was a woman, fifty-three years old, who for some years had suffered from a painful swelling situated in the right lobe of the liver. An exploratory puncture revealed the presence of a small quantity of fluid resembling that of a hydatid cyst. Although after the puncture the swelling diminished, Terrillon opened the abdomen on the right side by an incision parallel to the false ribs, exposed the tumor, and placed an elastic ligature around it. At the end of seven days the sphacelated portion with the ligature was removed. The wound, of which the base was formed of hepatic tissue, was separated from the peritoneal cavity by firm adhesions. Cicatrization was complete at the end of the sixth week.—*The Medical Press*, September 10, 1890.

The Microbe of Alopecia—Recent researches at the Institut Pasteur have been made by DRS. VAILLARD and VINCENT in regard to a form of baldness occurring in soldiers, which is very similar to, if not identical with, alopecia areata. Their report, published in the *Annales* of the Institut, show that the malady, in this particular instance, is caused by a micrococcus which, when cultivated and inoculated in lower animals, produces an analogous baldness. Hitherto dermatologists have strongly inclined to the belief that most of the cases of alopecia areata are forms of a tropho-neurosis, no microorganisms with an apparent causative relation having been discovered. The fact, however, that there are on record several cases with histories pointing very directly to contagion, has raised doubts as to the correctness of that explanation.

Massage in the Treatment of Dyspepsia.—DR. CSÉRI, of Budapesth, publishes an account of a mechanical plan of treating chronic dyspepsia which he has lately been carrying out with excellent results. The plan consists mainly in suitable dieting, and in a peculiar kind of massage. The author practises the latter when the stomach is full—about two or three hours after dinner. Frequently changing his mode of proceeding, he strokes and kneads the stomach from the fundus toward the pylorus, first gently and superficially, then more energetically, for ten or fifteen minutes, the patient lying on his back with his legs drawn up, and breathing with his mouth open. During the last few minutes the massage is extended to the bowels. The manipulation is neither painful nor disagreeable, but is very well borne. After the massage the patients experience a feeling of warmth and comfort; occasionally they are sleepy, but the fulness and sensation of weight have generally disappeared. The immediate result of this kind of massage is that the stomach is freed from gas, thus producing a great feeling of relief. The time chosen for the massage is when part of the already chymified ingesta begins to enter the duodenum from the healthy stomach. In dyspepsia the stomach is generally sluggish, and either the quantity or quality of its secretion is impaired, and consequently chymification or peristaltic motion, or both, are insufficient. It is also known that mechanical stimulation of the stomach may increase its secretion, and the author considers himself justified in concluding that massage thus increases the process of digestion. He also finds that at the same time muscular power increases and that the massage mechanically helps to advance the stomachic contents into the duodenum. The rapid cure of pains and general malaise after eating in cases of nervous dyspepsia is easily explained by the fact that the manipulation dilates the pylorus, so that after a few days it offers no impediment to the passage of the food.—*The Lancet*, September 20, 1890.

Toxic Effects of Creolin.—BOREHMEYER reports the case of a child who received a severe contused wound of a finger, which was treated by applications of a solution of creolin (one and one-half per cent.). On the fourth day the finger was covered with vesicles containing a yellowish liquid. On changing the dressing the eruption disappeared, but returned when the creolin was again used. WACKEY publishes an account of 17 surgical cases dressed with creolin. In 10 union by first intention occurred, but in 7 the creolin produced eczema, erythema, and vesicular eruptions, and desquamation in large patches. At the same time the patients had more or less constitutional disturbance, and an examination of the urine showed that the toxic symptoms were attributable to the presence of phenol. It would seem that children are especially susceptible to the deleterious effects of phenol and its derivatives, and hence are more readily affected by creolin than adults are.—*Therapeutic Gazette*, September, 1890.

Socin's Zinc-paste Dressing.—VON NOORDEN (*Brun's Beiträge z. klinisch. Chirurgie*) has found Socin's zinc-paste an admirable dressing after operations for harelip. The paste is composed of:

Zinc oxide . . . . 50 parts.
Zinc chloride . . . . 5 to 6 parts.
Water . . . . 50 parts.

When exposed to the air it dries very rapidly, forming a firm crust. It should be freshly prepared for use.

After completing a harelip operation, the suture-line and vicinity are disinfected and thoroughly dried, then the paste is spread over the entire upper lip, by means of a brush or spatula, and is reinforced with a very few thin layers of cotton. If the wound extends into the nostril, the dressing should also extend into the opening, but, of course, without blocking it. The nasal secretions will not soften the paste. In from four to six days the dressing may be changed to remove the sutures, and, if not already partly loosened, it can be clipped off. A fresh application is then made, and allowed to remain until it crumbles. The paste has also been used in small wounds of the face and scalp, after herniotomy, extirpation of labial cancer, and even after cœliotomy.—*Annals of Surgery*, September, 1890.

The External Use of Aristol.—POLLAK, of Prague, has had excellent results with the external use of aristol in the treatment of a case of strumous enlargement of the right lobe of the thyroid. He used an ointment prepared as follows:

R.—Aristol . . . . 45 grains.
Potassium soap . . 7½ drachms.
Ether } of each . . 75 minims.—M.
Alcohol }

In a case of epididymitis applications of vaseline containing ten per cent. of aristol also caused a rapid disappearance of the swelling.—*Monatshefte f. Praktische Dermatologie*, September 15, 1890.

Treatment of Eczema and Acne.—According to *Le Semaine Médicale*, September 3, 1890, UNNA recommends the following ointments for the treatment of eczema and acne.

R.—Lanolin . . . . 5 drachms.
Liquid chloride of calcium 10 "
Oil of cade . . 2½ "
Zinc ointment . . 7 "

This ointment is employed in cases of chronic eczema of a pruriginous form, accompanied by profound infiltration of the skin.

R.—Zinc ointment . .)
Lanolin . . . } 2½ drachms.
Liquid chloride of calcium)
Precipitated sulphur . 45 grains.

The following ointment may be used in cases of acne:

R.—Lanolin . . . .)
Lard . . . . |
Liquid chloride of calcium } 2½ drachms.
Oxygen water . . |
Precipitated sulphur .) 1 drachm.

The action of the oxygen water in this last prescription is for the purpose of removing the comedones commonly found in the face of persons suffering from acne. Wherever rapid decoloration of these comedones is desired the following may be used:

R.—Oxygen water . . 5 to 10 drachms.
Vaseline . . . . 5 "
Lanolin . . . . 2½ "

THE MEDICAL NEWS.

A WEEKLY JOURNAL
OF MEDICAL SCIENCE.

COMMUNICATIONS are invited from all parts of the world. Original articles contributed exclusively to THE MEDI-CAL NEWS will be liberally paid for upon publication. When necessary to elucidate the text, illustrations will be furnished without cost to the author.

Address the Editor: H. A. HARE, M.D.,
1004 WALNUT STREET,
PHILADELPHIA.

Subscription Price, including Postage.
PER ANNUM, IN ADVANCE . . . . $4.00.
SINGLE COPIES . . . . 10 CENTS.
Subscriptions may begin at any date. The safest mode of remittance is by bank check or postal money order, drawn to the order of the undersigned. When neither is accessible, remittances may be made, at the risk of the publishers, by forwarding in *registered* letters.

Address,　　LEA BROTHERS & CO.,
NOS. 706 & 708 SANSOM STREET,
PHILADELPHIA.

SATURDAY, OCTOBER 11, 1890.

SYPHILITIC DISEASE OF THE HEART.

THE power of the syphilitic poison to impress itself upon all the tissues is so well recognized, that *a priori* no objection can be raised to the recognition of a specific cardiac affection due to that virus. If, indeed, the blood be the medium of communication by which the toxic agent—microbe or ptomaïne, or whatever it may be—is diffused throughout the organism, it would seem most natural that the heart itself should suffer in a large proportion of cases. Specific inflammation of the heart-muscle, as well as of the peri- and endo-cardium, and even syphiloma of the heart are sometimes noted in autopsies. No such importance, clinically or pathologically, has yet been attributed to this especial form of syphilitic disease as would have been given it were the heart as vulnerable to this morbid agent as are the mucous membranes, the skin, the bones, the abdominal viscera, the vessels, and the nerves. Indeed, cardiac disease due to syphilis seems to be far less frequently encountered than gross vascular lesions—aneurism, cerebral thrombus, or rupture of weakened vessel-walls.

PROFESSOR ZAKHARINE, of Moscow, according to an extract from his clinical lectures (*Revue Générale de Clinique et de Thérapeutique*, August 20, 1890), believes that the infrequency of cardiac syphilis is not real but apparent, and complains of the want of proper attention to the subject on the part both of clinicians and of pathologists. Especially, he says, have the syphilitic lesions of the cardiac nerves and vessels been neglected. His indictment of the clinicians, moreover, is more severe than that which he brings against the pathologists. "Among the causes of cardiopathies," he says, "syphilis is indeed enumerated—they speak of gummous myocarditis; but on the other hand, not one word is said of the semeiology of syphilis of the heart, so that the perusal of treatises on internal pathology leaves the impression that cardiac syphilis is merely a 'find' of the autopsy, and pertains more to the domain of anatomy than to that of the clinic. One seeks in vain for an answer to the questions, Under what clinical form does syphilis of the heart present itself? How shall it be treated?" The number of personal observations reported toward filling this lacuna in clinical studies is ten.

The acknowledgment is candidly made that, as a rule, syphilis of the heart is characterized by a great complexity of symptoms referable in part to alcoholism, gout, chronic arteritis, gastro-intestinal troubles, and syphilitic lesions of other organs. Moreover, the cardiac symptoms are exceedingly variable, comprising continuous dyspnœa, with palpitation and a sense of oppression, paroxysms of cardiac asthma and of thoracic angina, œdema, and effusion into various cavities. The heart is usually enlarged through hypertrophy of the left ventricle; the pulse is feeble, rapid, and irregular; and frequently there is a systolic murmur.

Now in all this there is nothing at all characteristic, and the further fact is admitted that the diagnosis is to be based upon the antecedents of the patient; whereupon the institution and success of specific treatment—sodium iodide internally, and mercurial inunctions—confirms it. Notwithstanding the success of the treatment, there remain "objective signs of enlargement of the heart, and perhaps a slight systolic murmur beneath the sternum."

There is this to be observed, however, in the report of Zakharine's cases, that the administration of the ordinary cardiac remedies, digitalis and the like, was without influence; while amelioration began with the institution of specific treatment. Furthermore, neither valvular lesions nor alterations of the integrity of the orifices were manifested by objective signs in any instance.

The cases are divided on the basis of their symptomatology into three groups: myopathic, neuropathic, and mixed. Both mercurial inunctions and the internal use of the iodide are considered indispensable in treatment. The inutility of digitalis and its congeners has already been remarked. Two additional therapeutic measures are considered : the institution of a strict milk-diet, and the use of blisters over the præcordium. The milk-diet is recommended because it lessens the gastro-intestinal troubles and increases diuresis, while indirectly, by its diminution of ascites and meteorism, it removes some of the provoking causes of dyspnœa and angina. It is also supposed to diminish the fatty deposit over the heart by causing increased absorption ; but no proof is forthcoming in support of this theory. The soothing effect of præcordial blisters, while marked in cases of peripheral neuritis of the thorax, especially angina and intercostal neuralgia in the gouty and rheumatic, is but insignificant in syphilis of the heart.

While this subject is an important one, and we believe that it does deserve more attention than it has received, yet there seem to be two points overlooked by the author. The one, that inquiry is always made by the careful physician into possible syphilitic taint, hereditary or acquired, in the class of cases described, and if it is found, specific treatment is at once instituted—the cardiac complications being assigned, not the prime *rôle* the author would give, but being looked upon as part and parcel of a general infection. Secondly, it is a fact, although not a well-known fact, that sodium iodide and potassium iodide in small doses are extremely useful agents in the treatment of irregularity of cardiac action not due to syphilis.

Furthermore, in our own hospital experience with broken-down, alcoholic, syphilitic subjects, the general nervous, cardiac, vascular, and visceral changes are in general so far advanced that no therapeutic measures can do more than palliate. While, as to diagnosis, if one is willing to ignore the fact that both the whole organism and the organism as a whole are diseased, he can pick out any system he pleases, nervous, circulatory, respiratory, secretory, or any other, to bear the brunt of his nosological discrimination.

LAPAROTOMY THE WRONG WORD.

ALTHOUGH medical science is being continually purged of names which through long usage have been almost sanctioned, there yet remain a number of terms which are so distinctly erroneous as to make a change in their employment necessary. Within the last ten years the term "laparotomy" has come to be employed by the profession whenever it is desired to indicate that entrance has been made by the surgeon to the abdominal cavity through the belly-wall in any of its parts—whether the incision be made about the umbilicus, high up under the diaphragm, low down over the pubis, or, indeed, when it is made over either groin.

Our attention has been called to this point more particularly by an interesting little pamphlet, published by DR. R. P. HARRIS, of Philadelphia, who is so well known as a statistical authority upon abdominal operations, particularly those connected with diseases of females. Dr. Harris shows that the term "laparotomy" signifies an incision made into the flank and not into the anterior wall of the body, and suggests that in its place we employ the term "cœliotomy" to designate all operations in which the anterior belly-wall is opened.

Dr. Harris's suggestion as to the employment of this new term is not based upon mere dogmatic name-making, but is sanctioned, as he carefully shows, by the entire history of medicine and by the employment of the word "koilia" by the Greeks.

Every one who has been accustomed to employ medical terms for any length of time, finds it difficult to change the nomenclature to which they have become accustomed, and we fear that it will be a long while before Dr. Harris's scholarly attempt at correction of present errors is fully appreciated and followed. While a multiplication of medical terms is anything but desirable, it is equally necessary that the terms we do use should be correct, and we hope that "cœliotomy" will be employed hereafter by writers upon these subjects, and that laparotomy will be confined to indicate the operation in which the lateral portions of the abdominal cavity are operated upon.

THE EFFECT UPON THE EAR OF PASSING PROJECTILES.

IN the August number of the *Archives de Médecine et Pharmacie Militaires*, SURGEON-MAJOR NIMIER raises the interesting question of the causation of injuries to the ear by the near approach of flying projectiles, citing several instances of such lesions from the report on the Franco-German war, in three of which the drum-membrane was ruptured and in all more or less impairment of hearing resulted. He gives two possible explanations, the first of which is a modified view of the effect of the " wind of the ball," to which excessive potency used to be ascribed; the other, that the sonorous vibrations are the damaging agency. Without means to decide between the two, he inclines to the latter view, and quotes some of the experimental researches that have been made in gunnery as to the aërial disturbances coming into play under the circumstances. While these furnish some interesting and curious points which make the view to which he inclines possible, it is hard to see how they can do more.

The question principally concerns the military surgeon, for the effect under consideration is too remote and unimportant, in most of its aspects, to interest the gunnery expert, and the amount of experimentation bearing upon it has not been large. Beyond the " blast" region near the muzzle of his gun, the gunner is interested only in the influence of the atmosphere in retarding and deflecting his shot. Yet very interesting studies have been made both in this country and abroad in the photography of the projectile in rapid flight, and it has been found possible to secure pictures of the aërial waves set in motion by its passage. It has thus been shown that a cushion of condensed air is present in front of the shot, that waves stream off both from its pointed head and its sides, and that in the partial vacuum which is left behind it a series of undulations follow which may be visible even to the unaided eye. Probably as the result of this last phenomenon, the point has been noted that a shot moving with a velocity far in excess of the usual speed of sound, carries with it the noise of its discharge, until its flight is retarded to less than 1140 feet a second, when the sound-vibrations moving with their normal speed outstrip it for the remainder of its course. The sonorous vibrations conveyed to the ear by a close-passing shot at high speed are not only those of its own flight, but have the added influence of the discharge. Yet it is too much to believe that these are at all able to cause a rupture of the drum-membrane, much less to knock down and stun a man, as in some of the recorded instances; and it seems " far-fetched " to ascribe the deeper labyrinthine damage to the accompanying sonorous vibrations, rather than to the more palpably potent " wind." To this latter we need not ascribe the power to tear off limbs or effect such gross lesions as were once charged to it; but experi-

ment has shown that it is unquestionably a noteworthy force, quite capable of producing the injuries under consideration.

Probably the same phenomenon occurs near the path of the shot as is at times noted near the gun. The discharge forces the air away from the muzzle in a powerful wave which acts in all directions, though chiefly in the line of fire; but this is followed by a counter-wave of air rushing inward to replace that which has been disturbed. Glass broken by the concussion of heavy guns is not infrequently found to have fallen outward; and there are instances of the same effect when the drum-membrane has been ruptured and a flap turned outward. A passing shot has doubtless both a compressing and a suction effect upon the air in the auditory canal; and the damage is more probably due to the rapid alternation of these two forces than to the direct power of either, although they seem sometimes sufficient to throw a man down.

The persistent impairment of hearing after such an accident is a common result of even slighter injuries, such as a light blow upon the ear. Most aural surgeons have seen instances of permanent tinnitus and lessened hearing which dated from a slap, a shout, or even the kiss of a child upon the ear, and seemed to be due to labyrinthine concussion. Scepticism cannot always find any other cause as probable; and as a kiss has been known to rupture the drum-head (doubtless previously diseased), there is reason to accept the possibility of far-reaching effects from seemingly insignificant and invisible injuries.

Other effects incidentally mentioned by our author, may have no little influence on the function of the ear. He refers to several instances of epileptic seizures and other profound nervous disturbances which have had their origin in the terrific turmoil of battle and have proven both severe and lasting. Aside from the hysterical losses of sensation, there is room for much damage to the organ of hearing under the circumstances; and anyone who has made his recruit's obeisance to the shell which went screaming past him, has doubtless felt that there was a physical shock in the hurtling vibration to which it gave rise even when at a distance. Here the sonorous vibrations alone come into consideration; but it must remain almost impossible to discriminate between their physical and their mental effect, and consecutive impairment of hearing must seem rather a remote and indirect result.

A NEW MEDICAL MAGAZINE.

WE have received a copy of Vol. I., No. 1, of *The Journal of the State Medical Society of Arkansas*, which is published at Little Rock, Dr. Lorenzo P. Gibson being its editor.

The journal is well printed, on good paper, and seems to fulfil all that its friends could wish for it, its chief reason for existence being the idea of publishing a medical journal which would represent medical thought in that part of Arkansas, and afford an avenue of publication for the proceedings of its parent, the State Medical Society of Arkansas. We hope it may prove a great success.

REVIEWS.

A MANUAL AND ATLAS OF MEDICAL OPHTHALMO-SCOPY. By W. R. GOWERS, M.B., F.R.S., etc. Third edition, revised throughout, with numerous additions and additional illustrations. Edited with the assistance of MARCUS GUNN, M.D., F.R.C.S., etc. Philadelphia: P. Blakiston, Son, & Co., 1890.

THE second edition of Dr. Gowers's work on Medical Ophthalmoscopy bore the date 1881, since which time so much advance has been made in ophthalmic science that a third revision has been long desired. In the meantime, too, Dr. Gowers had issued his splendid work on nervous diseases, in which he gave evidence that he was well aware of the many pathological relations between the eye and the nervous system, and of the great value of ocular symptoms in the diagnosis of nervous diseases. In this third edition of his Ophthalmoscopy, further proof that the work has undergone a competent and thorough revision is afforded by the appearance of Dr. Gunn's name upon the title-page.

This excellent and almost unique treatise needs no praise, and contains so much of value that minor criticisms will not be construed either as hypercriticism or as detracting in the least from the value of the book as a whole. One may, therefore, the more freely express a regret that so many inelegant and even ungrammatical sentences have been carried over to this edition. Any page will furnish examples. One has frequently to read a sentence several times to detect the exact meaning conveyed by a slovenly and slipshod arrangement of words. For instance, and by no means the worst:

"They always indicate irregularities in the retina in which the vessels lie, commonly swelling, as in retinitis and retinal œdema."

"The aggregations of lymphoid cells which may occur in the nuclear and molecular layers, adjacent to an inflamed disk in tubercular meningitis, have been regarded as such, but their tubercular nature is uncertain."

An instance of revision and not rewriting is afforded by the recommendation, carried from the second edition, to use atropine for dilatation of the pupil, followed by the subsequent and new mention of the preferable agents, homatropine and cocaine. The paragraph in reference to atropine should have been left out, and the use of atropine, simply as a dilator of the pupil, condemned.

A great improvement in the present edition consists in the insertion in the text, and in connection with the subjects to which they refer, of the figures representing the minute anatomy of the tissue under consideration. The cuts themselves have been reproduced by a new process, and are much improved. New illustrations have also been added, and usually they are excellent, though that on page 5 illustrating opaque nerve-fibres conveys a very misleading idea of the more common appearance of this peculiarity.

Under tobacco- and alcohol-amblyopia no mention is made of the possible (or impossible) differential diagnosis of the two, nor of the relative influence of either the alcohol or the tobacco in producing an identical lesion and train of symptoms. Uhthoff's noteworthy work is referred to under the heading of Chronic Alcoholism (wrongly credited to the *Ophtalmic Revue* instead of to *Graefe's Archiv*), but under Tobacco-poisoning it is not mentioned.

Among the substances causing visual disorders should have been included a number of toxic alkaloids, such as mytilotoxin, vanillin, etc.

The appendix contains excellent and much-needed advice upon the methods of sketching the fundus oculi.

THE JOHNS HOPKINS HOSPITAL REPORTS. REPORT IN GYNÆCOLOGY. I. By HOWARD A. KELLY, M.D. Johns Hopkins Press, September, 1890.

THIS report, the first one which has been published in this branch of medicine by Johns Hopkins University, is typical of the gynæcologist who contributes most of the articles to its pages, showing as it does not only his possession of operative ability, but a wide knowledge of the literature and technique necessary to the successful operator in this branch of medicine.

The pamphlet is illustrated by several very good views of the operating-rooms, and is printed in handsome style in large type.

We congratulate Dr. Kelly upon the contents of this volume, as showing what he has done since he left Philadelphia, and we consider him fortunate in that he has so convenient an opportunity as these reports for the publication of the results of his work.

CORRESPONDENCE.

NEW YORK.

To the Editor of THE MEDICAL NEWS,

SIR: This summer has seemed more than usually dull in medical circles, possibly owing to the very large number of physicians who have taken the opportunity to enjoy a European trip, and at the same time attend the International Medical Congress. Besides this, the season has not been marked by the usual amount of sickness, and the absence of long periods of intensely hot weather has had a most beneficent influence on the infants who were trying to fight their way through "the second summer." Of course, there has been plenty of summer diarrhœa, but not much true cholera infantum, thus tending to confirm the opinion held by many students of pædiatrics, that it is long-continued, rather than intense heat, that favors the occurrence of this very fatal malady. Some philanthropists might be disposed to argue that the improvement in health was due to the labors of the many free physicians, who were sent out under various auspices to look after the health of those who occupy the most crowded and poorest districts of the city; but this, I cannot believe, is an adequate explanation. Medical charity has been dispensed with the same prodigality which in recent years has won for New York an unenviable reputation among the medical profession, and called forth many earnest protests; but those who are best acquainted with the workings of the charities know how feeble is their influence, and how little real progress is made. To preach the gospel of cleanliness in an Italian tenement is to strike terror to the hearts of its occupants, or to heap ridicule upon one's own head; while to insist upon a carefully-regulated diet for a sick infant among the poor Polish Jews means, to them, feeding the baby with lady-fingers and bananas. This season our tenement-house people have not only been supplied with free medicine and medical attendance at their homes, but they have been given beef-tea, milk, infant-foods, and that most costly luxury —ice. They have been taken on numerous day excursions, have been sent to the seashore until their sick children regained their strength, and have even been fed and clothed at the expense of their more fortunate fellow-citizens. All this is most praiseworthy if kept within proper limits, but to the physicians who are brought in actual contact with the beneficiaries of this charity, there is much food for earnest thought. It is exceedingly common for these people to declare solemnly that they have not even a few cents with which to buy the medicine, but it is the rarest to hear any such objection if the physician prescribes whiskey. With all the wealth of medical talent of New York City laid at their feet, it is not surprising that the dwellers in our tenements have learned to select their medical attendants, and they not uncommonly dismiss their family physician who has only a plain "M.D.," in order that they may be treated by Professor ——— of "the College."

The various medical schools have been thoroughly renovated, and each is straining its resources to the utmost to rival its neighbors. The Medical Department of the University is about to celebrate its fiftieth anniversary. During the half century of its existence it has conferred the degree of M.D. upon five thousand eight hundred and thirty-two matriculates. The Faculty have adopted a most commendable measure this year— namely, the requirement of a preliminary examination as a condition of matriculation. The University was the first in New York to adopt the method of clinical teaching by dividing the class into small sections. The College of Physicians and Surgeons has adopted the same plan at the Vanderbilt Clinic, and last year more than one hundred thousand patients furnished the material for this purpose.

The Sloan Maternity Hospital, which is upon the grounds of the College of Physicians and Surgeons, has established a very active obstetric service, about nine hundred deliveries having taken place there in the two and a half years since the hospital was opened. A few years ago, a practical knowledge of obstetrics could be obtained by only a very few medical students; now, in addition to the hospital just mentioned, there has been recently opened for the special purpose of private in-struction, an institution known as the "Midwifery Dispensary." It is situated near the populous down-town districts on the east-side, and is managed by several men who have had large experience both in the teaching and practice of obstetrics. A salaried resident physician and a limited number of students who reside at the institution, are always ready to answer calls, and as the cases are attended at their homes, the students have excellent opportunities to learn something of the difficulties that present themselves in private practice, and which are almost unknown in a well-appointed maternity hospital.

CHICAGO.

To the Editor of THE MEDICAL NEWS.

SIR: The fall term of the College of Physicians and Surgeons was opened on the evening of September 23d, at the college building, with music, dancing, and a banquet. The introductory address was delivered by Dr. C. C. P. Silva. The names of 125 students have been enrolled, with promise of several more.

Dr. William M. Tomlinson, of our city health department, in comparing the mortality reports of last year, says that Chicago is the lowest. The figures are as follows: Brooklyn, 23.76; New York, 22.79; Philadelphia, 20.82, and Chicago, 17.44.

An assistant health commissioner will shortly be appointed to succeed Dr. Dixon, but as yet the name of the new appointee has not been made known. The salary is $2500.

The property-owners in the vicinity of Cook County Hospital have sent in a strong protest against the erection of a city morgue in the hospital grounds.

It is said that there are several young physicians in Chicago who have no office, but travel about like doctors in the olden times. They go to drug stores at different hours to meet their patients, who pay very small fees, but by this means avoid the necessity of going to a hospital. It is perhaps a good thing for the sick who cannot afford to have doctors come to the house, and is certainly a new way to build up a practice.

Dr. Joseph Zeisler was elected a member of the German Dermatological Society, while in Berlin attending the International Medical Congress.

It is rumored that preparations will shortly be made to revive the *Chicago Medical Journal and Examiner*, of which Dr. S. J. Jones was formerly editor.

Dr. John A. Benson, Medical Superintendent of the Cook County Insane Asylum, who had charges of mismanagement and the improper employment of patients preferred against him, for contract work at Dunning, was recently exonerated by the commissioners.

Professor H. D. Garrison, in a lecture a short time ago, stated that the crumpled and crushed form of the human ear was originally caused and is now maintained by the habit of lying on the side of the head, and that the habit has resulted principally from the increasing weight of the brain. The question originally seemed to be whether man's ancestors would profit most by large brains or by symmetrical and perfect acoustic apparatus, and nature by selection had promptly decided in favor of a large brain.

The disciples of the new cult, known as "orificial surgery," are all homœopaths. They recently held a meeting here to effect permanent organization, and here-after they will convene annually. One of the most promi-nent of these *oriphysicians* is to deliver a special course of lectures on *orificial surgery* this winter, and all persons interested in this branch may attend for a small fee and receive enlightenment on the formation and removal of pus-pockets.

A clinical society is soon to be formed, known as the Chicago Clinical Society, with Dr. William T. Belfield as its first president.

The opening exercises of the Chicago Medical College and the Rush Medical college took place on September 30th, in their respective amphitheatres. Professor F. C. Schaefer delivered the introductory lecture of the former college, and Professor J. H. Etheridge that of the latter. Professor Roberts, of the Northwestern University, of which the Rush Medical College is a part, spoke briefly, saying that there had been a gratifying increase of attendance in all the departments. He estimated that there are about fifteen hundred young men being educated in the various departments of the university.

Rush Medical College starts out this year with about five hundred students, or nearly one hundred more than were registered at the opening term of last year.

In connection with higher medical education the following extracts from the annual announcement of this college are of interest:

"No student who desires to meet the requirements of the various State Boards, should hereafter enter upon the study of medicine without an ample preliminary education, and the mental discipline its acquirement insures. Such preliminary education should include the study of selected works on English literature, rhetoric, logic, mental science, the fundamental principles of algebra and geometry, and the elements of physics. A knowledge of the rudiments of Latin is essential, since this in a measure removes the difficulty of acquiring the technical language of medical science. After the years 1890-91 no graduate, unless he has studied medicine four years, and taken three courses of lectures of at least five months each, as required in Illinois (and six months each in Iowa), can begin the practice of medicine in these States without passing a rigid examination before the State Board of Health."

The Chicago polyclinic, profiting by the experience of the successful special course given last Spring, has made extensive provision for the accommodation of a large number of practitioners. A spacious amphitheatre, a well-appointed dissecting-room, and laboratories have been erected; and the teaching corps has been strengthened by several valuable additions.

The special course will comprise three distinct series of clinics and demonstrations, as follows:

1. Abdominal and pelvic surgery, with illustrations upon dogs and cadavers, by Professors Senn, Fenger, Parkes, Belfield, and Etheridge.

2. Clinical lectures and demonstrations, in the amphitheatre, in the various branches of medicine and surgery, by Professors Hoadley, Colburn, Hotz, Ingals, Church, and Fütterer.

Professor Moreau R. Brown will perform intubation and demonstrate the technique of the operation; and Professor Charles F. Stillman will give clinical instruction in orthopædic surgery and exhibit recent appliances for the treatment of deformities and diseases of joints, and demonstrate their uses. Professor P. S. Hayes will deliver a course of lectures on electro-therapeutics and the Apostoli method of treating uterine fibroids.

Dr. William G. Eggleston, formerly assistant editor of the *Journal of the American Medical Association*, is, and has been for some time, editorial writer on the *Chicago Herald*.

Cupid cut a large swath at the recent International Medical Congress, said a prominent physician of this city. According to a Berlin paper, one of the results of the Congress was the publication of four hundred engagements of marriage.

One of the ward clubs, of Chicago, has selected for County Commissioner, Dr. J. R. Brandt, who was consulting physician to the Cook County Insane Asylum and Infirmary for three years, and attending physician to the Cook County Hospital for two years. We believe that it will accord with the interests of Cook County if one of the county commissioners is a physician, for the reason that he is well qualified to look after the Insane Asylum, Infirmary, and similar medical institutions.

Professor Walter S. Haines, of Rush Medical College, recently made a chemical analysis of portions of the body of Mrs. Hattie Pettit, for whose alleged poisoning, her husband, the Rev. William F. Pettit, is to be tried at Crawfordsville, Indiana, on October 4th, and has reported to the State's attorney that he discovered strychnine in the parts examined.

American physicians, said a prominent doctor recently, seem to have a mania for prescribing the waters of European medicinal springs, and in consequence many wealthy individuals cross the water, who might, with equal benefit to themselves, patronize American springs. If American physicians would study our medicinal waters and be more patriotic in their recommendations, the health resorts of this country would be more thoroughly appreciated.

The wife of a well-known physician of Chicago recently took charge of her husband's accounts, and when she had gathered a sufficient sum of money she bought eighty acres of land on the South Side of the city, paying $600 per acre. Recently she sold the entire tract for $1,000 per acre, having made exactly $32,000 in three months. Her husband never saw the property nor gave the matter of its purchase or sale any attention.

BALTIMORE.

To the Editor of THE MEDICAL NEWS,

SIR: The College of Physicians and Surgeons, rejoicing in a new hospital and new lecture-halls, welcomes its students to more perfect facilities for laboratory studies which are now considered so essential.

The Johns Hopkins Hospital moves steadily onward in its well-chosen path, offering special courses of study which have been eagerly sought even by established practitioners among us. This institution is now beginning to find its true place in our city. It is useless to deny that the relations between it and our medical men were not cordial during the early months of its existence. It was opened with a grand flourish of trumpets, and the daily papers began at once to publish the most extravagant accounts of "wonderful" operations and cures ascribed to the different professors, and no physician or surgeon in private practice knew at what moment his patients might be spirited away by enthusiastic friends to be treated " better " in the wonderful new hospital wards. Later the professors took offices in our prominent streets, and added private practice and consultation to their hospital duties. The physicians of Baltimore, supposing that these newcomers, of wide reputation and introduced to the public in such an imposing way, would be rivals in both general and consulting practice, naturally could hardly repress certain doubts as to their own future or a feeling that the proceeding was not quite " fair play."

At present, however, there are prospects of harmony. The newspaper notices of extraordinary operations and successes have become infrequent or have ceased to appear, whether in consequence of the earnest remonstrances which have been made with the johns Hopkins Hospital authorities I am not prepared to say. Personal acquaintance with some of the new professors has shown that they will be a very agreeable addition to our medical circles. The fact that septicæmia and death are not strangers to the new hospital wards has had a somewhat soothing effect on the enthusiasm of the public, and we have learned that while the newcomers must be respected as equals they need not be feared in the fields of either operative work or general medicine.

The dispensary nuisance, which caused an outcry from East Baltimore practitioners, seems to have been somewhat controlled by the care which the Johns Hopkins physicians have shown in the exclusion of well-to-do patients. It is said that such patients are noted at the first visit, and that their pecuniary position is at once investigated by a special agent of the dispensary.

The University of Maryland School of Medicine has endeavored to keep pace with the other schools by extensive repairs of its old buildings and by additions to them. It has also engaged excellent trained nurses for the hospital, and established a training-school in which young women may obtain careful instruction in nursing.

Baltimore has at length begun to follow with earnestness the example of her northern sister-cities in the employment of specially trained nurses in private practice. Many excellent nurses have already been induced to come here from northern training-schools, and others have been obtained from our own hospitals, but the great and increasing demand for educated nurses, without whom the practitioner must always work at a disadvantage, can never be fully met until our own training-schools begin to supply the deficiency.

The Medical and Chirurgical Faculty, which last year took vigorous steps toward the position of the State Medical Society, will soon hold its semi-annual session in one of the towns on the other side of the Chesapeake. It is very earnestly hoped that this society will so unite in itself the divergent interests of the profession that at some early date it may take the lead in securing some remedy for the great and shameful abuses in the department of public medicine. A medical law which shall repress quackery and restrain our colleges from graduating uneducated students is sadly needed. In connection with this it may be stated that the movement toward a lengthened curriculum, to which our colleges appeared

to give consent, is likely to end, at least in those institutions where such a change is most needed, in mere talk.

The State Board of Health is making itself useful in resisting the careless pollution of our smaller water-supply at Lake Roland, which lies in a section of the country that is in some respects desirable for summer residence, but which is annually visited by epidemics of dysentery and typhoid fever.

It can hardly be said that our city Health Department is any more efficient under its new Commissioner than it was before he entered with such apparent zeal upon his duties. We have now, it is true, a very imperfect list of cases of contagious disease occurring each week printed neatly upon the back of the health report, but the health-force is still unfitted for its work, and physicians often appeal in vain for the correction of conditions which threaten the health of families and neighborhoods. As was honestly said by one who controlled a sanitary appointment in the city " the offices are for the benefit of the Democratic party," and woe be to the Health Commissioner who attempts to replace an efficient party-worker by an efficient sanitary agent. It is probably true that if physicians stood up persistently against such shameful abuses and showed the public what is done in other cities and what might be done here, they would ultimately win in the contest, but each concerns himself with his own personal advancement, and the politician gets the spoils. It is strange that, where there is such overcrowding of professional ranks, physicians do not claim as a natural right these sanitary posts, which yield a fair income and which are in Great Britain, if I mistake not, filled by medical men or by medical students licensed under the special diploma of " Sanitary Graduate," after a careful education in sanitary matters.

Now that women have so sturdily claimed the medical privileges of the johns Hopkins it is said that the homœopathic fraternity will try to secure the same privileges. Whether this is true or not, I do not know, but it is not at all improbable. Unfortunately for themselves, that body of practitioners has just experienced a serious schism, and its members differ greatly in regard to the degree of infinitesimality which is necessary for the cure of disease.

The medical societies will shortly begin work for the winter. The Clinical Society met on October 3d. It is the largest medical society in the city and does excellent work. The Medical Association and the Medical and Surgical Society are somewhat smaller; the Academy of Medicine is a feeble but respectable relic of the past; the Obstetrical Society is composed of a very active body of workers; the Society of the Woman's Medical College has but a local interest; and, youngest of all, is the johns Hopkins Hospital Society, which is composed of the hospital and dispensary staffs, and does work of a high order.

NEWS ITEMS.

The Act to Regulate the Practice of Medicine and Surgery in New Jersey.—The following is an abstract of the Act to Regulate the Practice of Medicine and Surgery in New Jersey, approved May 12, 1890:

1. The Governor shall appoint a State board of medical examiners, consisting of nine members, who

shall be persons of recognized professional ability and honor. The board shall be divided into three classes: the members of the first class holding office for one year, those of the second class for two years, those of the third class for three years. Further, the board shall be composed of five regular physicians, three homœopaths, and one eclectic, and no member shall be in any way connected with a medical college.

2. The board shall hold meetings for examinations at the capital, Trenton, on the second Thursday of January, April, July, and October of each year.

3. All persons commencing the practice of medicine or surgery in New Jersey shall apply to the board for a license; and such applicants shall be divided into three classes—first, those who have been graduated from a legally chartered medical school not less than five years prior to date of application for a license; second, all other graduates; third, medical students taking a regular course of medical instruction. Applicants of the first class shall submit to examination upon materia medica and therapeutics, obstetrics and gynæcology, practice of medicine, surgery, and surgical anatomy; those of the second and third classes, upon anatomy, physiology, chemistry, pathology, materia medica and therapeutics, histology, hygiene, practice of medicine, surgery, obstetrics, and gynæcology, diseases of the eye and ear, medical jurisprudence, and upon such other branches as the board may deem advisable. The questions for the examination of the first and second classes shall be the same in branches common to each class. The board shall not license applicants of the second and third classes after january 1, 1892, until satisfactory proof is furnished that the applicant has studied medicine and surgery for three years, is of good, moral character, and more than twenty-one years of age. Applicants of the third class, after they have studied medicine and surgery for at least two years, may be examined upon anatomy, physiology, chemistry, histology, pathology, materia medica and therapeutics; and if the examination is satisfactory the board may issue a certificate that the applicant has passed a final examination in these branches, and such certificate, if presented when making application for license to practise, shall be accepted in lieu of an examination in such branches.

4. All examinations shall be in writing, and the questions must be, except in materia medica and therapeutics, such as can be answered in common by all schools of practice. If the applicant intends to practise homœopathy or eclecticism, the members of the board of those schools shall examine the applicant in materia medica and therapeutics. The fee for examination shall be fifteen dollars for applicants of the first class and twenty dollars for those of the second and third classes.

5. The board may, by a unanimous vote, refuse to grant, or may revoke, a license for the following causes: persistent inebriety, the practice of criminal abortion, conviction of crime involving moral turpitude, or for publicly advertising special ability to treat or cure diseases which are considered incurable.

6. This act shall not apply to surgeons of the United States army, navy, or marine-hospital service, or to regularly licensed physicians or surgeons called from other States to attend cases in New jersey, or to any person now entitled to practise in New jersey.

7. Any person shall be regarded as practising medicine or surgery who shall append the letters M.D. or M.B. to his or her name, or prescribe any drug or other agency for the cure or relief of any injury or disease.

8. Any person commencing the practice of medicine or surgery in New Jersey contrary to the provisions of the act shall be deemed guilty of a misdemeanor, and, upon conviction, shall be punished by a fine of not less than fifty dollars or more than one hundred dollars, or by imprisonment for not less than ten or more than ninety days, or by both fine and imprisonment.

Rules for Conducting Examinations.—1. Each candidate shall present certificates of age, moral character, preliminary education, and time and place of medical studies.

2. All examinations shall be written with ink upon paper furnished by the secretary.

3. The examinations shall continue for two days, the sessions of the first day being from 9 A. M. until 1 P. M., from 2 until 6, and from 8 until 10 P. M.; those of the second day being the same, except that the evening session will be omitted. The final meeting, for the adjudication of the results, shall be held at 8 o'clock P. M. of the second day.

4. A general average of at least seventy-five per cent. shall be necessary in order to secure a license, provided that in no one branch the candidate receives an average of less than thirty-three and one-third per cent. In the latter case, should his total average in all the branches be over seventy-five per cent., the candidate may be immediately granted a second examination in the branch upon which he failed.

5. Each candidate shall sign a pledge that he has neither given nor received any information concerning the examination or used any unfair means. Any candidate found guilty of violating his pledge shall be rejected.

6. No fee will be returned to a candidate after he has commenced his examination. A rejected candidate may be reëxamined within one year without an additional fee.

Corrigendum.

THE PRODUCTION OF IMMUNITY FROM HOG-CHOLERA.

In the article on the production of immunity from hog-cholera (THE MEDICAL NEWS, October 4, 1890), the author would prefer Conclusion 3 to read as follows:

"The sucholotoxins and sucholo-albumins *should be* given in small doses *at intervals*. This, however, is not absolutely necessary, as the experiments show that the proper quantity of substance given at one time will also produce *immunity*, though not so satisfactorily as when the system is gradually accustomed to the poison."

OFFICIAL LIST OF CHANGES IN THE STATIONS AND DUTIES OF OFFICERS SERVING IN THE MEDICAL DEPARTMENT, U. S. ARMY, FROM SEPTEMBER 30 TO OCTOBER 6, 1890.

CRAMPTON, LOUIS W., *Captain and Assistant Surgeon* (Fort Sheridan, Illinois).—Is granted leave of absence for one month, to take effect about October 1, 1890.—Par. 2, *S. O. 80, Division of the Missouri*, September 30, 1890.

By direction of the Secretary of War, leave of absence granted JOHN L. PHILLIPS, *Captain and Assistant Surgeon*, in Special Orders No. 164, July 16, 1890, from this office, is extended two months.—Par. 3, *S. O. 228, A. G. O., Washington*, September 29, 1890.

PROMOTION.

MORRIS, EDWARD R., *Assistant Surgeon.*—On September 17, 1890, to be Assistant Surgeon with the rank of Captain, in accordance with the Act of June 23, 1874.

THE MEDICAL NEWS.
A WEEKLY JOURNAL OF MEDICAL SCIENCE.

Vol. LVII.　　　SATURDAY, OCTOBER 18, 1890.　　　No. 16.

ORIGINAL LECTURES.

CHLOROFORM AND THE HYDERABAD COMMISSION.

The President's Address delivered at the Annual Meeting of the Southwestern State Medical Society of Ohio, Cincinnati, October 10, 1890.

BY J. C. REEVE, M.D.,

OF DAYTON, OHIO.

GENTLEMEN: I offer no apologies for occupying your time with some portion of the subject of anæsthetics, even if you are thereby taken again over well-trodden ground. Apologies might easily be found if needed. The differences of opinion and practice which prevail as to the two great anæsthetics are far greater than ever, and also exist among practical men as to remedies whose action is fully and clearly understood. Whenever this subject is opened, questions of immense practical importance present themselves—questions which, in the present state of our knowledge, are impossible to answer. The limited portion of the subject chosen for to-night not only needs no apology, but it demands attention. The experiments of the Hyderabad Chloroform Commission and the conclusions drawn from them constitute the latest phase in the history of anæsthetics. They demand examination not so much as a contribution to knowledge we already had, but because the results obtained by experiment differ so widely from those of other observers; because the changes of doctrine introduced are wide and sweeping; because the conclusions formulated are stated with a positiveness which challenges scrutiny. When I add that the teachings of this Commission, if accepted, increase the responsibility and add to the anxieties of everyone who administers an anæsthetic; that further, if any reliance is to be placed on clinical experience the teachings are fraught with danger to patients, I know that you will agree with me that they should be submitted to a close and searching examination.

The Hyderabad Chloroform Commissions owed their existence to the liberality of the Nizam of Hyderabad and the enthusiasm of Surgeon-Major Lawrie, a disciple of Syme and a warm supporter of the Edinburgh school. The investigations were made in a country where there are no restrictions upon experiments with animals, and the commissions had, therefore, command of ample material. By the first commission, held in 1888, 141 dogs were killed by chloroform inhalation, the symptoms, and especially the sequence of symptoms, being carefully noted. The chief conclusion reached was that "it is impossible for chloroform vapor to kill dogs by acting primarily on the heart, and this holds good no matter in what doses or in what manner the poisoning

is induced."[1] This experience is so diametrically opposite to that of others, it may be said to that of all experimental physiologists the world over, that it called forth strong comments, especially from the *Lancet*. The criticism led to the formation of a second Commission, and by the liberality of the Nizam, who gave £1000 for the purpose, Dr. Lauder Brunton was added to the Commission, and went to India and took part in the investigation. By this second commission about 600 animals, mostly dogs, were sacrificed. The mode of death was studied, but attention was principally given to the effect of chloroform inhalation upon the two great functions of respiration and circulation, and especially to determine which ceased first. The result is stated to have been invariable—in every instance the respiration stopped before the heart. This is the briefest possible statement of the work of the Commission, and it is the "practical conclusions" drawn from this work that I now propose to examine. In view of some of the names attached to these reports my effort may be deemed presumptuous. I can only say that the day is past when a name will cause acceptance of a doctrine which is not in accord with facts. We no longer live in the age when men were content to be wrong with Nature that they might be right with Galen.

You will see that of the two modes of study open to us as to the action of medicines—experiment upon animals and clinical observation—the Commission has pursued one and only one. My study of the subject has been, and must be to-night, solely in the other. I am not an experimental physiologist. I am not, therefore, about to occupy your time with details of "tracings" and of "blood-pressure." And inasmuch as the results obtained by the Commission fail to agree with those of other observers, their work must be submitted to other experimenters for reëxamination. This has already been done, and I refer you with pleasure to the excellent paper by Drs. Wood and Hare for a criticism upon this side of the subject.[2] My object is to compare the results obtained by the Commission with observations made at the bedside, and the conclusions arrived at by them with clinical experience. When experiment upon animals and observation upon man agree in results we are sure —very sure—of our position. When these two modes of study do not agree, however, there can be no hesitation as to which we are to follow. The bedside is the last court of appeal for the physician and surgeon.

Permit a few general observations upon the second Commission before proceeding to particulars.

1. The Commission was organized *for a purpose*, which purpose was plainly stated. The object was "to show

---

[1] Lancet, February 22, 1890.

[2] THE MEDICAL NEWS, February 22, 1890. See also : "Remarks on the Second Report of the Hyderabad Commission, by the Glasgow Committee of the British Medical Association." British Medical Journal, June 14, 1800.

by experiments upon dogs that in death from chloroform the respiration always stops before the heart."[1] Without commenting at length upon this, I suggest that delicate instruments of observation, kymographs or what not, will yield no reliable results if that more delicate instrument which directs and observes them, the human brain, be clogged in its action by preconceived opinions. The scientific method is to make the experiments first and the doctrines afterward.

II. The report throughout shows no recognition of the possibility of more than one kind of death under chloroform inhalation. The effort was to discover whether danger to life arises " from failure of the heart *or* failure of the respiration."[2] From one end to the other the tone of the report is that death by the respiratory function necessarily excludes death by the heart. They seem to be looked upon as mutually antagonistic, and there is no recognition of the possibility that death may occur by either channel, or that both functions may cease simultaneously. Nearly twenty-five years ago I made and published a careful study of all the then recorded cases of death under chloroform.[3] That study was made largely in regard to etiology, and when I still held the belief that death was almost always the result of faulty administration. I learned then that the symptoms in the fatal cases varied widely, and that there was more than one path to the lethal end. That death may occur from long continuance of the inhalation—an over-administration of chloroform—is certainly possible, but it could only be brought about in this way by gross carelessness or inattention, and it is doubtful if the record of any clearly-marked cases of this kind can be found. The following forms of death are, however, to be plainly distinguished in looking over the reports of fatal cases :

1. Sudden death during the stage of struggling or excitement, in which it is difficult to say just where the process commences. There is great excitement of the nervous system, tetanic contraction of the muscles of the chest, with suspended respiration followed by very deep inspirations, and sometimes general convulsions. The frequency with which death has occurred at this part of the inhalation marks it as the most dangerous stage of the process.

2. Death by paralysis of the respiratory centre, the heart having been observed to continue beating after respiration had ceased. Ten deaths occurred in this way out of forty carefully observed cases.

3. Death by paralysis of the cardiac centres. The pulse fails, the divided vessels suddenly stop bleeding, the heart ceases to act, while respiration has been observed to continue for a time.

4. Death by simultaneous cessation of respiration and heart-action.

Of the modes of death, that in which the symptoms on the part of the circulation preceded or predominated was so frequently observed that the doctrine became current that death under chloroform was always cardiac death.

III. The exceedingly small number of observations upon which the very positive doctrines and important

conclusions of the Commission are based. Not many more than one thousand experiments were made, and because a certain event did not happen in that number of experiments it is claimed that it never happens. The weakness of this point is recognized and acknowledged by Dr. Brunton himself.[1] Had the experiments been ten thousand instead of one, the argument would still be weak. There were 28,000 administrations of chloroform in one corps of the Confederate army without a death. The distinguished surgeon, Hunter McGuire, had 15,000 administrations, and then a death. *Per contra*, an English hospital had one death in 200 administrations. But here, as everywhere, the tendency is to draw conclusions solely from personal experience. Whenever the subject of anæsthetics comes up in a medical society someone is sure to arise with the oft-repeated formula : " This is my plan ; I never had an accident ; follow this plan, which is safe beyond a doubt." The " plan " is, usually, a glass of whiskey before the administration. There can be easily adduced from clinical records more than a dozen cases in which sudden death took place when an alcoholic stimulant had preceded the administration. There are several cases of death under ether when the same had been given. The personal experience of Surgeon Lawrie is certainly marvellous, and he may well argue from it. He tells us that for fifteen years he has administered chloroform from five to ten times daily.[2] Taking the mean, this would give over 40,000 administrations, a number which surpasses that of many army statistics and is more than half the number of inhalations during our war. That his good fortune in having this number of cases without a death was due alone to one point, as he claims, " watching the respiration," we cannot accept. There was no such single method followed as a safeguard in the Confederate army.[3] Still, Surgeon Lawrie's experience was with human beings.

IV. The rigid application by the Commission, of occurrences observed in animals to the human subject. This is the weakest point of all, and immediately called forth a host of protests. Because in dogs death under chloroform always takes place by the respiration it therefore must always do so in man, is weak reasoning. Yet there has been such reasoning all through the history of anæsthetics. Because, in the majority of cases, death occurred thus in animals was formulated the doctrine, which stood for a long time unquestioned, that in man ether-death is always by the respiration and chloroform-death is always cardiac. Sure of my ground clinically, and fortified by the high authority of Kappeler that " ether-death does not differ materially from chloroform-death," I stated in 1882 that " ether, in the human subject, may cause death as suddenly, as unexpectedly, and in the identical manner that chloroform does."[4] An

[1] Official report, Lancet, January 18, 1890.
[2] Lauder Brunton, International Congress, Lancet, August 16, 1890.
[3] American Journal of the Medical Sciences, October, 1867.

[1] International Congress, Lancet, August 16, 1890.
[2] Lancet, January 18, 1890.
[3] In 1882 (Holmes's Surgery, American edition) I suggested that *climate* might explain the differences of experience with anæsthetics. This explanation might apply between the northeastern and southern parts of our own country, and between England and India. But it entirely fails to explain the deaths that have occurred under chloroform in France and Germany, *provided*, that we know all the deaths that have occurred under chloroform in France and Germany.
[4] Holmes's Surgery, American edition, vol. iii.

eminent surgeon of Philadelphia questioned the truth of the statement, and in reply I published the clinical proof.[1] As this work was mentioned at the late International Congress and the proof accepted by Professor H. C. Wood in his address, it is to be presumed that the fact will be hereafter generally accepted. The truth is evident that the results obtained by experiment on animals cannot be absolutely and universally applied to man, and it is astonishing that men claiming to be scientists should presume to make such application. It utterly breaks down before such potent facts as that dogs may be killed by elaterium without being purged; that pigeons bear enormous doses of morphine; and that goats and rabbits eat belladonna with impunity.

I select now some particular doctrines from the " Practical Conclusions " of the Commission, which they present in the most positive manner for the guidance of the profession. Carefully reading over the fifteen paragraphs in which these conclusions are given, it is surprising how many of the conclusions were well known to the profession long before, and which are therefore neither new nor necessary. It did not need a commission to tell us that the recumbent position is necessary for safety—the danger of any other has long been recognized. It certainly was unnecessary to tell us that the respiration should be free and unembarrassed. A tyro in physiology would recognize that in a patient to whom respiration and circulation alone remained of life, any interference with breathing, as by resting on the chest to restrain struggling, or by shutting out the air with an impervious towel, would be highly dangerous. This danger has been recognized and warning was given far back and all along in the history of anæsthetics.

The especial doctrines taught by the Commission, repeated and emphasized, are that in the administration of chloroform the respiration is the only thing to attend to, death always taking place by that channel; that disturbance of this function always and first indicates danger;[2] that by watching the respiration danger can be foreseen and averted; that "the utmost attention to the respiration is necessary to prevent asphyxia or an overdose." (See II.) The ninth section reads: "The administrator should be guided as to the effect entirely by the respiration. His only object while producing anæsthesia is to see that the respiration is not interfered with."[3] This doctrine carries with it another: that it is *not* necessary to watch the pulse. This is boldly stated by Surgeon Lawrie: "The pulse is of no value as a sign of approaching danger."[4] This is the doctrine of Syme, of Lister, and of the Edinburgh school. In connection with this we are asked to believe two things, if we can: "Pallor and loss of pulse do not indicate that chloroform has any direct effect upon the heart, but that it has been given in such a way as to interfere with the breathing;" and, "If part of the chloroformist's attention is to be directed to the pulse an important element of danger

comes into the administration."[1] Lauder Brunton reiterates the statement.[2]

The number of competent observers who have testified to the falsity of these doctrines would be enough to settle the question. At the debate in the Medical Society of London which followed Dr. Brunton's address, several bore witness to the frequency of failure of the pulse and heart-action before respiration was affected. Three experienced chloroformists of London hospitals gave in print testimony to the same effect.[3] Two cases were detailed in which there was positive observation that respiration went on after the heart's action had ceased.[4] But I will adduce some testimony given to the profession many years ago, and give some clinical facts. The first three cases of death under chloroform all showed signs of sudden cessation of the circulation Of the 50 fatal cases given by Snow, 18 took place by cardiac paralysis and in 12 it is distinctly stated by the observers that respiration still continued after the heart had ceased to beat, or after decided failure of the pulse had awakened alarm.[5] Of 21 cases of dangerous symptoms observed by Anstie, in 16 a change of pulse, with sudden pallor, was most prominently noted, and was the first symptom.[6] You have had two well-marked cases of this kind here in Cincinnati under the observation of my friend, Professor Dawson: a sudden cessation of bleeding at the wound first called the operator's attention to the state of the patient.[7]

Permit me to detail, with the utmost possible brevity, three cases from an observer whose competence, accuracy, and honesty cannot be called in question:

CASE I.—Patient was a woman, aged twenty-five years; under no apprehension or fear. The administration was for flexion of a contracted extremity. Pulse was 96, respiration 24. After inhaling chloroform for five minutes, there were muscular contractions, and the pulse rose to 102. In seven minutes there was muscular relaxation; reflex action upon touching the cornea was almost abolished; pulse regular, 96. Administration continued, and at end of fifteen minutes the radial pulse became suddenly intermittent, and, at the same time, the face became pale. The patient respired at this time peacefully and regularly. The administration was immediately discontinued and the patient recovered.

CASE II.—A woman, aged forty years. Chloroform was given for the removal of a tumor from the axilla and she feared the anæsthetic very much. A physician experienced in administration watched the pulse and respiration. Soon after beginning the operation, and without any hæmorrhage, the three medical men present observed that the patient's countenance became deathly pale; the one watching the pulse announced its disappearance, and soon afterward respiratory move-

---

[1] THE MEDICAL NEWS, january 22, 1887.
[2] Lancet, February 15, 1890.
[3] Official report, Lancet, january 18, 1890.
[4] Lancet, june 21, pp. 1390, 1391. It is entirely just to quote Surgeon Lawrie because he was president of the Commission, and his article is essentially an exposition of the official report.

[1] Lancet, June 21. 1890, p. 1391.
[2] Lancet, February 15. 1890. p. 350.
[3] Dr. Buxton, Lancet, February 15, 1890, p. 373: Dr. Hewitt, Lancet, March 1, p. 515: Dr. Sheppard, Lancet, March 8, p. 598.
[4] Dr. Battle, Lancet, February 22. p. 434. See also Lancet, june 21, 1890, p. 1425.
[5] Snow on Chloroform: cases 9, 10, 12, 17, 25, 32, 33, 38, 43, 44, 48, 49.
[6] On Stimulants and Narcotics.
[7] Transactions of the American Surgical Association, vol. ii., 1884.

ments were no longer visible. Bleeding from the wound had entirely ceased. The mouth was easily opened ; there was no falling back of the tongue. This patient was rescued with great difficulty.

CASE III.—A woman, aged thirty-four years, with lupus of the face and arm of many years' standing. For this she had undergone seven curettings, each time under the influence of chloroform, and without any unusual symptoms from the anæsthetic. Chloroform was given for still another operation, by means of the Esmarch wire-mask. It is expressly stated that great care was taken not to interfere with the respiration, which, indeed, is quite impossible with this apparatus. Pulse and respiration were watched, and both remained regular and good up to the close of the operation. After the operation, and about two minutes after removing the chloroform, the patient suddenly began to draw the head slowly to the right, the face became corpse-like, the eyes opened widely so that the fully dilated pupils could be seen ; almost at the same time the pulse ceased, the respiratory movements became slow and superficial, and, after some seconds, entirely ceased. She was dead.

These observations are by Kappeler.[1] In the last case it is probable that the pulse and respiration ceased together, but the testimony is no less clear that the respiration does not always give warning of danger. The fact is, that, in the human subject, death by cardiac paralysis has occurred so much more frequently than that by respiratory paralysis that the doctrine became current that chloroform-death is always cardiac-death. The doctrine is false. Chloroform sometimes paralyzes respiration first, as ether sometimes first affects the heart.

You will have noted the sudden change of countenance observed in these cases; it is, of course, a symptom which cannot be seen in animals. In man it has so often been the first symptom to attract attention that it presents the strongest clinical claims to consideration. In the three cases of danger which it has been my lot to witness, this symptom was present, and first awakened alarm. Thus does a master-hand draw the picture : "Without warning, generally, also, without disturbance of the respiration, the countenance takes on a waxen hue, as if under the stroke of a magic wand ; the lineaments are decomposed, the cornea loses its lustre, and the fully dilated pupils become motionless ; the jaw falls. At the same time the radial pulse ceases, and the heart-sounds are imperceptible, or extraordinarily weak ; the opened arteries cease bleeding. With cessation of the heart's action, the respiratory movements terminate without cyanosis or dyspnœa, or a few sighing and spasmodic inspirations continue after the heart has ceased to beat." [2]

Looking at the clinical side of the subject, there is a striking concurrence of testimony as to the suddenness with which danger appears under chloroform, and as to symptoms on the part of the circulation, preceding all others. In view of its amount and character, it is incomprehensible that the doctrine could ever be held that the respiration always gives warning of danger, and that death comes always by that function. The

cases giving evidence upon these points are so numerous that there would not be time to detail them to-night. But, in view of the evidence adduced, and of a few well-marked cases detailed, how does the statement of the Commission appear, that "the fear of chloroform paralyzing the heart is based on the results of laboratory experiments rather than on clinical experience?" [1]

The second doctrine of the Commission which demands consideration is that death under chloroform is always from an over-dose. The official report warns against danger from an "over-dose." Surgeon Lawrie says that the experiments have *proved* that "death from chloroform is always due to an over-dose." [2] What is an over-dose of chloroform? . Evidently, when the patient inspires air carrying more than a certain small amount of chloroform vapor. Sudden death frequently occurs in animals breathing a supercharged atmosphere, and in man it has often followed a single deep inspiration. The necessity of care to avoid this danger is plainly stated by the Commission.[3] But this is not new. The danger of charging air with more than a small percentage of chloroform has long been recognized. It was taught by Snow, who believed that safety would be assured if the amount of vapor was kept down to four or five per cent. This doctrine underlies and sustains the use of all inhalers—instruments which mechanically prevent the presence of more than a certain amount of vapor. But it has not stood the test of clinical experience ; death has occurred with all sorts of inhalers, even in the hands of the inventors who had vaunted their efficiency.

There is another way in which a patient may get an over-dose of chloroform, namely, when the administration is continued beyond the limits necessary for the surgeon's action and until respiration and cardiac action cease. It is a form of death difficult, if not impossible, to find in clinical records. And surely it is not necessary to warn against a danger so evident as this, which could only be caused by gross maladministration. Yet, this the Commission does. "The anæsthetic should never, under any circumstances, be pushed till the respiration stops." [4] Surgeon Lawrie says that there is not the least danger if the inhalation "is stopped directly the state of the cornea shows that the patient is ' under.' " This he repeats in italics ; and again italicizes from Syme, as an infallible rule for the safe administration of chloroform, that "*we never continue beyond the point when the patient is fully under the influence of the anæsthetic.*" [5] Now, let us throw upon this doctrine the electric light of clinical experience. About fifty per cent. of the deaths under chloroform have taken place before the stage of complete anæsthesia has been reached! [6] Some of them have occurred at the very beginning of the administration, after an inhalation of only a few seconds. Within so short a space of time as that, death occurred in four of Snow's fifty cases, and in five more it took place within a minute. Need I adduce any more evidence that cessation of administration when

---

[1] Anæsthetica, Stutigart, 1880.   [2] Kappeler.

[1] Official Report, Lancet, January 18, 1890, p. 151.
[2] Lancet, June 21, 1890, p. 1390.
[3] Sec. V., Official Report.
[4] Sec. VII., Official Report.
[5] Lancet, June 21, 1890, p. 1391.
[6] Sansom: Chloroform, 1865, p. 65. American Journal of the Medical Sciences, May, 1890, p. 506.

the cornea is rendered insensible will not obviate danger? And how do these early and sudden deaths bear upon the preceding doctrine that death is always by the respiration? Can death within a minute be caused in the human subject by any interference with respiration?

The last and most important doctrine of the Commission is that there is "no doubt whatever that, if the above rules be followed, chloroform may be given in any case requiring an operation with perfect ease and absolute safety." The only new rules laid down, it will have been observed, are the one positive, that the respiration alone should be watched, and the one negative, that the pulse should not be watched. The inference from this position of the Commission is that all deaths have been the result of bad administration. Surgeon Lawrie does not avoid the issue. There is never the least danger, he says, "when the chloroform is properly administered;"[1] and he describes a death as caused by the administrator, which bears no likeness whatever to what is seen in life, and is in strong contrast to the graphic picture drawn by Kappeler. It is against this doctrine and its corollary, so untenable in the light of clinical experience, so dangerous to patients, so momentous in their bearing upon the conscience and the material interests of the profession, that I most solemnly and earnestly protest. It is but just that when a man loses a patient under an anæsthetic, he should be required to show that due care was observed and all precautions taken: but to hold that the death is *prima facie* evidence of want of skill or carelessness is a monstrous doctrine. See where it carries us—to the unavoidable conclusion that many of the best surgeons of the world have caused deaths which might have been avoided; and that men who led in the study of this subject, who have devoted their lives to it, did not know how to administer the remedy properly. Simpson, and Snow, and Clover, and Kappeler, all had deaths—therefore, they violated the rules of safe administration.

I protest, in the interest of patients, against the doctrine that chloroform can be administered with absolute safety. If this procedure is to be looked upon as no more dangerous than giving a drink of whiskey and water, as has already been claimed, there will be a more frequent recourse to it, and lives will be sacrificed in consequence. The doctrine cannot be accepted without ignoring a vast amount of evidence, both experimental and clinical—evidence which outweighs all theories and all doctrines, no matter whose names may be appended to them. And, beside the few cases detailed to you to-night, even if there were no more, how does the statement appear, that "the fear of chloroform has arisen not from clinical observation, but from the results of experiments upon animals having been wrongly interpreted."[2]

No theory in science deserves a moment's consideration which does not cover all the facts. Now, the Hyderabad Commission has formulated in the most positive terms a theory of death under chloroform without any consideration of a most important class of cases—cases which, with our present knowledge, defy explanation, yet without a consideration of them no study of death

under anæsthetics can be complete. I allude to those in which the dangerous symptoms came on some time after the inhalation had ceased. Every administrator of chloroform should bear in mind the "residual air" of the lungs, which is to the tidal air as more than five to one. Of course, this residual air being charged with chloroform, the effects of the anæsthetic will deepen after the tidal air has ceased to carry more vapor into the lungs. But in the cases referred to, danger set in at a period too remote to be accounted for in this way—several minutes after the administration had ceased, breathing having continued long enough to change the air in the lungs several times. In Kappeler's case, given above, two minutes had elapsed. In case 50 of Snow's collection, the surgeons washed their hands, returned to the bed, and, seeing that the patient was all right, left the ward, to which they were hastily recalled to see the patient die. So important is the bearing of these cases upon the doctrines considered to-night that I will give a brief report of three of them.

CASE I.—Adult male. Operation under chloroform for fistula in ano, Cincinnati Commercial Hospital, Dr. Thomas Wood, operator. After the operation the patient *aroused sufficiently to answer one or two interrogations.* The order had been given to remove him from the amphitheatre when he was seen to gasp, and death rapidly followed in spite of artificial respiration. *At least three minutes* elapsed from the time the administration ceased until dangerous symptoms set in.[1]

CASE II.—Another Cincinnati case, on the testimony of a medical man present at the operation. Young adult male. Operation under ether for extirpation of eyeball. The operation was completed and the patient in good condition. The surgeons were engaged in examining the specimen when suddenly their attention was attracted to the man and he was found to be in a most dangerous condition, and was rescued only by vigorous measures.

CASE III.—I administered the A. C. E. mixture to a middle-aged man, upon whom my colleagues of St. Elizabeth's Hospital performed an operation on the bones of the leg. The operation had continued some time; all was going on well with the patient. I closely observed the pulse and respiration. So long a time had elapsed since I had held the sponge over the mouth and nose that it needed replenishing. The "sister," who held the bottle for me had gone away and placed it on the dresser several paces away. I walked to it deliberately, added the anæsthetic to the sponge, and returned, but was horrified to see the aspect of death on the man's face. No respiration was visible; no pulse to be felt. Quicker than can be told, his head was lowered, the tongue pulled out, and the best attempts possible were made at artificial respiration. After a time, which seemed an age, and when there seemed no more ground for hope, he drew a breath, and then slowly recovered.[2]

I have selected these cases, from among others of the same kind, because they occurred here close to you; because they concern three different anæsthetics, and because of their great importance. The Commission

---

[1] Lancet, june 21, 1890, p. 1390.
[2] Official Report, Lancet, january 18, 1890; and Lauder Brunton, International Congress, Lancet, August 16, 1890.

[1] Cincinnati Lancet and Observer, 1871.
[2] It may be of interest to state that a few weeks afterward I again administered the A. C. E. mixture to this patient. I had no hesitation in doing so after a hypodermic injection of morphine and atropine, and there was no trouble.

would doubtless say, in regard to my case, that my attention was withdrawn; that had I been "watching the respiration" the dangerous symptoms would not have occurred. But, before leaving the side of the table, I had ceased administering the anæsthetic for more than two minutes. And this important class of cases receives no consideration from the Commission. They merely allude to them as those "in which dangerous failure of the heart *is said to have occurred* some minutes after the administration of chloroform had ceased."[1] This is thrusting facts aside without examining them. What bearing do these cases have upon the doctrine of the Commission that there is no danger in the administration of chloroform if only the respiration be kept free and unobstructed? Can such a doctrine exist in view of these cases?

There is a doctrine, however, with which these cases harmonize. It is one that I presented several years ago, which further study has not caused me to abandon.[2] That doctrine is, that all anæsthetics are uncertain and irregular in the manifestation of their effects, and chloroform more so than any other.

A careful study of the whole subject shows that death cannot always be foreseen or averted. It has taken place in the hands of the most experienced administrators, in institutions where every precaution was taken and every means of rescue at hand. It has occurred with inhalers and without, to patients of all ages and when in the best possible health. Disaster has come when the anæsthetic was given for the most trivial operations, before surgical proceedings have commenced, during their progress, after their completion, and after the inhalation had ceased. A like sudden and unexpected death has been of frequent occurrence in animals, according to all experimenters, except the Hyderabad Commission.

In view of all this clinical and experimental evidence, and of the concurrent testimony of the best authorities of the world,[3] can we accept the doctrine that chloroform is a safe remedy? I disclaim any partisan feeling in the matter. If any man, after making a careful study of the clinical evidence, and in view of the disadvantages of ether, and of the fact that it, too, has its death-roll, shall elect chloroform as an anæsthetic, I have no denunciations for him. But for myself, such a study convinced me that it is uncertain in its action and more dangerous than other agents at command. Nothing in professional life ever caused me so much pain as the forced abandonment of this anæsthetic. And now I believe that if the doctrine of the Commission prevails, and if there be in consequence a more general resort to chloroform there will be disaster as the consequence.

I would devote some attention to the logic of the Commission's report, but lack of time will not permit. For the same reason I cannot enter upon some points of great practical interest. I should especially like to compare the results of the Commission with those obtained by Professor H. C. Wood, and with recorded clinical observations, and to show that in regard to shock under chloroform, experiment upon animals and bedside experience do not agree.

I ought, perhaps, to dwell upon the assumption of the Commission that watching the respiration and resorting to means for its continuance, will always carry the patient safely over the danger.[1] I am saved the trouble by adducing a single case, published in the same number of the same journal with one of the reports of the Commission. The patient, a woman aged twenty-four years, had taken chloroform several times; was in good health; and had no fear of the operation or the anæsthetic. The administrator had given chloroform about 700 times; Skinner's inhaler was used with twenty drops of the anæsthetic. Immediately upon adding a fresh supply of chloroform the patient suddenly stopped breathing. The tongue was drawn out and artificial respiration by Sylvester's method instituted and continued for half an hour. It was in vain; she was dead. An autopsy showed that all the organs were healthy, and gave evidence that the heart continued to act after breathing ceased.[2] Here, then, side by side with the report of the Commission, is a case of death by the respiratory function, in which measures of rescue were immediately resorted to by experienced men in a hospital, without result. There is sometimes a grim irony in facts.

I will conclude by giving a series of "practical conclusions," derived from studies of the subject by experiment upon animals, which do agree with observations upon the human subject. And I consider it a matter of no slight congratulation that they were presented at the late International Congress by one of our countrymen, Professor H. C. Wood, in his address on Anæsthesia.[3] They have been lately published in nearly all the journals, but they will bear repeating. The closest examination fails to detect any flaw in them, or to find any point which is not supported and which cannot be substantiated by clinical records:

1. The use of any anæsthetic is attended with an appreciable risk, and no care will prevent an occasional loss of life.

2. Chloroform acts much more promptly and much more powerfully than ether, both upon the respiratory centres and upon the heart.

3. The action of chloroform is much more persistent and permanent than that of ether.

4. Chloroform is capable of causing death either by primarily arresting the respiration, or by primarily stopping the heart, but commonly [sometimes] both respiratory and cardiac functions are abolished at or about the same time.

5. Ether usually acts very much more powerfully upon the respiration than upon the circulation, but occasionally, and especially when the heart is feeble, ether is capable of acting as a cardiac paralyzant, and may produce death at a time when the respirations are fully maintained.

6. Chloroform kills, as near as can be made out, proportionately four or five times as frequently as does ether.

---

[1] Official report, Lancet, January 18, 1890.
[2] Holmes's Surgery, American edition, 1882, vol. iii. p. 542.
[3] Ibid.

[1] Lauder Brunton, International Congress, Lancet, August 16, 1890.
[2] Lancet, February 22, 1896, p. 416.
[3] THE MEDICAL NEWS, August 9, 1890.

ORIGINAL ARTICLES.

PROPHYLAXIS OF TUBERCULOSIS.[1]

BY C. W. STROBELL, M.D.,

OF MIDDLETOWN SPRINGS, VERMONT.

TUBERCULOSIS, according to reliable statistics, is responsible for one-seventh of all deaths that annually occur in this country. It is a disease before which we, as physicians, have thus far stood wellnigh powerless, the subject's doom being sealed in our minds simultaneously with the confirmation of the diagnosis. It is in vain that alleged specifics and much-vaunted discoveries are tried. In vain have gaseous enemata, oxygen inhalations, superheated air, and nauseous fish-oil flashed spasmodically upon our therapeutic horizon, momentarily lighting up the gloom with a fitful glare, only to plunge us into deeper therapeutic darkness.

In order that we may be thoroughly in sympathy with our subject, and fully appreciate the rapid and salutary changes which the theories concerning the pathology of tuberculosis have undergone, let us briefly review its literature since 1865, previously to which investigators were groping in a dense theoretical fog. Villemin, in 1865, startled the medical world by the artificial production of tuberculosis, exciting renewed and intense interest in the pathology of the disease. He inoculated animals by inserting tuberculous matter beneath the skin through a small incision. One month later it was found that, with few exceptions, general tuberculosis had set in. Artificial tuberculosis, it was ascertained, could be easily generated in rabbits, guinea-pigs, oxen, sheep, goats, and monkeys. Cats and dogs proved not very susceptible, and in the case of a cock and a dove the experiments entirely failed. Villemin also produced tuberculous infection by injecting a watery suspension of tubercle into the bronchi. These researches constitute the first link of the chain of brilliant experiments that are rapidly guiding us to a solution of this problem in pathology.

With regard to the material inoculated in the later experiments Gee[2] says:

"Villemin used fresh tubercle, but soon afterward Andrew Clark and Waldenburg succeeded in rendering rabbits tubercular by inoculating them with materials other than tubercle. It was next found that not only animal tissue, but even the vegetable, such as a cotton seton, or a piece of cork, would set up tuberculosis. And lastly, the fact was discovered that a simple wound into which nothing was inserted would suffice to generate tubercle in rabbits, guinea-pigs, and certain other animals. However, Sanderson, in 1868, showed that of all the means of producing artificial tubercle by inoculation, none is more certain or more active than the material

taken from the diseased glands of a living animal already infected. The dose required is almost infinitesimal. If a diseased gland is squeezed into a little distilled water in a capsule, and the slightly turbid liquid injected, results are certain. Both Sanderson and Wilson Fox, in 1868, discovered that when non-tubercular matters are inoculated they become encapsuled by cheesy matter formed beneath the skin, so that the difficulty of explaining the subsequent tuberculosis is not so great as it seems at first. The tubercles follow, not the material inoculated, but the inflammatory products which surround it. Cohnheim inferred that the infectious matter was always caseous pus. But the inflammatory products around the wound of inoculation are not always cheesy, although they are usually so.

"Therefore the infectious virus which excites the general tuberculosis is not introduced from without, but is generated by the animal itself. The animal must possess a tubercular diathesis, and if this is present any kind of inflammation, set up in any way, may call forth tuberculosis."

This summing up of the status of the case in 1884 is interesting when viewed in the light of recent developments, for close upon the heels of these investigators came Klebs, Aufrecht, and Baumgarten, with the theory of the bacillary form of the virus. Schüller and Toussaint described it as a micrococcus.

The announcement of the discovery of the specific bacillus of tuberculosis by Koch was at first received with incredulity, and in some quarters with prejudice, which, however, disappeared as the confirmatory evidences multiplied, until to-day there seems to be no reason to doubt the specificity of Koch's bacillus, although as yet the precise action or manner of infection does not seem clear, *i. e.*, does the bacillus mechanically infect by its presence, as in the case of a cotton seton and various organic and inorganic materials, or by its secretions? This question is of vast importance regarding the therapeutics of the disease, for, could the view be proven (and in my opinion it is the true solution) that the secretion of the bacillus is the virus, then there opens before us a glorious prospect of being able to cure tuberculosis by neutralizing the virus. Already has Koch's discovery borne practical fruit in the prophylactic measures we are enabled to apply intelligently.

¶The pleura, peritoneum, arachnoid, and even the pericardium may be the seat of miliary tuberculosis; but it is generally noted that the lungs are the organs first attacked, and that it is extremely rare for tubercle to exist in any organ without being also present in the lungs.

The *Medical World*, June, 1890, states that:

"Tubercle bacilli are found in phthisis tuberculosis, scrofula, lupus, and pearl disease. In enteric disease they can be detected in the dejecta; in tubercular disease of the urinary apparatus, in the urine; in tubercular meningitis, in the nasal secretion; in phthisis they infest the expired air, the sputa, the secretions of laryngeal and pharyngeal ulcers, and the pus of anal fistulæ. In

---

[1] Read at the semi-annual meeting of the Vermont State Medical Society, June, 1890.

[2] Quain's Dictionary of Medicine, 1884.

16*

scrofula they swarm in the pus of diseased joints, and in the discharges from scrofulous ears. They have also been frequently discovered in lupus vulgaris, which is now considered by many pathologists to be a tuberculosis of the skin. In all these instances they are capable of cultivation; and many of the lower animals can be inoculated, which tends to prove that the inception of tuberculosis depends upon the passage of the living bacillus from one organism to another, the peculiar pathognomonic changes being consequent upon either its mechanical presence or the virulent character of its secretions."

The next question that concerns us is, What is the primal source of the bacillus of tuberculosis? Investigations thus far point very strongly to the bovine species as responsible for the disease in the human family. As evidence of this origin we will cite the case of one of our foundling homes, where an endemic of acute miliary tuberculosis broke out with great fatality. It was at length suspected that the dairy attached to the institution was the source of contagion. Investigation revealed that three-fourths of the cows were infected with tuberculosis. The milk was condemned as unfit for the use of the infants, and given to the swine, of which there were twenty-five or thirty. It was observed that with the withdrawal of this milk a marked improvement began in the health of the infants, which continued so far as tuberculosis was concerned. But there is a sequel to this, namely, that the swine that were given the rejected milk sickened, emaciated, and finally died. The order was given to kill all the cattle and swine upon the premises, which was followed by thorough disinfection and a complete restocking.

Although innumerable cases may be cited of the infection of certain of the lower animals by man through the ingestion of his excretions in various forms, there is not one instance, so far as I know, of such infection of an animal of the bovine species, which is probably due to the purity of their food. So that in the latter animals the bacillus seems to arise spontaneously.

Admitting, then, the bovine theory of the origin of tuberculosis, let us briefly enumerate the methods of infection beginning with the originators. Infection from the cow may be from either the meat, the milk, or the sputa. By the ingestion of tuberculous meat and milk man is infected, provided that a proper soil exists. By hereditary predisposition, and the ingestion of tuberculous milk and sputa, calves are infected, and propagate the disease in the herd.

Infection from man to man ranks next in importance, and this is either directly by the ingestion of sputa; or indirectly by the use of tuberculous pork and poultry. To the omnivorous habits of our barnyard fowls and of swine, is due the fact that they are very susceptible to this disease.

The house-fly, too, is by no means innocent, as shown by the experiments of Drs. Spillman and Houshalter.[1] Flies that had been seen to enter spittoons containing the sputa of phthisical patients were caught and placed in a bell-jar. On the following day several of them were dead. An examination of the abdominal contents and the excrement of these flies showed the presence of many tubercle bacilli. The authors point out the wide dissemination of the disease which may take place in this manner. It was clearly shown by Professor Dixon, of the University of Pennsylvania, that calves and pigs fed upon milk infected with tubercle bacilli, became tuberculous. The gastric secretions of the dog are said to be a greater defence against the successful invasion of the bacilli than are the similar secretions of man, but a healthy dog which Professor Dixon fed for several days on the meat of a tuberculous cow soon began to lose flesh, and died a few weeks later of tuberculosis.

Dr. Henry Behrends, a noted Hebrew physician and scientist of London, regards the freedom of the Jewish people from phthisis as due to the religious rules concerning the choice and killing of cattle, and the sale of meat. Dr. Behrends[2] writes that of 13,116 beeves slaughtered for the Hebrew trade in London in six months, only 6,973 came up to the peculiar Jewish requirements, and that the average rejections for five years had been 40 per cent. But the rejected beeves are often used by the Christian butchers. He also makes the astounding statements that in a large practice of over thirty years he has never met with a case of consumption among the members of the Jewish faith, and that other Hebrew physicians have had a similar experience.

The prevention of the disease seems possible by two simple measures. First, the devitalization of the sputum of consumptives, for the desiccated tubercle bacillus retains its vitality. Second, the legal inspection of all dairies at regularly stated periods, and the slaughtering of cattle for food purposes under the supervision of a regularly qualified and legally appointed veterinarian, who shall issue a certificate upon "proof-meat," and be held responsible for the wholesomeness of such meat.

As regards the sputum, devitalization should be secured almost immediately after being expectorated. Destruction by fire is the most convenient, safe, and certain method of devitalization. The patient should expectorate upon pieces of newspaper, which, upon receiving the sputum, are twisted and dropped into a receiver, which should be emptied into the fire as often as every three hours; or the papers may be immediately dropped

---

[1] New York Medical Record, November 12, 1887.
[2] Medical World, February, 1890.

into the fire. In view of the results of the experiments with the house-fly referred to above, it is unsafe to employ a sputum-cup during summer, or at any time in fact, as its contents are not, as a rule, thrown into the fire, which is the devitalizer *par excellence*. The sputum-cup is usually emptied into the slop-jar or out of the window, and in places where the bacillus has the best opportunity to find a favorable soil for its propagation. Kissing must be interdicted, as the bacillus may be deposited upon the lips and face, thus eventually finding access to the system.

Bovine tuberculosis when occurring in our Vermont herds is never noticed by the law, as is pleuro-pneumonia, but only by the farmer when he observes that a certain animal "is not doing well," is "off its feed," or "running down." What is his course in such a case? Invariably the animal is "stuffed" and given only limited exercise until sufficiently presentable either to sell to the butcher, or to slaughter at home, the meat being peddled (in the majority of cases by wholly innocent farmers) to unsuspecting consumers. The farmer will not allow any stock to "run-down" on his hands if he can prevent it; and, moreover, who of the consumers is to tell whether the cervical glands were enlarged or the lungs or other viscera tuberculous, since these parts are not, as a rule, offered for sale?

It has been said that cooking will devitalize the bacilli, but this was disproved by the experiments of Professor Gerlach, who cooked meat known to be tuberculous from fifteen to thirty minutes, fed it to animals, and produced consumption in two-thirds of all those experimented upon. I have personal knowledge of certain animals with swollen cervical glands, scrofulous joints, and emaciated frames that are being milked daily, part of the milk being consumed by the family, the remainder going to cheese factories, where, according to Professor Gerlach, the degree of heat to which the milk is subjected in the cheese-making process is not sufficient to devitalize the bacillus. Then as to the milk we drink: who, in the absence of official inspection, is to tell us whether it is sound or not? Surely not the farmer, who is ignorant of the existence of this germ. It may be said that the milk can be sterilized by boiling, but here again we are doomed to disappointment, for Professor Bollinger, of Munich, has demonstrated that tuberculous milk even when boiled will produce consumption.

What abominations are sold in the form of canned goods can only be surmised, as the Government makes no provision for their supervision. But the country is waking up to the importance of this question. The Government spends $500,000 per annum in the work of exterminating pleuro-pneumonia in our herds, but not because the disease can be transmitted to man. A much larger sum could be profitably expended in the extermination of tuberculosis, for it is clear that, in many cases, this disease, which kills one-seventh of the human race, is carried to man in infected meat and milk. Not long ago, in Oregon, all the cows in a noted and valuable herd were killed, because they either had tuberculosis or had been exposed to the disease. This action of Oregon is in the right direction, and should be followed by all the States. The great remedy for tuberculosis is to instruct and urge our Board of Cattle Commissioners (who have the requisite power granted them by the statutes) to ferret out all cases of tuberculosis among our herds with a view to its extermination, just as is done with pleuro-pneumonia. And, as already mentioned, the slaughtering of all animals for food purposes should be under the supervision of a veterinary pathologist. In connection with this the methods of inspection practised by the Jews is of interest. According to Behrends:

"Kosher meat, as the passed-inspection Hebrew meat is called, is thus prepared under the inspection of the proper official, often the rabbi himself, certainly one familiar with pathological appearances. A perfectly sound and presumably healthy animal is selected and thrown, and a keen, sword-like knife, three feet long, is pushed once across the throat, and then drawn forcibly back toward the operator, the animal then being hung up by the heels until thoroughly drained of blood. That oft-quoted jugular vein is, of course, severed, and so are the large arteries, by those terrible cuts, for the knife goes to the bone. Every organ is then carefully examined for traces of disease, especial attention being paid to the lungs, which must be non-adherent to the chest or to each other in any lobe, and must be fully inflated, then cut into and examined for foci of disease. The larger veins and arteries must then be dissected from the meat, for it is along them that abscesses are usually found, if found at all. If a defect is found at any of these points the meat is rejected as unsuitable for Jewish use. Poultry and fish have to pass a rigid inspection, and there are other stringent regulations regarding the treatment and cooking of even the passed-inspection food articles."

Associating this with his above-quoted forceful exposition of the immunity from consumption of the adherents of the Jewish faith, we are impressed with the importance of this matter.

This ancient custom of the Jews must be appropriated by us for our own preservation, and to insure the perpetuity of our race.

The advocacy by the *British Medical Journal* of a wider use of goat's milk is timely, and of great importance as regards infant-feeding, especially as cow's milk in cities is seldom free from a suspicion of infection or adulteration. The goat, on the other hand, does not have, or very rarely has, tuberculosis, is easily kept, and is a vigorous and healthy animal, thriving under almost any condition, while, as physiology teaches, its milk is nearest, in its several constituent properties, to human milk, therefore the best substitute.

In conclusion, let us urge our representatives to

arouse the Government to act in this vital matter, so that as speedily as possible it shall guarantee that our meat is " Kosher."

TWO CASES OF ACROMEGALY.[1]

By J. E. GRAHAM, M.D.,
PROFESSOR OF CLINICAL MEDICINE AND MEDICAL PATHOLOGY IN THE UNIVERSITY OF TORONTO.

IT has been well said that he who gives a name to a certain series of signs and symptoms not previously classified confers a benefit on science.

In 1884 Fritsche and Klebs published a long article, entitled " Ein Beitrag zur Pathologie des Riesenwuchses," in which an exhaustive description of a case is given, together with a list of similar cases published under various names.

It was not, however, until after 1886, when Marie published his first paper, and introduced the term *acromegaly*, that the attention of the profession generally was drawn to this disease. Since that time a number of cases have been reported, and some progress has been made in its etiology and pathology. I might here refer to the exhaustive article of Erb, published in the *Deutsche Archiv für klinische Medicin*, 1889.

Marie' gives a summary of cases published up to that time. In this list are eighteen undoubted cases, four probable ones, and six which, although published as acromegaly, Marie did not consider as examples of that disease. Two cases reported on this continent were not included in this list.

A case has also been published by Drs. Holschewnikoff and von Recklinghausen.[3]

Dr. Henry Waldo,[4] of the Bristol Royal Infirmary, reported a case which was of an acute form, lasting but six months. On post-mortem examination it presented some gross brain-lesions, which were very interesting and which will be referred to subsequently. The short duration of the case, the absence of marked enlargement of the head and face, the normal size of the inferior maxilla, and the peculiar condition of the skin, all make it doubtful whether this ought to be included in the list of genuine cases, or whether it is not a trophic neurosis which Virchow would describe as a partial acromegaly.

My attention was drawn to a letter in the *Medical World*, written by a physician in Missouri, in which the description of a patient is given who is probably suffering from acromegaly.

Of the cases published on this continent, one by Dr. Wadsworth[1] appeared under the heading " A Case of Myxœdema, with Atrophy of the Optic Nerves." Marie includes this in his list of genuine examples. To my mind, the case presented many symptoms of myxœdema as well as those of acromegaly. Changes of the skin and subcutaneous tissues were described such as are found in cases of myxœdema, while the enlargement of the bones would place it under the head of acromegaly.

The second case was reported by Dr. Adler[2] to the New York County Medical Society, and appears to have been a good example of the disease as described by Marie. The striking peculiarity of the case was a widespread enlargement of the lymphatic glands. There was no distinctive sign of myxœdema present.

The third case was published by Dr. O'Connor,[3] and is also a genuine case of the affection. " An extreme infiltration of the lining membrane of the cheeks and soft palate," is described, but whether this resulted from a simple hyperplasia of the connective tissue, or from an infiltration of mucin, is not clear—possibly the latter, as the doctor thought " some purely myxœdematous symptoms were undoubtedly present."

It would thus appear that three cases have already been reported on this continent. So far as I know, the two now to be described are the fourth and fifth in the order of publication.

In August of last year Dr. Osler, who was then on a visit to Toronto, drew my attention to a case in the Toronto General Hospital, under the care of my colleague, Dr. Burritt, which Dr. Osler considered to be a case of acromegaly. The patient was afterward transferred to me.

I am, therefore, indebted to Dr. Osler, who made the first diagnosis, and to Dr. Burritt, for some of the earlier notes of the first case.

The second patient I had frequently seen, and at once considered him an example of acromegaly, after the first had been shown me.

The following notes of the first case were made partly in August, 1889, but principally in April of this year:

CASE I.—G. B., aged forty years. Born in Canada. When young he suffered from severe attacks of asthma, which ceased when he was about seventeen years old. When twenty he had an attack of bronchitis, which was probably complicated by asthma. This lasted about a year, and his physician was apprehensive of tuberculosis. He,

---

1 Read before the Association of American Physicians, May, 1890. As this paper has already been published in the Transactions of the Association of American Physicians a word of explanation is necessary. The MS. was handed to Dr. I. Minis Hays to be given to THE NEWS, and was withheld by him until two weeks ago, when this office was notified of the fact by Dr. Graham.
2 Brain, July, 1889.
3 Virchow's Archiv, January, 1890.
4 British Medical Journal, March 22, 1890.

1 Boston Medical and Surgical Journal, January 1, 1885.
2 Ibid.
3 American Journal of Homœopathy, 1888.

however, recovered, and has not since been troubled with asthma. At twenty-two years of age he suffered from malaria, which continued for six months. He then lived in a miasmatic region.

From that time up to the commencement of the present illness he enjoyed good health. He was a strong, well-built, athletic man, but thinks that he worked too hard on the farm. At the age of thirty-five years he married. His wife died three years ago. He had one child that died in infancy of some intestinal trouble.

Family history: His father, a native of England, died aged seventy-five years, and for years previous to his death suffered from chronic rheumatic arthritis. His mother died at sixty-five, of an obscure disease of the bowels. He has eight brothers and two sisters, all living and healthy. He knows of no case similar to his own in the family.

When about thirty-five years old he complained of severe pains in the left side of his face, which were thought to be of neuralgic character. He had several teeth extracted, which did not, however, give him any relief. Some months after this he noticed a prominence of the left malar bone, and an enlargement of the left ramus of the inferior maxilla. The presence of the malar enlargement was brought to his attention by a physician whom he occasionally saw, and who told him that a tumor was forming on the left side of the face.

About three years ago, two years after the commencement of the pains, he noticed a general enlargement of the face, and at the same time of the hands and feet. The pains have continued without intermission for the last five years. They are of a dull aching character, and are often accompanied with dizziness and an indescribable feeling of distress in the head.

Three years ago he noticed that his sight was failing, first in the left, then in the right eye. This diminution of sight has steadily progressed up to the present time.

He has suffered much from chronic constipation, and from hæmorrhoids, which frequently bleed. His appetite has always been good. He has been in the habit of drinking large quantities of water, and has taken spirits moderately.

He has at times had polyuria, which would last for a month or so. Of late, weakness and shortness of breath are noticed after moderate exertion.

At the commencement of this illness he weighed 180 pounds. He now weighs 212 pounds, and is about five feet nine inches in height.

Present condition: Patient is pale and sallow. The face, hands, and feet are noticeably large in proportion to the rest of his body. He walks slowly and heavily, with his shoulders stooped, owing to a curvature of the spine. His face is much enlarged, and elliptical in shape. The skin of the face, of a sallow color, is loose, movable, and soft, and can be pinched up in large folds. There is no appearance anywhere of a deposit of mucin such as occurs in myxœdema.

Length of the face from the top of the forehead to the tip of the chin, 245 millimetres. Breadth between the malar prominences, 160 millimetres.

The forehead is low and receding. The supra-orbital arches are very large, especially the left one. The prominence of the eyebrows gives the eyes a somewhat sunken appearance. The malar bones are much enlarged, the left one being more prominent than the right. The nose is very voluminous, but is uniformly enlarged and not pugged. The upper lip is elongated and somewhat thickened. The superior maxilla is enlarged at the upper part. The alveolar surface is about the normal size, except at the posterior part of the left side. The inferior maxilla is everywhere enlarged, and is set forward, so that there is about a third of an inch between the teeth above and below when the mouth is closed. He says that before the disease began he could bite a pin in two. He has had some teeth extracted, and others are decayed. The tongue is enlarged, and presents a red furrowed appearance. The raphe is deep, and deep furrows branch out on each side.

The enlargement and position of the inferior maxilla give to the lower part of the face a heavy appearance. The lower lip is long, thick, and protruding. The chin is long and heavy. His beard does not grow nearly so fast as before the commencement of his illness.

The ears are uniformly enlarged. The cranium does not appear much larger than normal. The neck is not much increased in circumference, measuring 410 mm.

The right lobe of the thyroid can be felt with great difficulty, but no other part of the gland.

There is a slight forward curvature of the spine in the lower cervical and upper dorsal regions, and a corresponding lordosis in the lumbar region.

The hands are broad, flat, and fleshy. On grasping his hand it feels soft, and is so large that it cannot be properly held. The right is slightly larger than the left. Part of the index finger of the right hand was lost by an accident at the age of three years. The metacarpal bones are especially lengthened. The carpal joints are much enlarged and flattened, especially those of the index and middle fingers. At the side of the metacarpal bone of the little finger there is a mass of soft tissue, but not out of proportion to the fleshy condition of the rest of the hand. The palmar lines are deep and well marked. The skin presents a yellowish appearance, and is loosely attached to the subjacent tissue. The nails are short and broad, and present transverse markings; some of them are curved, so as to be sunken in the centre and turned up at the edges.

The forearms are normal in size, measuring in circumference, midway between the wrist and elbow, right 280 mm., left 260 mm. The elbows are somewhat larger in proportion: circumference over the head of the radius when the arm is straight, right 300 mm., left 281 mm. The arms midway between the elbow and shoulder joint measure: right 315 mm., left 300 mm. The scapulæ are not enlarged.

The feet are also increased in size; he is now obliged to wear boots three sizes larger than he wore five years ago. The feet are elongated and fleshy, but not particularly flat; there is no large mass of flesh found at the side of the metatarsal bone of the little toe, as was found in Marie's cases.

The feet measure antero-posteriorly, right 257 mm., left 269 mm. Circumference of the heel and instep, right 370 mm., left 385 mm. Greatest circumference of the foot, right 310 mm., left 290 mm. From these measurements it will be seen that the feet are uniformly enlarged. The toe-nails are short and broad.

The ankles measure, right 270 mm., left 260 mm. The legs, midway between the ankle and knee, measure, right 365 mm., left 352 mm. The knee-joints are slightly enlarged. Both patellæ enlarged. The thighs, midway between the knee- and hip-joints, measure, right 535 mm., left 530 mm.

The trunk does not present such abnormal conditions as will be described in the report of my second case.

The clavicles are much thickened, especially toward the sternal ends; the scapulæ are not enlarged and the sternum is not prominent; marked dulness is found over the upper third of the sternum. The chest measures over the nipples 1020 mm.; the abdomen over the umbilicus 930 mm.[1]

His respirations are diaphragmatic in character.

April 27, 1890. His pulse is 78; temperature normal; respiration 17. His heart is normal in size; but there is an accentuation of the second sound. The lungs are normal. There is no enlargement of the liver or spleen.

About a year ago he passed large quantities of urine, but he thinks it is now normal in quantity. The following analysis was made by Dr. Caven: Reaction strongly acid. Color normal. Specific gravity 1021. Albumin about one-seventh by measure. No sugar. Pus-cells in considerable number. Abundance of oxalate of lime crystals. No casts.

There is a chain of indurated and slightly enlarged lymphatic glands along the posterior margin of the sterno-mastoid muscle on each side. A similar condition is found in some of the glands in the posterior part of the neck. There is no evidence of any other changes in the lymphatic system.

The organs of generation are normal in size, but for the last three years he has had very little sexual feeling. A double varicocele is present.

He has a deep bass voice, which he says does not at all resemble that of five years ago. He could then sing and whistle with ease, now he cannot call out loudly, and can sing and whistle with difficulty.

The patient is much troubled by a thick mucus which collects in the back part of the mouth. There is much thickening of the mucous membrane of the posterior nares; this, in all probability, is the predisposing cause of the occasional deafness from which he suffers. His appetite is always good, and he is not often troubled by indigestion.

The tendon- and skin-reflexes are normal. Muscular power of the arms not much diminished. Last fall he had more than the ordinary strength of the forearm; at the recent examination his grasp was not so strong.

He complains of hyperæsthesia over the left side

[1] For a complete table of the measurements in this case see Transactions of the Association of American Physicians, 1890.

of the neck and head, also over the gums on the left side. There are no abnormal sensations in the extremities. He has a dull aching pain in the forehead, face, and teeth, from which he says he is never free.

The following account of the condition of his eyes was sent me by Dr. Reeve: Vision very imperfect; right eye, $V. = \frac{8}{cc}$: left eye, $\frac{10}{cc}$: and reads 14 Jaeger. Double temporal hemianopsia. Color-sense defective for green. Pupils of normal size and respond well to light and accommodation, but do not dilate well. Right pupil almost, if not quite, unaffected by a pencil of light from the temporal side; left pupil more influenced. Gray atrophy of optic nerves, not post-neuritic. Retinal arteries not more than one-half normal size, and veins small. Divergent strabismus. No present diplopia.

His hearing is at present fairly good; taste and smell normal.

He is not intellectually bright, and says he cannot do business as well as formerly.

He believes that he has improved during the winter months, but his appearance is not nearly so healthy as when he was last in Toronto.

The history of my second case was obtained partly from the attending physician, Dr. Leslie, and partly from the relatives of the patient. Although I had frequently seen him, I was never called to visit him professionally. He was sensitive about his condition, and did not like to have it referred to.

CASE II.—Mr. T., aged fifty-seven years, bank clerk, born in Edinburgh, came to Canada when he was twenty-three years of age. Nothing was at that time noticeable about his figure. He was a strong, well-built, large-boned man, about five feet ten inches in height. Shortly after his arrival on this continent the enlargement of his head and face commenced, and at twenty-eight years of age the change was so marked that his mother, whom he then visited in Scotland, scarcely recognized him, and expressed great astonishment at his appearance. So far as can be recollected the enlargement of the hands and feet began at the same time as that of the head. A gradual increase in the size of the extremities went on for years. Of late, the change in the form and size of the trunk was more noticeable.

During the last five years of his life he did not do any work. He had ample means, and seemed disinclined to enter into business. He was morbidly sensitive about his appearance, and did not care to talk about it, even to his physician. He was of an amiable, affectionate disposition, and spent most of his time at home. He was unusually bright and cheerful, fond of reading, and he talked with much intelligence.

The changes in the extremities may be described as follows: His hands were much enlarged, broad, and flat. The carpal joints were enlarged, so that he could not wear an ordinary finger-ring. The flatness and broadness of the hand were especially noticeable when he placed it with the palm downward on the table. A soft enlargement by the side of the fifth metacarpal bone could then be more especially seen.

His nails were short, broad, and small compared with the size of the fingers. He kept his nails closely cut, a circumstance which gave them a still shorter appearance. The right hand was considerably larger than the left.

His wrist was enlarged, measuring 9 inches in circumference.

There was nothing noticeable about the forearm and arm, except that during the latter years of his life they became much emaciated.

The feet were also enlarged, but not unshapely. The toes were elongated and flattened. (The sole of his slipper measured 12 inches in length by 4 in breadth.)

There was nothing noticeable about his legs and thighs, except a considerable enlargement of the knee-joints.

His head was much enlarged. Circumference, as shown by his hat-band, was 24 inches. His hat measured 8½ inches antero-posteriorly by 6½ transversely.

The face was elliptical in shape. The forehead was low and sloping. His son, who is now twenty years of age, has a similarly-shaped forehead. The eyebrows were prominent, and the skin over the forehead much wrinkled.

His nose was uniformly enlarged and slightly pugged.

His lips were thickened and enlarged, the lower being much more prominent than the upper.

The upper and lower jaws were much enlarged. He had a long, fat chin, which at ordinary times rested on his chest.

His neck, short and thick, seemed to be set on the upper and anterior part of the trunk. It was much arched behind and was marked by large, thick folds of integument, which were separated by deep furrows. His ears were also much enlarged.

His shoulders were much increased in size, and one was more forward than the other. There was a marked curvature of the spine in the upper dorsal region. The distance along the spine from the collar of the coat to a line drawn between the upper border of the axillæ, a measurement which tailors make, was 15 inches. The usual length of such a measurement is 7 or 8 inches.

The sternum was very prominent toward the upper extremity, and the ribs were flattened on each side. The circumference of the chest over the nipples measured 47½ inches.

Besides the kyphosis, there were lateral curvature and lumbar lordosis. The latter was very marked.

He at one time complained a good deal of toothache, and eleven years before his death had all his teeth removed.

His sight was good up to the day before his death, when he became almost totally blind. His hearing was acute, as were also his taste and smell.

He had a deep bass voice, which was slightly husky. He could never call out loudly, but always whistled when he wanted to attract the attention of any one at a distance. About the beginning of the year 1889 he caught cold, from which he was some time in recovering.

During the following winter months his family noticed that he slept more than usual. He would come down to breakfast, after a long night's sleep, looking pale and worn, and would fall asleep in his chair two or three times during the day. This tendency to somnolency increased during the early part of the summer.

The first time he consulted Dr. Leslie was about five years before his death. He then wished to obtain a certificate to exempt him from jury duty. He stated that he was nervous, and that he could not hear or speak well.

He afterward occasionally consulted the doctor about severe headaches from which he suffered. They were of the nature of migraine, and often lasted one or two days. He could not take much exercise, as he became easily tired. His appetite was always good, and he complained frequently of thirst. His urine was examined in January, 1889, and was found to be free from albumin and sugar.

On January 29th, he called on the doctor, complaining of pain in the calf of his right leg. He had been on his feet more than usual, and he was troubled with varicose veins. The pain was thought to be due to phlebitis. The limb afterward became red and swollen, and an abscess formed, which was lanced on July 11th. After a free discharge of pus, the patient improved until the 14th, when he became delirious. He afterward sank rapidly, and died on the 16th, apparently from acute septicæmia.

Measurements:

Circumference of chest over the nipple, 1162 mm.

Circumference immediately above the crest of the ilium, 1062 mm.

Distance from the collar of the coat to a line drawn across the upper margin of the axillæ, 387 mm.

Circumference of neck, 462 mm.

Circumference of wrist, 231 mm.

Circumference of head, 612 mm.

Circumference of right-hand at metacarpo-phalangeal joints, 216 mm.

Length of index finger, 127 mm.

Length of ring finger, 136 mm.

Length of little finger, 107 mm.

Length of thumb, 105 mm.

Length of foot, 301 mm.

Breadth of sole, 110 mm.

Circumference of foot, 262 mm.

These measurements are not quite accurate, as they were made from the patient's clothing.

In the cases just described remarkably similar signs and symptoms were present.

The differences will first be noted:

In the first case there was loss of sight from optic neuritis, a condition not present in the second. The latter patient appeared to be in a more advanced stage of the disease, as shown by the changes in the spine and thorax—changes which became more pronounced in the last five years, and which were present to only a limited degree in the first patient. The disease began at an earlier age in the second case and lasted twenty-three years. In the first it began at thirty-five, and from present appearances he will not 'live as long. Albumin was found in the urine of the first and not in that of the second case.

In each case there was a marked increase in the size both of the face and the extremities, and this enlargement was due not only to involvement of the soft parts, but of the skeleton as well. In neither case was there any myxœdematous condition of the skin or subcutaneous tissue.

The face in each case was elliptical, the cheek bones were prominent, the superior and inferior maxillæ were enlarged, the lips were thickened— the lower one more than the upper. The upper alveolar process in the second patient was much more enlarged than in the first.

In each patient the hands were increased in size and there was marked enlargement of the carpal joints. There were enlargement and lengthening of many of the bones and an increase of the connective tissue. The same description will apply to the feet.

In each case there was gradual lessening of vitality, although the mental faculties remained, to a great extent, unimpaired. In the second patient this diminution of vital force was more marked during the last six months of his life.

Each patient suffered from severe aching pains about the face and head. The first patient was a plain farmer of fair education, whereas the second was a well-educated man.

There can be little doubt that both cases belong to that class described by Marie under the name of acromegaly. That they were not cases of myxœdema is evident from the following facts:

1. The dimensions of the bony skeleton were in many parts much increased, whereas in myxœdema the soft parts are alone affected.

2. The face in myxœdema presents a round, full-moon appearance. In each of these cases the face was elliptical.

3. In myxœdema there is a distinct waxy-like condition of the skin and subcutaneous cellular tissue. There is also a thickened and scaly condition of the integument. In neither of the cases described was there thickening of the skin, and only in the first was there any discoloration.

4. In neither case was the mental condition present which is so marked in myxœdema. The first patient is engaged in selling horses, a business which cannot be carried on without a good deal of shrewdness.

The osteitis deformans of Paget is excluded, as in that disease the head is enlarged and the face retains almost its normal size. In the cases described the enlargement existed principally in the face. The deformities of the long bones which exist in osteitis deformans were not found in these cases. The latter disease begins after the age of forty years, while in the histories narrated the disease began earlier in life. There was more symmetry in the enlargement of the bones in the cases described than there is in osteitis deformans.

In gigantism we have a condition in which the extremities are enlarged only in proportion to the general stature. The face is not elongated and the lower jaw is not hypertrophied, or set forward, as has been described.

The leontiasis ossea of Virchow is excluded, as in these cases there were no well-defined bony tumors, but there was hypertrophy of the hands and feet— a condition not found in the disease described by Virchow.

Marie, I think, properly excludes localized hypertrophies, such as that of one extremity, or unilateral hypertrophy of the face, from cases of this affection. It is possible that these dystrophies may be produced by localized lesions of trophic centres similar to the general lesion which may hereafter be found in acromegaly ; such, for instance, as has been found in von Recklinghausen's case. In the case just described, as well as in the twenty-two reported by others, there is a distinct clinical history, as well as pathological conditions, which separate them from all previously described diseases.

Although, in my opinion, there is little doubt of the existence of acromegaly as a distinct disease, it seems, in some cases, to have a close relationship to myxœdema. For instance, in Wadsworth's case, which is put in the list of genuine examples by Marie, there was a waxy condition of the skin, as well as an enlargement of many of the bones of the skeleton. The same condition is described in the report of Tresilian's case. From this it would appear that, although in most cases of acromegaly the skin simply undergoes the same hypertrophy as the subjacent soft tissues, there are cases in which a myxœdematous condition is found in addition to the hypertrophy of bones and soft parts.

In studying the possible connection between these two affections two sources of error must be guarded against. Cases may have been described in which the skin and subjacent tissues were myxœdematous, and in those cases the waxy condition was not really due to a deposit of mucin. Again, as Virchow suggests, in cases of genuine myxœdema the bones may be enlarged to a considerable extent without the enlargement being noticed, because of the thick covering of integument and connective tissue infiltrated by mucin.

On account of the small number of post-mortem examinations made in cases of acromegaly, there is much obscurity as to the true nature of the affection. I regret very much that in this respect the report of my second case is so defective.

In one of Marie's cases Broca described the changes in the skeleton as follows: "The spongy tissue is especially the seat of hypertrophic changes, so that the following statement may be considered as representing the reality: In the skeleton of acromegaly hypertrophy shows itself in the bones of the extremities and in the extremities of the bones."

With regard to the morbid anatomy, Marie comes to the following conclusions: "Until proof to the contrary is brought forward, I shall cling to the belief that these three anatomo-pathological characters manifest themselves not only with a remarkable degree of frequency, but may even be looked upon as constant, viz., hypertrophy of the pituitary body with enormous dilatation of the sella Turcica, persistence of the thymus, and hypertrophy of the cord and the ganglia of the sympathetic system."

Klebs mentions prominently the enlargement of both the veins and arteries, and particularly the increase in the size of the valves in the veins. In some cases the thyroid gland has been either atrophied or diseased, whereas in others it has been found normal.

Since the publication of Marie's paper, in which the foregoing statement appeared, the few autopsies made have been on cases of doubtful diagnosis. The case described by Holschewnikoff and von Recklinghausen, previously referred to, presents some points of great interest. The patient died shortly after admission into the hospital, and the clinical history is, in consequence, defective. The autopsy was made in 1886, before Marie had published his first paper.

The measurements, with the exception of those of one hand, were not made in detail, nor was the appearance of the head and face elaborately given. The case is described as one of "syringomyelia and peculiar degeneration of the peripheral nerves, combined with trophic disturbance (acromegaly)." It presented the peripheral and central lesions of syringomyelia, together with the peculiar enlargement of the bones found in acromegaly.

The study of this case would direct one's attention to the spinal cord as the probable seat of the primary lesion in acromegaly. Unfortunately, as von Recklinghausen states, the spinal cord has not been carefully examined in any of the autopsies so far reported, and until such examination has been made much doubt will surround the pathology of this affection.

In the case reported by Dr. Waldo, and already referred to, the patient was fifty-four years of age, and the disease had lasted six months. The post-mortem examination revealed cavities in the brain, the probable result of embolism. There was also valvular disease of the heart. The condition of the spinal cord could not be stated.

In this case endocarditis, rheumatism, and embolism appeared in combination with hypertrophy of the bones and soft parts of the extremities.

From the comparatively slight opportunities the writer has had for the study of this affection, he is inclined to agree with Marie that acromegaly is a general disease presenting sharply-defined features which separate it from other pathological conditions. It would be difficult to find two cases of any chronic affection which present greater similarity of symptoms than those just described.

A point of importance in etiology might be here mentioned. Virchow, in referring to the connection said by some authorities to exist between this disease and the development of the organs of generation, gives it as his opinion that there is no evidence of any special relationship between them. It will be noticed on reading over the histories already published, that in the male there are frequently sexual weakness and even impotence, and that in the female a cessation of the menstrual function follows shortly after the commencement of the disease.

In the first of my cases there was a distinct loss of sexual feeling after the second year, while in each case the disease began shortly after marriage. In both instances, again, children were begotten while the disease was in progress.

In the first case no form of treatment proved of any avail. The second did not receive any special medication for the disease.

THE NERVE-SUPPLY OF THE SENSE OF TASTE.

BY JOHN FERGUSON, M.A., M.D., L.R.C.P.,
DEMONSTRATOR OF ANATOMY IN THE UNIVERSITY OF TORONTO.

PROBABLY few questions have been more discussed and disputed than that of the nerve-supply of the sense of taste. It is an interesting if not instructive task to look over the matter that has been written upon the subject. During the past ten years much good work has been done, but much still remains to be cleared up. It is quite generally admitted that the lingual branch of the fifth nerve and the gustatory branches of the glosso-pharyngeal carry the nerve-fibres of taste to the tongue and palate. The question, however, that for a long time hung in dispute was whether these nerves were the real supply to the parts of taste, or whether they carried nerve-fibres from some other source. It is to aid in clearing up this doubt that this contribution is offered.

One of my patients had complete loss of taste on the left side of his tongue extending to the tip. This condition had lasted two years. The most carefully conducted tests with bitter, sweet, acid, and saline solutions and with electricity failed to elicit the slightest existence of taste on the left side of the tongue.

The posterior part of the tongue, the fauces, and palate retained the power of taste, and a ready distinction could be made between sweetness and sourness. The region of the circumvallate papillæ could detect the metallic taste of a galvanic current from two cells.

I informed my patient of the great interest that centred in the case, and he agreed to permit an autopsy upon himself if he should die within my reach. As he had phthisis with cavities in the lungs the opportunity for a post-mortem examination did not seem very remote, nor did it prove so.

The autopsy revealed a small exostosis in the scaphoid fossa pressing upon the posterior opening of the Vidian canal, and by pressure destroying the Vidian nerve. The nerve-degeneration following this pressure could be traced along the main course of the Vidian, and thence along its two branches, the carotid and the petrosus major. This latter enters the geniculate ganglion of the facial. The degeneration could be readily followed until the point was reached at which the chorda tympani is given off. The process of degeneration here left the facial and followed the chorda tympani throughout its length. This condition of secondary degeneration was traced from the chorda tympani to the lingual branch of the third division of the fifth nerve, and thence along the lingual.

In the above case we have complete proof that the nerve-supply of taste for the tip and anterior part of the sides of the tongue comes from the fifth nerve, and enters the superior maxillary division of the same nerve. The course must then be from the superior maxillary nerve into the spheno-palatine ganglion, thence by the Vidian, through the Vidian canal to the gangliform enlargement of the facial, along this to the chorda tympani, through the chorda tympani into either the lingual, a branch of the third, or inferior maxillary of the fifth.

It will also be seen that the Vidian is not a motor root passing from the facial to the spheno-palatine ganglion, but a sensory nerve of the special sense of taste passing from the spheno-palatine ganglion of the second division of the fifth nerve to the seventh or facial.

Another important deduction from a study of this case is that the nerve fibres of taste for the back of the tongue, the fauces, and the soft palate cannot be carried by the chorda tympani; for although the chorda tympani was degenerated, yet the taste, as stated, was retained over the posterior part of the tongue, the fauces, and palate.

In cases, then, of disease in the middle ear, causing loss of taste on one side of the posterior part as well as of the tip and sides of the tongue, we must look for some other explanation than disease of the chorda tympani. For the elucidation of this problem I submit the following case:

It is that of a young man who has had otitis media, with caries, for about ten years, caused by an attack of scarlatina. On making the most careful examination as to the condition of taste, it became evident that there was complete hemiageusia.

Now, the only nerves that could have been involved in this case were those of the middle ear, the chorda tympani, and the tympanic plexus. The first case clearly proves that loss of taste in the back of the tongue and palate is not due to destruction of the chorda tympani, and therefore it must be due to disease of the tympanic plexus.

Now it is known that complete destruction of the root of the fifth nerve destroys the sense of taste on the side involved. We have already traced the course from the fifth nerve to the tip and side of the tongue, and it remains to trace the course from the fifth to the back of the tongue and palate.

The chorda tympani has been excluded as not having any part in the sense of taste of the back of the tongue and palate; and yet disease of the middle ear may destroy taste in these parts. Returning to the fifth nerve for a moment, we can trace the course as follows: From the main root into the inferior maxillary or third division, from this to the otic ganglion, and then by the small petrosal to the intumescentia of the facial, then into the tympanic plexus, and finally through this plexus to the glosso-pharyngeal, and back of the tongue and palate.

Disease of the root of the fifth nerve causes loss of taste. The channels by which the root of the fifth nerve can become connected with the middle ear are the Vidian nerve and its branch, the great petrosal from the spheno-palatine ganglion, and the small petrosal from the otic ganglion. Disease in the middle ear, like disease of the root of the fifth nerve, may cause total hemiageusia. And thus it is that middle-ear caries must destroy the taste-path of the great and small petrosal nerves. Following the course from the middle ear we notice that the tympanic plexus is connected with the glosso-pharyngeal, and through this with the back of the tongue and palate. The connection of the tympanic plexus with the glosso-pharyngeal nerve is established by the tympanic branch that joins the petrous ganglion of the glosso-pharyngeal.

But this is not all the evidence that can be submitted to prove that the sense of taste must come from the fifth nerve. In another case bearing upon this question there was every reason to believe that there was pressure of syphilitic origin on the left side of the medulla. The paralysis of the glosso-pharyngeal, spinal accessory, and vagus on the side of the disease, together with paralysis on the opposite side of the body, was extreme. Now if the glosso-pharyngeal nerve contained at its origin fibres of the special sense of taste, this would have been lost, which was not the case. Indeed, the sense of taste over the back of the tongue and palate was quite good. Here we have conclusive proof that the root of the glosso-pharyngeal nerve does not contain any fibres of the special sense of taste.

The route for the sense of taste, so far as the glosso-pharyngeal is concerned, would be from the root of the fifth to the third division of the fifth, then to the otic ganglion, from this by the small petrosal to the ganglion on the seventh, thence to the tympanic plexus, again by the tympanic branch to the petrous ganglion of the glosso-pharyngeal, and by this latter to the back of the tongue, fauces, and palate.

RUPTURE OF THE VAGINA AND ESCAPE OF THE FŒTUS AND PLACENTA INTO THE PERITONEAL CAVITY.

BY GEORGE B. TAYLOR, M.D.,
OF BARCLAY, PA.

THE patient, Mrs. S. J., was thirty-nine years old and born in Ireland. Her previous pregnancies were normal and the labors moderately easy.

When first seen by the writer she had been in labor twelve hours, under the care of her mother and a friend. Her pains were short and frequent and caused much suffering, "but were not the right kind." The woman was enormously fat, the pendulous abdomen almost resting upon the thighs when in the sitting position. Thus far during the labor she had been either sitting, leaning forward in a chair, or kneeling by the bedside to increase the pains.

External examination showed an umbilical hernia, the capacity of the sac probably being about one quart. The abdominal walls were lax and contained a large amount of subcutaneous fat. The uterus was anteverted to such a degree that with the woman erect its axis was approximately horizontal and with the fundus directed obliquely to the right. When upon her back this obliquity was increased. The vagina was unusually capacious and relaxed, especially in the upper portion. The pelvis was wide and roomy. Two fingers in the vagina were just able to reach the presenting part of the child. The cervix was dilated to about the size of a silver dollar and its margin was rather thick, fleshy, and soft. The membranes had ruptured and the head, with the encircling cervix, was resting on the pubic bone. Nearly one-half the area of the presenting part was inaccessible to the exploring fingers, and was in front of and above the pubes. The position, not positively determined, was probably left occipito-anterior.

After endeavoring to replace the womb in its proper position, with somewhat doubtful success, owing to the thickness of the abdominal walls, and directing the woman to remain upon her back, I was called from the room and detained about fifteen minutes. On my return I found the patient on her knees again by the side of the bed. I insisted on her immediate return to bed; objecting to this, as she said her pains were getting stronger since she arose, she unwillingly and clumsily climbed upon the bed, and while upon her hands and knees was seized with a severe pain, almost immediately followed by a second of still greater severity and longer duration. During the latter part of this pain she assumed a position on her knees and elbows, with her face buried in the pillow—in fact, almost the knee-chest position. The pain suddenly ceased with the sensation of "something giving way," but there were no evidences of shock or anything to indicate what had actually occurred.

During the preparation for another vaginal examination she had continuous, slight, colicky pain about the umbilicus, with one or two, not severe, uterine pains. With two fingers in the vagina the os could not be reached. Passing in the entire hand the uterus was found well contracted and entirely empty, as after the completion of an ordinary labor. The aperture of the os was transverse with a shallow notch on the right side. Passing behind the cervix the finger-tips came in contact with the smooth peritoneal covering of the sacral prominence. There was a large rent in the vagina passing posteriorly half-way to the vulva, and anteriorly to the cervico-vaginal junction and gaping widely at the sides. The rent gave the impression that the tissues had parted transversely across the vaginal vault and then longitudinally in or near the median line toward the vulva. The rectum was empty. Baring the arm to the shoulder the hand was passed behind the uterus into the abdominal cavity. The intestines were flaccid with little or no distention. The feet of the child were found beneath the spleen, the head lying in the left inguinal region, in front of and facing the left uterine appendages. The feet were brought down by traction and the head elevated by external manipulation, and delivery by the feet was accomplished with little difficulty. The child—dead, of course—weighed twelve pounds. The cord was cut and followed into the abdominal cavity up to the fundus and over and in front of the uterus. The placenta was beyond the reach of the hand and where the head of the child had been, from whence it was lifted by means of the cord and remove through the vagina.

The vagina was irrigated with a 1-to-40 carbolic solution. A long tube was inserted into the peritoneal cavity, and a stream of boiled water passed through it. No clots were found, and the amount of blood lost was trifling—probably not more than two ounces. Antiseptic precautions were used as far as possible before and after delivery, the surroundings and attendance being such as to render them for the most part futile.

It should be stated that there was no other physician nearer than seven miles, and that the case occurred on a cold winter night. Hence, I delivered the woman without professional counsel. Dr. Ladd, of Towanda, saw the patient in consultation twelve hours after delivery, and by digital examination found the condition of the vagina, etc., as stated above. After delivery the temperature gradually rose, reaching 102° on the second day, but in the next twenty-four hours falling to nearly normal, where it remained. The pulse (100 one hour after delivery) never regained its normal rate or character, and progressively lost force and volume until the seventh day, when the patient began to have "fainting spells," or "weak spells," in one of which on the tenth day after delivery she died. These attacks were probably cardiac dyspnœa, and death was doubtless due to heart-failure from afebrile sepsis.

During the extraction of the child the surface of the uterus, so far as accessible, seemed perfectly normal, the only uterine injury noted being the slight laceration or notch on the right side of the os. No force was used by the manipulating hand— an old laceration of the perineum, the relaxation of the soft parts, the size of the pelvis, and the extent of the vaginal laceration furnishing plenty of space. There was at no time prolapse of the intestines.

REMARKS.—The cause of the accident in this case depended on no one condition, but upon a combination of circumstances, the chief and immediate determining factor being the posture assumed at the time the child was expelled from the womb. The favoring conditions, more or less dependent upon one another, were the non-engagement of the head and its lodgement at the brim, uterine anteversion, looseness of uterine attachments, relaxation of the vaginal walls, pendulous abdomen, and gravity acting upon the uterus and its contents.

It might be here noted that the "functional lordosis," produced by obesity, must be a powerful factor in causing and maintaining anteversion of the pregnant uterus, and, as in this case, the projecting lumbar spine may have some influence in directing the whole organ forward, and lodging the head and cervix upon the pubic bone.

During the interval between the first examination and the patient's return to bed the stronger pains no doubt rapidly dilated and retracted the os, and gravity still further tilted the fundus anteriorly, producing by flexure over the pubic bone a narrowing of the antero-posterior vaginal diameter and longitudinal tension of the posterior vaginal wall. The head, fixed on the pubes, could not advance, and, as the os still further retracted, the tension and flexure became more pronounced. In labor, as the head passes from the os uteri, it may by flexion be directed to the pelvic inlet, and there engage, or if the flexion is antero-lateral it may pass around the brim to the iliac fossa. The resultant line of the expulsive and resistant forces falling within the circumference of the superior strait determines the first event in normal labor. In the present case this resultant was directed externally to the circumference, and this with the inclination of the fundus toward the right, directed the head toward the iliac plane, backward, outward, and to

the left, at the same time causing antero-lateral flexion of the head, and forcing it along the iliac plane toward the outer border. The head then burst through the inelastic friable walls of the vagina, when, free from resistance, aided by gravity, and impelled by the uterine forces, the child underwent spontaneous version, and slipped without hindrance into the peritoneal cavity. Or, it is not impossible that the vaginal wound was produced by the retraction of the cervix over the head, the head then passing into the iliac fossa, the shoulders emerging from the uterus, the anterior one being caught on the inner border of the pelvic brim, until at last, in the height of a pain, and when the woman dropped her head into the pillows, the uterus passed along the anterior abdominal wall toward the chest, released the shoulder, and was immediately emptied by the powerful pain. The sensation of something giving way undoubtedly occurred at the time the child passed into the peritoneal cavity. The afterbirth was probably expelled by one or two slight pains, which occurred during the resumption of the dorsal position. The positions of the child and placenta in the abdomen, as described, occurred while the patient was placing herself upon her back after the rupture.

This case has been reported at some length, for the reason that several of the writer's local professional friends seemed disposed to doubt the possibility of such an accident, and explained the case as one of rupture of the uterine neck and lower segment, extending to the vagina. The case occurred three years ago, in the second year of the writer's practice, and inasmuch as both previously and subsequently to this incident his obstetrical practice considerably exceeded that of the average general practitioner, he feels justified in believing his observations of the case correct, and in asserting that the above is not only a possible but a probable mechanism in such cases. Moreover, medical literature affords indubitable evidence that rupture of the vagina, with escape of the fœtus into the abdomen, has occurred in labor at full term.

It might be added that this case is analogous to rupture of the uterus as usually occurring, substituting the dilated os for the contraction-ring, and the upper portion of the vagina for the thinned and stretching lower segment. The various obstacles which cause a uterine tear are here represented mainly by the impingement of the head upon the brim.

The New York Polyclinic.—The curators of the New York Polyclinic announce that hereafter they will refuse to matriculate all persons who have not been graduated by some recognized medical college, or who have not obtained a legal permit to practise medicine, after two full years at such college.

INFANTILE VULVAR HÆMORRHAGE.[1]

BY THOMAS E. MC ARDLE, A.M., M.D.,
OF WASHINGTON, D. C.

IN the present report it is my purpose to place on record two cases of infantile vulvar hæmorrhage. Comparatively few cases are mentioned in general or special medical literature, and the text-books are almost completely silent upon the subject. I would have been surprised, not to say alarmed, when my attention was called to my first patient, if the subject had not been made familiar to me by a recent case in the practice of a medical friend.

Each of the few medical writers who have reported cases has offered a different theory of the cause. I have no theory at all to advance, and have only to say in regard to some of the explanations of this phenomenon that hæmorrhage from the infantile male genitalia would be as frequent as from the female if the theories were correct. We know, however, that rare as the phenomenon is in the female, it is much less frequent in the male infant.

CASE I.—On September 25, 1889, at 2 o'clock in the morning, I delivered Mrs. T. of her fifth baby, a girl. At my visit on the morning of September 30th, the nurse informed me that the infant had passed blood with every movement of the bowels since the preceding morning, and I was shown five napkins which were considerably stained with blood. I immediately examined the child and discovered that the hæmorrhage came from the vagina, and not from the bowels. At the time of the examination there was about a half-teaspoonful of blood in the vagina and between the labia. This blood was bright-red, and the napkin was stained by it, showing that the flow was continuous. The anus was perfectly clean and healthy.

Borated absorbent cotton was ordered to be used and perfect cleanliness enjoined. At the end of the fourth day the hæmorrhage ceased, and the child has since continued perfectly well.

CASE II.—On April 10, 1890, I delivered Mrs. C. T. of her first child, a girl. The labor was tedious, but in other respects normal. Five days later, at the morning bath, blood was discovered coming from the vagina of the infant. The same treatment was adopted as in the preceding case, and in four days the hæmorrhage ceased.

It will be observed that in each infant the hæmorrhage occurred on the fifth day after birth, lasted four days, and did not return.

The blood came from beyond the hymen and trickled between the labia. Whether it came from the vagina or uterus I am, of course, unable to state with any degree of accuracy, but it is my opinion that it came from the uterus. There was no malformation discoverable in either case. Both are

bright and happy babies, perfectly well nourished, and have passed through their first summer without any difficulty.

707 TWELFTH STREET, N. W.

MEDICAL PROGRESS.

Intubation of the Larynx in Croup.—D'HEILLY (*Archiv f. Kinderheilkunde*) reports thirteen cases of intubation for croup, the symptoms being such as usually require tracheotomy, namely, persistent dyspnœa, recession of the epigastrium, and commencing asphyxia. The youngest child was nineteen months old, the oldest four years. Two of the children were too near death to be benefited by any treatment; of the remaining eleven, only two were saved. In spite of this high mortality the author formed a favorable opinion as to the value of the procedure. It involves no loss of blood and no wound, it can be carried out easily, and serious and unexpected accidents are not likely to occur. An unsuccessful intubation can be repeated, and, if continually unsuccessful, tracheotomy can be performed. Neither shock nor rise of temperature attends the operation, and the air is not cold when it reaches the lung as it is when inspired through a tracheotomy tube.

On the other hand, the tube is frequently obstructed by false membrane, when it must be quickly removed and as quickly reintroduced. American authors recommend that the patient be allowed to cough the tube out, but this was never observed in d'Heilly's cases. Another objection to intubation is the difficulty of swallowing that it produces, which of necessity interferes with nutrition. Especially is this difficulty experienced in the administration of liquid food, which may be inspired and cause pulmonary disease. Feeding through the nose by means of a catheter may obviate this difficulty, but is attended with others.

The author thus summarizes the conditions in which the method may be used:

1. In very young children in whom tracheotomy offers only slight chances of recovery, and in whom even a slight loss of blood would be harmful.

2. In mild cases of croup which seem likely to continue as such and for which tracheotomy is a severe remedy.

3. In very severe cases of toxic diphtheria in which the patient is already much weakened.

4. In cases of croup following measles, in which tracheotomy is never successful. Intubation in such cases offers a slight chance of success.

5. In all cases in which tracheotomy is impossible or dangerous.—*Archives of Pædiatrics*, October, 1890.

Treatment of Profuse Menstruation.—The following prescription for the treatment of profuse menstruation is quoted by the *Southern Practitioner:*

℞.—Dialyzed ergot	.	.	10 drachms.
Glycerin	.	.	5 "
Salicylic acid	.	.	30 grains.
Distilled water	.	.	2½ ounces.—M.

One teaspoonful of this should be diluted with three teaspoonfuls of water, and injected into the rectum once daily.

---

[1] Read before the American Association of Obstetricians and Gynecologists, September, 1890.

The Treatment of Alopecia Areata.—This malady, which is probably due to the presence of the parasite, microsporon Audouini, is treated in the following manner by QUINQUAND :

The general treatment consists in the employment of cod-liver oil for three or four weeks, and after this the administration of from 5 to 6 drops of Fowler's solution daily. The local treatment consists in washing the parts thoroughly with soap, and immediately after applying to the affected surface the following mercurial solution:

R.—Biniodide of mercury . . 3 grains.
Bichloride of mercury . . 15 "
Alcohol . . . . 1½ ounces.
Water . . . . . 8 ounces.—M.

Following this, friction is to be made with the following liniment:

R.—Balsam of Fioravent } of each 4 ounces.
Camphorated spirit }
Tincture of nux vomica . 1½ drachms.—M.

Mixture for the Treatment of Myringitis.—

R.—Crystallized acetate of lead . 1½ grain.
Tincture of opium . . 20 drops.
Distilled water . . . 10 ounces.—M.

Make into a solution, and three times a day drop 10 minims into the ear. If this produces a considerable exudate in any portion of the tympanic membrane, it should be followed three times a day by 5 drops of pure glycerin, and syringing with warm water.

Multiple Abscesses in Nursing-infants.— According to COUDER, Bouchut was the first to make a study of this disease, and he believed it to be due either to conditions of the puerperal state, to syphilis, or to scrofula. Syphilitic abscesses should be regarded as merely softened gummata, and scrofulous abscesses are usually of tubercular origin. Couder cannot believe that all other cases are attributable to the puerperal state, and considers that there are others of unknown origin. Among the latter cases should be included those in which the mothers of the patients suffer from inflammation of the milk-ducts, pus being withdrawn by the infant in the act of nursing. Such cases may be considered instances of benign purulent infection, and the condition is an indication for withholding the breast from the child.

Abscess may also occur through infection of the umbilicus, hence in all cases the infant's umbilicus as well as the mother's breasts should be treated antiseptically.— *Archives of Pædiatrics,* October, 1890.

Antisepsis in Obstetric Practice.—In the Section of Obstetrics of the recent International Congress, a paper by DR. GALABIN, upon the use of antiseptics in midwifery was read. The excellent results of antisepsis in obstetric practice are ascribed by this author chiefly to the use of corrosive sublimate as a disinfectant for the hands, and for the purpose of irrigating the vagina both before and after labor. The rate of mortality in English maternities since the introduction of corrosive sublimate has fallen from 10 per 1000, to 2 per 1000. In the London General Maternity the patients are confined on horsehair mattresses that are disinfected if the case should become septic. For vaginal irrigation a 1-to-2000 sublimate so-

lution is used for two or three days, and after that a weaker solution. Before an examination, the hands are disinfected with a 1-to-1000 sublimate solution and lubricated with a 1-to-1000 solution of sublimate in glycerin. In normal cases in private practice he thinks a single injection of 1-to-2000 sublimate solution sufficient.

SLAWJANSKI, of St. Petersburg, said that in Russian maternities antisepsis is universally employed and has reduced maternal mortality to 0.28 per cent., and that if the method is properly carried out the presence of students has no effect upon the mortality.

PRIESTLY, of London, ascribed the good results of antisepsis in obstetric practice less to the antiseptics used than to the extreme cleanliness. He believed that sublimate solutions as weak as even 1-to-4000 could produce harmful effects.—*American Journal of Obstetrics,* September 1890.

Curetting the Uterus for Endometritis.—The operation of curetting the uterus for endometritis has been performed by BOUILLY seventy-five times since 1887. The procedure is particularly adapted to cases which are uncomplicated by polypi or myomata, and it may also be used in cases in which there is a certain amount of disease of the uterine adnexa. The principal indications for the operation are hæmorrhage, leucorrhœa, and pelvic and sacral pain before or during menstruation. Pain alone is not, however, a sufficient indication. In twelve of Bouilly's cases the operation was done without an anæsthetic, but such a plan is not usually advisable. Dilatation by means of laminaria tents should precede the operation for forty-eight hours. Before curetting, the vagina should be irrigated and the uterus drawn downward. If the endometritis is purulent the operation should be followed by an intra-uterine application of tincture of iodine or of carbolized glycerin ; if it is hæmorrhagic, chloride of zinc should be used. For a few days subsequently the vagina should be kept tamponed with some antiseptic material.

No accidents followed any of the author's operations, and in many of the cases the pain ceased at once or soon after. If there is extensive tubal disease no benefit can be expected from the operation.—*Annals of Gynecology and Pædiatry,* September, 1890.

Prophylaxis of Acute Rheumatism.—HIRSCH (*Centralblatt für klinische Medicin,* September 13, 1890) believes that to prevent recurrences of acute rheumatism it is frequently necessary for the patient to change his residence. It has been observed that the disease is especially likely to occur in certain houses or groups of houses, a fact that is strongly suggestive of the specific nature of the disease.

Injections for the Relief of Labor-pains.—In the *Revue Général de Clinique et de Thérapeutique,* September 3, 1890, the following prescription is given for this purpose, it having given satisfaction in the hands of BOUSQUET, of Marseilles:

R.—Antipyrin . . . 75 grains.
Hydrochlorate of cocaine 1½ "
Distilled water . . 5 drachms.

This is to be injected into the vagina in the earlier stages of labor.

THE MEDICAL NEWS.

A WEEKLY JOURNAL
OF MEDICAL SCIENCE.

COMMUNICATIONS are invited from all parts of the world. Original articles contributed exclusively to THE MEDICAL NEWS will be liberally paid for upon publication. When necessary to elucidate the text, illustrations will be furnished without cost to the author.

Address the Editor: H. A. HARE, M.D.,
1004 WALNUT STREET,
PHILADELPHIA.

Subscription Price, including Postage.

PER ANNUM, IN ADVANCE . . . . $4.00.
SINGLE COPIES . . . .   10 CENTS.

Subscriptions may begin at any date. The safest mode of remittance is by bank check or postal money order, drawn to the order of the undersigned. When neither is accessible, remittances may be made, at the risk of the publishers, by forwarding in *registered* letters.

Address,   LEA BROTHERS & CO.,
NOS. 706 & 708 SANSOM STREET,
PHILADELPHIA.

SATURDAY, OCTOBER 18, 1890.

TETANUS.

EXCLUDING the older ideas of tetanus, those of the existence of a condition of toxæmia or of an organic nervous derangement, the first valuable suggestion as to the real nature of the disease was published by Carle and Rattone in 1884. In this instance a patient, becoming affected with tetanus from a small acne-pustule, died in the hospital of St. Maurice, in Turin, three days after the inception of the disease. Two hours after his death, the experimenters removed under antiseptic precautions the pustule with the inflammatory zone about it, and suspended it in sterilized water. This solution they injected into the cellular tissue about the sciatic nerve in rabbits, and failed to produce the symptoms of the disease in only one out of twenty-four instances. The blood from the same individual injected into other rabbits did not transmit the disease; and the rabbits in control-experiments, inoculated with septic materials from other cases, presented no tetaniform phenomena.

In the same year Nicoläier published the results of a series of experiments which aroused considerable interest in the scientific world. In the course of a number of experiments of another nature this investigator succeeded in obtaining an experimental form of tetanus; and after a long series of further experiments, advanced the theory of its infectious nature, and described a specific microörganism—a bacillus.

Retaining in view the fact that an infectious disease should, under favoring circumstances, present an endemic and epidemic character, and the capability of transmission from one organism to another, MM. VERHOOGEN and BAERT have recently published an article upon the nature and etiology of tetanus, addressed to the Royal Society of the Medical and Natural Sciences of Brussels. These authors cite the well-known endemic character of the disease in our Southern States, Cuba, Ceylon, a number of the Pacific islands, and in other localities, and quote a large number of circumstances that suggest the occasional epidemicity of the affection as met in man and some of the lower animals. Among a number of clinical and experimental occurrences suggesting the probability of the transmissibility of the malady, and the likelihood of the agent of transmission existing in unclean instruments, Thiriar's experience is narrated. This operator was unfortunate enough to lose ten cases of major operations by tetanus before he determined the seat of the infection to exist in his hæmostatic forceps, the thorough sterilization of which by a high temperature was happily followed by a complete cessation of the undesirable sequences.

The coincidence of tetanus with such infectious diseases as scarlet fever, erysipelas, pneumonia, or malaria, is suggestive of its similar character.

The general course of the disease; the indefinite symptoms preceding its outburst and covering the probable period of incubation; the elevation of temperature; the occurrence of epistaxis; the existence in many cases of a cutaneous eruption resembling that of erysipelas; the nephritic symptoms and renal changes; and the enlargement of the spleen, are all characteristics of the usual course of an infectious disease.

To prove the specific nature of a malady, two series of conditions must be established: first, that the infectious agent be found in the affected organism, that its presence alone, introduced either directly or after previous cultivation, gives rise to the disease and to no other form of infection, and that no other morbific agent may induce the same result; second, that in whatever different forms the disease may present itself, these differences must constitute but secondary phases, and there must always exist a simple and unique type.

Several investigators have claimed as specific to tetanus the germs of their own discovery; but it seems probable that the bacillus first described by Nicoläier should be regarded as best fulfilling the required *rôle*. This bacterium measures three micro-millimetres in length and one in diameter, presents a terminal elliptical spore, is anaërobic, and, under certain circumstances of growth and temperature, possesses rotary motility.

In connection with this subject of the specific cause of the disease should be mentioned the occurrence in the tissues and fluids of the bodies of those dead from tetanus and in the cultures of Nicoläier's bacillus of several forms of toxines, isolated and described by Brieger under the names of tetanine, tetanotoxine, and spasmotoxine, alkaloids having the power to induce tetaniform symptoms when injected in animals. Such a discovery associated with the inability to obtain cultures of the bacillus from parts of the body other than the immediate vicinity of the infected wound, make it probable that the action of the germ is entirely local so far as its life-functions are concerned, although by the elaboration of these alkaloids its further influence is the general one seen in the phenomena of the affection. Such a conclusion is, perhaps, as yet unwarranted, since the absolute proof of the specificity of Nicoläier's germ is thus far wanting. That it exists in various tetanogenous substances, as the pus of the tetanic focus, and in virulent dust, is amply proved; although, on account of its anaërobic character and other special properties of growth, it is somewhat difficult to obtain in a state of purity. Obtained in such condition, it is a matter of fact, proved by a number of successful inoculations, that it possesses the power of producing the disease.

This same power is, however, claimed for several other microörganisms, although no absolute proof in these latter instances has entirely excluded the presence of Nicoläier's germ from the microbes experimented with, and there are on record numerous inoculations with Nicoläier's bacillus that failed to produce the disease. That such failures should exist, is not, however, unexpected. The complex conditions of growth, and the exclusion of air from the focus of inoculation, necessarily render a large proportion of the attempts unsuccessful. Intravascular inoculations would be apt to fail from the free access of oxygen in the blood, and the consequent destruction of the germs; free hæmorrhage from

the point of inoculation would likewise tend to prevent success, and the failure to exclude the air by the rapid formation of lymph about the focus could be expected to lead to no results.

The frequent association in one focus of pus-forming bacteria with the bacillus of tetanus adds another confirmatory suggestion to the present views of the history of this germ; the pyogenic forms demanding oxygen for their growth, and consuming the limited amount present, thus favoring the conditions for the best development of Nicoläier's germ and offering a convenient soil for its growth.

Granting the probability of a specific nature to the microörganism mentioned, and in view of its localized growth, and its production of tetanogenous alkaloids, what is the mechanism of its action in the production of tetanus? As the sites for its best development, large, open, suppurating or hæmorrhagic sores could not be regarded as affording the proper conditions; but small, quickly-scabbing wounds, or deep, slightly-suppurating punctures, or abscesses almost healed, offer the exclusion of air and the further requisites for its fullest activities. During the period intervening between the time of inoculation and the manifestation of the characteristic phenomena, there probably occurs a gradual increase in the numbers of the microörganisms, and there is elaborated a slowly increasing amount of the special alkaloids described. At first, through the eliminative action of the skin and kidneys, these toxic principles are expelled from the body as rapidly as formed; but with their constant increase, favored perhaps by a temporary failure of these organs of elimination, they finally accumulate sufficiently to render their influences manifest, particularly upon the nervous system. Confirmatory of such a view are the successful attempts in the treatment of tetanus by certain French physicians by the administration of sudorific doses of pilocarpine. The usual treatment of the spasms of tetanus, too, are clearly based upon the idea of the presence in the organism of substances exciting reflex motor spasms, chloral tending to diminish the recognition of afferent impulses and the bromides to decrease the force of the motor explosion following.

PAROXYSMAL HÆMOGLOBINURIA.

ONE of the most interesting conditions with which clinical medicine has to deal and to which it has paid particular attention during the last few years, is paroxysmal hæmoglobinuria, either when dependent upon malarial poison or when due to other causes not so clearly defined; and though the studies of Saundby, Murri, Barlow, and others have all tended to throw light upon this question a number of interesting experiments recently published by Dr. S. Monckton Copeman, in the London *Practitioner* for September, 1890, seem to afford conclusive evidence as to some of the causes of its occurrence.

In these studies Copeman found, by a series of careful researches, that exposure to cold in persons susceptible to this condition readily produced hæmoglobinuria, and in this he is interestingly in accord with Johnson, Mahomed, and Ralfe, who have all shown that cold will produce temporary albuminuria.

As the result of his studies Copeman concludes that the essential pathology of paroxysmal hæmoglobinuria appears to consist in the ready breaking-down of corpuscles of lessened resistance under the influence of cold, and the after-appearance in the urine of the products of such destruction; this ready breaking-down of corpuscles being apparently the final result of an imperfect power of production in the blood-forming organs, caused in turn by the baneful influence of syphilis, or possibly malaria or gout.

The details of Copeman's work are very interesting, and anyone interested in this rather uncommon ailment should certainly read his paper.

REVIEWS.

A MANUAL OF MODERN SURGERY FOR THE USE OF STUDENTS AND PRACTITIONERS. By JOHN B. ROBERTS, A.M., M.D. Illustrated. Philadelphia: Lea Brothers & Co., 1890.

THIS book of eight hundred pages may be said to represent in a very thorough manner and in a comparatively small space the status of the surgery of the day without presenting to its readers such advanced thoughts as to engender uncertainty in its assertions; and yet all the opinions expressed are sufficiently progressive to make the purchaser feel that in following the advice given he is doing all that the most carefully-trained surgeon could do for his patient. The illustrations, which are very frequently scattered through the entire volume, are, like the text, up to date and unusually well executed. The chapter upon "Injuries to the Nervous Centres" is, we think, a very good one. We notice with interest that in an article upon tetanus, Dr. Roberts makes the somewhat guarded statement that this disease is occasionally contagious, evidently not believing that every case is capable of influencing other cases near it.

At the same time the author very properly states that the weight of professional evidence points to the disease being due to a microörganism.

The chapter upon "Diseases of the Abdomen and Pelvis" is very thorough, and notwithstanding the rapid advances made in this portion of surgery is well up to date.

If intrinsic value is the chief factor in making a book sell rapidly, Dr. Roberts's book cannot fail to be a great success.

A TEXT-BOOK OF COMPARATIVE PHYSIOLOGY, FOR STUDENTS AND PRACTITIONERS OF VETERINARY MEDICINE. By WESLEY MILLS, M.A., M.D., D.V.S. Illustrated. New York: D. Appleton & Co., 1890.

PROBABLY no more enthusiastic searcher in the field of comparative physiology can be found in the English-speaking race than Dr. Mills, who, in addition to his laborious researches upon this subject, has within the year past placed before the profession of medicine and veterinary medicine two volumes which are of very great value, and which show that we have on this side of the Atlantic a rapidly-increasing appreciation of the usefulness of a thorough grounding in studies concerning animal life, by those who intend to devote their lives to medicine.

Dr. Mills has, we think, discovered a popular need in the present book, for it is one which medical students, as well as veterinary students, would do well to purchase, and we hope that it will become as widely used as it deserves to be.

The illustrations are unusually well selected and appropriate, presenting to the eye views which impress upon the mind the statements of the text.

SOCIETY PROCEEDINGS.

PHILADELPHIA COUNTY MEDICAL SOCIETY.

THE VICE-PRESIDENT, JOHN B. ROBERTS, M.D., IN THE CHAIR.

Stated Meeting, September 24, 1890.

DR. JOSEPH P. TUNIS read a paper on

RIB-FRACTURE FROM MUSCULAR ACTION,

in which he reported two recent cases and gave a complete review of the literature of the subject. Although some surgeons have denied the possibility of fracture of a rib from muscular action, most admit that it does occur. Of the one hundred and thirty-three cases collected by Gurlt, the majority had some condition present which rendered the ribs easily broken. Any condition which lowers the normal resistance of the bone-structure, such as osteomalacia, rickets, cancer, syphilis, scrofula, advanced age, or atrophy from continuous confinement, etc., must predispose to fracture. "In short, all diseases dependent upon cachexia more or less predispose to the occurrence of fracture," says Hamilton. When some such cause is present the existence of a fracture from muscular action can be readily accounted for. There are, however, numerous cases on record in which such accidents have occurred in healthy individuals, the determining cause of fracture being muscular action, and the mechanism varying with the anatomy of the affected bone. If these conditions are true for other bones, why may they not be equally true for the ribs?

The ribs offer three factors favorable to fracture: First, their shape; second, their position—firmly attached at the vertebral, and more or less free to move at the sternal end; and third, the powerful muscles attached to their bodies. They are "elastic arches," it is true, and capable of considerable movement; but their elasticity has its limit, and their movements are dependent upon the muscles attached to them. Of these muscles the diaphragm seems to be the most favorably situated to produce rib-fracture. Centrally attached by its crura and ligaments to the vertebral column, it is connected at its circumference "on either side, to the inner surface of the cartilages and bony portions of the six or seven inferior ribs interdigitating with the transversalis." Take, for example, the ninth rib. If the diaphragm should contract, it would draw the anterior third of this bone toward the vertebral column, the other two-thirds being held more or less firmly *in situ* by the serratus magnus, attached posteriorly, the internal oblique, the transversalis, and the intercostals. This contraction of the diaphragm continuing, if sufficiently powerful, would fracture the bone like a bent bow at the point of least resistance. Has the diaphragm sufficient force to accomplish this? It has sufficient force to free the throat or bronchi from irritating material; almost approximates the sternum and the vertebral column in dyspnœa, and often demonstrates this power in membranous croup. It can forcibly eject the contents of the stomach, or cause great distress, and even death, from obstinate hiccough. Well supplied with blood, exercised day and night, we may with some reason believe that, suddenly exerting all its force on three or four ribs, one or more may fracture. Certain it is that the ribs to which the diaphragm is attached are those most frequently fractured.

Above the sixth rib other muscles enter into the mechanism of fracture. In the case which Dr. C. B. Nancrede has reported, and in Dr. Bird's case, where the second rib yielded under unusual muscular strain, the pectoralis minor seems to have been the most probable determining cause, as this muscle is attached to the third, fourth, and fifth ribs, often the second, and is inserted into the coracoid process of the scapula. If the scapula were firmly held in place by the powerful muscles attached to it, the pectoralis minor would be in a position to act with the advantage of leverage. This muscle, or the serratus magnus, would draw the anterior third of the bone away from the vertebral column, directly opposite to the movement of the lower ribs under the action of the diaphragm. Thus, the mechanism of a large number of the cases may be explained.

The first case reported by Dr. Tunis was that of a woman, in whom inherited syphilis was suspected, who fractured a rib by a violent paroxysm of coughing.

The second case was observed by Dr. Edward Martin. The patient while lifting a very heavy stone heard a distinct crack and felt an acute, knife-like pain in the left side. On examination the sixth rib was found broken at its sternal end.

Dr. Tunis then briefly described all the cases that have been reported, and concluded with the following deductions:

1. Forty cases having been reported, we may reasonably expect to hear of others, and perhaps to see them ourselves.

2. Of these accidents, more than one-fourth have occurred in individuals of apparently sound constitutions.

3. The left side is most often affected, and either the middle or anterior third of the rib is the usual position of the fracture. Of forty-nine fractures, only five have occurred above the sixth rib. The great majority have been among the lower six (omitting the twelfth).

4. The exciting causes have been: Coughing, muscular effort, sneezing, and vomiting. The determining cause has been the action of the muscles, unless thirty-four observers have been deceived by the testimony of patients who could gain nothing by such deceptions.

5. Herard reports the youngest example of this accident—a woman, twenty-two years old. Its non-occurrence at a younger age is probably due to the great elasticity of the ribs in youth.

6. Of these forty cases, two died of some intercurrent affection. The remaining thirty-eight made a complete recovery in the usual time.

7. More men have suffered than women, and the average age has been forty-eight years.

Dr. Tunis considers that the difficulty and the doubts which have attended the diagnosis of many of these cases ought to disappear, as more examples of this accident are reported. Already, by the consent of the majority of surgeons, and by the evidence of accumulated cases, the possibility of rib-fracture from muscular action, even in persons of sound constitution, seems sufficiently proven.

DR. JOSEPH PRICE then read a paper entitled

CERTAIN CAUSES OF MAJOR PELVIC TROUBLES, TRACEABLE TO MINOR GYNECOLOGY.

Dr. Price said that the popular cry for "conservatism" and preliminary treatment of cases requiring operation is not a scientific plea, but in most instances a *personal bid* for indulgence by those who try to accomplish something, without acknowledging on the one hand that there is little or nothing to encourage them in their work, so far as results are concerned; and on the other, that there is abundant proof that manifold and really major surgical affections arise merely from treatment recognized as orthodox from the standpoint of minor gynecology. Dr. Price said that he did not hesitate to put minor gynecology in a causal relation with a vast amount of the necessary major pelvic surgery.

First among these causes may be mentioned the Emmet cervical operation. Like many other surgical operations, this, when first described by its distinguished originator, was done by every surgeon, without the least consideration of its contra-indications. Very many minor tears of the cervix, in which only a cosmetic effect is obtained by operation, are made distinctly worse by operative interference. In many cases the pain becomes insufferable, from the lighting up of a dormant or unrecognized pelvic trouble, and an operation is required to undo the mischief of an unnecessary cervical closure. This fact has been recognized by Emmet himself, and he has counselled the careful selection of cases in order to escape these disastrous results. Where there is preëxisting pelvic disease, even though slight, no cervical operation should be attempted unless absolutely required by the condition of the patient.

Another operation which has met with much approval from some men, and which is apparently sometimes' successful, is the forcible dilatation of the cervix. It is clear that where there is antecedent inflammation of the pelvic viscera, that is of the genito-urinary system, such an operation as surgical dilatation of the cervix cannot be free from danger. In order to relieve dysmenorrhœa by this procedure, the condition must evidently be due to stenosis of the os or cervix. The question here arises, Can the cause of dysmenorrhœa be determined? Dr. Price thinks that in some cases it can, but that in many women in whom a stenosis would be expected, there is no difficulty whatever attending the menstrual flux. This being the case it is evident that a diagnosis cannot be made without a careful study of all the symptoms.

Again, in many women the causes of this condition are complex. It will not do to lose sight of this, and conclude that because a flexion exists dilatation will remedy menstrual pain. It is to be remembered that if there is coëxisting pelvic inflammation dilatation will increase it, and, under certain conditions, cause it if absent. Rapid dilatation of the cervix is a traumatism, and is attended with all the dangers of septic absorption as is any other violent procedure, and where traumatism incident to natural causes is confessed to be the cause of so much subsequent mischief, it should not be *expected that operative injury can be harmless.*

This conclusion, reached inferentially, Dr. Price said, has been abundantly confirmed practically on the operating-table by much of his later pelvic work. In a number of cases with a history of preceding dilatation, the after-operation shows an exceedingly complicated and inflammatory condition. Some of the dilatations were done during preëxisting disease, which was made worse by the interference, while others were done on uncomplicated cases to relieve the dysmenorrhœa, and resulted in the establishment of a disease in which operation was necessary to save life.

Judged simply by its remoter effects, the operation of rapid dilatation is a dangerous one, and results oftener in subsequent harm than in lasting good. The surgical injury to the cervix is, in many of these cases, more pronounced than the tears of the cervix which are closed by Emmet's operation.

Simple closure of lacerations of the cervix in cases of pelvic disorder, almost certainly exacerbate the symptoms. The necessary inflammatory action set up in the suture-tract is transferred along the lymphatic or venous channels to the seat of the earlier inflammation, until a pelvic peritonitis is kindled or rekindled, which at last entails abdominal section. The minor gynecologist, who has no regard for or appreciation of the relation of the commonly advocated general closure of perineal and cervical tears to major surgical complications, cannot but be a great factor in the causation of the same.

That the inconsiderate use of the uterine sound has been responsible for much inflammatory pelvic trouble is scarcely to be disputed. This is not because the sound is of itself a dangerous instrument, but because it is used by every tyro as an instrument of diagnosis. If used at all, it should be in the hands of those with whom its application, by reason of their skill, will be exceptional, and in the hands of the non-expert its use should be forbidden. The indiscriminate use of the sound and electrode is the most serious mechanical objection to the employment of electricity. Every sitting for the electrical treatment is prefaced by the use of the sound, and necessarily followed by the introduction of an electrode of some form. This is by a class of men who, usually, have had no previous gynecological training or education whatever. In such hands such methods can only be harmful, and we are now reaping the fruits of their work in a class of pelvic operations not surpassed in the complications presented. In the same category with the sound may be placed the curette. Dilatation, with curetting of the uterus, have been the cause of a long series of major operations.

Another class of cases coming under this head are those in which many intra-uterine applications have been made with such agents as nitric acid, chromic acid, and nitrate of silver. For a woman to have undergone a routine treatment with these caustics, and to have escaped pelvic inflammatory trouble, is little short of a miracle.

Dr. E. E. MONTGOMERY, in discussion, fully agreed with what Dr. Price had said with regard to the frequency of troubles necessitating major operations which result from the various methods of procedure in minor gynecology.

The practice of performing Emmet's operation at once upon cases in which a slight laceration is found has justly led to its discredit, although the operation is undoubtedly of great benefit in properly-selected cases. No case in which the presence of inflammatory conditions has not been eliminated or cured by proper methods is suitable for the operation.

Dr. JOHN C. DA COSTA thought that Dr. Price was not quite right in attributing the major pelvic troubles to gynecological treatment, for, in most cases, we may infer that the pelvic trouble already existed, and the practitioner made a mistake in treating the uterus rather than the uterine appendages. In regard to Emmet's operation, Dr. Da Costa said that it was often carelessly done on improper cases and without previously preparing the patient.

The uterine dilator he considers a very valuable instrument, but one that must be used with great care.

Dr. JOSEPH HOFFMAN referred to a case in which the uterus was perforated by a curette as an illustration of the dangers of the operation.

Dr. WILLIAM E. ASHTON said that if we have the pelvis perfectly free from disease, and if the uterus is strongly anteflexed and perfectly movable, and upon the introduction of the sound we find that there is a point of intense pain at the internal os, we shall find in a certain proportion of cases that good results are obtained from dilatation.

Dr. J. M. BALDY said that he was recently called to operate on the cervix in two cases in which he had been informed that the lacerations were very bad and that the women were suffering much. On examination, the tears proved to be comparatively slight, and needed no interference. There are some cases in which a cervix operation at first sight appears justifiable. These are cases in which the cervix is torn to the vaginal vault; but even if the cervix be torn on both sides to the vaginal vault, if there is not eversion and erosion, or much scar-tissue, there is no reason for operation.

Dr. C. P. Noble said that he was glad that the matter of the uterine sound had been brought up, be-cause he was convinced, as the result of his experience, that the less the uterine sound is used the better for the patient. In most cases but little information is gained. Recently a case passed through his hands in which pregnancy was suspected. The patient afterward fell into other hands, the sound was passed three inches and the patient was supposed not to be pregnant; but sub-sequent events showed that she was seven months preg-nant.

NEWS ITEMS.

The State Board of Medical Examiners of New Jersey.—The following questions were presented to the candidates who appeared before the first meeting of the State Board of Medical Examiners in Trenton, on October 9 and 10, 1890.

It is proper to state that two hours were allowed for replying to each set of questions, and that a general average of 75 per cent. was required to obtain the license:

Section I. Materia Medica and Therapeutics. (Regular.) Dr. Newell.

1. What is glycerin?
2. Name three antiseptics.
3. Write a prescription for acute diarrhœa in a child ten years old.
4. Name two cardiac stimulants and their doses.
5. Name two cardiac sedatives and their doses.
6. What is an emmenagogue?
7. What is iodine?
8. Name three cathartics.
9. Name three laxatives.
10. Write a prescription containing a salt of bismuth.

Section I. Materia Medica and Therapeutics. (Homœopathic.) Dr. Worthington.

1. Explain the theory of " Similia similibus curantur."
2. Give mental symptoms of pulsatilla.
3. Differentiate the skin symptoms of apis mellifica and rhus tox.
4. Give the antidote to ignatia amara.
5. What are the urinary symptoms of lycopodium?
6. Describe the characteristic cough of spongia tosta.
7. Differentiate the throat symptoms of mercurous iodatus rubrum and crotalus.
8. Give the heart symptoms of glonoinum.
9. What are the laryngeal symptoms of kali bichro-micum?
10. Give abdominal symptoms of baptistia tinctora.

Section II. Obstetrics and Gynecology. Dr. Brown.

1. Give signs of pregnancy, stating the period at which each appears.
2. Give treatment of placenta prævia.

3. Give diagnosis between ascites and pregnancy at the seventh month.
4. Give treatment of post-partum hæmorrhage.
5. What is the difference between accidental and un-avoidable hæmorrhage?
6. What are the indications for craniotomy?
7. Give causes of delay in labor.
8. Give differential diagnosis between ovarian tumor and retroflexion of the uterus.
9. Give causes, symptoms, and treatment of pruritus vulvæ.
10. Give causes, symptoms, and treatment of dysmen-orrhœa.

Section III. Practice of Medicine. Dr. Watson.

1. How would you make a physical examination of the thorax?
2. How often, what and how much, would you feed a four months' old bottle-fed infant, in twenty-four hours?
3. Give the complications of pertussis.
4. Give the complications and sequelæ of scarlatina.
5. Give the complications and sequelæ of typhoid fever.
6. Describe a case of cirrhosis of the liver.
7. Give the differential diagnosis between hæmoptysis and hæmatemesis.
8. Give the differential diagnosis between empyæma and pleurisy with effusion.
9. Describe a case of acute meningitis in the adult.
10. Describe a case of acute Bright's disease in the adult.

Section IV. Surgery and Surgical Anatomy. Dr. Hendry.

1. Describe briefly how you would investigate a surgi-cal case, and by what method you would write a history of such a case.
2. Inflammation: (*a*) definition, (*b*) symptoms, (*c*) lo-cal effects, (*d*) constitutional effects, (*e*) What is an acute abscess? (*f*) How is pus formed?
3. State briefly your views with regard to the germ-theory of putrefaction as applied to antiseptic surgery.
4. Supposing that in a case of retention of urine from an enlarged prostate, you could not succeed in pass-ing the catheter by the natural passage, what pro-ceeding would you adopt?
5. State the diagnostic characters of carcinoma of the mamma. What are the circumstances which warrant extirpation?
6. State the diagnostic symptoms of the diseases and injuries of the hip-joint.
7. Describe the operation for tying the external iliac artery.

Section V. Anatomy. Dr. Uebelacker.

1. Describe the knee-joint.
2. What muscles are attached to the humerus?
3. Describe the diaphragm.
4. Describe the cæcum and its valve.
5. Describe the pulmonary artery.
6. Describe the pulmonary vein.
7. Describe the circle of Willis.

8. What are the valves of the heart and their functions?
9. Describe the kidneys.
10. Describe the great sciatic nerve.

SECTION VI. PHYSIOLOGY. DR. ATWELL.

1. What is the reaction of the gastric juice, and from what element is this reaction maintained?
2. Describe the mechanical action of the stomach in the process of digestion, and state what produces it.
3. What is the difference between a secretion and an excretion? Give types of each.
4. Describe the process of oxygenation of the blood, and where does it take place?
5. How does the pulse of a child at the age of one year compare with that of a man at the age of forty years?
6. Where are the distinct seats of motory and sensory properties in the spinal cord?
7. Describe the innervation of the heart.
8. What do you understand by the term reflex action? Give an example.
9. What are the reaction and specific gravity of normal urine, and what is the average quantity for an adult in twenty-four hours?
10. What fluids emptied into the alimentary tract have assigned to them the power of emulsifying and digesting fats?

SECTION VII. CHEMISTRY. DR. TIESLER.

1. Explain the three principal modes of fermentation: alcoholic, acetous, and lactic.
2. How many acids of phosphorus are known?
3. What constitutes a sulphide? A sulphite? A sulphate?
4. What do you understand by an element? A molecule? An atom?
5. What is phenol?
6. Name two oxides of hydrogen.
7. How do alkalies and alkaloids differ? Give an example of each.
8. How is nitric acid prepared?
9. What is the difference between calomel and corrosive sublimate?
10. Explain H_2O, H_2SO_4, CO, CO_2, Fe, As_2S_3.

SECTION VIII. HISTOLOGY, PATHOLOGY, AND DISEASES OF THE EYE AND EAR. DR. WAGONER.

1. Give the composition of the blood.
2. In what does human blood differ from that of the frog?
3. Describe the mucous membrane of the stomach.
4. Give the condition of the mucous membrane of the stomach in chronic inflammation thereof.
5. Give the condition of the lung in the second stage of acute lobar pneumonia.
6. What results from embolism of a cerebral artery?
7. Give the treatment of acute conjunctivitis.
8. What are the operations for cataract?
9. Give the prominent symptoms of acute catarrh of the middle ear.
10. What are the sequelæ of purulent inflammation of the middle ear?

SECTION IX. HYGIENE AND MEDICAL JURISPRUDENCE. DR. WORTHINGTON.

1. In the physical examination of water what points are to be noted?
2. Are disinfectants more efficacious in the sick-room when used in solution or fumigation?
3. Which is the most powerful disinfectant?
4. How is air vitiated by respiration?
5. In preparing a gallon of a 1-1000 solution of corrosive sublimate, what quantity of the drug is required?
6. In a case of suspected infanticide, what are the most important tests to determine whether the child was or was not born alive?
7. About how soon after death is complete rigor mortis found?
8. What diseases simulate poisoning by arsenic?
9. Differentiate idiocy and insanity.
10. Give all the causes of sudden death.

The Medical Examining Board of Tennessee.—The medical practice act of Tennessee, resembling that of New York, has gone into effect; and the State Board of Examiners, containing representatives of regular medicine, homœopathy, and the eclectics, has been appointed. The hydropaths were left out, and Dr. J. F. Woodward, of McMinnville, who is one of that school, has vented his indignation in a picturesque circular, taking the appointing powers to task for the omission.

Number of Medical Students in Philadelphia for the Session of 1890--91.—The following list of the number of medical students who have so far matriculated in Philadelphia regular schools up to date is of interest.

Medical Department University of Pennsylvania:

First year	220
Second year	186
Third "	165
Fourth "	4
Total	**575**

Jefferson Medical College:

First year	212
Second year	175
Third "	135
Total	**522**

Medico-Chirurgical College, total, 123.

Woman's Medical College has no information to give until November 1st, or until all the students will have registered.

It is generally estimated that about 30 more men will matriculate at the Jefferson, and 20 at the University.

The number of students at the Hahnemann School is 206.

Vaccination in France.—The special committee appointed by the Academy of Medicine, at Paris, to inquire anew into the prophylactic value of vaccination, have made a report strongly in favor of the adoption of laws that will make vaccination and revaccination compulsory in France.

OFFICIAL LIST OF CHANGES IN THE STATIONS AND DUTIES OF OFFICERS SERVING IN THE MEDICAL DEPARTMENT, U. S. ARMY, FROM OCTOBER 7 TO OCTOBER 13, 1890.

By direction of the Secretary of War, ARTHUR W. TAYLOR, *Captain and Assistant Surgeon*, is relieved from duty at Fort Wingate, New Mexico, to take effect on the expiration of present sick-leave, and will report in person to the commanding officer Fort Adams, R. I., for duty at that station, relieving J. J. Cochran, Captain and Assistant Surgeon. Captain Cochran, upon being relieved by Captain Taylor, will report in person to the commanding officer Camp Eagle Pass, Texas, for duty at that station, relieving Paul Clendenin, First Lieutenant and Assistant Surgeon. Lieutenant Clendenin, on being relieved by Captain Cochran, will report in person to the commanding officer Fort Brady, Mich., for duty at that station.—Par. 8, *S. O. 232, A. G. O., Washington, D. C.*, October 3, 1890.

By direction of the Secretary of War, WALTER REED, *Captain and Assistant Surgeon*, is relieved from further duty at Mount Vernon Barracks, Ala., and assigned to duty as Attending Surgeon and Examiner of Recruits at Baltimore, Md.—Par. 7, *S. O. 233. A. G. O., Washington, D. C.*, October 4. 1890.

By direction of the Secretary of War, leave of absence for three months is granted ROBERT J. GIBSON, *Captain and Assistant Surgeon*, to take effect on being relieved from duty at Fort Trumbull, Conn., by Henry M. Cronkhite, Major and Surgeon.—Par. 12, *S. O. 232, A. G. O., Washington, D. C.*, October 3. 1890.

By direction of the Secretary of War, C. N. BERKELEY MACAULEY, *Captain and Assistant Surgeon*, is relieved from duty at Fort Supply, Indian Territory, and will report in person to the commanding officer Fort Lewis, Colorado, for duty at that station.—Par. 2, *S. O. 233, A. G. O., Washington, D. C.*, October 4, 1890.

By direction of the Secretary of War, ROBERT B. BENHAM, *Captain and Assistant Surgeon*, will proceed from Fort Hamilton, N. Y., to Mount Vernon Barracks, Ala., and report in person to the commanding officer of that post for temporary duty, relieving John J. Cochran, Captain and Assistant Surgeon, who will return to his proper station.—Par. 8, *S. O. 232, A. G. O., Washington, D. C.*, October 3, 1890.

By direction of the Secretary of War, RUDOLPH G. EBERT, *Captain and Assistant Surgeon*, is relieved from duty at Angel Island, Cal., to take effect upon the arrival at that post of William H. Gardner, Major and Surgeon, and will then proceed to Vancouver Barracks, Wash., and report to the commanding officer of that post for duty.—Par. 15, *S. O. 232, A. G. O., Washington, D. C.*, October 3, 1890.

By direction of the Secretary of War, ALLEN M. SMITH, *First Lieutenant and Assistant Surgeon*, is relieved from duty at Fort Snelling, Minn., and will report in person to the commanding officer Fort Assinniboine, Montana, for duty at that station, relieving Paul Shillock, First Lieutenant and Assistant Surgeon. Lieutenant Shillock, upon being relieved, will report in person to the commanding officer Fort Custer, Montana, for duty at that station, relieving William R. Hall, Captain and Assistant Surgeon. Captain Hall, upon being relieved by Lieutenant Shillock, will report in person to the commanding officer Fort Schuyler, N. Y., for duty at that station, relieving Norton Strong, Captain and Assistant Surgeon. Captain Strong, on being relieved by Captain Hall, will report in person to the commanding officer at Fort Meade, South Dakota, for duty at that station.—Par. 8, *S. O. 232, A. G. O., Washington, D. C.*, October 3, 1890.

By direction of the Secretary of War, VAN BUREN HUBBARD, *Major and Surgeon*, is relieved from duty at Columbus Barracks, Ohio, and will report in person to the commanding officer Fort Spokane. Washington, for duty at that station, relieving Henry S. Turrill, Captain and Assistant Surgeon. Captain Turrill, upon being relieved by Major Hubbard, will report in person to the commanding officer Madison Barracks. N. Y., for duty at that station, relieving John D. Hall, Major and Surgeon. Major Hall, on being relieved by Captain Turrill, will report in person to the commanding officer Fort Canby, Wash., for duty at that station.—Par. 8, *S. O. 232, A. G. O., Washington, D. C.*, October 3, 1890.

By direction of the Secretary of War, the following changes in the stations and duties of officers of the Medical Department are ordered:

STERNBERG, GEORGE M., *Major and Surgeon*.—Is relieved from duty as Attending Surgeon and Examiner of Recruits at Baltimore, Md., and as a member of the Army Medical Board appointed to meet in New York City, N. Y., and will repair to San Francisco, Cal., and take charge of the Medical Purveying Depot at that place, as Acting Assistant Medical Purveyor, relieving B. J. D. Irwin, Colonel and Surgeon. Colonel Irwin, on being thus relieved, will report in person to the commanding general Department of the Columbia, for assignment to duty as Medical Director of that Department, and as Post Surgeon, Vancouver Barracks. Wash., relieving William E. Waters, Major and Surgeon, now Post Surgeon, and temporarily in charge of the Medical Director's Office. Major Waters, on being thus relieved, will report in person to the commanding officer Fort Custer, Mont., for duty at that station.—Par. 8, *S. O. 232. A. G. O.*, October 3, 1890.

By direction of the Secretary of War, CURTIS E. MUNN, *Major and Surgeon*, is relieved from duty at Angel Island, Cal., and will report in person to the commanding officer Fort Monroe, Va., for duty at that station, relieving John Brooke, Major and Surgeon. Major Brooke, on being relieved by Major Munn, will report in person to the commanding officer Fort Leavenworth, Kansas, for duty at that station, relieving Alfred A. Woodhull, Major and Surgeon. Major Woodhull, on being relieved by Major Brooke, will report in person to the commanding officer Fort Sherman, Idaho, for duty at that station.—Par. 8, *S. O. 232. A. G. O., Washington, D. C.*, October 3. 1890.

By direction of the Secretary of War, WILLIAM C. BORDEN, *Captain and Assistant Surgeon*, is relieved from duty at Fort Sam Houston, Texas, upon the arrival of C. C. Byrne, Lieutenant-Colonel and Surgeon, and will report in person to the commanding officer Fort Davis, Texas, for duty at that station, relieving Peter R. Egan, Captain and Assistant Surgeon. Captain Egan, upon being relieved by Captain Borden, will report in person to the commanding officer Fort Warren, Mass,. for duty at that station, relieving George McCreery, Captain and Assistant Surgeon. Captain McCreery, on being relieved by Captain Egan, will report in person to the commanding officer Fort Clark, Texas, for duty at that station, relieving Charles M. Gandy, Captain and Assistant Surgeon. Captain Gandy, on being relieved by Captain McCreery, will report in person to the commanding officer Fort Shaw, Montana, for duty at that station.—Par. 8, *S. O. 232, A. G. O., Washington, D. C.*, October 3. 1890.

By direction of the Secretary of War, WILLIAM H. GARDNER, *Major and Surgeon*, is relieved from duty at Washington Barracks, District of Columbia, to take effect upon the arrival of Joseph K. Corson. Major and Surgeon, and will report in person to the commanding officer Angel Island, Cal., for duty at that station.—Par. 8, *S. O. 232, A. G. O. Washington, D. C.*, October 3. 1890.

By direction of the Secretary of War, HENRY M. CRONKHITE, *Major and Surgeon*, is relieved from duty at Fort Lewis, Colorado, and will report in person to the commanding officer Fort Trumbull, Conn., for duty at that station, relieving Robert J. Gibson, Captain and Assistant Surgeon. Captain Gibson, on being relieved from duty by Major Cronkhite, will report in person to the commanding officer Fort Sam Houston, Texas, for duty at that station.—Par. 8, *S. O. 232, A. G. O., Washington. D. C.*, October 3, 1890.

By direction of the Secretary of War, the leave of absence granted LEONARD WOOD, *First Lieutenant and Assistant Surgeon*, in Special Orders No. 74, August 30, 1890, Department of California, is extended one month.—Par. 7. *S. O. 232, A. G. O, Washington, D. C.*, October 3, 1890.

BAILY, JOSEPH C., *Lieutenant-Colonel, Assistant Medical Purveyor, and Medical Director of the Department of Texas.*—Is granted leave of absence for one month.—Par. 3, *S. O. 86, Department of Texas*, October 3, 1890.

By direction of the Secretary of War, JAMES A. FINLEY, *Captain and Assistant Surgeon*, is relieved from duty at Fort Totten, North Dakota, and will report in person to the commanding officer Jefferson Barracks. Mo., for duty at that station, relieving William D. Crosby, Captain and Assistant Surgeon. Captain Crosby, on being relieved by Captain Finley, will report in person to the commanding officer Fort Pembina, North Dakota, for duty at that station.—Par. 8, *S. O. 232. A. G. O., Washington, D. C.*, October 3, 1890.

BYRNE, CHARLES C., *Lieutenant-Colonel and Surgeon.*—Is relieved from duty as Attending Surgeon at the Soldiers' Home, near this city, and will report in person to the commanding officer Fort Sam Houston, Texas, for duty at that station.—Par. 8, *S. O. 232, A. G. O., Washington, D. C.*, October 3, 1890.

APPOINTMENT.

VOLLUM, EDWARD P., *Colonel and Surgeon.*—To be Chief Medical Purveyor, with the rank of Colonel, August 28, 1890.

PROMOTIONS.

IRWIN, BERNARD J. D., *Lieutenant-Colonel and Assistant Medical Purveyor.*—To be Surgeon, with the rank of Colonel, August 28, 1890.

FRYER, BLENCOWE E,. *Major and Surgeon.*—To be Assistant Medical Purveyor, with the rank of Lieutenant-Colonel, August 28, 1890.

COWDREY, STEVENS G., *Captain and Assistant Surgeon.*—To be Surgeon, with the rank of Major, August 28, 1890.

THE MEDICAL NEWS.

A WEEKLY JOURNAL OF MEDICAL SCIENCE.

| VOL. LVII. | SATURDAY, OCTOBER 25, 1890. | NO. 17. |

ORIGINAL LECTURES.

PHANTOM TUMORS—ABDOMINAL DROPSY—OVARITIS—FIBROID TUMOR OF THE UTERUS.

*A Clinical Lecture
delivered at the Hospital of the University of Pennsylvania,
September 24, 1890.*

BY WILLIAM GOODELL. M.D.,
PROFESSOR OF GYNECOLOGY.

Reported by LEWIS H. ADLER, JR., M.D.,
RESIDENT PHYSICIAN OF THE EPISCOPAL HOSPITAL; LATE RESIDENT
PHYSICIAN OF THE UNIVERSITY HOSPITAL.

GENTLEMEN: The first case that I present to you is one of a kind that often puzzles physicians. The patient is past the age of forty-nine years; her youngest child is over twelve years of age. An enlargement of the abdomen has been present for seven years, and she has intermenstrual pains. In order to ascertain her condition, I shall examine her first without an anæsthetic and, finally, under ether.

Phantom tumors occurring in this region, on superficial examination resemble genuine tumors and are very deceptive, but usually they will be found to be resonant on percussion.

In this case there is a prominent and resonant abdominal tumefaction, but I find that I can come to no positive conclusion until the woman is etherized. If there be a tumor, the intestines clearly lie above it. When she came to my office, a short time ago, there was even more distention than now, owing, perhaps, to greater flaccidity of the abdominal walls, and, consequently, to their greater distention by the bloated intestines.

Before proceeding further with the case, I shall have the patient removed from the clinic-room and anæsthetized, in order to be more certain in rendering my decision. If there be no fluctuation, there is no liquid; and if in front of the tumor there is a resonant mass, due to the accumulation of fat and gas, the only way for us to dispel this doubt, or, at least, to lessen greatly the difficulty of the diagnosis, is to use ether, for, the presence of the gas being mostly a nervous phenomenon, it is largely dispelled by this means.

Phantom tumors most frequently occur in women at the time of the menopause. Many physicians make the mistake of imagining women with such an enlargement to be pregnant, and are surprised and mortified to discover their error. A case will occur somewhat in this manner: A woman approaches the age of forty-five years; she loses her periods; fattens, and her abdomen becomes distended with gas. She at once concludes that she is pregnant, and announces the fact to her husband and intimate friends. Those in the secret patiently await the advent of labor and hold themselves in readiness to congratulate her upon the Benjamin of her old age. The family physician defers his summer vacation, and everything, even down to a handy pincushion, is ready for the little stranger. But, lo! when the expected time arrives all are wofully disappointed. Days and weeks pass by, but still no child is born. The whole affair was due to fat and gas. If the woman had been examined under ether, such a failure in diagnosis would not have been made. Nor is this mistake of imagining themselves pregnant, when they are not, confined alone to human females. A bitch will make all preparations for her expected litter, and be disappointed for exactly similar reasons.

Phantom tumors are provoking, as well as deceptive, to physicians. A woman goes from one to another, and is not benefited. The reason is because she is not anæsthetized and examined *per vaginam* by the double touch. Sir James Y. Simpson, the distinguished gynecologist, now dead, meeting in his practice one of these patients who had thus, without etherization, been going from one doctor to another, put her under the influence of an anæsthetic, and that, too, in the presence of her sister, who was also allowed to examine her abdomen. As the patient recovered consciousness, she still contended that she was pregnant, when her sister contradicted her by saying: "Hush, Hettie, hush! ye ha' nae chiel in your wame, for I felt your back-bane."

In the patient before you, as her bowels move freely, the abdominal swelling cannot be due to any obstruction in the intestines, because where fæces can pass, gas can pass. As I previously stated, this distention is often due to nervousness. I had a patient who used to come to my office for examination, upon whose abdomen I could have beaten a "reveille." When she was etherized, the distention wholly disappeared.

In the present case Dr. Taylor is doing the percussing for me, as my fingers are engaged in holding the abdominal wall. I grasp the abdominal walls firmly in my hand, and when the woman becomes thoroughly etherized, and consequently entirely relaxed, I shall be able to obtain even a better hold. While I am so engaged, Dr. Taylor elicits no fluctuation in the portion of the abdomen remaining below and finds no evidence of a tumor.

I also thought that an abdominal hernia might be the cause of all this woman's trouble. There is sometimes a natural separation of the recti muscles, allowing a protrusion of the intestines, which constitutes what is known as ventral hernia; and, moreover, this affection sometimes follows ovariotomy.

The rule by which you are to guard against mistakes is to insist upon the use of the *double touch*, as well as the examination *per vaginam*. By these means I am enabled in many cases to outline accurately the size of the included uterus.

In the present case, by passing two fingers of the left hand into the vagina and then meeting them with the fingers of the right hand placed on the outside of the abdomen, I find that the left ovary is doubtlessly enlarged; the other ovary may also be in the same condition. But this condition will not account for the largeness of the abdomen, which is to be explained not alone by omental fat, and by the thickness of the abdominal walls, but also by their flaccidity and distention by large quantities of gas.

The treatment upon which I should like to put this woman is that of asafœtida in large doses—not one or two grains, but nine grains, three times a day, before meals, in three-grain *sugar-coated* pills, so that she will not taste them after they are swallowed. After three days, this trouble of tasting the medicine generally ceases, and she would then be able to take twelve grains three times a day if needful.

Now, in this case there are some, but not sufficient, indications to perform abdominal section. In former times the exploratory incision was done even more than it is nowadays, in order to arrive at a positive diagnosis; but this is not necessary at present, owing to the introduction of anæsthetization as a preliminary step to a thorough examination. Therefore, you will have learned another golden rule by which you may be guided in your practice, and that is : if a woman with an enlarged, resonant, but not fluctuating, abdomen comes to you, act upon the supposition that there is no tumor present, but only gas. If you then err it will be on the safe side.

ABDOMINAL DROPSY.

Physicians sometimes mistake pregnancy for tumors, because they are liable to meet with cases of pregnancy when they are not expecting them, and when they ought, morally, not to occur, even among the higher classes. In such cases always inquire about the menstruation, and if it has ceased, always think first of pregnancy as being the cause of its stoppage. If the case be one of dropsy, it has its cause somewhere in the great tripod of life—the heart, the liver, or the kidneys—and means a constitutional trouble with constitutional disturbances. We get in such cases, resonance. Why ? Because the intestines are floated upon the fluid, unless they be bound down by old inflammatory adhesions, or unless the belly is so distended that a wide space exists between the intestines and the abdominal wall, which space is filled with fluid.

OVARITIS.

The next patient is twenty-three years old. She has been married for three years and has an abdominal growth. She complains of a pain in the left side of the abdomen, running down the inside of the thigh, along the course of the genito-crural nerve. Such pain is sometimes due to ordinary sciatica, but it is not so in her case. Her menstruation is painful and profuse, which may mean something or nothing.

I now begin our examination, in which I use my finger, not the speculum, which, as a rule, should be reserved for treatment only, for upon one's finger one can acquire a degree of sensitiveness, of education, which must always remain strangers to any instrument. Upon making this examination, I find what is called a *sickle-*

shaped cervix. The womb is pushed over to the left by a tumor on the right side, which is round, not in the form of a sausage, like that of a prolapsed and enlarged tube. Therefore, it is an ovary, and, if it arises from a constitutional cause, a cold, a peritonitis, or any of the exanthemata, as it does in this case, the other ovary is most apt to be affected, and both will have to be removed. This, while it is a painful operation, is not a very dangerous one.

Such constitutional manifestations of cold often follow exposure, especially such indiscretion as sitting upon cold steps at night during menstruation.

After marriage the great cause of ovaritis is the contraction of gonorrhœa from the husband. Then there may be much inflammation, an abundant exudation of plastic lymph, and the organ becomes bound down by adhesions to adjacent structures, causing upon each movement of the woman sickening pain similar to that sometimes experienced in the analogous organ in the male. The other ovary, not primarily the seat of any germs, may be all right.

FIBROID TUMOR OF THE UTERUS.

Double touch proves the gynecologist. I know of a doctor, well posted on general medicine, who, when a woman came to him for treatment for some obscure pelvic trouble, after an imperfect examination, simply inserted a pessary into the vagina. It is needless to say that, even as a palliative measure, it was a failure. A rule, then, for you to remember henceforth is that if a physician does not know how to examine a woman by the *double touch*, he knows nothing about gynecology. A recent graduate, whether from this or any other firstclass college, can do more in a case like the patient I now bring before you than many of the older physicians who did not have an opportunity to learn these methods of diagnosis at college, and who since have not thoroughly kept up with the subject.

This woman is forty years of age, and has been married for many years. Seven years ago she miscarried and gave birth to a dead fœtus. For five years subsequent to this abortion she had no menstrual flow. Whenever you meet an abortion, no matter where, the question that should first come into your minds is : Can this be due to syphilis ? Examine both the man and woman, if possible, asking not only whether they ever had syphilis—for they may not know what that means— but whether they have ever had a sore on their privates, or the mucous patches, eruptions, and other manifestations of the disease, upon the other parts of their bodies. In this case, the first thing that strikes us in our examination is that the nymphæ are very much enlarged. If she were unmarried, I should think first of self-abuse, though I should not be certain that this was the cause. You can see that these nymphæ are flattened and elongated. In the Hottentot women they extend nearly to their knees, and, are considered ornamental.

I now pass in the uterine sound, and, in doing so, resort to the "master's wrinkle." This consists in introducing the instrument into the cavity of the uterus by pressing the handle down, raising it, and then depressing it, when in it goes. We have here a large fibroid of the uterus. I think there is also a smaller fibroma to the right of the uterus—a sub-peritoneal fibroid.

What is to be done in such cases? Now, as this is a tumor that rarely kills, the question is whether the woman is suffering sufficient pain or annoyance for me to operate. The uterus might be removed; but this is hardly ever needful in such cases. The operation generally resorted to is oöphorectomy, because by this means the monthly flow of blood to the organ is stopped, and the tumor ceases to grow, from lack of nutrition. If, however, you refuse to operate, or the patient be afraid to run the risks incident thereto, you can put her on the two medicines, ammonium chloride and fluid extract of ergot —say, ten grains of the former, which is the great absorbent, and from fifteen to twenty drops of the latter, which, by cutting off the blood-supply from the tumor, cause it to cease to thrive and will gradually make it lessen in size. These medicines are to be taken three times a day, and preferably at meal-times, lest from the action of ergot on the vasomotor nerves, nausea and digestive disturbance be occasioned. Again, fibroid tumors being flesh tumors, not cystic, they increase slowly in comparison with fluid tumors until the change of life, when they either cease to increase or lessen in size. If the change of life is deferred until later, these tumors may become fibro-cystic, and sometimes cancerous; but, as I have never met with an instance of the latter in my practice, when women become nervous and question me on the subject, I hoot at the idea. If, on the other hand, a woman with a fibroid tumor be not well-off pecuniarily, so as to live a life of ease, nor free from pain, I generally advise the removal of her ovaries. In this case I shall put the woman upon the above-mentioned medicines until I can more thoroughly study her case.

These three cases, then, are of great interest, because they are intensely practical. The first teaches the lesson that phantom tumors are to be studied most carefully, and that, too, with the woman under ether, as well as that the great medicine for phantom tumors is asafœtida.

The second case is one of ovaritis, following scarlet fever, in which, as both organs are nearly always affected, the treatment consists in double ovariotomy.

The third case is that of a uterine fibroid, which can be treated either by laparotomy or by the medicines, ammonium chloride and ergot, always remembering that, if the woman can be tided over the years of her menstruation, the tumor will then cease to give trouble and decrease in size, even if it does not entirely disappear.

ORIGINAL ARTICLES.

SOME OF THE DIFFICULTIES MET WITH IN ABDOMINAL SURGERY, AS ILLUSTRATED BY CASES FROM PERSONAL RECORDS.[1]

BY A. VANDER VEER, M.D.,
PROFESSOR OF DIDACTIC, ABDOMINAL, AND CLINICAL SURGERY IN THE ALBANY MEDICAL COLLEGE, ALBANY, N. Y.

I HAVE thought it well to present these cases that to myself have suggested many anxious thoughts and some misgivings. It has seemed to me wiser to

[1] Read before the American Association of Obstetricians and Gynecologists, Philadelphia, September 17, 1890.

do this than to offer a series of cases covering a number of months since my last records were given to the profession. It would be far more pleasing to offer a full report of all cases operated on, but such a report would necessarily contain a number of simple cases, without interest in diagnosis or treatment. It is also true that in presenting these cases as I do, the cynic and the iconoclast may visit upon me an undue amount of criticism. This is something, however, that can be taken care of in the future. What I desire, is to bring out the strong fact that the reading and thinking public, the intelligent classes, have been led to believe that the surgeon can successfully do almost any operation within the pelvis and abdomen.

Is this true?

As one doing considerable abdominal surgery in a large section of the country, I must, looking at the subject from one standpoint, answer the question in the negative. Looking at it from another standpoint, I can most earnestly answer it in the affirmative. The factors that will ever enter into the latter answer are the early recognition of abdominal disease by the family physician, and also the desire to call the surgeon early, if only to make a diagnosis.

The negative answer is one with which the public is greatly concerned. What can we promise to the friends of the patient whose case, either from traumatism or acute or chronic conditions, becomes one for abdominal surgery? We know that the accumulated experience of the past few years has thrown upon this subject an immense flood of light; but more is needed. This paper is offered with the hope that as the subject emerges from discussion it may be clearer to us all.

CASE I.—Miss S. M., aged twenty-four years, a domestic. Admitted to the Albany Hospital, September 17, 1888. She gave the history of a tumor first noticed eighteen months previously, and which was diagnosed soon after as being entirely within the pelvis. Her menstruation had been fairly regular, but during the past six months the tumor had grown quite rapidly, giving her more pain, and she was losing flesh so rapidly as to alarm her friends. Up to this time she had opposed an operation.

On careful examination the tumor was found to fill the pelvis and to extend to the umbilicus, and was somewhat sensitive and movable as the patient was turned from side to side. No ascites. Tumor was hard and elastic. Cervix well defined, but the body of the uterus could not be outlined.

Diagnosis: Probable fibro-sarcoma of the broad ligament. Exploration by abdominal section was advised with a view to remove the growth if possible.

Operation, September 27, 1888: The tumor was found to occupy about the position described above, and was entirely connected with the left broad ligament, with many deep adhesions within the pelvis and about the sigmoid flexure.

No abdominal adhesions of importance. A number of ligatures were applied to the points of adhesion, and the pedicle, made from the broad ligament and the adhesions, was secured by a Staffordshire knot. The pelvis was cleansed by sponging and no serious oozing appearing; the abdomen was closed without drainage in the usual manner.

The patient rallied from the operation and did well until the beginning of the third day, when nausea began, followed in twelve hours by vomiting. Rectal injections, small doses of calomel, and one-drachm doses of sulphate of magnesium failed to produce any movement of the bowels, and but little gas passed. Patient did not suffer very severe pain, but there was considerable distention of the abdomen from intestinal gas. The vomited material at first was spinach-like; a few hours before her death it became more fæcal in character. The patient died about 4 P.M., October 2d, death beginning with cold hands and feet.

I thought that she died from traumatic peritonitis, but the autopsy showed that a coil of the ileum had become attached to the sigmoid flexure, where the adhesions had been separated, and had doubled upon itself, causing obstruction of the bowels, which was the true cause of death.

This was in October, 1888. Who will deny that, had I opened the abdomen on the third day, found the point of obstruction, loosened the adhesions, and flushed the abdominal cavity with hot water, the patient would have recovered? Again, in all such cases, especially where we have reason to believe that the growth is a sarcoma, or a true carcinoma, with adhesions, is it not better to flush the cavity and to leave it filled with the fluid, not using a drainage-tube, in order that the intestines may continue to float some time after the operation?

CASE II.—Mrs. H. M., aged thirty-one years, married, the mother of three living and healthy children, of which the oldest is aged six years. Family history good. Father died at the age of fifty-three years of paralysis, though he occasionally suffered from stomach trouble. Mother living at the age of sixty. Three brothers and four sisters living.

The patient began to menstruate at the age of fourteen years, and was regular up to seven months ago, when the flow ceased. When nineteen years old she had an attack of what was termed dyspepsia, and was very ill for two months. Since then she has had similar attacks about once a year, lasting from two to three months. They are always accompanied with more or less pain throughout the abdomen. Her last child was born in July, 1887, and since then she has had more or less nausea, with vomiting, and has gradually lost flesh.

About the latter part of July, 1888, she noticed an enlargement in the abdomen a little to the right of and above the umbilicus. Her family physician had called three or four consultants, and the consensus of opinion was that she had carcinoma of the pylorus.

She was admitted to the Albany Hospital, November 20, 1888. She was much emaciated. There was little intestinal distention, except about the ileo-cæcal region. Above this point could be felt a hard mass, nearly circular in outline, and about the size of two fingers. She had been much constipated at times, but whenever her bowels could be moved and kept moving she felt much better. When she vomited it was first the food or drink that she had recently taken, then a dark, greenish-looking fluid, at times becoming fæcal in appearance and odor. Stomach not distended.

I believed that she had a malignant growth implicating some portion of the intestine near the ileo-cæcal region.

An exploratory section was advised with the understanding that if possible the growth should be removed. I was also prepared to do an intestinal anastomosis if that became necessary.

Operation, November 23, 1888: A section through the right linea semilunaris was made, the patient having been previously prepared. There was found a projecting tumor near the junction of the ascending and transverse colon, from which adhesions extended around the gut, entirely closing its calibre. The tumor seemed to pull down and hold the intestines quite firmly in the lumbar regions. I loosened these adhesions and, believing the tumor to be malignant, concluded that it was best to make the operation as short as possible; hence after exploring the pyloric end of the stomach I closed the wound. Though very weak she bore the operation well and returned to a fairly good condition within twelve hours.

The wound closed perfectly, and the patient had a number of good fæcal movements in the few days following the operation. She vomited occasionally, and at times there would be traces of blood with the mucus from the stomach, but no substance resembling fæcal fluid was ever observed. After the tenth day she was able to take more food than at any time for a year previously. At times she complained of distress about the stomach, saying that it was distended with gas, and that she still felt the old indigestion. At times she would feel much better, and she gained sufficiently to walk about her room. At other times for a day or two she would frequently vomit a dirty, brownish-looking fluid. She could not take solid food with comfort. Bowels would move each day with the aid of a mild enema. During her convalescence she occasionally took anodynes, but not to any extent. Cocaine often relieved the gastric distress, as did various other remedies.

She returned to her home, December 19th, much improved in her general health. To her husband, herself and friends I stated that she had a malignant growth which it would not be safe to undertake the removal of, and that the occasional unpleasant symptoms were probably due to secondary deposits in the walls of the stomach. At her home, as her family physician, Dr. Popen, informed me, she remained very comfortable for weeks. At times the tumor was more distinct than at others. At one time, for a few days, she seemed so well that her husband came to my office and asked me frankly if it were not possible that a mistake had been made in the diagnosis. But gradually the vomiting of mucus, and especially recently-taken fluids, became more serious, and she finally died of exhaustion.

Autopsy, made by Drs. Popen, Marselius, and Macdonald, revealed an hour-glass contraction of the stomach near the cardiac end ; bands of adhesions closing the stomach so completely that only a probe could be passed through the stricture. These adhesions were very firm. The entire intestinal tract was normal. The supposed malignant tumor proved to be a displaced kidney, firmly adherent in its new position, but normal. I think it not improbable that at one time this was a floating kidney, that at times it produced sympathetic disturbance of the stomach, that she had many attacks of acute gastritis, occasionally accompanied with local peritonitis, and that in one of these latter attacks the kidney became fastened by the new adhesions.

Should I have discovered the hour-glass contraction of the stomach at the time that I made the section ? If I had, is there much probability that I could have loosened the adhesions? The latter I believe could have been done by making an anastomosis of the lower end of the duodenum or upper portion of the jejunum with the cardiac end of the stomach. But would we have been justified in doing this in the face of our supposed malignant tumor?

CASE III.—Mrs. L. R., married, no children, family history of tuberculosis. She has some cough, and marked dulness over the apex of the left lung.

Admitted to the Albany Hospital, November 10, 1888. One year ago she noticed an enlargement on the right side of the abdomen, which has gradually increased, and she now presents a well-marked ovarian cyst. Operation was advised to relieve the patient of her anxiety, in the belief that she had sufficient strength to recover.

Operation, November 12, 1888: The pedicle was very short and was ligated with soft Chinese silk, which I had previously used in similar operations, but in this instance the wax had been removed, which made the silk very soft, pliable, and easily handled. This patient did well until the end of the third day when she began to show symptoms of septic peritonitis and died soon afterward.

Autopsy: The ligature was found completely softened, loosened, and very friable. There had been some hæmorrhage, but not extensive, from the pedicle and the whole peritoneal cavity was filled with pockets of pus.

It is possible that the general constitutional condition of this patient may have had something to do with the causation of the peritoneal complication, but undoubtedly the imperfect ligature acted as the exciting cause.

There is no doubt that the patient would have been benefited by reopening the abdomen on the fourth day, washing it out, putting in a drainage-tube, and, if necessary, controlling hæmorrhage. The case has been a warning to me not to make use of this kind of ligature.

CASE IV.—Mrs. G. T., aged fifty-one years, has had one child and several miscarriages. Her family history is good. She first noticed an enlargement of the abdomen some five years ago, but it has become more marked during the past two years, and especially during the past year and a half. She has lost much flesh.

The patient has passed through much family affliction, losing her only child at the age of twenty years, and her parents soon after. Her menstruation has usually been regular, but at times very excessive. During the past year the flow has not been so great and has occurred every two or three months only.

In the past three years she has had a number of attacks of local peritonitis accompanied with much pain, and has been obliged to take morphine freely, having taken for a long time previously to the operation, eighteen grains in the twenty-four hours. Her physician had made the diagnosis of ovarian tumor, and this I had only to confirm, though believing that it was possibly complicated with a fibroid of the uterus.

The case was plainly a multilocular tumor, and could be easily defined when I first saw the patient with Dr. L., and while agreeing with him as to the necessity of an operation, yet I was anxious to postpone it if possible until the weather became somewhat cooler. However, she was losing ground, and while she had previously opposed an operation, it was now evident to her that her only hope was in an operation. She was anxious to be tapped, but this we positively declined to do, assuring her that it could do little good, there being evidences of many cysts. Her face presented the appearance so characteristic of ovarian disease.

Her condition grew so serious that we concluded to do the operation. We prepared a room in her own house, and secured two of my best trained nurses. The patient's friends were opposed to the operation, and some of my acquaintances thought I was foolish to operate on so serious a case.

Operation, August 28, 1889: The tumor was composed of more cysts than I had ever seen, and their contents, in color, consistence, etc., were as varied as possible. There were adhesions to every organ within the abdominal cavity. These were loosened by a sponge and the fingers, and much time was consumed in applying ligatures. A long and tedious operation resulted in the removal of a tumor weighing fifty-six pounds. (The patient's average weight in early life was ninety pounds.) The abdomen was thoroughly flushed with hot water, which was allowed to remain. A glass drainage-tube was placed in the lower end of the incision. For three days the hæmorrhage was considerable, and at times so serious as to give me much anxiety. I then suggested to Dr. Macdonald, my assistant, who had remained with the patient at night, to inject a solution of the subsulphate of iron through the tube. Hæmorrhage then ceased, oozing grew less and less, and the tube was removed on the ninth day. The patient for forty-eight hours required large doses of morphine, after that less, and in time she reached a very small dose, and I think that the habit is now broken. She made a good recovery, and to-day herself and friends are more than grateful.

What anxiety would have been spared me, as the operator, had she submitted to an early operation.

CASE V.—On the evening of October 14, 1889, I received a telegram requesting me to come about twenty miles in the country to see a case of intestinal obstruction, and, if necessary, to operate. I was tired and the last evening train had left, but my assistant, Dr. W. G. Macdonald, responded to the call, and found the patient a laborer, aged forty-two years, with such surroundings that it seemed impossible to do any operation there. Accordingly, he was brought to the Albany Hospital early on the morning of October 15th.

Patient was well developed, and weighed about 160 pounds. Previous health good. At the age of seventeen years he developed a left inguinal hernia, which had not given him much trouble until three years ago, when his usual truss failed to retain it. He then grew careless, often going without any truss. On October 5, 1889, the bowel escaped quite freely, but he lay down in his usual position, and thought that he replaced it. After a hearty dinner of beans, etc., he was taken with vomiting, and had to give up work. Vomiting continued for two days. He did not have severe pain until the third day. No movement of the bowels could be obtained either by injections or medicines. On October 9th, there was no appearance of a hernia, but much soreness on the left side. The fourth day pain and vomiting ceased, and the abdomen became greatly distended.

When I saw him on the morning of October 15th he presented an anxious appearance, sunken eyes, cold extremities, cyanosis, subnormal temperature, husky voice, restlessness, and every symptom of approaching death. His pulse was 140 to 150.

It is in this condition that we are too often called to see cases of abdominal surgery.

My first impulse was to make an incision directly over the seat of his old hernia, and look for the trouble there, but I finally concluded that about the only thing I would be able to do would be enterostomy.

Operation: I made the median section, giving very little ether, and passed in two fingers on either side, but did not detect any trouble at either of the rings. I then brought out at the opening what I believed to be a fold of ileum, incised it, emptied out a great quantity of gas and liquid fæces, and attached it to the walls of the abdomen. The patient was then placed in bed with artificial heat around him, and was given stimulants by the rectum and hypodermically. He was also given aromatic spirit of ammonia, digitalis, and nitrite of amyl. Although the operation did not occupy more than eighteen minutes, it was for some time a grave question whether he would rally at all. In a few hours he became conscious, expressed himself as greatly relieved, and at the end of twelve hours warmth returned in the extremities, with all the other evidences of good reaction.

The fistulous opening continued to discharge freely liquid yellow fæces. A milk diet was given at first, but as it seemed to pass somewhat quickly from the opening solid food was ordered. This, the patient stated, afforded him more satisfaction, and controlled his hunger.

He now rapidly improved, and gained in flesh, but no movement of the lower bowel could be obtained. On October 28th, an unsuccessful attempt was made to force water, *per rectum*, through the fistula.

November 1. Senn's apparatus for the injection of hydrogen gas was used. It acted well, but only the large intestines could be dilated. The dilatation ceased abruptly in the neighborhood of the ileo-cæcal valve.

I now determined to do a more thorough operation, and to find the point of obstruction and its nature, and then, if thought best, do an intestinal anastomosis. I made the incision to the right of the median line, about as we would for removal of the appendix, but extended it somewhat higher. I found strong adhesions implicating the ileo-cæcal region and a portion of the ileum. These were so firm that I thought it unwise to disturb them. I discovered that the portion of the small intestine that I had opened to form the fistula was very near the lower end of the ileum. I, therefore, thought it best to attach the loop nearest to, and just above the fistula, to the beginning of the ascending colon, which was done without much difficulty by means of Senn's bone-plates and Lembert's sutures. The portion of the ileum just below the fistula, together with the cæcum, was entirely collapsed, and with the adhesions, the appendix, etc., formed a dense mass. All this was "side-tracked" by the anastomosis. The wound was closed and dressed in the usual manner.

Patient rallied well. Pulse 100, full and strong. Fistula began to discharge eight hours after operation.

On the second day he complained of dyspepsia, and pain from the distended abdomen.

On the third day he passed gas, and a slight amount of fæcal matter *per rectum.* At 7 P. M., on this day three superficial stitches were removed. The wound looked well despite the fact that on two occasions the discharge from the fistula had run over the seat of operation. The wound was cleansed and painted with a solution of iodoform in collodion.

On the eighth and ninth day there was a slight fæcal discharge from the rectum. He took a small amount of general diet.

On the eleventh day an enema was followed by two solid movements. Fistula continued to discharge.

On the fourteenth day glycerin suppositories were given, and caused a large movement.

19th. An attempt was made to freshen the edges of the fistula, which had grown very small, yet discharged occasionally, very much to the annoyance of the patient. The operation was almost successful, and was repeated on November 20th. The fistula then closed, so that his passages became natural.

The patient now began to worry about going home, whether he would be able to support his family, etc. He was apparently doing well, his appetite was good, and he slept well.

December 4. He began to show signs of restlessness, and while not complaining of pain in the abdomen, he suffered from severe pain which began in the left groin and darted down the thigh. There was also pain in the back. The left leg was cold, the posterior tibial artery could not be felt, and he had all the symptoms of arterial embolism. The limb was wrapped in warm applications. His temperature suddenly went up to 105°, and the pulse to 150. Stimulants by the mouth and rectum and hypodermically were employed. He continued restless, passed into a condition of collapse, became delirious, and died on the 5th at 2 A. M.

Autopsy: Rigor mortis not marked ; body emaciated ; the recent wound in good condition. Abdomen opened in the line of the old fistulous wound. About one drachm of pus was found at the most dependent portion of the last wound for closing the fistula. No recent peritonitis, but evidences of old peritonitis. Extensive adhesion of intestines among themselves, and to the abdominal wall on the right side. The portion of the intestines where the anastomosis had been performed was removed, and union was found to be perfect. The opening connecting the intestines admitted the end of the little finger. Bone-plates entirely absorbed. All the other organs apparently healthy.

This case has caused me much thought. I am convinced that had I attempted any more prolonged operation at the time he was brought in he would have died on the table. Who will deny that his chances in an operation would have been decidedly better had he been seen in consultation in the early part of the attack? What can we do in such cases, in which, when we are called, the conditions of shock and collapse are so decided? This case also impresses us with the danger of repeated irritations of an old hernia. Adhesions will form, and are often present when we least expect them. Consider, however, that the adhesions were on the side opposite to that of the hernia.

Case VI.—Mrs. G. H., aged thirty years, married at the age of eighteen years, and the mother of five children. She began to menstruate when twelve and a half years old, and was regular from that time until her first pregnancy, which occurred two months after marriage. She then had four children in rapid succession. Her first child weighed nearly twelve pounds, and the labor was somewhat tedious. She states that she took large quantities of ergot, and that her pains at the end of the confinement were very severe.

The patient first came under my care in June, 1883, for uterine trouble. Previously a plump, handsome girl, she now had the anxious expression and the general appearance of much past suffering.
17*

I found a laceration of the perineum, a badly-lacerated cervix, and the uterine appendages much thickened and very sensitive. The uterus was much enlarged and completely retroverted, cervix swollen and tender, with the evidences of pelvic peritonitis.

The usual hot-water treatment, local scarification of the cervix, tampons of glycerin, and rest were employed. The diet and bowels were carefully regulated. After four months' treatment she began to improve, but at this time her children sickened and two of them died, which depressed her very much. Later her treatment was renewed, and when the local tenderness and inflammation had sufficiently subsided I made an effort to have her wear a suitable pessary, but this instrument always did more or less harm.

During the latter part of 1885 she began to have quite severe hæmorrhages. Her menstruation would begin gradually, then come in gushes, and exhausted her very much. There were no evidences of a tumor. I curetted the uterus thoroughly, and brought away considerable granular detritus, which was followed by a decided improvement in her symptoms.

Again an attempt to wear a pessary was made, but the result was not encouraging. She had now at her home a very intelligent family physician, and as there had been some return of the hæmorrhage in May, 1886, I advised him to curette the uterus, and to get along as well as possible without the pessaries. This treatment was carried out and she did improve somewhat, so much so that in April, 1887, I operated on the laceration of the cervix. This was followed by an improvement in all her symptoms. Just previously to this operation she acquired the morphine-habit, which was very difficult to overcome.

About three months after the operation she began to show symptoms of a tapeworm. This caused much mental depression, but medicine finally expelled the tænia.

After this she had more hæmorrhage, and was curetted again, with excellent results. The uterus remained in good position, and was nearly normal in size. Soon after, she became pregnant, which caused great depression and a return to the secret use of morphine or codeine. The infant was born in August, 1888. She had the best of care and did well, but after the puerperium her strange actions disturbed her physician and friends. It was evident that she was taking anodynes. She frequently made costly and unnecessary purchases, and at public gatherings she had one or more seizures in which she became unconscious.

Her physician and husband again consulted me as to what had best be done. I advised that she be sent to some private hospital, and an effort was made to place her under the treatment of Dr. S. Weir Mitchell, but owing to his absence this was found impossible. At last she was brought to the Albany Hospital, where we succeeded in stopping the anodynes.

During the previous six months she had been irregular in her menstruation and suffered much. On examination I found the tubes thickened, the ovaries very sensitive, and the uterus markedly retroverted. After consultation, and with the full and earnest endorsement of her husband, it was thought wise to make an abdominal exploration, discover the true condition of the appendages, and, if necessary, to remove them, bring the uterus into position, and attach it to the abdominal walls. In view of the supposed diseased condition of the tubes I did not approve of doing the Alexander operation.

October 30, 1889. The patient being in the best condition mentally that I had seen her in for months, and much improved physically, after proper preparation, assisted by my calleagues, I operated. Pyosalpinx was found. One ovary was cirrhosed, the other very much enlarged and in a condition of cystic degeneration. The pampiniform plexus on each side was enormously enlarged. The appendages were included in the Staffordshire knot, and removed in the ordinary way. I did not have much trouble in bringing the uterus into position and attaching it to the under surface of the abdominal wall in front, but this was a fatal step in the operation, as the result will show.

The operation was done at 11 A.M., and occupied about half an hour. There was no hæmorrhage of importance, though I tore a considerable number of adhesions on the left side. In closing the wound no drainage-tube was introduced.

I left her at noon, fully recovered from the operation, and expressing herself as feeling very comfortable. At 1 o'clock I found her sleeping, and apparently comfortable, but she looked pale and her pulse was rapid and weak. I suspected hæmorrhage, and opened the lower end of the wound, when a flow of blood told but too well what was going on. I immediately opened the incision and found that the ligatures had failed to hold the large veins, from which a serious hæmorrhage had occurred, filling the pelvis and extending up into the abdomen. With the assistance of Dr. Townsend, we secured, after much effort, the bleeding vessels, but our patient was moribund. Rectal injections of hot whiskey were employed, and warm milk was injected into the median basilic vein, but all did little good, and at 3 P. M. she was dead.

My reflections on this case have been of the saddest. I think that we undertook too much; at least I should have secured the plexus of veins in sections when fastening the uterus in position. It may be said that the house physician, who was in charge, as well as the experienced nurse who was present, ought to have discovered the patient's condition and reported at once to me; but she was so comfortable as entirely to disarm them.

CASE VII.—Mrs. M. E. N., aged forty-five years, widow; admitted to the hospital, May 6, 1890. Family history good. Patient was well and strong up to twenty years of age, when she was treated for "womb trouble." Since then she has taken more or less medicine.

Menstruation began at the age of thirteen years. At times it was painful, and the quantity irregular. She married at the age of twenty-two years, but has had no children or miscarriages. Never had any acute disease, and always worked hard. Between seven and eight years ago, after having had vague, indefinite symptoms for some months, she noticed a hard, round bunch low down in the abdomen. When first seen this was the size of a cocoanut, but increased and now fills the abdomen, spreading out in all directions. The tumor is hard and dense, but never caused severe pain. Patient has lost strength, but not flesh. Menstruation unchanged. Bowels regular. She urinates a little more frequently than is natural.

She came to the hospital saying that she was unable to work and was anxious to have the tumor removed. When told that it implicated the whole uterus, and that if an operation was done all would have to be removed, she replied : "I cannot live long as I am ; I will take all the risk ; you do the operation."

The tumor was movable, yet presented so formidable an appearance that I declined to operate, and for two months made use of electricity and ergot, the tumor constantly increasing. It became such a burden as to make it almost impossible for her to get about, and on June 23d, I did a supravaginal hysterectomy. I was obliged to make an incision from the ensiform cartilage to the symphysis pubis, but found no adhesions. Using a corkscrew I lifted the tumor directly out of the abdomen, but was distressed to observe enlarged veins, as in the previous case. I placed around the neck of the tumor Tait's rope écraseur, isolated and tied the veins in sections, and removed the tubes and ovaries separately. I then removed the uterus with the tumor. The pedicle formed was about half the size of my wrist. I at first endeavored to control the hæmorrhage with a Staffordshire knot, but this was not sufficient. I then tied the vessels separately as they appeared in the stump, and tied the stump in sections by the lock-stitch. I then brought together the peritoneum over the stump and broad ligament, shutting the latter out from the peritoneal cavity. Silk alone was used for the ligatures and ¿utures. A long, glass drainage-tube was introduced well down in the cavity of the pelvis at the lower end of the incision, and the longest incision that I have ever made was closed in the usual way.

For five days there was a free, bloody discharge from the tube ; after that only stained serum. The tube was removed on the twelfth day. On the twenty-first day her temperature ran up and indicated pus-formation. Examination on the next day confirmed what the nurse suspected during the night, namely, that an abscess had empted into the vagina. Vaginal douches were used daily, and a careful watch kept up for escaped ligatures, but none were found. Aside from the abscess the patient made an uninterrupted recovery.

PEROXIDE OF HYDROGEN AND OZONE [1]

BY PAUL GIBIER, M.D.,
DIRECTOR OF THE PASTEUR INSTITUTE OF NEW YORK.

SINCE the discovery of peroxide of hydrogen by Thenard, in 1818, the therapeutical applications of

[1] Read before the International Medical Congress, Berlin, August 7, 1890.

this oxygenated compound seem to have been neglected both by the medical and the surgical professions; and it is only in the last twenty years that a few bacteriologists have demonstrated the germicidal potency of this chemical.

Among the most elaborate reports on the use of this compound may be mentioned those of Paul Bert and Regnard, Baldy, Péan, and Larrivé.

Dr. Miguel places peroxide of hydrogen at the head of a long list of antiseptics, and close to the silver salts.

Dr. Bouchet has demonstrated the antiseptic action of peroxide of hydrogen when applied to diphtheritic exudations.

Professor Nocart, of Alfort, attenuates the virulence of the symptomatic microbe of carbuncle, before he destroys it, by using the same antiseptic.

Dr. E. R. Squibb,[1] of Brooklyn, has also reported the satisfactory results which he obtained with peroxide of hydrogen in the treatment of infectious diseases.

Although the above-mentioned scientists have demonstrated by their experiments, that peroxide of hydrogen is one of the most powerful destroyers of pathogenic microbes, its use in therapeutics has not been as extensive as it deserves to be.

In my opinion, the reason for its not being in universal use is the difficulty of procuring it free from hurtful impurities. Another objection is the unstableness of the compound, which gives off nascent oxygen when brought in contact with organic substances.[2]

Besides the foregoing objections, surgical instruments decompose the peroxide; hence, if an operation is to be performed, the surgeon uses some other antiseptic during the procedure, and is apt to continne the application of the same antiseptic in the subsequent dressings.

Nevertheless, the satisfactory results which I have obtained at the Pasteur Institute of New York, with peroxide of hydrogen, in the treatment of wounds resulting from deep bites, and those which I have observed at the French clinic of New York, in the treatment of phagedenic chancres, varicose ulcers, parasitic diseases of the skin, and also in the treatment of other affections caused by germs, justify me in adding my statement as to the value of the drug.

But it is not from a clinical standpoint that I now direct attention to the antiseptic value of peroxide of hydrogen. What I now wish is merely to give a full report of the experiments which I have made on the effects of peroxide of hydrogen upon cultures of the following species of pathogenic mi-

crobes: bacillus anthracis, bacillus pyocyaneous, the bacilli of typhoid fever, of Asiatic cholera, and of yellow fever, streptococcus pyogenes, microbacillus prodigiosus, bacillus megaterium, and the bacillus of osteomyelitis.

The peroxide of hydrogen which I used was a 3.2-per-cent. solution, yielding fifteen times its volume of oxygen; but this strength was reduced to about 1.5 per cent., corresponding to about eight volumes of oxygen, by adding the fresh culture containing the microbe upon which I was experimenting. I have also experimented upon old cultures loaded with a large number of the spores of the bacillus anthracis. In all cases my experiments were made with a few cubic centimetres of culture in sterilized test-tubes, in order to obtain accurate results.

The destructive action of peroxide of hydrogen, even diluted in the above proportions, is almost instantaneous. After a contact of a few minutes, I have tried to cultivate the microbes which were submitted to the peroxide, but unsuccessfully, owing to the fact that the germs had been completely destroyed.

My next experiments were made on the hydrophobic virus in the following manner:

I mixed with sterilized water a small quantity of the medulla taken from a rabbit that had died of hydrophobia, and to this mixture added a small quantity of peroxide of hydrogen. Abundant effervescence took place, and, as soon as it ceased, having previously trephined a rabbit, I injected a large dose of the mixture under the dura mater. Slight effervescence immediately took place and lasted a few moments, but the animal was not more disturbed than when an injection of the ordinary virus is given. This rabbit is still alive, two months after the inoculation.

A second rabbit was inoculated with the same hydrophobic virus which had not been submitted to the action of the peroxide, and this animal died at the expiration of the eleventh day with the symptoms of hydrophobia.

I am now experimenting in the same manner upon the bacillus tuberculosis, and if I am not disappointed in my expectation. I will be able to impart to the profession some interesting results.

It is worthy of notice that water charged, under pressure, with fifteen times its volume of pure oxygen has not the antiseptic properties of peroxide of hydrogen. This is due to the fact that when the peroxide is decomposed nascent oxygen separates in that most active and potent of its conditions next to the condition, or allotropic form, known as ozone. Therefore it is not illogical to conclude that ozone is the active element of peroxide of hydrogen.

---

[1] Gaillard's Medical journal, March, 1889.

[2] The peroxide of hydrogen that I use is manufactured by Mr. Charles Marchand, of New York. This preparation is remarkable for its uniformity in strength, purity, and stability.

Although peroxide of hydrogen decomposes rapidly in the presence of organic substances, I have observed that its decomposition is checked to some extent by the addition of a sufficient quantity of glycerin; such a mixture, however, cannot be kept for a long time, owing to the slow but constant formation of secondary products having irritating properties.

Before concluding I wish to call attention to a new oxygenated compound, or rather ozonized compound, which has been recently discovered and called "glycozone" by Mr. Marchand.

This glycozone results from the reaction which takes place when glycerin is exposed to the action of ozone under pressure—one volume of glycerin with fifteen volumes of ozone produces glycozone.

By submitting the bacillus anthracis, pyocyaneus, prodigiosus, and megaterium to the action of glycozone, they were almost immediately destroyed.

I have observed that the action of glycozone upon the typhoid-fever bacillus, and some other germs, is much slower than the influence of peroxide of hydrogen.

In the dressing of wounds, ulcers, etc., the antiseptic influence of glycozone is rather slow if compared with that of peroxide of hydrogen, with which it may, however, be mixed at the time of using.

It has been demonstrated in Pasteur's laboratory that glycerin has no appreciable antiseptic influence upon the virus of hydrophobia; therefore I mixed the virus of hydrophobia with glycerin, and at the expiration of several weeks all the animals which I inoculated with this mixture died with the symptoms of hydrophobia.

On the contrary, when glycerin has been combined with ozone to form glycozone, the compound destroys the hydrophobic virus almost instantaneously.

Two months ago a rabbit was inoculated with the hydrophobic virus which had been submitted to the action of this new compound, and the animal is still alive.

I believe that the practitioner will meet with very satisfactory results with the use of peroxide of hydrogen, for the following reasons:

1. This chemical seems to have no injurious effect upon animal cells.

2. It has a very energetic destructive action upon vegetable cells—microbes.

3. It has no toxic properties; five cubic centimetres injected beneath the skin of a guinea-pig do not produce any serious result, and it is also harmless when given by the mouth.

As an immediate conclusion resulting from my experiments, my opinion is, that peroxide of hydrogen should be used in the treatment of diseases caused by germs, if the microbian element is directly accessible; and that it is particularly useful in the treatment of infectious diseases of the throat and mouth.

STUDIES IN THERAPEUTICS: BERBERIS AQUIFOLIUM.

BY JOHN AULDE, M.D.,

MEMBER OF THE AMERICAN MEDICAL ASSOCIATION, OF THE MEDICAL SOCIETY OF THE STATE OF PENNSYLVANIA, OF THE PHILADELPHIA COUNTY MEDICAL SOCIETY, ETC., PHILADELPHIA.

NOTWITHSTANDING the glowing reports which appeared more than ten years ago in such journals as the *Therapeutic Gazette*, relating to the valuable properties of this drug, but little progress has been made by it toward a permanent place in our materia medica. True, it is one of the important ingredients of the preparation known as Cascara Cordial, and enters into the composition of the compound syrup of red clover (Syr. Trifolium Compound), but at present it does not occupy a position which is well adapted to promote its general use. The literature upon this subject which I have lately examined (*Pharmacology of the Newer Materia Medica*, George S. Davis) appears to be more highly colored than the qualities of the drug warrant, although I have no doubt that excellent results followed its use in the hands of those who estimated its clinical position ten or more years ago. My own experience with the drug covers a period of several years in private and in dispensary practice, and my estimate will be based upon my own work and clinical observations; although, of course, I have been guided in its administration by the reports of others, to whom I desire to give proper credit, although I cannot mention their names, nor can I attempt to enter upon a discussion of the claims which have been put forward in regard to the action of the drug in the numerous classes of cases treated.

Inasmuch as this remedy is comparatively a new one to many younger practitioners, it is advisable to give some information in regard to the source and character, together with a brief reference to the physiological actions of the drug.

Berberis aquifolium (Pursh), variously known as holly-leaved barberry, mountain grape, and Oregon grape-root, belongs to the natural order Berberidaceæ, and is found on the Pacific slope of the United States. At least one of the active principles is an alkaloid, berberine, which exists in other plants also, and occurs in the form of an amorphous powder, soluble in hot water and alcohol, but insoluble in ether. In addition to this alkaloid the plant contains resins, and when the fluid extract is combined with water, the water should first be rendered alkaline, else the alkaloid will be precipitated. The dose of the fluid extract, which is the product I have investigated, ranges from 5 to 20, or even 30 drops three times daily ; and, as a rule, it is best dispensed in combination with a little glycerin or an alcoholic preparation. A discussion of berberine, the alkaloid, properly belongs to the study of Hydrastis canadensis.

Pharmacology.—The taste of preparations containing berberis alone is that of a simple bitter, but it is not especially disagreeable ; to the writer it resembles very much the taste of the bark of fresh elders, such as boys use in making whistles. It is far less objectionable than either nux vomica or cinchona preparations, and can readily be given to children. Taken into the mouth it has the effect of slightly increasing the flow of saliva, but small doses cause no burning sensation in the stomach. When ingested with food, or shortly after, the flow of gastric juice is augmented, if we may judge by the increased activity of the digestion under those conditions, and a stimulating effect appears to be produced throughout the alimentary tract. My impression is, that in some cases through its influence upon the intestinal glands, a more healthy condition is established, owing to the more rapid elimination of waste-products.

The character of the cases in which it is used with curative effect would lead to the supposition that berberis is an active agent in promoting tissue-change. This may possibly be due to the lack of actively poisonous properties, such, for example, as those that we find in nux vomica ; certainly the exhibition of moderately small doses produces effects which are extremely satisfactory in the treatment of numerous affections, and I am inclined to believe that these beneficial effects are largely due to the eliminative properties of the drug acting upon the liver and the kidneys, and to its stimulating action upon the glandular appendages of the intestine. Still, it cannot be regarded as a drug which has a depressing action upon the organism ; on the contrary, the general action of berberis, when taken for a considerable time (one or two weeks), is practically that of a tonic.

Its *antagonists* include astringents and remedies which depress the system or interfere with digestion. Its *synergists* may be said to embrace all drugs and remedial agents which improve the general tone, whether they accomplish this by a process of rebuilding, as iron and arsenic, or by causing the elimination of poisonous or diseased materials, as in the case of iodine and mercury.

Unlike nux vomica, cinchona, and simple bitters generally, berberis produces an effect upon the system which is, as a whole, excellent, although apparently not marked. After medicinal doses no changes occur in the circulation or in the temperature of the body. Respiration remains unchanged, and the general effect upon the muscular system appears to be that of a tonic. The beneficial effect upon the digestive system, the blood, and the secretions, is quite perceptible. If there is constipation the movements of the bowels become more regular, and, with appropriate regulation of the diet, the stools become of good consistence and color, an influence which the blood quickly feels. The consequences are that the complexion clears, muscular strength is augmented, and along with a slight increase in the activity of the urinary organs and the skin, berberis may be said to be an ideal alterative. That it is an important alterative, I have the best evidence ; but that it will take the place of others I doubt, although combinations can be made with berberis as an ingredient which will surpass many of the products in use at the present time. In looking at the alterative action we must not forget that a remedy, to be alterative, must act as a tonic ; and to act in this manner it must be laxative, diuretic, and diaphoretic—properties which are characteristic of the drug under consideration to a degree sufficient to warrant its more general use by members of the profession in general practice.

Therapeutics.—For convenience it is desirable to study the applications of the remedy in the treatment of disease by grouping the different affections in which the drug may be used with the expectation of obtaining good results. First upon the list should be indicated that class known as the " blood diseases," which includes syphilis and scrofula. In each of these diseases the remedy has been highly extolled, although I cannot speak from personal observation of its value in the former. With attention to diet and hygiene, and alternated with other drugs which may be classed as hæmatinies, I have seen remarkably good results follow the use of berberis in scrofulous disorders, and even in cases with a tendency toward scrofula. The general practitioner will, of course, understand that no one remedy is sufficient to overcome the diathesis in these cases, but I fully believe in the utility of berberis in restoring the functions to their normal condition.

In my experience, which has been comparatively limited, not having used the drug in more than twenty-five cases of various disorders, the best results have followed its use in the treatment of derangements of the alimentary tract, with or without constipation. The symptoms calling for its exhibition are very much the same as those which are so well known as indicative of indigestion, namely, coated tongue, fœtid breath, and a general feeling of malaise, with little or no appetite. The special indications, however, which I have thought demanded berberis, may be summarized as follows : Long-continued gastric and intestinal indigestion, not very severe, but occasionally lighted up by some indiscretion of diet or exposure to inclement weather, or over-exertion. The patient has become thin, but not emaciated, and does not suffer much inconvenience from constipation, although there may be slight rectal irritation from hæmorrhoids. If the patient be a woman all these symptoms will be more distinct than if a man, and in addition there may be some uterine trouble. This complication is very common about the climacteric, but it in no-wise forms a contraindication to the use of the drug. The following case will illustrate this fact more fully:

Mrs. S. is, for all practical purposes, an invalid, having been under treatment for about two years, and during three or four months she has been con-fined to her bed. She is now forty-two years old, and her eldest child is aged thirteen years. She has passed through the hands of four physicians during her illness. There is decided derangement of all the functions, and she has become very much depressed physically. Brooding night and day over her misfortunes has caused her to suffer occasionally from melancholy, and she thinks it would be im-possible to live had she not access to a bottle of medicine containing chloral and bromide, which her last physician prescribed for her. In order to avoid any complications which might arise from having two kinds of medicine, I scratched off the label from the bottle containing the anodyne mix-ture. As I did not purpose giving her any medi-cines of that nature I thought that that was the best method of "tapering off."

Beginning in the mouth, this patient had some derangement of the whole alimentary tract. She suffered from stomatitis, from dyspepsia, from fer-mentation of food in the intestines, from obstinate constipation, and from hæmorrhoids. In addition, there were more or less ovarian pain and tenderness, almost constant headache, and cardiac irritability.

The treatment consisted in regulating the diet, and prescribing remedies for the purpose of remov-ing the most conspicuous symptoms, and in the course of a few weeks she was sufficiently improved to be placed on tonic treatment, the most active constituent of which was fluid extract of berberis aquifolium, 20 drops three times daily.

This patient first came under observation during the past winter, and as a result of the final prescrip-tion, containing berberis, she gained so much that treatment was discontinued at the end of two months. Since then she has gone to housekeeping, and through patients whom she sends me from time to time I learn that she is quite as well as she has been at any time for many years.

Another patient, a woman of more than sixty years, who had long resided in a malarious section in the South, consulted me about the same time as the preceding case, and was placed on berberis after anti-malarial treatment had arrested the disease. A few weeks only were required to correct the ailments which had been brought about by the malarial complication.

A favorite formula with me is the following:

℞.—Fluid extract of berberis aqui-
    folium . . . . ⎱ of each, ½ ounce.
    Glycerin . . . . ⎰
    Tincture of prickly ash with Jamaica rum, 4 ounces.
    Dose, a tablespoonful in water after meals.

Both xanthoxylum and berberis possess valuable antiperiodic properties, and when we have to con-tend with complications the appropriate remedies will readily suggest themselves. Thus, when we have to deal with a torpid condition of the liver, podophyllum, or euonymus will be considered, while if there be constipation some preparation of aloes, or, preferably, cascara, will be indicated. When a diuretic influence is sought, small doses of hyoscy-amus may be added, and in cases of marked debility nux vomica will be the proper remedy. Occasion-ally it will be found that a special cardiac tonic is demanded, and in such cases strophanthus should be used. I recall a case of this character which occurred during my connection with the Medico-Chirurgical Hospital, which illustrates in a striking manner the value of the drug.

A drayman, aged sixty-one years, had suffered for a long time from general weakness and loss of appetite. He had been treated for nervous pros-tration, for senile heart, and for fatty degeneration of the heart, but no improvement had attended the efforts of his physicians. Upon examination I de-cided that he was suffering from the effects of tobacco-poisoning and from gastro-intestinal catarrh, and prescribed for him 5 drops of the tincture of stro-phanthus with 20 drops of the fluid extract of ber-beris aquifolium and a little syrup of rhubarb, to be taken after meals three times daily. In a week he was improving so rapidly that no change was made in the treatment.

Through the kindness of Messrs. Parke, Davis & Co. a quantity of the drug was placed at my com-mand in the dispensary, and was used with good results in a large number of cases.

The treatment of chronic rheumatism by the ex-hibition of the foregoing combination is in many cases rewarded by permanent relief, and it is also efficient in all glandular enlargements and in chronic hepatitis.

In the treatment of numerous skin affections, especially those of the scaly variety, along with appropriate diet and local measures, berberis will often prove effective when other approved methods of treatment fail to afford more than temporary relief.

By ridding the system of objectionable material, stimulating the activity of the glandular system and promoting digestion, berberis becomes a valuable aid in the treatment of various forms of phthisis, when the disease is not too far advanced. By re-lieving the congestion of the pelvic viscera, and keeping the bowels in a healthy condition, it answers a valuable purpose in the treatment of diseases incident to women, and with the addition of the tincture of prickly ash, there are few of such cases that will not be decidedly benefited by the use of berberis.

1910 ARCH STREET.

VAGINAL LITHOTOMY.

BY ROBERT REYBURN, M.D.,
PROFESSOR OF PHYSIOLOGY AND CLINICAL SURGERY IN THE MEDICAL
DEPARTMENT OF HOWARD UNIVERSITY, WASHINGTON, D. C.

ON May 5, 1888, I saw at my office, in consultation with Dr. Seifritz, Mrs. R., aged thirty-two years, white, and the mother of two children.

The patient had suffered for nearly two years before coming under the care of Dr. Seifritz from irritation of the urinary bladder and other symptoms which had been, by the several physicians who attended her, attributed to uterine disease.

Dr. Seifritz, on making a careful examination, had discovered a calculus in the bladder, and believing it to be of moderate size we determined to attempt its removal *per urethram.*

The patient was placed under the influence of chloroform and the urethra was fully dilated, so that the index finger could be introduced, and the bladder thoroughly explored. The calculus was readily found, and an attempt was made by long forceps to remove it from the bladder through the urethra, but it was too large to be removed in this way without great danger of lacerating the canal.

Dr. Bigelow's admirable apparatus for crushing and removing the stone not being at hand, I determined to remove it through the vagina. Introducing the forefinger of the left hand into the bladder through the urethra, the calculus could be plainly felt, and drawing it downward I pressed it firmly against the lower surface of the bladder, when I could feel it impinging upon the roof of the vagina. Keeping my forefinger pressed upon the calculus I made an incision about two inches in length through the roof of the vagina and coats of the bladder, directly upon the calculus, and thus removed it.

The operation was a simple one, and as easy as the opening of an ordinary abscess. Silver sutures were inserted so as to coapt accurately the edges of the wound, and were passed through the roof of the vagina, also including the walls of the bladder. After rallying from the operation the patient was sent to her home in a carriage.

The temperature on the day following the operation reached 102°, but after a few doses of antipyrin it fell to normal, and remained so.

The after-treatment consisted of washing out the bladder morning and evening with a one-per-cent. solution of boric acid.

For two weeks after the operation the patient suffered from incontinence of urine, due to the dilatation of the urethra, but this gradually lessened, and three weeks later the symptom had entirely disappeared. The sutures were removed on the twelfth day, and at that time the incision had entirely closed.

One month after the operation the patient was well, and has continued so.

The calculus was of the phosphatic variety, weighed 2 drachms and 20 grains, and measured one inch in its short diameter and one and a quarter inches in its long diameter.

Of course, it is hardly necessary to say that under ordinary circumstances the proper treatment of such a case would be litholapaxy. In a limited number of cases, however, the operation of vaginal lithotomy is useful, and is one of the easiest operations in surgery.

Professor E. L. Keyes[1] says:

"The operation is safe and successful. The mortality, according to Aveling's statistics, collected in 1864, is about three per cent.—one out of thirty-five cases. Vidal had thirty cases without a death, but complained that fistula often followed. Agnew credits forty-eight operations to American surgeons, with two deaths. In both these cases the stone was very large."

It will be seen, therefore, that the mortality of this operation is less than that of any of the other operations for stone.

The danger of the operation is the formation of a permanent vesico-vaginal fistula. My own belief is that this will rarely or never occur if the bladder is fairly healthy, and if irrigation with boric acid or other antiseptic is used.

APPENDICITIS PERFORATIS.

BY L. SCHOOLER, M.D.,
PROFESSOR OF THE PRINCIPLES AND PRACTICE OF SURGERY AND CLINICAL
SURGERY IN THE IOWA COLLEGE OF PHYSICIANS AND SURGEONS,
DES MOINES, IOWA.

APPENDICITIS is caused by foreign bodies or concretions of fæcal matter entering the appendix, the orifice of which is uniformly smaller than the canal itself. In health small portions of fæcal matter enter and escape from the appendix without causing irritation, and possibly foreign bodies, such as cherry-stones, seeds, etc., occasionally do the same, though the larger, firmer, and more irregular bodies are less likely to escape. When retained, they excite a catarrhal inflammation of the mucous membrane, which has the effect of still more tightly closing the only opening by which escape is possible. Suppuration and ulceration follow, and may cause perforation.

The symptoms of perforation are not always well defined. Those pertaining to the acute termination of the disease are the most distinct, and consist of sudden collapse, shock, or intense pain, with the sudden occurrence of all the symptoms usually present in violent forms of peritonitis. In this method of termination the pus is poured directly into the abdominal cavity. If there is chronic inflammation the symptoms will correspond to the

---

[1] International Encyclopædia of Surgery, vol. vi. p. 298.

character of the inflammation, and if there is burrowing of pus, as described by some authors, the
symptoms may be so obscure that great difficulty is
experienced in arriving at a conclusion as to the
exact origin of the inflammation.

While the latter method of termination has been
described, its occurrence is extremely doubtful. All
descriptions of the symptoms and progress are very
unsatisfactory, on account of the lack of positive
proof that pus burrows under the pelvic fascia.

The most frequent termination, or rather a process
which admits of a termination in the hands of the
surgeon, is the one in which the inflammation of the
tissues surrounding the appendix is of the constructive variety. In this variety a tumor can usually be
discovered in the right iliac region ; the appendix
is firmly attached to the abdominal parietes ; there
is circumscribed peritonitis ; the inflammation has
advanced before the suppuration, and the exudate
is abundant and completely encapsulates the collection of pus. In this form the appendix will be
found in the centre of the pus-cavity in a state of
either acute or gangrenous inflammation. There
will also be found a perforation midway between the
two extremities of the organ, and frequently, perhaps in one-half of all cases, the foreign body or
fæcal concretion may be found. Careful examinations in the future will undoubtedly greatly increase
the number of cases in which these bodies may be
found.

Great confusion exists with reference to all inflammations of the right iliac region, owing to the
indefinite or meaningless terms, *typhlitis, perityphlitis*, and that added by Musser, *paratyphlitis*. The
first is supposed to indicate an inflammation of the
cæcum, the second an inflammation of the connective tissue posterior to the appendix, and the third
an inflammation of the walls of the appendix. The
first is objectionable because meaningless—*cæcitis* is
more definite, and is anatomically correct. The
second, *perityphlitis*, is not applicable unless the
connective tissue exists, which is not admitted by
anatomists. The third, *paratyphlitis*, is used to
indicate an inflammation of the walls of the appendix, and were it not for the fact that the inflammation always has its origin in the interior, and
involves the mucous membrane, the term might be
of some value. In the present state of pathological
knowledge, and in view of the fact that the appendix is an organ subject to characteristic diseases,
a nomenclature based upon anatomical considerations is certainly preferable to the old terms that
have given rise to so much confusion, and have
confounded colitis and cæcitis with appendicitis.

When the collection of pus is small the difficulties
of diagnosis may be great, and in some instances
percussion may give increased resonance rather than
dulness. When the disease is chronic, there may
remain for a long time a small amount of pus, with
no tendency for the sac to rupture. In such cases
the collection may amount to a pint or more.

Even though the last method of termination is
greatly to be desired, it is not free from dangerous
complications. The originally circumscribed inflammation of the peritoneum may become general,
and if treatment is unduly postponed, obstruction
of the bowels may occur. The following case is
cited in illustration :

On September 8, 1888, I was requested by
Dr. Charles H. Plunket to see H. W., male, aged
eight years, who was said to be suffering from intestinal obstruction. I found him complaining of
paroxysmal attacks of pain, and occasionally vomiting small amounts of fluid. The pulse was 120,
and temperature normal. He was sleepless, though
morphine had been freely administered. The abdomen was tympanitic and countenance somewhat
anxious. Dr. Plunket's diagnosis was confirmed,
although the pain in the right iliac region caused a
suspicion of appendicitis—in fact, the history was
that the patient had returned from school three days
previously on account of pain in that region. The
abdomen was too much distended and tender to
permit of a very careful examination.

I saw him again on September 9th, when his condition was the same, except that there was general
peritonitis. I advised anæsthesia for the purpose of
diagnosis, which was consented to. A small tumor
was discovered in the right iliac region, and also
fulness on the left side, which was most apparent to
the touch *per rectum*.

Appendicitis, and general peritonitis, with obstruction, was diagnosed, and abdominal section
advised. I saw the patient again, September 10th,
when there was no change, except that he was more
exhausted than on the previous day.

Operation, September 11 : Chloroform being administered, an incision three inches in length was
made in the median line, which permitted a considerable quantity of fluid to escape. Two fingers
introduced into the cavity readily detected extensive
adhesions, and a small tumor at the site of the
appendix, adherent to the abdominal wall. Although
the manipulations were gentle, the wall of the sac
ruptured, and about two ounces of foul-smelling pus
escaped into the abdomen. The appendix was
found to be ruptured in the middle, and was at
once tied off. Further examination revealed firm,
adhesive bands just above the cæcum, causing complete obstruction. These were broken with the
fingers, and the ragged edges trimmed with scissors.
A similar condition was found at the sigmoid
flexure on the left side, and the same means were
adopted for the relief of the obstruction. When
these bands were severed there immediately escaped
from the rectum a large quantity of fluid fæcal matter,
which was estimated at thirty-two ounces, while the
escape of flatus was very free.

The small intestines were bound together throughout their entire extent, the inflammatory exudate

being abundant, but not firm. As there were no
evidences of further obstruction the intestines were
not disturbed. The cavity was thoroughly irrigated
with water at a temperature of 110° F., until, apparently, all pus was removed, a drainage-tube was
then inserted, and the wound closed. The discharge through the tube was slight, and had entirely
ceased at the end of forty-eight hours. The tube
was then removed, and the patient made a good
recovery.

Antiseptic precautions were taken at every step of
the procedure. In washing out the abdominal
cavity, water that had been boiled and filtered
three times was used.

The median incision in this case was certainly the
best, as it permitted a thorough exploration of the
abdominal cavity, and the easy manipulation of the
adhesive bands for the relief of the obstructions.
In cases without obstruction or other complications
an incision a little to the inner side of the prominence of the tumor is proper.

The rule applicable to other collections of pus is
also applicable to this disease, viz., early evacuation.
Aspiration has been favorably reported upon in some
cases, but in these there must have been some cause
other than a foreign body. No special after-treatment is required. If the entire abdominal cavity is
opened, as in the above case, thorough irrigation
and the insertion of a drainage-tube, preferably a
glass one, are imperative. No antiseptic should be
used in washing out the abdominal cavity.

If there is a tendency to gaseous distention of the
bowels a saline cathartic is admissible. Pain will
rarely be so intense as to require the use of opiates.

HOSPITAL NOTES.

*ALOPECIA AREATA—RHUS-POISONING—DOUBLE
SYPHILITIC INFECTION—SEBORRHŒIC
ECZEMA.*

*Abstract of a Clinical Lecture
delivered at the New York Post-Graduate Medical School.*

BY ROBERT W. TAYLOR, M.D.,
PROFESSOR OF DERMATOLOGY AND SYPHILOGRAPHY.

CASE I.—The first case to which Dr. Taylor directed
attention was one of alopecia of about a year's duration,
in a woman with good general health. The disease
formed a rather large heart-shaped patch on the occipital
region and the vertex, and two smaller ones on the
temporal region. The smaller spots had made their appearance during the last six months. The disease was
rather more extensive on the left than on the right side.

The lecturer said that in this disease there are usually
no prodromal symptoms, such as itching or anæsthesia.
After a round patch has formed, other patches develop
in the vicinity of the first, and then fuse together, often
resulting in a large denuded area. But, in this case,
there were little islets of apparently healthy hair left.
As the process goes on, the patch will undergo a very

perceptible atrophy, and the margins of such denuded
areas are sufficiently thickened to be detected by the
touch. Very often the entire scalp is ultimately involved
and sometimes every vestige of hair disappears from
the entire body. In these extreme cases, it is not uncommon to find also that the nails fall off.

The prognosis of these cases is a question of great
interest, and there are several points to be considered:
1. The general nutrition of the patient. Hairs are
epithelial structures, and their nutrition depends upon
that of the whole body.
2. The duration of the disease. If the duration has
been more than one year, the prognosis is not good;
and when it has lasted for from three to five years, absolute baldness is almost inevitable.
3. The amount of atrophy of the skin. There is a
peculiar color of the skin of these patches, not unlike
that of an old billiard-ball. When an examination of
the patch with a magnifying glass shows much atrophy,
the prognosis is bad; and when the follicles are decidedly funnel-shaped, there is no possibility of the
reproduction of the hair.

Dr. Taylor said that the nature of this disease has
been a "bone of contention" for many years. just at
present, the theory of its parasitic origin is popular, and
among those holding this view is von Schlen, who was
the first to proclaim it, and Dr. Robinson, of New York,
who claims that it is due to the development of some
peculiar micrococcus in the deep lymph-spaces, causing
so much inflammatory change that the hair-follicles
atrophy. The neuropathic theory supposes that it is due
to impaired innervation and consequent malnutrition of
the hair. Some are more conservative, and believe that
there are two distinct forms—one of parasitic and the
other of neuropathic origin. Dr. Taylor thinks the
neuropathic theory the most plausible one. Whatever
may be the opinion of its origin, the profession in
America is not yet quite prepared for the statement
made by a recent French writer in regard to "prophylaxis"; for, in this country, there are no observations
which would make us look upon the disease as in any
way contagious.

Treatment.—On the ground that it may possibly be a
parasitic disease, it is well to get rid of every nidus of
contagion, so the hair, if practicable, should be cropped,
the scalp thoroughly shampooed and cleansed, first with
alkaline washes and afterward with a 1-to-1000 or 1-to-2000
solution of bichloride of mercury. The following lotion
may be well rubbed into the scalp several times a day:

R.—Tincture of cantharides . . 1 ounce.
    Tincture of capsicum . . ½ "
    Water, sufficient to make . 8 ounces.—M.

Two drachms of cologne water may be added to this
mixture.
Later, it may be necessary to change the treatment,
for these cases are very obstinate. The scalp may be
blistered with cantharidal collodion, or with a mixture of
half an ounce of oil of mustard and two ounces of sweet
oil. Dr. Taylor said that he had tried electricity, but
had found it utterly useless. Cod-liver oil and other
tonics are often indicated.
Improvement will be shown by the appearance of
lanugo; but these will, in turn, often fall out.

CASE II.—This patient was an Italian laborer, who had an abundant vesiculo-bullous eruption on the back of the fingers and hands, but not in the inter-digital spaces. It was also abundant on the anterior and posterior aspects of the wrists, and about the penis and scrotum. It was evident that there was some local cause.

The patient had been working upon a railroad near New York, and, on questioning, the case was found to be one of poisoning by some species of poison-oak, which, even in midwinter, may give rise to such attacks of dermatitis. Dr. Taylor spoke of a very severe and persistent case of this kind which he had seen many years ago in the hospital, and which had been repro-duced upon the patient, and upon one of the orderlies, with the dried twigs of this hardy shrub.

Treatment.—The first essential in the treatment of all cases of inflammation of the skin, such as acne, eczema, rhus-poisoning, is to secure thorough cleanliness. It is not sufficient to plaster the affected part with an oint-ment. Patients with ivy-poisoning usually have much pain and burning, and to relieve these symptoms the parts should be soaked in hot water made alkaline with a little borax. This application is very soothing. After the soaking, apply absorbent cotton thoroughly saturated with lead-and-opium wash. After two or three days, a little carbolic acid may be added. The vesicles will soon begin to dry up and form crusts, and then the simple zinc ointment containing balsam of Peru and a little camphor for the pruritus, will be all that is re-quired.

CASE III—The next patient, an English woman, thirty-seven years of age, presented a history of unusual interest, on account of its rarity. Eleven years ago, there was an eruption on the body, followed by nocturnal headaches and slight alopecia. She is not definite as to the presence of a sore on the genitals. The eruption was followed by large ulcerating and serpiginous ulcers on the face, neck, and limbs, and by a syphilitic inflam-mation of the muscles of the right arm and leg, which crippled her for three years. This syphilitic process, which attacks the biceps, calf muscles, and the masseters, is a diffused inflammation of the connective tissue, and was first described by Notta. It causes an immobile contraction of the muscles, and is called syphilitic mus-cular contraction. The eruption left numerous large scars upon the body and extremities. Four years ago, she had a bubo in the right groin, which lasted four months. Seven months ago, she began to have pains in the arms and legs, and, five weeks later, an eruption appeared over the entire body, and still exists. About this time, headaches became severe, and there was much alopecia. She denies having had sexual intercourse for ten years until within about a year, but the hospital records show that, four years ago, she had a sore on the right labium minus. The present eruption first appeared as a papular and pustular syphilide, occurring even on the scars of the previous eruption. There is general glandular enlargement.

It is the rule to find only one attack of syphilis in a lifetime, but, like smallpox, measles, and various other infectious diseases, syphilis may occur more than once, although these exceptions are much more rare than in the other diseases mentioned. There are only about forty-four authentic cases of it on record, four of which were reported by Dr. Taylor. There have been, un-doubtedly, very many more, but they were not recog-nized, or, if recognized, not reported. With our im-proved methods of treating syphilis, a cure is possible, and a person once cured is liable to a second infection.

CASE IV.—A baby, five months old, next claimed attention for a seborrhœic eczema, which first appeared about one month ago, on the leg, and had the appear-ance of an ordinary chafe. This was powdered and washed, as usual, until it developed into a genuine eczema. The head is covered with greenish crusts, and the eruption on the neck is oozing and of a decided salmon-color. There is a patch on the buttocks, which, if left untreated, will spread to the popliteal region. There is not so much thickening as in the other forms of eczema, and it oozes a gummy, greasy secretion.

Treatment.—Cleanliness is, of course, all-important. Next to this comes the diet, which, in this case, has been condensed milk. Good cow's milk, properly sterilized in Arnold's sterilizer, should be substituted. No internal medicine is required. Locally, for such a delicate skin, resorcin is better than sulphur. To cleanse the parts after the application of the ointment, wipe them with a lotion composed of one part of bay-rum and three parts of water. The ointment most suitable for this case is as follows :

B.—Resorcin . . . . . . 20 grains.
Powdered starch } of each 2 drachms.
Oxide of zinc ointment } of each 2 drachms.
Petroleum ointment . . . ½ ounce.

The quantity of resorcin may be increased or dimin-ished according to the amount of stimulation produced.

MEDICAL PROGRESS.

Irrigation of the Intestine in Dysentery.—DR. H. A. FAIRBAIRN (*Brooklyn Medical Journal*, October, 1890) gives unqualified praise to the treatment of dysentery by irrigation of the large intestine. To be of use, the enemata should be large and repeated every two, three, or four hours. The quantity of water should be, for an adult, about three or four pints, at a temperature of from 100° to 105°. If possible, the water should be distilled, or at least boiled.

Dr. Fairbairn has not found it necessary to use any medicament in the water. As to the instrument used, he prefers a handball-syringe, believing that the pressure from a fountain-syringe is dangerous. The author also suggests that in chronic dysentery the walls of the bowel may be so much weakened that unless the pres-sure is very slight rupture may occur.

Medical Treatment of Fractures.—DR. DE VABONA Y GONZALEZ DEL VAILLE, of Havana, discusses, in a graduation thesis, the advantage of prescribing phos-phorus in various forms to patients suffering from frac-tures. He carried out a series of experiments on dogs and fowls, by breaking the femur by means of an osteo-clast and dressing the limb in splints. He then divided the animals into two groups, to the first group adminis-tering phosphorus, to the second no drugs being given.

The results were that the callus was more abundant in animals treated with phosphide of zinc than in those treated with phosphide of calcium, or in those to which no phosphorus was given.

These results were confirmed by observations in the surgical wards of a hospital, where it was found that patients with fractures who took from one-eighth to one-fourth grain of phosphide of zinc daily made exceptionally good and rapid recoveries. The only unpleasant effects produced by this treatment were, that one out of the eighteen patients on whom it was tried suffered from slight diarrhœa, and in another the pulse became slow and hard.—*Lancet*, September 27, 1890.

Ectopic Gestation Occurring Twice in the Same Patient.—

MR. G. ERNEST HERMAN (*British Medical Journal*, September 27, 1890) reports the case of a woman upon whom he operated for a ruptured ectopic gestation in January, 1887, removing the right tube. She again came under his care in May, 1890, with a clinical history and with physical signs that indicated a second ectopic pregnancy. The abdomen was opened by an incision in the line of the former one and the remaining tube was removed and found to contain a fœtus about one-third of an inch in length. The clinical history indicated that pregnancy had lasted about three months, and the size of the fœtus showed that it died at about the end of the first month.

Treatment of Labor delayed by Rigidity of the Cervix.—

DR. W. S. PLAYFAIR, in a discussion by the Section of Obstetrics of the British Medical Association, said that in 1874 he had directed attention to the value of chloral in labor. Since that time he has used it constantly with the best results and without trouble from rigidity of the cervix. Under the use of this agent the pains become longer, steadier, and more efficient, and the patient falls into a somnolent condition, dozing quietly between the pains, which are not lessened or annulled, as is so often the case when chloroform is used. More important than all, the wild stage of excitement which is so frequent in cases of rigid cervix is calmed, to the relief not only of the patient, but of the practitioner. It is not necessary to administer large doses; fifteen grains, repeated in twenty minutes, by either the mouth or the rectum, produce an effect that usually lasts for several hours. Possibly a third dose may be required, but never more. Another good effect of this drug is that when the expulsive stage is reached, the patient being already in a state of partial anæsthesia, much smaller quantities of an anæsthetic are required than would otherwise be the case.

Dr. Playfair also referred to the use of quinine, which, he said, acts rather as a general stimulant and promoter of vital energy than as an oxytocic, but that in cases of labor with feeble, ineffective pains in the first stage, one or two doses of fifteen grains often have a marked effect in strengthening the pains.

DR. ROBERT BELL said that the employment of strychnine in small doses for two or three weeks before labor has a wonderful effect in promoting uterine action. In labor delayed by rigidity of the cervix, although he has had good results from the use of chloral, he now uses tincture of gelsemium in from five- to ten-drop doses,

repeated at intervals of twenty minutes.—*British Medical Journal*, September 27, 1890.

The Treatment of Syphilis by Calomel Plasters.—M. QUIN-

QUAND (*Annales de Dermatologie et de Syphilographie*) recommends for the treatment of syphilis a plaster containing calomel and applied over the region of the spleen. The plaster is composed of diachylon plaster 300 parts, sublimed calomel 100 parts, castor oil 30 parts. The skin having been washed with soap, the plaster is spread on a piece of muslin about four inches square and applied. It is removed at the end of eight days, and after eight more days is again applied and is allowed to remain for the same length of time. This process is repeated indefinitely. In the case of patients who are engaged in manual labor, the plaster should be renewed in four or five days after being removed.

M. Quinquand has assured himself, by examinations of the urine, that mercury is absorbed when used in this way, and from it he has obtained as good results as from any other method of treatment. He considers this plan a particularly safe one, salivation being avoided, while a very small amount of mercury is constantly passing into the circulation.—*London Medical Recorder*, September, 1890.

Aristol in Blepharitis and Keratitis.—In the *Revue Géné-

rale et de Clinique et de Thérapeutique*, September 18, 1890, the following directions are given for the use of his new remedy in the affections named above. The advantages claimed for aristol are its lack of odor and its efficaciousness. Employed in the following ointment, it has been found useful both in papular and ulcerative keratitis and in ulcerative blepharitis :

R.—Aristol .   .   .   .   . 15 grains.
Vaseline ⎱ of each .   .   . 75 "   —M.
Lanolin ⎰

Apply a small portion of this daily to the surface which is affected. This ointment is not intended to displace the use of boric acid solutions, but may be employed in lieu of yellow precipitate.

Post-partum Hæmorrhage.—KÜSTNER (*Deutsche medi-

cinische Wochenschrift*) writes that hæmorrhage occurring immediately after delivery arises either from injuries or from the physiological utero-placental wound. Hæmorrhage from the laceration of the external genitals should be checked by compression or by sutures; hæmorrhage from laceration of the cervix should also be checked by sutures, drawing the uterus to the vulva by means of vulsellum forceps. To prevent atonic post-partum hæmorrhage, slow extraction of the child, besides waiting for the normal expulsion of the placenta, is recommended. Under no circumstances should attempts at placental expression be made during the physiological period of uterine relaxation (fifteen minutes), but we should wait until a number of spontaneous after-pains have occurred. To stop atonic hæmorrhage, Küstner recommends preparations of ergot, cornutin, heat, and bimanual irritation of the uterus. If these measures fail, he advises tamponing the uterus with iodoform gauze. The latter method he has used with satisfaction in eight cases, and believes that it is particularly useful when the source of the hæmorrhage cannot at once be determined. In such cases the entire genital tract should be tamponed.

In the *Journal of the American Medical Association*, June 12, 1890, an editorial writer calls attention to the value of the faradic current in the treatment of post-partum hæmorrhage, and doubts the necessity of tamponing the uterus in cases of doubtful diagnosis.— *Archives of Gynecology*, October, 1890.

Epsom Salt in the Treatment of Acute Dysentery.—SURGEON A. W. D. LEAHY, of India (*Lancet*, October 4, 1890), has treated 103 cases of acute dysentery by the administration of a saturated solution of sulphate of magnesium, to which was added a small quantity of dilute sulphuric acid. In the early stages of dysentery this treatment, the author has found, is remarkably efficient; the temperature falls, mucus and blood disappear from the stools, which become copious, fæculent, and bilious; tenesmus ceases; the skin acts well, and the patient sleeps after the first few doses. The more chronic the case, the less apparent are the advantages of the treatment.

The method is carried out as follows : A drachm of the saturated solution of the salt with ten drops of dilute sulphuric acid are given every one or two hours, until the stools become more copious, fæculent, and free from blood and mucus, the temperature falls, and the pain and tenesmus cease. When the stools are normal in character and are reduced to two or three in the twenty-four hours, an ordinary astringent mixture with opium or cannabis indica is usually all that is necessary to complete the cure.

The advantages of this method over the usual ipecacuanha treatment are, that it has no depressing effect; that it produces neither nausea nor vomiting; and that it quiets and soothes the patient. It probably prevents the formation of ulcers by its influence upon the hyperæmia of the bowel.

Solution for the Eczema of Dentition.—

  ℞.—Hydrochlorate of cocaine   2 grains.
     Bromide of potassium . 15 "
     Pure glycerin } of each . ½ ounce.—M.
     Distilled water }

Rub thoroughly together, and apply to the parts with the soft part of the finger. If insomnia is present, owing to the itching produced by the eruption, a teaspoonful of a syrup made up as follows will be found useful :

  ℞.—Bromide of potassium . 7 grains.
     Syrup of orange . . . 1 ounce.—M.

For the cure of the condition, an ointment composed of oxide of zinc, 1 drachm, and vaseline, 3 drachms, may often be employed with advantage.

An Ointment for Carbuncle.—

  ℞.—Ichthyol .   .   . 1 drachm.
     Camphorated lard . . ½ ounce.—M.

This salve is to be applied three times a day around the inflamed area, and if the surface has become broken the tissues are to be touched with nitrate of silver. It is said that the ichthyol diminishes pain, favors the resolution of the swelling, and aids in cicatrization.

Subcutaneous Injections of Water.—PROFESSOR SAHLI (*British Medical Journal*, September 20, 1890) practises the subcutaneous injection of water containing 0.73 per cent. of sodium chloride in the following conditions :

1. In uræmia complicating the course of either acute or chronic nephritis. In such cases the injection of a quart of the solution once or twice daily is, as a rule, followed by rapid abatement of the symptoms, particularly if, in addition, digitalis is administered.

2. In the typhoid state, in which frequently after the first injection delirium ceases, the pulse becomes stronger and fuller, and the tongue more moist.

3. In Asiatic cholera, cholera nostras, and infantile diarrhœa.

4. In poisoning, particularly by substances that are eliminated by the kidneys.

5. When the use of fluid by the mouth is objectionable, as in cases of perforation of the stomach or bowels, peritonitis, etc.

6. In acute anæmia from hæmorrhage.

Sahli believes these injections "wash out" the system by inducing profuse diuresis and the elimination of solids with the urine ; dilute the body-juices and the poisonous substances that may be contained therein ; furnish water to dehydrated tissues, and raise lowered blood-pressure by filling the vessels.

The injections are given by means of a hollow needle the size of a knitting-needle, antiseptic precautions being carefully observed. One quart of the solution can be injected in from five to fifteen minutes, and the best situation is the subcutaneous tissue of the abdomen.

Mixture for Diphtheria.—KOUZNETZOW recommends the following as a local treatment in diphtheria :

  ℞.—Concentrated alcoholic }
     solution of menthol   } of each 1½ drachms.
     Concentrated alcoholic }
     solution of naphthalin }
     Spirits of turpentine   } of each 3   "
     Glycerin   }

This is to be painted over the surface which is involved.—*Le Semaine Médicale.*

The Treatment of Hydrocele by Incision.— DR. SMIGRODSKI (*Bolnitchnaia Gazeta*, No. 12, 1890) reports fourteen cases of hydrocele treated by Volkmann's method. The ages of the patients varied between ten and sixty years. After incision the cavity of the tunica vaginalis was washed out with weak sublimate solution, the irrigation being continued during the dressing. In some cases the entire cavity was plugged with iodoform gauze, but, as a rule, small plugs of the gauze or fine drainage-tubes were inserted in the angles of the wound, the remainder of the incision being closed with both deep and superficial sutures. The plugs or drainage-tubes were removed in a few days, the sutures in from four to ten days. In the majority of cases primary union was secured, but where the walls of the sac were very thick the union was by granulation. As a rule, some swelling of the testicle on the side corresponding to the operation was observed. In one case a superficial abscess developed during convalescence, but all the cases were cured.—*Annals of Surgery*, October, 1890.

THE MEDICAL NEWS.

A WEEKLY JOURNAL
OF MEDICAL SCIENCE.

COMMUNICATIONS are invited from all parts of the world. Original articles contributed exclusively to THE MEDICAL NEWS will be liberally paid for upon publication. When necessary to elucidate the text, illustrations will be furnished without cost to the author.

Address the Editor: H. A. HARE, M.D.,
1004 WALNUT STREET,
PHILADELPHIA.

Subscription Price, including Postage.

PER ANNUM, IN ADVANCE . . . . $4.00.
SINGLE COPIES . . . .   10 CENTS.

Subscriptions may begin at any date. The safest mode of remittance is by bank check or postal money order, drawn to the order of the undersigned. When neither is accessible, remittances may be made, at the risk of the publishers, by forwarding in *registered* letters.

Address,   LEA BROTHERS & CO.,
NOS. 706 & 708 SANSOM STREET, .
PHILADELPHIA.

SATURDAY, OCTOBER 25, 1890.

THE ETIOLOGY OF TETANUS.

REFERRING again to the etiology of tetanus (see THE MEDICAL NEWS, October 18, 1890) the experiments of DR. E. O. SHAKESPEARE, of Philadelphia, are of considerable interest and importance. Although failing to discover tetanic microörganisms in the nervous system of tetanized animals, Dr. Shakespeare was able, by placing in contact with the central nervous system of healthy rabbits solutions of the spinal cords of tetanic cases, to produce in a short time the characteristic symptoms of the disease, while the subcutaneous injection of the same material proved absolutely innocuous. Further, the exclusion of the tetanogenous source by extirpating the infected sore or amputating the member in which it occurs, confirms the idea of a local activity with the manifestation of general influences from the elaboration of poisonous matters which circulate in the fluids. ·

Some observers are disposed to deny the infectious nature of tetanus, and consider the experimental form of the affection as not identical with the clinical variety. These differences between the experimental and clinical varieties are in the shorter period of incubation and more rapid course of the former, in the number of failures by inoculation, the lack of specificity of Nicoläier's

bacillus, and in the failure of the ordinary antiseptic measures to check the course of the affection. However, the period of incubation in the experimental form is short, probably because of the relatively large amount of the virus inoculated. The point of manifestation is not constant in either the clinical or the experimental variety, the muscles of the back of the neck and of the jaw being usually first affected in the former, while in the latter the muscles of the part inoculated are perhaps more often the seat of the first symptoms. The shorter duration of the course of the experimental form is also to be expected because the virulence of the virus is so marked that fatal results are induced the more quickly. The failures to induce the disease by inoculation are explicable by the complexity of conditions of the proper growth of the microörganism in the animal economy. The positive refutation of the objection that Nicoläier's germ is not specific is, perhaps, at the present unattained ; but the failure of the usual antiseptics in relation to the development of the affection simply bespeaks the great resistive power of the microbic cause to the action of the antiseptics. Nor should the fact of the occasional curative effect of operations upon nerves, as by cutting or excision, or stretching, lead to the conclusion that the fault exists in ·organic change of the nerve. The statement of its causation by violent emotional disturbances is to be regarded with considerable doubt, since, in the instances found in literature by MM. Verhoogen and Baert, the moral factor was invariably a·sociated with injury and the opportunity for the ordinary traumatic form to occur.

Following the course of discussion thus outlined, MM. Verhoogen and Baert finally come to these conclusions:

"That tetanus is a disease of an infectious nature, presenting all the ordinary characters of a zymotic affection, both in its genesis and in its general course and symptoms.

"That the disease is also of a specific nature, arising from the action of a microbic cause constantly found in cases of tetanus, capable of inducing tetanus, and no other form of infection, upon introduction into the organism."

In connection with the above. the recent efforts of Peyraud to establish a tolerance for tetanus infection is a matter of interest. Recognizing the similarity between the action of strychnine and the alkaloids isolated by Brieger, this investigator has attempted, by the introduction of strychnine into the economy by inoculation, to produce the effects of a vaccination, so to speak. Although the experiments as recorded would seem to be in general successful, the investigations leave much to be desired.

The local occurrence of the bacillus about the infected sore giving rise to general effects only secondarily, the question of the protective power of a previous attack of tetanus, and more especially the improbability of the identity of strychnine with the toxic principles evolved by the microörganisms in the animal economy, render extremely unlikely the existence of a protective influence by the vaccination of such vegetable alkaloid.

REVIEWS.

DICTIONARY OF PRACTICAL MEDICINE. Edited by J. K. FOWLER. Philadelphia: P. Blakiston, Son & Co., 1890.

THIS rather modest rival of Quain's larger book resembles it very closely indeed, not only in the general appearance of its pages, but also in the character of its articles. The names of the contributors are most of them so prominent that it is useless to attempt to mention any of them without mentioning all.

The editor has been fortunate in his selection of the authors, obtaining in nearly every case writers who are recognized as authorities on the subjects of which they treat. For those who do not care to purchase the much larger book of Quain, or who wish comparatively recent information concerning medical subjects in a somewhat narrow space, the book will certainly prove of value, and we heartily recommend it as one which will give a full return for the money invested in its purchase.

FAMILIAR FORMS OF NERVOUS DISEASE. By M. ALLEN STARR, M.D., PH.D. With illustrations, diagrams, and charts. New York: William Wood & Co., 1890.

IN writing this comparatively small book Dr. Starr has certainly done the average member of the medical profession a favor, for the title of the work shows that it is the "familiar forms of nervous disease" which are described; not the rare disorders, seldom met with, but the forms seen by the ordinary practitioner in every-day life. Further than this, the book is so copiously illustrated by practical cases that the information it contains is directly applicable to the general practitioner's needs. Dr. Starr's labors in this field have already placed him in the position of one of the leading neurologists of the country, and we can scarcely imagine that anyone can be found who would be better qualified to prepare such an aid to his medical brethren.

There are quite a large number of excellent prescriptions at the end of the book, and the illustrations are unusually clear in representing pictorially the statements in the text.

OINTMENTS AND OLEATES, ESPECIALLY IN DISEASES OF THE SKIN. By J. V. SHOEMAKER, A.M., M.D. Philadelphia and London: F. A. Davis, 1890.

THE labors of Dr. Shoemaker in the introduction of the preparations with which this book teems are so well known by those who are interested in skin diseases that it is only necessary for us to call the attention of our readers to the facts that the oleates have been received with very considerable professional favor on both sides of the Atlantic, and that the first edition of Dr. Shoemaker's book has been sufficiently popular to call for a second edition after the lapse of a few years.

To the physician who feels uncertain as to the best form in which to prescribe medicines by way of the skin the book will prove valuable owing to the many prescriptions and formulæ which dot its pages, while the copious index at the back materially aids in making the book a useful one.

THE PHARMACOLOGY OF THE NEWER MATERIA MEDICA, EMBRACING BOTANY, CHEMISTRY, PHARMACY, AND THE THERAPEUTICS OF NEW REMEDIES. Detroit: George S. Davis, 1890.

THIS series of contributions to our knowledge of the action of some of the drugs which have been introduced into medicine during the past few years, is very valuable to every physician who desires to keep pace with the medical progress of the day; and we doubt not that Mr. Davis's venture in its publication will be well received by the profession. Although the parts will appear every month, and their issuance will extend over at least two years, the subscription price for the entire work is but $2.00.

We cordially recommend the series to our readers, and do not know of another investment which will bring so much information for so little money.

MANUAL OF HYPODERMIC MEDICATION. By DRS. BOURNEVILLE AND BRICON. Edited by G. ARCHIE STOCKWELL, M.D. Detroit: George S. Davis, 1890.

THIS is a little book with which, in other forms, some of our readers are doubtless well acquainted. It is certainly useful in giving the physician accurate information in regard to the branch of therapeutics of which it treats, but we cannot quite agree with some of the American editor's notes. Thus, he says, in a foot-note, that "the theory that injections made into one part of the body will be absorbed more rapidly than in another is absurd, since, as all injections obtain their effect by absorption into the circulation, it is evident the differences that may arise from locality are frequently inappreciable." Every one knows that in some portions of the body absorption occurs much more rapidly than elsewhere, by reason of a close network of lymphatics or bloodvessels; so that an injection into the forearm is certainly absorbed much more rapidly than is one which is sent into the broad of the back. Most of the additions made by Dr. Stockwell add considerably to the value of the book, and he has certainly increased its usefulness by adapting it to Americans, and made it more serviceable than the mere translation of the book would be capable of being.

SOCIETY PROCEEDINGS.

AMERICAN RHINOLOGICAL ASSOCIATION.

Eighth Annual Meeting,
held in Louisville, Kentucky, October 6, 7, and 8, 1890.

The Association convened at the Galt House and was called to order by the President, Dr. Arthur B. Hobbs, of Atlanta, Ga., at 3 P.M., who then delivered the

ANNUAL ADDRESS.

He said that the Association had met to exchange views, to profit by one another's experience and observations, and for the advantages of social intercourse.

Conservatism should not be too rigidly adhered to in the advancement of science, and in order that one may be a successful specialist in any branch it is necessary that he should have had some experience in general practice, and have studied all the branches of medicine.

DR. EMMETT WELSH, of Grand Rapids, Michigan, contributed a paper entitled

THE RELATION OF NASO-PHARYNGEAL DISEASE TO CATARRH OF THE MIDDLE EAR,

in which he said that the relationship existing between naso-pharyngeal disease and catarrh of the middle ear is intimate and inseparable. The ear depends upon a healthy condition of the nares and naso-pharynx for the healthy performance of its functions, and patients presenting themselves for the treatment of ear-disease always give a history of catarrh of the nose and throat. Therefore it is essential not only to become familiar with the speculum, the rhinoscopic mirror, the catheter, Politzer bag, etc., but also to detect the diseases of the nares and naso-pharynx, their inflammations and obstructive lesions, and to understand the treatment of such conditions.

A spur upon the septum may excite tinnitus aurium, when, of course, treatment of the ear alone would be useless.

Repeated attacks of subacute otitis are often directly referable to some mechanical obstruction or inflammatory condition of the naso-pharynx, but how often do we find that this is not detected and that treatment is directed to the ear only. This is best illustrated by children who suffer from recurrent attacks of otitis media; when the membrana tympani is found inflamed, the child breathes with difficulty and chiefly through the mouth, and an adenomatous growth is discovered in the vault of the pharynx.

DR. T. H. STUCKY, of Louisville, Kentucky, then read a paper on

TONSILLAR HYPERTROPHY, ITS INFLUENCE ON NASAL AND AURAL INFLAMMATION,

in which he said that of all the diseases of the upper air-passages, he knew of none more conducive to the production of serious after-effects than tonsillar hypertrophy.

As to the etiology, very little is found in current literature. The exanthemata, diphtheria, and frequent attacks of pharyngitis seem to be etiological factors. Sex is not without some influence in producing the affection, for out of 1000 cases recorded by Morell Mackenzie, 670 were males and 327 females. Some cases follow acute attacks of quinsy, hereditary or acquired syphilis, granular pharyngitis, etc. As a rule, after the age of thirty years spontaneous cure takes place, it being the natural tendency of the gland to atrophy after this age.

It is immaterial whether the hypertrophy be due to the engorgement of the crypts, to either an active or passive hyperæmia, or to a true inflammatory hyperplasia, the indications for treatment are important.

Where there is simple hypertrophy due to an acute catarrhal inflammation, applications of the mild astringents have proven in the author's experience of little benefit.

The rheumatic character of acute tonsillitis or hypertrophy is accepted by many, and salicylate of sodium at the commencement of the attack, in ten-grain doses every hour or two until one drachm has been taken, will abort many attacks. On account of the nausea frequently produced by this drug Dr. Stucky has used the effervescent salicylate of lithium with equally satisfactory results, and without causing nausea.

For simple acute hypertrophy the treatment should be constitutional; locally, astringents may be used. When the tonsils are soft the galvano-cautery is very effective, a few deep cauterizations being made twice a week. The author has introduced the galvanic needle its full length into the tonsils at several points about one-eighth of an inch apart, with excellent results. The galvano-cautery snare, if there is a history of hæmorrhagic diathesis, is a valuable addition to the armamentarium of the rhinologist. Morell Mackenzie recommends the use of "London paste," applied once or twice a week over various parts of the organ; but this method Dr. Stucky considers slow and painful. Where the organ is fibrous, dense, and hard, tonsillectomy should be resorted to. While the danger from hæmorrhage is reduced to a minimum, the time, suffering, delays, and inconveniences which are overcome by ablation render it, in his judgment, the operation for speedy relief, and should always be performed if the hypertrophy is dense. The gallo-tannic gargle of Morell Mackenzie is an excellent application to check the bleeding. The cold wire snare is painful and slow, and will eventually be superseded by the galvano-cautery. If the uvula and soft palate remain relaxed after tonsillectomy and the use of astringents, amputate the uvula. The ear-symptoms, if acute, generally subside rapidly. After removing the tonsils, special attention should be directed to the condition of the nasal passages. If long-standing hypertrophies exist, remove them by the cautery or other means.

Simple inflation of the Eustachian tube by the method of Politzer or Valsalva will often relieve the patient after a few repetitions, but these methods should never be used unless the nasal passages as well as the vault of the pharynx have been thoroughly cleansed. If there is no marked change in the tympanum the method of Delstauch—massage—will prove of service.

SECOND DAY.—MORNING SESSION.

DR. E. R. LEWIS, of Indianapolis, Indiana, read a paper entitled

NASAL CAUTERIES.

He has discarded every form of caustic paste in the treatment of nasal hypertrophies. In the treatment of posterior hypertrophies, chromic acid can be easily and safely used by means of a guarded porte-caustique, and the practitioner who is not provided with the apparatus of a specialist and yet is called upon to treat nasal hypertrophies, will do well to use chromic acid in preference to any other caustic. Nitrate of silver is to be condemned in nasal treatment.

In Dr. Lewis's practice the galvano-cautery has taken the place of all other nasal cauteries. The galvano-cautery does its work neatly, aseptically, and, when properly used, painlessly and bloodlessly. For all nasal operations, except the removal of large growths by the loop, a small storage-battery is the most useful and convenient battery. The storage-battery in his office is kept constantly charged by four cells in the cellar beneath. It can be easily detached and taken out of the office and used for days without being re-charged. For the loop a larger or double battery is necessary, but even in that case the battery can easily be carried in the hand.

In the use of the galvano-cautery Dr. Lewis gave the following cautions:

1. Adopt preliminary treatment even if there is not much congestion or hyperæmia. The results are always more satisfactory after preliminary treatment of a few weeks, and the work to be done by the cautery can be better gauged.

2. Cauterize in the anterior portion and use the edge of the knife—not the flat surface—sinking it in as far as seems necessary and drawing it forward. It is best to keep the knife moving to prevent the tissues from sticking to it.

3. After the cauterization spray the parts thoroughly but gently with soothing solutions such as oil of vaseline, with a little eucalyptol in solution, followed by warmed Seiler's solution and finally oil of vaseline and eucalyptol. The oil may also be medicated with iodol.

4. Never cauterize both sides at one sitting.

5. Introduce the electrode while cold, apply it to the posterior part of the hypertrophy, then establish the circuit and draw the knife forward, the maximum heat having been determined by the rheostat. A bright-red heat gives the best results. Dr. Lewis never uses a black heat; a dull-red heat is apt to make the knife stick; a bright-red heat, even if inclining to white, seems the best. It must be remembered that the electrode is cooled by the secretions and tissues. The thumb should be removed from the button before withdrawing the electrode.

6. The parts should be treated gently for several days after cauterization, the secretions being removed with as little irritation as possible. If the other side is to be cauterized a week should be allowed to intervene, if possible, before doing it. The anterior part of the hypertrophy should be cauterized first, and the remaining portions at subsequent operations. Sometimes after a satisfactory cauterization of the anterior part, the posterior part can be easily removed with the snare, whereas it would have been very difficult to use the snare on the entire hypertrophy.

Apply cocaine by means of cotton on a probe, using a fresh ten-per-cent. solution. The cotton is gently applied to the anterior part of the swelling, held in position for a few seconds, then gently and slowly pushed back. Care is taken to have the sides and lower part of the hypertrophy well moistened by the solution, although the cotton must not be so saturated that the solution will run into the throat or drop on the floor of the meatus. In a few moments the parts are ready for the cautery. There is absolutely no pain; rarely is there a drop of blood; and after-pain is very unusual.

In a few cases slight nausea is felt at the close of the application of the cocaine, or during or after the use of the cautery. In such cases if a little wine or brandy is given the disagreeable feeling will pass off.

Dr. J. G. CARPENTER, of Stanford, Ky., followed with a paper on the

NASAL AND PHARYNGEAL MANIFESTATIONS OF SYPHILIS,

in which he said that primary syphilis, including the development of the chancre and infection of the adjacent glands, is infrequent in the nasal and pharyngeal chambers, though more frequent in the mouth and upon the lips; consequently it is the secondary form of syphilis and its sequelæ which chiefly concern the rhinologist.

The presence of the initial lesions of syphilis in the nasal or pharyngeal chambers causes swelling of the mucous membrane, pain, fever, infection of adjacent glands, and, in the nasal chambers, difficult nasal respiration.

Syphilitic rhinitis may result from heredity; the local lesions of secondary syphilis found in the upper air-passages may begin as a catarrhal inflammation, a rhinitis or pharyngitis, a local circumscribed erythema, or as a papular, pustular, or tubercular deposit. The epithelium of the mucous membrane rapidly becomes softened, disintegrated, and abraded, leaving one or several erosions that are quite painful and sensitive, and at first are bathed in a mucous secretion, which soon becomes muco-purulent or purulent as the ulcers enlarge and disintegrate.

In the treatment of syphilis of the nose and throat it is very important to arrest the disease as early as possible in order to prevent destruction of tissue and consequent deformity of the nose, palate, pharynx, and larynx. The anterior or posterior nares or Eustachian orifices may be occluded by adhesions.

The continuous use of mercury for from one to three years in small tonic doses, insufficient to produce tenderness of the gums, ptyalism, or relaxation of the bowels, is the most appropriate treatment for the permanent cure and eradication of the disease. The protiodide, the bichloride, and the biniodide of mercury stand at the head of mercurial preparations. External applications to the groins, axillæ, and thighs are adjuvants of the greatest importance in the treatment of syphilis.

The local treatment of syphilitic lesions of the naso-pharynx and larynx should consist in mild antiseptics and soothing applications to disinfect, soften, and wash away the morbid secretions and crusts.

For the treatment of the sequelæ of syphilis, such as caries, and necrosis of the bone and cartilage of the naso-pharynx and larynx, the same surgical rules hold good as in other localities, viz., to remove the dead bone, prevent further disintegration, and render the wound aseptic.

AFTERNOON SESSION.

DR. JOHN NORTH, of Toledo, Ohio, contributed a paper on

NASAL HYPERTROPHIES,

in which he said that the term nasal hypertrophy is frequently applied to every condition of the nasal mucous membrane in which there is thickening of the membrane and narrowing of the lumen of the nasal cavities, not dependent upon anatomical abnormalities or tumors.

DR. North divided hypertrophies into (1) chronic hyperæmia, (2) simple hypertrophy, (3) hypertrophy with hyperplasia, (4) hyperplasia, and (5) neoplasms.

In hyperæmia we have a superabundant supply of blood to the parts, dependent upon some derangement —paresis—of the vasomotor nervous system.

Simple hypertrophy is due to hyper-nutrition. There is no increase in the relative number of tissue-elements, but simply overgrowth of existing elements, dependent upon increased supply of nutrient pabulum.

Hypertrophy with hyperplasia may be due to hyper-nutrition from hyperæmia or congestion and inflammation produced by various causes.

Hyperplasia is caused by hyper-nutrition, congestion, and inflammation. In nasal hyperplasia there is no overgrowth of the tissue-elements. The increase in the thickness of the membrane is due to the organization of the products of inflammation thrown out from the vessels in the stage of congestion and exudation. Atrophy usually follows hyperplasia of the nasal mucous membrane.

Neoplasms usually appear upon the posterior part of the turbinated processes; the surfaces are rough and irregular.

In the treatment of true hypertrophy all that can be done by sprays of medicated vaseline is to cleanse the membrane and protect it from further irritation, permitting nature to cure the case. Prompt and permanent relief can be obtained by the removal of a small portion of the excessive growth. In these cases Dr. North prefers chromic acid, because it can be applied to a small portion of the membrane; and because it is circumscribed in its action, and the cicatricial tissue that it produces, continues to shrink for a considerable time. He finds the membrane in a better condition several months after the operation than it was at first. A spray of medicated vaseline should be used during the entire treatment.

In cases of hyperplasia the local application of iodine in vaseline is of the greatest importance. Neoplastic growths are easily removed by the snare, chromic acid, or electro-cautery. Constitutional treatment should never be neglected in any case.

DR. CARL H. VON KLEIN, of Dayton, Ohio, read a paper entitled

ADMINISTRATION OF MORPHINE BY THE NOSTRILS.

Dr. von Klein has administered morphine through the mucous membrane of the nose in more than one hundred cases with very satisfactory results. It is simply snuffed into the nasal chambers, and the dose is divided into two equal parts. He has found that this mode of administering morphine is the most satisfactory, and that the drug is more prompt in its action than when administered either by the mouth or hypodermically.

DR. A. B. THRASHER, of Cincinnati, Ohio, in a paper on

NASAL REFLEXES,

said that the multiplicity of symptoms attributed by modern rhinologists to nasal reflexes has caused not a little opprobrium to fall upon the specialist.

Among the affections attributed to intra-nasal lesions are: Asthma, hay-fever, cough, spasm of the glottis, gastralgia, dyspepsia, tumefaction and redness of the skin of the nose, œdema of the conjunctiva, conjunctivitis, photophobia, epiphora, asthenopia, glaucoma, scotoma, salivation, cardiac palpitation, disorders of smell, taste, hearing, and sight, huskiness of the voice and aphonia, exophthalmic goitre, rheumatic pains, vertigo, chorea, epilepsy, melancholia, agoraphobia, aprosexia, neurasthenia, migraine, cephalalgia, neuralgia, nocturnal enuresis, many uterine disorders, affections of the genito-urinary mucous membrane, etc.

Many of these affections are not true reflexes, but are caused by changes in blood-pressure, or by extension of inflammation by continuity of tissue. The specialist should carefully examine the nose, but he should also be a general physician and search the entire system for the often obscure *causus morbi*.

Dr. Thrasher reported two cases of salivation due to intra-nasal disease. He thought that in these cases the cause of the nasal reflex was twofold. Primarily, a diseased condition of the respiratory tract of the nose. Secondarily, an abnormal irritability of the central nerve-ganglia. This affection of the central nervous system may have been caused by repeated irritation of the intra-nasal tissues, or by some extra-nasal irritation.

In reflex diseases arising in the nose, vasomotor paresis, very different from active inflammation, is generally present, although it may be masked by acute inflammation.

The immediate exciting cause of the reflex may be a mechanical, chemical, or thermal irritant.

There is at times some difficulty in making the diagnosis, as the severity of the reflex is not in proportion to the amount of nasal disease. Sometimes the local application of cocaine will abolish the reflex; or again, it may be excited by the irritation of a nasal probe: but these means are not always to be relied upon.

As a rule, constitutional as well as local treatment must be instituted.

It is apparent that in these reflex disturbances the specialist should be broad in his ideas, not viewing the whole world through his nasal speculum, and not expecting to see all bodily ailments reflected in his rhinoscope.

THIRD DAY.—MORNING SESSION.

DR. R. S. KNODE, of Omaha, Nebraska, contributed a paper entitled

WHAT SHALL BE OUR EXCIPIENTS IN NASAL SPRAYS?

which elicited a spirited discussion.

The subject of

HAY-ASTHMA

also came up for general discussion, which was opened by DR. A. DE VILBISS, of Toledo, Ohio.

CORRESPONDENCE.

LONDON.

*The Opening of the Medical Session—Dr. Broadbent's
Address at Leeds—Dr. Barlow's Introductory
Address—The late Dr. Matthews
Duncan.*

To the Editor of THE MEDICAL NEWS.

SIR : The first of October has come and gone and brought with it the usual crop of introductory addresses of varying degrees of merit. In London, King's College, owing to building operations, was obliged to forego its "introductory." The provincial schools have of recent years fallen into the habit of summoning eminent men to deliver the time-honored oration, and this year Sir James Paget held forth at Liverpool, Sir Spencer Wells at Manchester, and Dr. Broadbent at Leeds. It is a matter of some difficulty nowadays for the lecturer to know whom he is supposed to be addressing, the new students, the old ones, or those who have already entered upon the active duties of their profession.

Sir Spencer Wells assumed that the latter formed the bulk of his audience, and delivered a weighty address on national sanitation, which of course gave him an opportunity to say a good word for cremation, of which he is one of the chief champions in England. Dr. Broadbent, on the other hand, addressed himself to the new students, and gave them much excellent advice. He began by expressing his dislike of the increase in the length of the curriculum, and thought that the old and shorter course had turned out excellent practitioners. Speaking of lectures, he said : " It is the fashion to decry lectures, but I will venture to say that there are very few courses of lectures which do not teach more than is found in books, and very few men who will not find something to learn from lectures after most careful reading. The subject is a living one in the lecturer's mind, and it will be set forth with greater emphasis of the important points than is possible in print; but if you really want to profit by a lecture you must have read up the subject so that it is familiar to your minds." Speaking of the importance of clinical work in the wards and of the familiarity with the physiognomy of disease thus to be obtained, he said : " Knowledge of this kind cannot be conveyed in books or imparted by a teacher. It is by the eye that you have to be guided when a case first comes before you, and you can see how important it is to have at once a clue to the nature of the malady. Books and lecturers can, it is true, tell you what to look for, but you must look for yourselves, and from the moment you enter the hospital you should

make it an object to fix in your minds the indications of disease apparent in the face. You should say to yourselves when you first see a case, ' Now, what is the matter with this man ?' and every time you see him later you should ask yourselves, ' Does he look better or worse ?' When you are in practice you will have to answer this question every day both to yourself and to the friends of the patient, and the confidence you inspire (and, indeed, your own usefulness) will greatly depend on the promptitude and justice of your answers. Perhaps the most valuable feature of the old apprenticeship system, now dead and buried, was, that observation of a patient's appearance and attention to what he said about himself were enforced."

Two other pieces of advice he gave to those about to become clinical clerks which they will certainly do well to bear in mind; one was that they should keep notes of all the cases under their own care, either a copy of the ward notes or an abstract of them, and the other was that they should read up in the text-books the disease illustrated by each case. There is no doubt that the chief cause of failure in students of the present day is their unwillingness to learn to think for themselves ; they want to be taught everything, and seem to believe that when they have taken the history and " present state" of the patient allotted to them they have done their share, and that the physician in charge of the case ought to do the rest.

Against this idea and the modern system of preparing for examinations Dr. Barlow raised his voice in his introductory address at University College, for whereas formerly, he said, it was only the stupid and the lazy who were crammed, now many feel themselves obliged to resort to cramming in order to get through their examination. Amongst the reasons for this change he thought perhaps that the teaching was not sufficiently catechetical, and he admitted that the standard of the examinations has been considerably raised ; but what he chiefly objected to was the modern system of allowing a man to pass his examination piecemeal. He felt very strongly that if a man was not able to pass in all the branches of his subject at the same time he ought to be rejected, and if it could be shown that the standard of the examinations was too high, this should be lowered. Like Dr. Broadbent, he disapproved of the old system of apprenticeship, and warned his hearers that medical education was yearly becoming more exacting, and the strife for competency and even livelihood more severe.

During the summer vacation the death of Dr. Matthews Duncan has deprived St. Bartholomew's Hospital, and, indeed, all London, of one of the foremost clinical teachers. He possessed in a high degree that essential quality of dogmatism, without which none can become a successful teacher. In private life he was, I believe, most genial, but in his work the uncompromising way in which he formed and adhered to his opinions often led people to think him harsh. The best bit of luck that ever happened to him was when, some fourteen years ago, he was passed over for the professorship of his own specialty in Edinburgh, for this left him free to accept the invitation which he received almost directly afterward to join the staff of St. Bartholomew's Hospital. This in itself was more than compensation for the disappointment he had just experienced, and he also at once stepped into the front rank of London consultants. He was for some years on the General Medical Council, but the qualities which stood him in such good stead in the lecture theatre and at the bedside were not so well appreciated there, and he must have felt that he had not the weight which his position in the profession might reasonably have entitled him to expect. His term of office at the hospital had nearly expired, and curiously enough amongst his papers was found a letter tendering his resignation and dated December, 1890. Speculation is rife as to who will be fortunate enough to be his successor, for the post of physician, accoucheur, and lecturer at St. Bartholomew's Hospital is one that anybody might be proud of.

LOUISVILLE.

To the Editor of THE MEDICAL NEWS,

SIR : The meetings of the American Rhinological and the Mississippi Valley Medical Associations, recently held in Louisville, were successful, both from a scientific as well as from a social standpoint.

Many able papers were read and on the evening of October 9th, Liederkranz Hall was filled to its utmost capacity with the laity and medical students, who came to hear Dr. John A. Wyeth's address on "The Medical Student." The address was an excellent one and was interspersed with numerous incidents of the author's career as a physician and surgeon. He read from manuscript, and used but few gestures, standing with his right hand in his trousers pocket, and holding his manuscript in his left hand. Dr. Wyeth is a very entertaining speaker, and his address was frequently interrupted by applause of the heartiest nature.

He said that he had passed through the varying experiences of a checkered career. He had, in accordance with the suggestion of the Litany, done those things which he should not have done, and had left undone those things which he should have done. He had been in many places where he had no business to be, but never in his life had he found himself in a position where he had so little business to be as in Louisville, trying to deliver an address to the best brains of the profession in the Mississippi Valley.

He further said that were he to launch forth with some pet problem in surgery, the obstetrician would find it convenient either to "talk shop" to anyone who would sit still for a minute under the infliction, or else walk out to the nearest instrument-maker and order a pair of forceps after his own model. The ophthalmologist would close his eyes and swear that the reader of the paper had a mental strabismus not amenable to any treatment except amputation of the head at the occipitoatloid articulation. The aurist would grow deaf to his enthusiasm, and the neurologists present might possibly forget themselves and speak to each other—an accident which has not so far occurred in the records of the New York profession. The practitioner in general medicine would surely grow weary, and all of the listeners might go to sleep, except the gynecologists—who never sleep. They might not find anything of special value in his theme, but the live gynecologist is not for a moment going to take his "weather eye" from the others of his group.

A few words relative to Dr. Wyeth's rather remarkable career may not be amiss. He came to Louisville about thirty years ago. He was eventually graduated, returned to his home and hung out his shingle. But somehow or other the people became very healthy, or else took their ills to some one else. The occasional "nigger" or two, with a "misery" in his chest or shaking with ague, would drop in on the new doctor, but that was all. Paying patients ignored his very existence.

He stood it for a time, and then, it is said, took to steamboating, a calling in which youth is no barrier to success. He followed a river-life for several years, just how many we are not able to ascertain, when the old "fever" returned and he wanted to be a doctor again. At that time he heard of the feats of surgery performed in New York, and thither he directed his steps. Again he matriculated, and again was graduated, this time with a view to follow surgery exclusively. Unlike his experience in Mississippi, he did not lack for patients in New York. Difficult cases of surgery in hospital and private practice became the rule instead of the exception with him. His fame began to spread, first in New York, then from city to city, until it became national—may we not say international? In the meantime he married the daughter of the famous Marion Sims, which also contributed to bring him into prominence. On Wednesday, October 9th, he returned to Louisville, the first time since he was graduated from the gloomy old building at Eighth and Chestnut Streets, thirty odd years ago. He left here a raw recruit in the ranks of the medical professsion; he returned as one of the most distinguished surgeons in the country.

Immediately after the conclusion of Dr. Wyeth's address, the visiting and local physicians attended a reception given in honor of the Association by Drs. D. W. Yandell and W. O. Roberts. Dr. Yandell's house was brilliantly illuminated for the occasion. The reception hours were from nine to twelve o'clock, and during this time there was an almost constant stream of visitors going and coming. The occasion was an enjoyable one, and every guest was pleased with the hospitable treatment received.

Dr. W. H. Wathen gave a formal dinner at his residence, in honor of Dr. Wyeth, at which the following gantlemen were present: Drs. W. P. King, of Kansas City ; R. Stansbury Sutton, of Pittsburg ; William Porter, of St. Louis ; John H. Rauch, of Chicago ; John H. Hollister, of Chicago ; Frank Woodbury, of Philadelphia ; George Hulbert, of St. Louis ; and E. S. McKee, of Cincinnati.

Dr. Wyeth demonstrated at the University of Louisville his operation of bloodless amputation at the hipjoint on a cadaver, after which Dr. J. W. Heddins performed Macewen's operation for the radical cure of hernia.

Dr. T. H. Stucky, of Louisville, banqueted the members of the American Rhinological Association.

The banquet tendered to the visiting physicians of the Mississippi Valley Medical Association was a very elaborate one. The tables were handsomely decorated for the occasion, and more than two hundred guests were present.

Dr. D. W. Yandell acted as toastmaster. In front of

his chair was a large bank of colored chrysanthemums, from which extended, on either side, through the centre of all the tables, a pathway of vines and flowers. Around the room each window was filled with potted plants and shrubs, while the tables themselves, with baskets of fruits, presented a most inviting appearance.

The first page of the *menu* was ornamented with a skull and cross-bones, flanked on either side by a hypodermic syringe and a scalpel.

While on such occasions men are liable to become "inebriated with the exuberance of their own verbosity," yet the responses to the various toasts at this banquet were very humorous and instructive. If outsiders had heard the speeches, we feel confident they would say that doctors, as a whole, are as good after-dinner speakers as are members of the bar or any other profession.

A word of praise, in conclusion, is due Dr. I. N. Bloom, Chairman of the Committee of Arrangements, for the clever and excellent manner in which he handled and placed the many guests, and looked after their comfort generally. It was not a small task by any means, but it was most gracefully and creditably performed.

MONTREAL.

To the Editor of The Medical News,

Sir : The importance of Montreal as a medical centre is indicated by the statement that it has a population of 240,000, contains four medical schools, three veterinary schools, and a school of pharmacy, three general hospitals, a women's hospital, and numerous homes and dispensaries available for medical teaching. The two lunatic asylums on the island do not as yet furnish regular clinical instruction.

The terrible catastrophe by fire at the St. Jean de Dieu Asylum is doubtless still fresh in the minds of the readers of The Medical News. The buildings have been rebuilt, and are again occupied, the management remaining in the hands of that wonderful woman, Sister Thérèse. The contract system, still in vogue, is held by many of the medical profession to be unsatisfactory. The Protestant Hospital for the Insane has recently been opened. It is on a fine site on the banks of the river, about three miles southwest of the city proper. The splendid new Victoria Hospital, at the base of the mountain, the munificent gift of two of our citizens, is progressing favorably, and it is expected will be completed within a year.

The medical schools opened on the first of October. The fifty-eighth session of the Medical Faculty of McGill University was opened by Dean Craik. His address was largely a retrospect of medical teaching in general, and at McGill in particular. In the teaching staff the principal changes are the retirement of the veteran surgeon, Fenwick, who is succeeded by Dr. T. G. Roddick, and the addition of Dr. James Bell to the chair of clinical surgery, as lecturer. Dr. Fenwick retires to the well-earned *otium cum dignitate* of the Emeriti staff after thirty years of active work in connection with the university. Two hundred and sixty-five students are already in attendance, of whom seventy are freshmen. The veterinary school, under Dr. McEachran, has been affiliated, and is now designated the Department of Comparative Medicine. The twentieth

session of the Medical Faculty of Bishop's College was opened without any formal address. Thirty students were enrolled. This faculty has just made arrangements for the admission of women, the only medical school in the Province which has done so, and several female students have taken advantage of the opportunity. Separate dissection-rooms and cloak-rooms are provided, but in most of the branches co-education goes on. At Victoria and Laval the instruction is in French, and at the first of these one hundred and eighty students are in attendance, while Laval has seventy-five. All attempts at amalgamation of these two schools have so far failed. Both are more or less thoroughly under Roman Catholic clerical domination, and the nursing in the Hotel Dieu and Nôtre Dame, the hospitals in which their clinical teaching is done, is by the nuns.

The Victoria school presents the curious anomaly of an essentially French and Catholic faculty affiliated with a Methodist university, viz., the Victoria of Coburg. The College of Pharmacy has opened its twenty-third session in a new and commodious building on Palace Street. The lectures here are duplicated in French and English. Both professors of materia medica are medical men. Sixty-five students attend.

Our medical societies also resumed their work with the beginning of October. At the last meeting of the Medico-Chirurgical Society Dr. Roddick showed a remarkable case of fragilitas ossium. The patient, a healthy and wellformed lad as to trunk, upper extremities, and head, of thirteen years, had already suffered *twenty-eight* fractures of the lower extremities: nine of the left thigh, fifteen of the right, and two of each leg. The first occurred at the age of eighteen months. The boy was one of several children, the rest of whom showed no abnormality. The family history also was good. The little fellow did not suffer much pain, and had become so accustomed to the accidents that latterly he had applied his splints himself without medical aid. The limbs were much distorted and worse than useless, the right femur being ununited. He drags himself around on the buttocks by means of his hands. Dr. Roddick has decided to amputate.

Among the pathological specimens presented the same evening, was one showing bacillary tubercle on the cardiac valves, from a case of general tuberculosis in an infant. Dr. Johnston, the pathologist, stated that this condition was very rare.

Dr. T. E. D. d'Orsennens, the *doyen* of the Montreal School of Medicine and Surgery, and of the profession of the city, is to be banqueted at the St. Lawrence Hall on the evening of the 16th inst., on the occasion of his jubilee of medical practice. It will be an interesting event, as the fatherly Professor of Obstetrics is held in great esteem, alike by his French and English *confrères*.

BOSTON.

To the Editor of The Medical News,

Sir : Since the last letter from Boston a few changes that may be of interest to your readers have occurred. The City Hospital has now grown to large dimensions, having had 6715 in-patients and 13,605 out-patients during the year 1889. This growth has necessitated the building of a new surgical wing and a department for infectious diseases, and the addition of three surgeons to the staff. Presumably the three out-patient surgeons will be appointed to the house-staff. The only changes as yet announced, however, are that Dr. Burrell has gone into the house, and that Dr. Munks has been appointed to the out-patient service. The contagious-disease department is an isolated building with its own set of servants, nurses, house pupils, and physicians. The latter are drawn in turn from the general staff for short periods of service, during which time they do no other work in the hospital. Excellent rules to guard against the danger of those on service carrying contagion have been adopted.

. Several changes have also been made in the dispensary staff. A large number of patients are treated in the dispensary, but its great value in the education of the younger physicians does not seem to be appreciated. During last year there were 24,456 out-patients and 15,122 district patients treated. Curiously enough, the medical school makes but little use of this large amount of material for teaching purposes, presumably because the staff are supposed to be young men. In reality few are under thirty, and the average age is about forty years.

The triennial catalogue of the Massachusetts Medical Society shows a total of 1587 active members, of whom only about thirty-four are women. One-half of the women practise in Boston, while the city directory gives about 140 women in the list of physicians. No conclusion as to the quality as a whole of the women doctors can be drawn from these figures, since many of the most prominent have not joined the State Society.

The Medical Library is still in its old building, and probably will be for some time to come. A report just issued gives $29,263 as the assets of the library, $5371 as the income, and $4711 as the expenditure.

The Medical Department of Harvard University appears to be in a flourishing condition, the new students considerably outnumbering those of former years. The new laboratory, now approaching completion, is three stories high and sixty feet long, extending to the east of the main building. The basement is given up to store and animal rooms, the latter being large, light, and well ventilated. The ground floor is devoted to the bacteriological department; it has a large general workroom and special rooms and closets for coats, glassware, thermostats, sterilizing apparatus, library, chemical work, etc., besides a room for the instructor and four smaller ones for special workers. The old quarters in the main building are to be retained for undergraduates. The two upper stories are divided into rooms for the pathological department and photography.

THE MEDICAL SOCIETY OF VIRGINIA.

To the Editor of THE MEDICAL NEWS,

SIR: With your kind permission I would like to correct a few errors in the reported abstract of my remarks before the Medical Society of Virginia, and which are found on page 349 of THE MEDICAL NEWS. I am reported as saying that puerperal malarial fever is a common complication or sequel of labor, and that it is often followed by rheumatism.

The tenor of my remarks was that malarial fever did complicate the puerperal state in certain cases, but I did not mean to say that it did so frequently. In an illustrative case of puerperal malarial fever which I narrated, I mentioned that *acute articular rheumatism* followed that fever, and I further stated that I had occasionally seen acute rheumatism as a complication of the puerperal state. In regard to the removal of the uterine appendages, I insisted that they should be ablated only when restoration to health could be accomplished in all probability by no other procedure. My remarks in reference to ectopic gestation were also misapprehended, possibly by my want of lucidity. I did not say that Mr. Tait had confounded *hæmatocele* and *hæmatoma* with extra-uterine pregnancy. I stated that Mr. Tait in discussing the relations of tubal pregnancy to hæmatocele did not distinguish between a free effusion of blood into the peritoneal cavity and retro-uterine hæmatocele in the true signification of the term, and consequenttly introduced elements 'of confusion; and further, that an escape of blood into the connective tissue of the broad ligaments should not be called *extra-peritoneal hæmatocele*, but *hæmatoma*. Very respectfully,

GEORGE TUCKER HARRISON, M.D.

NEWS ITEMS.

Diphtheria in Connecticut.—At Taftville, Conn., a village of French-Canadians, who work in the cotton-mills in or near that town, diphtheria has been allowed to spread by very imperfect sanitation. The disease was not known to exist in the place in the early summer, but appeared about three months ago, and it is reported that not less than fifty cases, with many deaths, have occurred. The habits of the villagers are secretive and opposed to ordinary sanitary regulations. Moreover, they dwell in large tenements, and are very much crowded. The same vehicles that are used at funerals are used for social purposes, and are not disinfected. Very few infected articles have been destroyed. One man, who lost four of his children by the disease, was in the habit of peddling milk from house to house during the time that his children were ill with the disease. In one house the health officer found the bodies of three small children, victims of diphtheria, upon a single bed. In another house, a child was sick with the disease, while five other children of the family were attending the village school. In adjacent villages a few cases of diphtheria have been observed, and were traced to the epidemic in Taftville.

The Loofah Bandage-material.—A writer in the *Chemist and Druggist* says that possibly the most important application of the "loofah," or towel-gourd of Egypt, will be in the manufacture of surgical bandage-stuffs. Bandages made of this material are already offered for use. In Germany soles for slippers are made from the loofah, and it is claimed that these soles are extremely elastic and are washable; they are constantly dry, and will keep the feet cool in summer and warm in winter. The loofah also makes an admirable undercloth for the saddle, as it rapidly absorbs moisture.

Mississippi Valley Medical Association.—The meeting of the Mississippi Valley Medical Association at Louisville, on October 8th, 9th, and 10th, was the most numerously attended and successful of the sixteen meetings of the Association. There were more than eighty papers on the programme, which was completed on the third day by a rigid observance of the limit-rule in reading papers and in discussion. The only thing which marred the occasion was the illness of the President, Dr. Joseph M. Matthews, of Louisville. He received a wound several weeks ago which resulted in blood-poisoning, and, although his condition was much improved, he was able to preside at but few of the sessions. He worked hard during the summer for the success of the meeting, and was keenly disappointed that he was prevented to a great extent from participation in its scientific and social pleasures. An entertainment at the Blind Asylum, for the visiting ladies, was highly appreciated by those so fortunate as to attend. The ladies' reception at the Galt House brought forth the beauty and chivalry of the Falls City in hosts, and more than one bachelor doctor left his heart or a part of it behind him. This was followed by a banquet to two hundred and forty guests at the Galt House, from which the last stragglers found their way some time before daylight in the morning.

The Southern Surgical and Gynecological Association.— This Association will hold its annual meeting at Atlanta, Ga., on November 11, 12, and 13, 1890, under the presidency of Dr. George J. Engelmann, of St. Louis. From the preliminary programme which has been issued, as well as the standing of the Association, there will undoubtedly be an unusually interesting meeting held, and members of the profession who can manage to be present, and who are interested in these branches of medicine, will be amply repaid for the trouble of going to Atlanta.

Obituary.—DR. MONTROSE A. PALLEN, of New York, died October 1st, aged fifty-four years. He was a native of Vicksburg, Miss., and was educated for the priesthood in the Catholic Church. He preferred medicine, however, and was graduated in 1856 by the medical department of the St. Louis University. During the late war he was medical director in the Confederate army, under General Hardee, and filled other important medical positions. About sixteen years ago he removed from St. Louis to New York to take the chair of gynecology in the University Medical School. For the past four years Dr. Pallen was compelled to abandon the more active parts of his professional pursuits, on account of frequently recurring attacks of angina pectoris, but acted as resident physician to the Albemarle Hotel, where he lived a retired life, and where his death occurred. Dr. Pallen had travelled extensively, and was a highly cultivated and an exceptionally generous man.

—— DR. PETER HOOD, a highly-honored London practitioner, died recently in his eighty-second year. He is said to have been one of the reformers who stayed the hand of phlebotomy, especially in diseases of children, early in the present century. His writings were much sought after at one time, his book on gout and rheumatism having passed through three editions. He advocated the treatment of cancer by means of testa preparata, or oyster-shell, for the purpose of superinducing a premature calcification of the nutrient and involved arteries of the invaded tissues, a method of treatment that was practised to a limited extent in this country.

OFFICIAL LIST OF CHANGES IN THE STATIONS AND DUTIES OF THE MEDICAL CORPS OF THE U. S. NAVY FOR THE TWO WEEKS ENDING OCTOBER 18, 1890.

BRAISTED, WILLIAM C., Detroit, Michigan.—Appointed an Assistant Surgeon in the U. S. Navy.

WALES, P. S., *Medical Director.*—Detached from temporary duty as a member of the Medical Examining Board.

AMES. H. E., *Passed Assistant Surgeon.*— Detached from temporary duty as a member of the Medical Examining Board.

HERNDON, C. G., *Surgeon.*—Ordered to Naval Hospital, New York.

PERSONS, R. C., *Surgeon.*—Detached from Naval Hospital, New York, and await orders.

SCOTT. H. B., *Passed Assistant Surgeon.*—Ordered before the Retiring Board.

PRICE, A. F., *Surgeon.*—Detached from Naval Dispensary, Washington, D. C.

ANDERSON, FRANK, *Passed Assistant Surgeon.*—Ordered to Naval Dispensary, Washington, D. C.

WHITE, C. H., *Medical Inspector.*—Ordered to hold himself in readiness for duty on the U. S. S. "San Francisco."

BRAISTED, WILLIAM C., *Assistant Surgeon.*—Ordered to the Army and Naval Hospital, Hot Springs, Ark.

SPRATLING, L. W., *Assistant Surgeon.*—Ordered to hold himself in readiness for orders to the U. S. S. "San Francisco."

SIEGFRIED, C. A., *Surgeon.*—Ordered to the U. S. Training-ship " New Hampshire."

BLACKWOOD, N. P., *Assistant Surgeon.*—Detached from duty in the Bureau of Medicine and Surgery, and granted leave of absence.

STONE, L. H., *Assistant Surgeon.*— Detached from the U. S. S. " New Hampshire," and wait orders.

EDGAR, JOHN M., *Passed Assistant Surgeon.*—Ordered to hold himself in readiness for duty on the U. S. S. "San Francisco."

GARDNER, J. E., *Passed Assistant Surgeon.*—Detached from the "Albatross," and wait orders.

BRIGHT, GEORGE A., *Surgeon.*— Detached from temporary duty at the Naval Academy, and placed on waiting orders.

AYRES, J. G., *Surgeon.*—Detached from temporary duty at the Naval Academy, and placed on waiting orders.

LUMSDEN, GEORGE P., *Passed Assistant Surgeon.*—Detached from the U. S. S. " Boston," and granted three months' leave.

AUZAL, E. W., *Passed Assistant Surgeon.*—Detached from the Naval Academy, and ordered to the U. S. S. " Boston."

SMITH, HOWARD, *Surgeon.*—Ordered to appear before the Retiring Board at Mare Island, Cal.

OFFICIAL LIST OF CHANGES OF STATIONS AND DUTIES OF MEDICAL OFFICERS OF THE U. S. MARINE-HOSPITAL SERVICE, FROM SEPTEMBER 8 TO OCTOBER 4, 1890.

HUTTON, W. H. H., *Surgeon.*—Detailed as Chairman of Board of Examiners, October 2, 1890.

LONG, W. H., *Surgeon.*—Detailed as a member of Board of Examiners, October 2, 1890.

PURVIANCE, GEORGE, *Surgeon.*—Granted leave of absence for thirty days, September 10, 1890.

GODFREY, JOHN, *Surgeon.*—Detailed as Recorder of Board of Examiners, October 2, 1890.

WHEELER, W. A.. *Passed Assistant Surgeon.*—To proceed to New Orleans, La., for temporary duty, October 3, 1890.

BANKS, C. E, *Passed Assistant Surgeon.*—Granted leave of absence for twenty days, October 3, 1890.

AMES, R. P. M., *Passed Assistant Surgeon.*—To proceed to New Orleans, La., for duty, September 13, 1890.

PETTUS, W. J., *Passed Assistant Surgeon.*—To proceed to Vineyard Haven, Mass., for temporary duty, October 1, 1890.

HUSSEY, S. H., *Assistant Surgeon.*—To proceed to New Orleans, La., for temporary duty, September 19, 1890. To proceed to Norfolk, Va., for temporary duty, October 3, 1890.

WERTENBAKER, C. P., *Assistant Surgeon.*—Granted leave of absence for twenty days, September 12, 1890.

PERRY, J. C., *Assistant Surgeon.*—Upon expiration of leave, to rejoin station at Mobile, Ala., September 29, 1890.

YOUNG, G. B., *Assistant Surgeon.*—To proceed to Memphis, Tenn., for temporary duty, September 13, 1890. To rejoin station, St. Louis, Mo., when relieved at Memphis, Tenn., October 3, 1890.

THE MEDICAL NEWS.

A WEEKLY JOURNAL OF MEDICAL SCIENCE.

Vol. LVII.   Saturday, November 1, 1890.   No. 18.

ORIGINAL LECTURES.

MACEWEN'S OPERATION FOR HERNIA—EXCISION OF A BUBO—WHITEHEAD'S OPERATION FOR HÆMORRHOIDS.

A Clinical Lecture,
delivered at St. Luke's Hospital, New York.

BY B. FARQUHAR CURTIS, M.D.,
ATTENDING SURGEON.

GENTLEMEN: This patient, who is a single man, forty-three years of age, first noticed a tumor in the left groin about twelve years ago, after a severe muscular effort. It grew to the size of a hen's egg, and then remained stationary for five years, when another muscular strain was immediately followed by the appearance of a similar tumor in the right groin. These tumors increased until they formed a mass about the size of a man's head. These large masses on examination proved to be double, oblique, reducible inguinal herniæ, and in March, 1889, the hernia on the right side was operated upon by the old method of simply dissecting out the sac, tying it high up, and leaving the pillars of the ring unsutured, to unite by adhesion, and closing the wound. In May of the same year, another surgeon operated on the left side by Dr. McBurney's method, and the patient remained in the hospital for a considerable time afterward. During this time he came under my care, and as his scrotum was exceedingly redundant, I amputated a portion of it, in August, and he was soon afterward discharged. Two months later, he tells us, both herniæ returned, *i. e.*, six months after the McBurney operation and eight months after the old operation, and he has been unable to wear a truss. He is naturally of a lax fibre, and is not a favorable subject for such operations; but he is extremely anxious to have something further done, particularly on the side where McBurney's operation was performed. Unfortunately, this is by far the most difficult side to operate on, owing to the matting together of the parts by cicatricial tissue, but I have decided to make the attempt, and shall perform the Macewen operation.

In this operation, as you know, the sac is exposed and if possible, dissected out without being opened. It is then doubled upon itself by means of a catgut suture passed through it, and is returned into the abdominal ring so as to make a mass between the fibrous tissues and the peritoneum. This mass is supposed to act as a pad, closing the internal ring. The two pillars of the ring are brought together by a peculiar form of suture to be hereafter described.

Having exposed the sac, you notice that I begin the dissection at its neck, as this is the part which is most easily recognized and most readily reached. The only serious danger is from injury to the cord; but by care-fully tearing through the soft parts with the fingers or forceps this danger, as well as the amount of bleeding, is reduced to a minimum. The abdominal ring is large enough to admit three fingers, and we must first insert a sponge into the ring to prevent the descent of the intestine. It is well to avoid frequent sponging of the parts, as this imparts to all the tissues a uniform red color, and greatly increases the difficulty of distinguishing between them.

Macewen's suture is first passed through the conjoined tendon on the inner side in a direction almost parallel with its fibres, entering about one inch above the pubic bone and emerging half an inch below. This gives a loop half an inch long, which includes the conjoined tendon. Each end of the silk is then passed through the external pillar at points opposite to the insertions of the suture in the conjoined tendon. In this way the two pillars of the ring are brought together and made to overlap slightly. This method of suturing the pillars I consider the best yet devised, and I think that it, rather than the plan of rolling up the sac so as to make it plug the canal, is the essential feature of Macewen's operation. The plug is of very doubtful efficacy.

I propose to modify the operation in this case by separating the cord and having it held to one side during the passage of the suture, so that the pillars are brought together from the pubic bone upward, and the cord is thus made to pass through the upper instead of the lower angle of the wound. This plan, I believe, is of Italian origin, and was suggested by the fact that excellent results are obtained when castration is added to the operation for radical cure, allowing complete closure of the external ring. Whether equally good results can be obtained by simply displacing the cord, is as yet uncertain. In this case as the ring is very large, I shall pass a second mattress suture half an inch higher than the first, but otherwise similar to it. The sutures should not exactly follow the direction of the longitudinal fibres, because they would cut completely through, and even with this precaution they cut considerably. As a rule, these herniotomy wounds do best when a drainage-tube is inserted for a few days, but notwithstanding the size of the wounds and the amount of laceration to which the tissues are subjected, they generally heal very kindly. It is interesting to note that there is rarely any complication, such as hæmatocele, orchitis, or epididymitis.

The operation is now completed. The sac was very adherent to the ring, and at the posterior portion of the neck required a very difficult and tedious dissection, during which it was torn, necessitating a complete removal of the sac, and thus modifying the Macewen method. The large opening in the peritoneum at the neck of the sac was brought together with a continuous catgut suture, taking care to bring the peritoneal surfaces into apposition; then the remains of the sac were cut off, and the pillars of the ring united.

As regards the general question of the treatment of hernia by operation, I would say that a reducible hernia which is easily retained by a truss is better without operation ; for the best statistics by all methods do not give more than fifty per cent. of permanent cures. There have been much higher percentages claimed for special methods by their authors or chief advocates, but it is suggestive that other operators cannot secure equally good results.

In this patient we shall make use of dressings which have been simply sterilized by steam, for after the previous operations the usual antiseptic dressings gave rise to a very troublesome eczema.

EXCISION OF A BUBO.

The next case which I present to you is that of a single man, twenty-four years of age, who comes to us with a mass of enlarged glands in the right groin. The only history of venereal trouble is that of an uncomplicated gonorrhœa three years ago ; nor is there any history of a traumatism which would be likely to lead to such a condition. The etiology then, is obscure, but no more so than is often observed in the case of adenitis in other situations.

The present swelling was first noticed twelve days ago, and was followed by pain and redness of the skin. At present the mass extends half an inch below and two inches above Poupart's ligament, and in its longest diameter, which is parallel to Poupart's ligament, it is about three inches in length. There is an indistinct sense of fluctuation in the middle portion, and it is probable that some suppuration has already taken place ; but in spite of this I think we can remove the entire mass and secure primary union. Such a result is much to be desired, for, you all know, that when these glands are allowed to go on to suppuration without removal, the process of healing is exceedingly tedious. Excision of such inflamed glands is much more popular now than formerly, the older surgeons fearing a wound of the femoral vein. Now that we know that the hæmorrhage from a wounded vein can be safely controlled by the lateral ligature or by a clamp applied in such a manner that it will not completely obstruct the venous current, this danger no longer deters us from operating.

The operation consists in making an incision in the long axis of the tumor, and turning back two flaps, proteeting the wound as far as possible from contamination with pus by covering it with pieces of iodoform-gauze. Constant irrigation during the operation does more harm than good, by spreading the purulent discharge over all parts of the wound, and should not be employed until the mass has been entirely excised. Having dissected the flaps free from the glandular mass, it is advisable to reach the cellular tissue at the extremities of the incision. As you see, pus has already broken through the capsule of the gland and infiltrated the subcutaneus tissue. We begin the removal of the mass at the upper and more accessible portion, lift it from the fascia, and working underneath the tumor, clamp the large vessels as they appear. Remarkably large vessels are often found supplying these inflammatory growths. Sometimes the glands just above the femoral ring are involved, and it is then a difficult matter to dissect them from the vessels. Having removed the large mass, a few isolated glands

are excised. The wound is now irrigated with 1-to-1000 corrosive sublimate solution, and, to secure a completely aseptic condition and at the same time to make slight pressure upon the interior of the wound, a strip of iodoform-gauze is introduced, over which the flaps are united. This gauze will be removed in twenty-four hours, and then properly-applied compresses will obliterate the cavity, and in all probability enable us to obtain primary union. Even if we should not attain this desirable result, the operation has greatly shortened the duration of the case ; for the healing process takes place much more promptly after excision of the glands than after simple incision and curetting.

EXCISION OF HÆMORRHOIDS.

The next patient is a man thirty-four years of age, who has suffered from symptoms of hæmorrhoids for ten years, having lost a considerable amount of blood from the anus during the last four years. His general health is otherwise good. A ring of large external piles surrounds the anus, and within this outer circle is seen a large mass of slightly-protruding internal piles. At the posterior edge is a narrow ulcerating cleft which passes through the entire thickness of the mucous membrane, but there is no sloughing.

The patient being under ether, in the lithotomy position, the buttocks are carefully shaved and cleansed, and the sphincter ani dilated. The bowels have been emptied by laxatives and by an enema given two hours before the operation.

The operation which we propose to do is that of excision, introduced by Whitehead, which is the best for such extensive cases of the disease as we find in this patient. The only disadvantages of the operation are the rather abundant loss of blood which it occasions and the prolonged manipulation. With antiseptic precautions the danger of sepsis is very slight, even if primary union should not be obtained, and if the operation is properly done the cicatricial contraction will never occasion stricture.

A shallow incision entirely dividing the mucous membrane around the circumference of the anus just inside of the white line which marks the muco-cutaneous junction, is made with a scalpel, and the greatest safeguard is secured against cicatricial contraction by keeping well within this line. In this case the line passes over the irregular surface of the external piles and is not easy to follow, but with a little care the incision is completed. Next the internal hæmorrhoids are drawn down with the fingers inserted in the anus, and the incision is deepened with a pair of blunt-pointed scissors, cutting somewhat into the hæmorrhoidal tissue, until the longitudinal muscular coat of the bowels is recognized. This is also divided close to the anus, by successive snips of the scissors, until the outer surface of the mucous membrane is recognized. The latter is then easily separated from the surrounding tissues as far as is necessary, and drawn down. The most difficult part to dissect up is, in the male, the anterior surface, toward the base of the bladder. Clamps are applied to the bleeding vessels and about half a dozen require ligatures.

In this case about an inch and a half of the mucous membrane was drawn down, including all the spongy diseased tissue, and then, beginning behind, it was divided beyond the limits of the diseased tissue with the scissors, only small portions being cut at a time, and the edge thus made being at once united to the edge of the external wound by a continuous, fine, silk suture. The principal bleeding vessels are usually found in the cut edge of the mucous membrane, but the hæmorrhage is easily controlled by the sutures. When the operation is completed a circular line of sutures is seen surrounding the anus. A large rubber drainage-tube about six inches long, wound with iodoform-gauze in the middle so as to make a spindle-shaped plug, is then introduced so that the thickest portion of the plug lies in the anus, and makes firm pressure upon the wound, thus preventing oozing of blood and favoring early union. The bowels are to be kept confined with opium for a week, if this can be readily done. If the bowels cannot be controlled, or if there is any objection to confining them, the stools should be made soft, but not fluid, and the anus and rectum carefully cleansed after each passage. The silk suture will be removed in ten days, unless it cuts its way out before that time. This patient has lost only a few ounces of blood, and although the operation has been rather tedious he is in good condition.

INTRACRANIAL LESIONS.[1]

BY W. W. KEEN, M.D.,
PROFESSOR OF THE PRINCIPLES OF SURGERY IN THE JEFFERSON MEDICAL COLLEGE, PHILADELPHIA.

THE programme proposes five questions for discussion. I feel that it will be better for me to leave the first two, concerning cerebral topography and the nature of the lesions, to the able neurologists who are to take part in the discussion, rather than to attempt to treat them so briefly and imperfectly as I should have to do in this paper. I shall, therefore, content myself with some observations on the last three questions, which are strictly surgical.

Before doing so, however, I desire to show to the members Mr. Horsley's new Rolandic-fissure meter, which I have lately obtained through his courtesy. Heretofore we have assumed that, as shown by Thane, the fissure of Rolando runs downward and forward at an angle of 67° with the middle line. Mr. Horsley's observations have convinced him that the angle varies with the shape of the head—that is tosay, with the cranial index. The higher the cranial index the greater the angle, the lower the index the lower the angle. Mr. Horsley assumes a standard for the cranial index of 75, as established by the caliper of Broca, and for the angle of the fissure of Rolando, 69° instead of 67°, and for every two integers of variation in the cranial index he assumes one degree of variation in the angle of the Rolandic fissure. Hence, if the cranial index is 77° instead of 75°, the angle for the fissure would be 70° instead of 69°, and if the cranial index is 73 the angle for the fissure would be 68°, and so on. Based upon this, he has devised the instrument which I show you, and which differs from the ordinary fissure-meters or cyrtometers in being provided with

means to rotate the arm representing the fissure of Rolando.

INDICATIONS FOR OPERATIVE INTERFERENCE.

In considering the indications for operative interference in the brain, we must bear in mind first, the peculiar physical characters and relations of the brain and the mechanical and physical disturbances to which it is subjected; and secondly, its functional disturbances.

The brain differs from all other organs of the body in its physical characters and in its relations. It is softer, and its functions are more easily deranged by pressure, especially if the pressure increases rapidly. Its texture is more delicate, and the continuance and undisturbed performance of its functions are more vitally important to the ordinary activities of life than are those of any other organ. It is also more closely and firmly encased than any other organ. It is perfectly true that other organs have an envelope of greater or less resistance and density ; for example, the eye is enclosed in the sclerotic, the testicle has the tunica albuginea, the structures in the palm are protected and to a certain extent enclosed by the palmar fascia, and the organs of the abdomen and pelvis, and those of the chest, are enclosed partly by bony and partly by muscular walls. If there is any increase in the contents, and, therefore, in the pressure within the eyeball, or within the tunica albuginea, either by inflammatory exudate, by suppuration, or by a new-growth, it is true that the envelope restrains them and produces compression, but the envelope will either yield or will be perforated with comparative ease ; and, besides, even should the organs be destroyed, this does not involve life. If there is any similar increase in the contents, and, therefore, of the pressure within the chest, abdomen, or pelvis, there is plenty of room for an exudate, for pus, or for a tumor to form, without producing fatal pressure on the contained organs. If an abscess forms under the palmar fascia it can escape either under the annular ligament into the forearm, or posteriorly between the bones, and so relieve the pressure.

In the brain it is different. Not only is it a delicate organ, the integrity and functions of which are destroyed to a greater or less extent by any pressure unless quickly relieved, but the bony case which protects it is so firm and strong that, as a rule, long before it can be perforated and the dangerous pressure thus relieved, the brain will be rendered incapable of performing its functions, or life itself be destroyed.

In the case of increased pressure, both the brain and skull vary very much in their behavior according as the pressure increases acutely or increases slowly. For instance, when we have a rupture of the middle meningeal artery or acute hydrocephalus, the pressure will quickly cause coma and death; but in a case of chronic hydrocephalus, and sometimes of tumor, the increase is so slow that the brain accommodates itself even for a number of years to a gradually-increasing pressure, and if the patient be young, even the bones of the skull will yield without producing a fatal result until after a long interval. These considerations must have great weight in forming our decision.

In addition to these mechanical disturbances there are certain functional disturbances not caused by increased pressure, and probably the result of microscopical, and

1 The opening of a discussion before the seventh annual meeting of the New York State Medical Association, held in New York October 22, 23, and 24, 1890.

even, as yet, undiscovered changes in the brain, which belong in another category.

Hence, in considering the question of operative interference from a clinical standpoint, the first great class of cases are those with *pressure-symptoms*, the second great class are those with what we may name, in default of a better term, *functional disturbances*.

In the first class, or *alterations producing pressure*, we may include abscess, tumor, effusions, and hæmorrhage. To these pressure-producing intracranial lesions (which are the only ones to be considered in the present discussion) should be added fractures attended by depression.

There is also another class of injuries, such as gunshot or other penetrating wounds, and lacerations of the brain-substance resulting from contusion, which produce very many of the symptoms that the lesions mentioned in the first class produce, as well as additional symptoms peculiar to these forms of wounds.

Among the *functional disturbances* may be mentioned epilepsy arising from traumatism and, therefore, usually attended by gross appreciable changes in the brain, though not necessarily by increased pressure; and, also, functional epilepsy in which there are no gross lesions. In the same class we should include inveterate headache, insanity, and other mental disturbances, and arrested development.

I will, therefore, briefly discuss, first, the indications for operative interference in the class of lesions attended by pressure-symptoms; and, secondly, the indications in those which are functional in character.

Lesions attended by increased intracranial pressure.— We can, in a few words, discuss the phenomena which attend intracranial pressure. First, the *intellectual function* suffers, and the patient becomes dull and stupid, and this stupor may gradually deepen into coma and total unconsciousness. Or, while consciousness is not affected, the faculty of speech may suffer, or ocular or auditory appreciation may be disordered. Secondly, there will be disturbance of *motility*, resulting either in paresis or paralysis of certain muscles or groups of muscles; for example, hemiplegia, monoplegia, or ophthalmoplegia. Thirdly, there may be changes in *sensation*, either over small or large areas. Fourthly, there will be changes in a majority of cases in the *optic disks*, and, possibly, in other parts of the eye-ground.

These phenomena will vary in detail, and will be more or less pronounced, according to the character of the case, and any one may be absent; but in no case can there be increased intracranial pressure to any extent without producing, wholly or in part, the picture I have so briefly drawn.

If to these pressure-symptoms we have added the phenomena peculiar to any one lesion, the diagnosis is well established. For example, in cases of tumor we will have the so-called cerebral vomiting, and, generally, headache and convulsions. In abscess we will very probably have a subnormal temperature and cerebral vomiting, a demonstrable cause in a long-standing otitis media, or a preceding severe fall or blow. In hæmorrhage from the middle meningeal artery we will have a history of a distinct traumatism, followed by that most important sign, an interval of lucidity, after which the coma will come on; while in ordinary apoplexy we have the age, atheroma of the arteries, and, what is usually equally impor-

tant, the absence of traumatism. Besides all these general symptoms, there will be the localizing symptoms, which are of the greatest value.

If any lesion which produces increased pressure— which pressure, if unrelieved, will prove fatal—can be located, and, with reasonable certainty, can be differentiated from other conditions which produce more or less similar phenomena, and if the location is such as to render it accessible, our duty is clear: we should open the skull and remove the cause of the dangerous pressure, just as we open the abdomen, the chest, or the palm to remove pus, an effusion, a clot, or a tumor. The head has been too long regarded as something apart, something different from other portions of the body. What I wish to urge is that it should fall into line with the other cavities of the body. Subject, as it is, to the same diseases and injuries, it must be subject also to the same rules for surgical interference; modified in detail, it is true, but in no wise differing in principle.

It is perfectly true that our means for making a diagnosis are, in the head, greatly limited, as contrasted with other parts of the body. For example: inspection, as a rule, reveals nothing, whereas inspection of the abdomen, chest, or palm reveals a great deal. We are cut off from the use of touch by reason of the hard bony skull. For a like reason percussion is almost valueless, and auscultation useless. But we have, on the other hand, changes in far-distant organs which do not exist with other lesions. The paralysis of the hand, the arm, or the leg helps us to recognize and locate the lesion in the brain with an accuracy which, though not unimpeachable, is becoming more and more marked from year to year. So, too, the alterations of sensation in distant parts, and the lesions of the eye-ground are often equally valuable and equally certain.

*Functional disorders.—*There are, also, certain functional disorders in which we ought to interfere, and can often do so with advantage, though the indications in this class are as yet far less clear than in the case of pressure-producing lesions. Our ability to decide this often difficult question is also gradually but surely increasing.

The indications for operative interference may be thus briefly summed up: The disease must be, first, a grave danger to life, growth, or mental development, or must so destroy the comfort of living that life is not worth having. Secondly, it must be established in each case that the ordinary medical means have been exhausted, and that nothing further can be expected from drugs, diet, hygienic care, etc. Thirdly, the danger to life from an operation must not be so great that we may not run this reasonable risk in the hope of great improvement. It has been amply proved of late years that trephining *per se* is not an especially dangerous operation, provided that it be carried out with modern antiseptic precautions. When we go beyond simple trephining and open the dura it adds a little, but not a great deal, to the danger. When we take a further step and excise a portion of the tissue of the brain the danger is increased, and may be even greatly increased, but not to such a degree as to prevent our taking the step if a great gain is to be reasonably hoped for, and if there is great danger of deplorable and probably permanent mental and physical loss and deterioration without such interference.

Exploratory trephining.—In both classes of disorders, however, there are a considerable number of cases in which we are in doubt, either of the character of the lesion, its extent, its location, or of its physical characteristics. In these cases the same rule should hold good in the head as in other parts. If the danger is great, and especially if the result without interference is almost sure to be fatal, as is so often the case, intracranial lesions must now fall into line with lesions elsewhere, and we should perform exploratory trephining in order to make a correct diagnosis, and if the exploratory operation shows it to be possible we should remedy the condition found. The vital importance of the brain and the gravity of its lesions, while they should make us cautious, should also make the rule of exploratory operation even more imperative here than elsewhere.

This rule, however, must be modified in one important respect in intracranial lesions. In the abdomen, for instance, we need not be absolutely sure of the location of the lesions, for when the belly is opened its entire cavity is at our command. In the brain the conditions are very different. Exploration is limited to the exposed area and its vicinity. Hence the location of the lesion should at least be *probable* before we operate. But the extreme gravity of these intracranial lesions should embolden us to operate when the location *is* probable. If we wait until it is ascertained with certainty we must wait till a post-mortem examination clears up the diagnosis.

I should be loath to give the impression that I recommend, even to the best surgeon, reckless or indiscriminate trephining. Each case must be carefully considered, all the facts elicited, and the possibilities, the advantages and the dangers weighed; and if, having done this, the possibilities of gain outweigh the probable dangers, exploratory trephining is clearly indicated.

THE TECHNIQUE OF OPERATIONS ON THE BRAIN.

Shaving.—Under this head I wish to insist primarily on the need of shaving the head in order to determine the existence, number, and position of any scars. I have almost never shaved a head without finding several scars, with perhaps the history of only a single traumatism.

I cannot better illustrate this, I think, than by briefly narrating the following history of a case, the result of which I have also the pleasure of showing you in the person of the patient himself.

W. A., aged fifteen years, weight ninety-seven pounds, was seen in consultation with Dr. B. A. Watson, in Jersey City, September 28, 1888. A little more than two years before, the patient fell from a swing on to a stone step, striking on the top of his head and cutting the scalp badly. He thinks he was not unconscious. The wound healed in four weeks. Two months after the fall his first epileptic fit occurred. The bromides reduced the number of the fits to about one in a month, but when not taking bromides he had a fit nearly every day, usually beginning in the hands, but on which side could not be determined.

On shaving his head four scars were discovered, the principal one, an inch and a half long, beginning at the fissure of Rolando, one-fourth of an inch to the left of the middle line, and extending on the right side to one and one-fourth inches to the right of the middle line, the direction being slightly oblique and backward. A second but smaller scar was found one and three-eighths inches back of the fissure of Rolando, and two and seven-eighths to the left of the middle line. A third, still smaller scar was found at the same distance back of the fissure of Rolando and three-eighths of an inch to the left of the middle line. The fourth small scar was just above and one inch to the left of the inion. The size of the scars was in the order in which they are named, all but the first being small. All of the scars were slightly tender, the tenderness being most marked in the third. Under this scar an obscure indentation of the bone could be felt. Naturally one would suppose that the largest scar was the one acquired at the time of the only known accident to the patient which was followed so promptly by epilepsy.

It will be noticed that the history of the fits gave no indication as to the location of the cortical lesion. There had been no motor phenomena in the legs, though the principal scar was over the leg-centre, nor had there been any sensory or mental phenomena, such as word-blindness, word-deafness, agraphia, etc. The eye-grounds were normal. I should also add that the boy had been kept in the hospital under Dr. Watson's observation, but on no occasion could a fit be observed.

In view of the difficulty of localizing any lesion by the symptoms, and of the tenderness of the scars, I determined to excise the scars themselves and examine the bone, and, if I found reasons to do so, to trephine at any point where the bone seemed to have been injured. If the bone was found normal I would only excise the scars, and await the result.

On September 28, 1888, the scars were excised. The bone appeared uninjured and nothing else was done. For a short time after the operation the fits were absent, but then returned, and for months there were from one to four a week. Observation in the hospital again failed to determine their character, but the mother was now quite confident that the right side of the body was more affected than the left. Moreover, the boy had developed homicidal and suicidal tendencies. Accordingly, on September 7, 1889, at his own and his mother's urgent request, I performed the following exploratory operation :

Though the largest scar was chiefly on the right side, the symptoms seemed to point to the left side of the brain as the region of the trouble. I therefore trephined at the left end of this scar, half an inch to the left of the middle line, as close as I deemed prudent to the longitudinal sinus. A one-and-a-half-inch button of bone removed showed nothing abnormal in the bone. In order to determine next whether there was a lesion of the skull on the right side under the scar, I took Horsley's dural separator and swept it carefully backward and forward, hugging the bone very closely with the advancing edge, lest I should penetrate or tear the sinus, and thus I worked slowly from the left side across the sinus and one and a quarter inches to the right side of the middle line. I found the manœuvre not difficult and perfectly successful. I separated the sinus from the bone, the adhesions of the dura being much greater there than on either side. I also loosened the dura on the opposite side, and determined by the separator that there was no irregularity on the under surface of the skull corresponding to the principal scar, as far as one and one-fourth inches to the right of the median line and one and three-fourths inches from the edge of the trephine opening. The history and this examination convinced me that the two small scars on the left of the trephine opening were possibly, if not probably, the site of the trouble.

Accordingly I exposed the brain under my first opening. Here the brain appeared normal. Biting away the bone in the direction of the lesser scars and opening the dura the brain was seen to be abnormal over an area an inch in diameter and corresponding to the second scar. The abnormal area was whitish, as from an old inflammation, with, at one point, apparently a small cyst. In front and to the left was a distinct area of redness one-third of an inch in diameter. The whole of the abnormal area also was slightly depressed. Unfortunately the battery which we had would not work at the moment when we wanted to use it, and I was unable to determine the possible motor value of the convolution. As nearly as I could judge, it corresponded to the supra-marginal, or possibly to the angular gyrus.

I then excised the abnormal part, which measured one inch antero-posteriorly, one and one-fourth inches transversely, and scant three-eighths of an inch in thickness. Immediately under this area, but half an inch deeper, I thought that I felt a spot of hardness which I removed with a Volkmann spoon. Examination of this afterward convinced me that my sense of touch was at fault, and that I had needlessly removed normal tissue.

The dura was now sutured, the large button and a number of small fragments of bone were laid upon it, and the wound was dressed as usual. The boy's highest temperature was only 100.6°, on one occasion, and in a week it fell to normal. His recovery was very rapid, a slight paresis of the right hand being the only apparent motor disturbance that remained.

Dr. Watson had the boy's eyes carefully examined, as I feared that I had injured the visual centre, or its radiating fibres, but there was neither ordinary blindness, word-blindness, nor apraxia.

Three months after the operation, I received a letter from the boy, expressing his thanks and adding that he had had no fits and was working for an express company. Since then he has followed the sea and been exposed to all its hardships. He has had no homicidal or suicidal tendencies. He has had only four attacks in nearly fourteen months, and the last one was more than three months ago. He has grown tall and robust. His hand is entirely well.

This case well illustrates the point I have made, that shaving the head is an essential preliminary to trephining. With the history of only one accident four scars were found, and the principal scar was evidently not the one corresponding to the cerebral lesion. In addition to this it shows that by the means I have described we can separate a sinus from the skull and reach across it to examine at least the bone, far away from the trephine opening.

Sublimate solution.—In connection with the preliminary preparation of the patient, I also desire to emphasize the fact that sublimate solution stronger than 1 to 2000, should not be used on the newly-shaven scalp. I have found that the ordinary 1-to-1000 solution pustulates the scalp; and even if there be no danger from it,

it is the source of great annoyance which may easily be avoided. When the brain is exposed I discard all antiseptics and use boiled water only, not so much on account of the possible danger of poisoning as because the antiseptic lessens the reaction of the cortex to the electrical current.

Hæmorrhage.—The position of the patient is important. Mr. Horsley always operates with his patient reclining, not very far from a sitting posture, and I think that it is a good one, as it diminishes hæmorrhage, and hæmorrhage and shock constitute the two great dangers of cerebral surgery. The preliminary use of morphine and ergot diminishes the calibre of the bloodvessels and is certainly of value. The application of antipyrine and cocaine (ten per cent. solution) is of undoubted value, I think, in checking general oozing, but I doubt if it is of any more value than the application of hot water ; and after all, it is not general oozing that troubles us so much as hæmorrhage from the large veins. Hence I think that both cocaine and antipyrine may be dispensed with.

For the arrest of hæmorrhage our chief reliance must be placed on the catgut ligature. With this the large vessels, and especially the large veins, should be double ligatured before division. After they have been cut it s very much more difficult to tie them. The hæmostatic forceps sometimes hold, but more commonly they tear away, which is followed by a renewed hæmorrhage, that is often controlled with great difficulty. The greatest care must be taken that the traction is equal upon each end of the ligature but that it is not too great—just enough to occlude the vessel and to retain their hold. To have room to cope with this formidable danger of hæmorrhage the opening in the skull must be ample. No vessel should be cut near the edge of the opening. If needful to cut it there the opening should first be enlarged by the rongeur forceps.

In addition to the ligature, hot water has yielded me very good results in many cases. But I am convinced that in at least one case I used the water too hot and produced cerebral disturbance which contributed to the fatal result. It should not be at a higher temperature than 120° F., if indeed so high.

Hæmorrhage from the superior longitudinal or from the lateral sinus is always alarming, and makes the operation speedily fatal, not only, I may even say not so much, from direct loss of blood as from the shock and the consequent loss of vitality of the nerve-centres. It recently happened to me to wound one of the large veins at its junction with the superior longitudinal sinus, in spite of the fact that I thought I was quite far enough away from that dangerous region. The reason for my being so unexpectedly near it was that in consequence of defective development the sinus was half an inch to one side of the middle line. I had recognized the defective development and had allowed for the displacement of the sinus, but as the result proved I had not allowed enough. The hæmorrhage was very severe, but was quickly controlled by a pair of hæmostatic forceps. During the later manipulations the forceps were detached, when another rush of blood came, and, although this, within a few moments, was controlled in the same way, the patient became moribund and died in fifteen minutes after the speedily-terminated operation, and about half an hour after the hæmorrhage occurred. The amount of blood lost was perhaps between eight and twelve ounces, an amount that the patient could have lost from the arm or from a wound in the scalp, without such direful consequences. Hence the large veins should be carefully avoided, especially near the middle line where they empty into the sinus, and if they must be divided it should be only after two ligatures have been applied.

Should the sinus itself be wounded one of three courses is open to us. The first, adopted by my friend Dr. W. J. Taylor during the past summer, is to seize the edges of the sinus by the hæmostatic forceps, and let the forceps remain *in situ* for two or three days. The second is to pack the sinus, as many surgeons have done, and in most cases successfully. The third is to tie the sinus with two ligatures, one on each side of the wound, as has been done in a few cases.

The last manœuvre, however, is much more difficult in abundant hæmorrhage following a wound of the sinus, than as a preventive of hæmorrhage when the sinus is to be deliberately cut across. The deliberate ligation of the sinus has been done a few times, once in a very remarkable recent case related to me by Mr. Horsley, in which he removed a large part of the frontal and of the squamous portion of the temporal bone, tied and divided the sinus and lifted the frontal lobes, thus gaining access to an aneurism at the base of the brain, pressing on the optic chiasm, for which he ligated both carotid arteries ; a surgical feat only equalled in its daring by the brilliancy of the diagnosis, which was verified by the operation. The patient, when I last heard, was recovering from the operation. Whether he will recover from the aneurism time only will show.

Not uncommonly after trephining, the cut edge of the bone bleeds very freely. To arrest this, Mr. Horsley informs me that he uses a paste or putty made as follows: Melt repeatedly one part of yellow wax and four of vaseline. Next, add carbolic acid one part to twenty of the wax and vaseline, and mix intimately. Then add sufficient white wax to make a mass that will be hard when cold, but that can be quickly softened by the fingers. With this (kept disinfected, of course) he " putties up " the vessels in the edge of the bone.

Drainage.—Whether drainage shall be employed, is an important question. In abscesses and other suppurative cases, continued drainage must, of course, be employed, but in ordinary operations I think the question must be decided in each case chiefly by the amount of hæmorrhage. If hæmorrhage has been arrested so that the wound is almost dry, drainage may be safely omitted. Mr. Horsley tells me that he has omitted drainage in all his recent cases. This is certainly the ideal operation, and the end toward which we all strive. In order, however, that we may do without drainage, the hæmorrhage must be checked to such a degree that only slight oozing if any remains when the wound is closed.

Exploring for abscesses.—As I have pointed out in former papers, the direction of exploration should not be obscurely described, such as " downward and a little inward and forward, etc.," but in a definite dirction from the opening—*e. g.*, in the direction of the external angular process, the opposite pupil, an inch above the opposite external auditory meatus, etc. The reader then can locate the abscess when he knows the point of departure, the

direction of the puncture and its depth. I have also given my reasons for preferring a grooved director to a needle in such exploratory punctures.1

Avoidance of shock.—I am persuaded by no little experience that in the head, more than in any other part of the body, we must bear in mind the lessons taught us by Dr. Cheever in his admirable paper on Shock, read before the American Surgical Association in May, 1888. He there urged that one of the important elements of shock was the time consumed in operation, and this applies especially to operations on the brain. A cerebral operation is always time-consuming, and this is especially bad in view of the prolonged anæsthesia. It is of the greatest importance, therefore, to abridge the time whenever it can be done.

Accordingly, I always raise the periosteum with the flap, instead of dissecting the two separately. Next, one of the most important elements in time is that required for trephining. The tendency has been of late to use very large trephines. I have commonly employed the one and one-half inch trephine, and I am persuaded that anything larger than this cannot be used with advantage. I have tried a two-inch trephine, but have found that it required a longer time than if I had made two or three one-inch trephine openings, and then bitten away the bone with the rongeur forceps to any further required extent. This arises from its becoming fastened in the bone, from the impossibility of adapting it well to the curved surface of the skull, and to the different thicknesses of the bone in different parts of its circumference. I have tried also to hasten the operation by using a surgical engine, but have found it not a practicable instrument. Mr. Horsley has recently devised an adaptation of the electric motor for working the trephine, with what success I do not know. The brace of a brace-and-bit has also been adapted to the trephine, with what advantage I cannot say. I am greatly inclined, however, to the opinion that the small trephine, one inch, or an inch and a quarter, and the later use of the forceps to bite away the intervening bridge, and afterward, if needful, still further to enlarge the opening, is the better practice, especially with a view to speed.

It is all-important also to use the battery in every case to identify the convolutions which are exposed, in order to determine in the human brain the motor value of the convolutions, if possible. In doing so, the graduated band of the fissure-meter should always be used to measure the distance of the convolution stimulated from the middle line, and from the fissure of Rolando or other well-recognized fissure. But while such determination of the motor value is important, it should not be made with too strong a current; the strength should be such as would freely move the operator's thenar eminence but no more. Nor should the time be wasted in repeated applications, further than is necessary to determine the facts. I mention the exact measurement to determine the situation of the stimulated area, because in a number of recorded cases, including some of my own, the value of such determination was practically lost by the inexactness with which the centres were located.

1 Transactions of the Tenth International Medical Congress, and THE MEDICAL NEWS, December, 1, 1889, and September 10, 1890.

18*

The dura may be sutured by either interrupted or continuous sutures, whichever will enable the surgeon to terminate the operation most speedily.

In addition to this the use of rest and of external heat from the very beginning of the operation, and of strychnine to prevent shock, and of alcohol, digitalis, and atropine to relieve it, have been forcibly advocated by Dercum,[1] and should certainly be tried.

Replacing the bone.—The question of closing the trephine opening by bone, is in my mind still a somewhat undecided one. In all the cases in which I have done it there is a flat surface instead of the normal arched contour of the skull. I have not been able to see, however, that it has produced any trouble, and it certainly acts as a valuable protective. In those rather obscure cases of headache and allied disorders, in which, perhaps, the chief value of the trephining lies in the alteration of intracranial pressure, the bone should not be replaced. In all other cases I have replaced it without any deleterious results, and I am inclined to think with advantage.

If the bone is to be replaced provision must be made beforehand for its care by placing it in a 1-to-2000 sublimate solution, and it should be the sole duty of one assistant to see that this is kept at a temperature of between 100° and 105° F., by means of hot water outside the cup or bowl in which the bone is placed. I have never had any trouble in replacing a disk as large as an inch and a half, and I prefer to do this than to spend time in chipping it up. But if the bone be greatly thickened it should not be replaced in mass, but either bitten into small pieces, or if the bone be diseased it should be rejected entirely. The suggestion of Senn to close the opening by means of decalcified bone is a valuable one, especially where there has been a prior loss of substance. It has also one marked advantage in that it can be better fitted to the opening than ordinary hard bone.

RESULTS.

These I will consider as to each disease or injury as briefly as possible. I shall not use the statistical method, but shall rather give the general conclusions I have reached, based both on my own experience and on a fairly thorough acquaintance with the literature of the subject. The topics, as announced, exclude from this paper the consideration of fractures of the skull, but I cannot help congratulating the profession on the development of cranial surgery in the treatment of these extremely serious injuries, and to urge that operative treatment shall be used more freely than formerly, not only with a view to the immediate saving of life, but to the prevention of later disorders, especially of epilepsy.

First, *Abscess.* No good surgeon will now hesitate to operate in a case of abscess of the brain. If there have been chronic middle-ear diseases or a serious local traumatism, followed by stupor and other evidences of intracranial pressure, paralysis of the oculo-motor nerves, choked disks, subnormal temperature and possibly hemiplegia, the surgeon should undoubtedly trepine, puncture, evacuate the abscess, drain and dress in the usual way. It is not so much a question of percentage as it is that every case which recovers is just

[1] THE MEDICAL NEWS, September 21, 1889.

one life saved which under the old method of treatment would inevitably have been lost. The question, "Where shall we trephine?" starts again the urgent cry for more accurate means of diagnosis, a cry that will not be suppressed until neurologists answer it satisfactorily.

Secondly, *Tumors.* Practically the same remarks will apply here as in abscess. Every case that recovers is a life saved from inevitable death in case we do not operate. The results have been on the whole, thus far, encouraging. Even very large tumors have been removed successfully, and a number of patients are still alive after several years. On the other hand, while a moderate number have died, there is again a not inconsiderable number that have suffered from a return of the original disease, and what is still more mortifying, there have been a number of tumors sought for and either have not been found, or have not even existed.

Here again we must ask most earnestly for the help of our neurological brethren, and happily we are not asking in vain. You will hear from some of them about to follow me the means for determining the location, the size, the number, and other characteristics of tumors and other intracranial lesions—means which become year by year more and more exact. We learn by our failures more than by our successes. Each case should be put on record, therefore, as a means of avoiding similar pitfalls. The technique of operation is now fairly satisfactory, though not yet perfect, and its dangers have been minimized, so that we no longer fear the operation. But what we need above all else to-day is a more accurate means of diagnosis.

Tumors will sometimes be met with that are too large for removal. It is extremely desirable that the neurologist shall be able to make a diagnosis of the approximate size of the tumor before the operation. But with our present knowledge it is too much to ask that this shall be done with absolute accuracy. Hence, unless it is almost certain that the tumor is too large it would be justifiable at present to attack it, for we may be mistaken, the tumor not being as large as had been anticipated and its relations with the brain much less intimate than had been supposed, and if so we may be able to remove it successfully : and if not, with modern methods in most cases the patient will recover from the operation, and in several recorded cases they have even been bettered by the attempted yet abandoned operation.

Again, it may be that tumors are erroneously suspected to be multiple, and hence not amenable to operation. Here, again, it is sometimes wise, inasmuch as tumor of the brain is a certainly fatal disease, at least to attempt the removal for the same reason as that just stated.

Tumors may be of such character that presumably they have infiltrated the tissues, so that a return will be certain after a very short interval. Here, too, we may be in error. Even in the case of a sarcoma, no infiltration may exist. I have lately had a case in point. Although the fall, which was the probable cause of the tumor, left no scar to mark the site of the blow, the diagnosis of the location of the tumor was exact. It was large, and the diagnosis had been that either one large tumor or two smaller ones existed. The nature of the tumor was doubtful but presumed to be tubercular, but the grounds upon which this diagnosis was made were not very certain.

The post-mortem examination showed that the tumor was large and situated in the area in which it was believed to exist, but even the slight manipulation for the removal of the brain produced auto-enucleation of the tumor. That it could have been removed by operation is very certain, and I have since deeply regretted that I declined to operate. The tumor was a sarcoma, and the microscopical examination showed that the walls of the cavity in which it was contained were not infiltrated with the sarcomatous growth. Whether, in spite of this, the removal would have been followed by permanent cure is doubtful, but the patient should at least have been given the chance.

Much doubt has been expressed as to the advisability of operating upon tubercular and syphilitic growths, but cases have been reported in which both were successfully removed. The argument in favor of operating on syphilitic growths is stronger than in the case of tubercular tumors, for the reason that tubercular tumors are more likely to be multiple than any other variety.

The depth at which a tumor lies is another important point. The deeper it is situated the less accessible it is to operation; and here, again, we must invoke the aid of the neurologists. I have operated on one case in which the evidence seemed to be pretty clear that the tumor was in the cortex of the angular and supra-marginal gyri. At the operation it was found to be underneath these gyri, but at such a depth as to render its extirpation impossible, and the patient died a few hours after the operation.

Perhaps the greatest opprobrium of cerebral surgery and the best proof of the need of more exact means of diagnosis is in the number of operations in which either no tumor was found, or it lay in a wholly different position from that which had been diagnosed. I have never yet operated upon a case in which no tumor existed, but in one case the tumor was believed to be in the cerebellum, and the post-mortem examination showed that it was in the floor of the third ventricle.

In one locality it is a question whether tumors, unless they are small and accurately diagnosed, can be removed with safety—namely, in the cerebellum. A few such have been operated on, but all proved fatal. In one case[1] I suspected a tumor and sought it, not by a formal operation, but by a slight opening in the skull and probing of the cerebellum, both through the exposed lobe and obliquely into the opposite lobe without any resultant injury. The post-mortem examination showed that the tumor was a soft sarcoma, and that my probe had passed through it without detecting its presence. But had I detected it and attempted its removal, the large vessels supplying it and its intimate relations to the fourth ventricle make it probable that the patient would have died upon the table. The structures in the neighborhood of the cerebellum and the fourth ventricle are so vital that I doubt whether we shall be able to cope with their dangers successfully, except, as I have said, in the case of small tumors, situated well back in the cerebellum and indicated by such symptoms that we can diagnose them accurately.

Epilepsy.—The most frequent disorder in which our advice is sought as to the propriety of operation is epi-

lepsy. In cases of traumatic epilepsy the results have been, on the whole, very encouraging. A considerable number of cases are on record, some of them very severe, in which the patient was entirely relieved of his dreadful malady; and, while idiopathic epilepsy has not yielded such good results, they have been sufficiently encouraging to warrant our persisting to operate in well-selected cases.

The results, I think, in general, may be summed up as follows. First: Taking one operator with another, a small percentage of cases will die from the operation. Secondly: In a small but somewhat larger percentage absolutely no result, good or bad, will follow recovery from the operation. Thirdly: In a large percentage of cases the patient, while not cured, will be benefited, the fits persisting, but with lessened frequency and violence. Fourth: Perhaps in twenty-five per cent. more or less the result will be practically a cure. If I may judge from the feelings of the parents and of the patients also, the opinion of those most interested is that the operation is justifiable, because the malady is so dreadful. Even if the patient is not benefited no harm is done, and whether he is benefited, cured, or dies, both he and his friends are content.

One thing especially should be noted. It has been used as an argument against operating that the removal of diseased tissue will result in a permanent paralysis, and that the patient pays dear for the cure; and that he may not only be cured but have the additional affliction of a useless arm or leg. This is not my experience. The paralysis which follows the excision even of a motor centre is only temporary. One of my patients whose hand was absolutely paralyzed immediately after the operation, had so far recovered between three and four months that he could play baseball; another is able to use his hand well though it is slightly paretic; and a third is scarcely conscious that his hand was ever affected.

Whether, as is most likely, this recovery of function is due to the development of the bilateral function of the corresponding centre on the other side, or whether, as seems less likely though not impossible, new cerebral tissue has been developed, is not certain. The recent experiments of Prus,[1] Salviati,[2] and Gilman Thompson[3] show that portions of the cerebral cortex can be successfully transplanted from one animal to another. Possibly this may hereafter lead us to a more perfect restoration of motor function, by a similar transplantation from an animal to man.

Hæmorrhage from the middle meningeal artery.—Hæmorrhage from the middle meningeal artery even without fracture is now an accident amenable to operation and not uncommonly with success. I would especially urge that if the clot is not found by the first trephining a second trephine opening should be made, as is advocated in the able paper of Krönlein.[4] The site of these openings should be, as he has indicated, first one inch behind the external angular process at the level of the upper border of the orbit, and, failing to find the clot, secondly at the same level and just below the parietal

---

[1] Transactions of the International Medical Congress, 1890.
THE MEDICAL NEWS, September 20, 1890.

[1] Annals of Surgery, vol. ix. p. 225.
[2] Wiener Medical Presse, No. 20, 1889, p. 838.
[3] New York Medical Journal, June 28, 1890.
[4] Deutsche Zeitschrift fur Chirurgie, Bd. 23, Hefte 3 u. 4, 1886.

boss. The two openings give access to the two branches of this vessel.

The accident, if untreated is necessarily a fatal one. The operation, while by no means always a success, has resulted most brilliantly in several cases, and its lesson is evident: that the surgeon should always at least endeavor to save life by trephining and ligature of the bleeding vessels.

Surgery of the lateral ventricles.—I have so recently and fully considered the question of the surgery of the lateral ventricles[1] that I need not here repeat what I have said in that paper, saving to urge that a trial be given to the method I have advocated, until its value or its worthlessness shall be determined.

Inveterate headache.—Cases of inveterate headache which have resisted all other known means and still make life unbearable are as yet in the category of undecided questions, judged by the results. Enough cases, however, have been recorded to show that trephining is well worth a trial until the value of the operation shall be determined.

Mania.—In mania following traumatism it is certainly right to attempt relief by a carefully conducted exploratory trephining. Should death follow, it is a relief from a condition worse than death, and should relief and cure follow, as has already been the fact in a number of cases, it is a brilliant triumph. The evidences of the site of the injury guide us to where to operate.

Arrested mental development.—In cases of imperfect mental development, from arrested growth or, as in the case of Hare and Felkin,[2] from a cyst following an injury, the result of operation has been such as to encourage us, but excepting those cases which follow traumatism I cannot look with great encouragement to the future of cerebral surgery in this direction. Whether the remarkable result of craniectomy recently recorded by Lannelongue[3] will show that we ought to give room for the growth of the repressed organ, must, in the absence of further evidence, remain for some time an open question. The same remarks apply to trephining for general paralysis.

DISCUSSION.

Dr. JAMES J. PUTNAM, of Boston, called attention to the relative value of certain signs of cerebral tumors, especially of such tumors as are a little outside of the familiar areas of the central, temporal, and occipital zones, and only infringe upon these, so that the symptoms would be liable to occur rather late in the progress of the case. It is generally admitted, he said, that monoplegias and localized hemiplegias are more valuable as localizing signs than monospasms and localized convulsions. A paralysis gives fairly positive evidence that the whole cortical area corresponding to a set of movements is destroyed ; whereas, a localized convulsion may be due to an irritative lesion in the tissues adjoining the area in question, or at a distance from it, or even to an unstable nutritive condition of the cortical area without gross lesions.

1 Transactions of the Tenth International Medical Congress, Berlin, 1890 ; THE MEDICAL NEWS, September 20, 1890.

2 Manchester Med. Chronicle, October, 1889.

3 Lancet, August 9, 1890, from l'Union Méd., Paris, July 8, 1890.

In accordance with a similar course of reasoning, the speaker said that a distinction could be drawn between the different localized paralyses on the one hand, and localized convulsions on the other. Those functions of the brain which are relatively highly specialized and complex in character, are more likely to suffer disturbance than the less highly specialized and complex functions. Thus, Hughlings Jackson long ago pointed out that, given an irritation of the arm- or in the leg-centre leading to an epileptic attack, the attack would be most likely to begin in the thumb or fingers in the one case, and in the toes in the other.

According to this statement, a localized convulsion or paralysis of the shoulder would have a greater localizing value than a convulsion of the muscles of the hand, and hence would indicate the presence of an irritative lesion of the shoulder-centre more surely than a convulsion of the muscles of the hand would indicate a lesion of the hand-centre. This the speaker believed to be true. Ordinarily an error in connection with this would not be of much importance, as the operation would in all probability be successful, and the mistake never be discovered. The mistake would be important, however, if the convulsions were caused by pressure transmitted from a considerable distance, or by œdema or anæmia. This occurred in a case of the speaker's, in which Dr. H. N. A. Beach had operated as a last resort for a supposed tumor of the frontal region. He was led to this diagnosis by the occurrence of repeated attacks of speechlessness, which were wrongly interpreted as motor aphasia, and by a twitching of the fingers of the right hand, associated with slight but distinct paresis of the extensors of the fingers. At the autopsy the tumor was found at the inferior parietal lobule just in front of the angular gyrus, and separated by a space of three-fourths of an inch from the motor area. In another case there were convulsive movements of the shoulder, not attended by loss of consciousness, and occurring only once late in the case. Had movements occurred several times, it would have been considered proper to operate, and had this been done, the tumor would have been found directly in the field of operation. The speaker wished to emphasize his belief that this shoulder convulsion might have been considered as a localizing sign of great value.

Direct and important physiological evidence also is not wanting in favor of the statement that the cortical areas corresponding to highly-specialized functions have a special irritability. Thus, Panett found that the visual centres in the case of a dog were more irritable to electricity than were the other areas ; so much so, that it was a disturbing element in some of his experiments.

A patient was recently treated at the Massachusetts General Hospital, in the service of Dr. A. T. Cabot, for a severe fracture of the occipital bone, leading, as the autopsy showed, to multiple contusions and small hæmorrhages with softening, over the surface of both hemispheres. The speaker carefully examined the brain, and found that the motor areas of the hands were not involved in the gross lesions ; and yet the night before the patient's death, although able to move his arms freely, he showed a striking paralysis of motion of the fingers, and especially of the extensors.

On these grounds, and in accordance with the principle he was trying to illustrate, Dr. Putnam suggested that spasm of the extensor muscles and paralysis of the flexors are probably more valuable than the reverse condition as localizing signs of the cortical lesion.

The *comprehension* of speech is certainly a more fundamental element of the language-function than the *power* of speech, for it is earlier and more readily acquired, and requires less subtle and perfectly-adjusted cerebral activity for its maintenance, and the so-called auditory aphasia or loss of the comprehension of spoken language is a more valuable localizing sign than motor aphasia. The doctrine of sensory aphasia would be more generally recognized were it not for the strong influence still exerted by Broca's remarkable discovery, which, in the minds of most medical men, chains every disorder of the speech-function to the notion of a lesion in the third frontal convolution. As a matter of fact, the function of speech is liable to betray the presence of cerebral disorders, either far from or near to the motor speech-area. Not only does the loss of auditory impressions entail aphasia, but the loss of visual impressions may have a similar effect.

The speaker then briefly referred to some interesting experiments on the effect of quickly recurring stimuli upon the irritability of different cortical areas.

Unilateral neuritis has been considered by some to be of significance as indicating the presence of a tumor of the opposite side of the brain; but, in Dr. Putnam's experience, and in that of a number of others whose cases he had found recorded, the reverse condition was present.

DR. CHARLES K. MILLS, of Philadelphia, said that the failures and errors in the present method of localizing intracranial lesions are caused as follows: First, by attaching too much importance to certain classes of symptoms, which are regarded as determinative of the site of the lesion, as, for example, the so-called signal or initial symptom. Secondly, by considering symptoms of late invasion only. Thirdly, by attaching relatively too much importance to motor localizing symptoms. Fourthly, by overlooking multiple or diffused lesions. Fifthly, by operating on incurable cases of arrested development. The so-called signal or initial symptom of brain-tumors, while of great value, has sometimes proved misleading. The motor signal symptom has been made use of in a large number of cases to guide the surgeon, and sometimes successfully, but almost as often unsuccessfully. It should be remembered that in every case of unilateral spasm and of monospasm, whether reflex, dural, nephritic, toxic or hysterical, the spasm really or apparently begins with an initial symptom in the limb or face. This may indicate that the beginning of the cerebral discharge occurs in the area of the cortex which controls the movement, but it would be unwise to operate with such an indication. Occasional conjugate deviation of the eyes and head has been used as a guide to operation, and is one of the errors into which a thoughtless neurologist might be led.

In making a diagnosis as to the existence of hæmorrhage, we must depend largely upon general symptoms. This is also true of the diagnosis of tumors, and still more true of abscesses. A number of mistakes have been made in trephining for tumor or abscess by the operator being too much guided by motor symptoms, which were really the result of the diffusion of the lesion to the motor areas.

In not a few cases of cerebral abscess, sensory or special symptoms might cause a decision in favor of operating, and at the same time might not properly guide the operator to the seat of the lesion. All active localized symptoms of the brain, the result of mastoid or aural disease, except, perhaps, word-deafness and left-sided affections, are the result of the extension of suppuration. Few physicians have escaped from mistakes in cases in which a large lesion either in the frontal or temporal lobe caused prominent motor symptoms by pressure, either upon the motor tracts in the capsule or upon the cortical areas and their tracts. In one case of this kind, all the symptoms pointed to brachial or crural monoplegia, due to tumor with intercurrent hæmorrhage. The autopsy showed a tumor with a large hæmorrhage, strictly confined to the right temporal lobe, but evidently causing great pressure. Several recorded failures were the result of overlooking the pressure of multiple or different lesions.

Operating in cases of tubercular disease of the brain, vessels, or membranes, has also been a source of error and cause of failure. It is, in most cases, an error to operate, guided by certain localizing phenomena, in the spastic and paralytic, congenital and early infantile affections. A careful review of the surgical operations guided by the rules of localization in whole or in part, show that probably the greatest success during the last few years has been in trephining for hæmorrhage. In traumatic cases failures have occasionally resulted, and for several reasons, chiefly because the fact is not fully considered that in many cases of depressed and non-depressed fractures hæmorrhages take place, not only at or in direct connection with the place of injury, but also at various positions more or less remote.

DR. JOHN B. ROBERTS, of Philadelphia, said that the impulse given to cerebral surgery by the wonderful results of the last few years, has been the means of saving life in many cases of traumatism, but he believed it had slain about as many of those who had been the subject of obscure lesions. It is well that the pendulum has swung the other way, and that cases are being selected with greater care and judgment. In cases of foreign body, such as gunshot wounds of the brain, it is generally agreed that operative interference is indicated, and that an exploratory trephining should be performed, not only for the removal of the foreign body, but also for drainage. which, after all, is often more important.

The speaker then referred to the importance of keeping the nose, pharynx, and similar channels leading to the seat of fractures of the skull as nearly aseptic as possible, for he thought that neglect of this precaution has been the cause of many cases of suppuration within the skull.

When symptoms of abscess are present, even if there are no clinical evidences of ear-disease, it is proper to open the mastoid process and search for a purulent focus before exposing the brain. If this should be found, it would make it almost certain that there was an abscess in some portion of the temporal lobe, and then an exploratory trephining would be indicated.

The jamming in the bone which occurs with the use of large trephines can be avoided by the use of the " segment trephine," which the speaker described some time ago, but much of the difficulty is frequently due to the fact that the trephine is not sharp. The ordinary trephine cannot be rendered surgically clean except by baking or steaming, but by employing the " aseptic trephine," which has no centre-pin, this difficulty can be overcome.

The results of these operations are often very brilliant, as in those reported by Macewen, of which one patient was living eight years after the removal of a tumor, and another one year after the removal of a tuberculous growth. The most unsatisfactory cases are those of epilepsy, except cases of traumatic origin, which are often treated most successfully by operation.

DR. JOSEPH D. BRYANT, of New York, in considering the question as to the present means of localizing intracranial lesions, limited the term *lesion* to abscess, hæmorrhage, depressed bone, and tumors of intracranial origin. He classified the means of localizing these lesions into topographical, physiological, and instrumental. The topographical means relate to the connection existing between the established landmarks and lines of the cranium that bear a positive relationship to the superficial parts of the encephalon, many of which parts have had definite functions already assigned to them. The physiological relate to the establishment of the site of the pathological process by studying the deviation of the function of a part from the normal as the result of a local disease or injury. The instrumental means are largely subsidiary, and their application is often more of an experimental than of a practical character. The speaker then described several cases bearing on the subject, and concluded with the following summary:

(1) That a small and presumably circumscribed injury of the brain at the upper end of the fissure of Rolando may excite a cerebral disintegration sufficient to involve the motor centres associated with this fissure, without causing notable constitutional symptoms. (2) That aspiration of the brain as a means of diagnosing the extent or situation of an abscess is of uncertain utility, even when a moderately large needle is used, and that the employment of the ordinary hypodermic needle for this purpose is entirely unreliable and misleading. (3) That extensive fissures may occur at some distance from the seat of the violence causing them, and that their existence may remain unrecognized unless carefully searched for. (4) That extensive and fatal complications may be caused at a considerable distance from the seat of an apparently innocent injury of the skull. (5) That when paralysis involving the motor areas of the brain follows an apparently trivial injury of the head, an operation at the seat of these areas is indicated if only for the purpose of exploration. (6) That the removal of a compressing blood-clot is not necessarily followed by improvement of the symptoms of compression, and that if the brain does not soon resume the normal relation with the skull, death will ensue.

In one of the cases cited, the patient immediately after being struck on the head with a bottle, lost the power of speaking his own name, but was able to write it as well as the name of his assailant. When admitted to the hospital, he had forgotten his own name, and that of many things. An examination of the injury disclosed a small circumscribed depressed fracture of the skull located near the lower end of the fissure of Rolando. On the following day the depression was elevated, and all the aphasic symptoms disappeared. This case impressed the fact that the effects of a circumscribed compression due to trauma may be limited to one motor centre only.

DR. THOMAS H. MANLEY, of New York, divided intracranial lesions into two classes, namely, those of extrinsic and those of intrinsic origin—those arising from violence or mechanical influence, and those resulting from pathological changes within the skull. Dr. Manley's remarks were chiefly confined to traumatic lesions, but with slight modifications they were applicable to intracranial new-formations. There may be grave symptoms, he said, from injuries of the head, without the bone being implicated; and, on the other hand, the bone is often shattered into many fragments and driven through the meninges and into the brain, and yet no single symptom indicative of cerebral disturbance be manifest. This is frequently observed in military surgery, and is often very conspicuous in young children. In general, in cases of depressed fracture, trephining is indicated and is readily performed, but if the fracture is situated over a sinus it may cause sudden and even fatal hæmorrhage. He thought it poor practice to replace the bone that is removed, for of all parts of the osseous system, the skull has the feeblest power of regeneration, and the union with the adjacent parts which seems to take place is probably not osseous.

The question of hæmorrhage is important, and he believed that in his fatal cases this was a prominent factor. As hematomata of moderate size are as readily absorbed here as in other parts of the body, in cases of intracranial lesions with intracranial hæmorrhage, trephining for displacement of the clot is not only unnecessary, but is illogical and dangerous. Within the last year he has trephined four children who had general traumatic meningitis ; two being trephined in consequence of the diagnosis of cerebral abscess. The brain-substance was deeply penetrated, but nothing was found, and the postmortem examination on the following day showed only general meningitis. The other two cases did not survive over forty-eight hours. The loss of blood, together with the lethal action of the anæsthetic, materially shortened their lives. He has found meningitis very prone to develop after cranial injuries in young children when antiseptics are used ; and since he has discarded them in these cases, and kept the head well covered with ice or cold lotions, it has been much less frequent.

When the use of the trephine causes much laceration of the brain-substance, the exposed part gradually disintegrates, and is absorbed, which may be followed by symptoms of impaired mental powers. When the area of destruction is small and unimportant, a young and healthy patient may completely recover.

Of all the organs in the body, there is none in which the effects of an anæsthetic are so evident, both by subjective and objective phenomena, as in the brain. When a patient enters the lethal stage during etherization the vascularity of the brain is enormously increased, as shown by the great increase of the volume, the convolutions rising and crowding into the aperture made by the trephine. As the ether is withdrawn the brain becomes less hyperæmic, and returns to its normal dimensions. One can easily understand that manipulations involving the brain under these circumstances must be always attended by serious difficulties, the vessels giving way under the most trivial disturbance, and cansing profuse hæmorrhage. Independently of the effects of the anæsthetic on the vascularity of the brain, is its influence on the nerve-centres, when the brain is injured or diseased; so that ether cannot be otherwise than harmful.

ORIGINAL ARTICLES.

THE CONTROL OF HÆMORRHAGE DEEP IN THE PELVIS, WITH THE REPORT OF A CASE OF OVARIOTOMY.

By CHARLES P. NOBLE, M.D.,
SURGEON-IN-CHIEF TO THE KENSINGTON HOSPITAL FOR WOMEN,
PHILADELPHIA.

At times it is desirable to have a method of controlling hæmorrhage deep in the pelvis, in addition to the usual methods of securing the bleeding point. Owing to the relative inaccessibility of the region, and to the fact that the hæmorrhage itself tends to obscure the field, it is often extremely difficult or is impossible to employ satisfactorily the ordinary methods of hæmostasis. When it becomes necessary to ligate fleshy pedicles, subsequent shrinkage of the tissue within the pedicle may permit bleeding. Also, when there are extensive raw surfaces on the broad ligament produced by the separation of densely-adherent tumors, or left after the removal of the ovaries and tubes disorganized by suppuration, and in certain cases of extra-uterine pregnancy, free oozing may occur, and is difficult to control by strictly local methods. In such cases stuffing the pelvis with gauze has been employed. In hysterectomy, with the intra-peritoneal management of the stump, and in myomectomy, the danger of secondary hæmorrhage is well recognized.

In such cases securing the ovarian and uterine arteries gives a control of the situation not attainable in any other way. In the case of oozing fleshy pedicles it is a necessary measure. The same is true of oozing raw surfaces on the broad ligaments. In case of active hæmorrhage, primary or secondary, in which the bleeding point cannot be readily secured, the ligation controls the hæmorrhage and gives time to secure the bleeding vessel. The method is particularly valuable when the broad ligament is fixed by exudate.

This procedure was brought to my attention by seeing Dr. H. A. Kelly employ it in several cases, and with very gratifying results. Since then I have adopted it twice with great satisfaction.

Mrs. X., aged thirty-seven years, has had three children and one miscarriage. Her health was good until January, 1890, when she had *la grippe.* Following this she suffered very much from bronchitis and dyspepsia, and rapidly lost strength, being finally obliged to go to bed. In March she came under the care of Dr. Minich, who, finding an abdominal tumor, referred the case to me.

I saw her April 7th, and found her a large, fleshy, very anæmic woman, with hurried, anxious breathing and quick, feeble pulse. The belly was enormously distended by a tense fluctuating cyst. Operation, after preparatory treatment, was advised, and she entered the Kensington Hospital for Women, April 14th. A severe cough with consolidation of the middle lobe of the right lung immediately developed. The temperature ranged from 99° F. in the morning, to 103° F. at night. Profuse night-sweats and orthopnœa prevented sleep. The condition of the lung, following *la grippe,* it was thought explained the general symptoms. Under stimulating expectorants, digitalis, stimulants and food, with counter-irritation over the chest, the lung slowly cleared up, the cough disappeared, and the appetite improved, but the septic symptoms remained the same. In spite of the entire absence of abdominal pain, no rational explanation of the sepsis was apparent except some inflammatory process connected with the cyst. Accordingly, notwithstanding the bad general state of the patient, section was made, under chloroform, May 10th.

On tapping the cyst fifteen quarts of puriform material were discharged. The cyst, which was non-adherent, was delivered and found to be deeply situated between the layers of the right broad ligament, and to require ligation over a surface of eight inches. A series of twenty-two interlocking ligatures was applied from the pelvic wall to the uterus, in the form of an arc owing to the deep development of the tumor.

The tumor was now cut away. As the tissues were very vascular, to provide further against hæmorrhage the ovarian and uterine arteries were ligated in their course. A ligature was passed through the broad ligament on one side of the ovarian artery, and back through the ligament on the other side of the artery, and the vessel was thus securely tied. A ligature was then passsd through the broad ligament close to the uterus, and again through the ligament to the distal side of the row of ligatures in the stump, and in this way the uterine artery was secured.

A sessile cyst of the left ovary (containing about a quart of fluid) with a broad attachment, likewise required a series of interlocking ligatures, fourteen in number. The left ovarian artery was tied in the same way as the right one. Hæmorrhage was in this way entirely controlled, and scarcely a drop of blood oozed from the extensive raw surface.

The extent of the raw surface was a source of anxiety, offering, as it did, such possibilities of intestinal adhesions. At the suggestion of Dr. Kelly the stump of the right pedicle was disposed of by stitching the raw surface of the broad ligament at uterine cosine, to the raw surface at the infundibulo-pelvic ligament. A few stitches along the anterior face of the broad ligament brought the raw surfaces nicely in apposition.

Very thorough douching completed the operation. Water had been freely used during the operation to wash away puriform material, some of which had escaped from the cyst. A drainage-tube was introduced and the patient put to bed.

The operation lasted two hours, the longest operation in my experience. Almost the entire time was consumed in introducing the ligatures, as the other steps in the *technique* required but a few minutes.

The patient steadily improved and all septic symptoms quickly disappeared. The drainage-tube was removed after thirty hours and the sutures after six days. On the eleventh day, symptoms of inflammation about the right stump appeared, and continued until pus was discharged through the incision on the twenty-first day. The subsequent history of the patient has been one of rapid recuperation.

The case is reported because of its bearing on the questions of pelvic hæmostasis and the manner of disposing of extensive raw surfaces. It is also of interest as a further illustration of how, under the most desperate circumstances, patients will recover, to encourage the surgeon to extend to others, under similar circumstances, the resources of surgery.

HYPERTROPHY OF THE PHARYNGEAL TONSIL AS A CAUSE OF DEAFNESS, WITH THE REPORT OF A CASE.

BY LAURENCE TURNBULL. M.D., PH.G.,
AURAL SURGEON TO THE JEFFERSON MEDICAL COLLEGE HOSPITAL,
PHILADELPHIA.

THE pharyngeal tonsil is a soft mass of lymphoid tissue, in health measuring not more than seven millimetres in thickness. It occupies the roof and the upper part of the posterior wall of the nasopharynx, reaching from the posterior margin of the roof of the nasal cavities to the edge of the foramen magnum. Laterally it extends into Rosenmüller's fossæ, and to the Eustachian tubes. It is always present, varying in size in different individuals, and occurs in folds which are either longitudinal, or form a regular network; more rarely it is a cushion with small round elevations.

The pharyngeal tonsil is covered with ciliated epithelium, and is composed of acinous glands and numerous follicles of lymphoid tissue, but differs from the true adenoid vegetations in not being pedunculated or giving to the finger the sensation of a soft, cushion-like mass.

The normal secretion from the pharyngeal tonsil consists of an absolutely transparent, somewhat viscid mucus of the appearance and consistence of the white of an egg, which becomes changed in diseased conditions. At the present day Luschka's idea of a normal pharyngeal bursa is abandoned, and it is only the morbid hypertrophied condition which resembles a bursa.

The simple form of hypertrophy of the pharyngeal tonsil is distinguished by characteristic features perceptible both to sight and touch. Explored by the finger a smooth, elevated, rounded mass is felt in the vault of the pharynx, encroaching upon the Eustachian tubes and upon the choanæ, so that the upper boundary of the posterior nasal fossæ cannot be defined. The sensation is entirely different to the touch, as I have before stated, from that which is felt when post-nasal growths are encountered.

When viewed in the rhinoscopic mirror in the case of a girl of sixteen years, it appeared as a solid rounded mass encroaching upon the Eustachian tube of the left side and pressing upon the orifice.

To the otologist the chief interest of the pharyngeal tonsil when diseased lies in its interference with the Eustachian tubes, which may be compressed by the growth. The following illustrative case had also a chronic rhinitis, with some enlargement of the faucial tonsil of the same side.

There was marked deafness on both sides, the hearing distance of the right ear was $\frac{9}{XXII}$, and of the left, the side on which the Eustachian tube was encroached upon by the tumor, $\frac{5}{XXII}$.

The membrana tympani of the right ear was retracted and dull; the auditory meatus was inflamed and irritated by an old ulcer near the edge, and was reduced in size by an old cicatrix following a perforation.

The Eustachian tube on each side was almost impervious to inflation by Politzer's method. There was also an ulcer in the left nasal cavity.

The treatment consisted of a cleansing spray to the naso-pharynx, an ointment composed of ten parts of nitrate of mercury to twenty of oxide-of-zinc ointment to the ulcer in the nose, and iodine and iodide of potassium dissolved in glycerin, to the faucial tonsils. To the enlargement of the pharyngeal tonsil, repeated applications of styptics were made. This treatment was kept up for weeks, with only partial reduction of the tumor, so that avulsion of the mass had to be resorted to.

After a month's treatment, the ulcer in the nose healed, the rhinitis was cured, and the ulcer near the membrana tympani had closed. By careful inflation and the use of a twenty-per-cent. solution of menthol in cosmoline, applied to the membrana tympani, at first every day for a week, then every second day, the membrane cleared so much that a partial reflex was secured. After that, inflations with air medicated by ether kept the parts free. The hearing was improved to $\frac{18}{XXII}$, while by the removal of the tumor and subsequent treatment the hearing became normal. No evil consequences resulted from the operation and cicatrization followed, while all traces of the tumor disappeared in a month after the operation.

AMPUTATION AS AN ORTHOPÆDIC MEASURE.[1]

By AP MORGAN VANCE, M.D.,

SURGEON TO THE LOUISVILLE CITY HOSPITAL, AND TO STS. MARY AND ELIZABETH HOSPITAL, LOUISVILLE, KY.

THE introduction of amputation as an orthopædic measure is out of the recognized lines of treatment, but as we are expected to relieve our patients of crippling and deformity, it is obvious that if amputation in some cases is the best, and often the only way this can be done, the operation may become orthopædic.

Even the most conservative among us occasionally meet cases in which the question at once arises, Would this patient be better off without this deformed foot or subluxated tibia? But, few of us have ever removed a useless limb in order to substitute a useful artificial one. In the past ten years I have had under my care a number of cases in which there was no doubt in my mind that amputation, performed only for convenience, was better than any other treatment. Possibly some will say, You should refer such cases to the general surgeon. But I think that the mechanical and special training of the orthopædist peculiarly fits him to deal with these patients. Who should be better able to determine the proper method to be used or the point of selection in given cases—the general surgeon or the orthopædist? The orthopædist, of course, for he should know all about the mechanism of the prothetic apparatus. The general surgeon learns how to do the operation by a given method, but rarely knows whether an artificial leg is made of cork, wood, or what not, or when doing an amputation, bears in mind the subsequent comfortable and useful adjustment of the prothetic apparatus. He rarely knows that it is absolutely necessary to have from four to six inches space above the ankle-joint for the attachment of an artificial foot, and consequently we often meet men struggling through life with stumps the result of amputation just above or through the joint. The same may be said of the knee. An amputation through this joint is an abomination to the artificial-leg maker and a never-ending trial to the patient.

At least three inches should be left for the proper adjustment of the apparatus. We daily meet cripples who would be rendered more comely, comfortable, and useful by means of an amputation and the fitting of an artificial limb. Particularly is this true of cases in which the knee can be saved, although the condition of some may be greatly improved by a thigh-amputation. Among those in which the knee can be saved will be found a few cases of old infantile paralysis (talipes), and adult cases of congenital talipes, in which painful bursæ

have developed, and life rendered unendurable from the pain caused by walking.

On the other hand, old subluxated knees, with ankylosed patellæ, flail-joints and great shortening, are not uncommon. I have known several of these cases that were converted from hopeless cripples into useful members of society by a proper amputation and the adjustment of an artificial limb.

The orthopædist is very frequently called upon to improve the condition resulting from the recognized, though barbarous, amputations through the tarsus, the only remedy for which is an amputation above the ankle-joint and an artificial limb.

The reason for these suggestions will be very apparent after an inspection of a modern artificial limb.

I will briefly report a few cases illustrative of the good done by amputation performed orthopædically.

CASE I.—A. E., aged twenty-one years, single, called on me for advice in regard to an extreme deformity of the feet. He was very tall and thin, and gave me the following history: His family was phthisical. His feet were perfect up to eight years of age, when they gradually began to turn outward. He can give no explanation of this except that a tendency toward the position was produced by a pair of boots which were too short for him, and turned over at the heels, thus putting the structures on the inner side of the ankle-joint on a strain. There was neither paralysis, nor disease of the bones. Efforts had been made to arrest the progress of the deformity, but they were of no avail.[1]

The patient was six feet and four inches high, as he stood on the ends of the tibiæ, and I estimated that at least four inches were lost by the deformity. There was ugly ulceration of the parts which were pressed upon in walking. I advised for his relief a double amputation below the knees, and the application of two artificial limbs.

Both of the amputations were done at the same time, May 28, 1887, by the method of antero-posterior flaps with circular incision of the muscles. There was no mishap during his convalescence, and July 20th, just seven weeks after the amputations, he walked out of the manufacturer's shop on two Bligh legs, assisted with only a stick, the first patient in the experience of the maker who had ever done this, even when only one artificial limb was required. The patient has gradually improved in walking, and when I last saw him, a year ago, he told me he had walked four and a half miles in an hour and twenty minutes, on a country road.

The method by which this man walked on his deformed feet being similar to that employed while walking on artificial limbs enabled him to manage the latter with greater ease than is usual. In adjusting the artificial limbs his height was reduced to five feet eleven and one-half inches.

After his convalescence he became a theological

---

[1] Read before the American Orthopædic Association, Philadelphia, September, 1890.

[1] Casts of the feet were shown to the members of the Association.

student at Hanover, Indiana, and now has charge of a church·in Southern California.

CASE II.—W. M., aged sixteen years, the subject of chronic hip-disease, with recent pathological dislocation.

After a subperiosteal excision of the upper end of the femur it was discovered that the whole of the femoral shaft was the subject of osteomyelitis. Amputation was done forty-eight hours subsequently by the following method : The bone having already been removed, subperiosteally, sufficiently far down to allow the application of the Esmarch bandage so that the tourniquet would come above the bone, the ·amputation was proceeded with by the mixed method—skin flaps antero-posteriorly, and circular incision of the muscles. No sawing of the bone was required, as the circular division of the muscles corresponded with the upper end of the bone so nearly that the limb slipped away without any difficulty. The boy gradually recovered, and reproduction of bone occurred in the stump, the whole of the periosteum being left in a tolerably fair condition.

This amputation, necessitated by force of circumstances, suggests this method as a practical one in all cases where disarticulation at the hip is necessary, as it permits the application of the Esmarch bandage and a bloodless operation. When the case was last examined two years and a half had passed since the amputation. Bone had been reproduced down to the end of the periosteum, and the joint was controlled by the muscles as if the original bone had never been removed. He uses an artificial limb, and I have seen him walk on rough roads with no more difficulty than is ordinarily exhibited by a patient when first trying to use an artificial limb.

CASE III.—Miss M. T., aged eighteen years, had an inflammation of the left knee at the age of three years. Upon examination there were found five inches of actual shortening, and great atrophy of the limb. The shortening was due to subluxation of the tibia and arrested development. She was unable to use the limb without the aid of a long splint extending to the hip and perineum, besides a five-inch patten. By the aid of these she could get about with great difficulty, and suffered from many painful exacerbations of the inflammation, due to falls.

Amputation above the knee was advised, and was performed, July 17, 1884. Within three months she had a Bligh leg adjusted, and since then she has been able to walk with comparative ease, and in comeliness and comfort is greatly improved.

CASE IV.—C. W., aged twenty-four years, single, gave the following history : When about six years of age he received a blow upon the right knee, which was followed by acute inflammation of the joint, the limb rapidly becoming flexed. Various surgeons treated him, and many attempts were made to straighten and keep straight the limb. In the course of time an abscess occurred, from which pieces of bone removed. For the last ten years or more he had walked by the aid of a crutch with a stirrup upon it.

On examining the patient I found his limb flexed to an angle of about ninety degrees, perfect bony ankylosis having taken place. It was much atrophied, although the muscles between the pelvis and thigh were well developed. The femur was bowed anteriorly from the weight thrown upon it while walking, the leg below acting as a lever.

The patient wanted his limb straightened, and after discussing the various procedures to bring about this result, we decided on the removal of a wedge-shaped piece of bone, including in the wedge the patella and part of the condyles of the femur and tibia—Buck's modification of Barton's operation.

On September 27, 1882, the operation was performed, the limb being straightened by force until the bony surfaces were in apposition. In order to accomplish this it was necessary to divide both hamstrings.

He took chloroform badly, which required the operation to be performed very rapidly, but no untoward symptoms followed after he was put to bed.

The patient was able to be about on crutches at the end of three weeks. In five weeks all dressings were removed, and the union was found to be bony. The external wound also had healed. There were two and three-fourths inches actual shortening.

This patient, in the eight years that have passed since the operation, has had no trouble, and walks ,well without a cane or crutch.

When this result was accomplished I felt that I had done a creditable piece of surgery ; but in the light of subsequent experience I now feel that in consideration of the greater danger of excision, and of the stiff knee and high shoe, that I would have done this man a greater service by amputating above the knee. Other cases might be instanced, but these are sufficient to illustrate the fact that amputation is often an orthopædic measure.

218 W. CHESTNUT STREET.

VERATRUM VIRIDE IN PNEUMONIA.

BY WILLIAM MARTIN, M.D.,
OF BRISTOL, PA.

IN the present age of scientific medicine the opinions of medical men differ as to the most rational and safe method of treatment of nearly all affections, and especially in the treatment of pneumonia do the views of physicians diverge widely.

In all the diseases which are acute in character and in which the crisis is reached in a few days, prompt medication is important, and without this promptness valuable lives may be lost. Some practitioners have no distinct plan of treatment in pneumonia, but rely on being able to combat symptoms as they arise ; thus the disease often gets beyond control.

The principal difference of opinion in the treatment of pneumonia is with reference to venesection, and the use of the so-called arterial sedatives. The old method of treating acute inflammations of deep structures by venesection is revived, and has its advocates, who announce great results and defy the profession to show equally good results by any other mode of treatment.

The majority, however, still practise the more recent method, that by the administration of remedies which have a sedative action on the circulatory system, of which the most valuable though not the most used is veratrum viride.

This drug is not used by many physicians because it has the reputation of being dangerous, and some who have used it may not have had good results simply because it was either not properly administered or because the tincture was not pure and of standard strength. When pure the tincture of veratrum is very efficient, and in the author's experience better results have been obtained by its administration than by any other plan of treatment. The best form to use in this disease is the pure tincture (Norwood's).

The dose should at first be small, gradually increasing until the physiological effects are produced, when, if the toxic symptoms are marked, it should be discontinued, and need not be renewed, except in rare cases. When the toxic point is reached such symptoms as depression, nausea, and, possibly, vomiting may develop, but these quickly disappear. Professor Bartholow[1] writes: "Notwithstanding the very formidable symptoms produced by large doses, fatal results have been extremely rare."

The principal effects of veratrum are reduction of the force and number of the heart-beats and lowered arterial tension. The drug may be carefully pushed so that the pulsations are reduced to but little more than thirty per minute without bad effects if the patient remains in the recumbent position. If depression, vomiting, and other symptoms appear, stimulation and a little morphine will soon produce reaction.

The best time to administer veratrum in pneumonia is in the first stage, but it is also beneficial in the second stage, the stage in which cases are usually first seen. The influence of the drug is similar to that of venesection, but is more precise, as the pulse can be reduced at will and at the same time lessened in force, thus reducing the blood-supply of the lungs, preventing further consolidation, and hastening resolution. In cases with feeble constitutions, such as inebriates, in which depression would be harmful, the results are better if the drug is not given in amounts sufficient to cause its physiological effects, and in these cases it is usually necessary to give ammonium carbonate with the veratrum.

It is very easy to find the proper amount for each patient if the drug is first given in small doses and increased gradually, for the effects will always be manifest before a lethal dose is given.

[1] Materia Medica and Therapeutics.

In cases with high temperature, rapid pulse, and labored respiration, the effects are marvellous: the temperature falls usually to normal, sometimes to a degree below; the pulse is reduced, sometimes to one-fourth of the previous rate; and the respirations become deep and quiet; while the patient, if vomiting does not occur, quietly falls asleep and awakens refreshed and better—the crisis is over.

By this method of treatment cases seen early may be aborted, and convalescence may be hastened in those seen in the second stage. Such local measures as may be indicated, should, of course, be used in combination with this internal treatment.

In a number of cases treated in this manner by the author, the average duration of the disease was remarkably short, especially in view of the fact that four were cases of double pneumonia and that one was phthisical.

Summarizing, we find that:

1. The administration of veratrum viride is the preferable method of treating pneumonia, and that the drug is best given in the form of a tincture, (Norwood's).

2. If the dose is at first small and gradually increased it is a safe medicament.

3. It should be given early, and if possible, in the first stage, though it is also of use in the second stage.

4. If used in cases with broken-down constitutions, as in inebriates, it should be administered cautiously. In such cases there is immediate danger from the depression, and the toxic effects should not be produced.

CLINICAL MEMORANDA.

THERAPEUTICAL.

Aristol.—The efficacy of the dry treatment by means of absorbent powders has been so frequently and positively manifested in cases of superficial wounds and ulcerations, that any substance which combines the qualities of a rapid absorbent, of a mild stimulant, and of a powerful antiseptic, is most valuable to the surgeon.

Many drugs for which these qualities are claimed have been recommended, and of all iodoform has been most generally accepted by the profession. This substance has, however, certain positive disadvantages. Its odor is penetrating and lasting, and to many patients intolerable. If applied to large surfaces the danger of toxic symptoms developing from absorption has been proved by numberless recorded cases. Hence, substitutes for this material are constantly being brought forward. Hydronaphthol and iodol promised well, and yielded good results, but after a comparatively brief trial their use was discontinued.

The latest substitute for iodoform is aristol, a combination of thymol and iodine. Aristol is a fine, absorbing powder, without unpleasant odor, and it is said never occasions toxic symptoms, nor causes undue irritation of a wound, being, moreover, a powerful antiseptic.

Bacteriological researches have not proved the antiseptic power of aristol. This, of course, does not conclusively settle the matter from a medical point of view, since iodoform is in the laboratory absolutely destitute of germicidal properties, though few doubt its efficacy in cases of suppurating wounds.

With a view to determining the applicability of aristol to the ordinary surgical affections encountered in dispensary practice, for it is here that the drug, if well approved, will mainly be of use, I directed one of my students, Mr. R. Pittfield, to record carefully the results of its employment as a dusting-powder in a comparatively large number of selected cases. It is difficult to tabulate accurately the results obtained in these cases, and no just judgment can be formed of the drug until its use is much more widespread than at present. In general terms it may be stated that the observed effects were very similar to those noted after the employment of iodoform. The wounds and open surfaces remained dry, granulations were slightly stimulated, and healing progressed favorably. Good effects were particularly marked in several cases of ulcerating gummata. In these there was pronounced improvement immediately upon substituting aristol for iodoform.

In but two cases was there any ill effect from the powder. In these granulations, which previously had been comparatively healthy, became highly inflamed and slightly sloughing, so that iodoform had to be used. As a result of the application of aristol to a variety of cases it would seem that the drug may be fairly ranked with iodol, hydronaphthol, and iodoform in so far as its immediate effects are concerned, that it is particularly serviceable in cases of ulcerative syphilis, and that it possesses the advantage of being devoid of disagreeable odor. As to whether it can by decomposing in foul wounds render septic products innocuous is yet to be determined, and upon this point will depend either its universal use or its relegation to the obscure position occupied by so many drugs which have been advocated from time to time.　　　　EDWARD MARTIN, M.D.,
Assistant Surgeon to the
Hospital of the University of Pennsylvania.

OBSTETRICAL.

Veratrum in Eclampsia.—The following case did not differ materially from the majority of cases of eclampsia, and it is chiefly to the treatment that I desire to call attention.

On May 22d, early in the morning, I was called to see Mary S., a robust negress about twenty years of age; primipara. She was unconscious, and both tonic and clonic convulsions were rapidly recurring. From her mother I learned that labor began on the previous evening, at which time the patient had a "fit," and that since then she had been unconscious. Several convulsions occurred during the night. As the least irritation would excite a convulsion, I gave half a grain of morphine hypodermically before making a vaginal examination. However, the morphine did not prevent a convulsion when I attempted to make the examination, so that I abandoned the idea of precipitating labor. The pulse was full and bounding, respiration labored and shallow, face and feet much swollen, and the kidneys not acting. Clonic convulsions became less frequent, but the condition of the respiration, skin, and pulse remained unchanged.

Although the symptoms indicated venesection, I was convinced that better results could be obtained from veratrum viride, of which I gave twelve minims of the tincture hypodermically, about two hours after the administration of the morphine. In a short time the pulse was reduced in frequency and became soft and compressible, the skin moist, and breathing less labored. I was told by the mother that the patient had answered twice when spoken to. The condition of the kidneys remained unchanged.

May 23. Condition was unchanged, except that a vaginal examination was made, which caused only twitchings of the muscles of the face and arms. Labor was advancing very slowly.

24th. The pulse increased in frequency and diminished in volume, and the skin became dry. I kept the patient quiet and gave morphine in small doses hypodermically. In the night the child was born. Hour-glass contraction followed, for which I gave chloroform, dilated the constriction, and removed the placenta. This operation caused convulsions.

The patient never regained consciousness, and died on the following afternoon. I was not present when she died, but from what the mother said I think that death occurred during a convulsion.

I am persuaded that veratrum is of greater utility than venesection, in cases where the symptoms seem to indicate the latter. Veratrum produces all the good effects of bleeding without the bad ones. It depresses, but does not exhaust the patient; it reduces the reflex excitability of the spinal cord, and it lessens very much, if it does not entirely check, the spasms. Pilocarpine should be used hypodermically, often enough to keep up free diaphoresis, and I believe that the fœtus should be removed as soon as it can be done without causing convulsions.

During the actual seizures, chloroform is our most potent remedy.　　　　JOHN H. AYRES, M.D.
ACCOMACK C. H., VIRGINIA.

MEDICAL PROGRESS.

The Uses of Hydroxylamine.—ROSENTHAL (*Deutsche medicinische Wochenschrift*, No. 35, 1890) has thoroughly reviewed the recent work on the uses of hydroxylamine. Comparatively few practitioners have employed the drug in the treatment of disease, and its effects have been chiefly observed in the management of skin affections. Thus, Eichhoff has used the drug in some parasitic and bacillary diseases of the skin. He has treated five cases of lupus, five of herpes tonsurans, and one of sycosis with the following ointment:

R.—Chlorohydrate of hydroxylamine　.　.　.　1½ grains.
Alcohol } of each　.　.　12½ drachms.—M.
Glycerin }

This mixture may be employed five times daily, but the parts treated must be previously washed with soap and water. Owing to the irritant and toxic properties of the drug, the solutions when first used must not be very strong. A case of lupus of the upper lip and nose yielded to this treatment in eight days, and at the end of four weeks the ulcers were entirely cicatrized. In the cases of herpes tonsurans the application of the drug was followed by eczema of the scalp, but the final results were good and were rapidly attained. Eichhoff thinks that good results may also be attained in psoriasis, parasitic and seborrhœic eczema, and in the eruptions of syphilis, and that subcutaneous injections may be employed in the treatment of leprosy.

Fabry observed twenty-four cases of psoriasis treated with hydroxylamine, and found that the action of the drug resembled that of chrysarobin and pyrogallic acid, with the advantage that it did not stain the clothing. Care, however, must be exercised in the employment of the drug, owing to its poisonous properties. Thus, the application of hydroxylamine in one patient, a woman, was followed by very marked albuminuria, which ceased with the suspension of the treatment. Fabry has employed the medicament associated with calcium carbonate, as follows :

R.—Chlorohydrate of hydrox-
　　ylamine　　　.　..　3 to 4 grains.
　　Alcohol .　　.　.　15 drachms.
　　Carbonate of calcium, a sufficient quantity to
　　neutralize.　　　　—M.

R.—Chlorohydrate of hydrox-
　　ylamine.　.　.　.　15 grains.
　　Water　.　.　.　.　2 pints.
　　Carbonate of calcium, a sufficient quantity to
　　neutralize.　　　　—M.

Blaschko advises an ointment of lanolin containing one or two per cent. of hydroxylamine. Such a preparation causes no pain and is well borne. Eichhoff has more recently employed a three-per-cent. ointment with success in one case of seborrhœic eczema, one of herpes tonsurans, and four of sycosis. Kantorowicz has also obtained good results with the employment of Eichhoff's formula. A case of herpes tonsurans was completely cured in twenty-four days. Groddeck has employed hydroxylamine in the treatment of twenty-five cases, with variable success. In solutions of a strength of 1 to 1000 the drug produced irritation, and in many cases it did no good. On the whole, he found hydroxylamine inferior to chrysarobin and pyrogallic acid, and, owing to its toxic properties, he thinks its use should not be extensive.—*La Médecine Moderne,* September 18, 1890.

The Treatment of Diphtheria by Inoculations of Erysipelas.—BABTSCHINSKI observed three severe cases of diphtheria which resulted in recovery after the spontaneous appearance of erysipelas. This led him to experiment with the treatment of diphtheria by inoculations with the cultures of the erysipelas microbes. Fourteen patients were treated by this method. The inoculations were made by means of scarification in the neighborhood of the submaxillary lymphatic glands. The symptoms of erysipelas showed themselves in from four to twelve hours, and as the erysipelas progressed the diphtheritic membrane gradually disappeared from the fauces, the lymphatic engorgement diminished, and the temperature fell. In two cases only was the treatment unsuccessful, and

in these, death occurred before the erysipelas developed. No additional treatment was used, and other cases of diphtheria occurring in the families of those inoculated were, without exception, fatal.—*London Medical Recorder,* September, 1890.

Tetanoid Convulsions probably Due to Infection of the Umbilicus.—MR. T. R. RONALDSON (*Edinburgh Medical Journal,* October, 1890) reports an interesting case of tetanoid convulsions in an infant. When the infant was nine days old, winking of the left eye and twitching of the same side of the face appeared, and with these symptoms swelling of the tongue. The spasmodic symptoms increased, and on the third day of the attack Mr. Ronaldson was called to attend the child. At this time the infant's appearance was that of health, and the only symptoms were the convulsive attacks, which were confined to the left side, beginning as tonic and ending as clonic spasms. On examination, the stump of the cord was found still attached to the umbilicus, and, though dry, had a putrefactive odor. There were no signs of inflammation around it. The remains of the cord were removed by means of scissors, and the stump was washed with bichloride solution and dressed with zinc ointment. The attacks, however, continued in spite of the administration of potassium bromide, chloral, and chlorodyne, and the application of twenty-per-cent. solution of cocaine, and nitrate of silver. On the seventh day of the attack the seizures became general, and recurred 204 times in twenty-four hours. On the thirteenth day, although the stump was rapidly healing, the umbilicus was excised. The fits at once diminished in frequency. On the fourth day after operation there were no seizures, but on the following evening they returned. The silkworm-gut sutures were then removed, after which the attacks diminished in frequency, although they did not disappear. Eight days later, sulphocarbolate of sodium, four grains every two hours, was prescribed, with the result that the digestion was upset and the fits became more frequent. Reducing the dose of sulphocarbolate, the convulsions gradually became less frequent, and none occurred after the thirtieth day following the operation. The child has since then remained in good health.

The excised umbilicus was examined by Dr. Edington, but no microörganisms were found.

Powder for Migraine.—The following powder is recommended in *La Médecine Moderne* for the treatment of migraine :

R.—Citrate of caffeine　.　.　1½ grain.
　　Phenacetin　.　.　.　2 grains.
　　Sugar of milk .　.　.　4　"　—M.

To be made into one powder. This dose may be repeated, if necessary, in the course of two hours.

Treatment of Gastric Ulcer.—In the *Revue Général de Clinique et de Thérapeutique,* the following summary of the treatment of gastric ulcer is given by ELOY. In cases where absolute intolerance of milk exists, predigested foods are to be employed, and the milk should be peptonized. Beyond the diet, four indications are to be combated—namely, gastralgia, flatulence, vomiting, and hæmorrhage from the stomach. For the pain in the belly it is recommended that the patient shall receive an injection of morphine and a hot application or a mustard-plaster to the epigastrium ; while if pain is due to the ingestion of food, we can resort to preventive measures only, which consist in the employment of liquid and unirritating foods, and the administration of five drops of the following mixture in a teaspoonful of water :

R.—Hydrochlorate of morphine 2½ grains.
  Cherry-laurel water . . ½ drachm.—M.

If constipation exists with the gastralgia, small doses of belladonna may be employed, or, as has been recommended by Bartholow, a powder consisting of 2 grains of subnitrate of bismuth and ¼ of a grain of sulphate of morphine, may be taken shortly before the meals. In some cases, however, small quantities of atropine may with advantage be substituted for the morphine. The following prescription may be found of service :

R.—Atropine . . . . $\frac{1}{10}$ grain.
  Subnitrate of bismuth . 1 drachm.—M.

Divide into ten powders, and take one at night and in the morning. If the vomiting is obstinate, small pieces of cracked ice may be held in the mouth and cold may be applied to the epigastric region by means of the ice-bag, while warmth is applied to the feet. Under these circumstances, too, subnitrate of bismuth is valuable. For the flatulence which is so commonly present in these cases, it is recommended that small amounts of calcined magnesia be ingested, or that a very small cup of coffee be taken three times a day. For hæmorrhage from the stomach the physician should administer ice, tannic acid, acetate of lead, and antipyrine. The acetate of lead, when prescribed, should be combined with morphine, but when tannin is used it is best associated with opium, as is shown in the following prescriptions :

R.—Acetate of lead . . 3 grains.
  Hydrochlorate of morphine 1 grain.
  Powdered white sugar . 1 drachm.—M.

Make into ten powders, and give two to five a day, or one every hour.

R.—Opium and tannin, of each 10 grains.
  Pure opium . . . 3 "
  Powdered sugar . . . 1½ drachms.—M.

This is to be divided into ten powders, and one powder is to be taken every one or two hours, or oftener, if necessary.

Antipyrine is often employed in hæmatemesis, because of the hæmostatic effect which has been noticed by Henocque, Huchard, and Arduin. It may be administered in powders of ten grains, one every hour for five hours, associated with cocaine. It is sometimes of great service when used as follows :

R.—Hydrochlorate of cocaine 1½ grains.
  Antipyrine . . . . 45 grains.—M.

Divide into five powders, and follow the administration of each by a tablespoonful of rum, as the alcohol favors the action of the antipyrine.

Tellurate of Potassium in Night-sweats.—According to *La Médecine Moderne*, October 21, 1890, tellurate of potassium has been found by NEUSSER to be valuable in the suppression and diminution of night-sweats. He employs one-third of a grain, in pill-form.

After the patients have taken this dose for a short time, it may be doubled without unfavorable results and with a good effect in reducing the quantity of sweat, provided the first dose has not been sufficient to control it. In rare cases the drug may produce dyspeptic symptoms. As a general rule, however, it has a favorable effect.

Local Anæsthesia for Slight Operations.—For operations upon small abscesses, opening fistulous tracts, or removing superficial growths, it is recommended that local anæsthesia be secured by atomization of the following solution :

R.—Chloroform . . . 10 parts.
  Sulphuric ether . . . 15 "
  Menthol . . . . 1 part.—M.

The anæsthesia which is thus obtained lasts from two to ten minutes.

Mixture for the Treatment of Smallpox.—According to *La Semaine Médicale*, the following is a useful mixture for the treatment of variola :

R.—Sublimed and washed sulphur . 2½ drachms.
  Glycerin } of each 6 "
  Water of orange flowers }
  Simple syrup . . . 5 "

Mix, and give a coffeespoonful to children, or a tablespoonful to an adult, every two or three hours.

The Action of Hypnal.—This drug, which is variously known as monochloralantipyrin or monotrichloracetyl dimethylphenylpyrazalon, has been recently introduced by certain European physicians as a valuable hypnotic and analgesic.

In the *Bulletin Générale de Thérapeutique*, September 30, 1890, FRÄNKEL has presented an exhaustive study, not only of the chemical constitution of hypnal, but also of its physiological action and the best modes for its administration. The conclusions reached by Dr. Fränkel are that the drug is useful in the insomnia produced by excessive pain, and not only in the sleeplessness which results from cough arising from bronchitis, but also in that due to tubercular disease, and in neuralgic insomnia. It possesses all the properties of both chloral and antipyrin, or, in other words, both relieves pain and produces sleep. The very nature of the compound almost of necessity makes it a useful remedy, since, as is known to most of the profession, chloral in ordinary doses has little effect upon pain, and antipyrin, while relieving pain, rarely produces sleep.

Hypnal being quite insoluble in cold water, the best way to administer it is in some mucilaginous mixture which will hold it in suspension, such as syrup of acacia : the following formula is given by BARDET for its administration :

R.—Hypnal . . . . 30 grains.
  Syrup of acacia . . 1 fluidounce.—M.

Dose : A dessertspoonful.

Or a very excellent formula is as follows :

R.—Hypnal . . . . 15 grains.
  Chartreuse . . . . 1 drachm.
  Water . . . . ½ ounce.—M.

The entire amount to be taken in one dose, or to be divided into several doses when given to children.

THE MEDICAL NEWS.

A WEEKLY JOURNAL
OF MEDICAL SCIENCE.

COMMUNICATIONS are invited from all parts of the world. Original articles contributed exclusively to THE MEDICAL NEWS will be liberally paid for upon publication. When necessary to elucidate the text, illustrations will be furnished without cost to the author.

Address the Editor: H. A. HARE, M.D.,
1004 WALNUT STREET,
PHILADELPHIA.

Subscription Price, including Postage.

PER ANNUM, IN ADVANCE . . . . $4.00.
SINGLE COPIES . . . . 10 CENTS.

Subscriptions may begin at any date. The safest mode of remittance is by bank check or postal money order, drawn to the order of the undersigned. When neither is accessible, remittances may be made, at the risk of the publishers, by forwarding in *registered* letters.

Address, LEA BROTHERS & CO.,
Nos. 706 & 708 SANSOM STREET,
PHILADELPHIA.

SATURDAY, NOVEMBER 1, 1890.

AN UNJUST PROSECUTION.

THE readers of the daily papers in and about Philadelphia who are at all interested in medicine or pharmacy noticed several weeks ago that two of the leading druggists of Atlantic City had been arrested and charged with the misdemeanor of selling adulterated drugs.

A complete explanation of the arrest lies in the fact that the State of New Jersey some time ago adopted the United States Pharmacopœia as its standard of drugs. This action is laudable so far as it goes, and we think it would be fortunate if the remaining States of the Union would stamp officially the product of the Committee of the Revision of the Pharmacopœia with their approval. That an act done with the best intentions may, however, result in legal absurdities, is represented by the case before us. The druggists, who were fined fifty dollars each, were in the habit of preparing their tincture of nux vomica from the so-called normal liquid of Parke, Davis & Co., which is an assayed fluid, the strength of which is governed not by the quantity of solid extract, as is directed in the U. S. Pharmacopœia, but by the amount of active principle or alkaloid which the drug contains.

The Dairy Commissioner of New Jersey having obtained samples of nux vomica, had it analyzed

according to the directions given in the last Pharmacopœia, with the natural result that the extract was not present in proper quantity, and upon the chemist's testimony the Justice before whom the druggists were taken at once administered punishment. That this punishment was unjust is, of course, at once evident to anyone who is familiar with the subject, and we would call attention to the fact that the authorities of the State of New Jersey could practically prosecute almost every druggist in that commonwealth for some similar breach of the letter of the law.

The advances which medicine and pharmacy have made in the last ten years practically prohibit the use of many impure substances, which owing to our lack of knowledge in 1880 seemed as pure as possible. Chief among these may be named saccharated pepsin, which everyone now knows is practically useless as compared to the pure pepsins which are manufactured by the leading firms in this country.

The ludicrous condition of affairs exists that for once honesty was not the best policy; for if the druggists who suffered had dispensed the officinal tincture of nux vomica the patients receiving the medicine would have received a more impure preparation than if the law had not been obeyed.

We earnestly hope that Governor Abbett will use his influence to have the present law either repealed or so amended that similar travesties on justice may not recur.

DR. BARTHOLOW'S RETIREMENT.

IN another column will be found the news of the retirement of Dr. Roberts Bartholow from the Chair of Therapeutics and Materia Medica in the Jefferson Medical College, and those who are interested in Philadelphia as a medical centre and in medical education throughout the country will hear with regret of the withdrawal of this eminent and brilliant teacher from the corps of active professors in this well-known school. Dr. Bartholow has always been one of the foremost in teaching the best and most advanced yet conservative employment of remedies for the cure of disease, and his precepts as enunciated in his works and lectures, have no doubt given encouragement and success to a large body of the profession, particularly in its younger element.

Dr. Bartholow having left a most lucrative practice in Cincinnati, was able to obtain in Philadelphia a foothold immediately upon his arrival, which his sterling worth strengthened from year to year, until its dimensions increased so greatly that he was forced to limit himself to consultations. We are assured that no one appreciates Dr. Bartholow's worth more than the trustees of the Jefferson College, and that his retirement was only decided upon after the most careful consideration.

A NEW JOURNAL OF NERVOUS DISEASE.

We welcome to our exchange list *The Review of Insanity and Nervous Disease*, which is a quarterly compendium of the current literature of neurology and psychiatry, edited by Dr. James H. McBride, of Milwaukee, Wisconsin, who has associated with him as collaborators Dr. Gray, of New York, Dr. Mills, of Philadelphia, Dr. Riggs, of St. Paul, Dr. Jones, of Minneapolis, and Dr. Bannister, of Kankakee.

After a careful examination of the pages of the first number we are forced to conclude that this is a publication which by reason of its able selection of abstracts is one to which every one who is interested in nervous diseases must subscribe, while the contents of this number are so uniformly good that the following issues will probably be equally worthy of praise.

SOCIETY PROCEEDINGS.

MISSISSIPPI VALLEY MEDICAL ASSOCIATION.

Sixteenth Annual Meeting,
held in Louisville, Kentucky, October 8, 9, and 10, 1890.

First Day.—Morning Session.

The Association met in Liederkranz Hall, and was called to order by the President, Dr. J. M. Mathews, of Louisville, at 10 A.M.

Dr. Frank Woodbury, of Philadelphia, read the first paper, which was entitled

INFECTIOUS DYSPEPSIA AND ITS RATIONAL TREATMENT BY THE ANTISEPTIC METHOD.

Dr. Woodbury said that in the present unsettled condition of medical nomenclature dyspepsia is as much entitled to recognition as a distinct disease as is consumption or chorea. Like the latter diseases, it is characterized by manifestations of nervous disorder, so that Cullen was not entirely wrong in considering dyspepsia as a neurosis belonging to the class of adynamiæ. Like pulmonary phthisis, its most marked symptoms are produced, the author believes, by the absorption of the products of parasitic microörganisms.

Abelous, a recent investigator of this subject, found sixteen species of microörganisms normally existing in

his own stomach, of which two species were micrococci, thirteen bacilli, and one was a vibrio.

Habitually laborious, painful, and imperfect digestion, when not symptomatic of other disease, constitutes dyspepsia; and when accompanied by fermentation of the contents of the stomach and general toxic symptoms, the result of microbian development, it may properly be called infectious dyspepsia.

The disorder is sufficiently prevalent and gives rise to enough discomfort and actual suffering not only to deserve our serious consideration, but also to enlist our best therapeutic skill. The excessive growth of microorganisms during digestion is favored by slow movements of the stomach and by a deficient quantity or defective quality of the gastric juice. Acid dyspepsia, or sour stomach, may, rarely, be due to excessive secretion of hydrochloric acid, but is generally caused by lactic, acetic, or butyric fermentation, produced by the bacteria in the stomach. The object of treatment in infectious dyspepsia should be to prevent the excessive development of microörganisms during the digestion of food. This is attempted (1) by the use of articles of diet which are not in a fermenting condition nor readily fermentable; (2) by adopting such hygienic and tonic measures as will invigorate the bodily powers, bring the gastric juice up to its normal standard of quality and quantity, and increase the muscular power of the stomach; and (3) by local antiseptic treatment, including the administration of drugs which retard fermentation, and especially by lavage or irrigation of the stomach with weak disinfecting solutions, or simply recently boiled water.

Dr. John H. Hollister, of Chicago, then read a paper on

HELP AND HINDRANCE TO MEDICAL PROGRESS,

and was followed by Dr. I. N. Love, of St. Louis, who, in a paper upon

COFFEE,

said that after an experience of five or six years he favored taking a cup of strong, black coffee, without cream or sugar, preceded and followed by a glass of hot water, every morning before rising, or at least one hour before breakfast. The various secretions are stimulated, the nerve-force is aroused, and the day's labor is easier, no matter how the duties of the preceding day and night may have drawn upon the system. Another cup at four in the afternoon is sufficient to sustain the energies for many hours. In this way the full effect is secured. The ideal food for brain-workers is hot milk, and if this regimen be followed and accompanied with at least eight hours of sleep in every twenty-four hours, the capacity for work is almost unlimited.

Dr. George Hulbert, of St. Louis, Missouri, read an interesting paper on

MECHANICAL OBSTRUCTION IN DISEASES OF THE UTERUS,

and submitted the following conclusions:

1. Normally we find the uterus in form and structure endowed with a capacity for menstruation far in excess of the demand.

2. In the pathological conditions considered as essen-

tial for mechanical obstruction we find that the conservation of force regulates the conditions so effectually that the capacity for menstruation is not abolished, and that the function is accomplished, unless there is *atresia*.

3. The phenomena believed to be dependent upon mechanical obstruction are not due to the forcible expulsion of retained fluids through the uterine canal, but are produced within the tissues, and are due to a disturbed rhythm of physiological forces caused by abnormal inervation, muscular action, and circulation.

4. The correct and rational interpretation of the testimony offered by symptomatology, pathology, and therapeutics removes mechanical obstruction from the domain of gynecology as a demonstrable fact, save in *atresia uteri*.

AFTERNOON SESSION.

The Association was called to order at 3 P.M. by First Vice-President Dr. C. R. Earley, of Ridgway, Pa.

DR. R. STANSBURY SUTTON, of Pittsburg, Pa., made (by invitation) some remarks on

THE SURGICAL TREATMENT OF UTERINE FIBROIDS,

and exhibited specimens.

DR. WILLIAM PORTER, of St. Louis, Mo., contributed a paper on

THE SELF-LIMITATION OF PHTHISIS,

in which he said that some time before his death Professor Flint promulgated the doctrine of the self-limitation of phthisis, and that this very interesting proposition was at one time freely discussed in various medical societies.

Dr. Porter said that after having carefully examined the facts cited in support of the proposition, he had no hesitation in asserting that there is not sufficient evidence to warrant us to accept the statement that phthisis is self-limiting, or that the element of self-limitation has a decided influence upon the result in any given case. He did not mean that all cases of phthisis necessarily die from the disease, but that when phthisis is firmly established there is nothing in the nature of the disease itself that indicates in any stage a fixed boundary—a line of demarcation as it were—but rather that all of its tendencies are progressive and downward.

DR. A. B. THRASHER, of Cincinnati, Ohio, then read a paper on

COUGH, ITS RELATION TO INTRA-NASAL DISEASE.

Cough, he said, is a reflex phenomenon due to the irritation of nerve-fibres in the bronchi, larynx, pharynx, nose, ear, stomach, etc.

A "normal" cough is for the purpose of freeing the air-tract from some foreign body. Irritation of the upper part of the trachea and of the ventricles of Morgagni most frequently produces cough, but irritation in many other locations may be referred by the sensory centres to this region, and thus give rise to cough. Inflammation of the cavernous bodies of the nose or of the septum has been known to cause a distressing cough that was mistaken for a symptom of tubercular disease. This is more apt to occur in persons of a neurotic temperament. The cough due to nasal disease may sometimes be recognized by its metallic ring and the absence of expectoration, and, as a rule, it can be provoked by touching the

irritable spot in the nose with a probe. Dr. Thrasher cited the three following cases illustrative of nasal cough :

Case I.—In this case there were no subjective symptoms of nasal disease. The cough had been present for three months and was not benefited by the usual cough-mixtures. The lower turbinated body was hypertrophied, and touching it with a probe provoked violent coughing. The cautery was applied, and in three days the patient was well.

Case II.—A young woman who had been coughing violently for three months. She referred the irritation to the throat, which had been pencilled and sprayed for some time, with no relief. Touching the posterior extremities of either lower turbinated body produced violent cough. Treatment was adopted as in Case I., with good results in two months.

Case III.—Cough had been present for six months and was not benefited by constitutional or local treatment. The seat of the trouble was found to be in the left middle and right lower turbinated body. Treatment similar to that of the other cases was followed by cessation of cough within a month.

A paper entitled

THE THERAPEUTIC USES OF CARDIAC SEDATIVES IN INFLAMMATION,

by DR. H. A. HARE, of Philadelphia, was read by title in the absence of the author.

EVENING SESSION.

DR. JOHN A. WYETH, of New York, delivered the public address, taking for his subject

THE MEDICAL STUDENT.

Dr. Wyeth said that the first or preliminary stage of a medical student's education is his academic life, the second his medical college life, and the third his post-graduate or practical life, which extends from the day he leaves his alma mater until his usefulness ceases. Practical training may be acquired in three ways, as follows :

1. Service as interne, preferably for a term of two years, in a general hospital.

2. Service in some post-graduate college where all departments of practical medicine are taught by instructors especially trained in their respective branches.

3. Service as an assistant to one or more well-qualified practitioners in general medicine.

SECOND DAY.—MORNING SESSION.

DR. H. C. DALTON, of St. Louis, reported six cases of

PENETRATING STAB-WOUNDS OF THE ABDOMEN,

in which abdominal section was performed.

Case I.—A negro, aged sixteen years, admitted to the City Hospital, St. Louis, July 23, 1890. Patient had been stabbed two hours previously with a long-bladed knife. The wound was at the free extremity of the twelfth rib. Several inches of omentum protruded, but the general condition of the patient was excellent; pulse 62, respiration 23, temperature 100°. An incision was made in the left linea semilunaris. Blood and fæcal matter were found in the peritoneal cavity ; there were two holes in the descending colon and one in the ileum, which were closed with continued iron-dyed silk sutures.

Discharged from the hospital, cured eleven days after admission.

Case II.—A man, aged twenty-one years, admitted August 21, 1890. He had received three stab-wounds an hour and a half before admission, one of which was an inch below the costal border and four inches to the left of the median line, and through this wound three inches of omentum protruded. The second wound was an inch above and two inches to the right of the umbilicus; and the third was in the seventh intercostal space in the right axillary line. A wound of the jejunum was closed by interrupted silk sutures. Four inches of the seventh rib were resected, the diaphragm was split f r three inches, and a wound in the liver was closed by one catgut suture. The diaphragmatic and cutaneous wounds were closed by continuous catgut sutures. Patient's temperature arose to 102° on the second day, after which he rapidly recovered.

Dr. Dalton laid particular stress upon the importance of carefully inspecting such wounds to the bottom, and severely condemned the method of trusting to the introduction of the finger.

He did not think that implicit confidence should be placed in Senn's hydrogen-gas test. ·

DR. M. T. SCOTT, of Lexington, Kentucky, reported a case of

GUNSHOT WOUND OF THE INTESTINE,

in which four perforations were made by a large bullet. Complete recovery followed abdominal section.

DR. J. B. MURDOCH, of Pittsburg, Pa., contributed a paper on

TORSION OF ARTERIES AS A MEANS OF ARRESTING HÆMORRHAGE.

There are two methods, he said, by which torsion may be applied: (1) limited torsion, and (2) free torsion. In the first method, two pairs of forceps are required. One pair grasps the vessel at its cut extremity, and pulls it from the sheath. The artery is then seized by the second pair of forceps at a point from one·half an inch to an inch above the cut extremity, the second forceps being held at right angles to the long axis of the vessel. The first pair is then given three or four sharp turns.

By the second method only one pair of forceps is required. It is the method recommended by Bryant as not being likely to injure the external coat of the artery.

The following is a table showing the number of arteries, divided in cases of amputation, in which torsion by the second method was resorted to at the Western Pennsylvania Hospital for the arrest of hæmorrhage :

Femoral	.	.	.	.	.	116 times.
Popliteal	.	.	.	.	.	18 "
Axillary	.	.	.	.	.	18 "
Anterior tibial	.	.	.	.	317 "
Brachial	.	.	.	.	.	81 "
Radial	.	.	.	.	.	45 "
Ulnar	.	.	.	.	.	45 "

Dr. Murdoch said, in conclusion, that the advantages of torsion as compared with ligation are: (1) The greater facility with which it can be applied. (2) Torsion is a safer method, being less liable to be followed by secondary hæmorrhage. (3) Healing is facilitated, because the wound is free from any irritating or foreign body.

DR. G. FRANK LYDSTON, of Chicago, then exhibited the skulls of a number of the most notorious criminals of the world, and made some very instructive remarks with reference to their peculiarities, shape, size, etc.

AFTERNOON SESSION.

DR. W. P. KING, of Kansas City, Mo., contributed a paper entitled

WIRING THE SEPARATED SYMPHYSIS PUBIS, SUPPLE-
MENTED BY A PELVIC CLAMP,

which will appear in full in THE MEDICAL NEWS.

DR. C. H. HUGHES, of St. Louis, Mo., read a very elaborate and profound paper, entitled

PSYCHOPATHIC SEQUENCES OF HEREDITARY ALCOHOLIC
ENTAILMENT,

which was followed by a paper on

UREA AND SEROUS MEMBRANES,

by DR. C. S. BOND, of Richmond, Indiana.

DR. ARCHIBALD DIXON, of Henderson, Ky., in a paper on

INGUINAL COLOTOMY,

said that the subject of colotomy, always one of interest, has, during the past decade, received much attention from the surgical world. As a measure to ward off imminent death, colotomy is demanded in all cases of obstruction in the colon, from whatever cause. For imperforate anus the operation holds a special position. It is intended to prevent impending death, but it may also be regarded as a cure for the disease. In many cases it is the first step in the process of cure. In a few words, it may be said that the indications to operate in any given disease depend, in the first place, on the chance which the patient has of getting well without operation; and, in the second place, upon the degree of probability that success will follow the operation. In cases of acute obstruction of the sigmoid flexure, or other part of the bowel, there is practically but one termination—death. No case of volvulus, whether of the large or small intestine, has as yet been known to recover under purely medicinal treatment. Here, then, the indication is as clear as the indication in hæmorrhage from the carotid —operation.

DR. EMORY LANPHEAR, of Kansas City, Mo., read a paper on

HYPNOTISM IN ITS RELATION TO SURGERY.

He reported a case of double talipes in which the subject had chronic Bright's disease which contraindicated the use of ether, and also had valvular disease, which prevented the safe use of chloroform. Dr. Lanphear hypnotized the patient, and operated at the first *séance*, contrary to the generally accepted idea that at the first *séance* a sufficient degree of anæsthesia cannot be produced.

Another case (reported by the permission of Dr. Shaw, of St. Louis) was that of a patient suffering from Jacksonian epilepsy due to a brain-tumor. He was hypnotized and trephined, the dura was opened, and a tumor weighing one and one-half ounces removed. The bone was replaced and the operation, lasting an hour, was completed.

DR. HAROLD N. MOYER, of Chicago, then read a paper on

THE HYPODERMIC USE OF ARSENIC.

He said that the hypodermic use of Fowler's solution has been recommended by various writers, among others, Hammond, who claimed that the dose which can be administered in this way is much greater than that which can safely be given by the mouth. Hammond has given as much as fifty drops of Fowler's solution as an initial dose. Again, he has often given the drug by the mouth until the eyes were puffed and vomiting was almost incessant, and then continued the arsenic in larger doses by hypodermic injection, with cessation of all gastric symptoms and the cure of the disorder.

In the case of a girl fourteen years old, suffering from chorea, the patient was placed upon the hypodermic use of arsenious acid, beginning with 3 minims of a five-per-cent. solution, and increasing every second day until three weeks after beginning the treatment, when she was receiving 13 minims at each injection, equivalent to about 36 minims of Fowler's solution. At the ninth injection she was discharged cured.

In the case of a woman who presented herself at the clinic in Rush Medical College with an enormous lymphadenoma of the side of the neck, after a few deep injections into the glandular mass the tumor began to diminish rapidly. When it had decreased one-half, the patient ceased attending and further observations could not be made.

Dr. Moyer's observations are in accord with those of numerous writers who have reported good results from the use of Fowler's solution in various forms of glandular enlargement, such as lymphoma, lymphadenoma, and Hodgkin's disease.

THIRD DAY.—MORNING SESSION.

DR. H. O. WALKER, of Detroit, read a paper on

PERINEAL CYSTOTOMY VERSUS SUPRAPUBIC CYSTOTOMY.

He said that in choosing an operation we should be governed (1) by its safety, (2) by its simplicity, and (3) by its applicability to the majority of cases.

For the removal of stone, litholapaxy undoubtedly stands preëminent, and can be done upon many patients past the age of three years, yet there are numerous restrictions to this method, such as stricture of the urethra, the large size of the stone, an enormous prostate, etc. There can be no question that when cutting has to be done the medio-bilateral method presents many advantages.

In looking up the literature of suprapubic operations since 1883, Dr. Walker found in the records of between three and four hundred operations, an average mortality of 30 per cent. A few operators have had a series of cases ranging from three to ten without a death. The most remarkable record in this respect is that of Dr. Hunter McGuire—twenty-one operations with but a single death. By the perineal method we find a mortality of from 5 to 9 per cent., rarely greater.

DR. EDWIN WALKER, of Evansville, Indiana, then reported

TWO CASES OF TUBAL PREGNANCY.

The first patient was twenty-seven years old, married for four years, and sterile. She had a history of uterine and tubal trouble before marriage. The menses were always irregular and were often missed for a month or two. She menstruated on June 29, 1890, but not in July. A few days after the missed period she began to suffer from severe pain in the right groin. On August 1st a sanguinous flow began, and an examination under ether revealed a soft tumor the size of a fist to the right of and behind the uterus. On August 17th the abdomen was opened, and the right tube, which was very large, was found ruptured. There was a large amount of clotted blood in the pelvis. The abdomen was irrigated with hot water and a glass drainage-tube used. The fœtus was not found. The operation was followed by some vomiting and pain, but recovery ensued without other bad symptoms. Drainage-tube removed on the third and sutures on the twelfth day. The highest temperature was 101.1°.

The author thinks that the present status of the question of operating is, that with such symptoms as were present in this case, abdominal section is the safest procedure to adopt.

DR. WILLIAM T. BELFIELD, of Chicago, in a paper entitled

A RÉSUMÉ OF EXPERIENCE IN THE VARIOUS OPERATIONS FOR CYSTITIS FROM PROSTATIC HYPERTROPHY,

reported 133 cases of operations upon the hypertrophied prostate, including eight of his own, as follows: Forty-one by perineal excision, mortality 9 per cent.; eighty-eight by suprapubic cystotomy, mortality 16 per cent.; four by combined perineal and suprapubic incision, none of which were fatal.

In fifty-six of these cases the patients had cystitis and had been dependent upon the catheter for periods varying from one to ten years. In all the cystitis was cured; in thirty-eight cases (two-thirds) the power of voluntary urination was restored and continued during the time of observation; in eighteen cases this function did not return.

Fifteen of the fifty-six cases were complicated with stone; excluding these, since it might be objected that the cure resulted from the extraction of the calculus rather than from the prostatic operation, there remain forty-one cases of uncomplicated prostatic operation. Of these, thirty-two (four-fifths) recovered the power of urination, and in nine this ability was not recovered.

DR. S. NORMAN, of Evansville, Ind., contributed a paper entitled

THE TREATMENT OF ORGANIC STRICTURE OF THE MALE URETHRA,

in which he said that in the practice of urethral surgery the operator cannot be too strongly impressed with the fact of the exquisite tenderness and sensitiveness of the urethra, and that the employment of the slightest amount of force in the introduction of an instrument should be regarded as a relic of barbaric surgery. When commencing the treatment by gradual dilatation, in sensitive patients, Dr. Norman always produces local anæsthesia by the injection of from twenty to thirty minims of a four-per-cent. solution of hydrochlorate of cocaine.

Relative to internal urethrotomy, he believes that if it is properly and thoroughly executed and if special care is exercised to maintain the patency of the canal until the wound is healed, recontraction is of rare occurrence. Authority is divided in regard to the propriety of performing internal urethrotomy in the bulbous or in the membranous urethra. Judging from the results obtained by Harrison, the combination of external and internal urethrotomy offers encouragement for the permanent cure of stricture. Dr. Norman has performed external urethrotomy without a guide only three times, but the results as regards the absence of recontraction were entirely satisfactory. External urethrotomy with a guide is a simple operation, can be performed with facility and rapidity, and promises more satisfactory ultimate results than internal urethrotomy performed in the deep urethra.

DR. L. S. McMURTRY, of Louisville, then made some impromptu remarks on

THE APPLICATION OF ANTISEPTIC METHODS IN MIDWIFERY PRACTICE.

He said that many medical practitioners can remember the time when the wards of certain hospitals were closed and undergoing renovation because puerperal fever had become epidemic, whereas a hospital to-day is the safest place in which a woman can be confined. A few years ago we were taught by Fordyce Barker that puerperal fever was an entity, a distinct fever, dependent upon a specific *materies morbi*. To-day we know that puerperal fever, so-called, is a septic peritonitis. A woman after labor is a wounded woman. She has undergone certain physiological processes, and has received injuries in the process of labor which open the lymph-channels by which she may be infected from without. There is no such thing as a woman having peritonitis without external infection.

To prevent this infection the vagina must be sterilized, the bed, the examining finger, and the nurse must be surgically clean, and the atmosphere as approximately aseptic as it is possible to make it.

The following papers were also read : The Advantages of Attending Medical Societies and of Reading Medical Journals, by Dr. T. B. Greenley, of West Point, Ky.; Internal Urethrotomy, with cases, by Dr. J. V. Prewitt, of West Point, Ky.; Was It Relapsing Fever? by Dr. A. D. Barr, of Calamine Springs, Ark.; Some Remarks on the Prevention of Myopia, by Dr. Francis Dowling, of Cincinnati, Ohio.

OFFICERS FOR 1891.

President.—Dr. C. H. Hughes, of St. Louis.

First Vice-President.—Dr. John H. Hollister, of Chicago.

Second Vice-President.—Dr. S. S. Thorn, of Toledo.

Secretary.—Dr. E. S, McKee, of Cincinnati.

Place of meeting, St. Louis, Missouri, on the third Wednesday in October, 1891.

NEW YORK ACADEMY OF MEDICINE.

HYDROPHOBIA :

Abstract of a Discussion by the Neurological Section of the New York Academy of Medicine, October 16, 1890.

The President of the Section, DR. LANDON CARTER GRAY, in discussing the clinical aspects of hydrophobia, said that the extreme variability in the period of incubation has given ground for the belief held by many competent observers that if such a disease as hydrophobia really exists, death may also occur as the result of fear, with symptoms closely resembling the true disease. The speaker thought himself justified in assuming that frequent mistakes are made in the diagnosis of rabies, the so-called dumb rabies being merely a symptom of purulent meningitis and meningo-encephalitis, and that very few cases of either rabies or hydrophobia—the latter term being used to signify the disease in man—have been observed in New York City or in this country. He believes that there is a disease running a fatal course in the dog and other lower animals, and that it is capable of being communicated to the human being and causing death, though the evidence of this rests mainly upon pathological and experimental findings.

DR. C. L. DANA said that there is no constant change to be found in this disease. The nerve-centres, which are the parts chiefly involved, are congested, and occasionally show hæmorrhagic and softened spots with subsequent evidences of increased vascular activity, exudation of leucocytes into the perivascular spaces, and, possibly, the beginning of a multiple focal myelo-encephalitis or of a focal necrosis. The symptoms are evidently not the result of organic changes in the nerve-tissues, but of a distinct poison—undoubtedly the product of microbic activity. In the light of Pasteur's scientific work this question of specific origin should be considered as proven. The speaker did not believe that there are authentic clinical records of a single case in which fear caused a disease similar to hydrophobia, or that there is a case of death from this hypothetical phantasm, although, possibly, tetanus or acute mania has followed bites in those predisposed by fright. He thought that Pasteur has demonstrated the fact that as a reliable prophylactic measure antirabic inoculations can be successfully employed.

DR. H. M. BIGGS then gave an elaborate description of the respective methods of inoculation and of the various emulsions used in the work both of Pasteur and Ferran.

DR. H. C. ERNST, of Boston, said that he regarded the results of Pasteur as among the greatest achievements of modern medicine. The speaker was converted to a complete acceptance of the theory after conducting a series of inoculation experiments. Nothing in medicine, he said, is more certain than the results obtained by inoculating healthy rabbits under the dura with emulsions of the spinal cord of hydrophobic rabbits.

As to the existence of a lesion pathognomonic of rabies, he did not think that this could at present be defined with scientific accuracy, but careful observations have demonstrated the almost uniform presence of a white-cell infiltrate in the walls of the minute bloodvessels in the medulla, engorgement of the veins, and occasionally peri-vascular hæmorrhages. What apparently are small miliary abscesses are also present. The condition has been aptly described by the term *miliary bulbitis*.

The speaker then gave the clinical histories of three cases of true rabies in man which had come under his personal observation, and which, taken with the fact that a large number of dogs were affected at or about the same period, pointed to the recent existence of an epidemic of rabies in Boston. One of the cases, cited in detail, was of special interest, because the patient between the paroxysms was able to describe his condition, and had been especially questioned as to whether he had any repugnance to water. This patient positively stated that he had no repugnance, but that any thought of deglutition caused an uncontrollable spasm of the muscles of the throat. The patient also said that he was perfectly conscious of his acts during the violent paroxysms, but utterly unable to control himself. Even while thus quietly describing his sensations a fit would come on, and the next moment he would be on the floor struggling with four or five men.

As to the value of preventive treatment, the speaker instanced the case of a boy who was bitten in August last by a dog which within fifteen minutes had also bitten several dogs, of which two died from rabies. The father of the boy becoming alarmed consulted the speaker. Inoculation was advised and submitted to twice a day, and no bad symptoms resulted. Before the boy's return home a third dog had succumbed to unquestionable rabies.

Whether there is anything in Pasteur's claims or not, one thing is certain: he has obtained a specific virus which can be transferred from one animal to another indefinitely, and always produces a sequence of practically identical symptoms. The experiments made by Dr. Spitzka were not carried far enough, although he produced in rabbits something similar to rabies.

While hardly wishing to be considered a champion of the Pasteur method if the statistics of the Institute were not reliable, Dr. Ernst said that he was still bound to believe in Pasteur's honesty of purpose. It is a significant fact that after the elimination of all cases in which an element of uncertainty exists, the mortality-rate for those treated by inoculation is only ninety-eight one-hundredths of one per cent. He expressed surprise at the statement that there could be no such condition as pseudo-hydrophobia or lyssophobia.

DR. R. W. BIRDSALL said that he had seen a number of cases of pseudo-rabies resulting from fright after a bite or scratch. These cases did not terminate in death, though he was not prepared to say that death from fright was impossible. The nervous shock received might set up a series of changes, such as motor paresis, œdema of the brain, and coma, resulting in death. He did not believe that we are yet able to refer the phenomena of true rabies to one variety of germ. The effects might be due to the presence of distinct varieties.

DR. H. P. LOOMIS said that he had considered the subject from a pathological standpoint only. His findings tallied very closely with those described by Dr. Ernst. Sections of the lower portion of the medulla showed congestion of the capillary vessels and giant-cell infiltration of the adventitia, but no capillary hæmorrhages or thrombi.

DR. BYRON, who has made extensive experiments both at the Carnegie and the Loomis laboratories, said that he had reached the conclusions that (1) inoculations of the specific virus of rabies under the skin are useless as a means of prevention, (2) that the results desired can never be produced by any process except subdural inoculation, and (3) that even then the effect is not inevitable. The question is a serious one and requires further research before any definite scientific conclusions can be formulated.

DR. E. C. SPITZKA said that he had made no experiments on rabbits, as intimated by Dr. Ernst, who had evidently not followed the points of the speaker's work. In the experiments made by himself on dogs by the introduction of various irritating substances into the brain, he had produced a bogus hydrophobia, but had never claimed that these were cases of true hydrophobia. He is now assisting in a series of elaborate experiments on rabies, the results of which cannot as yet be determined.

DR. L. C. GRAY, in closing, thought the discussion had proved (1) that there is among the lower animals a disease known as rabies, possibly constituting several diseases and due to different microörganisms; (2) that this disease is more frequent in the lower animals than is the similar disease in man known as hydrophobia; (3) that while this so-called rabies in animals occurs very often in this country, it occurs less frequently in the human being; (4) that very few medical men have seen cases of genuine hydrophobia; (5) that cases of pseudo-hydrophobia are by no means uncommon, and that death can result from the condition; and (6) that there is still considerable diversity of opinion as to the value of Pasteur's method, which should furnish material for discussion and incite to further experiment.

CORRESPONDENCE.

THE NERVE-SUPPLY OF THE SENSE OF TASTE.

To the Editor of THE MEDICAL NEWS,

SIR: I have read Dr. John Ferguson's extremely interesting article in your issue of October 18th, and think that the author is to be congratulated upon having been able to observe so demonstrative a case.

But while this case seems to prove very definitely that the loss of taste in this instance was due to disease of the Vidian nerve, the evidence that the glosso-pharyngeal nerve is not concerned in supplying the sense of taste is very much weaker. In an article by myself on "Paralysis of the Trigeminus and Its Relations to the Sense of Taste (*Journal of Nervous and Mental Diseases*, February, 1886), I summed up the facts in support of the gustatory functions of the glosso-pharyngeal as follows:

"1. By anatomical dissections the fibres of this nerve have been traced directly to the taste organs (Vintschgau).

"2. By the Wallerian and atrophy methods, Vintschgau and Honigschmied have found that after resecting the glosso-pharyngeal nerves in young rabbits the peripheral portions and the taste-buds atrophy and disappear (Hermann's *Handb. der Phys.*).

"3. The physiological experiments of Magendie, Panizza, J. Reid, Broughton, Valentin, Wagner, Stannius, Lussana, and others, show that after resecting the glosso-pharyngeals the sense of taste is partly or wholly destroyed.

"4. The clinical evidence that the glosso-pharyngeal has something to do with the function of taste is almost unanimous. In all cases of trigeminal paralysis reported, so far as I can find, there is either no loss of taste or loss of taste only on the anterior two-thirds of the tongue, Gowers's cases being the only exceptions to this rule."

Dr. Ferguson's statement that paralysis of the trigeminus always causes complete hemiageusia is, I think, decidedly contradicted by facts. My own case (*loc. cit.*) may be cited as an instance.

In *Brain*, January, 1886, Dr. Thomas Harris reports a case in which a tumor involved the right side of the pons, entirely destroying the fifth nerve and Gasserian ganglion on that side, and causing total hemianæsthesia of the face and tongue, without loss of taste.

On the other hand, I have collected (*loc. cit.*) several cases of paralysis of the glosso-pharyngeal with loss of taste resulting.

I might add that Dr. Ferguson's report is incomplete in this, that he did not trace the degeneration of the Vidian back to Meckel's ganglion and the second branch of the trigeminus.

This does not, however, seriously affect the very convincing evidence, so far as it goes, which his case furnishes. But there have been other cases which almost entirely contradict this one, and which especially invalidate the theory that the glosso-pharyngeal has no gustatory function.   Very respectfully,
CHARLES L. DANA, M.D.
50 W. FORTY-SIXTH ST., NEW YORK, October 22, 1890.

NEWS ITEMS.

Dr. Bartholow's Chair Vacated.—At a meeting of the Board of Trustees of the Jefferson Medical College held on Monday, October 27th, the Chair of Therapeutics and Materia Medica was declared vacant on the ground that Dr. Bartholow was mentally disqualified to hold the position. The most prominent candidates for the professorship are said to be Dr. S. O. L. Potter, of San Francisco, Dr. James C. Wilson, Dr. S. Solis-Cohen, Dr. Henry Morris, and Dr. T. J. Mays, of Philadelphia. The trustees adjourned after declaring the chair vacant, to meet on Monday, November 3d, to take further action.

Tri-State Medical Association.—The meeting of the Tri-State Medical Association of Mississippi, Arkansas, and Tennessee, has been postponed until November 19th and 20th.

The Saranac Lake Sanitarium for Consumptives.—Dr. J. Solis-Cohen informs us that he has received a letter from one of his patients in Dr. Trudeau's Sanitarium at Saranac Lake, reporting marked improvement in her own condition and in that of many other inmates. This patient was far from being a promising case, and the result speaks well for the system adopted by Dr. Trudeau.

To quote from this letter: "So far, I have seen no place equal to the Sanitarium—not even the fine hotels. It should have been called 'Paradise for Consumptives.'"

A Caisson-disease Hospital. — The *British Medical Journal* quotes from an engineering periodical a description of a compressed-air chamber, or cylinder, for the reception of workers in tunnels and others who suffer from caisson-disease. Mr. Moir, the engineer in charge of the Hudson River tunnel work, has devised for his men, several of whom have been severely affected, a "hospital" for caisson-cases. This so-called hospital is a steel-plate cylinder, eighteen feet long by six feet in diameter, and is divided into two compartments, one of which is an air-lock. Both chambers have been fitted up with beds and everything necessary for the comfort of the patients. The air-pressure is maintained by a pump, so arranged that it will furnish a constant supply of fresh air. The degree of pressure is not kept very high, seldom, if ever, exceeding thirty pounds to the square inch. This degree of compression promptly retards the progress of the trouble, if the early symptoms receive attention.

Obituary.—DR. COSMO BRAILLY, formerly of New York City, died at Hazlett, N. J., on the 5th inst., aged seventy-six years. He was a native of France and a graduate of the University of Paris, but he had spent nearly fifty years of his professional life in New York.

Corrigendum.

CHLOROFORM AND THE HYDERABAD COMMISSION.

In the address of Dr. J. C. Reeve (THE MEDICAL NEWS, October 18th) the third sentence should read : "The differences of opinion and practice which prevail as to the two great anæsthetics are far greater than ever prevail upon subjects fully and clearly understood."

OFFICIAL LIST OF CHANGES IN THE STATIONS AND DUTIES OF OFFICERS SERVING IN THE MEDICAL DEPARTMENT, U. S. ARMY, FROM OCTOBER 14 TO OCTOBER 27, 1890.

JARVIS, N. S., *Assistant Surgeon.*—Is granted leave of absence for one month, on surgeon's certificate of disability.—*S. O. 107, Department of Arizona.* October 14, 1890.

By direction of the Secretary of War, leave of absence for four months is granted JAMES E. PILCHER, *Captain and Assistant Surgeon.*—Par. 12, *S. O. 244, A. G. O.,* October 18, 1890.

By direction of the Acting Secretary of War, the retirement from active service, on October 12, 1890, by operation of law, of ANDREW V. CHERBONNIER, *Captain and Medical Storekeeper,* under the provisions of the Act of Congress approved June 30, 1882, is announced.—Par. 11, *S. O. 240, A. G. O., Washington, D. C.,* October 13, 1890.

GLENNAN, J. D., *First Lieutenant and Assistant Surgeon.*—Is granted leave of absence for one month, to take effect about the 31st instant. —Par. 1, *S. O. 146, Department of the Missouri,* October 23, 1890.

OFFICIAL LIST OF CHANGES IN THE STATIONS AND DUTIES OF THE MEDICAL CORPS OF THE U. S. NAVY FOR THE WEEK ENDING OCTOBER 25, 1890.

CORDEIRO, F. J. B., *Passed Assistant Surgeon.*—Detached from the U. S. S. "Nipsic," and granted three months' leave of absence.

HEFFINGER, A. C., *Passed Assistant Surgeon.*—Placed on the Retired List October 20, 1890.

THE MEDICAL NEWS.
A WEEKLY JOURNAL OF MEDICAL SCIENCE.

| VOL. LVII. | SATURDAY, NOVEMBER 8, 1890. | No. 19. |

ORIGINAL LECTURES.

PSOROSPERMOSIS FOLLICULARIS CUTIS.

A Clinical Lecture,
delivered at the New York Post-Graduate Medical School and
Hospital, October 8, 1890.

BY L. DUNCAN BULKLEY, A.M., M.D.,
PROFESSOR OF DERMATOLOGY.

GENTLEMEN: The patient whom I present to you exhibits very clearly the characters of a somewhat rare disease which has recently attracted considerable attention, and the nature of which has given rise to no little study and discussion. I trust, however, that before I have finished you will recognize that the disease has more than a scientific interest; that our remarks of to-day will stimulate you to a further study of the general subject involved; and that some practical good may result therefrom.

The clinical history of the patient before us is as follows:

Mr. M. L., a German, aged forty-nine years, enjoyed good health up the time of his entering the U. S. army, in 1862, in which he served for three years. About a year after entering the service, without any apparent cause, except an immersion in a river, after which he was sick for some time, small, dark lesions appeared upon the forehead and over the sternum, similar to those now present; and from that time, twenty-six years ago, he has never been free from the eruption, which has gradually increased in extent. These lesions began as small, reddish-brown points, or papules, which gradually enlarged, and gave a rough feeling on passing the finger over them; where they were most numerous they coalesced to a greater or less extent, forming patches of a dirty yellowish-brown color.

The increase of the eruption has been gradual, but at times more rapid, especially in the spring and fall, when he has fever, with pains in the bones (which may be malarial) confining him to bed; at these times the affected portions become swollen and red, and, he states, have been mistaken for erysipelas. This latter statement is, of course, of no importance, for we all know how commonly unusual eruptions of a congestive character are called "erysipelas" by those unacquainted with skin diseases. He cannot tell the date at which the various portions of the body became affected, but remembers that the forearms and backs of the hands were attacked about fourteen years ago.

He has two daughters, aged respectively fourteen and seventeen years, also a son twenty-four years of age, all of whom are healthy and free from any eruption. He has lost one child aged six weeks. His father and mother never had any eruption, and he has a brother aged fifty-four years, and a sister aged fifty-seven years,

living and healthy. Another brother died at the age of forty-three years of paralysis.

His present condition, as you see, is not very good. He has an anxious, careworn expression, and says that he is so nervous and weak that he cannot attend to any business. The skin lesions extend from the top of the head to the groins and upper thighs. The top of the head, which is bald, you will notice is almost covered with small, brown specks, filling the sebaceous orifices and giving a "nutmeg-grater" sensation on passing the finger over them. On the forehead the lesions are larger, varying from the size of the head of a small pin to that of a medium-sized flat bead; all are slightly raised above the surface, are either flat or rounded, and distinctly hard, though greasy; they are much the same on the cheeks, though here, as on other exposed parts, they are kept worn down by washing and friction. On the chest you see the disease most perfectly developed, and here, and on the abdomen, which is largely covered, the separate, hard, brown papules are more elevated, rougher, and of a darker color. On the back they are less thickly distributed, and on the forearms they are more closely set, forming patches. The groins and upper part of the thighs also exhibit thickly-developed masses of them, but nowhere do we find them so large or prominent as have been described in one or two similar cases; nor do we find a very distinct, fœtid odor which has been spoken of in other cases, although it is faintly marked here, and the patient says that at times it is much more perceptible.

The hands are rather peculiarly affected by the disease; on the backs there are single isolated papules, similar to those seen elsewhere, and also brownish, dirty patches, evidently made up of the papules, closely packed together. Notice also the nails, which are affected in a very remarkable manner. They are all greatly thickened, so as to be raised from their bed, and the thickening is in the centre, while the sides of some are atrophied, giving almost a claw-like appearance to them. All of them are, as you see, very fragile, both at the ends and sides, with furrows and fissures running longitudinally.

Observe, now, more closely the character of these papules, especially on the chest and arms, which appear at first sight to be firmly attached, and to form an integral part of the skin. They are quite easily raised with the point of a knife, without pain, and leave behind them a small depression, reddened, and somewhat resembling the surface left after picking out very small cups of favus; in some of them which I have thus dug out there is a little bleeding at the base. These small masses, then, seem to be rather loosely attached, and are evidently horny and fatty concretions seated in the orifices of the sebaceous glands opening into small hair-follicles. Some of these masses have already been examined under the microscope by my friend, Dr. Pollitzer, who reports the presence in them of the *psoro-sperms* which, according to the French observers to be referred to later, form the diagnostic feature, as they are the cause, of the disease. The wound on the head and one on the arm mark the sites where portions of the skin have been excised by us for further microscopical study, and you also see scars where portions have been removed by others on former occasions. I may here remark that this patient has been the subject of much observation and study by a number of physicians since I first treated him nearly ten years ago, and I may add that various opinions have been held as to the nature of his complaint. I am told that Dr. Lustgarten, of New York, first gave this patient's disease its present (and probably correct) name, and exhibited microscopical sections of the same at the recent Congress in Berlin.[1]

What, now, is this curious affection which has lasted for many years, and resisted varied and thorough treatment, even in hospitals? Although these cases are relatively rare, there are a number of them on record, and, as before remarked, the disease is worthy of study for many reasons.

At first sight this condition suggests an ichthyosis in which the lesions are separated and isolated, and we accordingly find that a similar condition was mentioned by Wilson[2] long ago, with the title *ichthyosis sebacea cornea*. Because of the evident implication of the sebaceous glands Guibout[3] afterward criticised Wilson, and, considering the condition as wholly inherent to the sebaceous glands, he gave it the name *acne sebacée cornée*. Next Lesser[4] considers the subject, and applies the name *ichthyosis follicularis* to the affection described by Guibout, and describes a case in a child, which he thinks is the same disease. Morrow[5] reports a case which is pretty certainly one of the affection under consideration, with the title *keratosis follicularis*, because he considered the nature of the affection to be a cornification of the products of the sebaceous glands and adjacent fine hair-follicles; still later White[6] reported a case of the same disease with the name *keratosis (ichthyosis) follicularis*, while Leloir and Vidal[7] very recently described it under the name *acné cornée*.

I have thus given you all that I know that bears on the subject previously to the studies of Darier[8] and Thibault,[9] which have turned our thoughts in quite another direction. These observers based their studies on two cases which appeared in the services of MM. Fournier and Besnier in the celebrated Hôpital St. Louis, of Paris. It is a little curious that just before they published their researches on the subject, one of these very cases was presented by M. Hallopeau,[10] one of

the physicians of the Hôpital St. Louis, before the Society of the Hospital, under the name "*acné sebacée concrète* with hypertrophy."

In examining the plugs or masses forming the papules, Darier, who is the head of the laboratory at the Hôpital St. Louis, found that the cellular elements composing them did not all behave under staining reagents exactly like altered epithelial cells, and under the microscope he found that there were other bodies which were foreign to the tissues under consideration I cannot, of course, give you all the details of his elaborate microscopical study, but will only tell you that he found certain round or oval bodies situated within the epithelial cells of the lower layers, which he believed to be of parasitic nature. I will give you very briefly Darier's own condensed statement of the appearance of these bodies as he described them at the International Congress for Dermatology and Syphilography in Paris, last year:[1] " The malady is due to special parasites, which appear in the form of round, nucleated bodies, surrounded by a dense membrane, and situated in the interior of the epithelial cells whose nuclei they compress. They are found in great abundance at the bottom of the sac formed by the dilatation of the follicle: the horny plugs themselves are to a great extent composed of the parasites, but they are transformed in this situation into hard and refracting particles."

The number of cases thus far studied is too few to permit of very positive conclusions either in regard to the mode by which the disease is acquired, or as to the exact relation of these bodies to the production of the disease. I may say, however, that these same psorosperm-like bodies have been found by Dr. Bowen both in the sections originally taken from the first case observed by Dr. White, already referred to, and also in a second case which he has recently reported[2] under the title *keratosis folliculosis (psorospermose folliculaire végétante)*, and, as already mentioned, in the plugs from the case now before you.

The exact nature of these bodies has not yet been fully determined. Darier believes them to be true parasites belonging to the order of sporozoaires, which are unicellular organisms belonging to the animal kingdom, and a subdivision of the protozoaires. This class includes (1) the gregarinæ, (2) the oval psorospermæ or coccidiæ (which is the one found in this disease), (3) the sarcosporidiæ, (4) the psorosperms of fishes or myxosporidiæ, and (5) the psorosperms of the articulates, or microsporidiæ. All these organisms live as parasites on other animals, and in certain cases give rise to fatal maladies. The coccidiæ, which alone interest us here, live almost exclusively in the epithelial tissues of vertebrates, where they are found even in the interior of the cells. They are distinguished from the other groups of sporozoaires, and especially from the gregarinæ, by several characteristics, such as the absence of movement at any period of their development, their intracellular location, their solitary encystment, and the relatively small number of spores formed in the cysts. The ovoid coccidia produce

[1] Annales de Derm. et de Syph., 1890, p. 707.
[2] Diseases of the Skin, London, 6th ed., 1887, p. 348.
[3] Nouvelles Leçons Clin. sur les Mal. de la Peau, 1879, p. 962.
[4] Ziemssen's Cyclop., Bd. xiv. S. 478.
[5] Journal of Cutaneous and Genito-urinary Diseases, 1886, p. 257.
[6] Ibid., 1889, p. 201.
[7] Traité Descriptif des Mal. de la Peau, Paris, 1889, p. 7.
[8] De la Psorospermose folliculaire végétante. Annales de la Dermatol. et de Syph., 1889, p. 597.
[9] Observ. clin. pour servir a l'histoire de la Psorospermose foll. végétante de Darier. Thèse de Paris, 8 Mai, 1889.
[10] Annales de Dermatol. et de Syph., 1889, p. 20.

[1] Comptes rendus, Cong. Internat. de Derm. et de Syph., Paris, 1890, p. 391.
[2] Journal of Cutaneous and Genito-urinary Diseases, january, 1890, p. 13.

cysts in the biliary ducts of the rabbit, and in the human liver and ureters[1] psorosperm cysts have been observed.

Before going further into the subject, and making what I hope will be practical suggestions, allow me very briefly to give the chief facts of the nine cases of this peculiar disease to which I have thus far found reference (including Dr. Morrow's and my own, and also three briefly alluded to by Dr. Boeck. of Norway).[2]

1. (Fournier, Darier, Thibault.) Male, aged forty-two years. a bookbinder, affected for seven or eight years; the disease beginning at first insidiously, increased more rapidly during the last two years. The eruption was general.

2. (Besnier, Darier, Thibault.) Female, aged thirty years, affected for three years only, and presenting clinically the same aspect as the preceding.

3. (White.) Male, American, aged forty-nine years. Eruption first appeared beneath the knapsack, after a long march, when in the army in 1862, twenty-seven years before the date of observation.

4. (White.) Female, aged twenty-one years, in whom the eruption slowly developed after she was five or six years old.

5. (Morrow.) Male. aged twenty-one years. a sailor. Eruption appeared about five years previously to observation, soon after beginning a seafaring life.

6. (Bulkley.) Male, German, aged forty-nine years. Disease appeared when in the army, twenty-seven years ago.

7. (Boeck.) Male, aged forty-seven years, who had had the disease sixteen years; numerous encysted coccidia in epidermis.

8. (Boeck.) Male, son of former case.

9. (Boeck.) Male, also a son of case No. 7. From these cases in the same family Boeck argues for the contagiousness of the disease.

You will notice the singular fact that Dr. White's first patient and mine were at exactly the same age when first seen, and that both of them acquired the disease in the army. But Dr. White's patient was an American, and this man is plainly a German, and the ages are really different. as the former case was observed considerably over a year ago. Moreover, on careful inquiry our patient denies that he is the one referred to by Dr. White, although, strange to say, he did see Dr. White, for the first time, only a few weeks ago. Finally, the description of Dr. White's case does not correspond to this.

I might add that Besnier, at the Clinical Society of the Hôpital St. Louis, when Hallopeau presented the case previously referred to, mentioned having seen still another case; and several writers cite the case reported in a thesis of Lutz,[3] as general hypertrophy of the sebaceous system, as one of the affection under consideration.

In regard to the true nature of this complaint, whether these bodies called by Darier *psorosperms* are in reality parasites, and whether they are the true cause of the disease, we unfortunately have as yet no means to determine absolutely. All efforts to cultivate these bodies have failed, nor has anyone succeeded in inoculating

animals with the disease, although several attempts have been made. The malady does not seem to be communicated by ordinary means, for three of the nine patients were married men, living with their wives, to whom the disease was not communicated. This, however, proves little, for tuberculosis may likewise exist under similar circumstances without infecting others, and it is only very recently that the contagiousness of the latter has been proved; also, tinea versicolor, known to be due to a vegetable parasite, is rarely communicated from husband to wife. But, as already mentioned, Boeck reported a father and two sons affected by the disease, which he considers proof both of contagiousness and of the coccidia as its cause. Unfortunately the cases were only detailed at a society meeting in Norway, and I have been unable to find a full account or description of them. Several able French and other microscopists and naturalists have agreed as to the parasitic character of the bodies referred to, and the evidence seems very strong that they are the producers of the disease in question.

But the most interesting and perhaps important part of the question lies in the fact that more or less similar bodies have been found in the tissues of several other maladies, which are quite distinct from the present one, and from each other, in their clinical features. So marked are these microscopical characters that Darier has proposed the name *psorosperms cutanées* to designate the group in which they should be placed. The first of these diseases is the so-called molluscum contagiosum with which all are familiar. This disease Neisser,[2] Darier, and others cited by them, believe to be due to the presence in the epithelial cells of similar parasites—the so-called "molluscous bodies" which have long been known; these resemble in a certain degree the psorosperms already described, and are thought to be identical or at least analogous to them.

These curious round bodies have also been found by Darier, Wickham[2] and others, in that peculiar form of epithelioma of the nipple known as Paget's disease; and Darier further states that Malassez, in 1876, "noticed in a large number of epithelial tumors, cellular bodies, granular or refracting, sometimes encapsuled, which presented certain analogies to the psorosperms of the rabbit," and that Cornil has reported having seen analogous organisms in certain cancers of the uterus.

Here, then, lies the real interest in the study of the disease before us, as well as the important and practical element previously alluded to; namely, the possible results which may come from a thorough investigation and knowledge of the effects in the tissues of an order of parasites, the psorosperms, which have been hitherto unrecognized—if, indeed, the assumption is correct that the three maladies in question are really caused thereby. And you will readily see, that if the observations in regard to epithelioma are correct a great step has been taken in the direction of discovering the cause of cancer. It has been recognized for some time that cancer is occasionally communicated from one person to another, which, to a certain degree, sustains the parasitic origin of the disease. The recognition of the causation of pus by

---

[1] Journ. of Cutan. and Genito-urinary Diseases. 1889, p. 318.
[2] Boeck: Monatshefte für prakt. Derm., Bd. xi. No 3, p. 132.
[3] Hypertrophie Gén. du Syst. Sebacée. Thèse de Paris, 1850.

[1] Viertelj. für Derm. und Syph., 1888. p. 558.
[2] Comptes rendus. Congrès Internal. de Derm. et de Syph., Paris. 1890. p. 385.

the various forms of micrococci has been prolific of good in surgery; the discovery of the bacillus in tuberculosis is working beneficially in the direction of the prevention of the spread of that disease, and may yield results in regard to treatment; and if it should be fully and positively determined that cancer is due to the presence of *psorosperms*, may we not hope for more rapid progress in its prevention and treatment than has hitherto been attained?

Thus, you see, gentlemen, that cutaneous pathology, always an interesting study, leads the way to investigations which may be of the greatest importance.

In regard to therapeutics, in the patient before us the discovery of the psorosperm in his tissues should give us a clue to a method of treatment which, theoretically at least, promises more benefit than he has received in the past; for, as you have heard, his disease has lasted about twenty-seven years, and he has never been much benefitted by treatment. It remains to be seen how much can be accomplished when treatment is directed against the parasitic element which we have assumed as the cause. Unfortunately, but slight results were obtained during the short time that the Paris cases were under treatment based on this view of the disease. But this need not deter us, for you can readily understand that there may be great difficulties in attacking a parasite *in situ*, and in this disease the bodies referred to are seated very deep in the skin, and penetrate even far beneath the horny plug that you saw me dig out. The existence of the bacilli of tuberculosis and leprosy is now established, but we have, as yet, no means of reaching them *in situ*.

In the present case I shall hope to make many trials of different local remedies in order to reach and destroy the parasite, and shall hope to show you the results. Mercury, iodine, and sulphur, in their various preparations, are the agents we will chiefly depend upon, and some of these covered by impermeable dressings should, I think, succeed in penetrating and destroying the organisms which we believe to exist in the tissues of this man.

ORIGINAL ARTICLES.

THE VALUE OF EXERCISE IN THE TREATMENT OF THE PELVIC DISEASES OF WOMEN.[1]

BY JOHN H. KELLOGG, M.D.,
OF BATTLE CREEK, MICH.

THE propositions which I shall undertake to maintain in this paper are the following:

1. That defective muscular development is a prime factor in the etiology of a large number of the pelvic disorders to which civilized women are subject.

2. That the mode of dress common among civilized women is a cause of deficient and asymmetrical muscular development.

3. That the dress commonly worn by civilized women is productive of such disturbances of the relations and functions of the abdominal and pelvic

[1] Read before the American Association of Obstetricians and Gynecologists, Philadelphia, September 16, 17, and 18, 1890.

viscera as directly lead to the production of functional and structural changes in the uterus and its appendages.

4. That properly-graduated exercises, with adjustment of the clothing that will permit free and unrestricted movements of every group of muscles in the body, are of great importance in the management of a large class of pelvic disorders.

The comparative immunity from the disorders peculiar to their sex, as well as from the pain and accidents connected with childbirth, of savage and peasant women, is a fact so well established that the presentation of new evidence is scarcely necessary. Personal study of this subject among Indian women of various tribes, including the primitive Yuma tribe, of New Mexico and Arizona, among Chinese women, and especially among. the peasant women of Italy, Germany, France, and England, has enabled me to confirm the observations of Engelmann and others who have given special attention to the question. During my study in European hospitals, I was forcibly struck with the comparatively small number of cases of chronic pelvic disease in women who from early childhood had been trained to muscular labor of a varied character. Such disorders as prolapsus uteri, posterior flexions and versions, and chronic inflammation of the uterus and its appendages are almost unknown among married women of this class who have led chaste lives. Among the peasant women of Europe, pelvic disorders are chiefly those which result from childbirth; and are largely attributable to the carelessness and stupidity of ignorant midwives and the inability to secure the necessary rest and care during the lying-in period. It is surprising to one whose gynecological observations have been chiefly confined to the better classes of American women, that the morbid conditions caused by mechanical injuries, such as lacerations of the cervix and perineum, give rise to comparatively little suffering in women who have a good muscular development. I have frequently seen German and French peasant women in whom the entire uterus, as well as a considerable portion of the bladder and rectum, had been outside of the body for many years as the result of injuries during childbirth or of imprudence afterward, who sought relief not on account of pain, but solely on account of the mechanical inconvenience. This freedom from pelvic diseases and from the extreme suffering which commonly accompanies these disorders in women of the higher classes, may fairly be attributed, in large part at least, to the excellent muscular development resulting from laborious lives.

The young peasant woman of Germany or Italy, who from early childhood has been accustomed to accompany her elder brother in the field, digging, sowing, reaping, threshing out the grain with a flail, or following the plow, is no more subject to diseases of the pelvic organs than is her brother. If she receives some slight injury to the cervix or perineum in childbearing, she does not thereby become a miserable invalid, and if she experiences any inconvenience, it is merely a mechanical one which she will probably consider scarcely worthy of attention. The peasant woman exposes herself to all sorts of weather without regard to her condition. Her bare feet are exposed to cold and dampness without reference to the approach or presence of the menstrual period. I have seen in that portion of England known as the Black Country, vigorous women old and young engaged in the laborious employment of brickmaking, handling and carrying for many hours each day masses of wet clay which the majority of American women could not even lift. The occupation of these women necessitates constant exposure of the feet as well as the hands to dampness; and yet I was assured by the women themselves, as well as by an intelligent local physician, that they seldom if ever suffer inconvenience from exposures which in many women would produce fatal results. The frugal dietetic habits of these women and their open-air life must have something to do with this exemption from the diseases peculiar to the sex; yet I think this remarkable immunity is more largely due to the unusually symmetrical and vigorous muscular development which they derive from their habits of life. This view is sustained by the anatomical and physiological importance of the muscles in maintaining the position of the uterus and its appendages in relation to the pelvis and to the other viscera of the pelvis and abdomen; and by the relative frequency of uterine displacements and other forms of pelvic disease in women of feeble muscular development who have apparently not been exposed to any cause sufficient to induce such disorders in a vigorous, healthy woman.

The maintenance of the uterus and its appendages in their normal position may be said to be wholly dependent on muscular structures. This may also be said of most of the viscera of the abdominal cavity. The pelvic floor which closes the common outlet of the pelvic and abdominal cavities is chiefly composed of muscles. The vaginal and rectal outlets are closed by muscles. The muscular structures which compose the pelvic floor are sustained by other muscular structures connected with the pelvic bones above. The so-called ligaments of the uterus which play so important a part in maintaining its position are largely made up of muscular fibres. The round ligaments are in part composed of voluntary muscular fibres. The anterolateral walls of the abdomen are chiefly made up of muscles which in a well-developed woman are exceeding strong and firm.

A study of the functions of the round ligaments, the results of which I presented at one of the meetings of the American Association of Gynecologists and Obstetricians, has convinced me that these musculat structures play a most important part in keeping the uterus in position, acting, not only as bands or "mooring-ropes," as Dr. Alexander calls them, but through the muscular contractility of which they are capable. The theory of their action the correctness of which I believe I have demonstrated, is that by contracting simultaneously with the abdominal muscles, they tilt the uterus forward, and thus prevent its being forced backward during violent contraction of the abdominal muscles, the uterus being drawn out of the current of downward pressure. The contraction of the muscles which compose the pelvic floor, when these muscles are properly developed, prevents abnormal lowering of the pelvic floor and of the pelvic organs. A weak, relaxed condition of these structures is usually found in women of feeble mscular development.

Uterine prolapse, retroversion, and retroflexion, and the various forms of ovarian prolapse which accompany these displacements are seldom met with among chaste unmarried women of savage or semi-civilized nations, but are very frequent among young women in America, and among the wealthier classes of all civilized countries. In this country, these conditions, when found in young women, are almost invariably attributed to some accident or imprudence in muscular exercise, such as jumping from a carriage, a fall on the ice, jumping the rope, walking too great a distance, lifting a pail of water, carrying a baby, or some similar circumstance. The baneful effects of stair-climbing have been dwelt upon by physicians as well as over-careful mothers. Not infrequently such light exercise as running a sewing-machine, or standing upon the feet behind a counter, has been charged with producing the worst forms of uterine displacements and other pelvic diseases. I do not say that such things never bring about uterine or pelvic diseases, but I have long been convinced that the causes mentioned above are of slight importance, and that back of them is an etiological factor of a general and fundamental character, the essential nature of which is deficient muscular development.

The mode of dress common among civilized women is productive of pelvic disease, not only by its mechanical effects upon the contents of the abdomen, but by its interference with the normal respiratory movements and the free action of the muscles of the back and abdomen.

In normal breathing, the shape of the chest is changed in the act of inspiration in such a manner that all its diameters are increased. The greatest increase, however, is in the longitudinal diameter due to flattening of the diaphragm, and in the transverse diameter of the lower part of the chest, due to the action of the inspiratory muscles, and according to Bruger, also in part due to the depression of the abdominal viscera by the contracting diaphragm. In normal respiration in children of either sex, and in both men and women of savage tribes, in which the dress of the two sexes is practically alike, the chief movements noticeable in inspiration are widening of the chest at its lower part and bulging of the abdominal wall. There is at the same time a rhythmical action of the muscles of the pelvic floor induced by the increased abdominal pressure which results from the flattening of the diaphragm.

That the respiratory movements are practically alike in adults of both sexes, I think has been fully established by the observations of Mays and others, as well as by my own studies upon Indian women of various tribes, Chinese women, Italian peasant women, and upon American women whose breathing has never been interfered with by tightly-fitting clothing.

The relation of corsets and tight bands to respiration has usually been studied solely with reference to their influence upon the lungs. The important relation of the respiratory process to the abdominal and pelvic viscera has too often been overlooked, although the disturbance of the normal relation existing between respiration and the circulation of the blood in the abdominal and pelvic viscera is undoubtedly of far greater importance than any interference with the respiratory process occasioned by constriction of the waist.

The effect of inspiration is to increase abdominal tension. This is accomplished by the flattening of the diaphragm, which is facilitated by the increase in the transverse diameter of the lower part of the chest induced by contraction of the serrati and other inspiratory muscles. The effect of abdominal tension is to hasten the emptying of the veins of the portal circulation, in which there is a natural tendency to retardation as the result of the resistance of the hepatic capillary system. In normal respiration, in which the intra-thoracic pressure is diminished by proper expansion of the chest cavity, this emptying of the portal circulation is also facilitated by a sort of suction which draws the blood from the abdominal viscera into the thoracic cavity. Thus, in normal respiration, there is a double action, the tendency of which is to accelerate the circulation in the abdominal and pelvic organs; and it is reasonable to suppose that the health of these organs must largely depend upon a continuous and efficient action of this pumping process which is so essential a feature in the maintenance of the blood-current.

The proper action of the chest may be aptly compared to that of a pair of bellows, the lower ribs to which the strong breathing-muscles are attached, representing the handles. The breathing-apparatus of a woman whose waist is constricted by a corset or tight band is nearly as much embarrassed as would be a pair of bellows with the handles tied together. The upper costal respiration so conspicuous in women who constrict the waist is not seen among savage women, nor in a woman whose respiratory organs have not been restricted by improper clothing. That this mode of breathing is quite abnormal might be inferred from the structure of the upper part of the chest, which is certainly not such as to suggest any considerable degree of mobility. This thoracic breathing is not only abnormal, but as I think I have already shown, it may produce disease. This is true of ordinary respiration, and is most emphatically true of forced respiration, such as is induced by singing or active muscular exercise, under the imperative demand for an increased supply of air. The respiratory muscles are then made to act with undue violence. In consequence of the constriction and the compression of the abdominal walls by the corset, the force is largely expended upon the organs of the pelvis, which are forced down out of position. The pelvic floor is more yielding than the rigid walls of the chest, and is depressed, thus laying the foundation for chronic displacement.

A civilized woman wearing the common dress, cannot expand her waist more than one-fourth of an inch when taking a deep inspiration. The expansion must occur somewhere, and the constriction of the waist forces the expansion to take place at either the upper or lower extremity of the trunk; the greater resistance of the upper ribs and the yielding character of the structures which form the floor of the pelvis cause depression of the pelvic floor to occur with lowering of all the organs which are dependent on it for support.

I have devised an instrument for the study of the influence of constriction of the waist upon the pelvic floor, which consists simply of a lever attached to an upright, and an adjustable support furnished with a vernier, against which one end of the lever plays while the other end rests upon the perineum. The fulcrum of the lever is so placed that the recording end of the lever has an amplitude of movement just five times that of the end placed against the pelvic floor. The instrument can be used with the woman either standing or lying. By the use of this instrument I find that lacing the corset as tight as it is ordinarily worn depresses the pelvic floor from five to twelve millimetres. I have sometimes observed a rise in the pelvic floor of fifteen millimetres immediately after the corset was loosened.

Dr. Trastour, an eminent French physician, has

clearly shown that what he terms the *statique abdominale* has an important relation to the health of the abdominal viscera. The relations of the several organs which occupy the abdominal and pelvic cavities are such that any considerable change in position necessarily results in disease. The stomach, dragged out of place, loses its natural tone, its walls become relaxed, dilatation occurs, and the patient suffers from all the distressing symptoms of gastric neurasthenia. The constant dragging upon the liver and the right kidney may displace these organs. Prolapse of the organs which normally occupy the upper part of the abdominal cavity necessarily compels the displacement of the organs beneath them, leading to what is termed by Glenard, and other French writers, *enteroptosis.* Prolapsed intestines become atonic, from the disturbance of the portal circulation, and not infrequently a pseudo-stricture of the large intestine is occasioned by the bowel folding upon itself, caused by the depression of its central portion, which is more easily dragged down than the ascending or descending portion. Obstruction leads to fæcal accumulation and dilatation. Such disturbances of the relations of the vsicera will be found in a large proportion of women suffering from pelvic disorders.

In one hundred cases of pelvic disease taken without selection and in the order in which they came under observation, I found disturbances of the normal relations of the abdominal viscera in ninety-four. The stomach and bowels were prolapsed in all of these cases. There was dilatation of the stomach in more than one-half of them. The right kidney was distinctly movable and had fallen below its normal position in thirty-seven cases. In twenty-seven cases the kidney had fallen so far below the normal position that it was freely movable. In three cases both kidneys were prolapsed. In four cases the liver was very considerably prolapsed; in three cases almost the entire organ was at the inferior border of the lower ribs. In one case, the spleen, which was four times its normal size, enjoyed the freedom of the entire abdominal cavity. When first noticed it was lying between the uterus and the bladder, and was at first thought to be a fibroid growth connected with the uterus.

In the six cases in which there was no disturbance of the relative positions of the abdominal organs, the patients had unusually well developed muscles and the pelvic disease was distinctly traceable to other than mechanical causes.

Mr. Lockwood, of St. Bartholomew's Hospital, London, has shown by elaborate post-mortem studies that hernia is accompanied with prolapse of the mesentery and the attached bowel to the extent of from four to nine inches, and in an address upon the subject he called attention to the influence of tight lacing in producing this prolapse in women.

I have made a large number of measurements of civilized and uncivilized women to determine the relations of the circumference of waist to the height, and other dimensions.

In one hundred civilized women, all eighteen years of age or over, the following are the average results:

	Height. (Inches.)	Waist (Inches.)	Percentage of height.
American women	61.64	24.44	39.6
English women (brickmakers who wear heavy skirts)	60.4	25	43.3
French women	61.6	28	45.4
Civilized Telugu women of India	60.49	24.65	40.6
Chinese women	57.85	26.27	45.4
Yuma women	66.56	36.84	55.2
Civilized man—American	67.96	29.46	43.3

A few words of explanation are necessary in order to present the full significance of the above figures. The civilized corset-wearing American woman has the smallest waist of any of the classes examined. The next in order is the Telugu woman, who suspends her clothing by a cord tightly tied about her waist. Dr. E. J. Cummings, of Ramapatam, Nellore District, India, who kindly made for me the measurements from which the above figures relating to Telugu women are deduced, tells me that it is customary with those women to draw the cord which suspends their clothing as tight as possible; yet the amount of harm done thereby does not seem to equal the mischief accomplished by the American corset. The women brickmakers of England doubtless diminish the size of their waists and produce considerable distortion of their figures by wearing the many heavy skirts suspended by bands drawn tight about the waist. Civilized man, next in the scale, has a much larger waist than civilized woman, yet does not equal in this respect the women who have had an opportunity to develop naturally. The measurements which I have made of savage men and women of the same tribe convince me that women naturally have larger waists in proportion to their height than men.

Properly-graduated exercises, with such an adjustment of the clothing as will afford opportunity for free and unrestricted movements of every group of muscles in the body, are a most important therapeutic means in the management of a large class of pelvic disorders. The exercises which I have employed are, in general, light calisthenics, consisting of free hand and body movements, and the use of wooden dumb-bells, Indian clubs, wands, chest-weights, and various gymnasium apparatus for bringing into play special groups of muscles, walking exercises, breathing exercises, and Delsarte. I also employ exercises with light iron dumb-bells, and light exercises on a

19*

trapeze, swinging rings, and horizontal bars, in suitable cases. The weight of the dumb-bells, clubs, and chest-weights, or other apparatus to be used, is prescribed for each patient, as are also the duration of the exercise and the number of strokes in the use of rowing-machines, and similar apparatus. The employment of a variety of apparatus, and of different forms of exercise, is important, as it not only encourages patients to take a larger amount of exercise than they otherwise would do, but enables them to do so without injury by bringing into play different groups of muscles or different combinations of muscular groups.

The exercise of lying upon the back, and alternately raising the legs from a horizontal to a perpendicular position is particularly valuable. Fixing the legs, and resting the body upon an incline adjusted at an angle suited to the patient, is another special exercise of value.

Resting in a horizontal position, face downward, sustaining the weight upon the elbows and toes, with the body held rigid and free from the supporting surface, is an excellent exercise to develop the muscles of the back and abdomen. This exercise may be varied by alternately raising and lowering the body, resting a few seconds in each position. Drawing the body up from a supine position to an angle of forty-five degrees, by catching the toes on the round of a ladder, is an exercise of great value for patients who are able to take it. It not only strengthens the muscles of the trunk, but at the same time empties the portal veins.

A breathing exercise which I have found of great value is the following : Placing herself in the genupectoral position, the patient takes a deep abdominal inspiration, then expels the breath by forcibly contracting the abdominal muscles, at the same time drawing up as strongly as possible the muscles of the pelvic floor. By this means the round ligaments, if they have not undergone complete degeneration, as well as the abdominal and perineal muscles, are vigorously exercised.

The passive and "active-passive" exercises of the Ling system of Swedish movements are also of great value in these cases, as I can testify after having employed this system for nearly sixteen years. Of great value, also, are manipulations of the abdomen, especially directed to the restoration of prolapsed viscera to their normal position. The circulation is accelerated ; prolapsed bowels, kidneys, liver, and spleen, may be restored to position, and thus by making room above, the prolapsed organs of the pelvis are encouraged to resume their normal positions. I have frequently seen excellent results from the employment of abdominal and pelvic massage in conjunction with general and special gymnastic exercises, and various forms of active and active-passive Swedish movements.

The good results of exercise are well shown by the following figures, which represent the gain in strength of the arm, leg, trunk, and respiratory organs respectively, as the result of physical training of the kind referred to. In one hundred women the average gain in two months was as follows :

Arms	.	.	.	. 16.2	per cent.
Legs	.	.	.	. 28.4	"
Trunk	.	.	.	. 28.1	"
Respiratory organs	.	. 28.6			"

The average gain of strength for four months was as follows :

Arms	.	.	.	. 51	per cent.
Legs	.	.	.	. 55.9	"
Trunk	.	.	.	. 54.9	"
Respiratory organs	.	. 46.6			"

The disproportionately greater gain shown in the longer period, clearly demonstrates the importance of time as a factor in a system of treatment of this kind. There must be time for the muscles to grow.

The great advantage of exercise in this class of cases is best appreciated by the study of individual cases. For example : I have frequently seen the aggregate strength of arms, legs, trunk, and respiratory organs, increased by three months of exercise more than 200 per cent., and I have many cases on record showing an increase of more than 400 per cent. In one instance the rate of increase was nearly 700 per cent.

A CASE OF FOREIGN BODY REMAINING IN THE EYE FOR TWENTY YEARS, FOLLOWED BY ABSCESS IN THE SCLERAL WALL.

BY B. L. MILLIKIN, M.D.,

OF CLEVELAND, OHIO.

ON March 18, 1871, E. M. O., then about ten years old, was struck in the right eye with a fragment of a musket-cap. which he supposed at the time did not enter the eye. However, the piece was not found. Following the injury the eyeball was greatly inflamed, and he was confined to his room for nearly three months. For two years after this the eye slowly improved, so that vision was pretty fair and he could readily read ordinary type.

The eye gave him no further trouble until about 1883, when he had a severe attack of inflammation which produced almost complete blindness. After this attack the eye again improved, and vision became fair, and he had no more serious trouble until the latter part of 1887, when the eye became painful and injected, and the sight failed.

I first saw the patient, February 28, 1888, when he gave me the above history, and stated that three or four days previously the eye had again become inflamed, and that he was then suffering great pain through the eyeball and the side of his head

Examination at this time revealed the following conditions:

In the cornea to the outer side of the pupillary margin and a little below the horizontal meridian, was a linear opacity extending outward and slightly downward, perhaps 2 mm. in length. Lying directly behind this and in the same direction was a slit in the iris, extending from near the pupillary border to the outer margin of the iris and so wide toward the periphery that the red reflex of the fundus was readily seen, and also the border of the lens. After several instillations of homatropine hydrobromate the pupil was well dilated, the dilatation being free in all directions except at the border near the slit, where the iris was attached to the anterior capsule. Both the ophthalmoscope and oblique illumination showed, directly behind the slit in the iris, an opaque track through the body of the lens, through which the foreign body had evidently penetrated. In the anterior portion of the vitreous, in the lower outer quadrant, was plainly seen, both through the pupil and the slit in the iris, a grayish-white body of considerable size and projecting into the vitreous. This had the appearance of an encysted body, being quite different from a sarcoma or other neoplasm. There was also a broad choroidal crescent and numerous floating opacities in the vitreous. The vision at this time in O. D. was $\frac{6}{XXXVI}$ and in O. S. $\frac{6}{VI}$.

Directly over the position of this body the sclera and conjunctiva were much injected, and painful on pressure. With slight pressure over this point the body could be seen to project farther into the vitreous. At no other portion of the eyeball was there any tenderness. Tension was normal. He was put upon instillations of atropine solution three or four times daily, and a boric acid collyrium, together with hot applications.

On March 7th he reported that four days previously he had had a very sharp attack of pain through the eyeball and side of the head, but that it subsided after two or three hours, and after that the eye continued to do well. The only change in the appearance of the eye noticed at this time was a peculiar discoloration over the seat of the foreign body as if the sclera was partially eroded.

After recovering from this attack there was no more trouble until September, 1889, when he had another severe inflammatory attack; but owing to my absence I did not see him again until November 27, 1889, when I found the eye in a state of active inflammation, and the vitreous showing numerous opacities, especially in the neighborhood of the foreign body. Under active treatment this attack slowly subsided.

Nothing noteworthy occurred until about the middle of December, 1889, when an enlargement of the sclera began to show itself directly over the position of the foreign body. This increased quite rapidly, so that by December 31st it was quite pronounced. It was somewhat irregular in shape, hard to the touch, and felt as if the sharp edge of the piece of cap might be forcing its way through. Pressure over this point produced much pain, while other portions of the eyeball were quite free from pain. No changes seemed to take place in the interior of the eye.

By January 14, 1890, the eye was free from general inflammation and had been so for some days, but the projection over the foreign body had increased. It was quite circumscribed, and there was no redness except in the immediate neighborhood of this projection. I believed that the piece of cap had become encysted, that gradually, from the repeated inflammatory attacks, the increase of connective tissue, and the action of the ciliary muscle it had worked its way through the retina and choroid and into the sclera, and that it would eventually cut through the sclera externally.

Following ordinary surgical principles the proper procedure seemed perfectly plain, viz.: to give exit to whatever was contained in the swelling. Under cocaine anæsthesia a needle was passed through the most prominent portion of the projection until it came in contact with a hard body. Then a triangular portion of the conjunctiva was dissected from the sclera at this point and a free incision made directly into the swelling. From this three or four drops of pus escaped, when the anterior walls of the sac collapsed.

With a spoon I then scraped out a number of black particles which were hard and under a lens seemed to be metallic. These, I have no doubt, were disintegrated portions of the piece of cap. As much as possible of the interior of this sac was removed with the spoon, forceps, and scissors. A needle was passed in two or three places directly through the sac and into the vitreous, in order to determine definitely if any hard substance remained.

The extreme thickness of the scleral wall at this point surprised me very much. It certainly was more than one centimetre thick, and notwithstanding the freedom with which I scraped out, and tore out with the forceps, and cut out, with scissors, the hard portions, I did not enter the vitreous or disturb it in the least.

Both before and during the operation the eye and its appendages were thoroughly washed with 1-to-5000 bichloride of mercury solution, and every precaution was taken to keep the wound clean. The cavity of the wound was freely washed with the bichloride solution, and the eyeball was dressed with a compress moistened with the same solution, and with a bandage. The pain from the operation, notwithstanding the very free use of cocaine, was considerable.

The patient recovered without a bad symptom. When an ophthalmoscopic examination could be made I found that the body in the vitreous chamber, previously so prominent, had entirely disappeared and could not be seen through the dilated pupil. By January 22d, all tenderness had subsided, except a slight amount over the wound. Vision = $\frac{3}{XXX}$.

Up to the present time there has been no pain and no tenderness, even over the point of the wound, where there had been tenderness on pressure for six or seven years at least.

At the present time, on looking well forward through the pupil, there is a slight whitish reflex, but this has not increased since the wound healed, and the opacities in the vitreous have slowly disappeared.

The scar externally is not noticeable, except on the closest scrutiny, and the condition of the eye is better than it has been for years. The patient, a merchant, is able to work steadily, and suffers no inconvenience whatever.

I have given a detailed account of this case because of the unusual features connected with it, and because I have not been able to find any report of a similar case in the literature at my command.

SALOL IN TYPHOID FEVER.

BY W. C. CAHALL, M.D.,
OF PHILADELPHIA.

DURING the past two years typhoid fever has been more than usually prevalent in the northwestern section of Philadelphia, and I have been impressed as never before with the fact that the ordinary treatment of this fever is very unsatisfactory. The patient is either vigorously treated with dilute acid, turpentine, or a mixture of tincture of iodine and carbolic acid, all of which, owing to the nausea they produce, are difficult and at times impossible to administer methodically; or, on the other hand, the patient is not treated at all, save when urgent symptoms develop.

At about the beginning of the increased prevalence of the fever in this city I was led, by reading reports of the use of salol for the *diarrhœa* of typhoid fever, to use it as a *specific* remedy in place of the tincture of iodine and carbolic acid mixture. Salol has the advantage of being acceptable to a sensitive stomach, so that its use can be systematically continued, an all-important feature of specific treatment. For a little more than a year and a half I have persistently treated every case of typhoid fever which has fallen into my hands with salol, rarely using anything in addition during the whole course of the fever, and so far with the most gratifying results.

Contrary to my usual custom, I have kept a strict record of every case of this fever that I have treated since beginning the use of salol. After eliminating all the cases in which, from their short, mild course, or from the absence of one or more of the characteristic symptoms of this fever, the diagnosis could be questioned, there remain sixteen cases, of undoubted typhoid fever.

It is not my intention to give a detailed history of each of these cases, but rather to give briefly the results of my observations on the whole.

The dose and mode of administering.—The dose of salol should be at least three grains every two hours, day and night, from the time the diagnosis is made until the morning temperature reaches normal. My experience has been that salol given in pill-form does not give as good results as when given in the form of a powder. This is probably due to the more rapid and complete absorption of the powder in the intestine.

The effects upon the symptoms.—The dry, rough condition of the tongue, so troublesome in this fever, was rarely seen in the sixteen cases, and if present, seldom lasted long.

Salol is insoluble in the saliva and is practically tasteless, hence, in the first few days of the fever, when the stomach is irritable and when there is nausea salol is easily taken, and in its quieting effects is equal to bismuth.

Upon the intestines the effects of the drug are marked; tympany disappears more rapidly than under the use of turpentine, and gives no further trouble throughout the course of the fever. Diarrhœa, no matter how excessive in the beginning, seldom requires any other remedy to control it, but progressively improves. Of hæmorrhage there were a few instances, but in no case was it repeated so frequently as to call for the classical "lead and opium" pill. Tenderness in the right iliac region was invariably present, but diminished without special treatment. Peritonitis supervened in no case. The rose-colored spots were present upon the abdomen and chest of all the sixteen cases, sometimes profusely, but in no case did I notice a second crop.

The effects upon the temperature were noticed within the first few days. Under ordinary treatment the temperature usually rises for the first ten days of the disease, but under the use of salol the temperature seldom rises after the first day of treatment, and after the first week steadily, and more or less rapidly, falls. In several cases the temperature reached normal by a fall of from two and a half to three degrees between evening and morning. In the first case in which this happened I confess that I passed a day of anxiety, fearing hæmorrhage. After the temperature reached normal there was a slight evening rise for two or three days, after which it remained normal.

The pulse does not increase in frequency to the end of the first week when salol is used, but remains full and seldom exceeds one hundred. In none of the cases was the action of the heart such as to require alcohol.

The only untoward effect of salol was the partial suppression of the urine in some cases, but in no case was it necessary to suspend the treatment. I have seen the same symptom produced by turpentine, but it is a point which should be carefully looked after, for in some cases the kidneys might be damaged by the carbolic acid which is set free by the salol. Albuminuria was no more frequent than is usually seen in cases of typhoid fever. All the cases are now in good health.

Complications.—One of the happiest features of this treatment was the infrequency of complications. With the exception of two cases of pneumonia, one of which developed when convalescence was almost established, and a few cases of slight hæmorrhage, there were no complications, and convalescence was invariably rapid and uninterrupted. This is probably largely due to the fact that salol does not disturb the stomach or interfere with digestion, so that the desired amount of nourishment can be given throughout the course of the fever, which cannot often be done when the stomach is continually disturbed by acid, turpentine, or the tincture of iodine and carbolic acid mixture.

Duration.—The average duration of the sixteen cases, not including the two complicated by pneumonia, was seventeen days. Some had a normal temperature at the end of the second week and a few in slightly over three weeks. There were no deaths.

Whatever the differences of opinion as to the cause of typhoid fever it is pretty definitely settled that, after a certain stage, the disease is a septicæmia, due to the ulceration of Peyer's glands. The natural tendency of the fever is to terminate about either the fourteenth or the twenty-first day, and when an intestinal antiseptic, such as salol, is used, which prevents the ulceration from infecting the system, the natural tendency to recovery is increased.

THE ANASTOMOSES OF THE PORTAL VEIN WITH THE SUPERIOR VENA CAVA, INFERIOR VENA CAVA, AND AZYGOS VEIN.

BY F. TISCHER, M.D.,
OF SAN FRANCISCO, CALIFORNIA.

AT the German Chirurgical Congress of 1889 Pietrzikowski spoke of the frequency with which pneumonia follows the reduction of incarcerated hernia, either when taxis alone is employed or when herniotomy is performed. Disregarding those cases in which there are concomitant chronic pulmonary diseases of old persons, such as emphysema and bronchitis) : those in which there are co-existing inflammatory processes in the herniotomy wound and peritoneum ; and those with complications induced by the inspiration of expectorated particles, such as lobar pneumonia, there still remains a series of conditions for which no plausible explanations exist.

Pietrzikowski maintains the view first promulgated by Gussenbauer, that pneumonia following the recent reduction of strangulated hernia has an embolic origin. The thrombi originating in consequence of the disturbed circulation in the capillaries and small veins of the constricted gut and its mesentery, must, after the restoration of the circulation following the reduction of the strangulated hernia, reach the circulation, and in this way give rise to emboli. As long as the thrombi remain uninfected they act only as temporary infarcts, but if they become infected in the intestinal wall the emboli must, of necessity, lead to inflammation of the pulmonary tissues.

In answering the question, What course must the thrombi, originating in the intestinal and mesenteric regions in the neighborhood of the portal vein, pursue in order to reach the lungs ? Pietrzikowski does not deny the possibility of small thrombi reaching the inferior vena cava through the capillary system of the liver and the hepatic vein. Larger thrombi, on the other hand, by avoiding the hepatic capillary system, can reach the lungs through the free anastomoses, between the portal vein and the inferior vena cava. Pietrzikowski makes no special mention of these anastomoses.

. Besides the above described anastomoses, others also are of interest. By cutting off the circulation in the portal vein, as occurs in hepatic cirrhosis and in thrombosis of the portal vein, there is the possibility of the formation of a collateral circulation by which the blood of the portal vein can still reach the vena cava. Of course, we must not overvalue the significance of this collateral circulation, as the clinical course of hepatic cirrhosis sufficiently demonstrates.

Further, these anastomoses appear to be the routes for the transmission of infectious matter which originates in ulcerative processes in the intestine, and causes pulmonary inflammations, as is sometimes seen in typhoid fever. Undoubtedly, the lobular pneumonia of typhoid fever is traceable, partly to the scanty expectoration of the bronchial secretion, and partly to the frequent inspiration of inflammatory products from the naso-pharynx. The occurrence of true lobar pneumonia in this disease can be explained as follows : The typhoid bacilli, having passed through the capillary system of the liver, are carried either to the lungs and there find a favorable soil in the catarrhal areas, or a detached thrombus containing typhoid bacilli originating in the infiltrated and ulcerated Peyer's patches passes by means of anastomoses of the portal vein directly to the lungs, and there is firmly lodged without having passed through the hepatic system. Of course, it is strange that in typhoid fever inflammatory areas seldom exist in the liver. notwithstanding that the main branch of the portal is the nearest route to this organ. One must admit that the liver is as unfavorable, a seat for the growth of typhoid bacilli as it is a favorable one for the poison of dysentery which causes suppurative hepatitis. In all probability the infected thrombi originating in

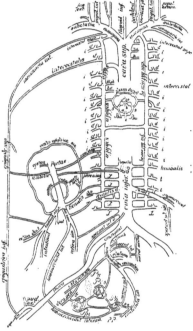

a. Vena medullæ spinalis anterior. b. Vena medullæ spinalis posterior. br. Vena bronchialis. c. Vena basivertebralis. co. Vena communicans obturatoria. d. ramus dorsalis Venæ intercostalis. he. Vena hæmorrhoidalis externa. i. Vena intercostalis. l. Vena lumbalis. ma. Vena mediastinica anterior. mp. Vena mediastinica posterior. p. Vena pericardiaca. pd. Vena pancreatico-duodenalis. Ph. Plexus hæmorrhoidalis. pp. Vena profunda penis. Ppi. Plexus pubicus impar. Psa. Plexus spinalis anterior. Psp. Plexus spinalis posterior. Pu. Plexus uterinus. Pvs. Plexus vesicalis. s. ramus spinalis. sp. Vena suprarenalis. th. vena thymica.

Peyer's patches, on their way through the anastomoses of the portal vein with the superior and inferior vena cava, occasion the pneumonia.

It may at this point be of interest to consider briefly these anastomoses, as shown in the accompanying drawing, prepared by the plan adopted in Henle's *Anatomy :*

The portal vein, as we know, gathers through its three main branches, the splenic, the superior mesenteric, and inferior mesenteric, and their tributaries, the blood of the stomach, small and large intestine, spleen, and pancreas. From the liver the blood is transmitted to the inferior vena cava through the hepatic vein.

The venous blood of the lower extremities and pelvic region passes through the iliac and hypogastric veins, that of the kidneys through the renal vein to the inferior vena cava.

The hemiazygos vein empties into the azygos vein at the level of the ninth dorsal vertebræ by means of a transverse branch. The azygos empties in the superior vena cava.

In the abdominal cavity the origin of the azygos and hemiazygos veins forms vertical branches connecting the lumbar veins, which empty in the inferior vena cava. The blood of the lumbar veins, therefore, goes partly to the inferior vena cava, and partly to the azygos and hemiazygos veins.

In the thorax the azygos and hemiazygos veins (including the posterior mediastinal and œsophageal) receive the blood of the intercostal veins. The rami dorsales of the intercostal and lumbar veins form the dorsal plexus around the bodies and processes of the vertebræ. They send the rami spinales into the vertebral canal, which receive the blood of the anterior and posterior spinal plexus, and these plexuses communicate through horizontal and vertical branches with each other, and with similarly named plexuses above and below. In the accompanying diagram they are represented in transverse section.

In the abdominal and thoracic portions of the spinal column are the following vertical routes, exclusive of the superior and inferior venæ cavæ: Azygos, hemiazygos, the vertical communications of the dorsal plexuses outside of, and of the plexus spinales anterior and posterior, within the canal.

In the anterior abdominal wall a vertical communication exists between the saphenous and internal mammary veins, which is due to the anastomosis of the inferior epigastric vein with the superior epigastric. From the internal mammary vein the blood is carried either to the anonyma brachiocephalic, or, through the communications of the internal mammary with the intercostal veins, to the azygos and hemiazygos veins.

It must also be noted that the renal veins are connected just as closely with the azygos and hemiazygos veins, and also with the lumbar veins, and with those of the superior intercostals, which, with the azygos and hemiazygos empty into the innominate brachiocephalic veins.

According to Professor Braune,[1] the veins of the thoracic and abdominal cavity have no valves.

The communications between the portal vein and the superior vena cava, inferior vena cava, and azygos vein, are as follows:

1. Communications between the mesenteric veins and those of the abdominal wall—superior and inferior epigastric veins. The blood may go either through the inferior epigastric to the long saphenous vein, and thence through the iliac to the inferior vena cava, or through the superior epigastric to the internal mammary, and thence into the superior vena cava.

2. In those cases in which the umbilical vein remains unobliterated the blood from the portal vein can reach the superior epigastric in an abnormal direction. From there the blood courses in the way described in sub-head 1, or through lumbar and gluteal branches. Bamberger states that the umbilical vein is not infrequently found unobliterated. When the umbilical vein remains open, and in hepatic cirrhosis, we have an obliteration of the portal vein, and a dilatation of veins, forming the caput medusæ, simultaneously takes place. When the umbilical vein is obliterated this dilatation occurs as the result of communications between the mesenteric and superior epigastric veins as described in sub-head 1.

3. Anastomosis of the internal hæmorrhoidal vein (a branch of the inferior mesenteric vein) with the hæmorrhoidal plexus. Through this vein many communications with the hypogastric vein are found—through the middle hæmorrhoidal vein, through the external hæmorrhoidal and internal pudendal veins, through the communicating obturator to the obturator, or through the vesical plexus.

4. Anastomosis between the mesenteric vein and inferior vena cava.

5. Anastomosis between the mesenteric and renal veins.

6. Anastomosis between the splenic and azygos veins.

7. Anastomosis between the small veins of the capsule of Glisson (branches of the portal vein), or between the coronaria ventriculi and the phrenic vein.

8. Anastomosis of the portal vein with the œsophageal, a branch of the azygos.

Finally, new anastomoses between the portal vein and the veins of the abdominal wall may be formed in the adhesions between neoplasms and inflamed viscera within the abdomen.

It would occupy too much of the reader's time to mention in this paper all the possible routes that can carry thrombi formed in the portal system to the

[1] Die Oberschenkelvene, 1871, page 8.

right heart, and from there to the lungs. These routes can be seen in the accompanying diagram.

In the diagram the liver and stomach are represented everted, so that the circle of the coronaria ventriculi, and that which the splenic makes with the gastro-epiploicæ, are above. Further, in order to make the anastomosis more clear, many of the veins are represented as short branches only. The plexuses in and about the spinal column are represented in transverse section at the level of the seventh dorsal vertebra; the communications of the intercostals with the internal mammary at the third intercostal space.

The relation, as represented in the chart, of the hemiazygos to the azygos is not the same in all cases. The hemiazygos more frequently empties into the upper portion of the hemiazygos accessoria, which carries the blood of the upper branches of the intercostals by a complicated route to the azygos, and, through the superior intercostal, communicates with the innominate vein. The lower vein, the hemiazygos, empties into the azygos at the level of the ninth dorsal vertebra. Usually, between the hemiazygos and the accessory hemiazygos a small branch carries the blood from one or more intercostal spaces to the azygos.

GENERAL PARESIS OF THE INSANE.

BY GERSHOM H. HILL, M.D.,

SUPERINTENDENT OF THE IOWA HOSPITAL FOR THE INSANE, INDEPENDENCE, IOWA.

THE symptoms of general paresis of the insane were first noticed and described about the year 1800. Esquirol described a typical case of the disease under the name of monomania. His pupil, Bayle, completed the study and gave an accurate description of the disease in 1825. Forty years ago general paresis had not been recognized in this country, but of late years the disease has made its appearance in all our institutions for the insane, and statistics show that it is increasing with alarming rapidity. For this reason, and because of the difficulty of early diagnosis, I have thought that the subject would prove interesting. Furthermore, the disease is important because it is not only incurable, but is sure to terminate in death within a few years.

I use the term *paresis* instead of *paralysis* because the loss of power is slight in the early stages and seldom in its course is any set of muscles or part of the body rendered completely powerless. As the name indicates, the characteristic feature of this disease is a paralysis that is general, but incomplete, occurring in a person whose mind is unsound. It is not my purpose to review the literature of this subject, but to state conclusions reached by my own experience.

Among thirty-seven hundred cases of insanity

treated at the hospital at Independence, there were forty of general paresis. There were seven cases in the first one thousand admissions, seven in the second one thousand, ten in the third one thousand, and sixteen in the last seven hundred. Although the disease was later in making its appearance in Iowa than in the eastern and more populous States, yet cases occur with increasing frequency. There were but two women among the forty cases admitted.

While one-third of the insane in Iowa are foreign-born, only one-fourth of the paretics were foreigners, therefore we cannot claim that the disease is imported.

The oldest paretic was fifty-nine years old when admitted to the hospital, and the youngest was twenty-six; the average age was forty-two years. Hence it will be seen that paresis attacks men while in their most active years.

Ten of the cases were single, and thirty were or had been married. While more than one-half of all our insane men are single, only one-fourth of the paretics are unmarried, consequently the disease is more likely to occur among the married than among the single.

The occupations represented by the forty cases are as follows: Merchants and salesmen, nine; mechanics, seven; laborers, seven; farmers, six; railroad men, four; hotel men, two; lawyer, one; editor, one; and insurance agent, one. One of the women was a dairyman's wife, and on account of her husband being an invalid she not only worked excessively, but was obliged to tax her faculties to the utmost in order to continue the business and support the family. The other woman was an artist, and her reputation for virtue was not the best.

So seldom does an insane woman have general paresis in our population, which is largely rural, that it is hardly worth while to include the sex in our statistical investigations.

Three-sevenths of our insane men are farmers, but only one-seventh of those having general paresis are farmers. While the same number of paretics were day laborers, there are only half as many laborers as farmers among the insane men. On the other hand, the proportion of professional railroad men and merchants who have paresis is large. This fact leads to a two-fold conclusion concerning the causes of this disease, namely, that business men are much more subject to it than those whose employment is chiefly manual labor; and that it is engendered by the vicissitudes and vices of city rather than those of country life. In a New York City asylum a few years ago, among sixteen hundred insane men two hundred and five were found to have general paresis. So far as my own observation extends, the disease is seldom brought on by purely intellectual pursuits.

With regard to education, I may say that paretics are seldom thoroughly educated, nor, on the contrary, are they often very illiterate. They are usually men of a nervous temperament, possessing an unusual amount of energy, disposed to tax their faculties and at the same time to find enjoyment in the indulgence of their animal appetites.

Among the predisposing causes heredity stands first in importance and frequency, and was discovered in twelve of the forty cases. In two there was a history of sunstroke, and in one a history of an injury to the head.

As to the exciting causes, the excessive and continuous use of stimulants is more likely to produce this than other forms of insanity, and the same may be said of excessive venery. More than half of my cases had used intoxicants freely; but several of the men who had formerly been intemperate had not used stimulants for a few years before becoming insane. On the other hand, in most cases of excessive sexual indulgence the habit existed when the insanity became apparent, so that it is impossible to determine whether this habit is the result of a morbid perversion of the appetite, and is only an early symptom of the disease, or whether it sometimes causes paresis. A history of syphilis was found in a few cases, and no doubt syphilis produces this as well as other forms of mental derangement. In men of limited capacity and education, whose minds are not well balanced, overtaxing the mental faculties produces paresis. In this as in other forms of insanity, several of the causes, both predisposing and exciting, are usually present in a case, so that it is difficult to decide which is the chief cause.

In persons having paresis it is usual to find the will or the emotional nature holding sway over the intellect.

Sleeplessness, impairment of the memory, an irritable disposition, changeableness in moods, carelessness in dress and in business affairs, with an inclination to do foolish things, are among the early symptoms; later the patient may have periods of excitement or anger, he may fail to distinguish between his own and the property of others, and may pilfer trifles which strike his fancy. Next he may be inclined to speculate or to assert that he has unlimited possessions. Some are disposed to make presents indiscriminately; others do not claim riches or manifest extravagance, but reveal a comfortable, complacent, self-satisfied frame of mind, although their actual pecuniary condition and their business or domestic relations may be most embarrassing. The tendency from first to last is to weaken all the faculties until the patient is too demented to take any interest in his own relatives and is unable to tell his name.

While these changes are taking place in the mind

the disease of the nervous system is making more or less rapid progress in the impairment of muscular power. The first change to be noticed is a tremor of the lips or facial muscles when efforts of speech are made, especially when the patient is excited; the tongue is unsteady when protruded, and hand-shaking may be done in an awkward and uncertain manner. In the course of time the gait becomes ataxic, the walk is unsteady or shuffling, a lack of endurance becomes apparent, and the patient is worn out by very moderate efforts at work. Hesitation in speech is generally noticed, and an inability to command names and ordinary words, hence conversation is fragmentary and desultory, and aphasia may be well marked. When inquiry is made from day to day and month to month as to the health of these patients, the stereotyped reply is "first-rate."

· Finally, these poor unfortunates become disorderly in their conduct, filthy and destructive in their habits, helpless and bedridden. Some of them have epileptiform or apoplectiform seizures, which in the early stages of the disease are usually short and fully recovered from, and the hemiplegia which may thus be brought about usually disappears in a short time. When the patient has icst his powers, both of body and mind, life ends after a prolonged period of unconsciousness.

In none of the cases admitted to our hospital had general paresis been diagnosed, although it might have been, in some instances, had the certificates required of the examining physicians a statement of the form of insanity.

The average duration of the disease in these forty cases, before they were sent to the hospital, was eight months; the shortest time it had existed was one week; the longest time before the patient was admitted was thirty months. In my opinion very few cases run their course without being sent to a hospital for the insane. At times they are lawless and too troublesome to be kept at home. In one-fourth of the cases there was a suspension in the mental manifestations of the disease so that such patients seemed quite natural for a time, and some were permitted to visit their homes for a few months. The average duration of the disease in twenty-five cases was two and a half years.

The morbid anatomy as it appears macroscopically shows a "wet" brain. The large quantity of cerebro-spinal fluid between the membranes and in the sinuses indicates atrophy of the brain-substance. In a few cases, however, in which the disease runs a rapid course, the brain is engorged with blood, completely filling the cranial cavity, and in such cases there is a diminution of the serum. The dura is somewhat thickened, the pia opaque and more or less adherent to the convolutions, especially upon the vertex. The arachnoid is also thickened and

opaque, and certain parts of it are marked by a granular roughness.

The brain itself is generally pale, flaccid, and diminished in consistence, except when the disease has run a rapid course and been characterized by active mental symptoms, when the cortical substance is likely to be dark and hyperæmic. The cerebellum is also hyperæmic, and less firm in consistence than natural. The membranes of the cord are in about the same condition as those of the encephalon.

There is necessarily great diversity in the appearance of microscopical sections on account of the varying conditions due to age, duration of the disease, a high or low degree of brain development, the effects of alcoholism, and of diseases in other organs of the body. The capillaries are usually dilated and sometimes filled with blood-corpuscles. There is hypertrophy and hyperplasia of the neuroglia, also granular degeneration of nerve-fibres and cells of the cerebral cortex and of the fibres of the subjacent white substance.

The disease usually begins in the medulla, is at first chiefly localized here, and later involves the cord.

RECAPITULATION.

1. As a rule general paresis affects men only.

2. Its victims are men in the full vigor of life, and generally from the middle classes of society.

3. It is usually caused by excesses, either in the use of stimulants, in venery, or in the application of body and mind to business affairs.

4. From its onset it is steadily progressive, is absolutely incurable, and runs its course in a comparatively brief period.

5. It has two separate sets of symptoms, muscular and mental.

THE PROFESSIONAL, MORAL, AND LEGAL RESPONSIBILITY OF THE OBSTETRICIAN IN CASE OF DEATH FROM PUERPERAL SEPTICÆMIA.

BY MANNING SIMONS, M.D.,
PROFESSOR OF SURGERY IN THE MEDICAL COLLEGE OF THE STATE OF SOUTH CAROLINA, CHARLESTON, S. C.

"THE professional, moral, and legal responsibility of the obstetrician in case of death from puerperal septicæmia," is a question that seems to have dawned upon the profession everywhere. The Chicago Medico-Legal Society 1 recently discussed the question "Whether the failure of a physician to accept and practise the precepts of antiseptic midwifery should make him legally liable and responsible if puerperal fever develops in his puerperal patient during his attendance upon her."

Dr. W. L. Richardson, of Boston, sounds the

---

1 March, 1888.

keynote of the public, and to some extent of the professional sentiment on this subject, when he says:

" Since the appearance of Koch's work on bacteria obstetricians all over the world have been endeavoring to find out how best to banish puerperal septicæmia from the lying-in chamber and maternity hospitals, and no one who has carefully investigated the subject denies that it can be banished, if the proper prophylatic measures are taken."

In these views of Dr. Richardson we recognize the prevailing idea that there is a large number of diseases the occurrence of which indicates either negligence or ignorance.

The list of such diseases is increased from time to time by the laboratory work of the pathologist and bacteriologist, and it becomes the duty of the practical, "every-day" doctor to apply to the new views and theories the test of the clinic.

It seems an opportune time to discuss this matter, for in a recent article Dr. W. T. Lusk says:

" There has likewise been, without doubt, an improvement in results among well-to-do classes. Among these there is a widely-diffused belief that puerperal fever is a preventable disease, and that for its occurrence the physician should be held responsible, and this leads to greater painstaking on the part of the latter, even when he is disinclined to accept deductions from modern scientific teaching."

Other medical writers go even further in this direction, and in illustration of this tendency to hold the obstetrician responsible for unfortunate results, we find in the address on obstetrics before the last meeting of the American Medical Association the following strongly-expressed opinion :

" There are a few simple rules pertaining to the subject of aseptic midwifery, and they must be scrupulously and delicately adhered to by every physcian who praetises the obstetric art. Failure to do this is to shoulder an awful responsibility, and the consequences of such neglect would be indefensible either in a court of morals or of law."

In order that such responsibility should rest upon the obstetrician, negligence or gross ignorance must be shown, or, to express it in the words of another :

" The surgeon must adopt the means and apply the skill well settled by the highest lights of his profession. He must possess and practically exercise that degree and amount of skill, knowledge, and science which the leading authorities have pronounced as the results of their researches and experience up to the time or within a reasonable time before the issue or question to be determined is made."

The first point, then, for us to consider, is the present state of professional opinion as to the causes of puerperal septicæmia.

All cases of puerperal septicæmia are certainly not alike either in their symptoms and course, in the mode of infection, or in the extension of the disease. It would be a useless task to endeavor to detail the theories that have been advanced to explain the facts, but it is almost a certainty that the general tendency is to attribute the occurrence of puerperal septicæmia to the entrance of disease-producing organisms, or of organisms capable of causing decomposition, and producing poisons chemical in their nature in the discharges of the parturient woman. The poisons are probably absorbed from the lesions in the genital tract, lesions which are liable to occur during the most natural labors. It is even held that it is possible for absorption of septic matter to take place through the unbroken mucous membrane.

We may recognize, then, two classes of cases of puerperal septicæmia :

First. Those in which the poison or septic material originates within the patient, so that she infects herself, the disease then being called *autogenetic.*

Second. Those in which septic matter is conveyed from without and brought in contact with surfaces in the genital tract that are capable of absorbing—the disease then being called *heterogenetic.*

According to the more recent theories, microorganisms are the ultimate cause of the disease in both of these classes.

In the first class there is probably that state called septic intoxication. In the second class there is a true septic infection.

In the first or the so-called autogenetic forms, the decomposition and putrescent changes in the retained coagula, portions of placenta, or membranes could not occur were it not for the presence of microörganisms, not necessarily pathogenic in theira nture ; whilst in the second class there are probably introduced peculiar pathogenic organisms, the manifold multiplication of which in the system produces the septic fever.

The cases of the latter class are characterized by a very short incubation, by a rapid course, and by the absence of such marked local lesions as are almost invariably met with in the class of cases first mentioned.

It is by no means certain that these poisons are always directly introduced by the fingers of the obstetrician or the nurse, but it is here that much of the responsibility lies. It is more than probable that the air loaded with germs in certain localities is itself a sufficient means.

This, in brief, is a summary of the present views upon the causation of puerperal septicæmia, and it remains for us to inquire as to what extent, if any, the application of the principles and details of antisepsis and asepsis has operated to reduce the amount and mortality of puerperal septicæmia.

According to Lusk, in a recent article, the ratio of deaths from puerperal septicæmia in New York

City has by no means kept pace with the increase of the population.

Not long since it was thought necessary in order to escape epidemics of puerperal septicæmia in hospitals, that lying-in wards should be placed in temporary buildings.

Now with the more modern plans of management it is found that whereas formerly these institutions furnished nearly one-sixth of all the fatal cases of puerperal sepsis, they, when properly equipped and organized, are the safest places for parturient women. This safety has been secured by modern methods of treatment based on recent observations.

According to the writer of the Address on Obstetrics, already referred to. "there are a few simple rules pertaining to the subject of aseptic midwifery." Our duty will be to enumerate these simple rules as taught by modern authorities. Our next inquiry, and that to which it appears to me discussion should be particularly directed, is as to which of these rules accord with the present state of obstetrical science, and which, therefore, should be accepted in order to avoid the charge of negligence or ignorance.

Before summarizing the present views I will call attention to the influence exercised by the surroundings of the patient in producing puerperal septicæmia independently of conveyance of the poison to the patient by the physician or nurse.

Among the factors to be considered with the surroundings of the patient are the water-supply, the public drainage, the plumbing, and the existence of diphtheria, scarlet fever, or erysipelas.

If these are admitted to be the means of causing puerperal septicæmia, and if it is also admitted that the essential causes of the disease are microörganisms which make their way by one means or another into the blood and tissues of the puerperal woman, then asepsis and antisepsis are properly applied to midwifery.

In treating of the prophylaxis of puerperal diseases we should consider :

First. The surroundings of the patient, including personal and public hygiene.

Second. The management of the patient herself, in order to insure asepsis.

Third. The preparations and precautions to be taken by the physician and nurse before entering upon the management of a case of labor.

It is not necessary for us to occupy ourselves with the matters included in the first class, for it can scarcely be claimed that the obstetrician is responsible for personal or for public hygiene.

The patient at the commencement of labor should receive a full bath, and after this a rectal injection. The lower abdomen, the inner surfaces of the thighs, the labia, and the anus are scrubbed with soap and water, then washed with pure water, and finally disinfected with a 1-to-1000 solution of corrosive sublimate. The vagina is douched first with soap and water, and then with a 1-to-5000 solution of corrosive sublimate. Most important is the management of the third stage of labor, in order to guard against the retention of clots, pieces of placenta, or membranes, in which decomposition may occur.

The Credé method of expelling the placenta is recommended, and ergot is given to secure thorough uterine contraction. and to prevent thus the formation of clots in the uterus when relaxation takes place, after the removal of the placenta.

In all cases after labor the vagina is douched with a bichloride solution, 1 to 5000.

In cases of protracted labor, of high forceps operation, of version, or of any manipulations by means of which air is admitted to the uterine cavity, the douche of sublimate solution, after preliminary vaginal irrigation, is carried to the uterine cavity. The external parts are dusted with iodoform and are covered with a piece of gauze freshly wet with 1-to-5000 bichloride solution, and over this is placed a pad of oakum. The dressing is changed once in six hours, at which time the genitals are scrupulously cleansed. During the puerperium no vaginal douches are given. These are the precautions as applied to the patient.

The third indication requires that the physician and nurse should, if possible, have taken baths. The physician should not have visited the deadhouse, or the wards of a hospital, or the rooms of private patients in which erysipelas, septic wounds or diseases, or the exanthemata are being or have been treated. The hands should be washed and disinfected before each examination during or before labor, and especial attention should be paid to the finger-nails, as the furrows around and beneath them are often the lurking-places of disease-producing matters. Examinations should be made as infrequently as possible.

These indications apply to the nurse with as much force as to the physician, and under no circumstances should the nurse be permitted to make a vaginal examination.

These, in brief, constitute the "simple rules" previously alluded to. But there is scarcely a point in these rules concerning which the opinions of all agree. Thus the pad of oakum over the vulva has been sneered at. The prophylactic douches have also been criticised, especially the ante-partum douches. On the other hand, it has been advised to irrigate the vagina during labor at intervals of two hours with a quart of corrosive sublimate solution. It has also been recommended that the vagina be first thoroughly rubbed with a preparation of creolin and mollin, and then irrigated for ten minutes with a creolin solution. There is also much difference of opinion as to the use of the douche during the puerperium, and the propriety of intra-uterine douches. It is recommended, however, by many that the bichloride solution be used, of a strength of 1 to 3000, and that an iodoform " bacillus " be introduced. Finally, to add to our confusion, we are reminded by Dr. William L. Richardson, of Boston, that corrosive sublimate douches are a most dangerous weapon.

The question that should be discussed, it seems to me, is, whether these rules should be observed in detail, in order that the obstetrician may escape the charge of negligence or ignorance, and if not observed, to what extent we should depart from them.

Considering the subject as I have endeavored to present it, as briefly as possible, one is impressed with the truth of the following words of an eminent jurist, " It will tend to encompass a most important and anxious profession with such dangers as to deter reflecting men from entering into it."

CLINICAL MEMORANDUM.

MEDICAL.

Two Cases of Vesical Calculus relieved by Buffalo Lithia Water.—CASE I. At three o'clock in the morning of January 2, 1890, I was called to see a woman who I found in a uræmic convulsion. This I controlled by inhalation of chloroform, and after securing diaphoresis I returned home.

Three hours later I was again called in haste, when I found her suffering from an attack of renal colic, which I relieved by a hypodermic injection of morphine. I then obtained from her the following history :

Age thirty-eight years ; a widow ; father living and healthy ; mother died of phthisis at the age of forty-one years. The patient had enjoyed good health until about two years ago, when she began to suffer from dyspepsia. She had been treated for ulcer of stomach, dyspepsia, inflammation of bowels, etc., but had never been examined for stone in the bladder. She had suffered from attacks of renal colic for the last eighteen months, which were increasing in frequency.

In the afternoon I was called again, and found that she was bleeding from the urethra. I examined the urine and found a large number of small calculi, and one the size of a pea, and angular, which, no doubt, had caused the bæmorrhage. I ordered her to take three drachms of solution of potassium citrate, and ten minims of deodorized tincture of opium three times daily, and Buffalo lithia water *ad libitum*. On January 5th I examined her for stone, and found a hard crust on both the anterior and posterior wall of the bladder. Washing out the bladder twice a week caused much improvement in the cystitis, and after the fifth week of this treatment I could not detect the crust, but found in the urine large fragments of calculi. Now, after using the lithia water for three months, the patient is in excellent health, the urine normal, and the cystitis entirely well. The potassium citrate and opium were not given after the second week.

I have used Buffalo lithia water in similar cases with very flattering results, especially in case's with marked lithæmia.

CASE II.—The patient, a soldier, aged sixty-one years, had suffered from cystitis, constant dribbling of urine, insomnia, and chronic diarrhœa, for nearly twenty years. He had been treated for stricture, and was at one time told that he had a stone in his bladder, although he was never examined with a sound. He finally permitted me to examine him for stone, under ether. After some difficulty in passing the sound, I found what I supposed was a large calculus. He would not consent to the operation of lithotomy, and in order to relieve him, I ordered potassium citrate and opium, and Buffalo lithia water *ad libitum*, as in Case I. ; for the diarrhœa, I gave the following mixture :

R.—Deodorized tincture of opium } of each 2 drachms.
Castor oil   .   .   .   . }
Turpentine   .   .   .   .   1 drachm.
Acacia   .   .   .   . a sufficient quantity.
Camphor water   .   sufficient to make 2 ounces.
Dose, one teaspoonful three times daily.

The bladder was washed out once a week with a solution of boric acid. The urine was frequently examined. On the first examination it contained an excess of urates, uric acid crystals, pus, and blood-corpuscles. After the fourth week the urine contained no pus or blood-corpuscles, but there was still an excess of urates. The patient's general health improved. At the beginning of the eighth week of treatment the urine was nearly normal, the dribbling had stopped, and the diarrhœa had diminished. At the end of the tenth week the irritability of the urethra and bladder was so much less that the sound could be passed without anæsthetization. The calculus was apparently very much decreased in size, but seemed harder. At different times I had noticed small crust-like concretions in the urine, which, no doubt, were from the calculus. It is a question whether the lithia water or the boric acid caused the stone to crumble.

At present the patient is in good health, with no dyspepsia, insomnia, or cystitis.

SAMUEL L. HANNON, M.D.,
200 " D" STreet, Washington, D. C.

MEDICAL PROGRESS.

Myxœdema and Cretinism.—BIRCHER (*Sammlung klinische Vorträge*, No. 357) believes that the secondary symptoms of myxœdema, namely, hypertrophy of the left ventricle, pallor of the skin, slow pulse, œdema, serous effusions, etc., are dependent upon the associated endarteritis, hepatitis, and nephritis, and that the latter are probably due to alterations of the kidneys. The nutritive fluids are changed, the blood is watery, the number of red corpuscles is diminished, and mucin is deposited in the tissues. The primary cause of all the symptoms is atrophy of the thyroid gland ; after total extirpation also a symptom-complex appears which resembles myxœdema in every particular. This operation-myxœdema begins with more severe symptoms, and runs its course more rapidly than the atrophic myxœdema.

The thyroid gland seems to be necessary to life, and, according to the author, apparently prevents the formation of mucin in the tissues, a function that cannot be assumed by other glands. If in a dog the thyroid is extirpated from the neck and the thyroid of another dog is implanted in the peritoneal cavity the animal will live, whereas if there is no implantation of the thyroid the dog will die. It is also possible that the gland, situated in whatever part of the body, supplies the organism with necessary fluids.

Bircher then describes the symptoms following total extirpation of the thyroid for goitre, as seen in five women. In three cases, soon after extirpation, serious symptoms of myxœdema became apparent but spontaneously disappeared. The fourth patient died with epileptiform convulsions soon after the operation. The fourth patient was a cretin, and after the extirpation the characteristic cachexia and tetanic and epileptiform symptoms appeared. Implantation of a piece of thyroid gland in the peritoneal cavity was followed by an improvement of all the symptoms, which, however, was only temporary. After a second implantation there was improvement again which continued, and the patient is now—three months after the implantation—well and able to work.

The author believes that the cretinoid degeneration is an infectious disease, the germs of which are found in drinking-water. Of its symptoms the most important and constant are hypertrophy of the thyroid and arrested growth of the bones, particularly those of the skull. There are three forms of the disease, namely, endemic goitre, the least serious ; endemic deaf-mutism ; and endemic cretinism (idiocy), the most serious. The author concludes his paper with the following propositions :

1. Myxœdema is a sporadic disease resulting from the loss of function on the removal of the thyroid and is a dyscrasia that chiefly affects the growing organism.

2. Cretinism is an endemic disease caused by long-continued infection, which causes hypertrophy of the thyroid, and if occurring during body-growth causes irreparable arrest of development. — *Centralblatt für klinische Medicin*, October 11, 1890.

Treatment of Prolapse of the Rectum.—MR. HARRISON CRIPPS (*Lancet*, October 11, 1890) contributes a very practical article on the treatment of prolapse of the rectum. In children, he writes, palliative treatment is often very satisfactory, provided that the condition is not caused by phimosis, vesical calculus, polypus of the rectum, etc. If the child is thin, good food and cod-liver oil should be given in order to restore the fat in the ischio-rectal fossæ, the absence of which doubtless facilitates the descent of the bowel. If prolapse can be prevented for two or three months a cure will probably be effected, and with this object in view great care must be exercised to prevent constipation. The stools must never be passed while the child is in a sitting position, but while lying upon its side at the edge of a bed. If, with the child in this position, while the fæces are passing, the mother will draw one of the buttocks upward so as to displace the anus from the median line, prolapse will almost certainly be prevented. The child should remain on its side for some time after the stool, and a pad, held in place by a T-bandage, should be worn for one or two

hours. If these measures are carefully carried out operative treatment will seldom be required.

In adults, palliative treatment seldom cures, although it may be tried before resorting to an operation. The patient should be cautioned against straining and should turn on the side as far as possible while passing a stool. Every passage should be preceded by an enema of eight ounces of warm water, and followed by a smaller enema —one ounce — of cold water. If there is superficial ulceration a drachm of tincture of catechu may be added to the last enema.

With regard to operative treatment, in a few severe cases complete removal of the prolapsed portion may be necessary, but before advising such a procedure, the risk of the operation and the probability of causing a stricture of the rectum should be considered. For these reasons complete removal should be reserved for cases in which other measures have failed, and usually linear cautery will be sufficient to effect a cure. This operation is performed as follows : The rectum having been emptied, the patient is etherized and placed in the lithotomy position, and by manipulation the bowel is protruded. With a hot iron four lines are then burned in the long axis of the bowel, one in front, one behind, and one on each side. Paquelin's cautery is not suitable for this purpose ; it is too hot when applied and cools too rapidly. The lines should commence within the apex of the protrusion and should terminate at the margin of the anus. They should be about one-fourth of an inch wide and deep enough to sear thoroughly the mucous membrane but not to destroy it. If dilated veins are crossed they should be tied on each side of the burn. The bowel should be returned as quickly as possible, or congestion and swelling may prevent replacement. If the bowel does not protrude at the time of the operation the cauterization may be performed with the assistance of a large duckbill speculum.

After the operation a rubber tube, seven inches long and one-third of an inch in diameter is passed into the bowel for five inches. Strips of oiled lint are then inserted and the space between them and the tube is packed with cotton dusted with iodoform. After forty-eight hours the dressing is removed, the parts are thoroughly washed, and a clean dressing is applied. After a few days the dressings may be dispensed with, but the tube should be kept in place for ten days or longer. The bowels should be confined by means of opium for ten days and then opened by a full dose of castor oil.

Anæsthetic Spray.—DR. B. W. RICHARDSON states that a solution of five grains of carbolic acid in five ounces of ether used as a spray is an excellent local anæsthetic. The anæsthesia produced appears before the skin is hardened by the cold—an advantage in cutting operations. If deep incisions are required a continuance of the spray upon the tissues causes very profound anæsthesia, and dissection can be continued without pain. The anæsthesia has the additional advantage of being more prolonged than that produced by other local anæsthetics, and there is little or no pain after reaction has taken place. The disadvantages of this spray are that in some instances the wound heals slowly and by granulation, leaving an ugly scar; and that in a very large wound there is danger of carbolic-acid poisoning. Dr. Richardson recommends use of the spray chiefly in cases of ulcerating cancer with pain and an offensive discharge.—*London Medical Recorder*, October 18, 1890.

The Uses of Keratin.—Drs. Unna and Beirsdorff recommend that drugs which irritate the gastric mucous membrane, such as digitalis, squills, salicylic acid, iodide of iron, etc., be given in the form of pills coated with keratin, or in capsules of the same substance. Drugs which diminish the activity or which neutralize the acidity of the stomach, such as tannic acid, nitrate of silver, and alkalies, should be given in the same way. A coating of keratin is also desirable when prescribing drugs that are required to act on the intestinal mucous membrane alone, and is especially valuable in the use of drugs which are given for the purpose of destroying intestinal worms, but which, if introduced into the stomach in the ordinary way, are absorbed to such an extent as to cause toxic symptoms, or to reduce their germicidal activity.

Keratin is obtained by treating shavings of horn with ether, alcohol, and an acid. It possesses the peculiar property of being insoluble in the stomach, but freely soluble in the intestines.—*Lancet*, October 18, 1890.

Menthol in the Treatment of Diphtheria.—For two years Wolf (*Wiener medizinische Presse*, October 12, 1890) has treated his cases of diphtheria by local applications of menthol mixed with sugar in the proportion of one or two parts of the former to twenty of the latter, with excellent results. The powder is applied by means of a large brush at short intervals. Frequently after removing the brush from the throat a shred of membrane is found attached to it. This is washed off, the brush is partly dried, dipped into the powder, and again applied, repeating the process until no membrane can be brought away. By the second or third day improvement is manifest, and a clean surface is soon found in place of the membrane.

"Boric-acid Massage" in Diseases of the Conjunctiva.—In the treatment of granular and follicular ophthalmia and similar conditions, Dr. W. M. Beaumont (*Lancet*, October 18, 1890) recommends rubbing the conjunctiva with finely-pulverized boric acid. The method is carried out as follows: First, the upper lid is everted in the usual way, and the boric acid is thickly sprinkled on the palpebral conjunctiva. The powder is then rubbed into the conjunctiva with the end of the index finger for five or ten seconds, after which the remaining boric acid may be washed away with a soft brush dipped in "lead lotion," or if there is not much discomfort it may be allowed to remain. The lower lid is then treated in the same manner. In some cases the first few applications cause pain, but after one or two applications tolerance is established. In the earlier applications pain may be prevented by instilling cocaine solution. The procedure may be repeated daily or on alternate days. The condition of the conjunctiva after two or three applications is that of healthy reaction. Dr. Beaumont then reports three cases of trachoma in which this method of treatment gave excellent results.

The Uses of Exalgin.—According to the Paris correspondent of the *Lancet*, M. Desnos has recently undertaken a series of researches upon the action of exalgin. He finds that its influence upon high temperatures is very slight, while as an anodyne its effects are marked. When amounts of from 7½ to 12 grains were given a sensation of vertigo was produced, and sweating, often profuse, was observed in many instances. The sweating was not infrequently localized or most marked over the seat of the pain for which the drug was given. Doses of 12 grains often produced very slight cyanosis. Generally, the drug was well borne by the digestive organs, and eruptions rarely occurred. The urine was usually decreased in amount, and always contained a considerable quantity of exalgin. To relieve pain a dose of 3½ grains will sometimes be sufficient, but 6 grains is an average dose. Twenty-one grains may be given in twenty-four hours in divided doses of 3 grains each. M. Desnos used the drug in various forms of neuralgia, renal colic, and in the lightning pains of tabes. The good effect in intercostal neuralgia was only slight, but in other varieties, including sciatic, and in the pains of tabes the relief was great. It was also of service in the one case of renal colic in which it was used.

An Epidemic of Sore-throat and Erysipelas Due to Infection by Milk.—In the *Glasgow Medical Journal*, October, 1890, is reported an epidemic of sore-throat and erysipelas occurring only in families that were supplied with milk from a certain farm. About eighty cases were observed. The most striking symptom was an intense inflammation of the fauces resembling erysipelas of the mucous membrane. In some cases true erysipelas of the skin developed. In two of the patients, who drank large quantities of the milk, there was a membranous exudate on the lips and tongue, but none on the tonsils or in the pharynx. The temperature was high (102° to 105°) during the first few days of the attack in every case. Convalescence was marked by extreme prostration. Paralysis was not observed and albuminuria was noted in only two cases. Three deaths occurred, all in infants under two years of age.

Unfortunately, no bacterial examinations of the milk were made, nor was there any search for ptomaïnes, but the connection between the epidemic and the milk-supply seems pretty clearly established.

Injection for Gonorrhœa.—The following prescription is quoted by the *Deutsche medicinische Wochenschrift:*

℞.—Antipyrine	.	.	.	.	1 drachm.
Sulphate of zinc	.	.	.	7 grains.
Cherry-laurel water ⎱ of each				2½ ounces.
Rose water ⎰				

Use as an injection.

An Ointment for Prurigo.—According to *La Semaine Médicale*, the following prescription is useful in the treatment of prurigo:

℞.—Resorcin	.	.	.	.	35 grains.
Precipitated sulphur	.	.	5 drachms.
Carbolic acid ⎱ of each	.			7 grains.
Salicylic acid ⎰				
Chloral	.	.	.	.	20 "
Vaseline	.	.	.	.	1½ ounces.

Use externally.

THE MEDICAL NEWS.

A WEEKLY JOURNAL
OF MEDICAL SCIENCE.

COMMUNICATIONS are invited from all parts of the world. Original articles contributed exclusively to THE MEDICAL NEWS will be liberally paid for upon publication. When necessary to elucidate the text, illustrations will be furnished without cost to the author.

Address the Editor: H. A. HARE, M.D.,
1004 WALNUT STREET,
PHILADELPHIA.

Subscription Price, including Postage.

PER ANNUM, IN ADVANCE . . . . . . $4.00.
SINGLE COPIES . . . . 10 CENTS.

Subscriptions may begin at any date. The safest mode of remittance is by bank check or postal money order, drawn to the order of the undersigned. When neither is accessible, remittances may be made, at the risk of the publishers, by forwarding in *registered* letters.

Address,   LEA BROTHERS & CO.,
Nos. 706 & 708 SANSOM STREET,
PHILADELPHIA.

SATURDAY, NOVEMBER 8, 1890.

POISONING FROM THE SURGICAL USE OF IODOFORM.

ALTHOUGH discovered in the latter part of the first quarter of the present century, iodoform was not very extensively used until about ten years ago, when Mosetig von Moorhof made known its virtues for surgical purposes. In late years its employment in the dressing of wounds, as an application to ulcers, and as an agent for the destruction of tubercle as met with in surgical diseases, has been very general. As is well known, the forms in which it is now used are: pure, as a powder; incorporated with gauze; combined with collodion; dissolved in ether, and in emulsion in glycerin or in oil. For injecting into cold abscesses, after their evacuation by aspiration, Verneuil is authority for the choice of the ethereal solution, the strength being five per cent., while the name of Mikulicz is associated with the ten-per-cent. glycerin emulsion, and Bruns has recommended a solution in olive oil of an equal strength. For this latter purpose, the treatment of cold abscesses, iodoform has proved itself a very valuable remedy.

It is, of course, chiefly due to its antiseptic properties, which are universally admitted, even though distinctly limited, that the drug has found favor. That it is not a substance to be applied with an unsparing hand, however, has been known for years; occasional reports of cases of poisoning caused by its use warning us that it must not be looked upon as wholly innocuous.

One of these unfortunate occurrences is reported by M. L. BAROIS (*Archives de Médecine et de Pharmacie Militaires*, No. 8, 1890). In this instance death was caused by the injection of about 55 grammes of a five-per-cent. ethereal solution into the cavity of a large cold abscess under the greater pectoral muscle of the left side. The amount of iodoform used was about 2.75 grammes. Symptoms of ether-narcosis immediately followed the injection, and were succeeded by the toxic effects of iodoform. The symptoms were chiefly cerebral, and continued for nine days, when death in coma supervened.

In addition to an excellent description of his observations in this case, the writer includes a review of the literature of the toxicology of iodoform, his investigation having yielded the discovery of forty-two reported cases, a table of which he presents. From his study of the question Barois found that the symptoms of poisoning make their appearance early and suddenly in the severe cases, and consist of mental depression succeeded by excitement, restlessness, and other signs resembling those of acute meningitis, such as hallucinations, etc. Periods of remission may occur, and gradual cure follow; or abundant sweats, a somewhat elevated temperature, dyspnœa, and a feeble pulse may develop, and a fatal termination is then to be expected. In the young and vigorous the latter are the symptoms which are most likely to occur, while in the old and in those of feeble constitution, the onset as well as the nature of the symptoms will be less intense, comprising anorexia and vomiting, mental depression, weakness of the limbs, and but slight disturbance of the temperature. In this latter type death has seldom been the result.

Search for the explanation of these calamitous effects of iodoform led to the institution of a number of experiments, and the results first obtained by Mundy and Mosetig von Moorhof at the bedside, and by MacKendrick and Binz in the laboratory, pointed to certain narcotic properties possessed by the drug. Hogyes, however, showed that in order to induce toxic symptoms in man it would be necessary to employ a very large quantity, 84 grammes, of the agent if the above theory were correct. A glance at the table given by Barois shows that disaster resulted from the application of much smaller quantities in all but five of the cases. From further experiments conducted by MacKendrick, Binz, and Hogyes, the following conclusions were reached: "First, iodoform given by subcutaneous injection is slowly decomposed in the fat; second, from a solution of iodoform in oil or fat, iodine is separated after several hours; third, the iodine set free forms albuminous clots, which disappear without leaving any traces in the tissues."

These results have since been confirmed, and both clinical and post-mortem evidence harmonize with them. It is iodine, then, which lies at the bottom of the mischief. Iodoform, readily decomposed in the presence of the subcutaneous fat of a wound, or in the tissues surrounding an abscess, liberates iodine, which, in the form of an unstable albuminoid compound, is taken up into the circulation and conveyed to the various organs of the economy, producing in them certain marked changes, as proved by the autopsies of the fatal cases. Before death evidence of its absorption is furnished by the excretion of iodine in the urine in the form of iodide of potassium. The pathological changes are a fatty condition of the liver, the kidneys, and the heart and other muscles, together with less significant lesions. The early appearance and the character of the cerebral symptoms in all the cases would lead us to expect more or less pronounced cerebral lesions to be found on inspection. Nothing more, however, is noted than "hyperæmia of the meninges and some arterial atheromatous lesions."

Two questions which are here pertinent are: First, how much iodoform, locally exhibited, is capable of producing toxic results? Second, in what form may it be applied with the greatest impunity?

The answer to the first of these, according to Barois, cannot be determined. In his fatal case the amount was but 2.75 grammes, while other observers have used much greater quantities without bad effects. Verneuil is said to be of the opinion that poisoning need not be feared when not more than 2.5 grammes are applied. In reply to the second question it may be stated that when incorporated with gauze iodoform may be used with greater safety than in glycerin, oil, or ether.

A glance at the table of the cases of fatal intoxication impresses one with the fact that a notable number of accidents followed operations upon the same anatomical region. Of the forty-two cases thirteen occurred after operations for cancer of the breast,

and one after opening an axillary abscess. Adding to these Barois's case we have a total of forty-three cases, in fourteen of which the poisoning resulted from the application of iodoform to the costo-mammary region.

The prevention of iodoform-poisoning will be best insured, first, by limiting the amount applied to that which has been shown to be the minimum fatal dose; secondly, by the exercise of especial care in patients suffering from certain classes of maladies, which, we may assume from our knowledge of the symptoms of iodoform-poisoning, would be easily influenced by the drug, such patients being those affected with cardiac, nervous, or renal diseases; thirdly, by being particularly cautious in the use of the agent in that region in which it has been shown to be peculiarly dangerous—the costo-mammary region.

As to the treatment to be pursued in these accidents, it is recommended that in addition to the removal of the cause—the suspension of the application—if possible, some unirritating alkali should be locally used, to neutralize at once the iodine set free, and prevent its entering into albuminoid combination; also that the alkalinity of the blood should be increased by the internal exhibition of alkaline salts, Vichy water, or bromide of potassium.

In conclusion, we allude to the fact that in the forty-three fatal cases above referred to, but a single one occurred in the practice of American surgeons. This case, reported in 1881, by Dr. Sands, of New York, was one in which colotomy had been performed for rectal cancer, the dressing consisting of powdered iodoform and iodoform-gauze, the amount of the drug used being 6 grammes.

Whatever its virtues, then, iodoform must be recognized as a positively dangerous substance when applied too liberally, and surgeons will best cope with the baneful results which it is capable of producing by putting into practice the principle of "an ounce of prevention," and restricting the amounts employed well within the limit of safety.

THE ETIOLOGY OF SQUAMOUS EPITHELIOMA.

THE occurrence of carcinomatous changes in chronic ulcerations of epithelial surfaces has long been appropriated by the adherents of Virchow's hypothesis of tumor etiology as direct evidence in favor of the correctness of the view of an irritative origin of such growths; and not infrequently such occurrences are offered as directly opposing the suggestions of Cohnheim as to the embryonal origin of neoplasms. In an article in the *North American Practitioner*, September, 1890, DR. VAN HOOK, after describing the clinical aspects of two cases of flat-celled carcinoma, arising, one in a chronic ulcer of the leg, and the other in the skin near a fistulous opening leading to an osteal necrosis of many years' standing, briefly reviews the pathology of such growths, calling attention to the paper of Boegehold, published in *Virchow's Archives*, in 1882. In the latter paper the writer, according to Van Hook, accepts as conclusive the well-worn theory of Virchow, setting aside Cohnheim's views as valueless for two reasons: " First, because these carcinomata arise in tissues of new origin, where no misplaced embryonal cells could exist; second, because the regenerative activity is here exhausted, whereas the Cohnheim theory demands an increase in this activity."

There are, however, certain suggestions arising from a study of the minute relations of the growth of these neoplasms to normal organization which are worthy of consideration, and which accentuate the incompleteness of the views of Virchow as explanatory of the growth of tumors. That the primary cause of the original wound was of a mechanical or chemical nature, can, in the majority of instances, be clearly demonstrated; but in attempting to explain how that irritation may induce the normal regenerative process to assume a pseudo-formative character, the mechanical theory is wholly inadequate. That any given irritation may excite cellular formation for the purpose of regeneration, or for the exclusion of the source of irritation, is the simple statement of a fact long observed; for the understanding of the manner of transformation of this normal formation into tumor formation further consideration must be invoked.

In the formation of new tissues in the healing of wounds of epithelial surfaces there may be uniformly observed an apparently undue proliferation of the epithelial cells. Near the margin of an ulcer or along the edges of a wound where the proliferation is most marked, minute examination at an early stage usually reveals a distinct line of separation between the forming epithelial cells above and the embryonal connective tissue in the deeper portions of the part; later, however, as if to gain a firmer hold upon the underlying structures, the epithelial layer is prone to send into the young connective tissue beneath, long, slender, branching prolongations, which persist for a considerable period after organization is complete. In this process of organization the new tissues are essentially embryonal in nature, and the process is entirely analogous if not identical, in the formation of the cells, in the character of the vascular supply and the mode of growth, to embryonic generation. Nor can the second objection of Boegehold be maintained. since the regenerative energy of the epithelial tissues, at least, is frequently evident even to superficial observation in these chronic ulcers by the heaped-up, irregular masses of epithelium distributed chiefly along the borders of the sores.

In the process of cicatrization it may be readily conceived that by the contraction of the newly-formed connective tissue, portions of these epithelial prolongations, retaining their vegetable energy and the functions of the dermal layer, may be entirely separated from the normal epithelium above. These islets of displaced growing epithelium, persisting in their penetrating tendency and in their squamous character, constitute the point of departure from the normal epithelial covering to the tumor of epitheliomatous type; and the presence of such actively-vegetating foreign tissue may give rise to the irritation necessary to the long continuance of the inflammation characterizing these chronic ulcers.

Viewed in this light, instead of militating against the proposition of Cohnheim that tumors are essentially accidents of embryonal procedence, the growth of these epitheliomata distinctly favors the verity of such an hypothesis. There exists in these cases a true displacement of cells of an embryonal nature by a species of invagination, which, although occurring in the adult, bears close analogy to the invaginations in the blastodermic layers in embryonic organization. While in many cases of chronic ulceration there seems to be a depression of the regenerative energy of the connective tissues, there is not, as Boegehold would suggest, any lack in the vegetative power of the epithelial elements. On the contrary, epithelial proliferation is as a rule excessive, as shown by the rapid closing of wounds in healing by first intention, and by the masses of epithelial tissue along the margins of an old ulcer; and it is not improbable that there should be regarded as an element in the tumor-growth in these cases, a failure of the normal resistance of tissue to tissue. connective tissue to epithelial, as proposed by Thiersch in relation to the epitheliomata of old age.

REVIEWS.

THE SCIENCE AND ART OF OBSTETRICS. By THE-
OPHILUS PARVIN, M.D., LL.D.   Second edition re-
vised and enlarged.   Philadelphia : Lea Brothers &
Co., 1890.

THIS excellent text-book has already found its way
into the library of so many practitioners and is so generally used by students that the second edition needs
but few words from the reviewer. Among the additions
noted is Hegar's sign of pregnancy, which is described
without comment and with which the author seems to
have had no experience. The method of treating
eclampsia by the hypodermic administration of morphine is referred to as being considerably used, but here,
too, our author refrains from expressing his opinion.
Of antisepsis in labor the author, naturally, writes in
more positive terms than in the first edition, and clearly
prefers creolin to either corrosive sublimate or carbolic
acid.

Were we asked to state the chief fault of Dr. Parvin's
treatise we would say that the author shows too distinctly
his respect for authorities and that he expresses his own
opinions too infrequently. For instance, in the section
on the resuscitation of asphyxiated infants, four methods of performing artificial respiration are described,
and the reader can only infer that Dr. Parvin prefers
Schultz's method. Some, however, may deny that this
absolute freedom from dogmatism is a fault, and unquestionably it possesses the advantage of requiring
students to form their own opinions, besides being discouraging to what has been aptly termed " mental lazi-
ness."

The most valuable features of the book are the
lucidity of the author's descriptions and a peculiar
charm of style which tempts one to read page after page
when, perhaps, the intention was merely to look up
some forgotten fact. As a whole, we believe that Dr.
Parvin's treatise is the best book on obstetrics for undergraduate students that has yet appeared, but that for
men in active practice there are one or two other books
equally good.

SOCIETY PROCEEDINGS.

NEW YORK NEUROLOGICAL SOCIETY.

Stated Meeting, October 7, 1890.

THE PRESIDENT, LANDON CARTER GRAY, M.D.,
IN THE CHAIR.

DR. W. B. PRITCHARD presented the brain of a patient
who died from tuberculous meningitis. When first seen
by the speaker, the patient was suffering from obstinate
insomnia and headache. A few days subsequently the
thermometer showed some elevation of temperature, but
this did not exceed 103° until shortly before death. The
mental disturbances were very marked from the beginning. There was complete loss of memory, right-sided
ptosis, difficulty, and finally loss, of speech, and the
rapid development of symptoms of complete bulbar
paralysis. The immediate cause of death was apparently
involvement of the vagus. There was decided right

hemiparesis. A very offensive purulent discharge from
the nose was present, and continued until the patient's
death. The autopsy revealed over the right parietal bone
a cavity with about the circumference of a dime, the
necrosis being presumably tuberculous in character.
Over the right eye were a linear scar and a depressed
fracture, but apparently the brain was not affected by
the fracture. At the base of the brain a thick tenacious
material was found. The medulla, pons, crura, and
cranial nerves were involved, and the dura over the convexity of both hemispheres was covered with an apparently tuberculous deposit.

DR. WILLIAM A. HAMMOND read a paper entitled,

CAN WE DIAGNOSE HYPERÆMIA OR ANÆMIA OF THE
CORD AND BRAIN ?

The reader said that for many years he had been
familiar with a group of symptoms which, from their
etiology and general characteristics, are indicative of
cerebral disturbance. About twenty-five years ago, after
considerable observation and many experiments performed upon the lower animals and upon man, he came
to the conclusion that these symptoms are the result
of an increased amount of blood in the brain. The
theory which he had advanced was, that natural sleep
was due to a comparatively anæmic condition of the
brain, normal wakefulness to an excess of intracranial
blood. Hence, persistent insomnia is necessarily a
pathognomonic symptom of cerebral hyperæmia. If
this symptom is associated with pain in the head, a feeling of distention, heat, vertigo, and hallucinations, and
is aggravated by the recumbent posture and by drugs
which increase the amount of blood in the brain, there
can be no doubt of the presence of cerebral congestion.
The reader had made many experiments with ergot, and
is convinced of its efficacy in diminishing the quantity
of intracranial blood.

In conclusion, he said that if a patient came to him
suffering from insomnia, pain in the head, vertigo, hallucinations, suffusion of the face, cephalic heat, &c., and
if the symptoms disappeared under the influence of such
remedies as the bromides, ergot, ice and douches of cold
water to the nape of the neck, cupping in the same
locality, nasal bloodletting, or spontaneous hæmorrhage,
he thought it evident that the patient was suffering from
cerebral hyperæmia.

In discussion, DR. M. ALLEN STARR said that while
he did not oppose Dr. Hammond's views, still his convictions at present were those expressed by Dr. Gray in
a paper recently read before the Neurological Society.
The symptoms explained by the assumed existence of
cerebral hyperæmia can also be produced by other
causes. Wakefulness, for example, is often noticed in
individuals who are very much exhausted, as in puerperal women after a severe hæmorrhage. He has also
observed it in patients who were anæmic. Therefore,
that wakefulness necessarily indicates a hyperæmic brain
is a theory which is hardly tenable. Certainly hyperæmia of the brain may, under certain conditions, be
diagnosed, but it is an open question whether this can
be done when only wakefulness is present.

As to drugs, he had been surprised to hear Dr. A. H.
Smith and Dr. Peabody state at a meeting of the Practitioners' Society last winter, that they had been treating

cases of supposed hyperæmia of the brain with nitro-glycerin and nitrite of amyl. These drugs, which are supposed to increase the amount of blood in the brain, were given upon the hypothesis that they dilated the entire arterial system of the body, and that the brain would thereby, to a certain extent, be relieved of blood. The reasoning at least appeared sound.

Dr. J. Leonard Corning thought that this reasoning was not scientific. If a patient complained of headache, and had a congested face and a pulse of high tension, and if the symptoms could be promptly relieved by pressure upon the carotids or jugulars, or by bandaging the legs, which should be assumed, congestion or anæmia of the brain? The speaker thought, congestion. If quinine or alcohol aggravated the symptoms, it would be certainly concluded that the trouble was congestion.

Dr. Gray then enumerated the conditions in which the symptoms described by Dr. Hammond might be found. Insomnia, he said, is common enough in mental diseases, worry, overwork, and constipation, and in many conditions in which there is nothing to show that there is hyperæmia of the brain. In the early stages of intracranial syphilis there is a condition somewhat of the nature of hyperæmia. But in Bright's disease, in which also there are hyperæmia and congestion, there is stupor. In some cases of insomnia it is possible to find a certain train of symptoms which would lead to the assumption of existing anæmia, and in others the symptoms would indicate hyperæmia. Experiments have recently been made on the brains of animals, the reports of which differ from those of other experimenters as to the cause of the increased volume of the brain during the waking period. It is an open question whether this increase is not due to cellular activity which increases the amount of blood.

As to the association of sleeplessness with the recumbent posture, of course the extended observations of the author of the paper deserve due consideration, but so also do the more limited observations of the speaker, who has not been able to verify the association.

The question is not as to the existence of cerebral hyperæmia or anæmia, but as to whether it can be clinically diagnosed. Flushed face may be dependent upon chorea, general paresis, or injury of the brain, and it is in such cases impossible to say whether the symptom was brought on by hyperæmia alone. The feeling of oppression and sense of fulness in the head are sometimes associated with errors of refraction, insufficiency of the ocular muscles, changes of climate, errors of diet, &c. To assume that in all these conditions there is hyperæmia of the brain, is assuming more than can be proved. It has not been demonstrated by any pathologist whether an increased amount of blood in the cellular tissue of the brain can exist without causing disease of the surrounding parts. It is strange that Dr. Hammond, after five months' study of the subject, cited no autopsies in confirmation of his theory.

Dr. C. L. Dana said that it is now generally admitted that there is such a condition as cerebral hyperæmia, and that it can be recognized in its acute forms. Such a state might be produced by drugs, certain neuroses, and trauma. The question is, What is the condition at the base of that functional disorder which has gone by the name of cerebral neurasthenia? Acute and chronic hyperæmia of the brain are conditions admitted to exist, but it is preferable to say "functional cerebral neuroses" or "psychoses" if the hyperæmia is a secondary process, which seems the inevitable conclusion if such cases are closely observed.

Many patients among the neurasthenics have symptoms of congestion of the brain; others of this class do not present the symptoms of typical cerebral hyperæmia. The hyperæmia of the brain is secondary to some disorder of the vaso-motor nerves, or to some functional condition involving the whole nervous system.

To state that sleep is produced by anæmia, and wakefulness by the return of the normal amount of blood to the head, is, the speaker thought, in the light of modern neurological studies, a theory unworthy of further investigation.

Dr. Hammond thought that his statements were not disproved. When Dr. Dana said that the neurologists of to-day ignored the theory of the physiological changes during sleep—a theory which the speaker might claim as his own—he thought that Dr. Dana was in error. He had stated that innumerable causes of headache existed, and it is only when it is associated with flushed face and vertigo, and when it is increased by a dependent position, that the diagnosis is certain.

CORRESPONDENCE.

MEDICAL LAW AND EXAMINATIONS IN MONTANA.

To the Editor of The Medical News,

Sir : Prior to the passage of House Bill No. 6, by the Sixteenth Legislative Assembly of Montana, in March, 1889, the restrictions regarding the requirements for the practice of medicine in Montana were few, and carelessly complied with. The Bill mentioned above is "An act to regulate the Practice of Medicine in the Territory of Montana, and to provide for the examination and issuing of certificates to persons desirous of practising the same, and for the punishment of persons violating the provisions of the Act."

There has been considerable consternation in the profession in Montana since this law went into effect, and a number of lawsuits have resulted. When the Act passed there were many undergraduates practising in the Territory, and the new law required all of these who had not been in continuous practice here for at least ten years, to appear before the Medical Board for examination. Those holding diplomas of reputable colleges were granted license to practise. The greatest " kick " is by physicians who came to Montana after the law went into effect, and who had been in practice in other States, and possessed good diplomas—yet were required to submit to an examination by the Board. But after becoming familiar with the manner in which the people have been preyed upon by the unscrupulous "quacks," the intelligent physician at once sees the necessity for such a law —both to the laity and the profession.

Section 1 of the law says : " The Governor, with the advice and consent of the Council. shall appoint seven learned and skilled physicians—who shall have been residents of the Territory of Montana for not less than two years preceding their appointment—not more than two of whom shall be from the same county—who shall constitute the Board of Examiners for the purposes of this Act." The Board consists of six regulars and one homœopath, who is the treasurer of the Board. Meetings for the examination of applicants and granting certificates are held on the first Tuesday of April and of October of each year, four members of the Board constituting a quorum.

The first meeting of the Board was held in Helena, October 7th, five members and about twenty-five applicants for examination and certificates being present. The members of the Board decided that each applicant should make affidavit in writing, of his age, the time spent in the study of medicine, the college by which he was graduated, and the date of his diploma. The examination was oral, each applicant going before each member of the Board. The questions asked, so far as your correspondent could learn, were straightforward and reasonable, strictly confined to the branches required by law, and well calculated to test an applicant's medical ability—"catch" questions being avoided.

For the benefit of those who are interested, I will give a *few* questions that were asked which may serve to remove the undue prejudice that exists against the law, and the persons appointed to execute it. In Anatomy, the following questions were asked: "What is anatomy? How many cavities in the heart? Where are the semilunar, the tricuspid, and the mitral valves? Describe the vomer, and tell where it is situated. What is the name of the principal artery supplying the stomach? Give the origin and insertion of the gastrocnemius. Name the coverings of the brain, and the situation of each. Where is the seminal vesicle? Name the different divisions of the alimentary canal."

In Physiology, the examination was as follows: "Describe the circulation of the blood. How many kinds of circulation are there? What is the function of the liver, and through what channel does the liver get its blood-supply? What are the principal constituents of the gastric juice? Name the five digestive fluids."

In Materia Medica: "Give the physiological action of aconite, the directions for its use, and the dose. What is opium? Which is the more powerful, hydrargyri chloridum mite or hydrargyri chloridum corrosivum? Give the dose of each. How much antipyrine would you give at a dose, and how often would you repeat it? What is the dose of phenacetin?"

In Practice of Medicine: "What is pneumonia? Name the different stages, and give the treatment of each. How would you treat sick-headache? Name the principal means used in examining for disease of the chest."

In Chemistry and Toxicology: "For what purpose is 'Fehling's solution' used? How would you recognize and treat a case of strychnine-poisoning? What are the symptoms and treatment of a case of arsenic-poisoning. In what way does a fatal dose of the mineral acids cause death?"

In Surgery, some of the questions were: "How would you treat 'Colles's fracture'? What do we understand by antisepsis? Name some of the indications for amputation. What is skin-grafting? How would you treat an extra-capsular fracture of the neck of the fémur?"

In Obstetrics: "How would you treat post-partum hæmorrhage? What are the indications for the use of forceps? How would you control convulsions occurring in the course of labor?"

Diseases of the Eye and Ear: "What is iritis, and what is the proper treatment? What is chemosis? How would you treat acute catarrhal conjunctivitis? How would you treat purulent conjunctivitis? Give the treatment for ulcer of the cornea. What is otorrhœa? Give the proper treatment of chronic discharges of the ear?"

Diseases of Children: "How would you differentiate measles from scarlet fever? Can you name an eruptive disease in which the temperature falls to normal when the eruption appears?"

Diseases of Women: "What is metritis? What is cervical endometritis? Give the treatment for the same. What do you understand ovariotomy to be? Name some of the tumors which develop in the female generative organs. How would you treat pelvic abscess?"

No two of the applicants were asked exactly the same questions, and the above questions are only some of those asked the writer and two other applicants. Three applicants were refused certificates, because they declined to submit to the examination and because they had not complied with the law in having attended three courses of lectures of at least four months each, and in being the possessor of a diploma from a reputable medical college.

Section 4 of the Act contains this clause: "In all cases of refusal or revocation the applicant, if he or she feels aggrieved, may appeal to the district court of the county where such applicant may have applied for a certificate." Some rejected applicants are taking advantage of this, and, of course, giving the Board unnecessary trouble.

The fee for the examination and certificate is fifteen dollars, and physicians coming to the State at any time may make application to any member of the Board for a certificate to practise, by presenting a reputable diploma and paying the fee, whereupon he will be granted a temporary certificate, good until the next meeting of the Board, at which time he must appear for examination. A few, defiantly refuse to comply with these provisions, and, against all such, the Board will be compelled to take legal proceedings.

Of the applicants, three were homœopaths and the remainder regulars. One member of the Board remarked that in no instance had he known an applicant to be asked whether he was a regular or irregular.

To my brother practitioners who are contemplating going before the Board and passing through the ordeal of an examination, I would say that my opinion of the Board is entirely different from that which I entertained previously to the last meeting, and that the examinations are perfectly fair.   G. T. McCULLOUGH, M.D.
MISSOULA, MONTANA.

RUSH MEDICAL COLLEGE AND THE NORTH-WESTERN UNIVERSITY.

To the Editor of THE MEDICAL NEWS,

SIR: Your Chicago correspondent made some very misleading statements in his letter published in THE

MEDICAL NEWS of October 11th. Professor Roberts never was connected with the Northwestern University, but he is the President of the Lake Forest University, and to that latter institution his figures referred. The Northwestern University never had or desired any connection with Rush Medical College. A short time ago, after the latter college had made for itself a reputation, and had a large patronage, Lake Forest University made advances to it and secured a union of interests. Lake Forest is twenty-eight miles north of Chicago, on Lake Michigan. The Northwestern University is located at Evanston, also on Lake Michigan. The main campus is just twelve miles from the Court House in Chicago. It has an endowment of over $3,000,000, and has enrolled this year over 2000 students. Dr. Rogers, who succeeded judge Cooley as Dean of the Law School of Michigan University, recently accepted the presidency of the Northwestern University. This University has in Evanston, the College of Liberal Arts, the Woman's College, School of Oratory, Conservatory of Music, Preparatory Department, and three theological schools. In Chicago are located the schools of medicine, pharmacy, dentistry, and law. At Evanston, and in the care of the University, is the large Dearborn telescope. For the use of scientific students in Evanston there is a large hall, with ample chemical and physical laboratories. In the College of Liberal Arts there is a course designed, whether wisely or not, especially for those intending to study medicine.

The medical department of the University is known among our profession as the Chicago Medical College, of which N. S. Davis, M.D., LL.D., is the Dean. This was the first medical school in the United States that established a graded course of three years, obliging students to pass examinations on the first year's work before taking a second. It was also one of the first medical schools in this country to insist upon a preliminary examination or a diploma from a literary school. Every person before graduation must have been a member of a clinical class of from four to eight, or perhaps ten, who receive special training in the diagnosis of such cases as are met with in office practice—this in addition to the general hospital and college clinics. The result is that a large proportion of the students are weeded out before the diplomas are granted.

A new building is to be erected by the Northwestern University on the south side of the city, for the schools of pharmacy and dentistry and for laboratories for the medical school. Very respectfully,

HENRY B. HEMENWAY, M.D.

EVANSTON, ILLS., October 15, 1890.

NEWS ITEMS.

Obituary.—DR. HENRY JACOB BIGELOW died at the age of seventy years, at his home at Oak Hill, Newton, Mass., shortly before noon on October 30th, and it may be truly said that in his death Boston has lost a surgeon who in his ability, originality, and ingenuity of Iuvention, has not been equalled in the past or present.

As long ago as 1844 he began to publish a number of surgical works which soon gave hiu a world-wide reputation, and an essay of his on "Orthopædic Surgery" obtained the Boylston Prize of Harvard University in

1844. He invented what is known as Bigelow's operation of lithotrity, the value of which is universally recognized. The French Academy of Medicine awarded him a prize for the operation in 1882, although the medical profession both in this country and abroad had long before recognized its value and resorted to it. Harvard University conferred the degree of LL.D. upon Dr. Bigelow in 1882, and he was made Emeritus Professor of Surgery in Harvard Medical School.

He retired from the practice of medicine in 1886. For a long period Dr. Bigelow was a sufferer from gastric and hepatic disease and his death was not unexpected by his friends.

The Recent Medical Examination in New Jersey.—Among the answers given to the New Jersey Medical Examining Board by applicants for license to practise were the following :

Question. Write a prescription for acute diarrhœa in a child ten years old.

Answer.

"R.—Tinctura opii . . . 1 drachm.
" catechu . . 5 drachms.
" kino . . . 2 drachms.—M.

" Take a teaspoonful every three hours."

Q. Name three cathartics.
A. " Compound cathartic pills, hydrar. cum creta, calomel."

Q. Describe a case of cirrhosis of the liver.
A. " Pain in the left side over the liver toward the back. . . ."

Q. Describe briefly how you would investigate a surgical case, and by what method you would write a history of such a case.
A. " I should investigate a surgical case under antiseptic precautions whenever practicable, and should write a history of such a case by the antiseptic system of surgery."

Q. What is an acute abscess ?
A. " A deep-seated, burrowing sore."

Q. Describe the operation for tying the external iliac artery.
A. " Etherize the patient, perform everything under antiseptic care, make an incision through the skin, fascia and connective tissue."

Q. Supposing in a case of retention of urine from an enlarged prostate, you could not succeed in passing the catheter by the natural passage, what proceeding would you adopt ?
A. " I should at once give diaphoretics, hydragogue cathartics, and apply warm poultices to the abdomen over the bladder. If all this should fail I should perform the operation of laparotomy."

Q. Describe the diaphragm.
A. " The diaphragm is perforated by several orifices. The œsophageal, aortic, venæ cavæ, and pharyngeal orifices."

Q. Describe the circle of Willis.
A. " In the fœtal circulation the blood pouring directly through the heart instead of the lungs forms the circle of Willis."

Q. What is the difference between calomel and corrosive sublimate ?

A. "Calomel contains but few corrosive and antiseptic properties. Corrosive chloride of mercury is a powerful corrosive agent and is a strong antiseptic."

Q. In what does human blood differ from that of a frog?

A. "The corpuscles in human blood contain a nucleus, and corpuscles in the blood of a frog contain no nucleus."

Q. Give the condition of the mucous membrane of the stomach in chronic inflammation thereof.

A. "In chronic inflammation of the stomach the mucous membrane presents, on inspection, a bright-red appearance. Large spots of mucous membrane is destroyed. The bloodvessels are congested. There is thickening of the mucous folds."

Q. Give the treatment of acute conjunctivitis.

A. "Apply eye-water every two hours. . . ."

Q. What are the operations for cataract?

A. "The operation for cataract consists in removing the cataract with a knife, which is done by introducing it into the eye back of the crystalline lens and removing that portion which is affected."

A Mohammedan Female Physician.—Dr. Razie Koutlairoff-Hanum, a young Mohammedan woman, who was born in the Crimea, recently passed a creditable examination as physician and surgeon at Odessa, and now enjoys the distinction of being the first woman of her creed to engage in the practice of medicine as understood by western nations.

A Hospital in Central Africa.—As an instance of the civilizing work now being carried on in the Congo Free State, may be mentioned the Bangala-station hospital, in the upper Congo basin, a little less than a thousand miles from the Atlantic coast. It was erected for the employés of the station, and contains forty beds, besides rooms for convalescent patients.

OFFICIAL LIST OF CHANGES IN THE STATIONS AND DUTIES OF OFFICERS SERVING IN THE MEDICAL DEPARTMENT, U. S. ARMY, FROM OCTOBER 28 TO NOVEMBER 3, 1890.

ARTHUR, WILLIAM H., *Captain and Assistant Surgeon.*—Is relieved from duty at Fort Bayard, New Mexico, and will report in person to the commanding officer Fort Grant, Arizona Territory, for duty at that post, relieving William B. Banister, First Lieutenant and Assistant Surgeon. Lieutenant Banister, on being relieved by Captain Arthur, will repair to this city, and report for duty to the commanding officer Washington Barracks, District of Columbia.—Par. 12, *S. O. 254, A. G. O., Washington, D. C.*, October 30, 1890.

WAKEMAN, WILLIAM J., *Captain and Assistant Surgeon.*—Is relieved from duty at Fort Bidwell, California, to take effect on the final discontinuance of that post, and will then report in person to the commanding officer Fort Huachuca, Arizona Territory, for duty at that station.—Par. 12, *S. O. 254, A. G. O.*, October 30, 1890.

WALES, PHILIP G., *First Lieutenant and Assistant Surgeon.*—Is relieved from station and further duty at Fort Huachuca, Arizona Territory, and assigned to duty at San Carlos, Arizona Territory, where he is now temporarily serving.—Par. 13, *S. O. 254, A. G. O.*, October 30, 1890.

So much of Par. 2, S. O. 208, A. G. O., September 5, 1890, as directed NATHAN S. JARVIS, *First Lieutenant and Assistant Surgeon*, to report for duty at San Carlos, Arizona Territory, is revoked. On the expiration of his present sick-leave of absence, Lieutenant Jarvis will report in person to the commanding officer Fort Bayard, New Mexico, for duty at that station.—Par. 13, *S. O. 254, A. G. O.*, October 30, 1890.

CONWAY, STEVENS G., *Surgeon.*—Is granted leave of absence for one month, with permission to apply for an extension of fifteen days, to take effect upon the arrival of Acting Assistant Surgeon A. P. Frick at Fort Marcy.—Par. 2, *S. O. 112, Department of Arizona, Los Angeles, Cal.*, October 24, 1890.

EDIE, GUY L., *Captain and Assistant Surgeon* (Fort Douglas, Utah).—Is granted leave of absence for one month, on surgeon's certificate of disability.—*S. O. 80, Headquarters Department of the Platte, Omaha, Nebraska*, October 27, 1890.

By direction of the Secretary of War, the leave of absence granted CHARLES B. EWING, *Captain and Assistant Surgeon*, in S. O. 131, Department of the Missouri, September 22, 1890, is extended fourteen days.—*S. O. 250, A. G. O.*, October 25, 1890.

By direction of the Secretary of War, the following changes in the stations and duties of officers of the Medical Department are ordered:

WOODRUFF, CHARLES E., *First Lieutenant and Assistant Surgeon.*—Is relieved from duty at Fort Gibson, California, and will report in person to the commanding officer Fort Missoula, Montana, for duty at that post, relieving Calvin De Witt, Major and Surgeon. Major De Witt, upon being so relieved, will report in person to the commanding officer Fort Hancock, Texas, for duty at that post.—Par. 6, *S. O. 249, A. G. O., Washington, D. C.*, October 24, 1890.

OFFICIAL LIST OF CHANGES IN THE STATIONS AND DUTIES OF THE MEDICAL CORPS OF THE U. S. NAVY FOR THE WEEK ENDING NOVEMBER 1, 1890.

STEPHENSON, F. B., *Surgeon.*—Detached from Receiving-ship "Wabash," and wait orders.

MARTIN, H. M., *Surgeon.*—Ordered to the Receiving-ship "Wabash."

STONE, LEWIS H., *Assistant Surgeon.*—Ordered to the U. S. S. "Pinta."

ARNOLD, WILLIAM F., *Assistant Surgeon.*—Detached from the U. S. S. "Pinta," and granted two months leave.

OWENS, THOMAS, *Surgeon.*—Detached from the Coast-survey Steamer "Blake," and wait orders.

BLACKWOOD, N. J., *Assistant Surgeon.*—Ordered to the Receiving-ship "Vermont."

BOGERT, E. S., *Assistant Surgeon.*—Detached from the U. S. Receiving-ship "Vermont," and ordered to the Coast-survey Steamer "Blake."

MOORE, A. M., *Surgeon.*—Detached from the U. S. S. "Kearsarge," and ordered to the Naval Hospital, Mare Island, Cal.

OFFICIAL LIST OF CHANGES OF STATIONS AND DUTIES OF MEDICAL OFFICERS OF THE U. S. MARINE-HOSPITAL SERVICE, FROM OCTOBER 6 TO OCTOBER 25, 1890.

HUTTON, W. H. H., *Surgeon.*—Detail as Chairman of Board of Examiners revoked; ordered to Washington, D. C., for temporary duty, October 14, 1890.

WYMAN, WALTER, *Surgeon.*—To inspect quarantine stations, October 14, 1890.

LONG, W. H., *Surgeon.*—Detailed as Chairman of Board of Examiners, October 14, 1890.

SAWTELLE, H. W., *Surgeon.*—Granted leave of absence for five days, October 13, 1890.

GASSAWAY, J. M., *Surgeon.*—Granted leave of absence for thirty days, October 11, 1890.

IRWIN, FAIRFAX, *Surgeon.*—Detailed as Recorder of Board of Examiners, October 14, 1890.

AMES, R. P. M., *Passed Assistant Surgeon.*—Granted leave of absence for thirty days, October 14, 1890.

WHITE, J. H., *Passed Assistant Surgeon.*—Granted leave of absence for thirty days, October 24, 1890.

PETTUS, W. J., *Passed Assistant Surgeon.*—To proceed to Vineyard Haven, Mass., for temporary duty, October 9, 1890.

PERRY, T. B., *Assistant Surgeon.*—Ordered to examination for promotion, October 9, 1890.

KINYOUN, J. J., *Assistant Surgeon.*—Ordered to examination for promotion, October 10, 1890.

CONDICT, J. A. W., *Assistant Surgeon.*—To proceed to Baltimore, Md., for temporary duty, October 18, 1890.

RESIGNATION.

AMES, R. P. M., *Passed Assistant Surgeon.*—Resignation, to take effect November 15, 1890, accepted by the President, October 14, 1890.

THE MEDICAL NEWS.
A WEEKLY JOURNAL OF MEDICAL SCIENCE.

Vol. LVII.	Saturday, November 15, 1890.	No. 20.

ORIGINAL LECTURES.

THE MORBID ANATOMY OF TYPHOID FEVER.

The Annual Address,
delivered before the Philadelphia Pathological Society.

BY ARTHUR V. MEIGS, M.D.,
PHYSICIAN TO THE PENNSYLVANIA AND TO THE CHILDREN'S
HOSPITALS, PHILADELPHIA.

MR. PRESIDENT AND GENTLEMEN: Permit me in the first place to express to you my deep sense of the honor which has been conferred upon me by being selected to deliver the annual oration before you on this occasion.

The conception that I have formed of what such an address before a pathological society should be, is that it should embody the results of some original investigation, or if that be impossible, should suggest some line of thought in which it would seem that research might lead to something of value.

In casting about for a subject worthy of your attention, it occurred to me that a consideration of the lesions found after death from typhoid fever might be of interest. It is not that I have very much that is new to present to you upon this subject, for both in the general treatises and in the special works upon pathology will be found an immense fund of information in regard to the various morbid conditions of the tissues and organs in this complaint. Rather is it because in the course of my professional career I have been impressed with the fact that the view seems very common among physicians that typhoid fever is a disease of the intestines alone. Clinical experience as well as pathological investigations have led me to look upon this view as an erroneous one. As I have studied the symptoms presented by my patients—epistaxis, an early symptom, often present before the abdominal conditions are pronounced, the hebetude or delirium, the subsultus, the eruption and sudamina, and the marked pulmonary conditions—I have been unable to rest contented with the view that the disease is seen in its true light when looked upon as primarily a disease of the intestines. Sometimes it has struck me that the reason the disease is commonly so considered, is because it is generally known among the laity as well as among professional men that it so often arises from drinking impure water, which is taken first into the alimentary canal, and from there starts upon its course of mischief. It would be as reasonable, however, to argue that strychnine in poisonous doses produces death by its effects upon the alimentary system because it is taken by the mouth, as that typhoid fever is truly a disease of the same system; though in each the poison commonly enters by the same avenue.

The importance of conditions other than intestinal ones in typhoid fever first forced itself upon me, so far as my recollection serves, rather from considering the disease clinically than from the grossness of the organic lesions. So much was this the case that two or three years ago I determined, as opportunities might arise, to make careful studies, both macroscopically and with the microscope, of as many of the organs and tissues as time and my ability enabled me to do.

It is the outcome of these investigations, as far as they have been made, that I want to present for your consideration. My results, of course, will be found to be far from perfect and there is room for further and almost unlimited study in the same line of thought, but so far as I shall make assertion of facts of observation I think you will find them to be true. When, however, I trespass into the fields of deduction you will, of course, do well to examine my logic and accept or deny my conclusions as the result may be.

With the object in view, then, of ascertaining whether other pathological changes besides the commonly-recognized ones in the intestines and mesenteric glands might be present, and be present perhaps with a greater or less degree of constancy, I have made careful search in some of my cases. The picture I wish to place before you cannot, I think, be better presented than by reporting somewhat in detail a case that was studied at considerable length.

There was admitted to the Pennsylvania Hospital, August 18, 1889, a man, twenty-seven years of age, who was born in America. He belonged to the laboring class, and said that he had never suffered from any previous illness except an acute attack of some kind when seven years old. He denied having indulged in excesses of any sort. Six days before admission to the hospital he ate watermelon and the next day was taken with abdominal pain; soon diarrhœa with a sense of heaviness and weakness of the legs came on. The day before coming to the hospital he had epistaxis, but he continued to work until his admission, though his appetite was poor and he had continual abdominal pain. He had also some cough and expectoration.

On admission his temperature was 103⅖° and there was some tendency to retention of the urine. The tongue was moist and coated with a white fur, but not tremulous. There was no eruption upon the abdomen.

Physical examination gave the following results: The first sound of the heart was soft (anæmic); the lungs were everywhere filled with bronchial râles; the hepatic dulness was of the natural extent, and the splenic dulness was somewhat increased. The treatment was four grains of quinine twice daily and ten drops of dilute muriatic acid three times daily. He continued to have fever, the temperature varying generally between 101° and 104°, and after the first two days in the hospital he had diarrhœa, with from one to five stools in twenty-four hours. After a few days the tongue became dry and the pulse running, and there was much subsultus. The treatment was changed, turpentine and whiskey being given ; still later, as he continued to grow worse, spirit of chloroform and tincture of digitalis were used. No characteristic eruption appeared, but he continued to fail, the temperature rose to 106° and he became excessively nervous and died, August 27th.

At the autopsy the following conditions were found. There were many pleural adhesions, especially to the diaphragm. The lungs appeared to be much congested, being intensely dark-red and in some areas almost black, and blood freely exuded on section. The heart looked natural except that it was soft and its lining was stained very dark red. The liver was rather large and firm, but not very dark or much congested. The bile-duct was patulous. The spleen was three times the natural size, firm in texture and intensely dark red on section. The kidneys were slightly enlarged, flaccid and dark-colored on section. The small intestine throughout half its length presented many typical typhoid ulcerations of Peyer's patches, besides an unusually large number of smaller ulcers scattered generally over the inner surface. The mesenteric glands were enlarged to an unusual degree and on section some of them presented small spots of softening, the contents of which ran out, leaving cavities. The colon was congested but otherwise normal. The spinal cord presented congestion of the vessels upon its surface, especially of its lower half, where the veins were very full. The cord itself, both the surface and on section, looked natural.

Microscopical examination of sections cut from the lungs, heart, liver, spleen, kidney, ileum, mesenteric gland, and the spinal cord was made.

The most marked change presented by the lungs was that over large portions of the sections the appearance was simply that of a mass of blood. Large quantities of red corpuscles, exhibiting their characteristic outline and of a yellowish color, and unstained by carmine, with many leucocytes of varying size and appearance scattered amongst them, covered whole fields under the microscope. The blood filled the air-vesicles, bronchi, and bloodvessels, and in places there were evidences of inflammation, the tissue showing round-cell infiltration, and there being some catarrhal-exudate cells. The bronchioles and tissue for a short distance around them were inflamed, the cells of the epithelial lining having undergone proliferation, and the subepithelial tissue being infiltrated, thickened, and containing vessels filled with clotted blood. The blood-clot in one vessel of the lung-tissue was variously channelled out, new vessels being in process of formation in it, if they were not actually already formed. The heart-muscle was, in some places, in a very good state of preservation, the cross-striæ being very sharp. In other parts the fibres were homogeneous or granular-looking. It seems likely that this was due to disease and not to faulty technique, for all the tissue was preserved, prepared, stained, and mounted under precisely similar conditions, if not at the same time, and yet the same section often showed the most marked contrasts. It seems that there was some endocarditis, for the endocardium appeared to be slightly thickened, and contained more than the natural number of nuclei.

That some myocardial inflammation, independent of the state of the muscle-fibres, was present, there can be no doubt, for there was a great multiplication of the red-staining nuclei which are naturally present in the intermuscular substance. In some areas there was a great deal of brown pigment in the muscle-fibres. Hæmorrhage into the substance of the muscle appeared to have taken place at one area.

In the liver the separation of the lobules from one another showed so plainly that it recalled the appearance of the liver of the pig. This must have been due to the presence of almost structureless fibrous tissue or exudative matter between the lobules. In many places the trabeculæ could be seen, but the secreting cells had disappeared, as though by some cause the cells had been removed or destroyed, leaving the supporting framework *in situ*. In spots the tissue was broken down, looking as though the area would have been a minute abscess if life had continued longer.

The spleen was generally of a yellowish color when thin sections were examined, and the tissue did not stain well with carmine. The most marked feature was that instead of being composed of the usual small lymphoid cells, a large proportion was made up of cells of from three to five times the diameter of an ordinary lymph-cell. These in many instances were multinucleated and resembled more closely the large exudative cells so common in the lungs in inflammatory conditions than anything else.

The kidney-tissue was disorganized, as is usual in persons dying of acute diseases in which the blood is broken down, the cells being swollen and granular and often loosened from their positions. A striking feature of the picture presented was that the Malpighian tufts were nearly bare, having shed much of their epithelium.

The ileum showed the ordinary conditions of infiltration and ulceration of Peyer's glands. There was thickening, and some of the follicles had been shed, while others were in process of shedding. The thickened portion of the lymphoid tissue was, as in the spleen, largely composed of multinucleated cells several times larger than ordinary lymph-cells.

The mesenteric gland that was examined was more than an inch in its longest diameter. The cavities which were mentioned as visible to the naked eye had no specially-organized walls, there being at the periphery merely an area of active red-staining cells which shaded off into the rest of the tissue. At one area was a spot the cells of which had stained intensely red, gradually shading off to the color of the surrounding tissue; this must have been an early stage of the same condition which at a later period produced the cavities. These, it would seem, could be described only as abscesses. The condition of the cells composing the gland was parallel with that of those of the spleen and of the cells in the lymphoid portion of the ileum. Instead of being the ordinary small lymphoid cells, a great proportion of them were large multinucleated cells like those that were so abundant in the spleen.

The spinal cord presented appearances of which it is not easy to give an adequate description. That it was not healthy seems to be beyond doubt, and yet none of the changes were very gross. The postero-median (Goll's) columns in the cervical portion were in worse condition than any other portion of the tissue examined. With the naked eye it could be seen in the sections that this portion of the cord had been stained a deeper red than the most of the tissue, and in it the nerve-fibres were not sharply outlined. The general impression was that there was too much neuroglia, which stained unduly red and seemed disposed to encroach upon the axis-cylinders. It appeared also as though the number of nuclei in the supporting tissue was increased. These appearances, of too much neuroglia, of being unusually red, and of the nerve-fibres not being as sharp in outline as natural, were present everywhere to a greater or less degree, but nowhere else to the same extent as in Goll's columns in the cervical portion. The central canal in the lumbar portion of the cord was quite widely open and the cells looked as though they had undergone proliferation. Sections were prepared from the cervical, dorsal, and lumbar regions, and were stained both with carmine and carminate of sodium, according to the method of Schultze.

This case exemplifies how extensive and grave may be the lesions in what was clinically an ordinary case of typhoid fever, in which all the usual symptoms were present except the rash. It would have been very easy for me in making the post-mortem examination to have stopped and rested satisfied after discovering the ulcerations in the ileum with enlargement of the mesenteric glands, and the usual so-called congestion of the lungs. This error I have often committed, and have thereby, I doubt not, overlooked again and again lesions as important as those of which I have given an account.

For my own part, I cannot see that we have more reason to consider typhoid fever a disease of the intestines because there seems to be invariably present a lesion of the ileum than we have to describe scarlet fever as a skin disease because one of its invariable manifestations is an eruption of the skin. Both are general diseases, and are more properly to be considered in the present state of our understanding of such things, as due to derangement of function. Amongst my records I have the notes of two cases of undoubted typhoid fever : in both of them post-mortem examinations were made, and there was found no enlargement of the mesenteric glands, it being recorded that the largest gland was not more than a quarter of an inch in diameter.

My case as described directs attention to a number of lesions that I think are both common (if not invariably present) and very important in the disease. It would have been improper for me to come before you to relate an account of one case alone and then generalize therefrom if I had made no further investigations, and it is to be understood, therefore, that any deductions I may make are the result of study in a number of cases, though in no other one was the study so extensive as in the one detailed at length.

Disease, or at least disorder, of the lungs is known to be a common accompaniment of typhoid fever, but I do not think it is ordinarily, if ever, given the prominence that belongs to it. Murchison says that he noted bronchitis in twenty-one out of one hundred cases, and that it may be one of the earliest phenomena of the disease. He says further that in a large proportion of the cases which terminate fatally within the first fourteen days death is due to bronchitis and hypostatic engorgement of the lungs. More commonly both these conditions supervene in the fourth week, and then they may lead

to a fatal result. Of pneumonia, he says that he noted it in thirty out of one hundred cases.

In cases in which I have made microscopical study of the condition of the lungs—and this was typically represented in the case I have narrated in full—the appearances could hardly be classified as those either of pneumonia or bronchitis, as those terms are commonly accepted. The appearances were rather those of hæmorrhage, for as has been already stated, the air-vesicles, bronchi, and bloodvessels were filled with red corpuscles and leucocytes. In some of my specimens I have found air-vesicles filled with blood alternating with others containing fibrinous exudative material, and again catarrhal exudate cells. Commingled with these appearances were found those of inflammation of the lung-tissue—round-cell infiltration—and there were also bronchi which were much inflamed. The impression left upon the mind by all this, however, was that an early lesion was the escape of blood from the vessels. The fact that organization and the formation of blood-vessels had taken place in the clots within the very bloodvessels themselves is exceedingly interesting.

The soft heart of typhoid fever, originally described by Stokes,[1] is recognized by everyone as an almost essential feature of the disease, though its precise pathology is even yet not as thoroughly worked out as is desirable. The changes are most accurately and graphically described by Stokes, and so far as gross appearances are concerned, nothing has ever been added to our comprehension of the condition. Of course, so long ago no knowledge of the pathological histology was possible, for microscopical work was as yet of the crudest description. Stokes described what he saw as follows : " The heart is little, if at all, altered in volume. It is generally of a livid hue, but this it may have in common with other internal organs, as is often seen in fever. It feels extremely soft, especially in its left portion, and the left ventricle frequently pits on pressure. Nothing remarkable is to be found as to the pericardium or endocardium, and the valves are unaffected. The principal change is found in the muscular structure, which is often infiltrated with an adhesive, as it were, gummy secretion. The left ventricle exhibits a singular appearance, for the traces of the muscular fibres are lost, and the external layer to the depth of an eighth of an inch, converted into a homogeneous structure, in which no fibre can be found. The color of this altered portion is generally dark, and it resembles the cortical structure of the kidney. In some cases this change occurs in patches varying in depth, and from a quarter to three-quarters of an inch in breadth."

This description leaves nothing to be desired so far as the macroscopical appearances are concerned. The histological changes as I have seen them are disorganization of the muscle-fibres, which are either granular in structure and contain much brown pigment, or are homogeneous ; great increase of the intermuscular nuclei, and sometimes hæmorrhage into the tissue. These

---

[1] It must be remembered that at the time Stokes made his observations the distinction between typhus and typhoid fevers was not yet made. This is evident from what he says in discussing the lesions in his book upon Diseases of the Heart and Aorta : " As to the intestines, we sometimes found ulcerations of the ileum, while in other cases no such lesion existed."

changes vary to almost any extent in different cases, healthy tissue alternating through the organ with diseased areas. The alterations of structure are probably not inherently irreparable, nature being capable under favorable circumstances of replacing the diseased by sound tissue. The result, therefore, the life or death of the patient, must depend, so far as the heart is concerned, upon the extent and situation of the change, complete recovery taking place in cases in which the disease has not progressed too far. The great increase of nuclei in the intermuscular tissue is a strange phenomenon, and in the present state of knowledge, somewhat inexplicable. It must be due to cell-multiplication either in the connective tissue or of the vascular tissue, the capillaries of the heart being always very rich in nuclei. Hæmorrhage into the tissue of the heart must have a most disastrous effect upon its functional activity.

The condition of the liver in some of the cases that I have seen was peculiar. The lobules were much more distinctly outlined than in the healthy state, and some evidences of degeneration and inflammatory action were present. In the *Transactions of the Pathological Society of London*, 1889, there is an article by H. Handford on "Hepatitis in Enteric Fever," in which he says: "But the most characteristic change, though so far as I have observed, not quite a constant one, is the presence of small rounded areas that stain imperfectly, that are infiltrated more or less thickly with leucocytes, and that are surrounded by a dense ring of cellular infiltration. . . . In other similar patches, which I take to be in a more advanced stage, the liver cells cannot be distinguished at all. . . . In yet a third variety there exist simply rounded aggregations of leucocytes, the smaller patches hardly distinguishable from commencing miliary tubercles, and the larger ones from the early stages of miliary abscesses." Accompanying the paper is a plate graphically representing the appearances, and both it and the description as quoted tally closely with what I myself have observed.

The spleen, everyone knows, is almost always enlarged in typhoid fever. The only thing that has struck me as at all peculiar in making microscopical examinations of that organ in typhoid fever is the appearance of the cells which I have mentioned in the description of a case, very large multinucleated cells constituting a large part of the organ. Cells of like appearance, as has already been mentioned, are very abundant in the mesenteric glands and in the glandular tissues of the ileum.

The kidney does not seem to take on any special characteristics, presenting merely the appearances commonly termed cloudy swelling, and in the few cases in which I have made examinations, the capillary loops of the glomeruli being to a considerable extent bared of epithelium.

The cavities, seemingly abscesses, in the mesenteric glands show how great was the destruction in these tissues.

Microscopical study of the condition of the spinal cord in typhoid fever does not seem heretofore to have been pursued to a great extent. Of late years, too, improvements in microscopical technique render possible a much more accurate and satisfactory examination of delicate tissues like the cord than was previously possible. That there was considerable disorganization of the

tissue in the case described is beyond doubt, and it presented itself in its highest degree in the posteromedian columns in the cervical portion of the cord.

It is interesting to contemplate and to reflect upon one phenomenon presented in the disease, namely, the tendency of the blood to escape from the vessels in so many parts of the body. Hæmorrhage into a tissue, though not necessarily destructive, is always to a greater or less degree injurious, and in typhoid fever it is common from the nose and from the ulcers in the intestines, into the lungs, and sometimes into the substance of the heart. The condition, too, of the spleen and mesenterle glands would seem to present something analogous to hæmorrhage, for they are much enlarged and engorged with blood, but the nature of lymph-gland tissue is such that with present methods of microscopical examination it is not possible to be absolutely certain whether there is any escape of blood from the vessels or whether it is still retained within their walls. The abundant presence of red blood-corpuscles in such tissues is of course perfectly patent to anyone who has ever examined them with the microscope.

The amount of red blood-corpuscles that commonly lie in the pulmonary alveoli after death from typhoid fever, and the way that they alternate with areas presenting the appearances of pneumonic inflammation and exudation, how the hæmorrhage occurred and what changes it may undergo, have seemed to me questions of the greatest interest. This question of hæmorrhage into the lung in typhoid fever, if not actually new, is, I think, capable of being presented in a somewhat new aspect. Every clinician knows how common a symptom in typhoid fever bloody expectoration is. The importance of the condition of the lungs and the frequency with which they are involved is the turning-point upon which will rest the question of death or recovery—a matter which can hardly be given too great prominence. It is from the consideration of these turning-points in acute diseases I think that most can be done for the science of therapeutics.

The common practice in typhoid fever is to direct our therapeutic measures toward what is called the antiseptic method, toward the old expectant plan, or almost alone toward feeding, and again another physician will place his chief reliance upon the supporting effect of stimulants. This may be well enough in most cases, but I am quite convinced that, often, careful observation of the lungs and watchfulness to foresee the advent of more serious lung involvement, and well-directed efforts made to bring about a cure through therapeutic measures applied to the lungs, will conduce very greatly toward reducing the mortality record from the disease. By constantly keeping in mind the fact that the lung condition is of the greatest importance, and by wisely changing our course of management and medication when we see that these organs are about to become involved, or that their condition is likely to become worse, even to the extent of neglecting or setting aside all other treatment and directing our attention to the lungs alone, cases may be saved which would otherwise be lost. This, at least, is my impression, after a good deal of experience with the disease.

My object to-night has been not to make a pretence that I had a finished treatise upon the morbid anatomy of typhoid fever to lay before you, but rather to call your attenion to such points of interest as, in my experience in the therapeutic management and pathological study of the disease, have come directly to my knowledge. For the disease is one which is so common that all physicians, whether they practise medicine or study pathology alone, are constantly called upon to deal with and to consider in its various aspects.

For my own part, I look upon it as a general condition, to be classed rather with diseases like smallpox or scarlet fever, which seem from their earliest stages to take hold of a large part of the system, though they have an invariable local manifestation, than with pneumonia, which begins locally in the lungs, and then by secondary involvement may invade other parts of the system to almost any extent. I am entirely unable, however the poison may have originally found entrance to the system, to see the reason for considering it to be truly a disease of the intestines. In many cases that I have attended there have never been, from beginning to end, any abdominal symptoms, no diarrhœa, no abdominal pain, no gurgling, no tympany—I have notes of cases in which, even from the beginning of the attack to the end in death, there was no loss of appetite. On the other hand, we all have frequently seen cases in which life was threatened or death occurred as a consequence of involvement of some other part of the system—the abdominal symptoms being, if not absent, at least so latent as to allow us to be quite sure that the threatened danger did not come from that quarter.

To show that I am not alone in such views as I have enunciated I will quote from an essay which seems to me a most admirable and suggestive one. In the Lumleian Lectures on Enteric Fever, by John Harley (*Lancet*, April 13, 1889), after discussing various *pros* and *cons* concerning the etiology of the disease, Harley makes the following statement: "From the foregoing considerations, I think it unreasonable to assent to the germ-theory of disease, and I can only regard it as another of the many instances in medicine and out of it where cause and effect have not been discriminated. Setting aside, therefore, this theory, I shall endeavor to prove that the disease under consideration is merely the effect of derangement of function." There is much more that is of interest in the essay, especially that it becomes evident as he unfolds his views that he tends to believe that typhoid fever may arise *de novo*. The germ-theory is of course the outcome and ultimate conclusion of the belief that the disease is local in the intestine.

There is another matter which I think is seldom given due weight in determining our prognosis in typhoid fever—the degree of our bodily perfection at the time we are attacked by any acute disease must largely influence our chances of recovery, and the degree to which our bodies are imperfect must render us more liable to disease. Does it not often happen that those who die of acute diseases had already in them some imperfection which took away the power to resist the depressing action of the acute process? Each attack from which we suffer and during which inflammatory processes take hold of any part of our tissues must leave us with a permanent mark—an imperfection—of greater or less degree. This thought is a very suggestive one and one which might perhaps be pursued with advantage to much greater length. In all cases of typhoid fever, therefore, we should, when dealing with them from the clinical standpoint, carefully try to ascertain if there was any preëxisting bodily imperfection which would make the prognosis more serious, and at our post-mortem examinations should seek equally carefully for the presence of lesions which were already present in the body before the attack came on.

Finally, let me recapitulate some of the points that it has been my desire to dwell upon and to elucidate.

1. The disease is in my estimation a general one, involving a large part of the system, and in no way a local disease of the intestine. This belief is supported by the many and extensive organic lesions found in the body after death ; and thus it would seem likely that Harley is right in his statement that the disease is due in the first place to derangements of function, and in rejecting the germ-theory of its origin.

2. The frequency of hæmorrhages in various parts of the body and their importance, I have dwelt upon and I wish to repeat my belief that hæmorrhage into the substance of the lung is most commom. This latter, if not a new observation, is a fact certainly not commonly known.

3. The observation that the spleen, mesenteric glands, and lymphoid tissue of the ileum are made up to a great extent of large multinucleated cells instead of the ordinary small lymphoid elements is a curious and interesting one and requires further study ; such study may possibly lead in the future to something which may have practical value.

4. Careful microscopical study of the condition of the spinal cord in the disease is much to be desired.

5. The attempt is made to show the need of a careful consideration of the previous condition of bodily perfection of persons attacked by the disease as having an important bearing upon prognosis.

6. We should be influenced in our treatment of typhoid fever to a great degree by the manner in which it takes violent hold of this or that portion of the organism. Our therapeutic efforts will be much more likely to be crowned with success by a careful consideration of this matter.

In conclusion, I repeat that my wish has been to make my essay suggestive rather than final, to point to threads which if followed to their endings may lead to an advancement of our knowledge of the pathological anatomy of typhoid fever, for such an advance will surely lead us in the future to a better treatment, if not to that which would be best of all, the prevention of the disease.

ORIGINAL ARTICLES.

THE TREATMENT OF ORGANIC STRICTURE OF THE MALE URETHRA.[1]

By SEATON NORMAN, M.D.,
OF EVANSVILLE, INDIANA,
LATE ASSISTANT SURGEON U. S. MARINE-HOSPITAL SERVICE.

I HAVE endeavored in this paper to portray the subject of the treatment of stricture in a light

[1] Read before the Mississippi Valley Medical Association, October 10, 1890.

interesting to the general practitioner as well as to the specialist in genito-urinary diseases. I have not treated my theme as exhaustively as I should have done had I prepared the article for an association of genito-urinary surgeons, and I have contented myself with the discussion of the most recent and most approved methods of treatment in organic stricture of the male urethra.

Dilatation, interrupted or gradual.—In view of the elastic and distensible character of the urethra, it has been the time-honored custom to begin the treatment of stricture by the passage of suitable instruments. The urethra is injected with carbolized olive oil, and the largest bougie that can be passed through the meatus is slowly and gently guided as far as the neck of the bladder. If the meatus is not sufficiently large to admit an instrument corresponding to the normal calibre of the urethra, a preliminary meatotomy immediately suggests itself. This process of dilatation is repeated daily, or every second or third day, as the indications demand, until the canal resumes its normal dimensions, or the more urgent symptoms of contraction disappear. It is unnecessary to state that when the stricture or strictures are located in the penile urethra only, the curved sound is not the proper instrument to employ. Either the ordinary straight steel sound or Weisse's *bougie à boule* will produce the necessary dilatation in this portion of the canal, and the introduction of an instrument into the bladder is not only in most instances unnecessary but absolutely injurious.

In the practice of urethral surgery the operator cannot be too strongly impressed with the fact of the exquisite tenderness and sensitiveness of the urethra, and the slightest amount of force in the introduction of an instrument should be regarded as a relic of barbaric surgery. When commencing the treatment by gradual dilatation, in sensitive patients, I always produce local anæsthesia by injecting from twenty to thirty minims of a four-per-cent. solution of hydrochlorate of cocaine. In the case of a stricture admitting a medium-sized sound, instead of injecting the carbolized oil it will be only necessary to lubricate the instrument, but in all instances in which we are dealing with a narrow or tortuous contraction, the passage of the sound will be greatly facilitated by the preliminary injection of oil.

Another point, which I think is not always fully appreciated, is, that we should never attempt to pass an instrument which will over-distend the stricture. I have seen the urethra rendered extremely sensitive and the process of dilatation delayed, sometimes for several days, by neglecting this simple precaution. As Brodie says, "The temper of the urethra varies as much as the temper of the mind," and the ulti-

mate success of any method of dilatation must largely depend upon a thorough appreciation of this fact.

Instead of the steel sound it is the custom of Reginald Harrison, one of the best writers on the surgical diseases of the genito-urinary organs, to employ the flexible *bougie à boule*, and in inexperienced hands I think that this is the best instrument, inasmuch as with it there is little danger of injuring the urethra, and scarcely the possibility of producing a false passage. The cases of stricture amenable to this method of gradual or interrupted dilatation are those of recent date, those in which the urethra will tolerate the occasional instrumental interference, and those in which the patency of the canal remains intact after the employment of suitable dilators.

Continuous dilatation.—Continuous dilatation deserves but a passing comment. Since the introduction of Bank's whalebone filiform bougies the necessity for continuous dilatation has become more and more infrequent. By using successive sizes of this valuable instrument the narrowest stricture can at one *séance* be so thoroughly dilated as to admit a small-sized bougie, or the ordinary urethrotome. Of course, tight and narrow strictures, through which it is impossible to pass even a filiform bougie, will occasionally be encountered, but these instances must be exceedingly rare. Surely no genito-urinary specialist can afford to exclude from his armamentarium instruments so important and useful as Bank's filiform bougies, as they will render him good service in every case of annoying and troublesome stricture.

Internal urethrotomy.—Since the fear of rigors and urine fever has almost entirely vanished from the mind of the genito-urinary surgeon the internal section of the constricting tissues has deservedly become the most popular operative procedure for the relief and cure of organic stricture. The antiseptic precautions, and the subsequent attention to urethral asepsis, first practised, I believe, by Reginald Harrison, have rendered internal urethrotomy one of the safest of operations. In no case in which the specific directions of Mr. Harrison were strictly adhered to have I noted a single chill, and the fever, when any occurred, was only such as might supervene upon the performance of any minor surgical operation. It has been experimentally demonstrated by Bouchard, and practically proven by Harrison, that the cause of urine fever is the absorption of the toxic elements of the urine by the freshly-made incision. If, then, by any means, we can succeed in maintaining the wound aseptic, the patient will suffer from neither rigors nor fever; the cut surface will heal with a cicatrix that is less contractile than the previous cicatrix, and the probabilities of permanent recovery will be greatly increased.

In discussing what I deem the most important and almost universally applicable operation for the radical cure of stricture, I will be pardoned for entering into the special details of the operation. The urethrotome that I now employ is Wyeth's modification of Otis's instrument, the only advantage of the Wyeth instrument being the cog-wheel attachment, which permits the incision to be made with greater accuracy. Dr. Gerster has recently brought before the profession a urethrotome for which he claims superiority because of the facility with which it can be separated into its component parts, and thus kept perfectly aseptic, but the Otis urethrotome can, I think, be rendered just as aseptic by boiling.

The urine in every case of stricture should be critically examined, and if the patient be suffering from suppurative disease of the kidney no operation should be advised.

As a rule, it is best to administer a general anæsthetic, unless it is against the especial request of the patient. It is a common custom with some surgeons to cocainize the part, and then to operate ; but one cannot have the same freedom of manipulation, and the patient's struggles will often interfere with the thorough application of the method.

For irrigating the urethra previous to the operation I use warm Thiersch's solution. Having injected a small syringeful of four-per-cent. carbolized olive ‚oil, I introduce the closed urethrotome beyond the deepest stricture. The instrument is then expanded until the resistance to the rotation of the screw is perceptible, and the knife is made to traverse the stricture from behind forward, and is slowly returned to its original position. The instrument is now still further expanded, and if any resistance still persists the cutting is repeated. I continue the dilatation to a calibre of 40, French scale, but rarely protrude the knife beyond the register of 30 or 32. A curved steel sound is then passed through the incision, the size of the sound corresponding to the normal calibre of the urethra operated upon. The sound usually employed for this purpose varies between 30 and 36 of the French scale.

After satisfying myself that all constricting bands have been divided, I introduce into the bladder a silk catheter or Tiemann's velvet-eyed soft-rubber catheter, draw off all the urine, and irrigate the bladder with warm Thiersch's solution. I then slowly withdraw the catheter until the solution escapes by its side from the meatus, so that the recent incision shall be rendered completely aseptic. The catheter is finally reintroduced just within the neck of the bladder, and secured in this position. The

urine is thus gradually drained from the bladder, and is received into a covered receptacle in the bed, or conducted by a rubber tube to a vessel beneath. The catheter is usually permitted to remain in place for forty-eight hours, the bladder and wound being irrigated twice daily. After the catheter is removed the patient is directed to inject one or two syringefuls of Thiersch's solution after each micturition.

When these precautions and directions were strictly adhered to I have never known a rigor or an elevation of temperature to ensue. I have observed a rise of a degree or a degree and a half above the normal temperature during the first twelve hours after the operation, but this I consider has no relation to urine fever.

If, as is claimed by Dreyfous, Sahli, and others, the urine can be rendered aseptic by the internal exhibition of salol—the salicylate of phenol—there will be no necessity for the retention of the catheter. But in all cases in which the stricture is complicated by cystitis it is well to have the catheter retained, so that the bladder may be kept entirely free from urine. In three cases in which I operated in this manner I can record most satisfactory results. Salol, I think, is worthy of a trial.

Internal urethrotomy performed in this manner is, I believe, a perfectly safe operation. As a routine practice I give immediately after the operation five or ten grains of the sulphate of quinine, and a hypodermic injection of a fourth or a third of a grain of sulphate of morphine. The opiate allays the pain and nervous irritability, but it is a question whether the quinine is really of benefit, unless, perhaps, the patient has recently suffered from malaria.

In most cases, in the evening of the third or fourth day, the patient should be directed to micturate, after which a medium-sized sound is passed through the incision, and followed by an instrument large enough to distend the urethra gently. The patient should retain his urine as long as possible, and should be instructed to inject one or two syringefuls of an antiseptic solution immediately after micturition. When the incision is thus kept aseptic and clean the wound heals kindly, and there is much less danger of subsequent contraction.

When there is more than one stricture, as is usually the case, the deepest is divided first and the others in succession from behind forward.

In regard to the location of the incision, whether upon the floor or the roof of the urethra, I am in the habit of cutting, when necessary, in both positions. In strictures of long standing, and in those in which the constricting band can be distinctly felt, I think it best to make the division first on the roof, and then, reversing the urethrotome, repeat the procedure on the floor of the urethra. The absorption and final disappearance of the organized tissues of the stricture are thus more likely to occur than when only the incision on the roof is employed.

The subsequent passage of sounds through the divided stricture is essential to the success of internal urethrotomy. As a rule, the sound should be passed every third day for a period of two or three weeks, and afterward once a week for two or three months. To obviate still further the probability of a recurrence of the contraction, it is best to pass the sound once every three months for one year.

I believe that if internal urethrotomy is properly and thoroughly executed, and if special care is exercised to maintain the patency of the canal until the wound is entirely healed, recontraction is of rare occurrence.

Authorities are divided in regard to performing internal urethrotomy in. the bulbous or in the membranous urethra. Judging from the results obtained by Harrison, the combination of external and internal urethrotomy offers encouragement for the permanent cure of stricture. I have had only three opportunities to perform external urethrotomy without a guide, but the results as regards the non-recurrence of contraction were entirely satisfactory.

External urethrotomy with a guide is a simple operation, can be performed with facility and rapidity, and promises more satisfactory ultimate results than internal urethrotomy performed in the deep urethra.

To enter into the details of the combined operations, as wall as to discuss the various operations for the so-called impermeable strictures, would increase the size of my paper far beyond its proper limits.

In conclusion, I wish to say that of the various scales that have been proposed for urethral instruments, only the French system is worthy of consideration. To have a urethrotome graduated in millimetres—and all of them with which I am acquainted are so graduated—and sounds corresponding to the English scale, is a manifest absurdity.

ACUTE DYSENTERY AND THE AMŒBA COLI.[1]

By ALFRED STENGEL, M.D.,
RESIDENT PHYSICIAN TO THE PHILADELPHIA HOSPITAL.

THE following cases of acute dysentery illustrate some points in the symtomatology and treatment of this disease, and furnished the material for some investigations into its etiology:

CASE I.—Mary D., seventy-three years old, has been an inmate of the hospital for many years, during which she has had various illnesses. She is known to have had albuminuria, with granular casts. On September 19, 1890, patient was seized with

[1] The cases reported in this paper occurred in the service of Dr. F. P. Henry at the Philadelphia Hospital.

dysenteric diarrhœa, severe and typical from the first. The stools were rather large and very frequent, and contained mucus and blood, but were unaccompanied by severe distress. There was fever, with great depression. The patient was given arsenite of copper, at the outset in doses of $\frac{1}{100}$ of a grain three times during the night, and in smaller doses every twenty minutes during the day. Ice suppositories, about the size of the thumb, were also used every three hours, but no relief was obtained. The stools became larger and more hæmorrhagic, the general depression increased, and the condition seemed more and more that of uræmia. Later, bismuth and astringents were tried, but without avail, and the patient died on September 22d, three days after the onset of the disease.

Autopsy showed a distinct ulcerative colitis and proctitis. No membrane was present, but small ulcers and much extravasated blood were found in the mucous membrane.

CASE II.—Patrick T., aged forty years, a laborer, admitted August 25, 1890. Patient was stout and healthy in appearance, but has used alcohol to excess, and has lived a life of hardship. He said that he had had diarrhœa for several weeks, and that he had been drinking heavily at the same time. When admitted he complained of great pain in the lower part of the abdomen, some pain in the legs and arms, great thirst and gastric irritability. The stools were very frequent, attended with much tenesmus, and consisted of stringy mucus, streaked with blood. The temperature was slightly elevated ; the pulse was rapid and weak. He was given bismuth subnitrate with paregoric and syrup of ipecacuanha every two hours. No relief was obtained from this treatment, which was continued two days. Later, acetate of lead and opium were given, with an occasional opium suppository. The latter proving irritating, and being discharged immediately after insertion, suppositories of ice were used instead, with great relief.

Under this treatment the tenesmus entirely disappeared, the stools became larger and free from blood and mucus, and the man's general condition improved. The temperature, however, made long daily excursions, reaching 102° or at night higher, and falling below the normal in the morning. As the diarrhœa still continued to be excessive and accompanied by considerable abdominal pain and tenderness, an astringent diarrhœa mixture was given, with no better result. The pains or cramps were sometimes unusually severe ; at such times the pulse became extremely rapid and small, the features pinched and blue, and the extremities first cold, then bathed in a profuse perspiration. Salicylate of bismuth in doses of 10 grains every two hours was next used, and under this treatment the patient slightly improved. There still remained excessive diarrhœa, with great weakness, and occasional pains which were sometimes severe, more often slight, and in spite of salicylate of bismuth, and, later, thymol, the case still remains in about the same condition. The temperature has made longer excursions, falling lower and rising higher than at first. The tongue is dry and coated, the pulse is weak and rapid, and the man is very weak, though not markedly emaciated.

CASE III.—Joseph Q., aged thirty years, a cigar-maker, was admitted to the wards on September 30, 1890, while intoxicated. Patient is an alcoholic, and has had malarial fever several times. He gave a history of having had diarrhœa for four or five days. The stools were very frequent, and accompanied by much tenesmus, soon becoming small. They contained mucus and blood, and were discharged involuntarily. On admission his temperature was 101⅖°, pulse 110, and respirations 18. The face was flushed, and there was considerable pain in all parts of the body. No disease of the lungs. The heart was acting very rapidly, and with a distinct galloping rhythm, especially marked at the apex. The urine was high-colored, and contained a trace of albumin, but no casts. The evacuations were very frequent and painful, and, as stated above, typically dysenteric.

Treatment with ipecacuanha and morphine was first adopted. Of the former, an initial dose of 30 grains, followed by 10 grains every two hours ; of the latter, small doses preceding the ipecacuanha were given. This treatment was continued for one day without inducing vomiting, excepting after the first dose, but without influencing the course of the disease. Ice suppositories were employed at the same time, but no good effects were derived from them. At the end of the day, treatment was changed to magnesium sulphate 40 grains, deodorized tincture of opium 5 minims, with syrup of lemon and water, every hour until four doses had been given, when the stools became large, dark, and free from mucus and blood. The mixture was then given every two hours during one day, when the changed character of the stool was fully established, and the pains were entirely relieved. Bismuth subnitrate and powdered opium were then used. A slight reappearance of the mucus required a temporary return to the magnesium sulphate mixture, but convalescence was fully established on the fifth day.

The fever in this case was moderate, but continuous, and the general condition was not much impaired, although there was some abdominal tenderness, especially on the left side.

CASE IV.—Emily F., aged seventy-two years, has been in the hospital for several months, suffering from chronic nodular rheumatism. She slept in a bed near that of Case I , and after the death of the latter her bed occupied the place made vacant. On September 28th, the patient began to suffer with diarrhœa, which soon became dysenteric. The stools were frequent, small, mucous, and bloody. There were much straining, abdominal pain, general depression, loss of appetite, and excessive thirst, but no elevation of temperature.

Salol in doses of 10 grains, combined with opium and ipecacuanha, was first tried, but gave no relief. Then the magnesium sulphate mixture was used, and after three or four doses the stools became large, brown, and painless, then less liquid, and less frequent, when bismuth and opium were substituted for the magnesium sulphate. For the great tenesmus which was a prominent feature in this case, ice suppositories were used with surprisingly good result. A temporary return of mucus in the stools required a return to the magnesium sulphate, but permanent relief was soon obtained, and the case convalesced. There was some abdominal tenderness in the left iliac region during the progress of the case.

CASE V.—Robert D., aged forty-eight years, is a stretcher-carrier in the receiving ward of the hospital, and is frequently called up at night. On the night of September 30, 1890, he was up several times, and became overheated. He had several loose, semi-liquid stools before morning, and on the next day began to have very frequent discharges, all of which were mucous and bloody, and were attended with much straining, and general as well as abdominal pain. There were slight fever, excessive sweating, loss of appetite, and great thirst.

On the morning of October 2d, the patient began to take arsenite of copper in doses of $\frac{1}{100}$ of a grain every two hours, but did not improve. Then the magnesium sulphate was used, and after a few doses the stools became painless and free, the general depression less marked, and mucus and blood disappeared from the discharges. The mixture was continued for a day longer, when bismuth and opium were substituted, and the case progressed favorably. In this case also there was a temporary reappearance of mucus in the stools, and some pain, but a few doses of the magnesium sulphate sufficed to relieve this. There was slight but continuous pain in the abdomen, especially in the left iliac region.

A summary of the important features presented by these cases may not be out of place.

The tendency of dysentery, especially in its less grave varieties, to begin with ordinary diarrhœa, is well illustrated in four of our cases, while the fifth case confirms the old observation that when overwhelmingly severe the disease is likely to be dysenteric from the start.

The character of the pain was similar to that which has often been observed, but the abdominal tenderness so prominent in four of our cases is not referred to in the text-books. This tenderness was slight in three of the cases, and excessive in one, was nearly constant, and was most marked in the left iliac region.

As to the propagation of the disease, it is interesting to note that in one patient in the same ward and adjacent to Case I., and in two other similar instances, mucous and slightly blood-tinged stools were observed (Cases III. and IV.).

Conclusions as to the effect of various plans of treatment can hardly be drawn from so few cases, but the observations may be of value in connection with those of others using similar methods.

In two cases ipecacuanha was employed—small doses in one, large in the other—but no change in the character of the stools or the course of the disease was observed.

Arsenite of copper, lately so much lauded in the

treatment of dysentery and diarrhœa, was used in three of the cases, first in minute then in larger doses, but no good whatever resulted, though at least one of the cases was favorable.

Salol was used in one case in doses of 10 grains, but was without effect. The mixture of magnesium sulphate with deodorized tincture of opium, syrup of lemon, and water, was given in three cases, after other measures had failed, and in each, after a very few doses, the character of the stools changed, the pain lessened, and no doubt the course of the disease was cut short. There was a tendency to relapse in each case, but a few doses of this mixture checked it, and convalescence was otherwise uninterrupted. Whatever the results that have been obtained by other remedies, certain it is that in these cases the magnesium sulphate served to alleviate suffering most promptly, and to check the progress of the disease.

In three of these cases suppositories of ice were used, in one after opium suppositories and enemata had been rejected. In two the results were most gratifying, the pain disappearing almost instantly. In the third, however, no effect was observed. It is difficult to say whether the number of stools was lessened by the ice, but when used at once on the occurrence of pain the interval between the stools seemed to be materially increased.

Renewed attention in this country has been called to the examination of dysenteric stools by a recent paper by Osler,[1] confirming the observations of Losch, Lambl, and Kartulis, who have found the amœba coli in the discharges of cases of ulcerative colitis, chronic diarrhœa, and dysentery, as well as in the abscesses succeeding such cases. Osler reports a case of chronic dysentery with abscess of the liver, in which examination of the stools and pus of the abscess revealed large numbers of the amœbæ. Our investigations have been confined to three cases (Cases III., IV., and V.), and in each the amœba was found in more or less abundance.

Macroscopically, the discharges of Cases III. and IV. were much alike—small, rather stringy, mucous, and blood-tinged. The appearance of the stools of Case V. was slightly different, being more lumpy, containing larger masses of blood, and more suggestive of a diphtheritic condition of the bowel.

Microscopically, there was but little difference. The stools of Case III. were examined on October 1st, the day after the patient's admission to the hospital. Large numbers of red corpuscles and pus corpuscles were found, besides many bacteria of different kinds, micrococci and bacilli, in active motion, predominating. Easily distinguishable from the other elements and very numerous, were the large

amœbaform bodies first described by Losch. They were conspicuous by their size, which ranged from 10 to 30 micromillimetres; by a more brilliant appearance of the protoplasm than was seen in the other bodies, by the constant active amœboid motions; and by the presence within them of both large and small vacuoles, or hyaline bodies. All portions of the mucous stools contained them, but they seemed most numerous in the small blood-stained masses. The protoplasm was granular and distinctly outlined, and contained large numbers of pigment granules in active motion. When at rest the bodies were round or ovoid, but long, finger-like prolongations were frequently extended, and the pigment granules were mainly aggregated at the extremities of these. Some of the amœbæ had distinct nuclei, and a few hyaline bodies or vacuoles.

Figure 1 represents the appearance seen on the first day.

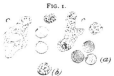

FIG. 1.

a. red corpuscles. b. leucocytes. c. amœba coli.

Subsequent examinations were made daily, or whenever mucus appeared in the discharges, with substantially the same results. On October 2d the number of amœbæ had already decreased, and the movements were much less active. Vacuoles now were more commonly observed, and were sometimes quite large, and a few were partially surrounded by pigment granules, as described by Osler. The number of vacuoles in each amœba varied from one to several. The movement of the protoplasm was slower and less evident, as was also that of the pigment matter.

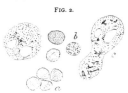

FIG. 2.

Figure 2 represents the appearances seen in the discharges of Case III., on October 3d, two days after the onset of the disease, and confirmed those previously made.

The organisms in Case IV. were smaller, the vacuoles more prominent, and the movement of the

---

[1] Johns Hopkins Hospital Bulletin, May, 1890.

pigment grains less active. The stool was some-what old, and was cold when examined. Subsequent examination showed less, but still quite numerous, amœbæ.

Figure 3 represents the appearances of the stools in Case IV. In this case the first examination, made four or five days after the onset of the disease, showed but few of the organisms, which, however, presented the same picture as those seen in Cases III. and V.

FIG. 3.

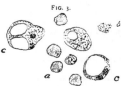

The attempt to stain the amœbæ with methyl-blue and fuchsine failed, but Kartulis says they can be beautifully colored with eosin.

On October 7th mucus taken from one of the large brown stools of Case IV. was injected into the rectum of a guinea-pig, but after eight days no result has been obtained.

AN INQUIRY INTO THE CAUSE OF ALARMING AND FATAL RESULTS FOLLOWING ATTEMPTS AT THE RADICAL CURE OF HYDROCELE.[1]

BY OSCAR H. ALLIS, M.D.,
SURGEON TO THE PRESBYTERIAN HOSPITAL, PHILADELPHIA.

I WISH to state at the outset that this paper is confined to the subject-matter embraced in the title, and that it has nothing to do with the anatomy, etiology, pathology, or diagnosis of hydrocele. Its purpose is to take up the three widely-accepted methods of dealing with hydrocele, viz., treatment by injections, by the seton, and by the open method; to give examples of casualties of a most serious nature that have attended each; and to present the reasons that have suggested themselves to the author for the too frequent occurrence of such accidents.

And first, let me state why I selected the subject. In the spring of 1882 an aged colored man was sent to the Presbyterian Hospital, suffering from retention of urine. His penis was withdrawn into the scrotal tissues, as is not infrequently seen when large hydroceles are present, but not, as sometimes happens, offering an obstacle to catheterization.

I was about to tap and inject the sac when my colleague, Dr. Porter, said to me, "I would be careful what I did to that man, as I lost a similar

[1] Read before the Philadelphia Academy of Surgery, October 2, 1890.

case not long ago." Scarcely realizing his statement, yet in deference to his suggestion, I simply tapped the hydrocele, and waiting for reaccumulation, tapped a second time in a fortnight, and injected alcohol. A few weeks later the patient left the hospital with a scrotal tumor, as we all supposed, undergoing the changes so commonly seen in the course of radical cure. A few weeks later I was sent for to see the man at his home. The scrotal pouch was crepitant, gas was escaping at one or more small openings, the general constitutional symptoms of septicæmia were present, and though I promptly laid open and depleted the tumor at many points, the old man gradually sank and died. Here were two deaths, and as I had been invited to prepare a paper for the Philadelphia Academy of Surgery, by its president, the elder Gross, I selected this subject.

I sent letters to one hundred and fifty physicians requesting them to give me a report of the disasters that had occurred in their practice from the radical treatment of hydrocele. About fifty replied, and from their answers I am enabled to present the following interesting data:

ABSCESSES—*from the employment of the seton.*

Dr. H. M. "I have had abscesses follow the use of the seton."

Dr. L. I. "In my practice two out of three had abscesses when I used the seton."

Dr. A. N. "With the seton only two abscesses occurred in twenty-eight cases. Of these one was in the scrotal tissues, the other occurred in the pelvis and broke into the bladder; ultimate recovery."

Dr. T. I. "I usually employ a drainage-tube. In one case it was withdrawn by the patient. I restored it and an abscess followed."

Dr. M. A. "I have had abscesses follow the use of the seton."

Dr. C. O. "In a double hydrocele, after failure with tincture of iodine, I employed the seton. Cure on one side with abscess, on the other without. In a case in which tincture of iodine had failed a cure was effected with the seton—and abscess."

Dr. M. C. "In three consecutive cases in which I employed silver wire I had abscesses."

ABSCESSES—*from injections of iodine.*

Dr. G. R. "I abandoned the tincture of iodine years ago on account of pain and abscesses."

Dr. B. T. D. "I have had repeated abscesses from the use of tincture of iodine—from one to two drachms."

Dr. W. E. "Twenty-five per cent. of my cases treated with the tincture of iodine have had abscesses."

Dr. D. N. "After injecting the tunica vaginalis testis I purposely scratched the lining of the sac with the canula. In this case a fearful abscess occurred in the scrotal tissues."

Dr. D. R. "I have had suppuration follow the use of tincture of iodine with no remedial effect."

Dr. L. E. "Abscesses and suppuration are no guaranty of a cure. Fifty per cent. of injections with tincture of iodine fail."

Dr. W. P. H. "I injected a healthy adult with tincture of iodine. Intense pain followed, with great local swelling and inflammation. Prompt measures were taken to control the inflammation, but an abscess resulted."

Dr. C. O. L. "I have found injections so unsatisfactory, so likely to give rise to abscess and sloughing, that I never resort to them any more."

SHOCK AND SEVERE PAIN.

Dr. T. L. "Out of ten cases treated with tincture of iodine three injections were immediately followed by excruciating pain ; and of the three, one was cured with abscess, and in two, though the injection produced agonizing pain, the result was a failure."

Dr. O. T. "Shock and extreme pain in the testicle followed an injection of the tincture of iodine. The shock and faintness lasted for more than an hour."

Dr. C. R. "I came near having a death in my office from injecting two drachms of deliquesced carbolic acid. Great shock and pain ; the patient became cyanotic and pulseless, and but for galvanism I think the man would have died. Still the hydrocele was not cured, and I was obliged to resort to the tincture of iodine to effect a cure."

HÆMATOCELE.

Dr. M. E. "I have had a hæmatocele follow the injection of dilute tincture of iodine, one-third strength."

Dr. H. A. "I was called to see a person suffering from a large hæmatocele. He had a few days previously been tapped and injected with tincture of iodine."

Dr. R. E. E. "I have had one hæmatocele follow tapping and injection with iodine."

ORCHITIS.

Dr. T. L. L. "Two cases of violent orchitis followed the injection of tincture of iodine, U. S. P."

Dr. A. S. H. "Orchitis with persistent hypertrophy of the testicle followed the use of the trocar and subsequent injection with tincture of iodine."

Dr. S. B. R. "I think epididymitis is a very frequent result of injections of tincture of iodine into the sac of the tunica vaginalis."

SLOUGHING OF SCROTUM.

Dr. G. A. R. "I have had the entire scrotum slough after injections of the tincture of iodine. In a second case the entire scrotum sloughed, and the sloughing process extended into the inguinal region—from the use of the officinal tincture of iodine. I have also had sloughing at the entrance and exit of a seton."

Dr. M. I. N. "I have had sloughing of the scrotum occur in my efforts to cure hydrocele."

Dr. K. I. N. "In a case of very large hydrocele that extended nearly to the patient's knee, there were sloughing and gangrene as the result of attempt at radical cure."[1]

Dr. W. A. R. "I have known sloughing of the scrotum to follow frequently the introduction of the seton."

Dr. P. I. L. "Gangrene of the scrotum and death occurred in a young child into whose tunica vaginalis I had inserted a single silk thread, and which I withdrew in twenty hours."

Dr. C. O. L. "I have witnessed sloughing of portions of the scrotum from injections."

Dr. M. A. R. "I have often seen sloughing of the scrotum after using the seton."

Dr. M. E. A. "Slight sloughing of the scrotum followed the injection of two ounces of port wine. It was left in the sac about twenty minutes."

Dr. C. R. "I had a case of hydrocele from which I withdrew three pints. Repeated simple tappings three or four times. Then I injected tincture of iodine, U. S. P. Sloughing of scrotum, exposure of both testicles, and narrow escape from death."

Dr. B. G. S. "When I was a medical student I witnessed the sloughing of the entire scrotum and narrow escape from death as the result of injection of tincture of iodine."

Dr. B. T. R. "Sloughing of the scrotum and pyæmia has occurred twice in my practice—once after injecting tincture of iodine, and once after the use of a seton."

Dr. A. L. L. "Sloughing followed the injection of iodine in a case in which a hæmatocele occurred, and to relieve which incision was employed."

Dr. S. T. O. "I have had sloughing follow excision of a portion of the tunica vaginalis testis."

Dr. R. O. S. "After injection with tincture of iodine the scrotum sloughed and the testicle perished. In this case the patient had hurt his scrotum the day before while riding a fractious colt."

Dr. L. E. A. "Sloughing and exposure of the testicle followed the injection of the tincture of iodine, two drachms. In this case the man went on a spree after the injection."

Dr. W. W. W. "My preceptor, a clinical teacher

---

[1] Treatment not given.

and eminent surgeon, came near losing a patient; after introducing a seton violent inflammation and extensive sloughing."

Dr. W. W. W. "My colleague in his practice had the upper part of the scrotum and cord slough away after the injection of a twenty-per-cent. solution of carbolic acid."

ALARMING SYMPTOMS—*developed in the course of treatment, with narrow escape from death.*

Dr. G. A. "I came near losing a case recently in the employment of my favorite method—the seton. The man certainly had a narrow escape from death."

Dr. W. I. R. "In a case under my care in which two flaxen threads were introduced, there were profound constitutional disturbance, high fever, profuse perspiration, and for a time matters looked very gloomy and threatening."

Dr. C. A. R. "In one case, where both testicles were exposed after using a silver-wire seton, the patient pulled through by the skin of his teeth. He had a most serious septic involvement, with numerous abscesses and prolonged tedious recovery."

Dr. B. G. S. "In one case, after injecting tincture of iodine my patient came near perishing, and escaped after sloughing of the scrotum."

Dr. J. W. H. "I saw a child five years old treated with the seton. Violent symptoms. The patient was alarmingly ill for several days. Belly became tympanitic and all the symptoms of localized peritonitis were present. In this case a single silk thread was introduced and permitted to remain twenty-eight hours. The operator was a practical hospital surgeon."

Dr. J. W. H. "I injected a robust fireman with deliquesced carbolic acid. Violent inflammation followed with vomiting, tympanites, high temperature and rigors. An abscess formed, free incisions were made, and the patient slowly recovered."

DEATHS.

Dr. T. I. F. "I have known a death to follow simple aspiration of a hydrocele, *i. e.,* emptying it with an aspirating needle without subsequent injection."

Dr. P. R. C. "Death followed incision of the scrotal pouch to relieve hydrocele, ten days after the operation."

Dr. L. S. P. "A death occurred in my practice in a case in which I employed a single silk thread. The child died from septicæmia and gangrene. The thread was only left in twenty hours."—Reported in the *Annals of Surgery.*

Dr. B. Y. R. "I have known death to follow the use of the exploring needle without injection."

Dr. O. H. A.[1] "Death from septicæmia followed the injection of alcohol."

Dr. W. G. P. "Death followed in about ten days after the injection of tincture of iodine in an old negro under my care."

Dr. A. N. D. "My preceptor lost a case from injecting the tincture of iodine. He was a famous clinical teacher and had had large experience in the treatment of hydrocele."

Dr. B. F. N. "I saw a case in a dissecting-room that I recognized as having been injected a short time before in a college clinic. The scrotum was greatly distended."[2]

Dr. R. O. C. "I have known death to follow ten days after the simple evacuation of a hydrocele with a small trocar."

Dr. S. E. X. "I have never had a death in my own practice from the treatment of hydrocele, but I witnessed one that occurred in the practice of a neighboring physician."

Dr. A. T. L. "When a medical student I witnessed death following the treatment of hydrocele."

Dr. W. R. R. "Two deaths have occurred in my practice from incision for the radical cure of hydrocele with thickened sac. One operation resulted in pyæmia, the other in gangrene of the scrotal tissues."

The following is a condensed tabular report of the cases:

Casualties.	Number of surgeons reporting.	Number of cases operated on.
Death[3]	12	13
Sloughing of scrotum	14	17
Abscesses[4]	14	...
Narrow escape from death	4	4
Pyæmia, with ultimate recovery	5	6
Hæmatocele	4	4

A glance at the list of casualties shows that abscesses are very frequent. Some of my correspondents attribute the occurrence of abscesses to their own carelessness. They think that the canula probably slipped, and that a part of the injection was thrown into the connective tissue of the scrotum. Such a mishap is possible, but not in any degree probable.

When a hydrocele is tapped two conditions should be borne in mind: one, *that the sac is tense and tough*—it is often distended almost to bursting. The second condition is that the trocar so universally

---

[1] Alluded to in the opening of the paper.

[2] This case is of doubtful value. My informant did not examine the scrotal tumor nor make an autopsy.

[3] Deaths: 1. mode of treatment not stated:
    3. from aspiration without injection.
    4, injections with tincture of iodine.
    1. injections with alcohol.
    1. from the use of the seton.
    3. following incision into the sac.

[4] For list of abscesses see body of paper.

used for withdrawing the fluid is a *blunt instrument;* hence, when it is thrust through such a dense, tough, tense membrane a hole is formed which, when the canula is withdrawn, will permit of the passage of fluids either way. This view is sustained by clinical observation. It is an almost universal experience that a puncture of the sac, whether by a surgical needle or by an extremely fine operating or hypodermic needle, will be followed by leakage until the sac is emptied. Some of my contributors have employed no other method than tapping for many years. It is plain, therefore, that the puncture permits fluids to pass *from* the sac. Again, it is clinical experience that hæmatocele may follow the puncture of the sac. In my own opinion, blood in a varying degree *always* pours into the sac after the withdrawal of the canula. If capillary vessels only have been transfixed the hæmorrhage will not be great; but if vessels of considerable size have been cut, a hæmatoma may be formed—as has been reported—the size of a fœtal skull at full term.

It seems, therefore, readily demonstrable that after the use of the trocar fluids may flow from the sac-walls into the sac-cavity, and from the cavity into the connective tissue. Hence, when my correspondents confess that abscesses occur from injecting the cellular tissue, and are due to their own carelessness, I dismiss the confession, since it admits too much and accounts for too little.

The graver conditions, reported by fourteen of my correspondents, of sloughing of the scrotum occurring after injections and the use of the seton, are to be explained by excessive inflammation. The swelling that arises, sometimes the result of recklessness on the part of patients, and sometimes due to the injected fluid or seton, transcends the limit of nutrition. The nutrient supply, never great in the scrotal tissue, is choked, and the tissues starve. The general sloughing is only an exaggeration of the milder and more controllable abscess.

But a class of mishaps of the gravest character remain to be disposed of—those cases in which septicæmia occurs. Every death, I believe, was from this cause, and the question arises, What is the pathology? It has long beeen a clinical observation that old hydroceles with hypertrophied walls do not collapse as do young and recent hydroceles. In all chronic cases the fluid, at first, flows from the canula in a full stream, but stops flowing long before the sac is empty. Now, many clinical teachers claim that the reason the tincture of iodine fails, is that the operator is not careful to empty the sac entirely before injecting it; the operator, therefore, kneads the sac, and in a few moments the fluid begins to flow from the canula in a stream. A repetition of the kneading process brings, after a few minutes, a second flow of fluid, and thus, by a little delay and patience, the operator entirely empties the sac. But alas, the patient must pay dearly for the surgeon's perseverance! The emptying of that thickened sac was possible *on one condition only,* viz., the introduction of an amount of air equivalent to the amount of fluid to be displaced. With an open canula in the hydrocele, just so much fluid escaped as the compression of the atmosphere could force out. The fluid from a tapped hydrocele flows out, not because the tissues of the hydrocele are contractile; the flow is due to atmospheric pressure, and when atmospheric pressure has a hypertrophied sac to deal with, the fluid ceases to run the moment that equilibrium is established. To act further on the walls of the sac and to drive out more fluid are impossible; hence, air enters the canula, and with it the tendency to a vacuum is overcome, and the fluid flows.

The injection is now thrown into a sac emptied, it is true, of hydrocele fluid, but filled *with air.* What follows? The injection lights up inflammation; new products are thrown out; heat, moisture, air, and decomposing blood, in a closed sac, offer a field for germ-proliferation second to none in the domain of surgery; and septicæmia, the result of putrid absorption, occurs.

The interrupted flow of fluid from an old hypertrophied hydrocele may be imitated by a glass bottle, to which an elastic India-rubber bladder is attached, with perforated rubber tube, extending throughout the bladder and to the bottom of the bottle. This apparatus represents a hydrocele upon which the atmosphere can act to a certain degree, but which cannot be wholly compressed. If the bladder and bottle are now filled with water and inverted, the fluid will flow in a stream until the rubber bladder is emptied; but the bottle, which cannot contract, remains full. But in a few moments air will enter the tube and run bubbling through the water in the bottle, when water will again flow through the pendant tube. It will flow for but a moment, since only a little air found its way through the tube, and only a little fluid can escape to equalize it; but, after a few minutes, more air will rush bubbling through the bottle, and be immediately followed by a jet of water from the tube. Thus, little by little, the bottle will be *emptied* of water *and filled with air.*

But, it will be asked, how about the three deaths from excision? Had I never had any experience with the open method I would be at loss to explain them, but experience has taught me that the best principles will miscarry when executed in a faulty manner.

In one of my cases of incision septicæmia developed and bid fair to do serious mischief, but when I extended the incisions to give dependent drainage, improvement promptly resulted.

Few surgeons, I am convinced, do their first open operation perfectly. The opened and emptied sac shrinks somewhat, the length of the incision is shortened, the sac becomes a cup for the retention of secretions, and serious, if not fatal mischief results. No experienced surgeon is satisfied with an opening that will admit " two finger-ends," yet such operations are performed and denominated *incisions*. The open method demands that the whole interior of the sac shall come under scrutiny ; that the excess of tissue in the sac shall be retrenched, unhealthy granulations, laminated fibrin, and all diseased tissue removed ; and that ample dependent and unobstructed drainage is established.

A few practical considerations will conclude this article. Most of the casualties reported occurred at a period when modern surgical views were unknown. Some of the accidents may be traced, no doubt, to want of care in the performance of the operation. The trocar and canula may be said to be unsurgical instruments, because they are uncleanly instruments, and the smaller they are the more unlikely they are to be clean. So, too, with a seton ; none but the modern surgeon would think of using sterilized silk, and there can be no doubt that uncleanly materials have often imparted a disease of greater magnitude than that which they were intended to cure.

If I may be permitted to express a preference for a mode of treatment I shall unqualifiedly endorse the open method. By no other method is anything like a diagnosis arrived at. True, before using the trocar care is taken that it be not thrust into a hernia or a sarcoma, but when the elimination is made and the surgeon is sure that fluid is present, if he be asked the cause of the fluid or the condition of the sac, the testicle, or the epididymis, he can reply with conjectures only.

By the open method the eye is enabled to see and the fingers to feel all parts of the sac, and if the operation is done with surgical skill and surgical completeness there will be no unpleasant sequelæ and no tardy recoveries.

The contributors[1] to this article were either men who had devoted their lives especially to surgery or men of large general surgical experience. Two inferences may be drawn from their contributions, namely :

That either their methods must have been very faulty and their results very unfortunate ; or, that the surgical treatment of this affection in the hands

---

[1] I have purposely withheld the names of my contributors. Some of them generously told me to make any use of their names and correspondence that I desired. But so long as the surgical faculties in our great colleges make no reports of their casualties I will not subject my contributors to the unjust aspersion that their sad results were attributable to lack of skill.

of the profession generally has not been honestly reported.

If it be said that the methods were faulty in preantiseptic days, it must also be confessed that all employed the same methods. If it be said that the operators were unfortunate, I reply that among the most unfortunate are names that add lustre to American surgery.

I shall let the reader form his own conclusions upon the *second* inference. For myself I will simply say that clinical assistants can give a longer list of disasters than clinical professors. I will not say in regard to this operation that surgeons would make a misstatement, but I am convinced that they have wonderfully short memories.

1604 SPRUCE STREET.

DISCUSSION.

In discussing this paper DR. WILLIAM HUNT said that his experience with the treatment of hydrocele has been so favorable that he had no adverse results to report. He recalled an abscess or two in hospital work, especially with the use of the seton, and while there were cases that have not recovered promptly after the use of iodine and carbolic acid, as well as after the open method of treatment, he recalled no untoward results. He asked Dr. Allis whether his record had any reference to the time before the introduction of antiseptic methods. Formerly, in the instrument-rooms of hospitals, there was no instrument so dirty as the trocar, because the essential parts were hidden from view ; and the question arises, How much did that have to do with the accidents noted ?

DR. WILLIAM G. PORTER said that he was much surprised to hear of the great mortality of operations for hydrocele. His own experience has been almost uniformly favorable, although he has had one case in which the injection of iodine was followed by death, in an old man. In that case the patient's age was apparently the only contraindication, and there were no symptoms of septic trouble, death apparently being due to exhaustion seventy-two hours after the operation.

The subject is one in which we are all interested, because all surgeons are constantly called upon to perform the operation. His preference is for iodine, and with the single exception mentioned he has seen no bad results from it, and can recall but one case in which it failed to cure.

Last spring he had an interesting case of hydrocele, in a child less than two years of age. Such cases he has almost always succeeded in curing by the external application of iodine and evaporating lotions, but in this case external applications had no effect. He then tried simple tapping, but this also failed, and after the fluid reaccumulated twice he used the seton, which was followed by cure. On account of the tender age of the patient, he was afraid to inject iodine.

He recently had a rather embarrassing experience, and one which he has not seen described. He was called to operate on an ordinary hydrocele, which he had examined by transmitted light, and which he was satisfied was a true hydrocele. He plunged a trocar into the centre of the sac without difficulty, but on withdrawing the canula, to his great consternation no fluid followed. He knew that the trocar had penetrated the sac, and he moved the instrument in various directions, but could not get a drop of fluid. He then ran a long probe through the canula in all directions, but still failed to get any fluid. He then tried to aspirate fluid by means of a long-nozzled syringe, but without success. Examining the swelling again by transmitted light, it was found perfectly translucent. On moving the trocar again, a drop of mucus-like substance came out and the fluid began to escape. He has not used the open method, as the injection of tincture of iodine has been satisfactory.

Dr. John B. Deaver said that his experience with the tincture of iodine was limited, but that he has operated on a large number of hydroceles by the open method, and has seen bad symptoms follow but once. He opens the tumor from the top of the scrotum to the fundus, and dissects out the parietal layer of the tunica vaginalis. The one unfortunate sequel occurred because he was in a hurry, and was not careful to see that all hæmorrhage was arrested. A hæmatocele followed, which broke down and suppurated. The patient was etherized, the broken-down clot removed, and the parts rendered aseptic and drained. The patient made a good recovery. Success in this operation depends upon perfect cleanliness, complete arrest of hæmorrhage, and draining. He always uses a large rubber drainage-tube.

While recently operating for the radical cure of hernia, he attempted to remove the entire sac, and disturbed the parts so much that in forty-eight hours the man had an acute hydrocele. Ten days later he successfully operated on the hydrocele.

He thought that the results recorded by Dr. Allis could in most cases be attributed to the introduction of germs by dirty instruments. In the use of tincture of iodine, if there is but one sac, the operation should be successful; but if there are two or three sacs not in communication with each other, the operation will fail.

His experience in the treatment of hydrocele in children is not large, but he has succeeded in bringing about a cure by tapping and scarifying the tunica vaginalis with the end of the canula. He has not done the open operation in children, although, should the occasion arise, he would not hesitate to do it. He would first try tapping and scarifying, unless these had previously been done. In cases of recurrent hydrocele he would do the open operation. The pain after the use of tincture of iodine is considerable, and epididymitis, or even peritonitis, might follow, but such results are not to be expected after the open treatment.

Dr. J. Henry C. Simes said that in the treatment of hydrocele his experience has been chiefly with tincture of iodine. During the past two or three years, in order to prevent the very severe pain which so often follows the injection of the iodine, he has injected through the canula two drachms of a five-per-cent. solution of muriate of cocaine, which is allowed to remain in the sac for a few minutes, and then drained off. The iodine is then thrown in, and it is a very exceptional occurrence for the patient to complain of pain. He has occasionally employed the open method, and with success, but the tincture of iodine has given such good results that he does not resort to the open operation until the iodine has failed.

Dr. J. Ewing Mears said that he was somewhat surprised at the results presented by Dr. Allis, and was disposed to think ample reasons were given by those who discussed the paper for the want of success and the results that have been reported. Unclean instruments and the failure to hold the canula properly in place, so that the fluid escapes into the connective tissue, are, without doubt, to blame.

He has practised all the methods of treating hydrocele. Formerly it was the custom to inject iodine and allow it to escape, and often the iodine was diluted. Then, principally under the teachings of Professor Agnew, a certain quantity of iodine was introduced and allowed to remain. He has never had untoward results after either method. In his experience the first has occasionally failed, but the second never. He has excised the sac, which is the accepted treatment in chronic hydrocele in which the tunica vaginalis has undergone changes and is much thickened.

There is no operation which he performs with more care, both in hospital and in private cases, than the injection of iodine in the treatment of hydrocele. He prepares the patient, and invariably keeps him in bed a week after the operation. The custom of some surgeons and physicians to inject a hydrocele sac in their offices and send the patient home is dangerous. His own results he believes have been influenced by the care he has taken. He is careful that the canula is clean, and even before the days of antiseptic methods he used hot water and other cleansing methods. Now he uses antiseptic methods in preparing the instruments before operating.

He would hesitate to accept the results reported by Dr. Allis as the results of properly-conducted methods of treatment.

In closing the discussion, Dr. Allis said that he had brought the subject before the Academy because every one in the medical profession is sometimes called upon to operate for hydrocele. His object was to let those who do not practise surgery know that this is a true surgical operation. Many, who would not dare to perform excision or incision, would tap; but he thinks that free incision is a far simpler operation than tapping, and infinitely safer.

In reference to Dr. Porter's case, in which a seton was used, Dr. Allis said that he had reported four cases in which the seton was used in young children. In one of his own cases a child had convulsions with other general symptoms twenty hours after the operation. It could not be determined whether the hydrocele or the seton caused these symptoms, for the child was in the teething period, and recovered from the operation, but he believed that the irritation of the seton had something to do with the symptoms. Dr. S. W. Gross had a case in which alarming reaction followed the use of a single silk thread. Dr. Pilcher, of Brooklyn, lost a case in which a seton had been used for twenty-four hours.

Dr. Allis said that more cases of abscess and sloughing have occurred from this operation than any of us think. The experiences of our hospitals and college clinics would show that the operation of injection is a serious one if we could learn the results. Even the elder Gross had cases of abscess and sloughing after the operation. One surgeon states that he almost had a death in his office from the injection of carbolic acid. Another states that he has had as much pain from carbolic acid as from iodine. Dr. Packard had said to the speaker: "I wish you would tell us how it is that we have the patient almost dying from the pain, and yet fail to cure the hydrocele." These are matters of common surgical experience.

Dr. Allis accepted all that Dr. Deaver had said. In some of the reported cases the operator states that he made the opening large enough to introduce two or three fingers, but such an incision is entirely too small in a hydrocele the size of a fœtal head. When it collapses it will close such an opening and unless a free incision is made there will be a well of pus to deal with.

In regard to the trocar, he had intended to mention uncleanliness as one cause of the sequelæ. Every one knows that the trocar is *par excellence* an instrument that is difficult to clean. After it is cleaned it should be passed through an alcohol flame, and even then there is reason to distrust it.

It is always a difficult matter to say what the origin of hydrocele is. One writer believes that twenty-five per cent. of the failures are due to disease within the sac, or of the testicle, or epididymitis. If the open method is employed the disease can be seen. No hydrocele should be injected if the fluid drawn off is not of a normal color. If the color is dark or chocolate, some injury has probably occurred, or there is some other disease.

The use of cocaine, original with Dr. Simes. is, doubtless, valuable.

All operations of this character should be done with scrupulous care as to cleanliness.

In conclusion Dr. Allis said that he thought no more important matter could be brought before the medical profession than the treatment of hydrocele.

THE TREATMENT OF TUBERCULOSIS.[1]

By LAWRENCE F. FLICK, M.D.,
OF PHILADELPHIA.

IN considering the treatment of tuberculosis it is necessary to keep constantly in view the anatomical construction and the physiological function of the affected part, and the etiology and pathology of the disease. Looking at the subject from these different standpoints the following principles can be laid down:

First. That whatever extraneous matter gets into the system enters through the medium of the blood, either by the way of the alimentary canal, by the lymphatic system, or by venous or arterial absorption, and that therefore the bacillus tuberculosis must find its way into the system in this way.

Second. That tuberculosis is strictly a local disease, no matter how many organs or parts may be affected, and that whatever the constitutional symptoms, they are always the result either of interference with the physiological action of some important organ or organs of the body, or of the absorption

of some foreign body, the product of tuberculosis, into the system.

Third. That tuberculosis is a specific infectious disease, which can only arise from some other case of tuberculosis, and that when it gets a foothold in any part of the body it can, and probably will, extend to other parts of the body.

Fourth. That tuberculosis has a predilection for those parts or organs of the body in which the circulation is sluggish, as a result either of inactivity of the organ or part, or because of former inflammation.

Fifth. That tuberculosis is always the same disease, whatever part of the body it may affect.

Sixth. That tuberculosis is frequently primarily situated in some unimportant organ of the body, and is overlooked until it affects either the lungs or the brain.

Seventh. That the gravity of the prognosis of tuberculosis is in proportion to the importance of the part of the body affected in carrying on the functions of life.

Eighth. That the improvement and curability of tuberculosis are dependent upon the amount of tubercular deposit, the location, the number of organs or parts implicated, the activity of the parts implicated, and upon the anatomical construction and the anatomical encasement of the organ or part.

Cases of tuberculosis, for the purpose of studying the treatment, can be divided into two classes, namely, those that are accessible to mechanical treatment, such as the use of the knife, caustics, and powerful germicides, and those that are not accessible to such treatment.

The cases of tuberculosis accessible to mechanical treatment are lupus, tuberculosis of the superficial glands, of the cartilages, tendons, joints, and bones, of the perineum and peritoneum, of the vermiform appendix, of the male and female reproductive organs, of the mucous membranes of the mouth, nose, throat, eye, and ear. The treatment of tuberculosis by the knife has at all times been looked upon as a doubtful procedure, and the awe with which it has been regarded by some seems akin to superstition. But this fear, like many of the superstitions of the past, was founded on observation of clinical facts which were inexplicable, but which, in the light of modern research, are easily understood. It was observed that after cutting into tubercular affections general tuberculosis frequently developed, to which the patient rapidly succumbed. We now know that this result is due to the absorption of tubercular matter into the circulation by the cut surface and its deposition in other parts of the body. With our modern knowledge of the infectious nature of tuberculosis it becomes imperative that the knife be not used unless the entire tubercular mass can be re-

[1] Read before the Philadelphia County Medical Society, November 12, 1890.

moved intact, and without reinoculating the patient. This can sometimes be done in tuberculosis of the superficial glands, of the vermiform appendix, of the reproductive organs, of the tendons, cartilages, bones, and joints, and in lupus. In tuberculosis of the accessible mucous membranes and in lupus, caustics and strong germicides are no doubt preferable to the knife. In tuberculosis of the peritoneum washing out and dusting the cavity with iodoform have given good results. It seems to me that where the tubercular deposit is confined to the peritoneum, repeatedly dusting with iodoform might be practised. In tuberculosis of the perineum good results are seldom obtained by the knife, and surgical interference had better not be attempted. Packing the sinuses with iodoform and constitutional treatment will give much more satisfactory results. In tuberculosis of the tonsils caustics are preferable to the knife.

The majority of the cases of tuberculosis come under the second class, namely, those which are inaccessible to mechanical treatment, or in which mechanical treatment is undesirable. For all such cases certain general laws can be laid down:

First. Whatever will sterilize the tubercular deposit without interfering with the nutrition of the body, will cure tuberculosis.

Second. Whatever tends to improve nutrition will help to cure tuberculosis.

Third. Whenever the tubercular deposit sets up excessive inflammation, rest is of primary importance.

The destruction of the bacillus tuberculosis is of course the principle underlying all treatment, whether it be accomplished by medicine or by nature's conservative methods. Throughout the entire civilized world there is at present great activity among medical men in search of a substance which will destroy the bacillus tuberculosis without interfering with the nutrition of the body. That such a substance exists, and will ultimately be discovered, can scarcely be doubted, now that science has indicated to us the way in which to proceed in our investigations. Even at the present time encouraging reports come from our own city, from Germany, and from France, which may soon be followed by the announcement that the discovery has been made. The experiments of Grancher, Martin, Dixon, and Koch, demonstrate that the development of the bacillus tuberculosis can at least be checked in organisms very similar to the human body, and these are the beginnings of a new line of study which may lead up to the discovery of the long-looked-for secret.

We have already in our armamentaria many drugs which will destroy the bacillus tuberculosis, either directly or by depriving it of its nutrition ; but they all interfere, more or less, with the nutrition of the body, or destroy the tissues when taken in large enough doses to produce the desired result upon the bacillus. Some of the drugs, however, in safe doses, will enable nature sufficiently to produce a cure. Prominent among the remedies which have been used as germicides in tuberculosis are iodoform, creasote, terebene, sulphuretted hydrogen, carbonic acid, boric acid, arsenic, mercury, tar, ethereal oils, chloride of calcium, salts of gold and silver, iodine, hydrocyanic acid, and the aniline preparations. Each of these has been praised and condemned, but, no doubt, each has merit in its way. My own experience is limited to a few of them, and to these I will confine my remarks.

Iodoform.—If there is any drug in the Pharmacopœia of which I can truthfully say that I believe it has curative powers over tuberculosis, it is iodoform. I have used it in a large number of cases for a period of four or five years, and I am quite sure that I can ascribe to its use improvement in many cases, and cure in not a few. Iodoform acts best in the early stage of the disease, before there is any breaking-down of the deposit, and before the circulation is entirely cut off. It can be given by either the mouth or the bowel, or through the skin. Sometimes it disagrees with the stomach, but just as frequently proves beneficial by preventing fermentation. I usually prescribe the drug in capsules with pepsin, pancreatin, and some bitter extract. When the tubercular deposit is in the pelvis I use the iodoform in the form of suppositories. One of the most effective ways of using the drug, however, is by inunction. I order it in cod-liver oil, in which it is soluble in the proportion of one part in fifteen, and direct that the body be thoroughly rubbed with the solution from half an hour to an hour once or twice a day. The benefits resulting from this method of using iodoform are most striking. I have experimented with the drug hypodermically, but am not as yet ready to make any report as to its use in this way.

Creasote.—Creasote has attracted much attention during the last few years as a specific for tuberculosis, and has been much discussed in the journals. It has been experimentally proved to be an excellent germicide, and has given good results clinically when administered in sufficiently large quantities. There is often difficulty in getting it into the system in large quantities. I myself have never been able to give it with any satisfaction except by inhalation, the drug being volatilized by hot air. In this way I have obtained most excellent results from its use, not, as I believe, by any local action upon the lungs, but through absorption into the blood. A good way to give it is dissolved in some hot liquid. When well diluted it is not so apt to disturb the stomach. Its administration should be begun in small doses, and gradually increased until very large quantities are taken.

Terebene.—Terebene is very similar in its action to creasote, but is much more pleasant to take. I have given it with advantage by inhalation, volatilized by hot air. It is a good substitute for creasote when the latter drug is decidedly objectionable to the patient.

Boric acid.—Boric acid is such an excellent germicide, and even in large doses is so harmless to the system that theoretically it should be an excellent remedy for tuberculosis. A year ago I gave it a fair trial, but while I saw some benefit from its use, it interfered with digestion to such an extent that I abandoned it. It seemed to be of most benefit in checking fever and night-sweats in the last stages of the disease.

Dr. Grancher, of France, has recently reported a series of experiments and clinical observations bearing upon the use of this drug in tuberculosis, which are quite encouraging. He did not find that it disagreed with the stomach.

Sulphuretted hydrogen.—Sulphuretted hydrogen figured very conspicuously a few years ago as a specific remedy for tuberculosis, but it did not earn for itself a premanent reputation. It was then looked upon as a new remedy, but in reality it had been used nearly a century previously under the name of the "cow-stable cure." Although it has some efficacy its application is so objectionable that it has properly been laid aside.

Carbonic acie, arsenic, mercury, the ethereal oils, chloride of calcium, salts of gold and silver, iodine, hydrocyanic acid, and the many germicide remedies, descriptions of which appear in the medical journals, has each had its champion, but my own experience is too limited with them to enable me to give an opinion. I find excellent use for mercury given at intervals, to prepare the system for other remedies, but I have never used it as a germicide. Arsenic receives great encomiums and no doubt deserves them, but I cannot join in the praises as I am not sure that I have seen any benefit from it. Iodine is a powerful germicide, and all of its preparations are no doubt more or less useful in tuberculosis; iodoform, of which iodine is the active agent, is however probably the best form in which to give the drug. Tar and hydrocyanic acid form the bases for many of the home-cures for consumption, and no doubt possess merit; but as with many of the other drugs mentioned, we probably do not yet know the most efficacious method of administering them.

The stock of germicide remedies for tuberculosis is already quite large and is constantly being added to. It is said that when there are many remedies for a disease there is no cure, but this is more apparent than real. Many roads may lead to a city, but some may take you there more quickly than others, and therefore many remedies may cure a disease but some may do it more speedily than others. Each of the germicide remedies for tuberculosis would no doubt cure the disease, could it be given in large enough doses without injuring the tissues, and some of them do cure the disease in the doses in which they can safely be given. May we not then confidently look forward to the discovery of new remedies in the near future, or methods of applying the old ones, which will always cure the disease, and in a comparatively brief time? Every remedy finds a field of usefulness in the hands of a well-informed, judicious physician; and when to them are added the many adjuvants, in the way of drugs, gymnastics, climate, etc., by which we can aid nature in her efforts to restore and maintain the integrity of the living organism, it can certainly no longer be said that tuberculosis is an incurable disease.

In all living organisms there undoubtedly resides a power to resist parasitic encroachment. In the human body this power has been supposed to reside in the blood and to be exercised by little bodies called phagocytes. Quite recently efforts have been made to impeach the phagocyte, but all seem to agree that the protective power resides in the blood. We certainly do know from clinical observations that in proportion to the excellence of nutrition, which is best indicated by a healthy condition of the blood, the system is capable of obstructing the inroads of disease. This is true of all diseases, but it seems to be especially true of diseases which have a long incubation period and which run a slow course. Persons whose nutrition is at *par* seem to have power to resist tuberculosis under ordinary exposure; and persons who have fallen victims to the disease seem to be able to cast it off or to resist its encroaches if their digestive and nutritive powers can be readily restored. Upon these two clinical observations much of the classical treatment of tuberculosis was wisely constructed, and whatever germicide remedies may be discovered, improvement in nutrition must always constitute the groundwork of successful treatment.

Inasmuch as the nutrition of the body is so dependent upon the digestive apparatus, the stomach is the first thing to be looked after in the treatment of tuberculosis. If there is any fault in the method of taking food, such as hurried and insufficient mastication, it must be corrected. The nature of the food taken ought to be carefully inquired into, with a view to ascertain whether it is sufficiently nourishing and whether it is suited to the idiosyncrasies of the patient; and if it is not suitable, the proper diet should be prescribed. If it is found that certain kinds of food cannot be digested by the patient, such foods should be given artificially digested. When the stomach is congested, as indicated by a large, heavily-coated tongue, a light diet should be insisted on and remedies prescribed to relieve the congestion, such as bismuth, bicarbonate of sodium, and magnesia. Small doses of iodoform sometimes act well in such cases. When the stomach and liver are sluggish, usually indicated by a rather pale, indented, slightly-coated tongue, pepsin and hydrochloric acid in some bitter mixture will give good results. When intestinal digestion is bad, pancreatin should be given. As soon as the digestive apparatus has been restored to good working order, forced nutrition should be adopted. Easily-digested food ought to be given at frequent intervals, and every precaution taken against burdening the stomach with indigestible food. All forms of starchy food which have been prepared in such a way as to imbed the starch globules in grease should be scrupulously avoided. Milk should form a large part of the diet, and should be taken at meals, between meals, and at bedtime. If milk disagrees with the stomach, the habit of drinking it can and should be formed by taking a small quantity at first and gradually increasing the amount. By perseverance the stomach can readily be trained to take from five to six pints of milk a day, in addition to one meal of solid food. Meat should be partaken of but once a day, and then in as large quantity as possible. Vegetables and fruit should be freely eaten, and a little light wine at or after meals will be of benefit. Cod-liver oil should be taken, beginning with small quantities and gradually increasing until a tablespoonful three times a day is tolerated, but the greatest care should be exercised that it does not disturb the stomach. The use of oxygen after meals, inhaled slowly for half an hour, will aid digestion and be of great benefit. Quinine, strychnine, and other tonics and stomachics may be given to stimulate the appetite. When the stomach becomes fatigued under this forced labor it should be permitted to rest for a few days, the same regimen being then resumed. During this time of rest it is well to give a dose of calomel, followed by magnesia.

Next in importance to attention to the digestive apparatus of the patient, is to see that he gets plenty of fresh air and the proper amount of exercise. Outdoor life is of the greatest importance, but it does not seem to make much difference where that outdoor life is obtained. The one thing to be kept in the mind of the physician in directing fresh air for his patient is home comforts. Unless the patient can command home comforts, do not send him away. Were every medical student compelled, as part of his education, to make the rounds of the health-resorts of the country on the same amount of money that the average health-seeker has at his command, fewer patients would be sent to health-resorts. Altitude and temperature have less to do with either the production or cure of tuberculosis than is generally supposed. The benefits of altitude can be artificially produced by compressed and rarefied air, and if the patient's mind be relieved from the classical errors about the pernicious influence of cold and moisture, he will be found to do as well in one climate as another, provided he protects himself properly by clothing and has the courage to go out in all kinds of weather. In reality, warm climates are more conducive to the development of tuberculosis than are cold.

Regarding exercise, the physician should be very explicit, as the tendency is to take either too much or too little. Outdoor life and exercise must not be looked upon as synonymous terms. As long as there is a disposition to fever or even to acceleration of the pulse, exercise had better be as nearly passive as possible. Gradually, as the disposition to inflammatory action decreases, and as the various organs of the body begin to perform their functions more normally, exercise may become more active and may be taken in larger amount. At no time, however, must it be carried to the point of fatigue. A good form of exercise is that of driving nails with a light hammer, or, when the patient becomes stronger, that of chopping wood. There is considerable advantage in exercising chiefly with the upper extremities. Pulmonary gymnastics are of great assistance in re-developing an injured lung, but they must not be practised until all disposition to inflammatory action has ceased. Pulmonary gymnastics and excessive exercise during the inflammatory stage are apt to cause the disease to extend, and to make the course of the case much more rapid.

In the acute stage of the disease, when the tubercular deposit sets up an inflammatory condition, bodily rest and remedies that will quiet the excited heart and allay excessive reflex irritation, form an important part of the treatment. During this stage the best place for the patient is in bed. When the tubercular deposit is in the pleura or lung, considerable benefit will be derived from strapping the affected side with adhesive plaster.

Digitalis has a very soothing effect in this stage, and will often contribute considerably to a cure. During the latter part of the eighteenth century it held the reputation among many of the best practitioners in England of being a specific for the disease. Beddoes, who probably saw as many cases of phthisis as any man who ever practised medicine, used the following strong language concerning digitalis in 1803:

" In cases of pulmonary disease, where the presence of tubercle was indicated by every symptom, and where they seemed ready to break out in open ulcers, I have verified the efficacy of digitalis; and I daily see my patients advancing toward recovery, with so firm a pace that I hope consumption will henceforth be as regularly cured by the foxglove as ague by the Peruvian bark. Could we have a single auxiliary for the foxglove, such as we have many substances for the bark, I should expect that not one case in five would terminate as ninety-nine in a hundred have hitherto terminated."

The only evidence of this great faith in the efficacy of digitalis as a cure for tuberculosis at the present day is found in the confidence still shown in the Niemeyer pill. I have myself used the drug largely in the early stage of the disease for five or six years, and my conviction is that the old faith was founded on correct observation, and that we have in digitalis a most useful remedy for the inflammatory stage of tuberculosis. For the reflex irritation and the resulting symptoms of cough and sometimes of vomiting when the tubercular deposit is in the lungs, and of convulsions and vomiting when the deposit is in the brain or its membranes, opium, bromides, and chloral are the chief remedies. Opium should be used only when it is absolutely indispensable, but when the reflex symptoms are such as to harass the patient, and to interfere with his progress toward recovery, and when no other drug will control them, opium should be unhesitatingly used in quantities large enough to produce the desired effect. In such cases the effect of opium is apparently magical, not only in restoring the confidence of the patient, but in improving his appetite and general condition. As soon as practicable, however, the dose should be decreased and the administration of the drug soon entirely stopped. Where there is bronchial secretion opium should be entirely eschewed. In such cases bromide of ammonium will sometimes act very well. For the reflex symptoms of tubercular deposit in the brain and its membranes, the bromides and chloral are indicated. For the elevation of temperature which is encountered during the inflammatory stage, rest in bed and the administration of digitalis are usually sufficient; but if the temperature is not reduced in a few days quinine, antifebrin, or antipyrine may be given. When the tubercular deposit is in the lung much benefit may be derived by counter-irritation, either in the shape of dry cups, fly-blisters, croton oil, or tartar emetic plaster. In the most acute stage, dry cups are preferable, inasmuch as they can be frequently applied. Fly blisters, whilst painful, are the most powerful external remedy at our command, and are especially useful when the inflammatory condition has reached the subacute stage. They should be repeatedly applied until all evidence of inflammation has disappeared. Croton oil and tartar emetic plaster may be used as substitutes for fly-blister if the patient is too timid to use the latter.

When tuberculosis has reached the stage in which symptoms are caused by the absorption of products of the disease, or because of the interference with the functions of diseased organs, the treatment necessarily becomes symptomatic. For the high temperature of sepsis the administration of large doses of quinine is the safest treatment. Antifebrin and antipyrine are too depressing to be given in this stage. Boric acid given in doses of from ten to fifteen grains every three or four hours is worthy of trial. For the sweats which follow the fever, usually called colliquative night-sweats, belladonna and aromatic sulphuric acid are the standard remedies, and are usually efficient. Agaricin has recently been attracting some attention as an excellent remedy for this condition, but I have had no experience with it. The patient should be cautioned not to use too many bedclothes at night, as sweats are sometimes aggravated thereby. It is also a good plan to sponge the body with warm alcohol.

For the irritative diarrhœa which frequently comes on in the latter stages of tubercular pulmonitis, without any involvement of the intestinal glands, a light, easily-digested diet, and bismuth, bicarbonate of sodium, and pancreatin are indicated. When the diarrhœa is due to tuberculosis of the intestinal glands it will be found difficult to control, but it can be temporarily checked by such astringents as catechu, tannic acid, and acetate of lead. A warm, dry application to the abdomen in the form of a hot bran-bag will be very soothing and beneficial.

The attacks of palpitation which are so distressing and which are apt to come on when there are large cavities in the lungs, I have found are almost instantly relieved by opium and digitalis. Great care must be exercised not to confound this palpitation with the dyspnœa accompanying extensive tubercular deposit and excessive bronchial secretion which it very closely resembles. In the latter conditions oxygen will give relief, and opium must be absolutely avoided. In these cases the reflex symptoms should be met by bromide of ammonium and counter-irritation.

In treating these various symptoms during the latter stages of tuberculosis it must always be borne in mind that they are mere symptoms and not the disease; and that in reality they are often the phenomena accompanying nature's frantic efforts to get rid of a foe. They must never be allowed to assume such a magnitude in the physician's mind as to make him forget his main purpose, namely, to cure the disease.

In conclusion, it may be well to say a word about the methods of medication in the treatment of tuberculosis. The methods usually employed are inhalation and administration by the mouth. Because of the anatomical construction of the respiratory system and its physiological action, and also because of the pathology of tuberculosis, medication by inhalation is restricted to those substances which exist in or can assume the form of vapor or gas, and which can at once enter the blood by endosmosis or be carried into it through the lymphatic system. Topical applications of remedies to a tubercular lung by way of the respiratory tract are useless, because the tubercular deposit is in the lung-tissue where it cannot be reached except through the circulation. All such plans of treatment, therefore, as the inhalation of hot air as a germicide, and of medicated vapors for their local effect, are based upon misconceptions, and can have no curative influence. Many substances can, however, readily enter the blood through the lungs, and inhalation is an excellent method of administering germicide remedies that can be converted into vapor or gas. The observation has recently been made that chloroform is very destructive to the bacillus tuberculosis, and very good results are reported from the daily inhalation of a small quantity of chloroform. This method of medication is as yet an unexplored field, but it promises well and is worthy of attention.

Medication by the mouth is the method most in use in the treatment of all diseases, and it is the one almost entirely depended on in the treatment of tuberculosis. In giving such substances as have the same physiological and therapeutic effect, in whatever chemical form they are used, medication by the mouth is by far the most convenient and most desirable method. Many substances, however, have different actions in different chemical forms, and with them, however destructive to germs they may be in the test-tube, we cannot know what their germicide and therapeutical powers will be after they have been acted upon by the salivary, gastric, and intestinal juices. It seems to me, therefore, that only such germicides should be administered by the mouth as do not have their therapeutical effect altered by chemical action before reaching the circulation. For drugs whose germicidal powers are changed by chemical action, intravenous injection, hypodermic injection, and inunction offer excellent methods, as in these ways the substances can be brought in contact with the bacillus tuberculosis without undergoing any chemical change. My short experience with inunctions convinces me that they are preferable to giving the drugs by the mouth. The entire question of medication is, however, as yet an open one, and offers an excellent field for clinical observation.

736 PINE STREET.

MEDICAL PROGRESS.

Cocaine Anæsthesia Obtained by Means of Cataphoresis.— DR. ARTHUR HARRIES (*Lancet*, October 25, 1890) writes that where local anæsthesia is required, cocaine hydrochlorate, administered by means of cataphoresis instead of hypodermically, should be employed. In a number of cases in which he adopted this method the anæsthesia was complete, and toxic symptoms of the drug were not observed. He uses a ten-per-cent. solution of cocaine, with which the flannel-padded positive electrode, corresponding to the size of the area to be anæsthetized, is saturated. The large negative electrode is soaked in salt solution and placed in a suitable position on the surface of the body. A continuous current of twenty-five milliampères is then passed for forty minutes. Dr. Harries believes that the causes of failure with this method are : That the currents used are too weak, and applied for too brief a time ; that the operator does not understand the apparatus ; and that a reversed current is used.

The Therapeutic Action of the Sulphate of Cinchonidine.— H. DE BRUN has recently made an elaborate study of the therapeutic action of the sulphate of cinchonidine in the treatment of the various types of malarial fever. He has carefully observed and recorded fifty-eight cases in private and hospital practice, especially at the Beyreuth Hospital. From the results observed he concludes :

1. That the sulphate of cinchonidine, administered in the amounts in which sulphate of quinine is usually given, is able to prevent the symptoms of paludal poisoning as effectually as the latter remedy. After one or two doses of the first drug the return of the paroxysms of intermittent fever is prevented.

2. The value of the sulphate of cinchonidine in malarial cachexia is doubtful. The drug arrests the destruction of the blood-cell, and rapidly diminishes the general ʻpaludal anæmia. It also causes the hæmatin of the blood to increase. It quickly reduces the size of both the congested liver and spleen, but is powerless if the enlargement is due to sclerosis. It also quickly relieves the pulmonary congestions of paludal origin as well as albuminurias dependent upon malarial congestion of the kidneys.

3. It is an excellent remedy in the treatment of intermittent neuralgias, and possibly may prove useful against other neuralgias due to common causes.

4. The sulphate of cinchonidine has often produced beneficial results in those cases where the sulphate of quinine has failed to do any good.

The superiority of the cinchonidine salt is also noticed, in that it is better tolerated by the stomach, and much less apt to produce ringing in the ears and vertigo.

5. The moderate price of the cinchonidine salts is another important consideration.—*Revue de Médecine*, September 10, 1890.

The Use of Sodium Salicylate in Pleural Effusions.— In 1883 Aufrecht recommended the administration of sodium salicylate in all cases of pleural effusion. TETZ (*Therapeutische Monatshefte*, No. 7, 1890), who has used the remedy for two years, states that his success completely confirms the views of Aufrecht. He considers that its action on pleural effusions is as striking as on rheumatism, and his experience has been that the average time of treatment is less than with other methods. Although it acts most promptly, and certainly in recent cases, he has seen collections of fluid of several weeks' duration yield to it—not only primary but also secondary pleurisies. As an example, he reports the case of a woman, about forty years of age, in whom a left-sided pleurisy had existed for two[?] and a half weeks. Ordinary treatment had very little effect, but on the day following the administration of sodium salicylate the effusion had diminished, and all traces disappeared by the fourth day. In another case of long-standing effusion for which paracentesis had been proposed, the use of the drug caused the accumulation to disappear rapidly.

In regard to secondary pleurisy, the author reports a case of tuberculosis with pleural effusion, in which the salicylate also caused rapid subsidence, the diagnosis being confirmed by an autopsy several months later.

Tetz gives the drug in fifteen-grain doses, at first four or five times daily, later three or four times daily for one week. He does not think that the action of the salicylate is that of a diuretic, but that it is a specific.—*Practitioner*, October, 1890.

Salipyrine.—GUTTMANN (*Internationale klinische Rundschau*, September, 1890) reports his results with the use of "salipyrine," a combination of salicylic acid and antipyrine. The compound is a white, odorless powder, with a slight burning taste, freely soluble in alcohol, but almost insoluble in water. Guttmann's conclusions are as follows:

1. Salipyrine reduces elevated temperature. In cases of continued high temperature, a dose of thirty grains should be given, followed by four doses of fifteen grains each, at intervals of an hour. The lowest temperature is reached in about four hours after the last dose, the fall being from 3° to 3½° F. More or less profuse sweating usually accompanies the fall,

2. In acute rheumatism salipyrine is as efficient a remedy as the other compounds of salicylic acid, but has no influence in preventing relapse.

3. In the treatment of chronic articular rheumatism the drug is also useful.

4. Salipyrine rarely produces disagreeable symptoms, even if given for two weeks in daily doses of ninety grains. In but one case was an eruption observed. This resembled the eruption produced by antipyrine, and disappeared in a few days.

5. The color of the urine is not affected by the administration of salipyrine, but the chloride of iron test shows the presence of a salicylate.

6. To reduce temperature, the dose of salipyrine should be twice that of antipyrine.

The Treatment of Partially-amputated Fingers.—ZATVAR-NITZKY reports the case of a boy who four hours before coming under observation, nearly lost the distal phalanx of his right forefinger by accidentally bringing it in contact with a circular saw. The end of the finger was still attached by a small cutaneous bridge. The author washed the injured part with sublimate solution, arrested hæmorrhage, dusted the wound with iodoform and carefully attached the plalanx to the stump by means of interrupted sutures and adhesive plaster, and applied antiseptic dressings and a splint. Complete union with good motion followed.

In considering such cases the author concludes that if there is much laceration or contusion of the soft tissues or comminution of the bone, union cannot be hoped for; but that if the injury is of the nature of an incised wound union may be obtained, even when several hours have elapsed since the accident, if the amputated part is not very cold and pale.—*Annals of Surgery*, October, 1890.

Disinfection of the Mouth in Diabetes.—DUJARDIN-BEAU-METZ (*Therapeutic Gazette*, October 15, 1890) refers to the fact that the majority of diabetics have a purulent inflammation of the gums, which may be the starting-point of systemic infection, and insists on the importance of disinfecting the mouth in such cases. The solution which has given him the best results for this purpose is the following:

R.—Boric acid . . . 6½ drachms.
　　Carbolic acid . . . 15 grains.
　　Thymol . . . 3½ "
　　Water . . . 1 quart.

Add to the above:

　　Spirit of anise . . . 3½ drachms.
　　Spirit of peppermint . . 10 drops.
　　Alcohol . . . 3 ounces.
　　Cochineal, sufficient to color.—M.

This should be diluted with an equal quantity of water and used freely after eating.

Management of Gonorrhœa.—LANG (*Wiener med. Wochenschrift*, October 2, 1890) discusses some of the causes of the prolongation and complications of gonorrhœa. One of the most important points in the treatment of gonorrhœa is, he thinks, the proper regulation of eating and drinking. In some cases attention to these is all the treatment that is necessary. The injection chiefly used by the author is a solution of sulpho-carbolate of zinc of a strength of from one-fourth to one per cent. Stronger solutions may be employed if a mucilaginous menstruum is used instead of water. It is important to pay attention to the size of the syringe. Patients, if not otherwise instructed, will often use a large syringe, and by injecting too much fluid injure the urethra. Lang uses syringes of three sizes holding respectively, one [and a half, two, and three drachms, and to each case orders the size which seems most suitable.—*British Medical Journal*, October 18, 1890.

Ammonium Acetate in the Treatment of Scarlatina.—VIDAL recommends large doses of ammonium acetate in the treatment of scarlatina, and believes that it will also be found useful in the treatment of other exanthemata. In three children suffering from scarlatina to whom he gave the drug in daily amounts of from 35 to 90 grains, the temperature rapidly fell and desquamation was established within four days. In the author's experience the earlier in the course of the disease that the ammonium acetate is given the better are the results.— *Wiener medicinische Presse*, October 5, 1890.

THE MEDICAL NEWS.

A WEEKLY JOURNAL
OF MEDICAL SCIENCE.

COMMUNICATIONS are invited from all parts of the world. Original articles contributed exclusively to THE MEDICAL NEWS will be liberally paid for upon publication. When necessary to elucidate the text, illustrations will be furnished without cost to the author.

Address the Editor: H. A. HARE, M.D.,
1004 WALNUT STREET,
PHILADELPHIA.

Subscription Price, including Postage.
PER ANNUM, IN ADVANCE . . . . $4.00.
SINGLE COPIES . . . . 10 CENTS.

Subscriptions may begin at any date. The safest mode of remittance is by bank check or postal money order, drawn to the order of the undersigned. When neither is accessible, remittances may be made, at the risk of the publishers, by forwarding in *registered* letters.

Address,   LEA BROTHERS & CO.,
NOS. 706 & 708 SANSOM STREET,
PHILADELPHIA.

SATURDAY, NOVEMBER 15, 1890.

THE TREATMENT OF RECTO-VAGINAL FISTULÆ.

IN *La Médecine Moderne*, October 9, 1890, is an article from the pen of PROFESSOR LE DENTU, the author who not long since gave us an excellent work on the *Surgical Diseases of the Kidneys, Ureters, and Suprarenal Capsules* (Paris, 1889, pp. 828). The occasion of Professor Le Dentu's article is the description of a new method of treating recto-vaginal fistulæ. The method consists of the dissection of a crescent-shaped flap, with its convexity tangent to the lower margin of the fistula, sliding this flap up so as more than to cover the fistula, and attaching its under raw surface to a crescentic denuded area, which includes the fistulous orifice. The sutures are held in place either by segments of a metal tube which, like perforated shot, can be compressed, or by sutures tied over a roll of gauze, in the manner of the old quill sutures.

While admiring the author's ingenuity and appreciating his success in the single case to which the method was applied, we cannot feel that we have here a means less difficult than other methods of treating these troublesome cases, and we believe that there is no treatment for recto-vaginal fistula which will always prove successful.

While we say that there is no *treatment*, we would insist that there are many *treatments*, each of which is excellent and suitable to various classes of case. In other words, we have grouped under the one name *recto-vaginal fistula*, conditions the repair of which may be either the simplest or one of the most difficult of gynæcological procedures.

Fistulæ resulting from cancer and syphilis are, as as rule, beyond the pale of relief, while the remediable cases, those arising from perforation of the recto-vaginal septum by pessaries, by trauma in childbirth, by ulceration, or by an imperfectly-united septum after the perineal operation for complete tear of the septum, present a host of different appearances, according as the fistula is high or low, transverse or longitudinal, large or small, a direct communication through which the rectal mucosa can be seen from the vaginal side, or communicates by a long sinuous track—all these as well as other factors are important and must be weighed, in determining the best plan for attacking a given case of recto-vaginal fistula.

Through the genius of Emmet, Simon, and others we already have a number of rational procedures, sufficient it would seem to cover all cases; thus we can operate upon the fistula through the rectum, or through both the rectum and the vagina, making a bevelled denudation ; or, in small direct fistulæ just above the vaginal orifice, the fistulous track may be dissected out through the vagina and closed from the vaginal side alone.

Splitting the perineum and recto-vaginal septum up to the fistula, cutting out the fistulous track and then sewing up the whole wound, has succeeded in some intractable cases situated near the posterior columna. The genius of success and the demon of failure in this work lie, we feel sure, not in the want of a new method which shall simplify—or shall we say complicate—everything, but more in the judgment exercised by the surgeon in his selection of one of the simple methods which we already possess ; in the dexterity with which a perfect and even denudation is made ; and above all, in the precision with which the sutures are applied—splitting the parts firmly, without constricting them, until the desired union takes place. The surgeon who understands how to use his sutures properly will not need to inject milk into the rectum at the end of the operation to learn if the fistula is closed, nor will he fear that accumulations of gas in the rectum or the passage of fæces will break his line of union.

What we here say of operations upon recto-vaginal fistulæ applies to all plastic operations in the vagina; it is not new methods we are in need of, but more dexterity and greater skill in applying the old methods. Let our surgeons be truly clever workers with their hands.

SOCIETY PROCEEDINGS.

TRI-STATE MEDICAL ASSOCIATION.

Second Annual Meeting, held in Chattanooga, Tenn., October 11, 15, and 16, 1890.

FIRST DAY.—MORNING SESSION.

The Association met in Turner Hall, and was called to order by the President, Dr. J. B. Cowan, of Tullahoma, Tenn., at 10 A. M. Prayer was offered by the Rev. Charles Hyde.

The remainder of the first session was devoted to introductions, miscellaneous business, and reports of the Executive Committee.

AFTERNOON SESSION.

DR. W. P. McDONALD, of Hill City, Tenn., contributed a paper entitled

REPORT OF A CASE OF CANCRUM ORIS OR GANGRENOUS STOMATITIS.

He was called to see the patient, a girl four years old, on August 5th. She had some fever, the tongue was coated with a brown fur, the surface being more or less fissured, and her general appearance indicated great depression. Her bowels were inclined to be loose, and her abdomen seemed to be somewhat tympanitic. He believed the case to be one of typhomalarial fever, and began treatment by a mercurial purge, which was followed by large doses of quinine and bismuth. This treatment was continued for two days, after which he ordered ten drops of syrup of the iodide of iron after meals, with quinine and bismuth in small doses three or four times a day. This treatment was continued for about ten days, when the patient had greatly improved.

Fourteen days after his first visit he was called to see the patient's mother, whom he found with nearly the same symptoms as those that the child first presented. During his absence from the city, another physician had treated an older daughter, who probably had the same disease. The little child was still improving, but her mouth remained sore. On examining the mother he found several small ulcers on the right side of the mouth, with a general inflammatory appearance of the gums and of the mucous lining of that side of the buccal cavity, with some bleeding from around the teeth. The trouble seemed at first to yield to a mouth-wash of chlorate of potassium and creasote, but on the seventeenth day of the illness the inflammation increased rapidly, the whole cheek became much swollen, and the mucous membrane dark and gangrenous. On August 24th a dark spot about the size of a dime made its appearance externally near the right wing of the nose. This rapidly enlarged, involving the wing of the nose and the adjacent tissues, and on August 25th it had involved the right side

of the nose to the inner canthus of the eye and the upper lip to the median line, and had rapidly spread on the cheek, reaching the point at which the zygomatic muscles cross the masseter. Both the upper and lower teeth on this side became loose and dropped out.

Careful investigation revealed a strumous diathesis in the family, but there was no history of tuberculosis.

According to good authorities, cancrum oris usually occurs as the sequel of other diseases. The statistics of Rilliet and Barthez show that out of 98 cases of this disease, 41 followed measles, 5 scarlet fever, 6 whooping-cough, 9 intermittent fever, 9 typhoid fever, and 7 mercurial salivation.

In Dr. McDonald's cases the questions are, Did the disease occur as a sequel of typho-malarial fever, or was it the result of mercurial salivation.

In discussing this paper, DR. E. T. CAMP, of Gadsden, Alabama, said that he had seen a case similar to the one reported, which he pronounced gangrena oris, the whole of one cheek being destroyed. There was evidence of mercury having been taken in the early part of the illness. The case terminated fatally within a few days. The patient was four or five years old and of the lower class.

DR. JAMES E. REEVES, of Chattanooga, contributed a paper entitled

"ON ALL SIDES A LEARNED DOCTOR."

The author introduced his subject by an earnest plea for higher medical education, stigmatizing cheap medical colleges with no facilities for imparting instruction as the greatest stumbling-blocks in the way of true progress.

He referred to the present tendency to make one-sided physicians, and maintained that the specialist should build on the broad foundation of the general practitioner in order to reach professional eminence.

EVENING SESSION.

DR. ANDREW BOYD, of Scottsboro, Alabama, read a paper on

FRACTURE AT THE ELBOW-JOINT,

and reported several cases. He said that after reduction there are but two positions in which to treat fracture at the elbow-joint, viz., the extended or straight, and the flexed position. The author thinks that the flexed position is the better, for the reasons (1) that in all cases there is danger of ankylosis, and it is much better to have a flexed ankylosed arm than a straight one; (2) that after the splints have remained in place from twenty-five to thirty days, the arm is atrophied and almost helpless; (3) that it is easier to overcome the flexor muscles than the extensors, and a patient can extend an arm with more ease than he can flex it.

MR. SYDNEY B. WRIGHT, of Chattanooga, read a paper on

EXPERT TESTIMONY,

of which the following are the most important points:

1. That the circumstances from which the conclusion is drawn should be fully established.

2. That all the facts should be consistent with the hypothesis.

3. That the circumstances should be of a conclusive nature and tendency.

4. That the circumstances should to a moral certainty

exclude every hypothesis but the one propounded to be proved.

5. That mere circumstantial evidence, unless the chain of circumstances is complete, ought in no case to be relied on where direct and positive evidence which might have been given is withheld by the opposite party.

DR. W. G. BOGART, of Chattanooga, reported a

CASE OF NEUROSIS,

in a girl aged seventeen years. The patient was constipated and had a coated tongue and fœtid breath. Her temperature was 103°; pulse 115. She had been growing more irritable and less communicative, and had suffered from sleeplessness, pain in the back of the head, and a general feeling of depression for several months. She was placed under treatment and seemed to improve. Six months later she was seized with convulsions, and still later she suffered from amenorrhœa.

An interesting feature of the case is that the patient passed three different varieties of worms. A small, black-headed worm, one-half inch long, which had decided vermicular movements; another, with a head like that of a pin ; and a third, a small thread-like worm two inches in length.

A paper on

NEURALGIA,

by DR. W. S. GAHAGAN, of Chattanooga, was then read by title.

SECOND DAY—MORNING SESSION.

The first paper was read by DR. J. C. SHEPARD, of Winchester, Tennessee, and was entitled

A FEW REMARKS ON THE FEVERS OF MIDDLE TENNESSEE AND THEIR TREATMENT.

He said that the great malarial period extended from the time of the settlement of the country up to about 1840, during which time all the fevers of the country were malarial and periodical. The great typhoid period commenced about 1840 and continued until near 1860. During this period malarial fevers were almost, if not entirely, unknown, and typhoid was everywhere dominant and every case was typical. About 1860 there was a return of malarial fever, but in connection with typhoid fever. This was the typho-malarial period, which continued for fifteen or twenty years.

About 1880 the characteristic symptoms both of typhoid and of malarial fevers commenced to disappear, and are still growing less frequent. This is the period of *fusion*. We now have only one fever, which is a continued fever, neither typically typhoid nor malarial, and not even typically typho-malarial. There is not now, and there never was, a continued malarial fever, *per se*, in Middle Tennessee.

Of treatment but little was said. Cold baths the speaker considered impracticable, and new antipyretics should be given with caution. He believed that too much quinine is used in the continued fevers of Middle Tennessee.

DR. L. P. BARBER, of Tracy City, Tennessee, followed with a paper entitled

A CONTRIBUTION TO THE STUDY OF THE CONTINUED FEVERS OF THE SOUTH,

in which he said that the nosology and etiology of the continued fever of the South are now justly attracting much attention, and form a subject upon which much is yet to be learned. Only a close and accurate study of the disease by competent observers, in many and different localities, a thoughtful comparison of these observations, and free discussion, will advance our knowledge of its nature, and shed light on the vexed question of its cause.

Encouraged by the recent vigorous inquiry and research in this direction, Dr. Barber began, some fifteen months since, to keep a record of all cases of fever that occurred in his private practice, and the comparison of the cases has helped him toward a decision as to the nosology of continued fever.

Dr. Barber then reported a large number of interesting cases, after which the two papers on continued fever were discussed.

DR. G. W. DRAKE, of Chattanooga, in opening the discussion, said that the human body is an aggregation of cells, and that among these cells are found, in various tissues, certain loose migratory and amœboid cells—phagocytes—which he would call the police force intended to protect the tissues against invasion. When the germs of typhoid fever attack Peyer's patches and the solitary glands, the migratory cells from the adjacent parts, and possibly from distant parts, rush to the conflict. The result is great destruction both of microbes and of phagocytes, and their putrefying remains produce *typhotoxin* and probably other ptomaïnes.

He believed typhoid fever to be produced by germs once external to the body, but expressed a "judicious scepticism" as to whether Eberth's bacillus is the *sole* cause, and its presence absolutely necessary in all cases.

DR. JAMES E. REEVES said that the malarial influence was undoubtedly slowly, but surely, travelling northward.

DR. J. A. LONG, of Long's Mills, Tennessee, related his experience in McMinn County, Tenn. The fevers there have the symptoms of typhoid fever, but there are many non-typical cases. Some are cases of typhoid in a malarial diathesis. He believed that a few cases of malarial fever continue because quinine is given in too small doses.

DR. H. BERLIN, of Chattanooga, presented some photo-micrographs as an evidence of the existence of microbes in these fevers.

DR. GEORGE A. BAXTER, of Chattanooga, suggested the use of salol and naphthol in the treatment of fevers.

DR. J. B. MURFREE, of Murfreesboro', Tennessee, thought it impossible for two fevers to exist at the same time in one person, and said that there is no typho-malarial fever. We have mild cases of typhoid as well as of other fevers. The use of antiseptics with proper nutrition and stimulation is the proper method of treating typhoid.

DR. REEVES asked Dr. Murfree if he thought typhoid was contagious.

DR. MURFREE said it was to a certain extent.

DR. P. D. SIMS, of Chattanooga, said : "Our fevers are not all either malarial or typhoid. We have another fever dependent upon filth. It may be called *sewage* or *drainage* fever. It is adynamic in type and is liable to take on most of the symptoms of specific typhoid fever. This is the fever now upon us, arising from the continued and increasing pollution of our water-supply from sewage sources."

DR. T. Y. PARK, of Peavine, Georgia, suggested that as these fevers present the symptoms both of typhoid and of malarial fever, it is convenient to use the term typho-malarial, as we cannot make the public understand the technical points of difference, and we cannot examine our cases for the microörganisms.

DR. GEORGE A. BAXTER, of Chattanooga, presented a paper on

SOME NEW USES OF SILICATE OF SODIUM.

The paper chiefly had reference to a jacket made by a new process of hardening the silicate, which it is claimed is an improvement on all other jackets, inclusive of the plaster-of-Paris, leather, woven wire, or watch-spring jackets now in use for the treatment of spinal injuries or disease. It is lighter, equally durable, equally immobile when on, and can be removed at any time and adjusted to any lateral pressure desired.

AFTERNOON SESSION.

DR. RICHARD DOUGLAS, of Nashville, contributed a paper on

ABSCESS OF THE LIVER,

which, he said, is the result of absorption of some morbid product from the intestine, or from some ulcerated surface. The bacteria enter the circulation and are deposited in the liver, where an abscess is formed. This may be without a rise of temperature.

Dr. Douglas then reported the following case : Four months after an attack of typhoid fever the patient had a chill, slight pyrexia, and a trace of jaundice, these lasting only a few days. There was a globular swelling in the right hypochondriac region ; the only local symptoms of which were dull pain and tenderness. The diagnosis was confirmed by aspiration. A free incision let out eight ounces of inodorous pus, and the patient recovered in four weeks.

DR. E. E. KERR, of Chattanooga, reported a

CASE OF GALL-STONES,

and was followed by

DR. J. B. MURFREE, of Murfreesboro', Tennessee, who read a paper on

UTERINE FIBROMA.

A uterine fibroma, he said, is a morbid growth developed within the walls of the uterus, and is composed of muscle-cells, fibro-plastic material, and cellular tissue, and is due to a perversion of nutrition. It is non-malignant and homologous in its structure. Pain, hæmorrhage, rectal and cystic irritation, indigestion, dropsy, and exhaustion are some of its results. The growths may threaten life by hæmorrhage, inflammation, septicæmia, or pressure.

The treatment is divided into four methods : (1) Symptomatic; (2) General (by medicines); (3) Electrolysis, and (4) Operative.

By the first method we simply treat the symptoms as they arise and ward off threatened dangers. Hæmorrhage is the most troublesome symptom, and is best treated by quietude, opiates, etc. The hot douche and the tampon are also useful. The general treatment is by the administration of medicines, which are powerless to cause the absorption of a fibrous tumor, and do no good, except to build up the general system.

Ergot is sometimes given to cause the death and expulsion of the tumor, but the speaker has no confidence in it.

The treatment by electrolysis has met with some success, and is worthy of trial. It is especially adapted to the interstitial variety.

Surgical treatment is resorted to for the permanent relief of uterine fibroma. It consists in the removal of the tumor by traction, torsion, excision, enucleation, excision, écrassement, or hysterectomy. When the tumor projects into the uterine cavity it is best removed by excision. When it is interstitial it should be treated by electrity. When subperitoneal it had better be left alone unless the woman's life is a burden and death is threatened, when it should be removed by abdominal section. Hysterectomy should never be resorted to as an ideal operation, but only as a forlorn hope. But conditions do arise when it is eminently proper and should unhesitatingly be performed.

In discussion DR. W. H. WATHEN, of Louisville, Kentucky, said that the more frequently he opens the pelvis the more often does he find that his diagnosis was not correct. Apostoli's method he considered dangerons in private practice, and to be successful in its application the operator must be the most exclusive of specialists. The tumor may be lessened in size, but there are few, if any, cures. A fibroma should not be interfered with unless it gives trouble.

DR. RICHARD DOUGLAS wished to emphasize what Dr. Wathen had said regarding Apostoli's treatment. From observation at his clinics and inquiries in the hospitals in Paris, he had not found any cases that were cured, but he had heard of two cases that died as the result of the treatment, one of these being in the practice of Dr. Keith, of London.

DR. L. P. BARBER, of Tracy City, Tennessee, said that Apostoli's method certainly promises much, notwithstanding the remarks of Drs. Douglas and Wathen. He saw something of the results of the treatment during the past summer, and Dr. Franklin H. Martin, of Chicago, told him that of about 200 cases only three had received no benefit. About fourteen per cent. received temporary benefit, eighty-four per cent. were symptomatically cured, there were a number of actual cures. Dr. Martin has had no deaths in all his experience with electricity, The result, to the unprejudiced, is certainly in favor of the proper use of electricity.

DR. MURFREE, in closing, said that he felt that much could be accomplished by Apostoli's method.

DR. W. H. WATHEN followed with a paper entitled

LAPAROTOMY *versus* ELECTRICITY IN ECTOPIC PREGNANCY,

in which he said that electricity, the only fœticidal means now recognized as orthodox by physicians who practise destroying the life of the fœtus, without abdominal section, in ectopic pregnancy, is no longer used for this purpose when the pregnancy has continued longer than three and a half or four months, and is seldom used after the third month. At this time the fœtus cannot be killed except by electro-puncture, and the complications and the deaths consequent upon this practice have been so numerous that the most radical advocates of electricity are afraid to introduce the electrodes into the gestation-sac. The use of electricity in extra-uterine pregnancy is practically confined to the United States, and while it is advocated by men of recognized ability and learning in obstetrics and gynecology, Dr. Wathen believes that very soon it will have no support.

The speaker then entered into an argument in favor of abdominal section, for the difficulty and sometimes the impossibility of diagnosing extra-uterine pregnancy in the early months are so manifest that it would be ridiculous to claim that in all the reported cases pregnancy existed ; while in the cases in which the abdomen is opened a positive diagnosis may be made by seeing the embryo, or the chorionic or placental villi. If the embryo or fœtus in an extra-uterine pregnancy is killed by electricity, a more or less diseased condition of the pelvic structures is left that endangers the health or the life of the woman, the dangers usually being increased as pregnancy advances. But if abdominal section is done, there is no obstructed tube or other pathological condition left, and if the woman recovers from the immediate effects of the operation she is entirely cured. Her life is no longer in jeopardy because of the danger of pelvic abscess, sepsis, or exhaustion following an effort to discharge the suppurating contents of the gestation-sac through fistulous tracks into the rectum, vagina, bladder, or through the abdominal walls. If we could eliminate the cases in which there was an error of diagnosis we would find that the mortality from the use of electricity and the bad after-results are far in excess of the mortality from abdominal section in the practice of experienced operators.

(*To be continued.*)

CORRESPONDENCE.

To the Editor of THE MEDICAL NEWS,

SIR : In your issue of October 18th, I notice, with regret, a foot-note to my article on "Acromegaly." The late publication of the paper was due to a misunderstanding on my part, and was not the fault of Dr. Hays.

Yours very truly, J. E. GRAHAM.
TORONTO, October 27, 1890.

NEWS ITEMS.

New York Academy of Medicine.—On November 20th the new building of the New York Academy of Medicine, which has just been completed, will be opened with appropriate ceremonies. Dr. Loomis will give an address of welcome, Dr. E. L. Keyes will deliver the anniversary address on the "New York Academy of Medicine," while Dr. Abraham Jacobi will speak upon the subject of "Our Library." Dr. Billings, Dr. Weir Mitchell, Dr. Fritz, and Dr. Fordyce Barker are also expected to be present and to speak. Invitations have been sent out to many of the prominent men in the different cities of the Union asking them to be present, and the occasion will undoubtedly be one of which both New York and the medical profession throughout the country may be proud.

Dr. Bartholow's Retirement.—Referring to the statement in THE MEDICAL NEWS of November 1st, as to the cause of Dr. Bartholow's retirement from the faculty of the Jefferson Medical College, it affords us pleasure to state that in the resolution of the Board of Trustees the only reason assigned is that his arduous and unremitting labor in the duties of his chair had rendered a period of rest imperatively necessary for him. If permitted, we would be glad to publish the correspondence of the Trustees with Dr. Bartholow, which bears emphatic testimony to the distinguished ability and untiring zeal with which he has for so many years discharged the duties of his position.

Uncertified Deaths in Great Britain.—The assertion was recently made on the floor of the British House of Commons that 15,000 persons die and are buried in Great Britain, each year, without a death-certificate having been given as required by law.

OFFICIAL LIST OF CHANGES IN THE STATIONS AND DUTIES OF OFFICERS SERVING IN THE MEDICAL DEPARTMENT, U. S. ARMY, FROM NOVEMBER 4 TO NOVEMBER 10, 1890.

By direction of the Secretary of War, BASIL NORRIS, *Colonel and Surgeon*, and GEORGE M. STERNBERG, *Major and Surgeon*, are appointed members of a Board of Officers to meet, at the call of the senior officer thereof, in San Francisco, Cal., to examine such officers of the Corps of Engineers as may be ordered before it, with a view of determining their fitness for promotion, as contemplated by the Act of Congress approved October 1, 1890.— Par. 5. *S. O. 261, A. G. O., Washington, D. C.,* November 7, 1890.

By direction of the Secretary of War, CHARLES T. ALEXANDER, *Lieutenant-Colonel and Surgeon*, and JOHNSON V. D. MIDDLETON, *Major and Surgeon*, are appointed members of a Board of Officers to meet, at the call of the senior officer thereof, at the rooms of the Board of Engineers, Army Building, New York City, to examine such officers of the Corps of Engineers as may be ordered before it, with a view of determining their fitness for promotion, as contemplated by the Act of Congress approved October 1, 1890.— Par. 4. *S. O. 261, A. G. O., Washington, D. C.,* November 7, 1890.

By direction of the Acting Secretary of War, leave of absence for four days is granted WILLIAM D. CROSBY, *Captain and Assistant Surgeon*.— Par. 1, *S. O. 259, A. G. O., Washington,* November 5. 1890.

LA GARDE, LOUIS A., *Captain and Assistant Surgeon*.—Is detailed as a member of a Board for duty in connection with the World's Columbian Exposition, and will report by letter to Major Clifton Comly, Ordnance Department, member of the Board of Control and Management of the Government Exhibit to represent the War Department.— Par. 1, *S. O. 260, A. G. O., Washington,* November 6, 1890.

BACHE, DALLAS, *Lieutenant-Colonel, Surgeon, and Medical Director Department of the Platte*.—Is granted leave of absence for one month.— Par. 6, *S. O. 82, Department of the Platte,* Omaha, Nebraska, November 1, 1890.

OFFICIAL LIST OF CHANGES IN THE STATIONS AND DUTIES OF THE MEDICAL CORPS OF THE U. S. NAVY FOR THE WEEK ENDING NOVEMBER 8, 1890.

EDGAR, J. M., *Passed Assistant Surgeon*.—Ordered to the U. S. S. "San Francisco," November 10, 1890.

SPRATLING, L. W., *Assistant Surgeon*.—Ordered to the U. S. S. "San Francisco," November 10, 1890.

WHITE, CHARLES H., *Medical Inspector*.—Ordered to the U. S. S. "San Francisco," November 10. 1890.

SCOTT, HORACE B., *Passed Assistant Surgeon*.—Placed on the Retired List, October 31, 1890.

ASHBRIDGE, RICHARD, *Passed Assistant Surgeon*.—Surveyed and sent to Hospital, Philadelphia, Pa.

KENNEDY, R. M., *Assistant Surgeon*.—Detached from Navy Yard, League Island, and ordered to the U. S. Training-ship "Richmond."

ATLEE, L. W., *Assistant Surgeon*.—Ordered to the Navy Yard, League Island, Pa.

EXTRA EDITION.

MEDICAL NEWS.

A WEEKLY MEDICAL JOURNAL.

Vol. LVII. No. 20.
Whole No. 981.   SATURDAY, NOVEMBER 15, 1890.   SUPPLEMENT.   Per Annum, $4.00.
Per Copy, 10 Cents.

KOCH'S DISCOVERY.

SPECIAL CABLE DISPATCH TO THE MEDICAL NEWS.

A FURTHER COMMUNICATION ON A CURE FOR TUBERCULOSIS.[1]

BY PROFESSOR ROBERT KOCH, M.D.,
OF BERLIN.

IN an address delivered before the International Medical Congress I mentioned a remedy which conferred on the animals experimented upon an immunity against inoculation with the tubercle bacillus, and which arrested tuberculous disease. Investigations have now been carried out on human patients, and these form the subject of the following observations. It was originally my intention to complete the research, and especially to gain sufficient experience regarding the application of the remedy in practice, and its production on a large scale before publishing anything on the subject; but in spite of all precautions, so many accounts have reached the public, and in such an exaggerated and distorted form, that it seems imperative, in order to prevent false impressions, to give at once a review of the position of the subject at the present stage of the inquiry. It is true that this re-

view can, under these circumstances, be only brief, and must leave open many important questions.

The investigations have been carried on under my direction by Dr. A. Libbertz and Stabsarzt Dr. E. Pfuhl, and are still in progress. Patients were placed at my disposal by Professor Brieger, from his polyclinic; Dr. W. Levy, from his private surgical clinic; Geheimrath Drs. Fräntzel and Oberstabsarzt Kohler, from the Charite Hospital; and Geheimrath v. Bergmann, from the surgical clinic of the University. I wish to express my thanks to these gentlemen.

As regards the origin and the preparation of the remedy, I am unable to make any statement, as my research is not yet concluded. I reserve this for a future communication.[1]

The remedy is a brownish, transparent liquid, which does not require special care to prevent decomposition. For use, this fluid must be more or less diluted, and the dilutions are liable to undergo

---

[1] Translated from the original article published in the Deutsche medicinische Wochenschrift, November 14th, 1890.

[1] Doctors wishing to make investigations with the remedy at present, can obtain it from Dr. A. Libbertz, Lueneburger Strasse, 28, Berlin, N. W., who has undertaken the preparation of the remedy with my own and Dr. Pfuhl's coöperation, but I must remark that the quantity prepared at present is but small, and that larger quantities will not be obtainable for some weeks.

decomposition if prepared with distilled water. As bacterial growths soon develop in them they become turbid, and are then unfit for use. To prevent this, the diluted liquid must be sterilized by heat and preserved under a cotton-wool stopper, or, more conveniently, prepared with a one half per cent. solution of phenol.

It would seem, however, that the effect is weakened both by frequent heating and by mixture with phenol solution, and I have therefore always made use of a freshly-prepared solution. Introduced into the stomach the remedy has no effect. In order to obtain a reliable effect it must be injected subcutaneously, and for this purpose we have exclusively used the small syringe suggested by me for bacteriological work. It is furnished with a small India-rubber ball and has no piston. This syringe can easily be kept aseptic by the use of absolute alcohol, and to this we attribute the fact that not a single abscess has been observed in the course of more than a thousand subcutaneous injections.

The place chosen for the injection, after several trials of other places, was the skin of the back between the shoulder-blades and the lumbar region, because here the injection led to the least local reaction—generally. none at all, and was almost painless. As regards the effect of the remedy on the human patient, it was clear from the beginning of the research that in one very important particular the human being reacts to the remedy differently from the animal generally used in experiments, namely, the guinea-pig. A new proof for the experimenter of the all-important law that experiment on animals is not conclusive, for the human patient proved extraordinarily more sensitive than the guinea-pig. As regards the effect of the remedy, a healthy guinea-pig will bear a subcutaneous injection of 2 cubic centimetres, and even more, of the liquid without being sensibly affected ; but in the case of a full-grown healthy man 0.25 cubic centimetre suffices to produce an intense effect. Calculated by the body-weight, one-fifteen-thousandth part of the quantity which has no appreciable effect on the guinea-pig acts powerfully on the human being.

The symptoms arising from an injection of 0.25 cubic centimetre I have observed after an injection made in my own upper arm. They were briefly as follows : three to four hours after the injection there came on pain in the limbs, fatigue, inclination to cough, difficulty of breathing, which speedily increased in the fifth hour, and were unusually violent. A chill followed, which lasted almost an hour. At the same time there were nausea, vomiting, and a rise of body temperature to 39.6° C.

After twelve hours all these symptoms abated, the temperature fell, and on the next day it was normal. A feeling of fatigue and pain in the limbs continued for a few days, and for exactly the same period of time the site of injection remained slightly painful and red. The smallest quantity of the remedy which will affect the healthy human being is about 0.01 cubic centimetre, equal to 1 cubic centimetre of the one-hundredth dilution. As has been proved by numerous experiments, when this dose is used reaction in most people shows itself only by slight pains in the limbs and transient fatigue. A few showed a rise of temperature to about 38° C.

Although the effect of the remedy in equal doses is very different in animals and in human beings, if calculated by body-weight, in some other respects, there is much similarity in the symptoms produced, the most important of these resemblances being the specific action of the remedy on the tuberculous process, the varieties of which I will not here describe. I will make no further reference to its effects on animals, but I will at once turn to its extraordinary action on tuberculosis in human beings. The healthy human being reacts either not at all, or scarcely at all, as we have seen, when 0.01 cubic centimetre is used. The same holds good with regard to patients suffering from diseases other than tuberculosis, as repeated experiments have proved ; but the case is very different when the disease is *tuberculosis*. A dose of 0.01 cubic centimetre injected subcutaneously into tuberculous patients causes a severe general reaction as well as a local one.

I gave children aged from two to six years onetenth of this dose, that is to say, 0.001 cubic centimetre—very delicate children only 0.0005 cubic centimetre—and obtained powerful, but in no way dangerous, reaction. The general reaction consists in an attack of fever, which usually begins with rigors, and raises the temperature above 39°, often up to 40°, and even 41° C. This is accompanied by pain in the limbs, coughing, great fatigue, and often sickness and vomiting. In several cases a slight icteroid discoloration was observed, and occasionally an eruption like measles on the chest and neck The attack usually begins four to five hours after the injection, and lasts from twelve to fifteen hours. Occasionally it begins later and then runs its course with less intensity.

The patients are very little affected by the attack, and as soon as it is over feel comparatively well, generally better than before. The local reaction can be best observed in cases in which the tuberculous affection is visible; for instance, in cases of lupus, changes take place which show the specific anti-tuberculous action of the remedy to a most surprising degree. A few hours after an injection into the skin of the back—that is, in a spot far removed from the diseased area on the face or elsewhere—the lupus begins to swell and to redden, and this it does generally before the initial rigor. During the fever the swelling and redness increase, and may finally reach a high degree, so that the lupus-tissue becomes brownish and necrotic in places where the growth was sharply defined. We sometimes found a much swollen and brownish spot surrounded by a whitish edge almost one centimetre wide, which again was surrounded by a broad band of bright red.

After the subsidence of the fever the swelling of the lupus-tissue gradually decreases and disappears in about two or three days. The lupus-spots themselves are then covered by a soft deposit, which filters outward and dries in the air. The growth then changes to a crust, which falls off after two or three weeks, and which—sometimes after only one injection—leaves a clean, red cicatrix behind. Generally, however, several injections are required for the complete removal of the lupus-tissue; but of this, more later on. I must mention as a point of special importance that the changes described are exactly confined to the parts of the skin affected with lupus. Even the smallest nodules and those most deeply hidden in the lupus-tissue go through the process and become visible in consequence of the swelling and change of color, whilst the tissue itself in which the lupus-changes have entirely ceased remains unchanged. The observation of a lupus-case treated by the remedy is so instructive. and is necessarily so convincing, that those who wish to make a trial of the remedy should, if possible, begin with a case of lupus.

This specific action of the remedy in these cases is less striking, but is as perceptible to eye and touch as are the local reactions in cases of tuberculosis of the glands. bones, joints, etc. In these cases swelling, increased sensibility, and redness of the superficial parts are observed. The reaction of the internal organs, especially of the lungs, is not at once apparent, unless the increased cough and expectoration of consumptive patients after the first injections be considered as pointing to a local reaction in these cases. The general reaction is dominant; nevertheless, we are justified in assuming that here, too, changes take place similar to those seen in lupus-cases. The symptoms of reaction above described occurred, without exception, in all cases in which a tuberculous process was present in the organism after the use of 0.01 cubic centimetre, and I think I am justified in saying that the remedy will, therefore, in the future, form an indispensable aid to diagnosis.

By its aid we shall be able to diagnose doubtful cases of phthisis; for instance, cases in which it is impossible to obtain certainty as to the nature of the disease by the discovery of bacilli or elastic fibres in the sputum or by physical examination. Affections of the glands, latent tuberculosis of bone, doubtful cases of tuberculosis of the skin, and similar cases will be easily and with certainty recognized. In cases of tuberculosis of the lungs or joints which have been apparently cured we shall be able to make sure whether the disease has really finished its course, and whether there be still some diseased spots from which it might again arise as a flame from a spark hidden by ashes.

Of greater importance, however, than its diagnostic use, is the therapeutic effect of the remedy. In the description of the changes which a subcutaneous injection of the remedy produces in portions of the skin affected by lupus, I mentioned that after the subsidence of the swelling and decrease of the redness the lupus-tissue does not return to its original condition, but that it is destroyed to a greater or less extent and disappears. Observation shows that in some parts this result is brought about by the diseased tissue becoming necrotic, even after but one sufficiently large injection, and at a later stage it is thrown off as a dead mass. In other parts a disappearance or, as it were, a necrosis of the tissue, seems to occur, and in such case the injection must be repeated to complete the cure.

In what way this process of cure occurs cannot as yet be stated with certainty, as the necessary histological investigations are not complete ; but this much is certain, that there is no question of a destruction of the tubercle bacilli in the tissues, but only that the tissue inclosing the tubercle bacilli is affected by the remedy. Beyond this there is, as is shown by the visible swelling and redness, considerable disturbance of the circulation, and, evidently, in connection therewith, deeply-seated changes in its nutrition which cause the tissue to die more or less quickly and deeply, according to the extent of the action of the remedy. To recapitulate, the remedy does not kill the tubercle bacilli but the tuberculous tissue, and this gives us clearly and definitely the limit that bounds the action of the remedy.

It can influence living tuberculous tissue only, and has no effect on dead tissue ; as, for instance, necrotic cheesy masses, necrotic bones, etc., nor has it any effect on tissues made necrotic by the remedy itself. In such masses of dead tissue living tubercle bacilli may possibly still be present, and are either thrown off with the necrosed tissue, or may possibly enter the neighboring and still living tissue under certain circumstances of the therapeutic activity. If the remedy is to be rendered as fruitful as possible this peculiarity in its mode of action must be carefully observed. At first the living tuberculous tissue must be caused to undergo necrosis, and then everything must be done to remove the dead tissue as soon as possible, as, for instance, by surgical interference. Where this is not possible, and where the organ-

ism is unassisted in throwing off the tissue slowly, the endangered living tissue must be protected from fresh incursions of the parasites by continuous applications of the remedy. The fact that the remedy makes tuberculous tissue necrotic and acts only on the living tissue, helps to explain another peculiar characteristic thereof, namely, that it can be given in rapidly-increasing doses. At first sight, this phenomenon would seem to point to the establishment of tolerance, but since it is found that the dose can, in the course of about three weeks, be increased to five hundred times the original amount, tolerance can no longer be accepted as an explanation. As we know of nothing analogous to such a rapid and complete adaptation to an extremely active remedy, the phenomenon must rather be explained in this way, that in the beginning of the treatment there is a good deal of tuberculous living tissue, and that consequently a small amount of the active principle suffices to cause a strong reaction, but by each injection a certain amount of the tissue capable of reacting disappears, and then larger doses are necessary to produce the same amount of reaction as before.

Within limits, a certain degree of habituation may be perceived as soon as the tuberculous patient has been treated with increasing doses, for so soon as the point is reached at which reaction is as feeble as that of a non-tuberculous patient, then it may be assumed that all tuberculous tissue is destroyed. Then the treatment will only have to be continued by slowly-increasing doses and with interruptions in order that the patient may be protected from fresh infections while bacilli are still present in the organism, and whether this conception and the inference that follows from it be correct, the future must show. They were conclusive, as far as I am concerned, in determining the mode of treatment by the remedy which in our investigations was practised in the following manner. To begin with the simplest case—lupus.

In nearly every one of these cases I injected the full dose of 0.01 cubic centimetre from the first. I then allowed the reaction to come to an end, and then, after a week or two, again injected 0.01 cubic centimetre, continuing in the same way until the reaction became weaker and weaker, and then ceased. In two cases of facial lupus the lupus-spots were thus brought to complete cicatrization by three or four injections; the other lupus-cases improved in proportion to the duration of treatment.

All these patients had been sufferers for many years, having been previously treated unsuccessfully by various therapeutic methods. Glandular, bone, and joint tuberculosis was similarly treated, large doses at long intervals being made use of. The result was the same as in the lupus-cases—namely, a speedy cure in recent and slight cases, slow improvement in severe cases.

The circumstances were somewhat different in phthisical patients, who constituted the largest number of our patients. Patients with decided pulmonary tuberculosis are much more sensitive to the remedy than those with surgical tuberculous affections.

We were obliged to diminish the dose for the phthisical patients, and found that they almost all reacted strongly to 0.002 cubic centimetre, and even to 0.001 cubic centimetre. From this first small dose it was possible to rise more or less quickly to the amount that is well borne by other patients. Our course was generally as follows: an injection of 0.001 cubic centimetre was first given to the phthisical patient, and from this a rise of temperature followed, the same dose being repeated once a day until no reaction could be observed. We then increased the dose to 0.002 cubic centimetre, until this was borne without reaction, and so on, increasing by 0.001, or at most 0.002 to 0.005, cubic centimetre.

This mild course seemed to be imperative in cases in which there was great debility. By this mode of treatment the patient can be brought to tolerate large doses of the remedy with scarcely a rise of temperature. But patients of greater strength were treated from the first partly with larger doses and partly with frequently-repeated doses. Here it seemed that the beneficial results were more quickly obtained. The action of the remedy in cases of phthisis generally showed itself as follows: Cough and expectoration were generally increased a little after the first injection, then grew less and less, and in the most favorable cases entirely disappeared. The

expectoration also lost its purulent character and became mucous. As a rule, the number of bacilli decreased only when the expectoration began to present a mucous appearance. They then entirely disappeared, but were again observed occasionally until expectoration completely ceased. Simultaneously the night-sweats ceased, the patients' appearance improved, and they increased in weight within from four to six weeks.

Patients under treatment for the first stage of phthisis were freed from every symptom of disease and might be pronounced cured; patients with cavities not yet too highly developed improved considerably and were almost cured, and only in those whose lungs contained many large cavities could no improvement be proved. Objectively, even in these cases the expectoration decreased and the subjective condition improved. These experiences lead me to suppose that phthisis in the beginning can be cured with certainty by this remedy. This statement requires limitation in so far as at present no conclusive experiences can possibly be brought forward to prove whether the cure is lasting.

Relapses naturally may occur, but it can be assumed that they may be cured as easily and quickly as the first attack. On the other hand, it seems possible that, as in other infectious diseases, patients once cured may retain their immunity; but this, too, for the present, must remain an open question. In part, this may be assumed for other cases, when not too far advanced; but patients with large cavities, who suffer from complications caused, for instance, by the incursion of other pus-forming microörganisms into the cavities or by incurable pathological changes in other organs will probably obtain lasting benefit from the remedy in only exceptional cases. Even such patients, however, were benefited for a time. This seems to prove that in their cases, too, the original tuberculous disease is influenced by the remedy in the same manner as in the other cases, but that we are unable to remove the necrotic masses of tissue with the secondary suppurative processes.

The thought involuntarily suggests itself that relief might possibly be brought to many of these severely-afflicted patients by a combination of this new therapeutic method with surgical operations (such as the operation for empyæma), or with other curative methods, and here I would earnestly warn people against conventional and indiscriminate application of the remedy in all cases of tuberculosis. The treatment will probably be quite simple in cases in which the beginning of phthisis and simple surgical cases are concerned, but in all other forms of tuberculosis medical art must have full sway by careful individualization and making use of all other auxiliary methods to assist the action of the remedy.

In many cases the decided impression was created that the careful nursing bestowed on the patient had a considerable influence on the result of the treatment, and I am in favor of applying the remedy in proper sanataria as opposed to treatment at home and in the out-patient room. How far the methods of treatment already recognized as curative, such as mountain climate, fresh-air treatment, special diet, etc., may be profitably combined with the new treatment cannot yet be definitely stated, but I believe that these therapeutic methods will also be highly advantageous when combined with the new treatment. In many cases, especially in the convalescent stage, as regards tuberculosis of the brain and larynx, and miliary tuberculosis, we had too little material at our disposal to gain proper experience.

The most important point to be observed in the new treatment is its early application. The proper subjects for treatment are patients in the initial stage of phthisis, for in them the curative action can be most fully shown, and for this reason, too, it cannot be too seriously pointed out that practitioners must in the future be more than ever alive to the importance of diagnosing phthisis in as early a stage as possible. Up to the present time the proof of tubercle bacilli in the sputum was considered more as an interesting point of secondary importance, which, though it made diagnosis more certain, could not help the patient in any way, and which, in consequence, was often neglected.

This I have lately repeatedly had occasion to observe in numerous cases of phthisis, which had generally gone through the hands of several doctors without any examination of the sputum having been made. In the future this must be changed. A doctor who shall neglect to diagnose phthisis in its earliest stage by all methods at his command, especially by examining the sputum, will be guilty of the most serious neglect of his patient, whose life may depend upon the early application of the specific treatment. In consequence, in doubtful cases, medical practitioners must make sure of the presence or absence of tuberculosis, and then only will the new therapeutic method become a blessing to suffering humanity, when all cases of tuberculosis are treated in their earliest stage, and we no longer meet with neglected serious cases forming an inextinguishable source of fresh infections. Finally, I would remark, that I have purposely omitted statistical accounts and descriptions of individual cases, because the medical men who furnished us with patients for our investigations have themselves decided to publish the description of their cases, and I wished my account to be as objective as possible, leaving to them all that is purely personal.

KOCH'S DISCOVERY.

THE cablegram which forms this extra edition is one which contains, in all probability, the seed of a discovery the extent of whose fruit cannot be grasped by the human mind, and which bids fair to surpass the triumph of Jenner in his warfare against smallpox. Unlike variola, which occurs in epidemics, the great white plague, consumption, has year after year, with far more fearful results, swept off millions of human beings, until every hamlet and village has learned to speak of it with bated breath.

It is not for us, knowing so little of the true nature of Koch's studies, to decide at this time as to the future of his methods. Not improbably many of the profession may be conservative enough to declare their utter lack of faith in all such work. On the other hand, there is the ever-present need in medicine of sufficient thoughtfulness to avoid following every new idea with feverish haste, and while we can regard the man and his work with pride, it behooves us to reserve our opinions until time discloses the more minute workings of his methods.

It also seems appropriate that the leading medi-·cal weeklies of each of the great Anglo-Saxon races, THE MEDICAL NEWS and *British Medical Journal*, should be the first to present this subject in an authoritative manner to their countrymen on the same day that the author publishes his original copy in the *Deutsche medicinische Wochenschrift.*

Removal of the Gall-bladder.—TERRIER (*Bull. de l'Académie de Médecine*) records his second cholecystectomy, both operations being successful. The operation has been performed only five times in France. Dr. Terrier's last patient was a woman aged fifty-years who had suffered from exceedingly severe attacks of hepatic colic for twenty-six years. The liver was enlarged, but the gall bladder could not be felt, and there was no jaundice until just before the operation, when the usual signs of biliary obstruction appeared. As these symptoms were not relieved by the usual remedies and as death seemed probable the abdomen was opened. The incision was made in the right linea semilunaris and the distended gall-bladder easily found. It was adherent to the omentum but was easily detached. About one pint of viscid, almost colorless, fluid was drawn off. A number of calculi were then removed with difficulty, after which the neck of the gall-bladder was ligated and the body and fundus removed. The abdomen was closed in the usual manner, a medium-size drainage-tube being inserted. After the operation a large quantity of bile escaped through the tube and there was much vomiting, but the patient made a complete recovery.

M. Terrier thinks that in cases in which the gall-bladder is very large the median incision would be preferable. The separation of the gall-bladder from the liver may be followed by free oozing which can be checked by pressure with a sponge or by the thermo-cautery. Large vessels can be lightly tied.—*British Medical Journal*, October 18, 1870.

Psorospermosis.—DR. BOECK (*Monatshefte f. praktische Dermatologie*, September, 1890) presented the following case of psorospermosis to the Society of Physicians of Christiania. The patient, a man aged forty-seven years, had suffered from the disease for sixteen years. Scattered over nearly the entire surface of the body was an eruption of papules, varying in size from a millet- to a hemp-seed, which were covered with epidermic scales. The case was a typical example of Darier's *psorospermose folliculaire végetante.*

Microscopical preparations were shown in which there were numerous encysted coccidia in the epithelium, especially in the stratum granulosum. Where the process was severe the epidermis became detached from the papillary body in such a measure that only single rows of cells covered the latter. Dr. Boeck also presented to the Society at a subsequent meeting two more cases of the disease, both the patients being sons of the patient mentioned above, evidence in favor of the contagiousness of the disease. The eruption in the sons occupied the same sites as in the father. Dr. Boeck said that the disease, when not of not of too long duration, was amenable to treatment, and that therefore treatment should be commenced early. In one of the recent cases pyrogallic acid ointment was applied with success ; in the other case no treatment had been adopted.—*British Medical Journal*, October 18, 1890.

Sunflower in Malarial Fevers.—DR. V. N. ZUBOVITCK (*Vratch*) has administered sunflower to a number of cases of malarial fever. He used the remedy in the form of a tincture of either the fresh flowers or the fresh bark of young stems. To an adult a liqueur-glassful was given three times daily, the administration being continued for two or three days after the complete cessation of the paroxysms. With others, Dr. Zubovitch finds (1) that the sunflower treatment is invariably followed by a complete and permanent cure in from three to ten days, even in inveterate cases in which quinine has utterly failed ; (2) that all types of malarial poisoning are equally amenable to this treatment ; (3) that during the administration of the sunflower no unpleasant symptoms of the drug are manifested other than occasional profuse night-sweats ; (4) that the tincture of the flowers seems to act more quickly than that of the bark.—*St. Louis Medical and Surgical Journal*, November, 1890.

Treatment of Epithelioma of the Face with Acetic Acid.—At a recent meeting of the French Society for Dermatology and Syphilography ARNOZAU reported eight cases of epithelioma of the face commencing in the sebaceous glands, that were treated by local applications of acetic acid. The applications were made with a piece of wood, a glass rod, or, if the disease was extensive, with a brush. In some cases the acid was used every second day ; in others, every day ; and in still others, several times daily. During the first sittings crystallized acetic acid diluted one-half or two-thirds with water was used ; later the pure acid was applied. The treatment causes sharp burning, which, however, is of short duration. The eschar produced by the acid at first adheres closely, then begins to loosen at the edges, and the applications should be continued until the crusts drop off and leave a healthy, granulating surface. The granulations then begin to cicatrize, and finally leave a small scar. The patient can carry out the treatment himself.—*Occidental Medical Times*, November, 1890.

The Removal of Freckles.—The *Pharmaceutical Record* quotes the following prescriptions for removing freckles:

R.—White precipitate ⎱ of each 1 drachm.
　　Bismuth subnitrate ⎰
　　Glycerite of starch . . 4 ounces.—M.

Apply every second day.

Or,

R.—Sulphocarbolate of zinc . 1 drachm.
　　Glycerin . . . . 2 ounces.
　　Alcohol . . . . 1 ounce.
　　Orange-flower water . . 1½ "
　　Rose water, sufficient to make 8 ounces.—M.

Apply twice daily.

THE MEDICAL NEWS.

THE LEADING MEDICAL WEEKLY OF AMERICA.

THE MEDICAL NEWS to-day presents to its great host of readers a practical illustration of the vast benefits they derive from ideal medical journalism. Modern methods of communication render it possible for a vigilant and complete organization to keep in touch with the most distant centres of medical advance, and possessing both these qualifications, THE NEWS publishes to its readers simultaneously with publication in Berlin, the authentic account of what is possibly the greatest discovery yet made or to be made by man. Should this discovery prove to be what the claims and character of Robert Koch warrant the world in believing, the effects on the destinies of mankind are inconceivable. It is the proud position of THE MEDICAL NEWS to be the leader in disseminating this intelligence throughout the length and breadth of America, not alone to its own subscribers, but in the interests of humanity to great numbers of accomplished physicians who have not hitherto seen the binding obligation of keeping themselves at all times posted on all that may concern their patients.

Tuberculosis, though the chief scourge of mankind, is only one of a vast number of ailments constantly under study by brilliant men in all parts of the globe, and it is the well-executed duty of THE MEDICAL NEWS to keep its readers armed at all points with the latest knowledge for use not only against this, but against all other diseases as well. Such enterprise is only rendered possible by the coöperation of vast numbers of readers, and each new subscriber increases the power of his medical newspaper for doing good to all his fellow-men, and at the same time derives personal benefits vastly disproportionate to the small outlay involved. Such an investment is in the highest sense profitable, bearing weekly dividends each exceeding the principal in quantity of value, and in quality only to be estimated by the benefits conferred by the most enlightened medical science upon present and future generations.

ORDER BLANK

LEA BROTHERS & CO PUBLISHERS, 706 & 708 Sansom Street, Philadelphia.

Enclosed find remittance for .... Dollars,
for which please send me, from date of receipt, to December 31st, 1891—

(1)—THE MEDICAL NEWS ($4 00)

(2)—THE AMERICAN JOURNAL OF THE MEDICAL SCIENCES ($4.00)

(3)—THE MEDICAL NEWS and THE AMERICAN JOURNAL OF THE MEDICAL SCI-ENCES ($7.50)

(4)—THE MEDICAL NEWS and THE MEDICAL NEWS VISITING LIST for 1891 ($4.75)

(5)—THE AMERICAN JOURNAL OF THE MEDICAL SCIENCES and THE MEDICAL NEWS VISITING LIST for 1891 ($4.75)

(6)—THE MEDICAL NEWS and THE YEAR-BOOK OF TREATMENT for 1891 (ready early in 1891), ($4 75)

(7)—THE AMERICAN JOURNAL OF THE MEDICAL SCIENCES and THE YEAR-BOOK OF TREATMENT for 1891 ($4.75)

(8)—THE MEDICAL NEWS. THE AMERICAN JOURNAL OF THE MEDICAL SCIENCES, THE MEDICAL NEWS VISITING LIST for 1891 and THE YEAR-BOOK OF TREATMENT for 1891 ($8.50)

Name ....

Town ....

ERASE WHAT IS NOT WANTED.

THE MEDICAL NEWS.

A WEEKLY JOURNAL OF MEDICAL SCIENCE.

VOL. LVII.　　　　SATURDAY, NOVEMBER 22, 1890.　　　　No. 21.

ORIGINAL ARTICLES.

INGUINAL COLOTOMY, WITH THE REPORT OF A CASE.[1]

BY ARCH DIXON. M.D.,

OF HENDERSON, KY.

ON June 19, 1890, I was requested by Dr. P. H. Griffin to examine a case of suspected fæcal impaction with consequent obstruction.

The patient, a man, aged twenty-two years, tall and spare, had a previous history of frequent and long-continued attacks of constipation, which yielded to treatment within a short time. On June 12th, Dr. Griffin was called to see him in one of these attacks, and found what he supposed to be a fæcal impaction in the sigmoid flexure. There was intense pain, radiating throughout the abdomen, and most marked in the left inguinal region. The usual remedies were prescribed, but without relief. On June 13th, in addition to calomel followed by castor oil, large enemata of hot water were used, which increased the pain and caused only a small discharge of fæcal matter. Opiates were given and purgatives administered each day with no relief, he having taken on the day previous to my first visit about a pint of castor oil and fully as much Epsom salt. I found him with a pulse of 140, temperature 102°, respiration 36; and with tympanites and general tenderness over the abdomen. Under a careful examination no tumor could be detected, but on passing the finger into the rectum a bulging of the bowel, with a teat-like protuberance extending below the sigmoid flexure, could be felt. The gut was entirely occluded. Dr. Griffin's attention was called to this fact, and colotomy was proposed as the only method of relief. The length of time which had elapsed since the obstruction began, nearly eight days, almost precluded the possibility of recovery, yet I deemed the operation a justifiable one if only to relieve pain. Dr. Griffin concurred in this opinion.

Two hours later, assisted by Drs. John Young Brown, P. H. Griffin, William A. Quinn, and medical student Arch Dixon, Jr., the operation was done. On making the usual incision the small intestine bulged through the opening, but was pushed back and retained by a flat sponge. Two fingers of the right hand were introduced, the rectum found and followed up to the sigmoid flexure, where a distinct tumor could be felt blocking the entire gut. Further examination by breaking adhesions and drawing the tumor through the

incision, which had to be slightly enlarged, showed that the obstruction was due to volvulus at the sigmoid flexure. The gut was twisted upon itself and lapped over like the end of a tobacco "twist." Adhesions had formed and were so firm that the lumen of the bowel was entirely destroyed, a solid tumor remaining in its place. The intestine was intensely congested, dark and purple, and near the tumor was almost black. The questions of stitching the colon to the edges of the incision and immediately opening the gut, or of resecting the tumor, closing the rectum, dropping it back into the cavity and stitching the other cut end to the incision, at once presented themselves. At this juncture, in manipulating the tumor and testing the firmness of the adhesions, a slight tear was made in the gut immediately above the tumor, through which a small quantity of liquid fæcal matter escaped. This decided the question. The colon was immediately clamped above and below the tumor (phimosis forceps covered with rubber tubing being used as clamps) about two inches above and one inch and a half below the tumor. The rectal end of the intestine was first cut, its edges were turned in and stitched with Lembert sutures of fine silk, dusted with iodoform, and dropped back into the cavity. The same procedure was followed above, entirely removing the tumor. The cut edges of the colon were carefully stitched to the walls of the incision. Upon removing the clamp there was a gush of liquid fæcal matter through the opening, which continued for a short time. The abdominal cavity was irrigated with hot water through the opening left for the removal of the clamp and sponge, until the water returned clear and pure. The opening was then closed and a pad of iodoform-gauze was placed over the artificial anus, and covered with borated cotton, the dressing being retained by a many-tailed binder, the use of which was suggested by my friend, Dr. L. S. McMurtry. The patient was then put to bed with hot bottles around him.

Reaction was fairly good, and on the next morning the man expressed his thanks for the relief afforded him, he having had no pain since the operation. His condition, however, was not promising. Pulse 140, temperature 100°, and respiration 36. Abdominal tenderness was not marked, but there was a condition of exhaustion, which gradually increased until death took place at 9.50 P.M., June 20th, thirty-one hours after the operation.

In regard to the treatment of this case before I saw it, comment is unnecessary. The questions are, whether under the circumstances. the operation was a justifiable one, and whether resecting the gut, closing the rectal end and dropping it into the

---

[1] Read before the Mississippi Valley Medical Association, Louisville. Ky.. October 9 1890.

cavity, and the formation of an artificial anus at the incision, after the manner of Madelung, were to be preferred to stitching the colon to the walls of the incision and making an immediate opening into the gut without regard to the tumor formed by inflammatory adhesions. Taking everything into consideration, the almost gangrenous condition of the bowel at the site of the obstruction, the tear through which fæcal matter had escaped, the doubt that the wall of the gut would hold the stitches, and the fear of leaving a gangrenous tumor within the cavity, all of which were strong arguments in favor of the graver operation. I feel justified in the course pursued, even if nothing more was accomplished than relieving the patient from the terrible agony which he was suffering.

Some general remarks on the operation of colotomy may not be out of place here, especially as there seems to be a difference of opinion among surgeons in regard to the superiority of the two methods—*lumbar* and *inguinal*.

During the past decade the subject of colotomy, always one of interest, has received much attention from the surgical world. The revival of Littré's operation, so long debarred by the dread of opening the peritoneum, has made it necessary to compare the merits of the extra- (so-called) and intra-peritoneal methods. Littré, in 1710, first proposed to open the sigmoid flexure for the relief of imperforate anus in children, but there is a doubt as to his having peformed the operation. At all events, the operation seems to have been forgotten until revived by Pilloré, of Rouen, in 1776, who operated by a different method, opening the cæcum by an incision in the right inguinal region.

In 1796 Callisen suggested an operation whereby the colon might be entered without opening the peritoneal cavity. He experimented on the cadaver and endeavored to expose the bowel where it was not covered by peritoneum, by a vertical incision in the left lumbar region; failing in this, he made an attempt to carry out his idea on the living subject.

To Amussat unquestionably belongs the credit of having first performed the retro-peritoneal operation, which was done upon the right side through a transverse incision, with the result of five successes in six cases.

In this country, Ashmead, of Philadelphia, did a left lumbar retro-peritoneal colotomy in 1842, being unaware at the time of his operation of Callisen's proposal.[1]

Until recently the operation has usually been a combination of the methods of Callisen and Amussat. Like Callisen's, it was done on the left side;

and like Amussat's, it was carried out through either a transverse or an obliquely transverse incision. The oblique incision, first recommended by Bryant, is now adopted by most surgeons.

Colotomy may be performed for any condition which obstructs the passage of the fæces through the colon, or under any circumstances in which it is advisable to place the bowel at rest. Obstruction may be produced by various causes, such as cancer of the rectum or sigmoid flexure, or of any other part of the colon; tumors of the peritoneum or of any abdominal organ, pressing on the bowel; volvulus of the sigmoid flexure, of the cæcum or of the ascending colon; and by fæcal accumulations and collections of foreign matter. Colotomy may be called for in cases of incurable ulceration of the bowel, however induced, if we have reason to believe that the irritation caused by the fæces and the movements of the intestinal walls contribute to the continuance of the disease, and also in cases of extreme dilatation, with atony of the colon, giving rise to frequent attacks of obstruction.

As a measure to ward off imminent death, colotomy is required in all cases of obstruction of the colon from whatever cause. For imperforate anus the operation holds a special position. It is intended to prevent impending death, and it may or may not be regarded as a cure for the disease. In many cases it is the first step in the process of cure. In every infant born with imperforate anus an operation in the anal region is first attempted; if this fails, colotomy is performed to prevent death. Later, an attempt may be made to cause the bowel to discharge through the anus. In a few words, it may be said that the indications to operate in any given case depend, in the first place, on the chance which the patient has to recover without operation; and, in the second place, upon the probability of success following the operation. To cases of acute obstruction of the sigmoid flexure, or elsewhere in the intestines, there is practically but one termination—death. No case of volvulus, whether of the large or the small intestine, has as yet been known to recover under purely medicinal treatment. Here, then, the indication is clear enough, as clear, Grieg Smith[1] says, as the indication in a case of bleeding from the carotid artery—operation.

But, in the case reported above, it may be said that while the patient had no chance of recovering without operation, yet there was no probability that success would follow the operation, owing to the length of time that the attack had lasted. But it was no fault of mine that the operation was not done sooner, and at the time of operating it was known that there was little, if any, chance of saving

---

[1] Greig Smith. Abdominal Surgery, Second edition.

[1] Loc. cit.

life, but that relief from the intense pain was certain. It, was under such conditions that the operation was proposed and consented to. It accomplished all that I expected, for, from the moment the patient came from under the influence of the anæsthetic until death took place, there was no pain.

Now as to the comparative merits of the two methods of operating. As I have said before, the operation of inguinal colotomy is not new; it was suggested one hundred and eighty years ago, but it was left to modern surgery to simplify the procedure, to lay down fixed rules for its performance, and to carry it almost certainly to a successful issue. The indications for its performance are the same as those for the lumbar method, which I am confident it will supersede. In a recent paper,[1] I find that so good a man as Dr. Mathews, the President of the Mississippi Valley Medical Association, in speaking of colotomy, uses the following language: "It is not the purpose of this paper to discuss the question *pro* or *con*, but it is safe to say, that with English and American surgeons, only one operation —lumbar colotomy—is looked upon as justifiable."

In view of the fact that such surgeons as Treves, Chavasse, Reeve, Kelsey, Cripps, the Allinghams, and others, advocate the *inguinal* in preference to the *lumbar* operation, this statement must be looked upon as rather sweeping. Dr. Mathews further says: "It does not seem at all plausible to say that with any method of operating, as much safety can be had in opening the peritoneum as in not opening it. If antiseptic surgery makes inguinal colotomy so very safe, why is it not logical to say that it also renders the lumbar operation doubly safe as compared with other ways."

Is it true that in the lumbar operation the peritoneum is never opened? On the contrary, is it not true that in a large majority of the cases the peritoneum *is opened?*

H. W. Allingham, Jr., in an interesting paper on the causes of failure to find the colon in the operation of lumbar colotomy, and the way to obviate them,[2] says:

"The difficulties sometimes met in finding the large bowel, and the occasional cases in which serious errors have been made, are known to all; and all will agree that unless one of the longitudinal muscular bands, which are invariably, and only, found in the large intestine, be seen, the intestine should not be opened from the loin. These bands are described as being situated: one on the anterior surface, another along the inner part, and the third at the posterior aspect of the gut. It is this posterior band that is looked for, and generally supposed to be seen when searching for the bowel in the lumbar region. It is thought by some authorities that these bands can be easily detected without opening the peritoneum; but this is not so, except in a very few cases.

¹ Medical Progress, July, 1890.
² Annual of the Universal Medical Sciences, vol. iii., 1889.

The author finds, from examination and dissection of over one hundred ascending and descending colons, that the bands are always more easily and distinctly seen when they are covered by the peritoneum, which makes them hard, prominent, and shiny; whereas, when the peritoneum is stripped from them, these characteristics are lost. He admits that in eight cases out of one hundred examined, one or two of these bands could be seen, but not very distinctly, on the posterior part of the intestine, although they were uncovered by peritoneum. When the peritoneum covers only about one-half or two-thirds of the circumference of the gut, it is generally reflected from the gut at the longitudinal bands to the walls of the belly. Thus, unless the peritoneum is stripped off, the bands are not visible. If an attempt is made to expose the longitudinal fibres, the peritoneum, owing to its being so firmly adherent to them, is frequently torn, and the peritoneal cavity opened, perhaps, unknown to the operator. It is argued, in favor of lumbar colotomy, that the large intestine can be reached without opening the abdominal cavity. This, of course, is possible, yet it is much more important to make certain that the large intestine is being opened by first seeing the longitudinal bands. *This, from the anatomical points mentioned, can only be done by opening the peritoneum.*" (Italics are my own.)

Moreover, Mr. Allingham, proves that only by finding the bands can the large intestine be known with certainty in most cases. His conclusions are strengthened by three cases, in which he operated on the right side in the dead subject, it afterward appearing that if he had not looked carefully for the longitudinal bands, the descending portion of the duodenum would have been opened instead of the large intestine, an accident that occasionally happens in operating on the living.

Again, the position of the colon may be an abnormal one. In one hundred cases Treves found it out of its usual position on the right side in twenty-six cases, and in the same number of cases he found it out of its usual position on the left side in thirty-six. In eleven cases out of sixty Allingham found it out of position on the right side, and on the left side in ten out of sixty. Thus the general average of anomalous positions is, on the right side, eighteen and one-third cases, and, on the left side, sixteen and two-thirds out of one hundred. From this it would appear that the normal position of the gut is less common than generally supposed. With the intestine in its normal position, and when a longitudinal band uncovered by peritoneum can be seen, all should go well in the lumbar operation. But when no bands can be seen, the safest distinction between the large and the small intestine is wanting, and in such cases Mr. Allingham considers it more advisable to open the peritoneum and search for a portion of the intestine with longitudinal bands than to run the risk of opening the small intestine under the impression that the peritoneum has not been opened, and that it is the large intestine which is being dealt with. Mr. Allingham further says: "The colon may be entirely surrounded by firmly-adherent peritoneum, and may have a comparatively short mesentery, in which condition it is absolutely impossible to reach it, or to see the longitudinal bands without first opening the peritoneal cavity." The colon was found by Mr. Treves to vary in length on the right side in twenty-six cases out of one hundred, and on the left side in thirty-six cases out of one hundred. Mr. Allingham observed the same variation in forty-nine cases out of sixty on the right side, and in fifty cases out of sixty on the left—a percentage on the right side of eighty-one and two-thirds, and on the left side of eighty-three and one-third. In cases in which the mesentery is very long, the intestine, though it may usually be in the loin, can so change its position that when operating on either side it may lie on the side of the belly opposite to that in which the incision is made. Thus absolute certainty that it is the large, and not the small, intestine, or the stomach, that is to be opened, is imperative. The presence of the appendices epiploicæ may inform the surgeon that he has found the large intestine, but these are not as important as the longitudinal bands, since the appendices may not exist on the piece brought to view. Mr. Allingham does not advocate lumbar colotomy when it is possible to perform inguinal colotomy, for the lumbar is certainly the more difficult operation, the patient runs greater risk, and recovers less quickly, and the after-results are not as satisfactory.

Kelsey says: "Allingham does not emphasize the point which he renders so plain, that when the lumbar operation is performed with these necessary precautions to make sure that the colon is the part opened, it loses its only supposed advantage over the inguinal—the non-interference with the peritoneal cavity."

Mr. Allingham gives the following reasons for thinking inguinal colotomy preferable to lumbar colotomy[1]:

1. The position of the patient is better at the time of operation, for himself, the operator, and the anæsthetist.

2. There is not so much tendency for the gut to fall away from the wound, either at the time of or after the operation.

3. The intestine is easier to find, chiefly because the incision is high. The results of five hundred post-mortem examinations are quoted to verify this statement.

4. The fæces do not pass below the artificial opening if a good spur is made.

5. There is less constitutional disturbance.

6. There is little or no suppuration.

7. The tendency for the opening to contract is not greater.

Chavasse, of Birmingham, advances the following reasons for prefering the inguinal to the lumbar operation: [1]

1. It is readily performed.

2. The patient is easily able to attend to his or her wants in connection with the false anus.

3. The patient is able to lie on his back without discomfort.

4. In malignant disease four or five inches more of the colon are left for the performance of its duties.

5. Being nearer the seat of the disease the operator is able to ascertain, if necessary, the precise limits of the growth.

As a matter of experience, Chavasse states that he has always found that the opening in the sigmoid flexure has been sufficiently remote from the neoplasm not to become implicated during life. Malignant disease of the flexure, except at its juncture with the rectum, is of rare occurrence. Up to the time of writing his paper he had performed inguinal colotomy thirteen times without a death.

Cripps[2] records the results obtained by him in 37 operations, 15 of which were lumbar and 22 inguinal, with 2 deaths, a mortality of more than 5 per cent. The mortality of colotomy has been very great. The analysis of 244 collected cases of lumbar colotomy made by Batt in 1884, gave a mortality of 32 per cent., while the inguinal operation gave a mortality of more than 50 per cent. These statistics, he thought, represented the results up to that period, but they are misleading as an indication of what may be expected of the operation at the present time. Batt regards colotomy as an operation of great delicacy, requiring accurate anatomical knowledge and manipulative skill. The preparation of the patient, the hygienic surroundings, and the subsequent treatment óf the wound all demand most careful consideration, and materially influence the result. His chief objections to the lumbar operation are as follows:

1. The absence of sufficient working space between the lower border of the last rib and the crest of the ilium.

2. Difficulty in the identification of the bowel in the limited space, as it is sometimes impossible to recognize the longitudinal bands, and numerous instances are recorded in which the small bowel, the duodenum, or even the stomach has been opened by mistake.

3. In fat or muscular patients, the difficulty owing to the depth of the bowel and its want of mobility, in fixing the colon to the skin without undue tension.

---

[1] Annals of Surgery, vol. vii. p. 460.

[1] Lancet, February, 1889.
[2] Annual of Universal Medical Sciences, vol. iii., 1890.

4. Abnormal deviations, rendering it impossible to find the bowel by this incision.

5. Inconvenience of the posterior opening for cleanliness and the adjustment of pads.

Inguinal colotomy obviates all these objections by affording a practically unlimited space in front, and an incision through which the bowel can be carefully inspected and identified by its longitudinal bands, by its convoluted surface, and by its appendices epiploicæ. The mobility of the sigmoid flexure and the laxity of the skin prevent the difficulty of fixing the bowel without undue tension. The ease with which thorough exploration of the cavity can be made through the incision removes all difficulties attending the abnormal course of the colon. This method also possesses the advantage of enabling the surgeon to verify the diagnosis by free exploration.

The objections urged against inguinal colotomy are that there is a tendency of the bowel to prolapse, and that it is unsuitable for urgent cases. The first objection can be overcome by drawing down the bowel to its full extent, and the second is believed to be more imaginary than real.

Madelung[1] recommends that the colon be completely cut through; the lower opening being closed and returned, the upper opening being sutured to the skin. At the meeting of the British Medical Association at Leeds, Mr. F. Marsh showed a patient on whom he had performed this operation with a very satisfactory result.

Cripps's operation is performed as follows:[2] The patient having been carefully prepared by a bath and by cleansing of the operative surface, an incision two and a half inches long and one and one-half inches from the anterior-superior spine of the ilium is made across an imaginary line drawn from the anterior-superior spine to the umbilicus (Fig. 1). In order to make the opening somewhat valvular, the skin should be drawn a little inward and the tissues divided until the peritoneum is reached; the peritoneum should then be picked up and incised to nearly the full length of the cutaneous incision. The colon being found, a loop of it is drawn into the wound, and, if loose folds of the sigmoid flexure remain immediately above the opening, it should be drawn down and passed through the fingers into the cavity at the lower angle. When all the gut has passed through the fingers, two provisional ligatures of stout silk are inserted into the longitudinal muscular bands opposite the mesenteric attachment, two inches apart. The bowel is now temporarily returned to the cavity, and the parietal peritoneum is sutured to the skin, on each side of the incision, by two

[1] International Medical Annual, 1890.
[2] British Medical Journal, April, 1890.

sutures of fine Chinese silk, one and one-half inches apart (Fig. 2), after which the bowel is fixed to the skin and parietal peritoneum by seven or eight fine sutures on each side—the last sutures, one at each angle, crossing from one side to the other in such a manner as to leave two-thirds of the circumference of the bowel external to the sutures. The sutures for the lower side should be passed through the lower longitudinal band, as this is a strong portion of the bowel. Those for the upper portion should be inserted close to the mesenteric attachment (Fig. 3). It is best to pass all of the sutures and then tie them with moderate tension in the order inserted. In urgent cases the bowel can be opened at once; in other cases, the opening may be delayed until the fifth or sixth day, when it is usually found covered with a surprisingly thick layer of lymph.

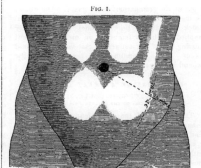

FIG. 1.

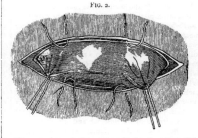

FIG. 2.

The provisional ligatures will be found useful guides, the bowel being opened the full length between them. The superfluous flaps on either side should be trimmed with scissors to the level of the skin. All sutures may be removed by the ninth day, or earlier if there is redness around them. If the bowel is not opened immediately, a piece of protective should be placed over it to prevent adhe-

FIG. 3.

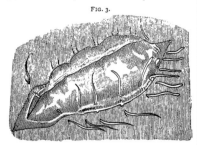

sions of the granulations to the gauze. The wound is then dressed antiseptically, with an additional thick pad and a broad flannel bandage firmly applied. This is important in order to prevent tearing out of the sutures in case vomiting should occur. During vomiting firm pressure upon the wound is of great value.

THE ABUSE OF A GREAT CHARITY.

BY GEORGE M. GOULD, M.D.,
OPHTHALMOLOGIST TO THE PHILADELPHIA HOSPITAL.

THE abuses of the out-patient departments of many of our city hospitals have become so manifold and so outrageous that public silence is no longer a virtue. Some definitive measure of therapeutics, either social, legislative, or surgical, must at once be devised and made effective.

In brief and in general the facts seem to be something like the following :

The motive in the hearts of the founders and supporters of hospitals was, and is, to aid the deserving poor, who have been visited by the misfortune of disease or physical injury, to have their diseases and wounds healed free of charge by the best medical skill. This must ever remain a most commendable charity, to be deprived of which would be sad for civilization. Few things speak so clearly of the highwater-mark in practical religion and morality reached by the modern world, and it is the unique honor of the medical profession which in this respect no other profession can rival, that this beneficent work is effected by the unselfish and unpaid labor of men who make no claim of merit or show of faith. The burden of this writing is an astounding proof that these noble men have been absurdly generous of their service, and have become the victims of their transcendent unselfishness. What explanation of the abuse under discussion I, or any other, may offer, whatever alloy of baser motives and intermix-

ture of sin may be proved, it will forever remain the glory and honor of medicine, and, indeed, of humanity, that in an age of sordidness and self-seeking so many men have given daily life-long service to humanity without money and without price, with a zeal equalled only by the early Christian missionaries, and with a modest quietness that even they could not rival. These facts may serve to paralyze the finger of shame or scorn pointed at the medical profession by any other, justifying rather a touch of pity at the tangle we have got ourselves into.

In the beginning a distinction should be sharply drawn. Of the in-patient departments, or hospitals proper, nothing disparaging may be said. Barring a few exceptional and curable abuses connected with them, they fulfil their duties with exceptional excellence. But many patients are able to visit the hospital for treatment, and without becoming the recipients of the further charity of bed and board, return at once to their homes and business. Such are called out-patients, and the rooms or departments where the treatment of such patients is carried out constitute the out-patient departments. The physicians and attendants of these departments visit them on specified hours and days, and usually have little or no other relations with the hospital. The out-patient department is thus seen to be an after-thought and outgrowth, sometimes a morbid excrescence upon the body of the true hospital, or in-patient department. When the out-patient is in truth too poor to pay for treatment, or when his disease, if neglected in any way, threatens the welfare of the community, it will at once be conceded that it is the community's right and duty to care for such a patient.

But, with this praiseworthy practice has grown up a most execrable abuse. There has of late been widely circulated a paragraph of some statistician to the effect that in 1889 there were 214,000 charity patients treated in one so-called "pauper city" of the Eastern States. In the great Northern and Central Hospital of England the number of out-patients treated in one year, three years ago, was, in round numbers, 10,000. In 1889 it was 15,563, 3,000 more than during the previous year. According to the *Scotsman*, out of a population of 236,000 in Edinburgh, 103,095 are relieved by medical charities, a percentage of 43. In Glasgow, the proportion is much less, showing that to local custom is largely due the difference in medical pauperization. Mr. Smith claims that in Manchester the abuse of medical charities has been reduced from 42.32 per cent. in 1880 to 6.89 per cent. in 1889. The most conservative medical journal we have, the *Lancet*, says that "everyone admits that the number of hospital patients has grown at a rate fourfold greater than that of the population." In our country no reliable statistics are at hand, but no one would deny that the *Lancet's* estimate is as low as it possibly could be made. The proportion is probably much greater. It cannot be contended that disease has increased to the same extent, because statistics indubitably prove that diseases are less numerous and less fatal than formerly, and that human life is being lengthened by medical science. We touch the quick and lay bare the root of the trouble when we find that a large proportion, if not a majority, of these hundreds of thousands of charity cases could pay for medical treatment were they not shamelessly pauperized by the unasked gratuity held out to them by these institutions. An innate vice of human nature seems to be the desire to get something without paying for it, and the kind-hearted must always be on the strictest guard that want is real, and suffering not assumed. The degradation of patient and of physician is in full operation, and what was once honorable both to give and receive has become alike dishonorable to receive and to give.

First, as to the patient. Due to the indiscriminating methods of the gift, it is fast becoming a settled conviction that the hospital is in some way a governmental or State institution. Most patients are surprised when told that the physicians who treat them never receive a cent from the city, the State, or from anyone. If told that all hospitals are built and supported by the gifts of kind-hearted people, the service is still considered as one to which they have a perfect right, and arrogant feelings are betrayed by every look, word, and gesture. Gratitude either to the unknown giver or to the physician is rarely shown, though this is frequently if not generally, due to the dictatorial way the patient is treated. To illustrate the manner in which the matter is viewed by the out-patient, I may allude to the case of a woman who had been in a hospital, but who could not afford the loss of time required by the hospital treatment. She did not object to paying me fifteen dollars for the three visits made at my office. The hospital she had gone to was one of the rare examples in which there is even a routine of questioning as to the patient's ability to pay for medical attention. She had been told by her friends to wear her shabbiest clothes, and in answer to any query to aver that she was unable to pay. This she did, and she laughingly added that it was the general custom of her neighbors to proceed in this manner. Every clinician has numberless recollections of similarly ludicrous or disgusting instances of how women come dressed far more richly than the doctor's wife could afford to dress, of absurd pretensions, and innumerable trickeries. That he is but getting his just due the patient learns to believe by the many subtle processes of self-deception and

21*

cunning whereby men always learn to justify lack of self-dependence. Custom and habit conclude the facile descent to Avernus. "What's the use of paying when we can get it for nothing?" is the unanswerable curbstone logic. No lesson of history and social science is more horribly true than that indiscriminate almsgiving is a crime against God and man, debauching alike both giver and receiver, and multiplying the evil it would thoughtlessly cure. The Roman senators had the mob's dreadful cry, *Panem et Circenses!* in their ears as Rome went to her death, and to our modern demagogic legislation we are adding morbid forms of private charity to teach men loss of self-control and self-help. To free medical advice, free treatment, and free drugs, it is even seriously proposed to add, to the out-patient's ruin, free lunches and free soup.

Not only morally, but medically, the practice has its baneful effect upon the patients. They flock to the hospital in such numbers that the visiting physician has often to treat, or pretend to treat, from thirty to seventy-five per hour. It is the acme of folly and nonsense. "Snap diagnoses" must be made and medicines delivered as if by machinery. Formulæ are kept printed and numbered and are hurried to the druggist, who has the compounds already made and labelled. Upon the appearance of certain symptoms, that might as well be ticketed No. 1, 2, 5, etc., formula 3, 6, or 8 is shot out as if by a nickel-in-the-slot machine, with the exception, of course, of the nickel justice. Every careful physician detests such things, and there is probably some shame in the hearts of everyone who finds himself doing them. A friend told me yesterday that a boy came to him who had made the rounds of several hospitals—there is a large class of folk descriptively termed the "rounders"—and who continuously complained of pain in the side. No other physician had had the time or conscientiousness to examine the boy thoroughly, but had given him salicylates for probable muscular rheumatism. My friend, with some reluctance at the loss of time, quickly had the boy's clothing removed, and at once found curvature of the spine! Possibly this may be an extreme and humiliating example, one not frequently occurring; but every hospital physician will tell you that such examples are entirely too frequent, and that the like may take place many times each day. In almost every case the out-patient cannot get the careful treatment that he should have, and that he would get if the physician's services were paid for. Moreover the patient who can run to the hospital every time he imagines himself to have even the slightest ailment, soon learns to neglect the simplest hygienic rules upon which health depends, quickly falling into habits of self-indulgence, over-reliance upon the doctor, chronic hospitalism, and querulousness.

To the physician, also, the injury is quite as plain. Men spend their early years and their own or parents' savings in laborious study and unflagging zeal to prepare themselves for a life-work that at best is full of arduous duty and toil, that offers no brilliant financial results and demands the best that its devotees can give. When they enter upon their career they find that the older physicians treat, free of charge, thousands and hundreds of thousands of patients who could pay something, and that the younger physicians who need encouragement and practice, and to whom these patients would naturally fall, are left to starve for years, until somehow, by the grace of God, the accidents of chance, or the wiles of scheming, they wriggle into a properly-compensated practice. It is brutally unjust to the young practitioner. It is also as entirely unjust to the suburban and country practitioner, who every day finds that his patients and neighbors have gone to the city hospital and have been treated for nothing. He well knows that he could have treated them more carefully and scientifically at home than the overworked city doctor (perhaps his college class-mate) can do in the over-crowded out-patient department. And he knows how able to pay these patients may be. It is highly ungenerous and selfish on the part of those who, having established their practice and feeling financially secure, are able to give an hour or two of each day to treating hundreds of patients without compensation for the poor satisfaction of vanity or to cull from many routine and uninteresting cases one that is rare and "interesting." It is but fair to state that this injustice is unparalleled in any other profession. There are no law hospitals or charity courts where legal advice and counsel may be had for the asking. The young lawyer is not at the outset of professional life met with such an outrageous indignity. Is health worth less to men than property and legal rights? Why should those who give their lives to medicine not be paid for their work?

Several strange and indirect evils result from these crowded out-patient departments. Students and young physicians are taught by conceit, example, and necessity to make hurried, "snap" diagnoses, to treat diseases by memorized prescriptions and the rule of thumb, mechanically, carelessly, and hastily. Every careful physician well knows how fatally un-scientific and full of errors such procedures must be. Disease is neither understood nor cured in that manner. Finally, it may be noted that the crowded out-patient room is a bad school of manners. Both ungentleness and ungentlemanliness are almost necessary. A mob of folk have to be handled in a great hurry, and dictatorial manners, harsh commands, and discourtesy are too frequently the result.

How and why has the abuse arisen? It may be accounted for as the combined result of several confluent causes, among which, as has been intimated, must never be forgotten the tender solicitude and unselfish kindness toward the sick on the part of medical men generally. But other reasons are not hard to find. First in importance is the carelessness of almsgivers and testators in failing to demand, and in vigilance to see, that their donations do not become a source of injustice to the medical profession and of corruption to the patient. The physician has never advocated payment for his own services, and the efficacy of the charities of the rich has always been dependent upon the greater charity of the physician. When once the necessity of carefully guarding against this abuse of kindness becomes generally recognized, almsgivers may be relied upon to correct the wrong. Men are kind, and are willing to relieve unmerited and even merited misfortune and suffering, but nothing more quickly shuts the hand and freezes the sympathies than the knowledge that the one you are helping secretly thinks you a fool for doing it, that the method of helping unwittingly increases the evil, and that kindness to one is a greater unkindness to another.

The trustees and managers of hospitals are often largely at fault. Every institution has something in its charter or regulations prohibiting the abuse and guarding against its happening. Subscriptions could hardly have been secured without such an understanding on the part of the donors. But whatever may be said to the contrary, and with some honorable exceptions, it might as well be frankly stated that these rules and regulations are widely ignored. Not one hospital in twenty even asks if the patient is or is not able to pay something for his treatment. And if asked, when the desired and to-be-expected answer in the negative is returned, the investigation is deemed at an end, though the answer is a manifest falsehood. Could human nature, under such circumstances, be expected to resist the temptation to lie? Some far more exhaustive and effective method of getting at the truth than people's own report of themselves has long been recognized as necessary in other forms of charity, and why not in this?

It may strike one as strange, but it is nevertheless a fact, that there is competition among hospitals as furious as it is foolish. The rivalry as to which can do the most good is but a step to that as to which can treat the greatest number of patients. It is a form of the struggle for existence prevalent everywhere, and, as everywhere, it is not always the fittest but the strongest and most unscrupulous that sometimes survives. I have been told that the statistics of hospital reports are by no means always to be trusted. There is a laudable and there is a foolish pride in relieving the poor. The managers and residents must justify their office and their hopeful promises. The "source of supplies" is not averse to entertaining the pleasing thought that he is doing a world of good, and that his gift has not been tied up in a napkin. Such things tend to increase carelessness, indiscrimination, and general sentimentalism. The bidding for patients in the general competition is not seldom frank and unconcealed. The yearly report that shows the greatest number and variety of patients makes the breasts of donor, superintendent, and physician swell with pride and their eyes snap with partisan satisfaction. How easy, under such circumstances, for the abuse to thrive and wax strong.

Sometimes, nay, generally, a "chromo is given with each purchase;" that is to say, most hospitals also dispense medicines without charge. Frequently it is right to do so, but frequently it is mere competition. How can one institution charge even the smallest fee for drugs when its rival does not? It would soon lose its "patrons."

Perhaps the best motive underlying the abuse, and coming the nearest to justifying it, is the desire for "clinical material" for teaching purposes. Hospitals that are not used by medical teachers cannot make this excuse; but they feel the rivalry of those that are so used, and bidding for patients becomes almost a necessity. Schools of medicine must be located in cities where clinical examples of disease are numerous and easy to obtain. Students must see and know disease in order to recognize it in the future in all its forms and to treat it intelligently. Every school of medicine must therefore have its hospital and stimulate its out-patient department to the degree required by this necessity. Whatever may work to this end without too great abuse and too much injustice to others may be conceded as right and necessary. It may even be admitted that a large number of patients must be attracted in order to glean the desired types and illustrative examples of certain diseases. And yet we speedily come to neglected discrimination and unnecessary abuse. For the honor of medicine and of the school there should be in every case attracted a leisurely and careful diagnosis and scientific therapeutics, and such schools should not allow themselves to be drawn into competition with the dispensary and the advertising hospital. There is too frequently an unseemly hunger for the curiosities, the exaggerated anomalies of disease—the "interesting cases." Lecturers are prone to show such cases for teaching purposes. They serve at once to command the students' attention and display the professorial erudition. But there can be no doubt that, for the students' good, the commonest types of disease are precisely those he should see and study most.

It is these that he will soonest and oftenest have to treat when in practice; and if he is well prepared the anomalous case will soon classify itself. The most common should be emphasized as the most "interesting."

Yet another source of the evil may be found in the desire of the visiting physician, whether teacher or not, to see a large number of patients, and thus to study disease in its infinite diversity. To this may be added his desire for increased operative skill and dexterity of hand to be gained by much practice, the perfected technique, the lessons to be derived from errors and mistakes, the confidence in self derived from a large experience, and the subtle self-flattery and self-satisfaction in handling large numbers of men and the awful issues of life and death.

And, since the whole truth were better frankly told, another, and possibly most active, though subtle, stimulant of the out-patient abuse is the desire of the chief and his assistant physicians to build up indirectly a private practice. It is well known that no medical man is permitted by the code of professional ethics to advertise. Let it become suspected that a physician is permitting the use of his name by the reporters of the daily papers to spread the knowledge of his skill and the fame of his cures, and at once a blight falls upon him. It is impossible thereafter to rehabilitate his reputation. He has taken a mean advantage of his more honorable brethren, and, as many a doctor who should have been a politician or a stock-broker has learned, medicine is not commercialism or politics. This fact puts the sordid ambitious doctor at a disadvantage in the race for professional fame; but without the strict preservation of this ethical principle, ambitious sordidness would soon gain limitless success and scientific medicine would be at an end. But the fact serves indirectly to multiply the number of the dispensaries and out-patient departments. The older men are in charge of the larger and better institutions, and, of course, "they never resign or die." The younger are handicapped, and, fretting under the fact, they manage to start rival dispensaries. In becoming the head of such a clinical department the visiting physician is able to spread the knowledge of his name through the district whence his patients come, and the practice at his office soon increases. By one means or another charity-patients at the hospital become pay-patients at the private office. The patient loses much time at the hospital, meets unpleasant people, sees unpleasant sights, is barbarously "bossed" about, etc. At the private office it is very different. The hospital becomes a "feeder" to the private practice in more ways than this. I have known it to be frankly admitted that this is the design and the habit, justification being found for the same in many ways. Whether acknowledged or not, and whether flagrant or subtle, the motive and its execution are all too prevalent. Sentiment—*vulgariter*, "the charity racket"—is "worked" to furnish the financial prerequisites of the undertaking, of which the secondary object alone is the alleviation of human suffering.

By inference I have suggested or alluded to some of the baneful results of the out-patient abuse. In part they may be recapitulated as follows :

1. Encouraging pauperism, dependence, and deceit in a large class of the community already too fatally prone to depend upon the State or charity instead of upon prudence or self-help. This is but one of several reasons that would justify summoning the case before the public as a jury.[1]

2. The abuse, if longer ignored, will soon reach such extreme exaggeration, that when the knowledge of its enormity finally bursts upon the community, all forms of related praiseworthy and necessary charity will be chilled, and the efficiency and usefulness of true hospital work rendered impossible from the lack of funds caused by the disgust of testators and of the charitable, at the misuse of their endowments and the abuse of their kindness.

3. A double injury—first to the patient from a hurried and routine diagnosis and treatment, and secondly to the physician, his science, and his skill, from not patiently studying disease, and not conscientiously applying the proper remedy.

4. The degradation of the profession by turning its practice into a sort of medical "free lunch counter," by encouraging envy and subtle methods of advertising, and by preventing the younger and the country practitioners from rising in their work, and depriving them of their proper *clientèle*. To these things may be added the multiplication and yet deeper abuse of one of the reactions already in full swing in every city, the custom of the doctor to own a drug store, and to give advice and prescriptions free, on condition that the medicine shall be bought at his store.

What is the cure ? A number of cures have been proposed, and the following have been, or are being tried :

1. That the competition idea be thoroughly car-

[1] A year ago I gave to the editor of a medical journal, a personal friend, a little article having the same general tenor and purpose as the present one ; but he refused to publish it on the ground that the abuse did not exist, and that even if it did exist, I would injure my standing among my professional brothers by calling in the public as witnesses of it. I replied that no one could love my profession better than I, and that the very veneration in which I held it nerved me to brave the possible scorn of a few interested or narrow-minded partisans. There can now be no doubt about the extent of the abuse, even *The Lancet* admitting and deploring it. It will certainly not be cured by ignoring it.

ried out—*à toute outrance*. This means that every practitioner who wishes, or who can, shall rent a room in as conspicuous place as possible—perhaps, get a church to give him the use of one for sentimental reasons, or a drug-store for financial reasons— and advertise to the uttermost the free treatment— and doctor. A beautiful spectacle [1]

2. The purgatorial plan—a compromise between heaven and hell—that is, out-patient departments where all who are treated are expected to pay something, as little as they must, as much as they will, or with a regular minimum fee of, say, ten to twenty-five cents. A variation of this plan is the medical club formed by a number of members who secure a physician's services at a low club-rate, either per visit or per annum. The design is favorable to the self-respect of the better poor, and gives the attendant some sort of financial justice. It has the excellent advantage of putting the relations of doctor and patient on some basis of mutuality, of encouraging courtesy, and of discouraging slipshod haste and treatment. It is open to the great liability of failure that purgatory itself is subject to—it is neither one thing nor the other. Those lost to self-respect will go elsewhere, and keep their money for beer and ribbons. Those who can pay a little will usually be able to pay a modest fee at the private office.

3. The establishment of charity days or hours at the private office, when all who come will be treated free of charge. This plan is open to all the objections that the hospital abuse suggests, and to many more besides.

4. The sliding scale at the private office, the fee depending upon the patient's circumstances, the lowest honorarium being demanded in the case of the very needy. Willingly or unwillingly, this plan is *de facto* largely pursued, assuring the sensitive poor a desired and desirable protection and privacy, and the kind-hearted advisers a privilege few like to deny themselves.

These four ways pertain to the individual judgment and action of each physician. But, as may readily be divined, the evil will never come to an end by individual action. The abuse is a huge and corporate one, and it has so slowly and blindly drifted to its present low level that only a wide knowledge and a combined harmonious action on the part of many can adjust and remedy it.

It would naturally seem that the pride and honor of the medical profession would spur to an activity of immediate and effective therapeutics. Just what should or will be the nature of such a remedy no single person would be sufficiently venturesome to say. But assuredly the remedy lies openly in the hands of medical men and medical societies ; assuredly one swift word from these sources would right the whole matter. That, so far, the Profession has made no effort in this direction, and that it so commonly denies the fact of the abuse, argues ill for its self-healing power. A fatal anæsthesia seems to characterize as well as mask the symptoms of the disease. The successful practitioner is satisfied with the *status præsens*, the unsuccessful is afraid or powerless. In the meantime the disease grows visibly worse. The sting in the sneer, *Physician, heal thyself!* has lost its hurt. It is well known that when ill a physician never treats himself, but calls in a brother practitioner. Perhaps, also, the rule would work well in the case now in hand. If so, and while awaiting a more concerted and effective method of therapeutics, it might not be amiss to prescribe a general prophylactic measure, a codicil to all wills and bequests running somewhat as follows :

"And I further direct that the fact of the acceptance of the stated moneys, bequests, and gifts, by the trustees of the above-mentioned hospitals, dispensaries, and charitable institutions, shall of itself be the warrant and guarantee upon their parts of a solemn promise that no patient shall receive medical treatment, advice, or medicines within or under authority of the same, who does not bring proof of his poverty and of his deserving from the Charity Organization Society, or who in some other equally certain and convincing way does not demonstrate that he is unable to pay for such medical advice, treatment, and medicines. And I further direct my heirs and executors to withhold the payment of all such bequests and gifts from those institutions whose trustees will not enter into such an agreement, or from such as may at any future time fail to carry out such agreement, or who, in any way, fail to exercise the most stringent care that the sick who receive the benefit of this bounty shall be needy, deserving, and worthy persons, the subjects of misfortune not by their own gross crime or fault."

Postscript.—Since the above was written, and just as it was sent to the printer, the *Lancet*, in a leading editorial, attacks the abuse, using much the same arguments as I have advanced. It says, *inter alia :* "The absence of any effective inquiry into the fitness of patients is monstrous. What would be thought of a poor-law system which gave relief without inquiry? It would be denounced as immoral and demoralizing. It is not otherwise with voluntary charities. . . Much efficiency may be dearly bought at the expense of the medical profession in the first place. and of the demoralization of the poor in the second. The wide disapproval of it has been too long disregarded by hospital governors, and we fear we must add. to some extent by medical teachers."

TREATMENT OF INFANTILE CLUB-FOOT PRELIMINARY TO OPERATION.[1]

By F. H. MILLIKEN, M.D.,
of Philadelphia.

THE purpose of this paper is to offer some suggestions regarding the treatment to be used in cases of club-foot before proceeding with the final operations of tenotomy and osteotomy. Not infrequently we hear of tenotomy, and even of osteotomy, being performed on the feet of infants not more than two or three months old. This is premature practice, and is attended with disadvantages which result from the fact that the muscles of the feet have not been used.

In a congenital, or in an early acquired case of talipes, the bones, tendons, and ligaments are distorted and displaced, and although tenotomy may be performed, and the feet twisted into their normal position, yet, as the members do not assume their proper functions until the child walks, it must remain for many months an open question whether a further resort to the knife may not be necessary. Although success is attained by careful surgeons who personally supervise the subsequent manipulative and mechanical treatment of these cases, it cannot be denied that relapses are more frequent among very young infants than among older ones who received surgical assistance at about the time they began to use their feet and legs.

The fact that a relapsed case of talipes is always difficult to correct should make us hesitate to perform a cutting operation until other and simpler means have been tried, but if resort to the knife is the only alternative, the operation should be performed at the age when the child would begin its efforts to walk. Although it is advisable to postpone cutting operations until near this time, other means should not be neglected, and, if possible, the child should be helped to use its limbs properly without any operation.

Happily, malformation of the limbs is readily recognized at birth, and no time need be lost in using such means as the surgeon may decide on as most suitable to the case, preliminary to the probable final resort—tenotomy.

At birth the tissues are soft and yielding, and with slight manual force can be helped into their proper places. A case of slight talipes can be relieved by daily manipulations, while the same case, if left to itself for several months, would have a tendency to permanent malformation. Owing to this condition, the machinery of the limb being thrown out of gear. the natural coöperative action of the different mechanical parts being altered, permanent lameness and deformity are established.

[1] Read before the American Orthopædic Association, Philadelphia. September 16. 1890.

Perhaps no better means could be suggested for correcting a case of infantile talipes than holding the child's foot in the correct position until a cure is accomplished. But, as in the nature of things, this is impracticable, the next best course must be adopted. The nurse must be *instructed* to manipulate the foot ten or twenty times a day, bringing it into a correct, or as nearly as possible correct position. Emphasis is placed upon the word *instructed*. It will not do to let the nurse merely see the surgeon manipulate the foot and then imitate the procedure as best she can. The surgeon must see that she understands how to grasp the child's foot, and that she knows in what direction to apply the force. A nurse lacking intelligence enough to understand the surgeon's directions is worse than useless, as illustrated by the following case :

A child under my care suffered from equino-varus with incurvation of the toes. The nurse was instructed to grasp the heel and ankle firmly with her left hand, and the anterior portion of the foot with her right hand. She was shown how to correct the incurvation, and by continuing the force bring the foot into a condition of valgus, if possible. In endeavoring to carry out the instructions, the woman grasped the child's leg above the ankle, took hold of the foot and gave it a wrench that bade fair to rupture the deltoid ligament.

In addition to manipulating the foot, the muscles that control it should not be neglected. Massage and the faradic current should be applied, and here, also, the surgeon must be vigilant to see that his directions have been faithfully carried out. Simple instructions to rub and knead certain parts are likely to be neglected, but if a liniment is ordered with which to do the rubbing, the nurse or mother will use it, and by noticing from day to day the diminution in the quantity of the liniment, the surgeon learns whether the rubbing is done.

Very little dependence can be placed on mothers to aid us in correcting the deformed feet of their children. The child's cries excite sympathy, and hence the manipulations are either abandoned, or are so gently performed as to be of little practical value. In view of this fact mechanical means must be employed to stretch the contracted tissues, and, after stretching, to retain the foot in the corrected position. Perhaps the simplest and most efficient appliance for this purpose is a plaster-of-Paris bandage. In the dispensary of the• Hospital of the University of Pennsylvania, nothing has given so much satisfaction, among infants under the age of one year, as the following method of treatment :

First, we stretch. to the utmost tension consistent with safety, the contracted tissues which are holding the foot in malposition. This is effected by a succession of efforts, using a sufficient amount of force to draw and adjust the parts to the desired position, and then easing off the strain, and repeating it again and again. Continuous tension would probably injure the tissues and prove less efficient.

The tolerance of the feet to the application of force is remarkable. I have frequently felt the tissues tear, and have heard them snap under my hands during my efforts to correct a deformity. This tolerance is most apparent in cases of obstinate and relapsed talipes, in which it is necessary to use powerful levers and wrenches to accomplish the desired result.

After correcting the deformity as far as is possible, by stretching and adjusting the parts, prominent points should be protected by pads of cotton, over which a flannel roller should be smoothly applied. Care must be taken to avoid creases and reverses in applying the flannel bandage, otherwise troublesome sloughs are likely to follow, necessitating an abandonment of the treatment for a time, or the substitution of another dressing. The same caution is applicable in making the first turns of the plaster bandage.

In applying the plaster bandage the turns should be made with a view to correct the deformity by making traction on the roller, *e. g.*, in a case of equino-varus, the bandage should begin at the external malleolus, run diagonally across the top of the foot to the ball of the great toe, thence under the sole to the little toe, and then with a long sweep to the middle third of the leg. This may be repeated until the entire leg and a portion of the thigh are covered. The knee should be bent, otherwise the child is liable to kick the bandage off. The greatest care should be exercised to hold the foot in a correct position while the plaster is setting. It should not be grasped by the hand, as the fingers leave indentations in the soft plaster, and these; when dry, are liable to cause sloughs by pressure on the delicate skin. The palm of the hand should be applied to the sole of the foot, and pressure should be made in a direction opposite to that of the deformity.

Hahn recommends a method by which the foot may be held in a corrected position while the plaster is hardening. One or two layers of plaster are first applied, when the cross-piece of a T-shaped board is placed on the sole of the foot, the ends extending beyond the heel and the toes. The upright of the T projects from the side of the foot. Several turns of the bandage are then made to cover and secure the board. A powerful lever is thus obtained. When the plaster has sufficiently hardened the projecting ends of the T may be removed by means of a saw. I have never used this method, but it seems an efficient one.

Bradford and Lovett in their excellent work recommend that the plaster dressing be renewed every two or three weeks. This, I do not think is often enough. Renewal once a week, or every ten days, gives the surgeon more work, but better results. When the dressing is removed it is advisable to wash the limb with soap and water, and then to rub it vigorously with alcohol, or better still, with fluid extract of hamamelis. Before re-incasing the foot in plaster the deformity must be still further reduced, and this treatment should be practised at each subsequent dressing. A decided improvement of the position of the foot will soon be apparent if the manipulations are properly performed, and more especially if the surgeon be not too timid to use sufficient force to bring the parts into their normal position.

The plaster-of-Paris dressing has been almost universally described as cumbersome, awkward, and unsightly. The criticism is just if the foot is encased in roll after roll of the plaster, but this is not necessary. My own practice is to use a bandage one and a half inches wide. Three, or at most four, layers for the foot, and three for the leg, are sufficient to hold the most obstinate foot in the corrected position. Over this a woollen legging or a stocking may be drawn. The toes should be exposed, thus enabling the mother to note any change in their appearance. If they become cold, or blue, the dressing should be removed at once, but this will not be necessary if the plaster is properly applied.

The plaster dressing is preferable to apparatus that correct the deformity by means of straps, for the reason that pressure is made on the entire foot, whereas, in the Scarpa shoe, and in others made on the same principle, traction is almost entirely confined to straps. These are liable to cause excoriations at the points of contact with the skin, necessitating the removal of the apparatus. Valuable time is thus lost. The only disadvantages in the use of plaster are that electricity, massage, and friction cannot be also employed. It has an advantage, however, possessed by no other appliance —that of not being tampered with or removed by the parents of the child.

Elastic traction is employed in cases of club-foot to aid the weaker muscles, and as a constant force tending to pull the deformed members into place. The well-known apparatus of Barwell may be used, but is objectionable because the urine of the child is liable to soak the dressing. The same principle is carried out by Sayre's shoe, which consists of an ordinary laced shoe, in which the "upper" is replaced by a ball-and-socket joint. This leaves the front of the shoe free to be acted upon by force. Two steel uprights extend from the heel to the upper third of the leg. An elastic strap is attached to the sole of the shoe and extends to a button which is riveted to one or other of the uprights near the knee.

Dr. Willard has introduced a shoe that is equally efficient and less expensive. Instead of a ball-and-socket joint, the shank consists of a piece of thin sole-leather, or of soft "upper" leather, thus permitting free movement in every direction. The brace used with this shoe is an improvement on the simple uprights. Greater leverage is obtained by means of a steel arm which is riveted to the stirrup of the uprights. This arm extends forward, upward, and outward, and has an eye at its free end. Through this eye runs a catgut cord, fastened below to the sole of the shoe, opposite the head of the metatarsal bone, and above it to a piece of elastic webbing. The apparatus is especially useful in cases of varus with incurvation. Another very simple and efficient apparatus, also introduced by Dr. Willard, consists of two pieces of printer's blanket, an elastic band, and two ordinary shoe-strings. The printer's blanket should be from two to three inches in width, and sufficiently long to encircle the foot, and the leg above the calf. The ends of the blanket are pierced with eyes, or lace hooks may be substituted, and the two pieces are laced to the foot and leg with the gum-side next to the skin. The elastic band is then fastened to the laces and stretched between the pieces of blanket. The strength of the bands should be adapted to the requirements of the case. The advantages possessed by this simple dressing are, that owing to the adhesive property of the gum it does not readily slip, and need not be so tightly laced as to interfere with the circulation of the blood. It does not absorb urine or fæces, or cause excoriation of the skin, and can be frequently washed without injury. Best of all, it permits manipulation and the use of electricity without disturbing the dressing. An ordinary shoe can be worn with this dressing, thus concealing it, a point which many mothers appreciate.

In private practice, and among people possessing a fair amount of intelligence, the traction principle is by far the best method of treating infantile club-foot; but in dispensary practice we meet with a different class. Here the directions are not faithfully carried out, and the cases often show little improvement. For this reason the fixed dressing is preferable for dispensary cases.

But neither the fixed dressing nor any other can be entirely depended upon to correct a case of severe club-foot, or to effect a permanent cure without a final resort to the knife. What is here advocated is preliminary treatment only. When the child shows an inclination to walk the proper time has come to perform tenotomy, and then the advantages of the previous treatment will be apparent. The plantar fascia will not require such extensive division: the divided ends of the tendons will not separate so widely, and the deformity can be reduced with comparatively slight force. Besides, with ordinary care there is no fear of a relapse, and the child will be equipped with a more efficient foot than it would have possessed had tenotomy been resorted to earlier.

RACIAL INFLUENCE IN THE ETIOLOGY OF TRACHOMA.[1]

BY SWAN M. BURNETT, M.D., PH.D.,
PROFESSOR OF OPHTHALMOLOGY AND OTOLOGY IN GEORGETOWN UNIVERSITY, OPHTHALMIC AND AURAL SURGEON TO THE GARFIELD AND TO THE PROVIDENCE HOSPITALS, DIRECTOR OF THE EYE AND EAR CLINIC AT THE CENTRAL DISPENSARY AND EMERGENCY HOSPITAL, PRESIDENT OF THE MEDICAL SOCIETY OF THE DISTRICT OF COLUMBIA, WASHINGTON, D. C.

No apology is needed to practical ophthalmologists for bringing forward even the most insignificant suggestion as to the nature, etiology, or treatment of so intractable and disastrous a malady as trachoma ; and the Committee of Arrangements of the Section of Ophthalmology of the International Congress but echoed this sentiment that prevails among the profession in making trachoma one of the principal themes of discussion. Vast as is the literature upon the subject, there is still lacking that which gives us grounds for positive opinions regarding the cause, pathology, and therapeutics of the disease.

The special point that I wish to emphasize and to which I would direct the careful attention of the profession is the essentially dyscrasic nature of the affection. This feature of trachoma seems to have been almost ignored by the majority of those who have dealt with the subject. The oversight can probably be accounted for by the great impetus given to the study of pathological anatomy in all its ramifications within the last three decades, and which has temporarily obscured that larger and more comprehensive view obtained by a study of the disease from the standpoint of its clinical manifestations and its natural history.

We have had many sections of the trachomatous conjunctiva, and bacteriological investigations without number, and yet it cannot be said that there is anything approaching unanimity of opinion as to the pathology or treatment of a disease which, probably next to ophthalmia neonatorum, produces more blindness than any other affection to which the eye is liable.

It is far from my purpose to intimate that these investigations have been valueless. Besides the accurate and positive information that they have given us as to the changes in the conjunctival tissue as a result of the disease, they have had, I think, the negative value of causing us to look outside of the eye for the original cause of the affection.

Trachoma is generally admitted to be an affection *sui generis*. Its course, and particularly its results, are such as are found in no other inflammatory affection of the conjunctiva. The total destruction of the mucous membrane and its conversion into cicatricial tissue are consequences that follow no other inflammation, no matter how severe or how long continued, except, probably, tubercular inflammation. In its course, behavior, and results the dyscrasia bears a stronger resemblance to tuberculosis than to any other morbid process of which we have knowledge, and that great clinician, v. Arlt, in 1854, first noticed the similarity of the two diseases.

Among the more recent changes of opinion, however, toward a wider conception of the nature of the morbid process, was the study of the geographical distribution of the disease by Dr. Chibret,[1] who honored the Congress with a contribution on the subject. The investigation of Farrovelli and Gazzaniga[2] on the geographical distribution of trachoma in the Province of Pavia, and those just published by Reisinger[3] on its distribution in Bohemia, are confirmatory in a general way of the results obtained by Chibret, who found that an altitude of one thousand feet gave a comparative freedom from the disease, and facilitated its cure when present. Other minor contributions from competent persons have confirmed these observations.

At the meeting of the International Ophthalmological Congress, held in New York in 1876, I called attention, for the first time, to the fact that the negro race in the United States seems to enjoy an immunity from trachoma. Further and careful observation among a large negro population since then have confirmed that statement in full. The material of my clinic in Washington is largely composed of negroes either pure or of mixed blood, and among about 6000 cases of eye-disease available for statistical purposes in that race which I have examined, I found but a single instance of genuine, unmistakable trachoma, and three or four of doubtful character. Occasional cases of this disease have undoubtedly been seen in negroes in America, but the experience of such careful observers as White, of Richmond, Va. ; Chisolm, of Baltimore ; Baldwin, of Alabama, and many others who have spoken to me verbally on the subject, is in all essential particulars in accord with my own.

This immunity cannot be attributed to elevation, since all the places mentioned are at or near the sea level ; nor to good hygienic surroundings, for the negroes, with the exception of some of the better class, live in over-crowded rooms, with every possible

[1] Read before the Ophthalmological Section of the Tenth International Medical Congress, held in Berlin, August 3–9, 1890.

[1] Comp. Rend. Copenhagen Congress, 1884.
[2] Annali di Otalmologia, An. xvii. Fasc. 1.
[3] Graefe's Archiv. B. xxxvi., Ab. 1, 1890.

facility for contagion and the spread of infectious disease. The only factor that can be considered is that of race, with its powerful influence in predisposing to or giving immunity from the operation of morbid processes. The influence of race is marked, and I presume will not be doubted by anyone. The negro is known to be less susceptible to malarial fevers and to scarlet fever than is his white brother, but more prone to strumous or scrofulous affections of all kinds. The Hebrew is generally supposed to be particularly liable to glaucoma, while the Irish are peculiarly susceptible to trachoma, and wherever they go they carry this predilection with them, even when the conditions of life are infinitely better than those of their native country.

My first acquaintance with trachoma and its results was in a part of Eastern Tennessee which has an altitude of from eleven hundred to fourteen hundred feet. Thére, among a force of workmen, chiefly composed of Irishmen and negroes, the Irish laborers would have trachoma, often in its worst form, while the negroes associated with them never had the disease. So that an altitude of seven hundred and fifty feet more than is sufficient to give immunity in Europe did not give security to these Irishmen. Farrovelli and Gazziniga also found that altitude was not the only factor, and that trachoma occurred in what was otherwise a very healthy locality.[2]

All of these observations point, it seems to me, to the fact that there must exist in the form of a dyscrasia a predisposition to the disease, just as tuberculosis almost always requires for its development the existence of what is generally known as a "tuberculous predisposition." Trachoma must be something more than a local disease, and it cannot be a purely contagious affection. In fact, there are some who doubt whether it is contagious at all.[1]

This diathesis, while it bears considerable resemblance in certain of its manifestations to tuberculosis and scrofula, must be quite distinct from them in other very important characteristics, for the negro race is very subject to the ravages of both scrofula and tuberculosis, scrofulous affections of the cornea and conjunctiva forming a large percentage of their ocular diseases.

The influence of this view of the pathology of trachoma upon our therapeutics must, it seems to me, be radical. We should cease to treat merely the local manifestation of the disease and should turn our attention to the diathesis lying back of it. We are not yet sufficiently acquainted with the

diathesis to enable us to indicate more than a few points that should be considered in its further study. Among these, climate and particularly altitude seem to be the most important, though it is probable that there are factors other than climate and altitude which will have to be considered. If these views are correct, the placing of trachomatous patients among the best possible hygienic surroundings becomes a matter of necessity.

JOINT-INJURIES OF THE UPPER EXTREMITIES.[1]

BY CHARLES D. BENNETT, M.D.,
OF NEWARK, N. J.

JOINT-injuries are always serious, even when the apparent and immediate damage is slight. So much of a person's usefulness is dependent on the free and natural movements of the joints, that any study of articular injuries, or any time spent in considering their treatment, cannot be thought wasted.

The results of treatment are always plainly shown in joint injuries. Vicious union of a fractured bone may usually be hidden by some device of dress, but a stiff joint or an unreduced dislocation is a permanent impairment of power and a disfigurement that cannot be concealed. And as all of our more delicate manipulations are performed by the upper extremities, so will a mistake in diagnosis or carelessness in treatment be here most apparent.

The cases recorded in this paper, gleaned principally from the records of St. Michael's Hospital, illustrate some of these conditions. They are reported, not because they are rare or peculiarly interesting, but because they are actual experiences, and afford some idea of what may occur in the experience of any practitioner.

CASE I.—H. D., forty-five years old, was brought to the hospital, September 10, 1877, by her attending physician, for an opinion. Four months previously she had fallen, twisting her arm under her.

The injury was treated as a sprain until about two weeks previously, when another physician was consulted, who doubted the original diagnosis, and brought her for examination.

Examination revealed a fracture through the condyles of the humerus and backward dislocation of the radius. The joint was firmly ankylosed, and the adhesions could not be broken up. She was sent away with the advice to let the arm alone.

CASE II.—C. B., aged ten years, came to the hospital, August 15, 1877. In the preceding June the patient, while wrestling, fell with his arm back of him, striking the elbow. On rising, he could not move the elbow-joint, and had considerable pain. He was seen by a physician, who did not recognize the injury, and who treated him with

---

[1] Professor George C. Kober, of Washington, who has had an extensive experience in Northern California, informs me that he has frequently seen trachoma at an altitude of 4700 feet, particularly among the Indians.

[2] Vanneman, Annales d'Ocul., January and February, 1889.

---

[1] Read before the Newark Medical and Surgical Society, October 16, 1890.

liniments. On admission a backward dislocation of the radius and ulna, with firm adhesions, was diagnosed. Under chloroform an unsuccessful attempt at reduction was made, which caused much swelling and pain. This, however, with the use of evaporating lotions, soon subsided, and the boy was discharged unimproved, with the joint firmly ankylosed at a slight angle.

CASE III.—A Sister of Charity, aged about fifty years, slipped, and catching at a beam above her, sustained an injury of her shoulder.

Her arm immediately became helpless, and painful on being moved. A physician, evidently believing the injury to be only a contusion, prescribed rest, evaporating lotions, and, later, rubefacients and blisters, but the immobility continued. Six weeks after the accident another physician saw the case, diagnosed a partial dislocation of the humerus, and attempted reduction. He claimed to have succeeded, although the disability continued.

Six weeks later the patient came to St. Michael's Hospital and an unreduced subclavicular dislocation of the humerus was diagnosed.

At a later consultation doubt was thrown upon this opinion, some of the staff believing that the lesion was a fracture of the anatomical neck of the humerus, and although measuring over the shoulder girdle and under the axilla showed one-half inch more than the other side, and the arm from acromion to olecranon was one-half inch shorter than the uninjured limb, the doubt prevailed, and it was decided that nothing could be done.

CASE IV.—A boy, aged thirteen years, sent to St. Michael's Hospital, May 24, 1889. While fighting he fell with his arm under him. On rising the arm was stiff and sore, and a physician who treated him for several days finally sent him to the hospital with a diagnosis of lateral unreduced dislocation of the elbow-joint.

On examination the elbow was found much swollen and presented all the evidences of an abscess on the inner side. The parts were so tender that nothing could be done until ether was given, when the abscess was opened, a large amount of pus let out, and the fact that no dislocation existed clearly established.

The wound healed well and the joint promised to be as useful as before, when the boy's natural disposition asserted itself and he eloped from the hospital. I saw him two months later when the joint-motion was considerably impaired.

CASE V.—C. B., aged twenty years, admitted to the hospital, June 19, 1886. On May 29th, she fell down a flight of stairs, striking on her head and on the anterior surface of her shoulder. She was treated by liniments and electricity.

Upon examination great tenderness over the tuberosities of the humerus, atrophy of the deltoid, and induration about the insertion of the deltoid were found. The elbow could not be raised from the side.

The tenderness and pain were relieved by soothing applications, and a few days later, the patient being under ether, a dislocation of the shoulder was reduced, and in a month she was discharged well.

These cases are instances of unfortunate mistakes. Three of the patients are permanently crippled, and their ability to maintain themselves and their families is seriously impaired. The injuries are not peculiar or unusually hard to diagnose, but the doubt that prevailed in Case III. illustrates the necessity of giving every joint-injury, however trivial, a thorough and painstaking investigation.

The two following cases are cited to show that when the proper diagnosis has been made, zeal in interference must be tempered by judgment, or the original injury may be rendered more serious:

CASE VI.—C. F. H., aged eight years, fell sideways with outstretched arm against a wall. He was immediately brought to the hospital, where the exact nature of the lesion was not determined. The arm was bandaged and the boy sent home. On the next day the diagnosis of partial inward dislocation of the forearm was made, but for some reason the application of a lotion was the only treatment prescribed, and the boy was directed to return when the swelling had subsided.

Two weeks later he returned, and under ether reduction was attempted, but failed. During the attempt fracture of the lower extremity of the humerus occurred. All efforts at reduction were abandoned, and the arm was extended and placed in splints. In two weeks passive motion was commenced, and ultimately a useful arm was obtained.

CASE VII.—T. S., aged thirty-one years, was brought to St. Michael's Hospital February 14, 1883. In the preceding October the patient had an attack of acute rheumatism confined to the left elbow, from which he recovered in about three weeks, with a stiff joint. Eight attempts to break up the adhesions, the patient being thoroughly anæsthetized, had been made, and resulted in acute suppurative arthritis, which opened through six sinuses. Patient was temperate and gave no history of syphilis or struma.

On admission the elbow was greatly swollen and inflamed, and around the joint the bones were enlarged. He had profuse night-sweats and was much emaciated. A poultice was applied to the elbow, quinine and iron were given, and amputation was advised.

The advice was not followed, but the patient's general condition improved, and in six weeks he left the hospital much better, but with a useless arm.

The cases that follow are recorded not merely because they were severe injuries and interesting in themselves, but also because they are fair types of a peculiar class of injuries—buffer accidents. Many similar cases come to St. Michael's Hospital, the injuries varying in degree from a slight bruise to the absolute destruction of a limb, for which amputation is the only treatment.

The crushing force exerted by two loaded cars coming in contact is immense, and in an arm caught between them the resulting cellulitis is always severe, and if sloughing occurs, it is always extended, and the injury is generally greater than is apparent.

Often, even where no wound or even abrasion can be found, the skin and subcutaneous tissue will, in two or three days, turn black, and a slough reaching from shoulder to wrist will form. Hence, in this class of injuries the prognosis should be very guarded, and the almost inevitable cellulitis watched for, and promptly treated.

Some of the cases reported here were possibly not joint-injuries at all, but as the crush included the joint as well as the adjacent soft tissues, and as it was necessary to treat the joints, the cases are included with the others.

CASE VIII.—P. H., aged twenty-two years, while coupling cars, had his arm caught between the bumpers. On admission to the hospital, October 9, 1889, the extremity from hand to shoulder was much swollen. Around the elbow-joint and the upper half of the forearm was a large, fluctuating swelling, probably a hæmatoma. There were extensive abrasions and large bullæ on the inner side of the forearm just below the elbow. Radial pulse faintly perceptible. Forearm could not be flexed on account of swelling and pain. Although there was no crepitus, fracture was suspected. Evaporating lotions were applied and the arm was placed in a straight splint. Six days later a small slough formed over the olecranon, which separated and left a healthy ulcer. The hæmatoma steadily diminished and the radial pulse became good. On November 23d an abscess which had formed on the anterior aspect of the forearm was opened. Joint-motion improved rapidly under passive movement, and on December 9th the patient was discharged well.

CASE IX.—T. J. C., aged forty years, admitted to the hospital, May 31, 1889. His arm had been caught between the bumpers while coupling cars, and from wrist to shoulder was swollen to about twice the natural size. No pulse at wrist. The swelling about the elbow, especially on the radial side, was very hard. It was impossible to determine whether a fracture was present. An evaporating lotion was applied to the arm and the hand was wrapped in cotton. A straight splint was used.

During the next four days little change took place except that the cellulitis lessened in intensity while the inner side of the arm from the axilla to near the elbow became black. On the fifth day the radial pulse could be faintly felt, and from this time the condition of the arm steadily improved.

The prominent swelling about the elbow, being mostly effused blood, diminished very slowly, and in consequence of the general cellulitis and the pain following any interference with the arm, passive motion could not be practised as early as usual and the joint became very stiff, but under patient treatment this lessened, and on June 26th the case was discharged with orders to report to the out-patient department.

This case was especially interesting in view of the long absence of the radial pulse. The parts seemed ready to slough and the question of amputation was fully discussed, but the final decision to wait proved to be a wise one. Just what arrested the blood-current in the radial artery could not be determined. The radial pulse never regained its former volume and even after entire recovery could be found with difficulty only. Over the upper part of the shaft of the radius and under the hæmatoma remained a hard mass which felt like callus.

Whether the radial was compressed by the blood-tumor, was pinched between the fractured parts of the radius, or had directly suffered in the original crush, was a point on which opinions differed, but there was little doubt that the artery had been practically obliterated and that the pulse was re-established by some anastomotic branch.

CASE X.—P. F., aged twenty-two years, admitted, March 13, 1889. While performing his duties as brakeman, his right arm and forearm were caught between the bumpers of coal cars, the injury being most severe about the elbow. On examination, the entire limb was found much swollen and very painful. Slight subcutaneous hæmorrhage was apparent near the elbow, and between the elbow and axilla, and a few bullæ were formed on the inner side of the forearm. No fracture was found.

The arm was placed on a straight splint and evaporating lotions were at once applied, but the crush had been so extensive that although the skin was not broken, its vitality was gone, and in a few days a slough formed that extended from the wrist to the axilla and included more than one-half the circumference of the limb.

Over the elbow anteriorly, the sloughing opened the joint and a probe passed directly between the ulna and humerus, detected bone that was rough and denuded of cartilage.

With such extensive and deep sloughing there was high fever, with delirium, and later, great depression. The man became very ill, life was in great danger and amputation through the shoulder-joint was seriously considered. But his general condition was too poor, and from the sloughing tissues healthy flaps could hardly have been obtained, so again the decision was to wait, and again the result was a good one. The cellulitis ceased to extend, the slough separated, leaving healthy granulations, the opening into the elbow-joint closed, and after three months the wound had entirely healed, leaving the arm with only slight motion between complete extension and flexion to a right angle.

CASE XI.—W. S., aged twenty years, a brakeman, admitted January 21, 1886. His elbow had been caught between the bumpers of two freight cars.

On examination, two small wounds were found, one on the inner and one on the outer side of the elbow-joint, both of which communicated with fractured bone. Under ether, the joint was found to be completely disorganized, the condyles of the humerus being separated from each other and from the shaft. The tip of the olecranon was broken off and many small fragments, including articular surfaces, were detected. The soft parts showed little bruising, both arteries could be felt at the wrist, sensation in the forearm and hand was perfect, but little blood had been lost, and there was little or no shock.

Excision of the injured joint was determined upon, and through a longitudinal incision over the olecranon the ends of the bones were turned out, the humerus was sawn just above the condyles, the ulna through the coronoid process on the same level, and the head of the radius was removed. The incision and wounds were closed with continuous silk sutures, a drainage-tube was inserted, a dressing of absorbent cotton applied, and the arm bandaged to a long anterior splint. There was no hæmorrhage and no ligatures were used. During the entire operation the wound was irrigated with corrosive sublimate solution.

For three days after the operation the patient was comfortable, but his temperature varied between 102° and 103°. On the fourth day the arm became very painful, considerably swollen and reddened, and cellulitis was evident from about three inches below the elbow to the shoulders. There was a very slight discharge. The arm was placed on a posterior splint, all dressings were removed, and the inflamed parts treated with evaporating lotions. Two days later the superficial cellulitis had diminished, but sloughs were forming along the incision and the wounds, and there was a free discharge of pus. The wounds were washed out daily with antiseptic solutions and all sloughs were gradually cleared away, among them a section of the ulnar nerve about five inches long.

The fever ceased, suppuration steadily lessened, and bony union was obtained. The man was eventually discharged well, with his elbow fixed in a slightly-flexed position.

An interesting point in this case was in regard to the sensation and motion along the course of the ulnar nerve. Of course, after the nerve sloughed the little finger was paralyzed, and sensation was lost in this finger and in the outer half of the third finger, but before his discharge the patient had some feeling in both fingers and slight return of muscular power. It seems hardly possible that five inches of nerve tissue could be replaced, especially in so short a time, yet in what other way could the return of sensation and motion be explained?

CASE XII.—William S., aged ten years, was admitted to St. Michael's Hospital, October 7, 1887. He had fallen from a tree, a distance of about twenty-five feet, striking the ground with the outstretched palm of the right hand.

He was brought to the hospital several hours later, when a compound backward dislocation of the wrist was found.

The extremity of the radius protruded one inch from the wound, and a longitudinal fracture, beginning at the articular surface and extending two inches up the shaft, held tightly one of the flexor tendons. The styloid process of the ulna was also fractured. The protruding end of the radius had been stripped of periosteum, and the wound, which exposed the entire wrist-joint, was full of blood and dirt.

The boy was etherized, three-fourths of an inch of the radius was sawn off, the tendon was released, the wound thoroughly cleansed with carbolic solution, a drainage-tube inserted and the arm put in Esmarch's interrupted splint, held by a plaster bandage.

The wound did very nicely. Only slight cellulitis followed, but there was considerable discharge, which necessitated dressing the wound every two or three days, this being done without removing the splint. Granulating tissue soon filled the cavity and the wound rapidly closed until only a small sinus remained on the palmar surface, through which dead bone could be felt with a probe. The boy was transferred to the out-patient department on December 6th. At that time the sinus remained as described, the dead bone was apparent but firmly attached, and there was considerable motion of the wrist-joint.

He continued a somewhat irregular attendant at the hospital until May, 1888, and when after an absence of six weeks he again appeared, the fragment of dead bone was loose, and by slightly enlarging the opening, a section of the radius, one inch in length, was lifted out, after which the sinus promptly healed and the boy was discharged well.

This was a very instructive case. The injury was severe, the joint was apparently totally destroyed, and amputation seemed the most rational treatment, especially as at the best only a stiff, deformed, and useless hand seemed possible. But when the boy was last seen he possessed every motion of the wrist-joint, although each was slightly restricted. He had perfect control of the fingers, had no deformity except a slight deflection of the carpus to the ulnar side, and, in brief, had almost as good use of the hand as before the accident.

This whole series of injuries, few though the cases be, and perhaps seemingly unimportant, well illustrate the care, patience, and judgment required in general surgical work. By a hasty diagnosis and brilliant operation the case may be easily disposed of, sometimes, however, with a stiff joint or missing limb which more care or less haste might have saved, and there is no doubt that in such cases the surgeon does better for his patient and for himself who adopts and adheres to the oft-quoted maxin, *festina lente.*

167 CLINTON AVENUE.

MEDICAL PROGRESS.

The Microörganisms of Intermittent Fever.—The researches of DR. CAMILLA GOLGI (*Archivio per la Scienze Mediche*) tend to show that not all the intermittent fevers are caused by the same microörganism. Dr. Golgi states that he has been able to demonstrate distinct differences between the hæmatozoon of tertian fever and that of the quartan type. Biologically considered, the tertian parasite completes its development in two days, while that of the quartan variety requires three days, and the amœboid movements of the former are more marked than those of the latter. Morphologically a distinct difference may be observed in the early stages of development; the amœbæ of tertian fever have more delicate protoplasm and a sharper contour than that of the amœbæ of quartan fever, while the pigment-granules and the bacillary forms are larger. Finally, segmentation takes place in a less regular manner in the tertian than in the quartan organism. Clinically, the destruction of the hæmoglobin in the red corpuscles is much more rapid in the tertian than in the quartan.

Prescription for Offensive Breath.—The following deodorant mouth-wash is quoted by the Paris correspondent of the *Medical Press and Circular*, October 1, 1890:

℞.—Bicarbonate of sodium ⎫
　　　Saccharin　　　　　　⎬ of each　1 drachm.
　　　Salicylic acid　　　　⎭
　　　Proof-spirit　.　.　.　. 6 ounces.

Add one teaspoonful to a cupful of water, and use as a mouth-wash.

An Analgesic Spray.—DR. DOBISCH, of Zwittau, recommends the following as a spray-solution in superficial neuralgias, especially those of the head:

℞.—Menthol　.　.　.　.　1 drachm.
　　　Chloroform .　.　.　.　10 drachms.
　　　Ether .　.　.　.　15　"　—M.

This, it is said, will freeze the skin in about one minute. If, in addition to the local effect, a moderate constitutional anæsthesia is desired, a small quantity of the mixture may be sprayed upon the nose and mouth for a moment, the head being covered by a canopy to confine the vaporized solution during a few inhalations.

Treatment of Eczema.—LUSTGARTEN recommends the following ointment in the treatment of eczema:

℞.—Oleate of cocaine　.　.　½ to 1 drachm.
　　　Lanolin　.　.　.　. 3 drachms.
　　　Olive oil .　.　.　. 5　"

This ointment he thinks is particularly valuable in eczema of the anus and genital organs. Two applications should be made each day and followed by the use of absorbent powders. Hot baths are very useful if prolonged. For pruritus of the anus, suppositories of the oleate of cocaine are often exceedingly useful.

Lotion for Sweats.—

℞.—Tincture of belladonna .　.　½ ounce.
　　　Cologne water　.　.　. 4 ounces.—M.

Bathe the affected parts.

Solution for Intertrigo.—

℞.—Bichloride of mercury .　.　½ grain.
　　　Distilled water　.　.　. 3 ounces.

Dissolve, and after solution is complete, wet compresses with the liquid and place them upon the affected parts, allowing them to remain there for an hour. This may be done three or four times a day when the intertrigo is very severe, but it should be remembered that there is some danger of the absorption of the drug and the production of ptyalism if this treatment is resorted to too frequently. Where intertrigo is so severe as to become gangrenous or diphtheritic, Wertheimer prefers to employ local antiseptics such as carbolic acid, and he also washes the parts with water, alcohol, or tincture of iodine. In cases where there is simply excoriation, diachylon ointment may be mixed with equal parts of olive oil and applied to the affected parts. The diseased area should always be kept perfectly clean and all exudation should be removed as rapidly as possible.

The Administration of Mercury to Syphilitic Infants.—Infants who are born syphilitic, or who contract the disease shortly after birth, improve so wonderfully in many instances under the use of mercury, that the following note from the *Revue Général de Clinique et de Thérapeutique* concerning this subject is of interest:

When the child is from five to six weeks of age, ELOY recommends that 5 to 20 drops of Van Swieten's liquid shall be given each day in milk. (Van Swieten's liquid consists of a solution made by the addition of 1 part of bichloride of mercury to 100 parts of alcohol and 900 parts of distilled water.) At the same time that this liquid is given internally, it is advisable to use inunctions of mercurial ointment, or, better still, to employ mercurial ointment diluted by lanolin, equal parts. After this ointment has been used for two or three days, it is best to administer a hot bath. Wiederhofer, of Vienna, considers that red precipitate in the proportion of 1 part to 100 parts of lanolin is even better than ordinary mercurial ointments for inunctions. Baths of corrosive sublimate are particularly valuable, the patient being immersed every third day for a varying length of time, according to the effect of the drug upon the general system. The bath is prepared by adding three grains of corrosive sublimate and fifteen grains of chloride of ammonium to one-half pint of distilled water. This is poured into a wooden or earthenware bath-tub just before the child is immersed in the warm water, which has already been placed there. When the child is older, that is six or seven months of age, the following prescription may be administered with advantage:

℞.—Biniodide of mercury　.　. 1½ grains.
　　　Iodide of sodium ⎫ of each　. 1 drachm.
　　　Distilled water　⎭
　　　Syrup of orange　.　.　. 6 ounces.

Of this give ⅓ a coffee-spoonful to a child of a year, and 5 coffee-spoonfuls to a child of from five to eight years. In other instances calomel and white sugar may be given, ⅙ of a grain of mercury being used for each dose. Sometimes the protiodide of mercury may be given in the same quantity in place of the calomel, and it is particularly useful in combination with the saccharated carbonate of iron in the dose of ⅕ grain, enough white sugar being added to give the powder proper bulk.

THE MEDICAL NEWS.

A WEEKLY JOURNAL
OF MEDICAL SCIENCE.

COMMUNICATIONS are invited from all parts of the world.
Original articles contributed exclusively to THE MEDI-
CAL NEWS will be liberally paid for upon publication.
When necessary to elucidate the text, illustrations will be furnished
without cost to the author.

Address the Editor: H. A. HARE, M.D.,
1004 WALNUT STREET.
PHILADELPHIA.

Subscription Price, including Postage.

PER ANNUM, IN ADVANCE . . . . $4.00.
SINGLE COPIES . . . . 10 CENTS.

Subscriptions may begin at any date. The safest mode of remittance is by bank check or postal money order, drawn to the
order of the undersigned. When neither is accessible, remittances
may be made, at the risk of the publishers, by forwarding in *registered* letters.

Address,   LEA BROTHERS & CO.,
Nos. 706 & 708 SANSOM STREET,
PHILADELPHIA.

SATURDAY, NOVEMBER 22, 1890.

THE LOCAL PARASITICIDE TREATMENT OF CANCER.

THE nature and general appearance of cancer,
more than of other tumors, suggest a microörganismal
original; and although there have been absolutely
no successful attempts at demonstrating such an
idea, the question must be considered as still *sub
iudice*. The present state of our knowledge by no
means admits the probability of such an origin,
but the enticing hope of a brilliant discovery is
sufficient to maintain the interest of investigators
and clinicians in the subject. Many eminent surgeons continue to apply some such substance as solution of chloride of zinc to the exposed tissues after
the ablation of a cancerous growth, to destroy a possible specific microörganism.

This idea of the microörganismal origin of cancerous growths is suggested to POUCEL, Surgeon to the
Marseilles Hospital (*La Semaine Médical*, September
10, 1890), by several successful results obtained by
him from interstitial injections of bichloride of mercury. This writer details seven cases of growths of a
cancerous appearance which were treated in this manner. In two cases of undoubted cancer of long standing and in persons of advanced life the treatment was
unsuccessful. Of the five successful cases, one, a
woman aged fifty-eight years, without syphilitic, tubercular, or cancerous antecedents, or acquired syphilis, presented a large nodular growth of the left breast,
with no retraction of the nipple or ganglionic enlargement. Several interstitial injections, the course
of treatment extending over several months, caused
the entire disappearance of the tumor, and the patient continues in a normal condition. Another case
was that of a woman with a tumor of the right breast,
which was large, hard, irregular, and ulcerating,
and with a retracted nipple, but no glandular enlargement in the axilla. After a number of injections of
corrosive sublimate the tumor disappeared, but the
patient died several months later in an attack of
angina pectoris, and no histological study of the
case seems to have been made. The third of the
five successful results was obtained in the case of a
retired army officer, who was afflicted with a suppurative periganglionic inflammation of the groin.
Upon incision there was found an enlarged, hard,
solitary gland in the inguinal chain. The patient
confessed to having had a hard chancre a number
of years previously and was placed upon antisyphilitic medication, but the growth increased in size,
became hard and nodular, and had the external
appearances of an old inguinal hernia. After twenty-
three days of bichloride injections (ten *séances*, injecting three milligrammes every two days), the swelling completely disappeared and has not recurred.
A fourth successful case, the son of the last patient,
presented several indurated glands in the groin,
which in Dr. Poucel's opinion were of the nature
of ordinary lymphadenomata and caused by toxæmia. They were of several years' standing, at first
indolent and soft, recently hard and increasing
rapidly in size in spite of internal medication—
chiefly iodide of potassium and quinine. A daily
injection of corrosive sublimate solution caused
their disappearance within eight days. The last
successful case was not under Dr. Poucel's direct
observation, and had been variously diagnosed by
surgeons as hæmorrhoids, syphilomata, and cancer
of the rectum.

Upon these seven cases rests Poucel's evidence
as to the parasitic nature of cancerous formations.
In two apparently unquestionable cases of cancer
death occurred, and from these, of course, no inferences can be drawn. Of the remaining five
diagnosis in three is confessedly weak, and apparently almost surely mistaken. Of the first two, while
the local disappearance of the growth was apparently accomplished, in one the death of the patient
within a short time from an attack of angina pectoris
coupled with the lack of an autopsy permits the

suspicion of the existence of metastatic foci, angina pectoris being no rare sequel to cancerous generalization. Of these seven cases the last one alone seems worthy of entire credence. It is unfortunate that no histological examinations were made in any of these cases.

The general history of the germicidal treatment of cancer is in accord with these results of Dr. Poncel, each successful report being counterbalanced by innumerable failures, and usually by the stigma of doubt. The local use in such cases of what are now known as antiseptic materials dates far back in the history of modern medicine; and in Philadelphia the local employment of corrosive sublimate in these neoplasms was recorded as early as 1793 (Senter, *Transactions of the College of Physicians of Philadelphia*, 1793, vol. i. p. 245). The use of interstitial or parenchymatous injections was first suggested by Broadbent (*Medical Times and Gazette*, 1866, ii. p. 572), acetic acid being employed for the purpose; and since then various reports have appeared extolling the merits of this or that substance as an injection-material. The vast bulk of evidence as to these methods has been decidedly against any special parasitic cause of the disease. Whether the present suggestion leads to definite results, of course further experience must decide, the evidence in hand being of little value in the face of the mass of contradictory testimony.

SOCIETY PROCEEDINGS.

PHILADELPHIA ACADEMY OF SURGERY.

Stated Meeting, November 3, 1890.

THE PRESIDENT, D. HAYES AGNEW, M.D.,
IN THE CHAIR.

DR. J. EWING MEARS reported a case of

OCCLUSION OF THE JAWS OF TWENTY-SEVEN YEARS' DURATION IN A WOMAN AGED THIRTY-FOUR YEARS.

He first read a letter from the patient's brother, a physician of Texas. The letter stated that the patient was badly salivated when six or seven years of age, and that there were considerable destruction of tissue and extensive adhesions. A physician divided all the adhesions and opened the mouth, but left the subsequent treatment to a timid nurse, and the result was a failure. When fifteen years of age and when the ankylosis was complete, she was taken to a prominent surgeon in Nashville, who failed to open the jaws. He said that he could not break up the ankylosis without endangering the maxilla at or near the angles. Her health was good but she could not masticate food. She had had a number of asthmatic attacks and several attacks of facial erysipelas which had promptly yielded to treatment.

On coming under Dr. Mears's care the patient gave a fuller history of her case. She said that the surgeon in Nashville had endeavored to open the mouth by continuous traction applied by means of a wire placed around the jaw. This failed and some years later she went to New Orleans to consult Professor Richardson, of the University of Louisiana, who sent her to Dr. Mears.

Notwithstanding the fact that the space between the teeth would just admit the point of a thin knife-blade, she had been doing duty as a teacher, talking through the teeth. She also presented a condition which has been noted in cases of the same nature, that is, non-development of the bones and soft tissues of the face. She was about five feet eight and one-half inches tall, and yet she had the face of a child—what Dr. Mears has designated as a "baby-face." This, both she and her friends had recognized. After the operation, as could be seen from a photograph, this appearance changed and she now has the face of a woman at her time of life.

Previously to operating the buccal space was entirely obliterated. There was simply an opening between the lips through which could be seen the incisor and canine teeth of the upper and lower jaw, but nothing more. The case was at once recognized as one of cicatricial occlusion. She was etherized, an incision was made through the cicatricial tissue on each side, and the mouth forced open. At the same time Dr. Mears removed nineteen teeth. Those of the lower jaw crossed under the tongue, those of the upper jaw projected in various directions, so that in the oral cavity proper there was scarcely room for the tongue. These teeth had irrupted after the jaws became occluded, and not being able to develop in a proper manner, had taken the positions described. The cavities made by the incisions were packed with five-per-cent. iodoform gauze. This dressing was removed in two days and fresh gauze inserted.

After the painful stage following this operation had passed, the second stage of the treatment was begun, and consisted in the passage of ligatures through the cicatricial mass. These ligatures were deposited as deeply as possible on either side by means of a long needle with an eye near the point, the ligatures being brought out on a line with the position of the last molar tooth. The ligatures consisted of heavy silk, carbolized and twisted, and were tied loosely. In conjunction with this, Dr. Mears used an apparatus which he devised some years ago for opening the mouth and for performing operations on the oral cavity. As was expected, some contraction followed the division of the cicatricial tissue. The object in passing the ligatures was to get a track or canal which, after a time, would be lined by mucous membrane and would permit division of the overlying tissues without reformation and reunion, as we treat webbed fingers or toes. In three weeks' time the tissues over the ligatures were divided and the ligatures were reapplied, using two on each side, one above the other. These were allowed to remain in place for three weeks, when the overlying tissues were again divided, and it was found that an opening of one and three-quarters inches had been secured. The use of the instrument was continued for some time after the patient's return to her home. The speaker then exhibited a photograph showing the result a year and a half after the operation. She reports that the opening is equal to one and a half inches, taken between artificial teeth.

Dr. Mears said that the result in this case was similar to those that he has secured in other cases in which he adopted the plan of treatment by ligatures. He has from time to time tried simple division of the tissues, but invariably the jaws have again closed. The plan of inserting ligatures is of course adapted only to this class of cases, and not to ankylosis or synostosis of the temporomaxillary articulation. All the incisions were made and the ligatures were deposited within the mouth.

The change in the appearance of the face is quite marked. The shape of the face in such cases is due in part to non-use of the muscles of the jaw, and in part to non-development of the bones. The speaker has reported other cases of this kind, one in which he opened the mouth of a gentleman, in whom the closure was of seventeen years' standing, and although he was thirty-two years of age he had never grown any beard. As soon as the man regained the use of the jaw the beard began to grow and the face was soon covered with hair. This can probably be explained by the increased circulation brought about by the use of the muscles.

In discussing this paper Dr. O. H. Allis said that the condition of the teeth to which Dr. Mears had alluded would hardly seem possible to one who had not seen similar cases. The person cannot keep the mouth in a cleanly condition. If a tooth ulcerates or becomes inflamed it is impossible for a dentist to remove it. The amount of suffering which such a patient must go through can hardly be described. He did not know of an operation that is a greater boon to such patients than that described by Dr. Mears. The speaker has performed it but once, and in this case he signally failed by the ordinary means, but with the assistance of Dr. Mears he secured a good separation of the jaws. In this case a portion of the jaw was removed.

In closing, Dr. Mears said that he cordially agreed with what Dr. Allis said. We can scarcely appreciate the condition of a patient with complete occlusion of the jaw. In some of his cases there was considerable danger from the condition. One patient, a boy, crowded a large quantity of pie between his teeth by the aid of a knife and a stick, so that he was in great danger of asphyxia. Patients dread any inflammation of the pharynx because of the impossibility of local treatment. In some of the cases, when emesis occurs, the vomited matter escapes through the nose. In all the cases there is a great deal of courage and a desire to be relieved, especially on the part of the women. In the case which was reported tonight, the patient lived on fluids. In another case the patient had worn away to a great extent the incisor teeth by rubbing pieces of meat on them in order to get the juice. These operations, he said, give as satisfactory results as any operation in surgery.

Dr. L. W. Steinbach then read a paper on

THE ENDOSCOPE.

The speaker said that he wished to direct the attention of the Fellows to the use of this instrument of precision in the examination of the interior of the male urethra.

The ideal method of examining the urinary passages,

or any other cavity, is that which makes them accessible to the eye; such a method has been perfected and is available to every one who cares to employ it.

The urethral speculum, or endoscope, in its simplest and best form, is a cylindrical tube, from four to six inches in length, and one-fourth of an inch in diameter, with a funnel-shaped expansion at its ocular extremity. It is made of hard rubber or polished metal, and for convenience of introduction is provided with a closely-fitting conductor, the rounded extremity of which forms an obturator to the visceral end of the tube.

The illumination is obtained by reflecting the rays of the sun, or of a gas- or lamp-light from a large concave head-mirror, bringing them to a focus on a level with the internal orifice of the endoscope.

No special preparation of the patient is requisite; he is seated on a chair with his back toward the source of light, the garments arranged to expose the pubic and scrotal regions only; the physician, sitting on a chair opposite, introduces the previously-oiled instrument in the manner of introducing a sound.

The penis is seized with the thumb and index finger of the left hand behind the glans, the remaining fingers are placed upon the pubes to steady the organ, whilst the right hand carries the endoscope with the thumb pressing upon the conductor to prevent it from slipping out. The instrument is guided along the centre of the urinary canal to a distance of four inches, which is sufficient to inspect any portion anterior to the verumontanum. When we desire to inspect the prostatic portion of the urethra or more posterior structures, an instrument six inches in length is required, and the patient must be placed in the recumbent posture to enable us to guide the endoscope under the pubic arch. It is necessary to have one or more long probes and a pair of slender forceps for the purpose of carrying absorbent cotton, which is used to remove secretions and deposits of the substance which is employed to lubricate the endoscope, and to apply medicines. The forceps are also used to withdraw pieces of cotton which occasionally slip from the probe. When we bear in mind that the mucous membrane of the urethra is arranged in longitudinal folds, and upon transverse section presents a stellate appearance, we at once understand the image which we behold when the conductor is withdrawn and the secretions removed.

The portion of the urethra seen at one time is necessarily small, but by gradually withdrawing the tube every part of the canal can be inspected. It requires practice and instruction to interpret properly the images that present themselves, but the reward is more than ample when we are able to recognize the different inflammatory stages, congestion, granulations, ulcers, cicatrices and polypi, and can apply our remedial agents in a rational manner directly to the portion affected.

The adverse criticism of this method, which in the hands of a few of its zealous advocates has developed into a science, comes mainly from those who have not taken the trouble to master the subject, or who abandoned it because of the complicated, costly, and unsatisfactory appliances which were deemed necessary.

In discussion Dr. John B. Deaver said that Dr. Steinbach had not referred to the Leiter electric-light endoscope, the instrument that the speaker was in the habit of using. This is a very satisfactory instrument, and with it the mucous membrane of the urethra can be seen with remarkable clearness. In one case, where divulsion had been practised, a teat of mucous membrane was left which was at once apparent to a gentleman who used the instrument for the first time. This case served to illustrate one argument in the speaker's paper opposing divulsion of strictures, read before the American Medical Association. He has been able to cure many cases of gleet in which he was unable to discover a stricture of large calibre with the urethrameter, which he considers the best means for discovering this most common cause of gleet, by making applications to the granulating membrane through the endoscopic tube.

A man was recently brought to him who, four days after suspicious intercourse, had localized pain one inch within the meatus and an induration along the floor of the urethra with slight discharge. In making the urethroscopic examination an ulcer was found which presented the appearance of a chancroid. There was also unilateral enlargement of the glands. The ulcer was touched with a fifteen-grain solution of nitrate of silver, and after three applications it was well. This could, of course, have been accomplished with the tube which Dr. Steinbach referred to.

A urethroscopic tube six inches in length, Dr. Deaver thinks, is not of much service without the incandescent lamp. With the lamp there is no difficulty in exposing the prostatic urethra, although there is some pain caused by the introduction of the instrument beneath the triangular ligament. In a number of cases he has satisfied himself of the presence of pathological conditions of the prostatic urethra, particularly in impotence, of which these lesions are the commonest causes and in which he has obtained satisfactory results from applications through the tube.

He calls the instrument a *urethroscope*, which he thinks is a better name than *endoscope*.

In closing, Dr. Steinbach said that he wished to indicate only one method of making these examinations. He has had ample experience with the instrument which Dr. Deaver mentioned. It is surprising that we do not use these instruments more extensively in the examination of the urethra, the deep urethra, and the bladder. In the University of Vienna there has been for the past ten years or more a chair, occupied by Dr. Grünfeld, devoted to this subject. They have daily clinics, and examine from twenty to one hundred patients. The professor in charge, while showing all the various instruments devised for this purpose, teaches his pupils to use the simpler forms and those which are cheap. When we wish to examine the bladder or some particular growth in the urethra, the electric light is probably better, but in ordinary cases the light reflected from the head-mirror answers every purpose. A four-inch tube is sufficient for most purposes. The longer tube is necessary for the deeper urethra and its introduction requires more skill. When we wish to examine the bladder it is necessary to have a glass obturator, to prevent the escape of urine through the tube.

Dr. Steinbach then showed one of the most recent forms of the electric-light cystoscopes and some of the simpler forms of urethroscopes, which he described.

TRI-STATE MEDICAL ASSOCIATION.

Second Annual Meeting,
held in Chattanooga, Tenn., October 14, 15, and 16, 1890.

(Continued from page 520.)

Second Day.—Evening Session.

The Association met in Stone Church, and was called to order at 7.30 p.m. An

ADDRESS OF WELCOME

was delivered by Dr. G. W. Drake, and was responded to by Dr. G. C. Savage, of Nashville.

This was followed by the President's Address, entitled

"THE DOCTOR."

The President said that the man who starts out to be a doctor must understand that the life is one of toil. The laggard, the indolent, the careless, or the sluggard never succeed. The doctor must be educated, not as that term seems to be understood in these days. Modern education, he feared, is too much a process of *stuffing* and *cramming*. The term education means more than this. To educate is to draw out, to enlarge, to expand, to develop, and to strengthen.

Third Day.—Morning Session.

Dr. T. Hilliard Wood, of Nashville, Tennessee, contributed a paper on

HYPERTROPHY OF THE TONSILS.

He said that the treatment of hypertrophy of the tonsils has been subject to many variations. If the enlargement be due to swelling of the mucous membrane or to engorgement and congestion of the tonsil, the application of astringents may be of service. The most useful local remedies are the subsulphate and perchloride of iron (about one part to six or eight parts of water or glycerin) and alum or tannin in powder. But where there is true overgrowth, the remedy must be of a destructive character, and escharotics, not astringents, must be used. For this purpose "London paste" is useful, and should be applied once or twice a week. This will produce a slough, and repeated applications will reduce the gland to the normal size.

Constitutional measures to effect reduction of the tonsils include remedies to combat the diathesis upon which the enlargement often depends, such as iodide of potassium, and cod-liver oil; the general tonics, such as the preparations of iron, and the simple bitters, are also useful.

With reference to operative treatment, excision by the tonsillotome is most popular, although the speaker prefers the bistoury and vulsella forceps. The operation is rendered painless by applying to the tonsil a solution of cocaine, and by injecting, with a hypodermic syringe, a few drops of the solution into the substance of the gland. As a rule, general anæsthetics should not be used.

To reduce to a minimum the danger from hæmorrhage, we have the comparatively bloodless operations by the cold snare, ignipuncture, and the galvano-cautery amygdalotome. Of these the galvano-cautery amygdalotome seems preferable, and is highly recommended by Wright, of Brooklyn. Ignipuncture is tedious, requiring repeated applications, and is attended by considerable pain. Moreover, it cannot be employed in the cases of refractory children.

In discussing this paper Dr. N. C. Steele, of Chattanooga, said that the amount of hæmorrhage during tonsillotomy depends upon the condition of the tonsil. He uses the bistoury in adults and the tonsillotome in children.

Dr. E. T. Camp said that he had been able to reduce hypertrophied tonsils without operation, by using iodized phenol locally, and general remedies.

Dr. George A. Baxter suggested painting the tonsil with flexible collodion.

Dr. Savage said that there were two indications for operating, viz.: Repeated attacks of tonsillitis and interference with breathing. He uses Mathews's tonsillotome and never applies cocaine. . From personal experience he knows that the operation is not painful.

Dr. Gahagan suggested cold food and drinks in cases of incipient tonsillitis.

Dr. Reeves thought that in removing the tonsils we leave cicatricial tissue which alters the quality of the voice. He uses tincture of iodine locally.

Dr. Willis F. Westmoreland, of Atlanta, Ga., said that the enlargement of the tonsils is due to exposure, hence the greater number of cases in males. He prefers the bistoury, and has abandoned cocaine because it increases bleeding. Ignipunctnre is too painful.

Dr. Frank Trester Smith, of Chattanooga, resorts to ignipuncture when he cannot get consent to excision. Bleeding may continue for a long time after the use of cocaine. The indications for operation are (1) difficult breathing, (2) unnatural voice, and (3) recurring tonsillitis. The voice after operation improves, as a rule.

Afternoon Session.

Dr. E. A. Cobleigh, of Chattanooga, read a paper entitled

A CASE OF REMARKABLE INJURY, WITH RECOVERY,

and exhibited the patient.

The patient while working in a well was struck by the sharp end of a heavy drill one inch in diameter, which fell about forty-five feet. The implement penetrated the back of the neck, ploughed through the tissues, and emerged from the right side of the chest, protruding about eight inches. The man stepped down from the platform on which he was working, supported himself against the side of the well, and called on a fellow workman to pull out the drill. A stalwart negro tried to do so with both hands, but failed. He mounted the platform and tried again by a steady pull, which did not budge the impaling instrument. He then resorted to a to-and-fro motion with the powerful leverage of the long handle, and was thus able to loosen and extract the drill from above.

The patient was now very imperfectly fastened to the well rope with a noose passed around him, and was drawn to the surface, placed in a chair and conveyed to an adjoining work-room. The patient is twenty-eight years old, five feet and eleven inches high, and weighs 185 pounds, having a magnificent physique.

Examination showed that the wound of entrance was situated one and one-half inches to the right of the spinous process of the fifth cervical vertebra, and that the drill had barely missed the spinal column. It passed downward and very slightly forward and to the right, leaving a rather smooth, oval opening with somewhat inverted edges, resembling the wound of entrance of a round shot, and not as large as one would expect from the size of the wounding instrument, yet sufficiently large for the cervical muscles and fascia to be plainly seen. The shape of the wound caused it to close like a valve, yet air was entering and escaping with a pink froth at nearly every respiratory effort. There was not much hæmorrhage.

From the neck the drill passed into the chest cavity between the scapula and the clavicle, without damage to either of these bones, impinged on the third and fourth ribs, which were fractured in the line of the wound—the fragments evidently being parted as by a wedge while the drill was *in situ*—then passed down on the anterior and outer surface of the fifth and sixth ribs without injury to either, and emerged by a large gaping and ragged wound, with everted edges, at the inferior border of the sixth rib, its centre being at the time of the examination two inches below and one and a half inches to the right of the nipple. There was only moderate bleeding from this wound, into the opening of which Dr. Cobleigh could introduce the tips of three fingers, and no air was escaping. The skin and subcutaneous tissues seemed to be absolutely deadened by the magnitude of the injury, and to have lost their normal elasticity. He passed two fingers into the wound, entering the pleural cavity under the broken ends of the lower fractured rib, which could be distinctly felt. Everything was torn and indefinite, the ends of the broken bone were removable, but he was not able to satisfy himself whether the subjacent lung surface was injured, though he thought it was. The length of the wound was fourteen and a half inches.

On withdrawing the fingers the wound closed by the collapse of its sides, which prevented profuse external hæmorrhage. There were intense pain and a marked degree of shock as shown mainly by the pulse, the mind remaining clear throughout. The integument, however, was quite clammy, and the patient complained a great deal of chilliness, but had no pronounced rigor. There were extreme rapidity and difficulty of respiration, and Dr. Cobleigh believed that the man would die in a short time, especially as the signs of depression were increasing fast, the pulse becoming flickering, irregular, and intermittent, and the mucous surfaces blanching.

Dr. Cobleigh regards the recovery of the case as remarkable and fit to be recorded with the celebrated "crow-bar" case of Maine, and with the later case of abdominal perforation by a railroad coupling-link which happened a few years ago in Kentucky.

Dr. Willis F. Westmoreland, of Atlanta, Georgia, read a paper on

MORBID REFLEX NEUROSES AMENABLE TO SURGICAL TREATMENT.

Dr. H. Crumley, of Chattanooga, presented a case resembling epilepsy, which was examined by many members of the Association.

Dr. J. R. Rathmell, of Chattanooga, reported a

CASE OF ABSCESS OF THE LIVER.

The patient had dysentery in july, and Dr. Rathmell was called to see him on December 17th. The abscess began to discharge through the lung on December 21st, and continued till February 27, 1890, when the patient died. No autopsy was made.

Dr. Townes followed with a paper on

DILATED CARDIAC HYPERTROPHY, WITH NEPHRITIC COMPLICATIONS,

illustrating his paper by specimens of the condition and by other specimens for comparison. Attention was called to the etiology, and especially to alcoholism and its effects upon the kidneys and liver. The weight of the heart shown was twenty-six and a half ounces. The kidney was an example of those termed by Formad, of Philadelphia, " pig-back."

In the treatment of this patient tincture of digitalis was administered, at first 10 drops, increasing later to 60 drops every hour. Then tincture of strophanthus was given, 20 drops, three times daily, and the heart-beats were reduced from 124 per minute to 47.

EVENING SESSION.

Dr. R. J. Trippe, of Chattanooga, reported a

FATAL CASE OF PERITONITIS,

which occurred in a muscular negro, as the result of a blow on the abdomen with a crow-bar.

Dr. C. H. Holland, of Chattanooga, reported a case of

PHLEGMONOUS ABSCESS

occurring in a man twenty-five years old.

Dr. J. H. Atlee, of Chattanooga, reported a

CASE OF OVARIOTOMY.

In May, 1889, he was called to see Mrs. L., white, aged twenty-one years ; married for two years without issue. Menstruation began at the age of fourteen years, and was regular. Immediately after marriage she noticed an enlargement in the left side of her abdomen, which gradually increased until it became so large as to impede locomotion and interfere with respiration.

Dr. Atlee diagnosed multilocular cyst of the left ovary, and decided to operate. Two weeks later, on the day appointed for the operation, he found her with a pulse of 120, a temperature of 103°, and very rapid respiration, and in the presence of these symptoms he thought it best not to operate. Upon the patient's solicitation Dr. Atlee performed paracentesis and drew off thirty pounds of a thick coffee-colored albuminous fluid, which presented, under the microscope, the ovarian cells of Drysdale. Ten days thereafter he removed by abdominal section a tumor weighing forty-five pounds, which in every way confirmed his diagnosis. Before removing the tumor he secured the pedicle, which was short and thick, with two ligatures, each ligature including one-half of the pedicle.

About the eighth week after the operation symptoms of cystitis, with difficult and painful urination, appeared. The urethra was found to be occluded with a foreign body which, upon removal, was identified as one of the ligatures used in tying the pedicle. About the sixth month after the operation cystitis reappeared, and gradu-ally increased in severity until the second ligature was passed from the bladder. This ligature Dr. Atlee now has in his possession. The patient has since remained in perfect health, and is now a strong, healthy woman.

Dr. Frank Trester Smith followed with a paper entitled

FLUORESCEIN IN THE DIAGNOSIS OF EYE-DISEASES.

Dr. J. E. Purdon, of Cullman, Alabama, contributed a very elaborate paper on the

DYNAMICS OF MEDIUMISM,

and arrived at fifteen conclusions after a long and careful study of the subject.

Dr. W. C. Maples, of Bellefonte, Alabama, read a paper on

SOME IRREGULAR FORMS OF EPILEPSY, WITH REPORT OF A CASE.

Dr. Maples thinks that the case reported was one of epilepsy, although in some respects it resembled hystero-epilepsy. His reasons for thinking it to be a case of epilepsy are :

1. The amount of fever. In hystero-epilepsy there is generally but little or no fever. Some authors assert that we may have a true hysterical fever, but the weight of authority is against that opinion.

2. The complete unconsciousness.

3. The biting of the tongue. Hystero-epileptics seldom or never injure themselves.

4. The facial expression and pupillary phenomena. The facial expression is generally calm and serene throughout a hystero-epileptic attack.

5. The absence of hysterical phenomena in the interval between the attacks.

6. The sex. Hystero-epilepsy rarely occurs in males.

Dr. J. D. Gibson, of Birmingham, Alabama, presented a paper on

URETHRAL STRICTURE AND ITS COMPLICATIONS.

He considers the acorn-pointed sound the most convenient and practical instrument for the detection of stricture.

Dr. Gibson said that if he were compelled to use only one instrument in the treatment of strictures, that instrument would be the sound. He believes that if it is properly used, there are very few strictures that cannot be relieved, and that the only cases in which a urethrotome is necessary are tight and unyielding strictures in the pendant urethra or at the meatus. Inexperienced men are apt to be disappointed in the use of the sound, simply because they try to go too fast ; the idea should be to dilate the stricture and produce absorption, not rupture.

Internal urethrotomy, while often abused, is a potent means of treating urethral stricture, it being especially applicable to old and firm strictures in the pendulous urethra and meatus.

Dr. P. S. Hayes, of Chicago, followed with a paper entitled

NOTES ON APOSTOLI'S METHOD IN THE TREATMENT OF UTERINE FIBROIDS.

He said that one of the most clearly demonstrated

facts of the Apostoli method is that by means of it all uterine hæmorrhages, not puerperal, can be arrested.

All observers recognize that the positive pole is the one to be connected with the intra-uterine electrode. The reason for this is, that in electrolysis, especially when the electrolyte—the fluid undergoing electrolysis—is blood, the clot formed around the positive pole is small and dense, while that around the negative pole is large and flabby. Knowing, as we do, that oxygen, chlorine, and the acids are liberated at the positive pole when electrolysis is performed on the tissues of the body, and also knowing that hydrogen and the alkalies are liberated at the negative pole, we have only to apply our knowledge of the action of the acids and alkalies on the blood to explain the observed phenomena.

The occurrence of uterine hæmorrhage does not contraindicate the use of the method.

One of Dr. Hayes's patients, suffering from menorrhagia, came to his office, stating that she was drenched with the discharge, the hæmorrhage having occurred when she was some distance from her home. Dr. Hayes used the intra-uterine electrode connected with the positive pole, and passed a current of from 60 to 80 milliampères for eight minutes. The patient went home, a distance of three miles, and was in bed the remainder of the day. On the next day she was about the house, and the flow had nearly ceased. This period was by far the least severe that she had had for several months, and the amount of time spent in bed was three-fourths less.

Officers for 1891.

President.—Dr. Robert Battey, Rome, Ga.

First Vice-President.—Dr. E. T. Camp, Gadsden, Ala.

Second Vice-President.—Dr. Richard Douglas, Nashville, Tenn.

Third Vice-President.—Dr. D. H. Howell, Atlanta, Ga.

Secretary.—Dr. Frank Trester Smith, Chattanooga, Tenn.

Treasurer.—Dr. S. B. Wert, Chattanooga, Tenn.

On motion, the Association adjourned to meet in Chattanooga, Tenn.

THE NEW YORK SOCIETY OF MEDICAL JURISPRUDENCE.

Stated Meeting, November 10, 1890.

THE PRESIDENT, LANDON CARTER GRAY, M D., IN THE CHAIR.

DR. E. C. SPITZKA read

A REPORT ON THE EXECUTION OF WILLIAM KEMMLER.

After alluding to the fact that the New York Society of Medical Jurisprudence had taken the first steps to bring about a reform in the methods of capital punishment, which had led rather prematurely to the passage of the law establishing electrothanasia as a substitute for hanging, Dr. Spitzka said that the chief objection to this new mode of execution was the complicated machinery necessary. He then vividly described the execution of Kemmler, already too familiar to the general public in many of its details, in order to show the favorable, as well as the unfavorable factors which entered

into this particular case. He has witnessed a number of hangings, but never before was he unable to recognize at once the condemned one, by his appearance or demeanor. Kemmler's manner was so calm and yielding that it was indeed necessary for the warden to introduce him to the assembled witnesses.

After quoting Kemmler's last words, which he said had been correctly reported only by Dr. Carlos Macdonald, he described how the doomed man assisted in the preliminary arrangements, including the application of the electrodes. When the awful moment came, his body was thrown into a tetanic spasm, and, in the speaker's opinion, death occurred in an infinitesimal part of a second. The spasm lasted for the seventeen seconds during which the current was applied, and involved every muscular fibril. so that there was not only rigidity, but also quivering. The violence was so great that it would be easy to believe, that were it not for the secure manner in which the man was fastened to the chair, the tremendous force of the muscular contractions would have caused many fractures.

During the first application of the current, a peculiar pallor appeared on the man's scalp and spread down to the head-band, and the intense purplish congestion of the capillaries which surround the naso-labial fold showed distinct post-mortem hypostatic congestion, bounded by a serrated line. When this congestion appeared Dr. Spitzka announced that the man was dead. Up to this time, of course, no one had dared to feel the pulse, or make an examination of the body by touch. It was evident that the other witnesses also considered the man dead, for they gathered around the table, and prepared to sign the legal document as required by law.

At this time the victim's pulse was absent, the pupils were insensible to light, and one cornea was flaccid. The marks of his suspenders, and of every fold in his clothing, were traced upon his body in a singular manner. During the muscular spasm the thumb of one hand was driven into the finger, and when blood oozed from this wound one of the witnesses exclaimed that life was returning. This immediately produced a panic among the spectators, and Dr. Spitzka, as he himself says, made the great mistake of ordering the current turned on a second time. Again the body was convulsed, but the contractions were more like those seen in a galvanized frog when the contractility is becoming exhausted. At the time Kemmler met his death it was probable that he was in a state of "expectant inspiration;" [1] hence the bubbling of air through the thick mucus which had collected in the mouth.

In cases of death by powerful electrical currents, or by lightning, the fluidity of the blood has been commented on, and it is well known that under such circumstances bleeding from an incised wound is no proof that life is not extinct. Dr. Spitzka thought that such a phenomenon could be reproduced even as late as the fourth or fifth day after death. His examination made after the final cessation of the current, showed the absence of the tendon and pupillary reflexes, and the hypostatic congestions already noted. Seven or eight seconds after the cessation of the current there were repeated explosions of intestinal flatus, followed in a few seconds by a profuse flow of urine. After the first application of the current there was an erection of the penis and an emission of semen. The erection seemed to be produced by the erector muscles rather than by the turgidity of the blood-vessels.

Dr. Spitzka said that his object in bringing this subject before the Society was to direct particular attention to the uncertainty of all the usually-accepted signs of death. In the examination just mentioned he found that on touching the convict's ear it became pale, but on relinquishing his grasp the color immediately returned. This phenomenon has been made the subject of a successful prize essay, in which it was stated that the absence of the sign is positive proof of death. Yet after this man's body had been completely dissected, and the lungs, heart, intestines, brain, and spinal cord entirely removed, the phenomenon was repeatedly observed. He has observed the same thing in a few other cases in which he made an examination very soon after death. In the present instance the fluidity of the blood might partially explain the persistence of this phenomenon.

In speaking of the arrangements of the apparatus at the Auburn prison the author criticised quite severely the placing of the switches, and especially of the voltmeter in a room separate from the execution-chamber, thus making it impossible for the official physicians to observe the voltage of the current. On this occasion the volt-meter did not work properly, and he believed it was not intended that it should do so; for at trials both before and after the execution, it failed to work well for more than a few moments. The only way the physicians could judge of the condition of the current was by the appearance of the incandescent lights.

As is well known, much opposition has been raised against the execution by electricity on account of the State's selection of the dynamo of a particular corporation. It is worthy of note that the first accidental death by powerful electric current, occurred in Buffalo three or four years ago with a current from a Brush machine; and it would have seemed natural for the State to select the machine which had first so unfortunately demonstrated its ability to kill. The State should have but one plant, centrally located, and provided with a dynamo especially constructed for the purpose, and capable of generating a current of about 3000 volts. This machinery should be under the charge of a thoroughly competent electrical expert. The neurologist or ordinary medical man knows very little about these powerful currents, and should only direct the selection and proper application of the electrodes. Dr. Spitzka said that a collar electrode could be so constructed that it would hold the victim firmly without strangling him, and while securing better contact and easier application than the head electrode, would avoid the only preliminary to which Kemmler objected—the shaving of the scalp. The spinal electrode is even worse than the head electrode. It is unnecessary to test the resistance of the convict's body before the execution. All that is required is to employ the highest obtainable voltage and to apply it for a brief period. This would lessen the probability of burning, avoid the revolting spectacle of convulsions long after life is extinct, and would convince the public that death was instantaneous. The great cost of this method of capital punishment will probably prevent its introduction into other States.

Notwithstanding the disadvantages mentioned, Dr. Spitzka said that the execution of Kemmler was a more decent and dignified vindication of the law than the cases of hanging that he had witnessed.

In view of the part taken by the Society of Medical Jurisprudence in this matter of reform in the execution of the death penalty, Dr. Spitzka thought it might justly claim to be in the advance guard of forensic medical progress.

In discussion, DR. CARLOS MACDONALD, who prepared the official report at the request of the Governor, said that he had but little to add to Dr. Spitzka's report. In criticising the medical witnesses of this execution, it should be remembered that their advice was sought in regard to only one matter—the duration of the application of the current; and that even about so important a matter as the application of the electrodes, they were not consulted. At the preliminary tests made some months previously to the execution, it was decided to use a helmet electrode, and also a form of chair which had been recommended by Dr. Macdonald; but for some unknown reason both of these decisions were changed. He considered the discarding of the helmet electrode a mistake, as experiments on animals have shown that the most effectual mode of application was through an electrode embracing the frontal region. The great error had been in not continuing the current a little longer, remembering that the probable voltage was not nearly so great as had been intended. It probably did not exceed 700 volts; while, judging from experiments on animals, it should have been 1000. He believed that with proper contact, such a current, if applied for from fifteen to twenty seconds, would invariably cause instant death. He went into the switch-room in the Auburn prison in the interval between the applications of the current, not knowing that it was against orders, and found the incandescent lamps burning dimly. He recognized Mr. Davis in the room, and asked him, "What is the matter with your current?" to which Mr. Davis replied, "There is something wrong down at the dynamo." He had no time to make further inquiries, for he was sent out of the room. He believed that if contact had been maintained five seconds longer in the case of Kemmler, no muscular movements would have been observed.

DR. SACHS spoke of the execution as a "scientific experiment," for the resistance of the body varies so enormously in different subjects, and in the same subject at different times, that there is necessarily the greatest uncertainty as to the results. The Commission appointed to investigate these points, did not consider the differences between the lower animals and human beings, and consequently their conclusions were mere guesswork. He was, therefore, surprised that the execution proved so successful.

The President, DR. GRAY, also spoke of resistance, and endorsed the views of the preceding speaker. He thought that in addition to these elements of uncertainty, there was another obstacle—i.e., the difficulty which would be encountered if the condemned man should struggle or resist.

The HON. WILLIAM BARNES thought that struggling would finally lead to the abandonment of electrothanasia for a method with fewer uncertainties; such, for instance, as the guillotine.

Dr. N. S. Brill, whose paper originally led to the reform in executions, said that there was less danger of bungling with electrothanasia, when carried out according to the suggestions already laid down, than there was in hanging ; and the former had the additional advantage that the execution was constantly under the control of the executioner to the time of the victim's death, while in hanging, the executioner, after springing the drop, has no control whatever.

CORRESPONDENCE.

"RHUS POISONING."

To the Editor of The Medical News,

Sir : Under the head of " Hospital Notes " in your issue of October 25, 1890, I notice a method of treatment advised for " Rhus Poisoning." I have had a very large experience with this form of dermatitis and have never seen the application of " lotio nigra " fail in any stage of the disease. This was suggested to me by Harold Williams, M.D., of Boston. The part or parts may be freely bathed with black wash or wrapped in absorbent wool or cotton previously soaked in the solution. Immediate relief of subjective symptoms follows and the objective signs rapidly disappear. I have never seen untoward symptoms. The only objection to the treatment is, that *the physician makes but one visit.*

Nantucket, Mass.   J. Alban Kite, M.D.

NEWS ITEMS.

The Hot-air Clinique of Paris.—A clinique was recently opened in the *Rue de la Chaussée d'Antin,* Paris, for the hot-air treatment of consumptives. Here men, women, and children who have phthisis or are predisposed to it may be treated free of charge. Ranged around the walls of the establishment are a number of small tables, on each of which stands an apparatus for heating the air by means of a large spirit-lamp. From each of the reservoirs issues a rubber tube terminating in a mouthpiece, through which the patients inhale the heated air. The mouthpiece is double-valved, so that the expired air passes out without mingling with that delivered by the apparatus.

The Study of Medicine in Thibet.—The Buddhist Lamas' University, in the Transbaikal Province of Thibet, has a medical course of ten years. According to *Nature,* a traveller named Ptitsyn has returned from that country with a collection of medical books and drugs illustrative of the knowledge and the methods of practice in Thibet. Mr. Ptitsyn remarks that he has found over one hundred diseases described in the Buddhist literature, and of these a mythical origin is ascribed to only two. Strictly medical subjects are not studied until the fifth year of the course, the first four years being devoted to the study of the languages and theology. The eighth year is devoted to astrology, and philosophy is studied in the last two years.

Liabilities of Patients.—Mr. A. M. Hurlock, an attorney of Baltimore, is engaged in an attempt to get a bill through the Legislature of Maryland, which shall render a married woman's estate liable for medical services rendered to herself or to her children. Every now and then rich or well-to-do women with worthless husbands obtain under the present law the medical services of the doctor without compensation, and we think that a law such as proposed will materially help in stopping one of the leaks which wastes the stream of nutrition running into the lean professional purse. We trust that he may be successful, and that his example may prove contagions. The principal section of the proposed bill is as follows :

Section 1. *Be it enacted by the General Assembly of Maryland,* That married women shall be jointly liable with their husbands for medical services rendered to such married women or their children, that they may be sued jointly with their husbands for such services, and that judgments obtained in such suits may be a lien on their separate property.

American Academy of Medicine.—The Constitution was altered at the last annual meeting so as to admit, in addition to those possessing the degrees of A. B. and A. M., those who can present evidences of preparatory liberal education equivalent to the same.

Dr. J. E. Emerson, Detroit, Michigan, Chairman of Committee on Eligible Fellows, will forward to any applicant copies of the amended Constitution and By-Laws, List of Members, and other information as to the Academy.

OFFICIAL LIST OF CHANGES IN THE STATIONS AND DUTIES OF OFFICERS SERVING IN THE MEDICAL DEPARTMENT, U. S. ARMY, FROM NOVEMBER 11 TO NOVEMBER 17, 1890.

By direction of the Acting Secretary of War, leave of absence for three months is granted Charles M. Gandy, *Captain and Assistant Surgeon,* Fort Clark, Texas.—Par. 10, *S. O. 266, Headquarters of the Army, A. G. O.,* November 15, 1890.

Walker, Freeman V., *First Lieutenant and Assistant Surgeon* (Fort D. A. Russell, Wyoming).—Is granted leave of absence for one month, to take effect on or about the 15th instant. —Par. 3, *S. O. 85, Department of the Platte,* November 11, 1890.

By direction of the Secretary of War, the leave of absence granted Stevens G. Cowdrey, *Major and Surgeon,* in Special Orders No. 112, Department of Arizona, October 24, 1890, is extended fifteen days.—*S. O. 163, Headquarters of the Army, A. G. O., Washington,* November 10, 1890.

By direction of the Secretary of War, the extension of leave of absence on account of sickness, granted Henry McElderry, *Major and Surgeon,* in Special Orders No. 214, September 12, 1890, from this office, is further extended two months, on surgeon's certificate of disability.—Par. 28, *S. O. 263, A. G. O.,* November 10, 1890.

OFFICIAL LIST OF CHANGES IN THE STATIONS AND DUTIES OF THE MEDICAL CORPS OF THE U. S. NAVY FOR THE WEEK ENDING NOVEMBER 15, 1890.

Owens, Thomas, *Surgeon.*—Ordered to the Museum of Hygiene at Washington, D. C.

Martin, H. M., *Surgeon.*—Detached from the Receiving-ship " Wabash," and ordered before Retiring Board.

Rixey, P. M., *Surgeon.*—Continued in charge of Naval Dispensary at Washington, D. C., until November 20, 1890.

Green, E. H., *Passed Assistant Surgeon.*—Promoted to Surgeon. November 10, 1890.

Smith, Howard, *Surgeon.*—Placed on the Retired List, November 10, 1890.

THE MEDICAL NEWS.

A WEEKLY JOURNAL OF MEDICAL SCIENCE.

VOL. LVII.   SATURDAY, NOVEMBER 29, 1890.   No. 22.

ORIGINAL LECTURES.

CRANIECTOMY FOR MICROCEPHALUS— THE LATER HISTORY OF A CASE OF EXCISION OF THE HAND-CENTRE FOR EPILEPSY.

*A Clinical Lecture
delivered at the Jefferson Medical College Hospital,
November 19, 1890.*

BY W. W. KEEN, M.D.,

PROFESSOR OF THE PRINCIPLES OF SURGERY.

GENTLEMEN : The first case that I shall show you to-day is that of the little boy upon whom I operated before you last December. At that time I removed the hand-centre from the cerebrum for the relief of epilepsy.[1] First, as a caution to you, I will tell you of a slight accident that occurred.

You will notice that the scar, instead of being pale as it should be, is somewhat red at one point. Shortly after the operation the boy disturbed the dressings, and I feared that the wound would become infected. A small abscess formed which was followed later by the extrusion of two of the small pieces of bone, which you will remember I replaced. The large 1½-inch button is in good condition. At the second dressing after the operation I wished to remove the strand of horsehairs which had been placed in the wound for drainage, but on taking away the gauze I did not find them. The dressings were then carefully examined, as I thought that the hairs might have been pulled out when the gauze was removed. I then searched for them upon the floor and then carefully and gently in the wound itself, but not finding them I came to the conclusion that the child had pulled the hairs out at the time that the dressings were disturbed and that they had been lost. The wound healed nicely, except at the place where the two fragments of bone came out, which united slowly.

All went well till last june, when the cicatrix became red and irritated and a little later a small sinus formed, in which the horsehairs were found and removed. They were probably cut too short, and when the child disturbed the dressings were pushed into the wound, remaining there from December until June without giving rise to any trouble. I have never before had such an occurrence, and I give you this history so that you may avoid the same accident. I once performed an operation upon a young woman who had been previously operated upon, and found in the seat of the old wound one of the horse-hairs which had remained there a year without giving rise to any irritation.

In the present case, in spite of the horsehair, which must have caused some irritation, the boy's condition is much better, although he is not completely cured. The fits have been, as a rule, far less severe and less frequent than before the operation and his disposition is very greatly improved. In fact, he is quite a different boy and more amenable to control, so that he can now play with other children. He is interested in matters of every-day life almost as much as one would expect in a child of his age. His vocabulary also is now quite large, and he is learning quiet kindergarten plays, which he would not have touched or looked at in his restless impatience a year ago.

How far this change in disposition is due to the operation and how far to the careful training of Miss Bancroft and Miss Cox, of Haddonfield, N. J., who have had him in their training-school for feeble-minded children, I am not prepared to say ; it is my belief, however, that it is largely due to the operation, as his disposition began to improve while still in the hospital, and especially after he went to his home.

For some weeks after the operation his hand was completely paralyzed, but later it gradually recovered and is now only slightly paretic. The bilateral function of the opposite cortex has reëstablished the function of the lost centre. He can feed himself without difficulty, and you would probably not have noticed the slight defect had I not called your attention to it.

CRANIECTOMY FOR MICROCEPHALUS.

The operation that I next propose to do is the first one of its kind which, so far as I know, has been performed in this country. It has been done only twice in Europe, both times by Lannelongue, of Paris. Lannelongue's first case was that of a microcephalic idiot, the history of which I will read to you.[1]

The patient was a girl, four years of age, born at term and without accident ; father aged thirty-eight years and mother thirty-five years, both in good health. No hereditary disease. Five brothers and sisters in good health.

The child's mental development was retarded. She could not take any food but liquids, and up to the age of three years had not walked nor even stood. Within the last few weeks before coming under observation she had babbled a few syllables but no words. Saliva escaped from the mouth constantly. She had the appearance of an imperfectly-developed child of two years. Her eyes were brilliant, but she did not seem to be interested in anything about her, nor could one engage her attention. She was constantly uttering inarticulate cries, and scarcely ever ceased moving. Her height was 77 cm. (30⅜ inches), the circumference of the thorax 45 cm. (17¾ inches). Her legs, while they could not support her weight, were always in active motion. There were no contractures or paralyses ; sensibility normal ; reflexes not increased ; no epileptoid manifestations. Head very much narrowed transversely and

---

[1] THE MEDICAL NEWS, April 12, 1890.

[1] L'Union Médicale, July 8, 1890.

prominent at the vertex. Nose well developed and aquiline. Forehead retreating and very narrow. Antero-posterior diameter of skull 155 mm. (6⅛ inches), bi-parietal 109 mm. (4¼ inches), bi-frontal 86 mm. (3⅜ inches).

Operation May 9, 1890: A narrow strip of bone was removed on the left side of the sagittal suture, as the left side was smaller than the right. The bone was removed a finger's breadth from the middle line and was 9 cm. (3 9/16 inches) in length and 6 mm. (¼ inch) in breadth. The dura was not opened. The incision in the scalp was made in such a manner as not to correspond with the incision in the bone. The periosteum was not replaced. Healing took place in a few days. During the operation, as well as for four or five days afterward, a serous liquid escaped in small drops from the surface of the dura mater.

Results: On June 15th, that is to say, in five weeks, the child was calmer, the incessant cries had ceased the day after the operation, she took notice of what went on about her, laughed and seemed very happy, comprehended what occurred, tried to talk and pronounced several words. She can now stand alone; she walks with regular steps, tottering a little when she hastens. She no longer drools. Her intelligence seems to have kept pace in its development with the physical improvement. She is now able to eat at the table. She has been under instruction, which may account in part for the improvement.

A second, similar, case, but more pronouncedly idiotic, was operated on June 20, 1890. The incision to the left of the middle line was the same, but another similar portion of bone was removed from the frontal on the left side, leaving a little bridge at the fronto-parietal suture. In other respects the operations were the same. Of course, the time was too short to judge of the result.

The history of the case upon which I am about to operate is as follows:

M. E., aged four years and seven months, was first seen by me on November 3, 1890. Three grandparents are living and in good health. Paternal grandmother had scrofulous glands in her neck. Her mother is aged thirty-three years, father thirty-five years, and both are in good health. She has one sister, nine years old, in good health physically and mentally. The patient's birth was normal and she was a breast-fed baby. At four or five months of age she weighed 25 pounds, at fifteen months 40 pounds, at three years 31 pounds, and at present only 30 pounds. She has never walked, but began to stand at about two years of age. When twenty-one months old she could say "baby," "pretty," "bye-bye," and other words, but since then entirely lost the power of speech. Two years ago she had twenty-four convulsions in one day, probably from teething, which was late; but these are the only convulsions she has had. Had measles and whooping-cough in rather rapid succession when about a year old.

Present condition: She is evidently a healthy but poorly-developed child. Her bones are small, and her head is very small and moderately prognathic, with defective development, most marked in the frontal region, and also in the occipital. Two photographs, one taken at twenty-one months of age, the other a week ago, show the greatest difference in expression, the earlier one being that of a bright, intelligent baby, the later showing a plainly idiotic face. There are no contractures or paralyses. She is constantly moving and wringing her hands, but evidently not from pain. She drools a good deal. The condition of her reflexes is hard to determine because of the constant movements and the want of intelligence. Her mother thinks that she knows her parents and sister. She watches strangers somewhat, but notices little else. Seems to be pleased by having her hat put on, as though she knew it meant that she is going out of doors. All the sutures are firm. The anterior fontanelle, which existed at birth, is entirely closed. Percussion gives a uniform sound all over the skull, and is not painful. She has "drowsy spells" from time to time, often several times a day, when her head falls over and she sinks down almost asleep, but awakens immediately and is as well as ever. These attacks last only two or three seconds. Her intelligence varies considerably; some times she is much brighter than at others.

Measurements: Height, 92.5 cm. (36⅜ inches); circumference of chest, 50 cm. (19⅝ inches); head, antero-posterior diameter, 15.3 cm. (6 1/16 inches), bi-parietal, 11.3 cm. (4½ inches), bi-auricular, 11.6 cm. (4 9/16 inches), bi-frontal, 9.5 c.m. (3¾ inches). Circumference of head, 43.5 cm. (17⅛ inches). The two sides of the head are of equal size. You observe that the head is very small, being about the size of the head of a child eleven or twelve months old.

The result of the examination of the eyes, which was made by my friend Dr. Hansell, is as follows: "The examination was difficult and prolonged on account of the constant movement of the hands and arms, and lack of intelligence preventing coöperation. The pupils responded to light and association, the pupil of one responding in contraction and dilatation to the alternate exposure to light and darkness. Media clear; fundus normal; nerves (optic disks) of good color. The internal squint, said to be present at times, was to-day absent. The patient seemed to have good vision."

The inherent cause of microcephalus we do not know. Formerly it was supposed to be due to premature ossification of the cranial sutures, but the examination of several such skulls has shown that while this may sometimes be the case, yet in the cases examined there was no abnormality in the bony development of the cranium. On the other hand, we know that the growth of the skull keeps pace with the growth of the brain within it; and if the growing power of the brain be weak, a slight resistance on the part of its osseous envelope may be sufficient to check and stunt it. Reasoning in this way, Lannelongue concluded that it was a rational procedure to attempt to remove at least a part of the force that was preventing this enfeebled brain from attaining a larger and more natural growth; and his operation was planned to effect this end. It is too early yet to pass judgment upon the operation as a remedial measure, for so far we have only the report of his two cases. It seems to me an experiment well worth trial. The operation itself, if it does not produce the hoped-for result, is at least little, if any, more dangerous than trephining; and, inasmuch as the dura is not opened, the real danger of the operation should be very small. Of course, the operation is only applicable to children.

I propose to do the operation with slight modifications.

Lannelongue's incision in the scalp was made parallel to the line of the sagittal suture, commencing in front of the lambdoid and extending forward to the coronal suture, then turning off at an obtuse angle downward on the forehead, with a bridge of bone at the coronal suture.

Instead of continuing my incision forward on the forehead as Lannelongue did, I shall there make a curved incision with the convexity backward and all in the hairy scalp. I shall then raise this flap of skin and under it cut out the bone, thus avoiding any scar on the forehead. The incision in the skin will not be in the same line as that in the bone, so that the wound in the cranium will be covered by the scalp. I shall leave no bridge of bone at the coronal suture. The object of the operation is to make the side of the head, as it were, into a bony flap, with an attached base below and a free border above. This flap can be readily expanded even by feeble force from within, and will allow the brain "elbow-room," so to speak, for development. I shall extend it into the frontal and occipital regions, so that these lobes, and especially the frontal, which is probably the seat of the intellectual faculties, may be able to enlarge. As the skull grows stronger and stiffer it will still have strength enough to prevent danger to life from ordinary blows or other traumatisms. It is a matter of indifference in this case upon which side the incision is made, as the cerebral development is symmetrical. A cast of her head has been taken, and at different periods of the child's growth other casts will be taken and the progress of the growth of the head may thus be determined. As the usual mode of making a cast by plaster cream alone is rather objectionable, and in the case of this child, indeed, impossible, I devised the following plan: The head was shaved and rubbed with a little sweet oil. A thin coat of plaster-of-Paris cream was then evenly applied to get a smooth surface. Upon this three or four layers of a common plaster-of-Paris bandage were put on as a "recurrent" bandage, followed by a thin layer of plaster-of-Paris cream, and so on ultimately until the mould was completed. If either the occiput or the frontal portion of the head is so prominent as to prevent the removal of the mould, it may be cut over these places before it dries, the edges of the cut being carefully restored to their original position immediately after removal. No cutting was needed in this case.

In my operations upon the brain I use sterilized gauzes instead of sponges. This gauze is steamed for three-quarters of an hour in a Sattegast steam sterilizer, without chemicals, as I prefer not to use corrosive sublimate in these cases. All the instruments are boiled in a Schimmelbusch sterilizer, and the water in the apparatus is kept boiling during the operation so that any instrument may be quickly sterilized if necessary. One per cent. of carbonate of sodium is added to the water to prevent rusting the instruments.

I have explained the operation to the father and mother of the child, telling them that it is only an experiment, but that I consider that there is little danger in it, and a possibility of doing her great good. Upon these grounds they at once consented to the operation.

Upon making my scalp incision I find that there is unusually little bleeding. I have at former times in operating upon the scalp placed an Esmarch narrow band around the head to prevent bleeding, but this is unnecessary. It adds to the length of what is always a long operation, and I find the hæmorrhage is easily controlled by hæmostatic forceps. The flap is pulled to one side, and I now carefully remove with a half-inch trephine a button of bone from a point about a finger's breadth to the right side of the sagittal suture, so that there is no danger of entering the superior longitudinal sinus. The dura is very carefully separated from the bone, and in this case I think is more adherent than usual. The instrument that I shall use in removing the bone is a pair of rongeur forceps, much more curved than ordinarily, and only one-fourth of an inch wide. In case of hæmorrhage from a branch of the middle meningeal I would quickly bite away the bone over the bleeding part with a forceps and pass a ligature under the vessel by means of a curved needle. The middle meningeal always requires to be ligated in this way. It runs in a tightly-stretched membrane and does not contract and retract like other arteries and thus easily and spontaneously cease bleeding. As the patient should have all the chances for recovery that are possible, I shall operate upon only one side to-day, thus reducing the danger of shock. She will be constantly under my observation; if her mental condition does not improve as much as I desire I shall operate later on the other side. The line of incision in the bone is now complete and extends to within three-fourths of an inch of the supraorbital ridge and backward nearly to the occipital bone, measuring six and one-fourth inches in length and one-fourth of an inch in width.

One rather large branch of the middle meningeal artery is seen crossing the cleft. The forceps are all removed and the flap is carefully inspected to see if there are any bleeding vessels. The hæmorrhage is usually stopped by the forceps, but in case I find any bleeding points I will pass a stitch under them, as I wish all bleeding to be completely arrested before the wound is closed. The periosteum is next cut away from the edges of the groove so that it will not cover it and cause union of the bone. A few strands of horsehair are placed in the groove and are cut sufficiently long to prevent danger of their slipping under the scalp in this case. These hairs will all be removed, except two or three, at the end of two or three days. In sewing up the flap I am careful to get absolute coaptation, so that there shall be no overlapping, as this would expose a surface which must heal by cicatrization. The wound is carefully dressed with sterilized gauze and she will be laid upon her right side to favor drainage. Now, gentlemen, the operation is completed, and we have only to await the future. Her mental traits have been closely observed, so that it may be readily seen whether there is any change in her intelligence.

[NOTE.—She was entirely well and all the sutures were out in five days. The operation took an hour and convinced me that it could be done in probably one-half that time by a proper pair of rongeur forceps. These I have had made, and I will report upon their usefulness in the future.—W. W. K.]

Deaths from Wild Beasts and Snakes in India.—According to the *Medical Press*, 1587 persons were killed by snakes and 385 by wild beasts in the Madras Presidency, India, in 1889. The number of cattle destroyed was 15,550.

ORIGINAL ARTICLES.

WHAT I HAVE LEARNED TO UNLEARN IN GYNECOLOGY.

BY WILLIAM GOODELL, M.D.,

PROFESSOR OF GYNECOLOGY IN THE UNIVERSITY OF PENNSYLVANIA.

EVERY earnest worker in any field of the inexact sciences finds himself compelled to unlearn as well as to learn. The errors which he discovers and weeds out will usually be traditional teachings—the legacies of our forefathers—for we get many of our opinions, as well as many of our diseases, by heredity. What I have thus learned to unlearn in the treatment of woman's diseases will be the burden of this paper.

To begin, then, I have learned to unlearn the grandmotherly belief that the climacteric is in itself an entity, and that, as such, it is responsible for most of the ills of matronhood, and especially for that of menorrhagia. True, it must be conceded, that as an entity it does seem to disturb the vaso-motor system, and through it to cause many severe perturbations, such as tinglings and numbness, and sweating of the skin, flushes of heat and shivers of cold, emotional explosions, and a large group of hysterical symptoms. It can also lay claim to being an important factor in the causation of insanity. Yet, contrary to the prevalent lay and professional belief, how rarely can true uterine hæmorrhages or other uterine discharges be traced to the climacteric as a cause in itself. Yet many a poor woman has lost her health, her life, indeed, by her own and her physician's traditional belief, that her hæmorrhages or other vaginal discharges are critical and due to the "change-of-life," as it is popularly called—a misnomer which too often leads to indolent diagnosis and slovenly therapeutics.

What physician of any practice has not been called in to see some wretched sufferer, whose health has been crippled for months, or even for years, by hæmorrhages or by other discharges from the sexual organs, which have been attributed to the "change-of-life" by her friends, or—what is more inexcusable—by the successive physicians whom she has consulted? To the shame of the latter, they may not have made even a digital examination; yet a polypus or a fungoid degeneration of the endometrium, or a uterine fibroid, or a cancer of the cervix has been found by a more alert man, who does not believe in climacteric omnipotency. Never can I forget a case—not the only one—of a beautiful woman, beloved by a large circle of friends and surrounded by every luxury that wealth could furnish, who was allowed by her physician to bleed almost literally to death. Why? Because a polypus, being at first intra-uterine, was not recognized, and because her age justified, in his opinion, the diagnosis of "change-of-life." This diagnosis having been made, no other vaginal examination was ever thought of by this physician. But when he was discharged and another one was called in, the latter found the polypus dangling in the vagina. She was bedridden and as translucent as alabaster when I twisted off the growth. The hæmorrhages did not return, but neither did her health, and she died a few months later quite suddenly and very unexpectedly.

In other cases, by the careless indolence of the physicians, begotten by this traditional belief in climacteric influences, I have been compelled to undeceive some poor woman and break as gently as possible to her, that the flow which she had joyfully accepted as a return of her monthly periods, and which she has mistaken for rejuvenescence, is the sure token of an incurable and far advanced cancer of the cervix.

I have learned to unlearn the teaching that woman must not be subjected to a surgical operation during her monthly flux. Our forefathers, from time immemorial, have thought and taught that the presence of a menstruating woman would pollute solemn religious rites, would sour milk, spoil the fermentation in wine-vats, and do much other mischief in a general way. Influenced by hoary tradition, modern physicians very generally postpone all operative treatment until the flow has ceased. But why this delay, if time is precious and it enters as an important factor in the case? I have found menstruation to be the very best time to curette away fungous vegetations of the endometrium, for, being swollen, then, by the afflux of blood, they are larger than at any other time, and can the more readily be removed. There is, indeed, no surer way of checking a menorrhagia or of stopping a metrorrhagia than by curetting the womb during the very flow. While I do not select this period for the removal of ovarian cysts, or for other abdominal work, such as the extirpation of the ovaries, of a kidney, of breaking up intestinal adhesions, etc., yet I have not hesitated to perform these operations at such a time, and I have never had reason to regret the course. The only operations that I should dislike to perform during menstruation would be those involving the womb itself—such as the removal of a uterine fibroid, or a partial or a complete hysterectomy, and the various operations for uterine cancer, etc. This exception is based upon the danger of hæmorrhage arising from the increased vascular tension and pelvic hyperæmia, which exist during menstruation. This is well shown in fibroid tumor of the womb, in which this increased vascularity causes a corresponding increase in the size of the tumor itself. For obvious mechanical reasons it would also hardly be wise to sew up the torn cervix of a menstruating womb.

I have learned to unlearn that anteflexion and anteversion in themselves—that is to say, as displacements merely, and without narrowing of the uterine canal—are necessarily pathological conditions of the womb. Text-books speak of them as such, and exhibit many ingenious forms of pessaries devised to rectify these so-called displacements. But very rarely indeed do I have to resort to them, and then only to a stem-pessary in anteflexions; for I find in almost every virgin or every barren woman that the womb in varying degrees is either bent forward or is tilted forward, and is apparently resting on the bladder. The mistake made, as I have more elaboratively shown in my *Lessons in Gynecology* is in attributing to this natural position of the womb the various forms of pelvic trouble, especially that of irritability of the bladder, to which women are so liable. But the sympathy between the brain and the bladder is a remarkably close one—so close, indeed, that some physiologists contend that "every mental act in man is accompanied by a contraction of the bladder." The irritability of the bladder thus becomes one of the first symptoms of nervousness, to which everyone is liable. Many a lawyer before pleading an important case, and many a clergyman before delivering a discourse, is compelled from sheer nervousness to empty his bladder. So it is with the lower animals, which, when frightened, micturate involuntarily. A nervous bladder is then one of the earliest phenomena of a nervous brain—for nervousness means a deficient control of the higher nerve-centres over the lower ones—a lack of brain-control. Now, a hysterical girl, or a woman whose nervous system has given way under the strain of domestic cares, consults the physician for such ordinary symptoms of nerve-exhaustion as wakefulness, utter weariness, a bearing-down feeling, backache, and, perhaps, above all, an irritable bladder. Upon making a digital examination, he usually finds the fundus of the womb resting on the bladder, where it naturally should rest. At once he jumps to the conclusion that the whole trouble is due to pressure of the womb on the bladder—viz., to the existing natural anteversion or to the anteflexion, as the case may be. Enticed away by the vesical lapwing from the bottom factor—the shattered nerves—he now makes local applications, and racks his brain to adapt or to devise some pessary capable of overcoming the supposed difficulty, heedless of 'the dilemma that the upward, or shoring, pressure of the pessary on the bladder must be greater than the counter, or downward, pressure of the womb, to which he attributes the vesical irritability.

In the lying-in chamber the fear of septicæmia will ever haunt me, but I have long since abandoned the idea cherished by that class of waistless and witless nurses, now happily obsolescent, that the parturient woman is to be swathed like a mummy and to be kept as immovable. What earthly harm can accrue to a woman after a natural labor if she turns over from side to side, sits up in bed, or even gets up to use the commode, if she feels like it, I cannot see. Natural labor is a physiological process, not a pathological one, but tradition has thrown around the lying-in bed a glamour of mischievous sentiment.

In relation to this let me express my disbelief that mammary abscess comes from "caked" breasts, or from breasts over-distended from a secretion of milk too great for the infant's needs. Mammary abscess, in the suckling woman comes, in my opinion, from cracked nipples, and from cracked nipples alone. In proof of this let me ask my readers if any one of them has ever had a case of mastitis after a miscarriage, or one of gathered breast following a stillbirth—always provided the breasts were let pretty much alone so far as pumping and sucking are concerned. Under these circumstances the unsucked and unpumped breast will swell up and grow painfully hard, but it will not inflame or suppurate. Let me not be understood as saying that an overdistended breast should not be relieved by sucking or by pumping; but the means employed for this relief must be so sparingly used, and at such long intervals, as not to crack the nipples. This immunity from mammary abscess after miscarriages and stillbirths is attributed by the physician to his local applications of belladonnâ, or of other milk-drying drugs. But it comes from the absence of the exciting cause of cracked nipples—the sucking child.

Long ago I came to the conclusion, that the womb, like the nose, has its own secretions; and that, because the cervical canal is stopped up with mucus, it is not to be treated any more harshly than a stopped-up nose. I was led to this belief from seeing very many cervical canals wholly closed up, even destroyed by the remedies applied to get rid of this mucus. Then again I found that, just as the nose secretes abundantly under the stimulus of the emotions, so the womb secretes more actively under a stimulus conveyed to impressionable nerves—so much so, indeed, that leucorrhœa is a common adjunct to nerve-prostration, and is then cured by the cure of its cause. This nasal analogy led me soon to think that even uterine catarrhs are not of such paramount importance as to merit heroic treatment, and that metritis and endometritis, in so far as symptoms are concerned, are often idle words. The mucus of a uterine catarrh is in quality very much the same as the mucus of a nasal catarrh, and its secretion is in itself no more weakening. It is not a disease in itself, but is merely the symptom of a disease. It is not, therefore, that highly vitalized fluid, the loss of which, according to the traditional belief of the great majority of physicians, and of all women, saps the very citadel of life, brings on decrepit and premature old age, and hastens its victim to an untimely grave. This widespread error is a relic of mediæval ignorance, which believed in the existence of two seeds—the male and the female semen—and their admixture to insure conception. Hence leucorrhœa has erroneously come to mean pretty much the same thing as spermatorrhœa—a belief fostered by cunning quacks, who know how largely sex and sexuality make up our being and influence our credulity.

As a corollary to this, let me add, that I have wholly freed myself from the belief that cellulitis is at the bottom of most female ailments, and that the hot-water douche is its cure-all. My experience teaches me that, save in some cases of active congestion or of acute inflammation of the pelvic organs, the hot douche is of questionable utility, and. that its indiscriminate employment has done far more harm than good, especially when continued for any length of time. I cannot withhold the opinion that from its use both ovaritis, salpingitis, and peri-uterine inflammation have actually been set up by the overheating and the subsequent chilling of the pelvic organs. The crucial test of surgical research which cannot be gainsaid has shown that cellulitis is almost a myth, and that what have long been deemed exudation tumors and inflammatory deposits in the areolar tissue, are tubal and ovarian lesions.

I have learned to unlearn the idea—and this was the hardest task of all—that uterine symptoms are not always present in cases of uterine disease ; or that, when present, they necessarily come from the uterine disease. The nerves are mighty mimes, the greatest of mimics, and they cheat us by their realistic personations of organic disease, and especially of uterine disease. Hence it is that even seemingly urgent uterine symptoms may be merely nerve-counterfeits of uterine disease. I have, therefore, long since given up the belief, which with many amounts to a creed, that the womb is at the bottom of nearly every female ailment.

Nerve-strain, or nerve-exhaustion, comes largely from the frets, the griefs, the worries, the carks and cares of life. Yet, although the imagination undoubtedly affects it, it is not a mere whim or an imaginary disease, as all healthy women and most physicians think ; but it is the veriest of realities. When some flippant talker or some slipshod thinker scoffs at nervousness as a sham disorder, I say to him : "Can the bribe of a principality keep you from blushing when

you are ashamed, or from blanching when you are afraid ? Under the flitting sense of shame or of fear these vasomotor disturbances are momentarily beyond your control ; and so they are in the nervous woman, whose vital organs are, as it were—not transiently, but—perpetually blushing and blanching under deficient brain-control over the lower nerve-centres."

Strangely enough, the most common symptoms of nerve-disorder in women are the very ones which lay tradition and dogmatic empiricism attribute to womb-disease. They are, in the order of their frequency, great weariness, and more or less of nervousness and of wakefulness ; inability to walk any distance and a bearing-down feeling ; headache, nape-ache, and backache ; scant, or painful, or delayed, or suppressed menstruation ; cold feet, and an irritable bladder ; general spinal and pelvic soreness, and pain in one ovary, usually the left, or in both ovaries. The sense of exhaustion is a remarkable one ; the woman is always tired ; she passes the day tired, she goes to bed tired, and she wakes up tired, often, indeed, more tired than when she fell asleep. She sighs a great deal, she has low spirits, and her arms and legs become numb so frequently that she fears palsy or paralysis. There are many other symptoms of nerve-strain, but since they are not so distinctively uterine, and, therefore, not so misleading, I shall not enumerate them.

Now, let a nervous woman, with some of the foregoing group of symptoms recount them to a female friend, and she will be told that she has womb-disease. Let her consult a physician, and ten to one he will think the same thing and diligently hunt for some uterine lesion. If one be found, no matter how trifling, he will attach to it undue importance, and treat it heroically as the peccant organ. If no visible disease of the sexual organs be discoverable, he will lay the blame on the invisible endometrium or on the unseeable ovaries, and continue the local treatment. In any event, whatever the inlook or the outlook, a local treatment is bound to be the issue.

Until my eyes were opened to the harlequin tricks of the nerves, I have repeatedly made the same mistake, and I now see it made over and over again by other physicians. To give but two recent instances out of very many :

Not long ago a lady was sent to me by a very intelligent physician to have a cervical tear repaired. She had been seen by several physicians, all of whom had treated her locally, and all had concurred in the opinion expressed by my friend. Her most pronounced symptoms were insomnia, unending weariness, excessive nervousness, great dread of being alone, severe bearing-down, painful locomotion, constant backache, and an extremely irritable bladder which gave her no peace day or night.

She had in addition most of the canonical uterine symptoms. Being sure that a comparatively trifling tear of the cervix could not give rise to so many exacting symptoms, although she herself attributed them to this cause, I closely cross-questioned her, and soon discovered the source of the mischief. After a rather difficult labor—her sole one—she had given birth to a still child. This was a great disappointment, yet she was convalescing naturally, when a great conflagration broke out in her city. After destroying most of this city it swept onward toward her house. Her valuables were hastily packed up, and she was bundled up ready to be carried away at a moment's notice. Fortunately the fire was put out at the second house from hers. Since then she had never been well.

It was not the cervical tear that had wrecked her health, but disappointed motherhood, and the noise, the tumult, the fear, the long-drawn-out agony of suspense.

The second case gave the following history :

She was aged forty-two years, and was the mother of one child, now twelve years old. She had sharp pain in the right ovary, burning aches in the left one, and difficult locomotion. A sensating of tingling, prickling, and stinging heat pervaded her whole left side. Her left eye had wavering vision, as if she were looking through heated air. The catamenia, formerly scant and painful, were replaced by an abundant leucorrhœa. Her bladder was irritable and needed emptying day and night. She was tired all the time, lay awake most of the night, and her sleep was troubled by distressing dreams. A well-known oculist had cut the muscles of her eyes, several physicians had treated her locally off and on for many years, and she was now sent to me to decide the question of the removal of her ovaries. The womb lay in the first stage of retroversion, there was some endometritis, and the left ovary was tender and reachable. Finding, as in the foregoing case, that her symptoms were out of all proportion to the local lesions, I suspected nerve-trouble, which her history confirmed. Ten years ago, while sailing with her husband across a lake, a storm overtook them. The boat filled with water and, after a desperate struggle, they barely reached the shore. Two years later her nerves, still much shaken by this narrow escape from drowning, received another shock. A burglar broke into her home, and her husband had, in her hearing, a fierce and noisy hand-to-hand fight with him. One more year passed, and she met with a railroad accident, in which twelve persons were killed. but she was uninjured. This final shock completely shattered her nervous system, and she was plainly suffering from a sore brain, and not from sore ovaries. In one word, it was the old, old story of wounded nerves counterfeiting a wounded womb.

I have learned yet another trick of the nerves: that when riotous from being under-fed, from overwork, or from lack of discipline, they billet themselves, like an insolent soldiery. on some maimed

organ and hold high revel there. For instance, a woman, hitherto in perfect health, may have an adherent or a dislocated ovary, or a torn cervix, or a narrow cervical canal, or a slight displacement of the womb—lesions which may have given her no appreciable trouble whatever. But let her nervous system become unstrung, and at once, through disturbances in the circulation both of the nerve-fluid and of the blood-fluid, there set in vesical, uterine, or ovarian symptoms, which may indeed reach so exacting a pitch as to demand a local treatment. Nor are the sexual organs the only ones thus affected. Every weakened organ in the body is liable to such functional outbreaks. The stomach rejects its food, the bowels either refuse to act or else they are very loose, the heart loses its rhythm and beats irregularly, the vocal cords relax and the voice cannot be raised above a whisper, and almost every sphincter muscle in the body behaves as if it were insane. I have known a woman in her nervous attacks to become as jaundiced as if she had the liver of a Strasburg goose. The yellow color was fugitive, but it lasted longer than the emotion that caused it. Even the eyes, which before may have exhibited to their owner no visual defect, now blink painfully at the light or may cause violent headaches, which glasses alone can allay. In the following case various organs were thus affected :

An unmarried lady in splendid health and with a magnificent physique, had unusual muscular strength, which she was fond of testing. One day, while wrestling with her brother, which she often did, she felt something give way in the pelvis, and shortly after this her health began to fail. Her monthly periods, hitherto painless, now gave her acute suffering, and a persistent leucorrhœa soiled her linen. The left ovary throbbed with a constant ache, walking became painful, the bladder grew irritable, and the stomach began to reject its food. From sluggish circulation, local congestions took place, particularly in the head and in the pelvis. Thus, when she stood up, the pelvic organs seemed to fill up with blood and painful pelvic throbs beat time with her pulse. From these she got relief by sitting with her knees raised up, or by lying with her feet higher than her head. Soon insomnia, photophobia, and dreadful headaches set in. These were followed by illusions when her eyes were closed, which vanished when she opened them. She heard imaginary conversations and saw unpleasant sights. She became morose and irascible, and kept much by herself; in one word, her mind hovered on that ill-defined borderland between sanity and insanity.

The wrestling episode and her many orthodox uterine symptoms misled every one, including herself, her family, and several physicians, who attributed everything to uterine disease and treated her accordingly. She had much local treatment of the usual kind. and more for supposed anteflexion. Getting no better. she travelled many miles to con-

22*

sult me. My examination of her revealed merely glairy mucus in the cervical canal, some tenderness over the left ovary, which was slightly displaced, and the natural anteflexion of a virginal womb. These lesions were too trivial to account for her lamentable condition, and I looked to her history for an explanation. This clearly satisfied me that she was suffering from nerve-breakdown. This diagnosis was a great surprise to her and to her mother, who accompanied her; but, notwithstanding her contrary convictions, she entered my private hospital. With the exception of a few douches of corrosive sublimate for the leucorrhœa, her uterine organs were let severely alone, and she was treated merely for her nerves. Her friends were greatly dissatisfied with this treatment, and at their instance a near medical relative wrote me a letter in which, after criticising my treatment, he urged upon my attention the wrestling match and the uterine character of the symptoms. At the end of six weeks she left me very greatly improved in every respect, but as her headaches still troubled her more or less, I asked Dr. de Schweinitz to examine her eyes. He found some astigmatism in one eye, and "the highest degree of hypermetropia which he had ever seen, excepting in two other cases." Suitable glasses remedied these defects, and she afterward progressively improved—so much so, that eight months later I received from her a most grateful letter of thanks. Further, the physician himself who had criticised my treatment of her, wrote me quite recently, that he was about to send me a patient with analogous symptoms, who had been unrelieved by a long course of uterine treatment.

Just as headache does not necessarily mean brain disease, so ovary-ache does not necessarily mean ovarian disease. Yet time and again—and I say this deliberately—have ladies been sent to my private hospital to have their ovaries taken out, when the whole mischief had started from some mental worry. Their ovaries were sound, but their nerves were not, and no operation was needed for their cure. So misleading, indeed, are the symptoms of a jaded brain or of other nerve-strain, under the uterine livery in which they are often clad, that I have recently known a jilted maiden to be treated by a cup-and-stem pessary, and a bereaved mother to be douched and tamponned and cauterized for a twelvemonth. Such cases, even when accompanied by actual uterine disease, are not bettered by merely local treatment. Nor are medicines by themselves of much avail. What they need is massage, perhaps electricity, and that freedom from care which strict seclusion gives. Hope should be infused into every case, and, above all, there must be imported into it the personality of the physician. It was not the staff of the prophet that awakened the dead child; but death was quickened into life when the prophet threw himself upon its body and breathed into it of his own intense vitality.

As the outcome of much that I have learned to unlearn, I have arrived at this very short gynecological creed: I believe that the physician who recognizes the complexity of woman's nervous organization and appreciates its tyranny, will touch her well-being at more points and with a keener perception of its wants, than the one who holds the opinion that woman is woman because she has a womb.

TUBERCULOUS DISEASE OF THE TARSUS [1]

BY JOSEPH RANSOHOFF, M.D., F.R.C.S.
PROFESSOR OF ANATOMY AND CLINICAL SURGERY IN THE MEDICAL COLLEGE OF OHIO, CINCINNATI.

AMONG the joints affected by the tubercular process, those of the tarsus are involved in about ten per cent. of all cases. If in the present paper, I nevertheless venture to limit my remarks to this somewhat neglected field of joint-surgery, it is for the following reasons: (1) Because in no other portion of the skeleton, with the possible exception of the wrist, is disease so liable to spread from part to part, assuming a progressive type and generally terminating only after a number of years with partial or complete loss of the affected parts; (2) because in tarsal disease the influence of age on the progress and termination of tuberculosis of bone finds an excellent illustration; and (3) because in disease of no other part of the skeleton are the questions of how and when to operate, if operation be at all desirable, more difficult to answer.

Tuberculous disease of the tarsus, as commonly encountered, presents itself as an infiltration limited for a longer or shorter period of time to a single bone of the anterior or posterior row. Even here it appears to have a preference for certain bones, the cuboid of the anterior and the os-calcis of the posterior row being, in my experience, most frequently primarily involved. The greater weight brought to bear on these bones in walking, and their position, exposing them to injury, may account for this preference which doubtless exists. The extent of the joint-connections of a bone or a part of a bone, which is the seat of the disease, becomes a direct index of the rapidity of its extension. Thus the most favorable cases of the appended table were those in which the disease was limited to the os-calcis and the posterior calcaneo-astragaloid joint. A further reason for limitation to the heel-bone is in the large surfaces below, posteriorly, and on either side which are uncovered by ligaments and, therefore, permit the early evacuation of abscesses, the absence of subligamentous tension preventing the spread of disease. Far less frequent is extension forward toward the calcaneo-cuboid joint or the anterior calcaneo-astragaloid joint and its prolongation between the

---

[1] Read before the Mississippi Valley Medical Association, Louisville, October, 1890.

astragalus and scaphoid. When the latter direction has been taken the disease may easily spread around the astragalus and involve the ankle, or, affecting the scaphoid, may extend into the common tarsal sac. It is not until late in the disease that such extension takes place. In the case of a boy of eight years the disease remained limited to the calcaneum, notwithstanding one curetting done in New Orleans and another by myself two years later. In another case the disease remained limited even after five years.

In disease of the anterior tarsus the process is less likely to be localized. Made up of small bones, covered on many sides by cartilage, ensheathed in short and unyielding ligaments, the anterior division of the tarsus is an admirable place from which the disease may spread from bone to bone and from joint to joint, until each of the many is involved. The synovial membranes, if not primarily affected, are early filled with fungoid growths. Therefore the tumefied spindle-shaped appearance of the foot usually gives evidence of the nature of the disease long before the presence of sinuses makes the diagnosis certain. Adding to the complications of anterior tarsal disease is the primary or secondary involvement of more or less of the metatarsal bones. In at least two of the cases of the accompanying table the disease began in the metatarsus and remained localized until curetting was done. In the last case, recently operated upon, it could not be determined whether the primary nidus was in the cuboid or fifth metatarsal. When the area of disease was exposed it was found that the whole of the fourth and fifth and part of the third metatarsal were implicated. Finally, cases like that of John A., of the table, are encountered, in which every bone and every joint of the anterior and posterior divisions is involved, and the ankle-joint itself has not been spared. The shapelessness of the foot, the multiplicity of the sinuses, and the extent of bone denudation, as demonstrated by the probe, leave no doubt as to the wide extension of the disease.

The question presents itself, Is tarsal disease ever recovered from without operative interference? Only twice have I witnessed so fortunate a result; once in the case of a child with multiple sinuses leading to the anterior tarsus, and once in an adult, seen with Dr. Ravogli, in whom a very tortuous sinus leading to the astragalus closed permanently, leaving the foot with practically perfect function.

With few exceptions cases of tarsal disease, when pronounced, follow a tedious course, not for months, but for years. Except in two of my cases, in which death resulted from general tuberculosis, from two to five years elapsed before the patients were restored to usefulness, and that minus one foot

or with a more or less deformed foot. If the chronological record of treatment of cases of tarsal disease be scrutinized, it will be found the same in each: Six months devoted to embrocations, massage, the ice-bag or immobilization; six months with confinement to room or bed and the opening of abscesses; six months or a year devoted to watching the results of repeated attempts to cure by curetting; six months or a year given to more or less complete excision or amputation, or both. The adult with tarsal disease is deprived of three or four years of usefulness, even if recovery ensues. But in adults a fatal issue is not at all uncommon, death resulting from general tuberculosis, toward the development of which it is more than probable that our efforts to relieve sometimes contribute.

Far less gloomy is the outlook in tarsal disease of children, since in them its tendency is greater toward localization. The resistance of the surrounding structures is less than in adults. Abscesses are therefore more readily treated, and, more than all, there is the inherent recuperative power of the tissues in early life. Curetting or the informal excision of the diseased part usually relieves the difficulty and sooner or later the child recovers with a useful foot. I have never seen a case of tarsal disease in a child that required amputation, nor do I know of such a case in the experience of my friends.

In the management of tarsal disease that of early life must therefore be nicely differentiated from that of adults. In the former orthopædic appliances, improved hygienic surroundings, and fresh-air treatment can be more readily obtained, and economy of time is not so important an element as later in life.

To curtail the miseries of an adult with tarsal disease, recourse may be had to the following measures:

1st. Scraping away the tuberculous infiltration, or *évidement* of the carious bone.

2d. To more or less formal excision of one or more of the bones of the tarsus; and,

3d. To amputation.

Is *évidement* or curetting of caries of the tarsus followed by recoveries? Certainly not often, except in children, and I have known it to do positive harm. I may be permitted to report briefly three cases in illustration:

CASE I.—Mrs. R., aged forty-two years, seen with Dr. Schneider in 1885, had for two years a sinus on the inner side of the foot leading to a carious astragalus. Though lame, she was fully able to attend to her household duties, and her general health was good. In April I scraped away what I believed to be all of the diseased portion of the astragalus and os-calcis. There was no septic infection, but the wound did not heal. During the summer, abscesses followed by sinuses, developed over the scaphoid. The patient was now confined to bed.

On October 8th, I made a formal excision of the posterior division of the tarsus, and of the cuboid and scaphoid. The wound again failed to heal. The continuous drain on the system, the prolonged confinement, and possibly the mechanical manipulation incident to the operation, induced pulmonary disease. On January 3, 1886, amputation of the leg was done. The wound healed kindly, but six months later the patient succumbed to phthisis.

CASE II.—R. M., a laborer. in the poorest circumstances, seen with Dr. Carr. No history of tuberculosis. He had been in a hospital for six months. There was fungous disease of the anterior division of the tarsus, but no sinus was present. The patient insisting on an early operation, I removed, by scraping, the greater portion of the cuboid bone. The wound failed to close. A rapid development of disease in parts untouched by the operation led me to make a formal excision of the entire anterior tarsus by lateral incisions. Five months later recurrence ensued, and within less than a year after the first operation the patient died of pulmonary phthisis. The opportunity for an amputation did not present itself.

CASE III.—Ed. R., aged eighteen years, a jeweller, after an attack of scarlatina, developed caries of the first metatarsal of the right foot and of the anterior tarsus of the left. When first seen sinuses had existed on the dorsal surfaces of both feet for two years, during which time, though quite lame, he followed his vocation. The first scraping was done May 8, 1888. On February 5, 1889, excision of the anterior row of the left tarsus, the cuneiform, and the first metatarsal bone of the right foot was performed. The latter wound closed. On January 3, 1890, amputation above the ankle was performed, on account of implication of the posterior tarsus and extensive infiltration of the soft parts. Recovery was speedy, and the patient was working at his desk four months later.

Difficult as the acknowledgment is, it seems to me certain that the operation of scraping caused injury to each of these cases by disseminating the tubercular disease. The operative technique may have been at fault, although to produce ischæmia I use only the Esmarch strap without the bandage. Scraping was not performed during the acute stages; incisions were made as large as needed, and every effort was made to remove all of the diseased structures. But *évidement* has failed me and the tubercular deposits left *in situ*, increased, and were disseminated after, if not as a direct result of, the operation. Experience justifies me in holding the view that curetting in the tarsal disease of adults is an operation replete with danger.

Far more encouraging are the results obtained from early and formal excisions, particularly if the disease be limited to only a part of the tarsal framework. Until the very admirable work of Kappeller, of P. H. Watson, and, last but not least,

of my friend Dr. Conner, the utility, not to mention the justifiability, of the operation was questioned. In the accompanying table cases are recorded in which one or several bones of the tarsus were excised with fair and even with good results; yet, as will be seen in several, probably because they were done at a later period, the final results were unfavorable. Excision, limited to one or two bones, is practically devoid of danger, and the early removal, particularly of the anterior tarsus, where the disease is oftenest found, leaves a shortened foot, but a limb of normal length.

Concerning the best method of operation there should, in my judgment, be no question. The unilateral or bilateral incisions, though they save the tendons, afford but a poor opportunity to inspect the field of disease, and if all of it is removed, it is largely due to good fortune. On the other hand, by a free incision directly across the dorsum dividing the tendons, an inspection of the entire field of operation is permitted, and every vestige of disease can be removed. If thought best, one or two longitudinal incisions can be made over the metatarsal bones, and as much of the bones as need be can be removed. In one case that was operated upon the wound healed by primary union, and three weeks after the operation there was good motion of the toes. This and another of my cases has caused me to doubt the necessity of suturing the tendons. Unless the tendons are looped before division, their suture after the excision is extremely difficult, the upper segments being so retracted in their sheaths that attempts to withdraw them generally fail. It is probable, however, that when tendon-suture is practised a more useful foot is retained. In England, Holmes and Wright favor this dorsal incision, and in Germany Bardenheuer reports nineteen such operations, yet in three of them death resulted from general tuberculosis.

But removal of the whole or a greater portion of the tarsus is attended by a very considerable danger to life. According to Conner, the death-rate under fifteen years of age is 6.67 per cent., between fifteen and twenty-five years 10 per cent., and over twenty-five years 27.27 per cent. The latter mortality is, in my judgment, greater than that of amputation through or above the ankle. Unfortunately, as against this increased risk of life and the greater duration of treatment from late excision, there is no proportionately increased guaranty of immunity from recurrence. Even with the advanced operation of Wladimiroff-Mikulicz, the hope that a definite cure could be obtained because the operation is performed in healthy tissue has been frustrated. In five of the cases of Fisher, four of Zesa's, and one of Rose's recurrence ensued.

From what has already been stated, it is evident

that the third operative recourse in tarsal disease, namely, amputation, should, in my judgment, be resorted oftener and earlier to than has usually been done. In other words, it appears to me that there is a limit to the usefulness of conservatism in advanced disease of the tarsus of adults, and that the preservation of a deformed foot is hardly worth the sacrifice of three or four years of active life. Here, as elsewhere, every case is a problem, the solution of which must be largely influenced by the sex, vocation, social position, hygienic surroundings, and general condition of the patient.

resulted in 2 of the cases from general tuberculosis, which might have been avoided by a primary excision, or more certainly, by early amputation.

THE TREATMENT OF CROUP WITH SPECIAL REFERENCE TO TRACHEOTOMY AND INTUBATION OF THE LARYNX.[1]

BY H. R. WHARTON, M.D.,

SURGEON TO THE CHILDREN'S HOSPITAL OF PHILADELPHIA.

A FEW years ago I read before the Philadelphia County Medical Society a paper upon "Tracheotomy in Diphtheritic Croup." Since that time

Name and age. Years.	Date.	Duration of illness.	No. of operations.	Curetting.	Result.	Excision.	Part removed.	Result.	Amputation.	Result.	Remarks
Arthur R., 4	1882	3 years.	3	2	Failure.	1	Astragalus and tibia.	Perfect.	...	.....	After failure of curetting and thorough drainage, excision was performed.
Herbert B., 8	1883	5 "	3	2	"	1	Os calcis.	"	...	......	
Jos. B., 11	1885	3 "	1	...	....	1	Cuboid and ½ of os calcis.	Good.	...	......	
Mrs. R., 42	1885	3 "	3	1	Failure	1	Posterior tarsus, cuboid, and scaphoid.	Failure.	1	Died.	Six months later.
Isaac S., 18	1886	5 "	2	1	"	1	Os calcis.	Good.	...	......	Jewish Hospital.
Allen P , 26	1886	2 "	1	...	....	1	Second metatarsal and cuneiform.	"	...	......	Railroad injury.
Thos. M., 40	1886	2 "	2	1	Failure.	1	Anterior tarsus.	Failure.	...	Died.	From phthisis.
Esther A., 7	1886	2 "	2	2	Success.	...	....	. ...	...	.....	Os calcis.
Aug. F., 4	1887	1 "	1	1	"	...	....	......	...	.....	Cuboid and 5th metatarsal.
Wm. Burns, 60	1887	1 "	1	1	Failure.	...	....	......	...	.....	Refused further interference; sent to infirmary.
Ed. R., 18	1888	4 "	3	1	"	1	Anterior row.	Failure.	1	Recovered.	
	1888	....	2	1	"	1	First metatarsal and cuneiform.	Good.	...	......	
Jos. L., 28	1889	1 "	1	..	......	1	Second metatarsal and cuboid	Fair.	...	.....	Railroad injury; sinus remaining three months later.
John A., 41	1890	3 "	4	2	Failure.	1	Whole tarsus, tibia, and fibula.	Failure.	1	Recovered.	Cincinnati Hospital.
Kate I., 23	1890	8 months.	1	...	......	1	Anterior tarsus and third metatarsal.	Good.	...	......	Jewish Hospital.

Conclusions.—Although the number of cases here tabulated is not large, a few deductions can be made. Of 30 operations made for tarsal disease there were 15 of *évidement*, of which but 2 were successful, and these were children. In 6 the curetting was followed by an exacerbation of the previous difficulty. Of the 12 excisions, 4 were primary, and in 3 the operations were made before sinuses had formed. In these primary operations the repair was more rapid than in those in which curetting had previously been done. Four of the excisions were failures, in 3 from recurrence of the disease, and in the fourth from the uselessness of the foot. While no deaths were directly attributable to tarsal disease, death

my experience with the operation has been considerably enlarged, and I have also had some experience with the more recently introduced operation of intubation of the larynx in the treatment of such cases.

I think that the vast majority of cases of croup coming under my observation were diphtheritic, but I have also seen a number of patients in whom the disease might be considered as true or simple croup, which seemed to me to be the result either of catarrhal laryngitis or of œdema of the larynx.

The symptom calling for operative interference

---

[1] Read before the Philadelphia County Medical Society, November 12, 1890.

in croup is a form of obstructive dyspnœa characterized by suppression of the voice, great difficulty of inspiration, lividity of the lips, depression of the supra-sternal and supra-clavicular spaces, sinking in of the lower part of the chest, inability to breathe while in the recumbent posture, restlessness and inability to sleep except at very short intervals. When these symptoms are present and are increasing, I think that some operative interference is urgently indicated.

I would here call attention to the dyspnœa which is often observed in patients suffering from diphtheria, pneumonia, capillary bronchitis, or congestion of the lungs, and which differs from the form of obstructive dyspnœa that I have just described in being accompanied with very rapid respiration, and in failing to present the symptoms so marked in obstructive cases.

These cases I am often asked to see with regard to the question of surgical interference, but in such cases there is manifestly no indication for operative treatment, as the dyspnœa results from diminished air-space in the lungs, and not from a localized obstruction high up in the air-passages.

Inability to sleep I consider an important symptom in deciding as to the advisability of operative interference, whether by tracheotomy or by intubation of the larynx. This is a clinical observation which I made some time ago, and which Mr. Hewitt explains as follows: During ordinary sleep the activity of the diaphragm is lessened, the centres which preside over it enjoying comparative rest, while in obstructive dyspnœa the patient, to a great extent, depends upon the increased action of the diaphragm, so that natural sleep is generally impossible, except at short intervals.

Although the symptoms of dyspnœa may be marked and increasing, if the patient is able to sleep for half an hour or an hour at a time, I am inclined to employ a method of treatment, which I will describe, before I resort to either tracheotomy or intubation.

When I see a case of croup comparatively early in the disease when the symptoms are not so urgent as to demand immediate operative interference, I also employ this course of treatment which, I feel sure, often averts the necessity of operative procedure. If the case be one in private practice, I have the patient put in a room in which there is a stove, and upon this is kept constantly boiling a large pan of water to moisten the air. If the room is heated by a furnace, I use a gas-stove or alcohol lamp to heat the water and accomplish the same purpose.

I give the patient internally:

R.—Carbonate of ammonium   .   2 grains.
    Syrup of senega   .   .   10 minims.
    Mucilage of acacia   .   .   2 drachms.—M.

To be given every two hours unless the patient vomits, in the event of which I diminish the frequency of the dose.

I also frequently employ a steam atomizer, in the receiver of which is the following solution:

R.—Sodium carbonate   .   1 to 2½ drachms.
    Glycerin   .   .   .   .   2 ounces.
    Water sufficient to make   .   4   "

This solution was first recommended by Mr. Parker, of London.

If the patient is old enough to be manageable he should inhale the vapor from this for a short time, at intervals of fifteen or twenty minutes. If the patient is unruly or so young as not to be able to inhale the vapor, I have the bed converted into a tent by the use of a few sticks and a sheet, under which the steam atomizer is kept in operation, the spray being directed as near to the mouth as possible. It is surprising how willingly a comparatively young or unmanageable child will take the mouthpiece of the atomizer into his mouth and inhale the vapor after he has once done so, and has experienced the relief which follows its employment. If there is reason to think that the case is one of diphtheritic croup the patient is given in addition either calomel in small doses, bichloride of mercury, or any other drug which may be considered advisable.

Of the utility of this form of treatment in the early stages of croup, I have the highest opinion, for under its use I have frequently seen cases which were beginning to exhibit symptoms of marked dyspnœa gradually improve and cough up pieces of membrane or masses of muco-purulent matter, and in twelve or twenty-four hours be entirely relieved of dyspnœa and subsequently make an uninterrupted recovery.

My experience therefore leads me to recommend some such form of treatment in the early stage of croup if extremely urgent symptoms are not present, and I do not feel that everything has been done before resorting to operation unless this plan has been instituted.

If in spite of the treatment which I have described the symptoms of dyspnœa become more urgent and assume the characteristics which I have previously pointed out, I then consider that operative interference is indicated, bearing in mind the fact that an operation—either tracheotomy or intubation—is only a mechanical procedure to relieve the dyspnœa. Personally I am not in favor of very early operation, for as I have before stated, under the treatment described I have often seen the dyspnœa relieved and recovery follow.

If the symptoms presented are of such a nature as to call for surgical interference to relieve the dyspnœa, I consider several points in deciding as to which operation to employ. If the dyspnœa has existed for some days and is increasing; if there are patches of false membrane on the pharnyx; and if the patient exhibits marked constitutional evidences of diphtheria, I am inclined to recommend tracheotomy in preference to intubation. If, on the other hand, the dyspnœa has existed for a short time only, and if there is no false membrane in the pharnyx or sputa, although the dyspnœa may have increased rapidly, I generally recommend intubation, for it is in these rapidly-increasing cases of dyspnœa that intubation is an especially useful procedure.

The reason of my preference for tracheotomy in cases of slowly-developing dyspnœa is that in these there is usually a well-organized membrane in the larynx and the trachea, which may extend below the lower end of the intubation tube, or which may be pushed in a mass before the tube, suddenly occluding the trachea and arresting the entrance or exit of air. So much do I fear this accident, which has occurred in the hands of some surgeons, that I never introduce an intubation tube without having at hand the instruments necessary to perform tracheotomy

I also explain to the parents or to the friends of the patient that the first operation may not relieve the patient, and that a second operation (tracheotomy) may be required, and obtain, if possible, their permission to perform the latter if it should be indicated. In cases in which there is a well-organized membrane the masses that loosen may be too large to pass through the comparatively small opening in the intubation tube, and if the tube is not forced out by the expiratory efforts of the patient or removed by the surgeon or nurse, death may rapidly ensue. For this reason I leave the string attached to the intubation tube in place for a few hours, to facilitate its rapid removal if the occasion occurs.

After a case has been intubated or tracheotomized, I do not relax the local or constitutional treatment which was previously instituted; I continue to use the alkaline spray already mentioned, and if the case progresses favorably I remove the intubation tube at the end of the third or fourth day; and if the dyspnœa does not recur I do not reintroduce it. If, however, the dyspnœa recurs in a short time I reinsert the tube, and again remove it in a few days; and the second attempt is, I find, generally successful. After removing the intubation tube I continue the use of the alkaline spray for a few days.

One of the most serious objections to intubation is the trouble in nourishing the patient due to the difficulty of swallowing fluids while the tube is in the larynx; but occasionally patients will be found who can easily swallow fluids. I usually order a diet consisting chiefly of semi-solids, such as soft-boiled eggs, corn-starch and rennet; and if there is difficulty in swallowing these, I depend largely upon nutritious enemata. Thirst can be allayed by swallowing pieces of ice. The stomach-tube may be used to introduce nourishment in case the rectum becomes too irritable to retain the enemata. In some cases by allowing the head of the child to be lower than the body, and giving liquids while in this position, it will be found that they can be swallowed without difficulty. I have found that hoarseness persists for some time after the removal of intubation tubes.

If, as sometimes occurs, intubation fails to relieve the dyspnœa, or relieves it only temporarily, I resort to tracheotomy, and I have had recovery follow in such cases. If tracheotomy becomes necessary, the operation may be performed while the intubation tube is in place, removing the tube after the trachea is opened, if it interferes with the introduction of the tracheal tube.

The details of the operation of tracheotomy are so well known that I will not repeat them. Another reason for my preference for tracheotomy in the slowly-developing cases of dyspnœa, is that by a free opening into the trachea the membrane can be removed, and if the obstruction is in either the trachea or the larynx, the opening completely relieves the dyspnœa and gives the patient a full supply of air, until the separation of the membrane in the larynx occurs.

A number of cases after either intubation or tracheotomy develop recurrent obstruction due to extension of the membrane to the bronchial tubes. or to the development of a broncho-pneumonia, and in such cases further operative treatment is useless. These cases are characterized by dyspnœa of the type I have previously described, rapid respiration being the principal feature.

I do not think that a larger number of cases can be saved by intubation than by tracheotomy; in my personal experience the larger proportion of recoveries has followed tracheotomy.

In conclusion, I would say that in intubation of the larynx we have added a valuable surgical procedure to our means of treating croup. I think it is especially to be recommended in those cases which I have described as cases of rapidly-developing dyspnœa in which the obstruction is probably due to a slightly-developed diphtheritic membrane, to œdema of the larynx, or to catarrhal laryngitis. I do not think that intubation of the larynx is an operation entirely free from danger. Intubation has the advantage of being a bloodless operation, and practically without pain, and for this reason the friends of the patient will often consent to intubation when they would refuse to have tracheotomy performed. The management of cases after intubation is comparatively easy. with the exception of the difficulty of nourishing the patient.

In very young children, in whom the results of tracheotomy are not so favorable, I think intubation should first be employed, unless some contra-indication exists.

Tracheotomy generally completely relieves the dyspnœa, and allows the surgeon to clear the trachea of membrane, and is, therefore, to be preferred in slowly-developing cases of dyspnœa in which there is apt to be present a well-developed diphtheritic membrane in the larynx or trachea. If carefully performed, there is comparatively little risk in the operation itself. Patients after tracheotomy have little difficulty in taking a full supply of liquid nourishment, which certainly is most urgently indicated in an asthenic disease like diphtheria, and it is in this disease that the operation is most frequently called for.

EPIDIDYMITIS CAUSED BY ABDOMINAL STRAIN.

BY EDWARD MARTIN, M.D.

SURGEON TO THE HOWARD HOSPITAL; ASSISTANT SURGEON TO THE HOSPITAL OF THE UNIVERSITY OF PENNSYLVANIA.

ALTHOUGH it is undoubtedly true that the vast majority of inflammations involving the epididymis are dependent upon the extension of gonorrhœal infection through the vas deferens, it is well recognized that epididymitis may be produced by a number of other causes; thus traumatism, gout, rheumatism, malaria, and tubercle may all provoke a local inflammation of great intensity in this region.

In addition the physician will occasionally meet cases in which the possibility of all these causes is positively denied, and yet in which the symptoms of an active inflammation of the epididymis are present. The patients usually ascribe this condition to a strain or a violent lifting effort.

It is certainly true of the writer, and probably of the vast majority of practitioners, that such statements have been received with absolute incredulity, and that the causative agent has always been regarded as a preëxisting gonorrhœa, since this affection is very commonly accompanied by a moral obliquity which seems to render a truthful narration of the history of the case impossible.

Lately, however, two cases have been observed in which the statements of the patient seemed so trustworthy that sufficient credence was given them to make a careful examination, and in one instance, at least, this was so thorough, that the possibility of all the predisposing and exciting factors mentioned above could be absolutely excluded. The history of this case is as follows:

J. T., a porter, aged thirty-six years, is a strongly-built man of medium height. His father died of consumption at the age of fifty-six years; there is no other case of this disease in the family. He has always been strong. He practised self-abuse in moderation until the age of twenty years, when he was married. From the period of puberty he has suffered from a certain amount of sexual weakness, involuntary emissions taking place on slight excitement. This was still noticed after marriage, though to a less extent than before. He has had no venereal disease. Five days before he appeared for treatment, in the evening following a heavy day's work, he suffered from pain located in the lower part of the left testicle, and at the same time swelling was observed. These symptoms steadily grew worse, the pain extending into the groin.

On examination, the right testicle and epididymis were found normal; the left testicle was slightly enlarged and was tender, but still soft and of normal consistence. The epididymis was hard, very tender, and about three times its natural size. The skin over this region was hot and red.

An examination of the urethra showed the absence of stricture; no pus could be detected upon the instruments when they were withdrawn. A careful microscopical search of the urine was made, but no pus or albumin could be found. Rectal examination showed a slightly-enlarged prostate, moderate pressure upon which produced a desire to urinate. The seminal vesicles could not be felt. The lungs were found to be normal on examination. The patient had not suffered from rheumatism or malaria.

Two days later the swelling had increased, involving the testicle, the pain on standing or walking was severe. A Langlebert suspensory bandage was applied; this gave the patient almost immediate relief and enabled him to resume his work. This treatment together with careful attention to the condition of the bowels was sufficient to accomplish a speedy cure.

In the other case observed, an opportunity to make an examination sufficiently thorough to exclude absolutely the presence of posterior gonorrhœa was not offered, hence it cannot positively be asserted that it was a case of strain-epididymitis, though the evidence on the part of the patient was as nearly conclusive as this can ever be.

In the case detailed above we have an instance of epididymitis not associated with any of the causes or conditions commonly recognized as factors in the development of the disease. Pain and swelling developed after a hard day's work; neither were especially marked at first, and the latter shortly involved the testicle to a moderate extent. Provided the examination of this patient was carefully conducted, this case alone would establish the possibility of inflammation of the epididymis and testicle following muscular effort, or what has sometimes been called primary epididymitis. This case is not, however, without ample corroboration.

Though little has been written in the English language concerning strain-epididymitis, the affection has been long recognized by French and German writers. Thus Velpeau distinctly alludes to it, and following him we have a long list of authorities—Vidal, Curling, Gosselin, Soulé, Richet, Delomme, Coutan, Hamilton, Le Dentu, Pellier, Wagner, Eng. lisch, Hublé, etc. All are practically agreed upon the point that independent of any distinct idiosyncrasy, violent inflammation of the epididymis may be excited by strong muscular effort, particularly when such effort calls into play the muscles of the abdominal parietes.

As to the mechanism by which such inflammation is produced there is a widespread diversity of opinion; thus by some it is held that it is due to pressure upon the vas deferens, others hold that it is due to pressure upon the veins of the cord, and still others that the injury is inflicted by violent contraction of the cremaster muscle, which by suddenly jerking the testicle against the pillars of the external ring, causes a bruising of the latter, often accompanied by a rupture of the veins. This is called by the French the *coup de fouet*, or whip-snap action.

According to Roux, the theory of compression of the cord and its veins is made probable by the existence of certain fibres which pass from the rectus muscle to the inner lip of the iliac crest. When the abdominal muscles are thrown into sudden violent contraction, these fibres participate in the motion and, in pressing the cord upward, pinch it against the fibrous circumference of the external abdominal ring.

The general consensus of opinion, however, and this is particularly the case with recent writers, strongly inclines to the theory that the cremaster muscle alone is the direct cause of the inflammation.

That this muscle is capable of very vigorous contraction cannot be doubted. Thus it is not rarely observed that direct trauma of the testicle is followed by marked retraction of this organ, so that it may be drawn into the inguinal canal, or even into the abdominal cavity. Even in severe pain, such as that which accompanies renal colic, the testicles are frequently found in close apposition to the external ring, while anyone can observe the contraction of the cremaster by noticing the motion of one or both testicles during the passage of a catheter. Certain cases of chorea of the testicle are at times observed when this organ is moved by the cremaster with considerable rapidity and violence.

Richet, while acknowledging the important *rôle* played by the cremaster, believes that the result produced by this contraction is due, in the main, to rupture of the veins produced by pressure upon them. The majority of writers strongly favor the "whip-snap" action of the cremaster, and the consequent bruising of the epididymis and testicle as the cause of the subsequent inflammation.

According to this theory, then the cause of this form of epididymitis and orchitis is precisely the same as is the case when a blow is received upon this region.

Experimentally, it is found that the violence of traumatic orchitis and epididymitis is directly proportionate to the amount of injury inflicted, and that where the trauma is at all severe there is nearly always extravasation of blood, not only beneath the fibrous tunic of the testicle and epididymis, but into the parenchyma of these organs, particularly of the latter. It is also observed that the inflammatory symptoms following direct violence do not always immediately appear.

In the form of orchitis and epididymitis under discussion, it would seem that much the same lesions occur as when these parts are bruised by external violence. That there is frequently extravasation of blood can at times be confirmed by examination. The inflammatory symptoms are marked, but come on slowly.

Although this theory as to the cause of epididymitis from muscular strain is almost universally accepted, there are several powerful arguments against it. In the first place, direct trauma, even when not of sufficient violence to excite marked inflammatory symptoms of the testicle or its appendages, is immediately followed by agonizing and unbearable pain. If the mechanism of a spontaneous inflammation were that described above, and according to the whip-snap theory the violence is just as direct as though the testicle had been struck with a club, the histories of reported cases should uniformly mention the presence of such pain. This symptom is, however, conspicuous by its absence. There is often observed a sharp, sticking sensation, or a pain of moderate severity, but never that which characterizes pain of the testicle.

Again, muscular fibres are not capable of indefinite contraction; they can shorten to a certain extent, but beyond this no diminution of their length is possible. By the time the testicle has reached the external ring, it would seem that the contractile power of the cremaster must have practically reached its extreme limit, and hence it is difficult to conceive how this muscle is able to exercise sufficient pressure upon the testicle to produce serious lesions by bruising it against the columns of the ring.

Upon the "whip-snap" theory alone it is hard to explain why the affection should exert such a decided predilection for the left side. Of Englisch's seven cases, in six the left testicle and epididymis were involved—the seventh was bilateral. In the case reported in this paper the left testicle was involved, and other observers concur in this observation.

There is, however, a theory, the *rationale* of which

is much more readily comprehended, and which would account for the appearances observed in at least the great majority of the reported cases.

The spermatic plexus of veins is peculiarly under the influence of intra-abdominal pressure ; the vessels are provided with but few and imperfect valves ; are feebly supported by the surrounding tissues, and hence are especially subject to disease. Thus varicosity of these veins is one of the most common surgical affections, and the effect of the contraction of the abdominal parietes and the diaphragm upon these dilated veins is so marked, that succussion on coughing, or straining in any way, is sufficiently distinct to simulate that of an omental hernia.

Given, then, a sudden and violent increase of pressure in these vessels, it is perfectly possible to conceive that rupture may take place, even though they be healthy; this is of course more probable if they are weakened and dilated. Such rupture would naturally take place in the cord, in the epididymis, or even in the substance of the testicle. And if the theory of venous rupture from pressure is correct, we would expect the left testicle to be most frequently involved, as veins of this side are most frequently varicose, and we would expect the pain first to be slight and gradually increase, as more blood was effused and inflammatory symptoms developed.

Now these are the very conditions which characterize inflammation of the epididymis following muscular effort, and on this basis we think we have sufficient explanation for the occurrence of this affection without attributing any causative *rôle* to cremasteric contraction, although the latter may play a subsidiary part.

One of Englisch's cases strikingly illustrates the probability of this theory. The patient, a laborer, nineteen years old, while working, suddenly felt a sharp sticking pain in the left scrotum ; at the same time there was a discharge of blood from the anus. Shortly the characteristic local and general symptoms of orchi-epididymitis developed. Here effort called into play the muscles of the abdominal parietes ; this increased the intra-abdominal pressure. As a result of this, there was increased tension upon the veins of the rectum or anus and those of the pampiniform plexus. Evidently some branch of the hæmorrhoidal plexus gave way under the strain, and there was free bleeding. Why it is necessary to ascribe the testicular symptoms to bruising of this organ against the columns of the external ring rather than to rupture of a vein, is not explained by Englisch.

From the cases of epididymitis under discussion it is necessary to separate carefully instances of inflammation dependent upon latent disease, such as tuberculosis and malignant tumor. Here it is

not uncommon for the patient to notice first some trouble about the testicle immediately after violent exertion, though such trouble has in reality existed for some time.

It is well recognized that gonorrhœal epididymitis or orchitis is peculiarly prone to appear in those who are forced to undergo severe and prolonged labor, and that this complication develops after the disease has invaded the posterior portion of the urethra ; hence an examination of the meatus for discharge is, in cases of absence of the latter, not sufficient to exclude gonorrhœa as the cause of the intra-scrotal inflammation. The urine must be carefully examined for pus, and, moreover, the urethra should be explored to prove the presence or absence of stricture.

The prognosis of epididymitis or orchitis following increased intra-abdominal pressure from muscular contraction is exceedingly favorable. The treatment consists in keeping the bowels open and in the application of those agents most powerful in causing absorption of blood-clot and inflammatory exudate, namely, moisture, warmth, and pressure. This is accomplished by a modified Langlebert bandage,[1] which I employ in all cases of epididymitis, and which has yielded uniformly satisfactory results. The bandage is made in the form of an ordinary suspensory-bandage, but less pouched than those found in the shops. The part covering the scrotum is made of mackintosh. A wedge-shaped piece is cut out from each side of this, and lacings are arranged so that the edges of this V may be brought together. The scrotum is enveloped in a thick layer of absorbent cotton, the suspensory-bandage is adjusted, and, finally, the lacings at the sides are drawn in until tight, uniform pressure is exerted on the swelling. The mackintosh prevents evaporation and keeps the parts moist, the cotton preserves the heat, and by means of the gores at the sides of the bandage the pressure can be accurately adjusted. Even in gonorrhœal epididymitis this dressing commonly enables the patient to resume his work in a few hours, and in the form of inflammation under discussion it is equally satisfactory in its effect.

From a careful study of the literature of the subject, the following conclusions seem justifiable :

1. Epididymitis, orchitis, or orchi-epididymitis, may develop as the result of violent or prolonged muscular exertion, without the intervention of any of the commonly recognized predisposing or exciting factors.

2. Such exertion as is accompanied by strong contraction of the muscular parietes of the abdomen is particularly liable to be followed by this form of inflammation.

[1] This bandage is made for me by Mr. Lenz, of Philadelphia.

3. It is commonly taught that this affection is due to a sudden and violent contraction of the cremaster muscle, which jerks the testicle upward and bruises it against the columns of the external ring.

4. The facts that the left epididymis and testicle are nearly always involved, that the first pain is usually slight, and that this affection commonly develops in those subject to varicocele, show that the inflammation is more probably due to venous bleeding occasioned by increased blood-pressure, which is in itself due to the increased intra-abdominal pressure resulting from contraction of the abdominal muscles.

5. This inflammation usually invades the epididymis, though the testicle also may become involved. The first symptom is pain of moderate severity, often felt in the inguinal region, which is followed by swelling that may not appear for a day or two. The symptoms run an acute course.

6. The treatment consists in careful attention to the condition of the bowels, and in the application of a Langlebert suspensory-bandage. The patient, after the swelling has reached its height, need not keep his bed.

CLINICAL MEMORANDUM.

MEDICAL.

Death from Intra-pulmonary Injection.—The following mishap, occurring among the treatment of phthisis by intra-pulmonary injection, is interesting. During part of the writer's term of service as house physician of the Buffalo General Hospital in 1888–89, a large number of cases of phthisis were treated by intra-pulmonary injections. The medicament used was a three-per-cent. solution of beechwood creasote in oil of sweet almonds. Of this about ten minims were injected at a time into a cavity or solidified apex. In most instances the immediate effects were very encouraging. The expectoration usually decreased, and the temperature, after the slight rise caused by the operation, fell, and continued for a time nearly normal. More than fifty such injections had been made with favorable results, when the following accident occurred:

The patient was well nourished, and under tonic treatment, and the disease seemed to be in abeyance. Three injections had been made, at intervals of four days, into the left apex, followed in each instance by decreased expectoration and marked diminution of evening temperature.

The fourth injection was made by the usual method into the right apex, and the patient immediately after the procedure resumed his duties about the ward. Twenty minutes later he was seized with violent dyspnœa, which gradually became worse. He had formerly suffered from asthma, and the present attack resembled an asthmatic paroxysm. The irritation caused by the drug on the peripheral endings of the vagus seemed to afford a plausible explanation in support of this diagnosis. The usual remedies for asthma were administered, but all failed to give relief. Auscultation was rendered impossible by the violent tossing and groaning of the sufferer. About an hour and a half after the injection the patient died.

At the autopsy the right lung was found entirely collapsed, and the pleural cavity filled with air. The needle in entering the lung had passed through tissue as thin as ordinary writing-paper into an emphysematous space, communicating with a small cavity, which in turn communicated with a bronchus. After the puncture the thinness of the wall prevented it from retracting sufficiently to act as a valve, and the inspired air must have passed almost directly into the pleural cavity.

Cases of pneumothorax have been reported, following intra-pulmonary injection; but all were slight, and ended in recovery. Only one death immediately following this treatment is recorded, and in that case death was due to acute suppurative bronchitis. Had the pneumothorax been diagnosed in my case at the outset of the attack it is possible that surgical interference might have saved the patient. The condition, however, was wholly unexpected, and was not recognized by any of the physicians who examined the case.

The slight benefits following this method of treatment are, in the writer's opinion, secured at too great a risk to make the procedure advisable.

ROBERT T. FRENCH, M.D.

213 ALEXANDER STREET, ROCHESTER, N. Y.

HOSPITAL NOTES.

PYELO-NEPHRITIS FROM CALCULI—GRADUAL DILATATION FOR CONTRACTED BLADDER —TRAUMATIC TETANUS.

Abstract of a Clinical Lecture delivered at Bellevue Hospital, New York.

BY JOHN W. S. GOULEY, M.D.,
VISITING SURGEON.

BEFORE presenting any patients, Dr. Gouley showed some specimens removed post-mortem from a case of prostatic enlargement and obstruction to urination, with the grave complication of a contracted bladder. He said that if the capacity of the bladder has become increased, no matter how thick the walls may be, there is a prospect that the patient will live a long time; but if its capacity is so diminished that it can hold only one or two ounces of urine, the prognosis is exceedingly bad.

The patient, from whom the specimens were removed, was admitted to one of the New York hospitals last June for cystitis, and was there subjected to the operation of suprapubic cystotomy. An India-rubber tube was introduced and secured in position, with a rubber bag attached to receive the urine. In September he was admitted to Bellevue Hospital. The man thought that the operation had given him decided relief; but this is doubtful, for a catheter retained so long in the bladder, acting as a foreign body, must have become encrusted with phosphates. After admission to Bellevue Hospital his bladder was irrigated once daily, but it was so irritable that not more than two ounces of urine could be retained. The urine was constantly voided through the urethra, in spite of the opening which had been made above the pubes for the purpose of draining the bladder.

The record states that there was no albuminuria, but there should have been some albumin derived from the pus in the urine. Absence of albumin in the urine does not, however, exclude even extensive renal disease. The patient became gradually more feeble and died during the preceding night. The kidneys, both of which were shown, were increased in size, the left being the larger. On section of the left kidney pus was found in its pelvis, and this, together with the condition of the cortical portion, afforded an excellent illustration of pyelo-nephritis. Searching a little further the cause of the existing pyelo-nephritis was found to be the presence of calculi in the renal pelvis, there being three stones of uric acid, one of which was five-eighths of an inch in diameter, the others were smaller. In the right kidney there was also pyelitis; but the pelvis was not so much distended, and there was no stone. The bladder was about the size of the prostate, and would hold scarcely two ounces of fluid.

The suprapubic operation was done for the purpose of draining the bladder, and yet there was no urethro-vesical obstruction, and the record shows that the urine was passed by the urethra from the time the patient entered the hospital till the day of his death. The operation was a conspicuous failure so far as draining the bladder was concerned. It is well known that where there is calculous pyelitis, and particularly where there is a pyonephritis, the most constant, and sometimes the only, symptom is referable to the bladder. The diagnosis of renal calculus is not easy, unless there is sufficient distention of the pelvis of the kidney to cause a tumor sufficiently large to be detected by the usual methods of physical examination. If a correct diagnosis had been made in this case the only proper operation would have been a nephrotomy, and had such an operation been performed it is likely that the vesical symptoms would have speedily subsided.

In cases in which there is no renal calculus, but simply a contracted condition of the bladder from some other cause, as, for instance, urethro-vesical obstruction from contraction or from prostatic enlargement, much can be done for the comfort of the patient, and in some cases a cure may be brought about by employing the method of gradual hydraulic dilatation of the bladder, just as a urethral stricture would be gradually dilated, substituting for the solid sound the dilating force of water. In carrying out this method of hydraulic dilatation the quantity which is daily injected into the bladder at each sitting is to be increased almost imperceptibly. In this way the twofold object of treatment is attained—namely, keeping the bladder clean, and at the same time increasing its capacity. After a number of weeks or months it is found that the bladder is capable of retaining very much more fluid than at first.

CASE I.—Dr. Gouley then showed a patient as an illustration of this treatment. He first came to the hospital about a year ago, and is now an out-patient. When first seen his bladder was very irritable, and would not hold more than one and a half ounces of fluid. He has been treated at intervals ever since. His general health is now good and his bladder is capable of holding seven ounces of the ordinary solution used for irrigation, which is equivalent to holding eight or ten ounces of urine. Vaginal cystotomy for the relief of a similar condition in the female has been very frequently performed in recent years, but

Dr. William M. Polk has stated that he has abandoned the operation, having found the method of gradual dilatation more satisfactory. Other gynecologists have also abandoned vaginal cystotomy and have substituted the more innocuous method of gradual hydraulic dilatation. This method of dilatation of contracted bladders is not new. It was recommended long ago by Civiale, but it does not seem to have been very generally adopted until lately. Fourteen years ago the speaker removed several villous tumors from the urethra of a lady already advanced in years, and supplemented the operation by dilatation of the bladder in the manner just mentioned. Before the operation urination was very frequent, occurring every few minutes, and so painful and distressing that her general health was rapidly failing. As a result of the treatment her bladder was able to hold five or six ounces of fluid and she is now enjoying a hearty old age.

CASE II.—The next patient was an old man, who is said to have had urethral stenosis, which was dilated so that it now admits a No. 12 sound of the English scale, and yet he urinates every half hour. This trouble, then, is not dependent upon the diminution of the urethral calibre, but upon the condition of the bladder. On passing a soft catheter there seems to be some sensitiveness of the urethra, but the bladder, as shown by the quantity of fluid injected, holds five ounces; hence, there is no indication for hydraulic dilatation, and the treatment should consist of sytematic efforts to keep the bladder free from pus by daily irrigation. The following solution is useful for this purpose:

R.—Bichloride of mercury . . 5 grains.
Ammonium chloride . . 15 "
Spirit of gaultheria . . . ½ ounce.
Sodium borate . . . 1 "
Glycerin . . . . . 8 ounces.—M.

Half an ounce of the above mixture and two and one-half ounces of peroxide of hydrogen solution with seven ounces of warm water may be used for irrigating the bladder.

Dr. Gouley then referred to a case of traumatic tetanus in the ward of his colleague, Dr. Charles Phelps, which he said is a rare disease in New York. The first symptom of the disease made its appearance a few hours before the lecture. The patient is a boy, about sixteen years of age, who ten days previously was caught between cog-wheels and sustained a severe injury of the left lower extremity. Both the popliteal and peroneal nerves were injured, the former so badly that its ends could not be brought together by sutures, as was done in the case of the peroneal. On his admission to the hospital an hour or two after the injury, the wound was found to be in an exceedingly filthy condition, and was cleansed as thoroughly as was possible. No untoward symptoms were noticed until this morning, when a slight trismus or " lock-jaw " was observed. So far there has been no laryngeal spasm. This patient had already been given repeated doses of Calabar bean. Dr. Phelps says that he has had two cases of recovery from tetanus which he is inclined to ascribe to the use of the Calabar bean. The lecturer said that he also had had two recoveries, in both of which the disease had progressed until the patients presented the classical picture so vividly portrayed in Bell's *Anatomy of Expression*, and yet they received only a little morphine and bromide of potassium. In one of these cases the patient, who was about thirty years of age, had a compound fracture of the forearm with a filthy wound; the other was a boy of nineteen years, who had a severe laceration of the foot. The speaker was once induced to amputate during the prodromic symptoms of tetanus, but this did not avert the fatal termination.

Tetanus is a rare affection in New York City, but it seems to be endemic near the eastern end of Long Island, and is quite common, particularly that form known as trismus neonatorum, in hot climates. Some very interesting researches have been made recently into the etiology of tetanus, the results of which lead the observers to the belief that tetanus is of microbic origin. Briéger has made cultures of the tetanus bacillus, and extracted in this way a ptomaïne to which he has given the name of *tetanin*, and this in solution, when injected hypodermically into small animals, has been found to produce symptoms similar to those of tetanus.

The patient before the class had neither opisthotonos nor emprosthotonos; but the slightest movement or excitement caused a facial spasm. One of Dr. Gonley's successful cases was in such a condition for three months that simply touching him was sufficient to bring on a severe spasm. In some of these cases it is necessary to resort to rectal alimentation; and if this mode of feeding be properly carried out it is not difficult to keep up a fair standard of nutrition. He once nourished a child of five or six years entirely by the rectum for thirty days. The fluid for injection should be simple—usually milk—and before each injection the rectum should be thoroughly cleansed by a simple enema. This is important; for after a while a hypersecretion of mucus follows this method of alimentation, and beef peptones and other articles of food may remain in the rectum and putrefy, until the stench of the evacuations is intolerable.

The facts which in this case the wound looks healthy and that the slough is separating, together with the mild character of the symptoms and the very moderate disturbance which the presence of so many persons seems to have produced in him, cause us to think that the disease may terminate favorably.

MEDICAL PROGRESS.

Evacuation of the Uterus after Parturition. — MME. GACHES-SARRANTE (*La Semaine Médicale*) believes that ergot should be used neither during labor nor after, as the uterus is never completely emptied during parturition, and the clots or shreds of membrane that remain may become sources of infection, and are a frequent cause of subinvolution. The author's practice is to empty the uterus completely in all cases by passing the hand into the cavity of the organ. This procedure she thinks is attended with little danger if the hand is aseptic and if care is taken to avoid wounding the uterine tissue. If the uterus is thoroughly emptied and washed out with sterilized water, hæmorrhage is immediately arrested and involution is rapid.

Treatment of Acne.—In a paper on the treatment of acne, DR. HENRY W. BLANC, of New Orleans (*Journal of the American Medical Association*, October 25, 1890),

lays particular stress on the importance of keeping the digestive organs in good condition by avoiding improper food and securing a movement of the bowels daily. The comedones and pustules should be opened regularly by a lancet and comedone-compressor, and it should be remembered that scarring is less likely to result from the disease if these measures are carefully carried out than if the pustules are not interfered with. As an application, sulphur has given the author better results than any other agent. As a lotion he prefers the following modification of the well-known *lotio alba :*

R.—Potassium sulphide ⎫
    Zinc oxide   ⎬ of each 2 drachms.
    Zinc sulphate   ⎪
    Glycerin   ⎭
    Rose-water sufficient to make 4 ounces.—M.

Apply to the skin after having thoroughly removed the oily secretion. This application produces a sensation of puckering and dryness of the skin. It is well to alternate this lotion with the following :

R.—Precipitated sulphur .   .   . 1½ drachms.
    Salicylic acid   .   . . 20 grains.
    Fluid extract of ergot .   . 2 drachms.
    Lanolin sufficient to make . 1 ounce.—M.

This should be applied morning and evening after having washed the face with water and Hebra's alcoholic soap-lotion. [Hebra's soap-solution is composed of green soap 4 ounces, dilute alcohol 2 ounces, spirit of lavender 1 drachm.] In some cases ichthyol and salicylic acid combined as follows are useful :

R.—Ichthyol .   .   .   .   . 6 drachms.
    Salicylic acid   .   .   .   40 grains.
    Vaseline .   .   .   .   2 ounces.—M.
Apply to the face night and morning.

During the treatment of acne it is important to avoid anything which irritates the skin, such as dust, frequent washing, and friction with a coarse towel. It is well to use a bland soap in order to remove the oily secretion of the sebaceous glands, or in its place the following lotion may be used :

R.—Boric acid ⎫ of each .   .   . 2 drachms.
    Glycerin ⎭
    Alcohol .   .   .   .   1 ounce.
    Ether sufficient to make .   . 3 ounces.—M.
This may be allowed to dry upon the face, and will not attract attention.

Therapeutics of Biniodide of Mercury.—DR. C. R. ILLINGWORTH, who has so persistently advocated the use of biniodide of mercury as an antiseptic, contributes another paper upon the subject (*Provincial Medical Journal*, November 1, 1890). The salt is prepared by dissolving bichloride of mercury in a solution of potassium or sodium iodide. Locally he uses the solution in the following diseases: Ophthalmia neonatorum, 1 to 3000; gonorrhœa, 1 to 5000 or 6000; hay-asthma, 1 to 1000; alopecia, 1 to 500; scabies, 1 to 400; ringworm, 1 to 4 or 5; ozæna, 1 to 3000 or 4000; otorrhœa, 1 to 2000 or 3000; pelvic abscess, 1 to 2000 or 3000; and in the strength of 1 to 2000 to disinfect the mouth and throat in scarlet fever and diphtheria. and the nose, eyes, and air-passages in measles and whooping-cough.

Dr. Illingworth considers the alterative action of the drug of even more importance than the antiseptic action, particularly in the treatment of inflammatory diseases of the serous membranes, such as meningitis, pericarditis, pleuritis, and peritonitis. For instance, in the meningitis of children he uses the following formula:

R.—Solution of bichloride of
  mercury (B. P.) . . 2 to 3 drachms.
Potassium iodide . . 7 to 15 grains.
Antipyrine . . . 15 to 30 ".
Syrup. . . . . ½ ounce.
Water sufficient to make . 1½ ounces.— M.
Dose.—One teaspoonful every one or two hours.

In addition to this, 1 or 2-minim doses of tincture of aconite may be given. If convulsions occur 1-grain doses of chloral may be given every hour for twelve hours. If the temperature is very high, Dr. Illingworth gives sodium salicylate 2 grains and aromatic spirit of ammonia 2 minims with each dose of the above mixture. Pleurisy he treats on the same general plan.

Treatment of Seminal Emissions. — According to the *Canada Lancet*, BUMSTEAD recommends the following to diminish the frequency of seminal emissions:

R.—Potassium bromid. ⎫
 Tinct. of chloride of ⎬ of each 1 ounce.
  iron   ⎭
 Water . . . . . 3 ounces.—M.
Dose.—One or two teaspoonfuls an hour after meals and at bedtime.

Methyl-violet (Pyoktanin) as an Antiseptic. — STILLING (*Therapeutische Monatshefte*) recommends mythyl-violet (sold by Merck under the name of *pyoktanin*) as an antiseptic, and believes that it also has the power to prevent the formation of pus. Pathogenic and other microbes, as is well known, have a great affinity for aniline colors and are rapidly killed by them. A 1-to-1000 solution of methyl-violet applied to the eye stains the conjunctiva, iris, and scleretic, but not the cornea, blue, which disappears within twenty-four hours. The drug is practically non-poisonous, although fatal to rabbits if introduced into the peritoneal cavity in large quantities. Stilling recommends a 1-to-1000 solution of the dye in corneal ulcers, blepharitis, conjunctivitis, phlyctenulæ, keratitis, and serous iritis. He also says that it will sterilize the pus of suppurating wounds and ulcers, and that it is useful as an injection in cases of empyæma and purulent peritonitis, and as an enema in typhoid fever and dysentery. Surgical instruments may be sterilized by washing with a 1-to-10,000 solution of the drug, and wounds, after operations, may be douched with 1-to-2000 or even weaker solutions.

GARRÁ and TROJE (*Münchener medicinishe Wochenschrift*) find that methyl-violet is not poisonous, but that it has no specific antipyogenous action. Their experiments apparently show that although a solution of 1 to 1000 inhibits the development of the cocci found in pus, it does not kill them even after an exposure of twelve hours.

M. BRESGEN speaks highly of the value of methly-violet in the treatment of diseases of the nose, and considers it especially useful in local suppurating areas of the nasal mucous membrane, such as occur after cauterization. It should be applied in solution until the tissues are of a deep-blue color, after which the nasal cavity should be plugged with methyl-violet wool for two hours. According to the author, the application diminishes suppuration and inflammation and relieves pain.—*British Medical Journal*, November 8, 1890.

The Curability of Acute Phthisis.—DR. MCCALL ANDERSON (*British Medical Journal*, November 8, 1890) divides acute phthisis into two forms, namely, acute (miliary) tuberculosis and acute pneumonic phthisis. In the latter form the disease exhibits, almost from the first, more or less extensive consolidation, most frequently of the upper lobes, leading to widespread destruction of the lung, and soon terminating the life of the patient.

Although acute phthisis is usually considered a fatal disease, Dr. Anderson has reported seven cases with five recoveries, all of which were treated by the following plan:

1. Two thoroughly-trained nurses, one for night the other for day, are indispensable. The patient must be fed upon fluid food both day and night, soup being avoided if diarrhœa is present. From two to ten ounces of whiskey daily are required in the beginning of the attack, but should be given in frequent small doses with the food.

2. At bedtime a subcutaneous injection of sulphate of atropine (from $\frac{1}{100}$ to $\frac{1}{60}$ grain) is given. This checks perspiration, acts as a sedative, indirectly helps to reduce the fever, and diminishes the secretion from the lungs.

3. Remedies to lower the temperature are given and are of the utmost importance. Some benefit is derived from permitting the patient to suck ice freely, from giving the food and drinks iced, from sponging the body with iced vinegar and water, and from using iced enemata, but our main reliance must be upon one or more of the following methods:

a. Niemeyer's antipyretic pill or powder (quinine 1 grain, digitalis ½ to 1 grain, opium ¼ to ½ grain) given every four hours, and increasing the amount of opium if there is diarrhœa. The effects of the digitalis must be watched, and if the pulse becomes very slow or the urine scanty the remedy must be omitted for a time.

b. The daily administration shortly before the time that the temperature tends to be the highest, of from ten to thirty grains of quinine, either in a single dose or in divided doses within an hour.

c. The application of iced cloths to the abdomen for half an hour every two hours so long as the temperature exceeds 100°. In applying the cold cloths the nightdress should be drawn up to the chest, a folded blanket placed under the patient, and the bedclothes arranged so that they cover the chest only, the remainder of the body being protected with an extra blanket. Two pieces of flannel are employed, each being sufficiently large, when folded into four layers, to cover the front and sides of the abdomen. One cloth is applied and covered with a dry piece of flannel, while the other is placed in a vessel of iced water by the side of the bed. The flannels should be changed at intervals of a minute.

Dr. Anderson, at the close of his paper, reports a case in which this treatment was carried out, the patient recovering.

THE MEDICAL NEWS.

A WEEKLY JOURNAL
OF MEDICAL SCIENCE.

COMMUNICATIONS are invited from all parts of the world. Original articles contributed exclusively to THE MEDICAL NEWS will be liberally paid for upon publication. When necessary to elucidate the text, illustrations will be furnished without cost to the author.

Address the Editor: H. A. HARE, M.D.,
1004 WALNUT STREET,
PHILADELPHIA.

Subscription Price, including Postage.

PER ANNUM, IN ADVANCE . . . . $4.00.
SINGLE COPIES . . . . 10 CENTS.

Subscriptions may begin at any date. The safest mode of remittance is by bank check or postal money order, drawn to the order of the undersigned. When neither is accessible, remittances may be made, at the risk of the publishers, by forwarding in *registered* letters.

Address,   LEA BROTHERS & CO.,
Nos. 706 & 708 SANSOM STREET,
PHILADELPHIA.

SATURDAY, NOVEMBER 29, 1890.

KOCH AND HIS DISCOVERY.

THREE things may be noticed as the result of the publication of his methods by Koch. First, an extraordinary professional and popular interest ; second, a flocking of medical men and consumptives to Berlin; and third, a gradually-increasing feeling of distrust both of the advantages of the so-called cure, and of the man for his refusal to reveal the secret of the preparation of the anti-tubercular fluid.

The popular interest shown is natural and proper, but the flocking of medical men to Berlin is probably useless—for those who remain behind will be kept informed of all points of interest by the cable, and those who go will be so lost in the rush that their identity will be overlooked, as the investigator and his assistants cannot supply and teach men by the thousand. Again, the trip to Berlin by consumptives is useless and absurd, both because of its dangers and ultimate uncertainty of relief, and by reason of the fact that the rule of "first come first served," so rigidly adhered to, forces a visitor to wait for weeks before he can be treated.

There is much to be said for and against Koch and his so-called cure, for there is a professional, a pecuniary, and a humanitarian side to the subject. While it is against professional ethics to hide from others anything which could be of benefit to the sick, it can be well said that anyone who makes so great a study and possible revolution in medicine should be allowed time to put every part of his work on an unalterable basis. On the other hand, if the daily papers are correct, Koch considers his work in this line finished, and is said to be preparing for studies on scarlet fever, diphtheria, and measles. This must be only partly if at all true, for the popular feeling would force both the government of Germany and the man to lend himself to the propagation of so great a boon to all nations.

In the first moment of excitement everyone felt inclined to believe much more of the possibilities of the discovery than even Koch professes to believe, and a careful and just perusal of his paper shows that he is as conservative and careful in his claims for it as in his researches. He particularly urges the necessity of remembering that all clinical tests have not been made, and still more positively points out that the remedy is of value in pulmonary phthisis only when the disease is in its earliest stages. No one who stops to think can believe otherwise, for regeneration of specialized tissues in man is practically never accomplished, and a lung once seriously involved or broken down cannot be replaced.

Without approval or condemnation it is proper for us to wait for more information. and at least to give Koch credit for a splendid attempt if not a glorious victory over disease.

The readers of THE MEDICAL NEWS can rest assured that they will be kept well informed of all matter pertaining to the subject that possesses official sanction, and that resort to full cable dispatches will be made, as in the issue of this journal for November 15th, should anything of particular interest be made public.

A LEGAL ERROR.

THE absolute inability of the ordinary jury to decide as to questions in which medical points are involved has, with unfortunate frequency, resulted in unjust verdicts and unfortunate convictions. Not only do juries reach verdicts which are as wonderful as they are wrong, but it is a notorious fact that even the judges seem to be unable to see the right side of a medical case and, in consequence, so charge the jury that there is little left for this body to do but to bring in the defendant as guilty.

Our attention is called to this subject particularly by an article which appears in the August and September numbers of *The Medical Standard*, of Chicago, detailing a case in which. for the purpose of making a diagnosis, and also with the hope of affording relief to the patient, who was suffering from marked dyspnœa, a physician introduced an aspirating needle in the axillary line between the sixth and seventh ribs to the depth of one and one-half inches. Immediately after the operation there was some evidence of collapse, which was combated by the administration of brandy and other stimulants; but after this time the patient gradually grew worse and died on the fifth day. Before his death, however, a homœopath was called in, who ultimately made an autopsy, assisted by two others of his own school. Having no love for the regular physician who had previously been in attendance, it was not difficult for these gentlemen to make the friends believe that malpractice had been resorted to by their predecessor, and the result was a trial in which the jury promptly brought in a verdict of guilty against the defendant, notwithstanding the judge's charge to the contrary. On the second trial the verdict was given against the defendant once more with damages at $50, the judge in this instance directing the jury to bring in a verdict *against* the defendant, stating that "expert evidence is a lower order of evidence, and ought not to overthrow positive and direct evidence of witnesses who testify to facts in conflict with such experts." Such an expression of opinion upon the part of the judge is opposed to that of the decision of the Supreme Court of Iowa, which decided that the expert evidence of physicians as to the nature, diagnosis, and treatment of disease is the highest order of evidence. However, this statement of Judge Couch in this particular instance applies with considerable force to the testimony of the homœopaths, which had much to do with the conviction of the defendant. They both stated that it was never proper to use the aspirating needle for the purpose of aiding in making a diagnosis, and one of them testified that he had never heard of such a thing. Further than this, it was asserted by these followers of Hahnemann that the diaphragm is not attached to the inner walls of the chest, is of no particular use, and has no function to perform.

At this distance it is not possible for us to decide as to whether the regular physician inserted an aspirator in such a way as to injure the liver and lung, but that death should have occurred as long as five days after this operation seems to prove that this simple procedure could scarcely have caused a fatal result, even if carelessly performed. Further than this, the post-mortem showed ample cause for death in the presence of far advanced diseased processes.

CORRESPONDENCE.

CHICAGO.

To the Editor of THE MEDICAL NEWS.

SIR : Since the foundation of St. Luke's Hospital, on February 17, 1864, until September 25, 1890. 9277 persons have been received and cared for as in-patients. During the last year 819 were admitted to the wards and rooms, and 2360 received medical advice and surgical treatment at the dispensary free of charge. While the hospital is free to those who cannot afford to pay, there are some rooms set aside for those who can afford to do so. Pay-patients can also be admitted to the wards. Of the 819 admitted in 1889 270 were pay- or part-pay patients, the amount paid into the treasury by them being about $9000. The number of days of hospital care given during the last year was over 24,000—16,140 days, or 67 per cent., being given to charity patients. This makes the average stay of the 819 patients nearly one month. The average cost of each patient per day, aside from the cost of repairs, was $1.465. The admissions from the Episcopal Church were 77 ; from other Christian bodies 515, of whom 219 were Roman Catholics. The expenses for the year were $38,980.77.

The Woman's Physiological Institute has for its distinctive object a series of free afternoon lectures on the subjects of hygiene and sanitary science. All women are cordially invited to avail themselves of the opportunity to listen to able and instructive physicians and educators who have gratuitously contributed their time and talents to this enterprise. A course of twelve lectures is given. Dr. H. A. Johnson lectured before the Institute a few days since, his subject being "The Chest."

The overcrowded condition of the Cook County Insane Asylum will be relieved in a short time, when four cottages, now being erected, will be ready for occupancy. These cottages will accommodate 300 patients. The Asylum was badly crowded when Dr. Benson took charge, and he has done much to lessen the inconveniences which formerly existed.

Dr. James A. Lydston, in a paper on the "Etiology of Cataract," recently read before the Chicago Medical Society, advocated the theory that there is a relationship between the functions performed by the crystalline lens during accommodation and the formation of cataract, stating that he believed that the proper maintenance of accommodation depended upon the tonicity of the ciliary muscle, which is brought about by the process of osmosis taking place between the crystalline lens and the aqueous and vitreous humors ; and that, if the tonicity of the ciliary muscle is impaired from any cause, degenerative changes will begin to assert themselves, and will be manifested by a more or less dense opacity of the lens.

Dr. Lydston further calls attention to the changes observed in the lens in advanced age, and believes that the osmotic process, upon which the lens depends for nutrition, is favored by the periodical contraction and relaxation of the ciliary muscle during accommodation.

Dr. D. W. Graham reported to the Chicago Pathological Society a very unique case of a foreign body in the stomach of a child twenty-two months old. The child was believed to have swallowed some unknown object, but whether it was more than a piece of bread or other solid food was not known. The child slept, and ate and digested its food as usual, and there were no marked symptoms except crying-spells which were severe and frequent, as if from colic. When six weeks had elapsed a small abscess formed in the left hypochondriac region close to the costal cartilage, at a point corresponding to the mammary line. The abscess was opened, and, after several days, a foreign body was discovered in the wound. Dr. Graham now saw the case, and found what proved to be a lady's hat-pin projecting into the wound. The pin could be easily pulled out for several inches, but was arrested by the head, which was too large to pass through the opening. Dr. Graham now proceeded to do what probably proved to be the simplest and easiest laparotomy and gastrotomy on record. A grooved director was passed along the shaft of the pin, by the aid of which the opening was enlarged with a probe-pointed bistoury sufficiently to allow a pair of strong-jawed hæmostatic forceps to be pushed in where the probe had been. The object of this was to force the head from the shaft of the pin. This was soon accomplished, when the shaft was easily lifted out. Some gas escaped, and enough of liquid and partially-digested food to show that the track led directly into the stomach. The glass head was passed with the fæces on the following day, in two pieces. The shaft measured five and one-third inches in length. The wound healed at once, requiring only one re-dressing. No stitches were used to close the wound. The stomach was firmly adherent to the abdominal wall, which rendered the problem of the method of procedure and the operation very easy.

Among the cases of unusual interest lately presented to the orthopædic class at the Chicago Polyclinic, was one of spasmodic wry-neck successfully treated by spinal traction and incision of the urinary meatus.

Professor Charles F. Stillman, in remarking upon the case, alluded to the profound effect upon the nervous system produced by some malformations of the penis, and cited a number of instances of locomotor ataxia and other nervous diseases which had been somewhat improved by complete division of the meatus when contraction existed. The patient above referred to exhibited a penis in which the meatus was entirely closed by membrane, and after its removal the canal was found to be normal throughout its whole extent. The patient had previously urinated through a small sinus in the frænum. A congenital pouch existed at the extremity of the penis, retaining a few drops of urine.

The patient was thirty years of age, and had always been nervous and irritable, but had had no serious illness until September, 1889, when the head exhibited a tendency, without known cause, to turn toward the right, with the chin elevated, which condition gradually grew worse, and was soon complicated with tremor and spasm. When first seen, in April, 1890, he had spasmodic tor-

ticollis, and for several months previously had been confined to his room.

The treatment consisted of exercise, during traction upon the spinal column on both the upright and recumbent curved boards, together with the operation already referred to, and was attended with entire success. The case was considered of interest because of the well-known obstinacy of these cases to ordinary remedies.

Dr. George F. Fisk recently read an interesting paper on the "Use of the Phonograph in Testing the Hearing," before the Chicago Medical Society. His method of using the phonograph in his own practice is to prepare the cylinder in the absence of the patient, speaking fifteen or twenty test-words in a loud and even voice into the machine. Such words the phonograph reproduces so that a person of normal hearing can distinguish them at a distance of from twenty to forty feet, according to the strength of voice used in recording them. No hearing-tube is used, simply the air-conduction in a quiet room. The patient is at first placed thirty or forty feet distant from the phonograph—beyond hearing-distance—and then gradually brought to a point where most of the words can be correctly repeated. The words heard, hearing-distance, name of patient, date, etc., are then recorded on the same cylinder, which is given to the patient for use at another examination or in consultation with another aurist. It is believed that the phonograph is the only instrument to test the hearing which fulfils the following conditions: (1) It makes use of human speech; (2) it is accurate and independent of the examiner; and (3) it makes a record capable of interpretation and use by other aurists.

In examining several phonographs with the same cylinder, and controlling the hearing-distance by two observers possessing normal hearing, no difference could be detected in the different machines. At present five accurate copies have been made of a given cylinder, but at great expense. If indefinite reproduction from a given cylinder (phonogram) shall in the future become possible, then aurists in different parts of the world can use the same tests, and their records and tests will become perfectly intelligible to one another, as is the case now with the oculists' records through the universal employment of Snellen's test-types.

ST. PAUL AND MINNEAPOLIS.

To the Editor of THE MEDICAL NEWS,

SIR: Nothing of very great interest to our profession has lately occurred in Minnesota. We have had our annual meeting of the State Society, at which the following officers were elected:

President, W. L. Beebe, M.D.; First Vice-President, W. D. Flinn, M.D.; Second Vice-President, F. E. Bissel, M.D.; Third Vice-President, J. E. Moore, M.D.; Secretary, C. B. Witherle, M.D.; Treasurer, R. J. Hill, M.D. Some interesting papers were read and cases shown, and as a whole the meeting was a very successful one.

Perhaps of the most interest to the profession at large are the results of our excellent State Medical Law as shown by the report of the Secretary of the State Examining Board, Dr. Arthur Sweeney. This Examining Board has now been in existence for three years, and although occasional difficulties have occurred in the administration of its duties, they have been of minor character and easily overcome.

Our first medical act was passed November 15, 1883. Under this act a State Medical Examining Board composed of the Regents of the University of Minnesota was organized. This board granted 1501 licenses, of which 1325 were granted to physicians with diplomas from recognized medical colleges upon registration of their diplomas; 33 to physicians after examination, and 143 (exemption certificates) to physicians who had practised in the State for five years prior to the passage of the act.

July 1, 1887, this act was repealed and the present act passed, on conviction that the act of 1883 was not an efficient barrier against making incompetent practitioners. The following are some of the interesting features of the act:

The Governor of this State shall appoint a board of examiners, to be known as the State Board of Medical Examiners, consisting of nine members, who shall hold their office for three years after such appointment, and until their successors are appointed.

Provided, That the members thereof first appointed under this act shall be divided into three classes, each class to consist of three. The first class shall hold office under said appointment for the period of one year; the second class for two years, and the third class for three years, from the date of their appointment.

It is further provided that no member thereof shall be appointed to serve for more than two terms in succession, and no member of any college or university having a medical department shall be appointed to serve as member of said board, two of which shall be homœopathic physicians.

The Board of Medical Examiners shall hold meetings for examination at St. Paul, the capital of Minnesota, on the first Tuesday of January, April, July, and October of each year, and such other meetings as said board may from time to time appoint.

All persons hereafter commencing the practice of medicine and surgery, in any of its branches, in this State shall apply to said board for a license so to do, and such applicant, at the time and place designated by said board, or at the regular meeting of said board, shall submit to an examination in the following branches, to wit: Anatomy, Physiology, Chemistry, Histology, Materia Medica, Therapeutics, Preventive Medicine, Practice of Medicine, Surgery, Obstetrics, Diseases of Women and Children, Diseases of the Nervous System, Diseases of the Eye and Ear, Medical Jurisprudence, and such other branches as the board shall deem advisable, and present evidence of having attended three courses of lectures of at least six months each. The clause requiring "three courses of lectures of at least six months each" applies only to those who have been graduated later than July 1, 1887. When desired, said examination may be conducted in the presence of the dean of any medical school or the president of any medical society of this State. After examination, the board shall grant a license to such applicant to practise medicine and surgery in the State of Minnesota; which license can be granted only by the consent of not less than seven members of said board, and shall be signed by the president and secretary of said board, and attested by the seal thereof. The fee of such examination shall be the sum of ten dollars. The board may refuse or revoke a license for unprofessional, dishonorable or immoral conduct. In all cases of refusal or revocation the applicant may appeal to the appointing power of said board.

The examinations are conducted with the utmost fairness and justice. Each applicant writes his name opposite a number in a book, which number he places on his paper. It is against the rules of the board that the Secretary, who conducts the examinations, shall reveal the name of candidate until the latter has been granted or refused a license.

The examination lasts for two and a half days, two hours being allowed for each subject. The papers are forwarded in a sealed box to the examiner. After the close of the examination the full board meets, the markings are submitted to the secretary, and the candidates are then voted on by numbers, after which the results are announced.

The following rules and regulations govern the conduct of the examinations:

I. Any applicant for examination and license to practise medicine in this State, who is a graduate of *over five years*' standing before making application for such examination and license, shall be considered an "old practitioner," and any such applicant who is a graduate of *less than five years* shall be considered a "recent graduate."

II. Applicants who are "old practitioners" shall be required to obtain a minimum marking of not less than *sixty-five* per cent. in each of the following subjects: 1. Practice of Medicine; 2. Practice of Surgery; 3. Materia Medica; 4. Obstetrics, and Diseases of Women and Children; and a minimum marking of not less than *thirty-five* per cent. in each of the following subjects: 1. Anatomy; 2. Chemistry; 3. Physiology; 4. Pathology, Histology and Preventive Medicine; 5. Diseases of the Eye and Ear; 6. Medical Jurisprudence.

III. Applicants who are "recent graduates" shall be required to receive a minimum marking of *thirty-five* per cent. in: 1. Practice of Medicine; 2. Practice of Surgery; 3. Materia Medica; 4. Obstetrics, and Diseases of Women and Children; and a minimum marking of not less than *fifty* per cent. in each of the following: 1. Anatomy; 2. Chemistry; 3. Physiology; 4. Pathology, Histology, and Preventive Medicine; 5. Diseases of the Eye and Ear; 6. Medical jurisprudence.

IV. No applicant shall be granted a license whose general average in all the subjects in which he is examined by this Board is less than *sixty-five* per cent., one hundred being the highest average possible for any applicant to obtain.

It will be noticed that the clause providing that to be eligible for examination, the applicant must present evidence of having attended at least three courses of lectures of six months each, excludes, as nearly as possible, applicants with an imperfect medical education. In spite of this clause, however, some of the answers to the questions are so ridiculous, and show such an utter lack of knowledge, as fully to impress anyone with the fact that some of our best schools sometimes send out very poor graduates. Dr. Sweeney, in his excellent *Register of Physicians*, states that since the passage of the act,

July 1, 1887, to July 5, 1890, "Thirteen examinations have been held, at which 205 candidates have presented themselves. Of this number 128, or 62.44 per cent., have been issued licenses, and 77, or 37.56 per cent., have been rejected. Of the total number of candidates, 62 had graduated five years prior to the date of examination, of whom 30 were licensed and 32 rejected. Two licenses granted by the former board have been revoked, it having been ascertained that the diplomas upon which the licenses were issued were fraudulent. One license has been revoked for unprofessional conduct in attending a patient while under the influence of intoxicants."

Under the old board of 1883 and the present one up to July 5, 1890, 1629 licenses have been issued.[1] On July 5, 1890, there were in active practice in the State 1191 physicians of all classes holding licenses, as follows:

Located.	Licensed on presentation of diplomas.	Exemption certificates.	Licensed on examination by the Board of 1885.	Licensed on examination by the Board of 1887.	Affidavits of exemption filed.	Exempt by practice prior to 1887.
Ramsey County . .	149	3	3	32	4	10
Hennepin County .	212	8	2	33	...	25
Balance of State . .	481	81	20	40	37	51
Total	842	92	25	105	41	86

Located.	Regular.	Homeopathic.	Eclectic.	Unclassified.	Total.
Ramsey County	149	34	4	14	201
Hennepin County	196	44	9	31	280
Balance of State	503	78	25	104	710
Total	848	156	38	149	1191

As the members of the Examining Board are chosen from the ranks of the profession not connected with any of the medical colleges, there is no chance of partiality in this direction. The board is a mixed body, composed of regular practitioners and homœopaths, the regulars being in the majority. Naturally some of the questions asked by men who are not teachers are sometimes peculiar, and some complaints are heard. As a whole, the results of the board's work have been eminently satisfactory to both applicants and the profession at large, and I think we can now say truly that Minnesota receives into the ranks of its medical profession only the better educated graduates from our best medical colleges.

------

[1] This table and the facts of this paper have all been taken from the Register of Physicians, issued by the Secretary of the State Medical Examining Board, Dr. Arthur Sweeney.

NEW YORK.

To the Editor of THE MEDICAL NEWS,

SIR: I have to chronicle an event of the greatest importance to the medical profession of this city, and one which it is confidently hoped will mark a new era in its history. I refer to the formal opening of the new building of the New York Academy of Medicine. Of course, there have been some grumblers, who, steeped in utilitarian ideas, could see no justification for this lavish expenditure for the new building, when, as they said, even on occasions of great interest, it was easy to find seats in the assembly hall of the old building. It is, unfortunately, true that the attendance at the meetings was often shamefully meagre, but the library had outgrown its bounds, and, more important than all this, those who had devoted much time and consideration to the advancement of the interests of the Academy, foresaw, with commendable wordly wisdom, that if the Academy desired to exert still more influence in public matters, it must place itself before the eyes of the public in a fitting position of dignity and honor; in short, it must show a proper self-respect if it would win the respect and esteem of others. This point was emphasized in the anniversary oration delivered by Dr. E. L. Keyes, when he said that if there were sermons in stones, then the very walls of the building had already delivered an address in a strain of far greater dignity than any to which he could aspire.

The new home of the Academy, which is at No. 17 West Forty-third Street, near Fifth Avenue, is a very accessible location, and is as nearly central as it was possible to obtain. Compared with the accommodations of this medical body in a room over a coal-yard, forty years ago, this new edifice is superb. It covers a plot, 75 x 100 feet, and has a basement, four full stories and two half stories. The front is partly of fine red sandstone and partly of brick, the apex of the gable being finished in carved stone-work. The main assembly hall with the adjoining banqueting hall is a memorial of the late Dr. Alexander Hosack, and is known as Hosack Hall. The smoking-room adjoins the assembly hall, and, by opening the dining-room and this smoking-room, one large hall can readily be obtained when needed for unusually large gatherings. Such an arrangement was particularly valuable on the evening of its formal opening, for upward of one thousand ladies and gentlemen assembled to do honor to the occasion. The second story is mainly occupied by the reading-room and library, with its abundant accommodations for the current medical periodicals, and a book-room capable of holding two hundred and fifty thousand volumes. The third and fourth stories contain small meeting-rooms for the Sections of the Academy, and for other societies; also rooms for laboratory work; and one provided with a skylight, so that Fellows who have not sufficient light in their offices may be able to photograph their cases. The building is finished in a beautifully fine and very dark antique oak; ventilation is secured by a revolving fan in the basement; and the illumination is by incandescent electric lights arranged on very tasteful fixtures.

The opening exercises, to which I have alluded, were held on the evening of November 20th. After the invocation by the Rev. Dr. Howard Crosby, Dr. Alfred L.

Loomis delivered the President's address, in which he spoke of the eminent men who founded the Academy, of its proud record for scientific work, and of its library of forty thousand volumes, together with the largest and best collection of journals to be found in the country. He said that, as there were well-organized sections in all the special departments of medicine and surgery, each Fellow might find a congenial place in which to work. They were under no obligations to the past, but under bonds to the future. The career of the physician of the future would be nobler and pleasanter, because he would have less of ignorance and prejudice to combat, but he would require a higher culture than his representative of to-day. In closing his address, he said: "So shall the congratulations, which we utter to-night, re-echo from these walls when other voices recall this day. Join with me, then, in thanksgiving to the Great Physician for what has been accomplished, and in this invocation, that those walls may not crumble or cease to shelter faithful, earnest, Christian men, until suffering humanity is free from its bondage to lust and excess, and is victorious in its struggle against the invisible arrows of disease." In the course of his oration, Dr. Keyes said that, "although the idea of founding such an Academy of Medicine was conceived and began to take shape in the latter part of 1846, it was not until December 12, 1874, that it secured a home of its own at 12 West Thirty-first Street. One of its important functions had always been the promotion of the public health, and how truly it had done its part in this direction was to be seen in the "existence of our efficient city Board of Health, which was conceived and formed in the bosom of this Academy in the interest of the citizens of New York." The membership of the Academy had reached nearly seven hundred, and the library, which was among the youngest, having been founded by donations in 1877, was already safely housed in a fire-proof home, and occupied the third place numerically in the medical libraries of America, and the fourth place among the purely medical libraries of the world. It was but natural that much should be said on this occasion in praise of the library, of which all New York physicians are justly proud, and, it is safe to say that that feeling was greatly enhanced by the description given by Dr. S. Weir Mitchell, of the miserable way in which the library of the French Academy was housed. When Dr. Mitchell asked why it was so poorly classified and arranged, he was told that they were "waiting for the Government to put up a new building." Surgeon-General John S. Billings, in offering congratulations on behalf of the medical officers of the army and other departments of the government, said that the central feature of this Academy was its library, and facetiously added that he would like to say a few things about the "*branch*" of this library in Washington." At that "branch," they are always ready to extend such courtesies to the profession as is possible, but their work in this direction had been somewhat misunderstood. About one year ago, the editor of a leading medical journal, of New York City suggested to a correspondent, asking for a certain kind of information, that he might obtain it for a small compensation by applying to the Surgeon-General at Washington. Dr. Billings said that he then had a very realizing sense of the great power of the

press, for he was immediately overwhelmed with all sorts of letters and inquiries. Dr. Reginald Fitz, of Boston, spoke of the principal library in that city, and Dr. Abraham Jacobi pictured the needs of " our library," and made an eloquent plea for financial aid for it. The venerable Fordyce Barker, who was introduced as one " whose Presidency marked a new era in the history of the Academy," was received with enthusiastic applause. In a few well-chosen words he offered his congratulations, and said that that auspicious occasion would have been long delayed had it not been for the zealous work of the President and of his immediate predecessor, Dr. Jacobi. Dr. S. Weir Mitchell, in offering the congratulations of the College of Physicians of Philadelphia, took the opportunity of calling the attention of the general public to the fact that what we are often pleased to style " our profession," is rather a guild or brotherhood, possessing a creed of morals including honor, chastity, brotherhood, and the largest charity ; the records of much of its work not being kept in the books of this world. As regards the charity of the profession, he thought the public generally did not understand that two-thirds of the most celebrated physicians of New York City gave three or four hours a week to free work among the poor. He was not aware that a similar custom existed among merchants or lawyers.

At the conclusion of the speeches, a collation was served in the banqueting-room. Letters of congratulations were read from well-known physicians in Chicago, New Haven, Boston, and elsewhere, and Oliver Wendell Holmes sent a characteristic letter, which was a fitting close to this memorable occasion. He said: "Academies have been too often thought of as places of honorable retirement and dignified ease : roosts where emeritus professors and effete men of letters, once cocks of the walk, could sit in quiet rows, while the fighting, the clucking, and the crowing were going on beneath them. But the academy which fulfils its true function is a working body. We look to this great and able body of men to guard the sacred avenues to the temple of science against all worshippers of idols. The medical profession will always have to fight against the class of wrong-headed and dishonest individuals and schools, as they call themselves. There are a certain number of squinting brains as there are squinting eyes among every thousand of any population, and there will always be a corresponding number of persons, calling themselves physicians, ready to make a living out of them. Long may it be before the wholesome barriers are weakened that separate the thoroughbred and truly scientific practitioner from the plausible pretender. I trust it will always be enough for a physician to be able to say, 'I am a member of the New York Academy of Medicine.'"

MILWAUKEE.

To the Editor of THE MEDICAL NEWS,

SIR : In the busy and generally uneventful round of professional life as it here exists, your chronicler for Milwaukee and vicinity finds comparatively little that is of interest regarding medical affairs. The subject at present uppermost in the professional mind here, as elsewhere, is the new remedy for tuberculosis. The leading men of the profession look upon the subject encouragingly, and hope that Koch may, in these latest investigations, add to his already brilliant reputation and furnish to the world an effective weapon against the "great white plague." Dr. H. M. Brown, of Milwaukee, left for Berlin on November 22d to study the subject in Koch's laboratory. Dr. Conway, of Chicago, has also gone, at the request of Professor Ingals, for the same purpose. Drs. Frank and McDill, of this city, are already spending the winter in Berlin, and will undoubtedly avail themselves of the opportunity to study and investigate the subject.

Apropos of the subject of laboratory work, the need of a good working bacteriologist and laboratory in Milwaukee often finds expression. The average general practitioner is not usually a man fitted for the work either by inclination or previous training : and the time, to speak of one item only, required for satisfactory work is so great that the man in general practice can accomplish little or nothing in bacteriology. It is hoped that a fund contributed by wealthy citizens and controlled as might be deemed wise by some local or State society, may place at our disposal a well-equipped laboratory under the direction of a skilled pathologist. At present morbid specimens are not infrequently sent to Washington, New York, or Philadelphia for examination. The private laboratory of Mr. Edward Allis, in this city, is an example of what can be done in the manner suggested above. The work done is purely biological and is under the superintendence of Professor E. O. Whitman. Issued quarterly from this institution and edited by the gentlemen named, is the *Journal of Morphology*, the scope of which is defined in its title, and its high scientific standing is attested by the favorable notices it has received from the highest authorities in biological science both in this country and in Europe.

During the late summer and fall typhoid fever has been more than usually prevalent, and more recently an unusual increase in the number of cases and deaths from diphtheria has been noticed. In one section of the city it was deemed advisable to close for a short time one of the public schools, and other special precautions have been taken by our Health Commissioner, Dr. Wingate, to limit the spread of the disease. Notwithstanding these facts Milwaukee still maintains its reputation as a healthy city, its death-rate per thousand being less than that of other neighboring cities of about the same or larger size.

The Emergency Hospital recently extended its field of usefulness by the addition of a maternity ward. It is hoped that this institution, which has already demonstrated its worth, may in the near future find a better habitation : for a new building and a larger equipment are needed.

The State Medical Society has just published its transactions for the current year. This is the twenty-fourth volume of proceedings and compares favorably with previous issues : the papers and discussions which it contains indicate a growing interest in the work of the society on the part of the physicians throughout the State. The society is still at work on the subject of State medical legislation, and the matter will probably again be brought up at the next meeting of the State Legislature. The meeting of the State Society for next year will be held at Madison. The officers of the society are : Dr. George D. Ladd, president ; Drs. F. E. Walbridge and B. T. Phillips, vice-presidents ; Dr. J. R. McDill, secretary.

ST. LOUIS.

To the Editor of The Medical News,

Sir : Our medical societies are now holding their regular weekly meetings again. At the St. Louis Medical, which meets in the hall of the public school board every Saturday evening, one or more papers are read and cases are reported more or less formally.

The subject of pyosalpinx has been attracting a good deal of attention in the societies for several weeks past, some very interesting specimens having been exhibited and the cases reported and discussed.

The Medico-Chirurgical Society is also holding its meetings every week instead of bi-weekly, as formerly, and the new society hall and reading-room are very convenient and pleasant. The question of lengthening the term of study preliminary to graduation from medical schools has attracted a good deal of attention here this fall, and the discussion has resulted in interviews of different professors of medical colleges by reporters of the daily newspapers. The Missouri School of Medicine (Medical Department No. 2, of the Missouri State University) has announced that after the current year a three years' carefully-graded course of study will be required of all applicants for graduation at that institution. The St. Louis school has enforced this rule for several years, beginning at a time when scarcely any of the Eastern colleges made that requirement.

The other three schools have not yet been able to adopt a three years' course.

A few days ago, after reading in one of the journals an obituary notice of Dr. Montrose A. Pallin, I chanced to pass the building which was his home when he lived here, and noticed upon it a sign with the words " The Montrose." In the rapid westward growth of our city the change from the fashionable residence to the boarding-house is the common fate of many handsome buildings ; but I do not remember another instance of the utilization of the name of a former owner to increase the popularity of a boarding-house.

There has been an unusually large amount of continned and typhoid fevers this fall instead of the ordinary intermittent malarial fevers which we expect at this season of the year. In one case which occurred under my observation a girl of sixteen years had a temperature of 106.8° on five successive days in the fourth week of a fever which continued six weeks before convalescence occurred.

The St. Louis Training School for Nurses graduated a class of seven a few weeks ago. The women who are carrying on this school have done an excellent work, and the graduates of the school, having had a two years' course of study and training, are admirably qualified for their work.

NEWS ITEMS.

Various cablegrams from Berlin all agree in supporting the opinion expressed in the editorial in this number of The Medical News concerning the uselessness of either doctors or patients travelling to Berlin at this time with the idea of obtaining any of the benefits which may accrue from the employment of Koch's antitubercular fluid.

Various regimental surgeons in different portions of the German army have been ordered to set aside soldiers under their care who are suffering from tuberculosis, in order that the service may be benefited as early as possible, but it is worthy of note that nearly ninety per cent. of the cases which are receiving injections of the antitubercular fluid are not sufferers from pulmonary tuberculosis, but chiefly from lupus and allied diseased conditions.

We are also informed through the cable that there are already hundreds of English doctors in Berlin who are permitted to see little and who have opportunity to learn less. They all agree in complaining bitterly of the scant courtesy which is shown them, and it is asserted by those who ought to know that the same treatment will be shown to the American doctors when they arrive.

Professor Koch has always been notorious for the seclusion which he insists upon, and to see him now is absolutely impossible. He has also practically limited the employment of his liquid to von Bergmann, Cornet, and Levy, all of whom in one way or another ·have placed the discoverer under personal obligations by favors done him in the past. So complete a monopoly have these men of the employment of the liquid that they have established numerous private hospitals in Berlin, in which they charge exorbitant prices, both for living expenses and medical attendance. Thus 'it is said that Levy charges every patient $25 for each visit, and that even with this extortionate price he treats nearly two hundred patients daily. The other physicians, it seems, are not far behind Levy in their charges, and physicians, students, and patients are endeavoring by every means in their power to obtain information which cannot be had. The number of consumptives who have flocked to Berlin from all parts of the Continent reaches several thousand, and it is supposed that at least 1700 of these have already been treated—none of them, of course, as yet with marked improvement in their condition. The fact that so many consumptives have applied for relief is said to be a source of much distress to Dr. Koch, who realizes better than anyone else apparently that his remedy is not a cure-all.

A Hospital at Long Branch, New Jersey.—The rapidly growing town of Long Branch, New Jersey, has for several years felt the need of an infirmary. This want has been met by the purchase, by the Monmouth Memorial Association, of a large hotel property, which can easily be converted into a well-appointed hospital. Dr. S. H. Hunt, President of the Association, has been chiefly instrumental in carrying the project through.

Physicians at Law.—Dr. Marcely, of Buffalo, N. Y., is suing Dr. Tremaine, of the same city, for $25,000 damages for libel. It is stated that Dr. Tremaine referred to Dr. Marcely in a Society meeting as a "notorious quack," and asserted that electrical treatment as an alleged radical cure for hernia was quackish practice. Both are regularly educated physicians, Dr. Tremaine being Emeritus Professor of Surgery in one of the medical schools of Buffalo.

Case of Aconite-poisoning.—A correspondent reports a case of aconite poisoning in a farmer in Nebraska, who, having obtained some tincture of aconite for the purpose of using it as a liniment upon his horse, made an application of the liquid to his own head in order to relieve a headache. He rapidly developed symptoms of aconite-poisoning, and died in about twenty-four hours.

Alvarenga Prize.—The College of Physicians of Philadelphia announces that·the next award of the Alvarenga Prize, being the income for one year of the bequest of the late Senor Alvarenga, and amounting to about $180, will be made on July 14, 1891. Essays intended for competition may be upon any subject in medicine, and must be received by the Secretary of the College, Dr. Charles W. Dulles, on or before May 1, 1891.

OFFICIAL LIST OF CHANGES IN THE STATIONS AND DUTIES OF OFFICERS SERVING IN THE MEDICAL ·DE- .PARTMENT, U. S. ARMY, FROM NOVEMBER 18 TO NOVEMBER 24, 1890.

MOSELEY, EDWARD B., *Captain and Assistant Surgeon.*— Is granted leave of absence for one month.—*S. O. 100. Department of Texas,* November 17, 1890.

By direction of the Acting Secretary of War, leave of absence for six months, on surgeon's certificate of disability, with permission to go beyond sea, is granted HENRY G. BURTON, *Captain and Assistant Surgeon.*—Par. 9, *S. O. 269, Headquarters of the Army, A. G. O.,* November 17, 1890.

By direction of the Acting Secretary of War, JOHN L. PHILLIPS, *Captain and Assistant Surgeon,* is relieved from further duty at Fort Crawford, Colorado, to take effect on his relinquishing the unexpired portion of his present leave of absence, and will report in person to the commanding officer Camp Guthrie, Oklahama Territory, for duty at that station. reporting by letter to the commanding general Department of the Missouri.—Par. 7, *S. O. 269, A. G. O.,* Washington, November 17, 1890.

By direction of the Acting Secretary of War, leave of absence from January 1, to March 24, 1891, inclusive, with permission to go beyond sea, is granted HENRY JOHNSON, *Captain and Medical Storekeeper.*—Par. 18, *S. O. 268, A. G. O., Washington,* November 15, 1890.

OFFICIAL LIST OF CHANGES IN THE STATIONS AND DUTIES OF THE MEDICAL CORPS OF THE U. S. NAVY FOR THE WEEK ENDING NOVEMBER 22, 1890.

AYERS, J. G., ·*Surgeon.*—Ordered to the U. S. Receiving-ship " Wabash."

EVANS, SHELDON GUTHRIE.—Commissioned an Assistant Surgeon in the U. S. Navy.

BATES. N. L., *Medical Director.*—Ordered as President of the Naval Medical Examining Board at Mare Island, Cal.

MOORE. A. M., *Surgeon.*—Ordered as a member of the Naval Medical Examining Board at Mare Island, Cal.

OFFICIAL LIST OF CHANGES OF STATIONS AND DUTIES OF MEDICAL OFFICERS OF THE U. S. MARINE-HOSPITAL SERVICE, FROM OCTOBER 26 TO NOVEMBER 15, 1890.

CARTER, H. R., *Passed Assistant Surgeon.*—Granted leave of absence for fifteen days, November 14, 1890.

GUITERAS, G. M., *Assistant Surgeon.*—Granted leave of absence for thirty days, October 29, 1890.

HUSSEY, S. H., *Assistant Surgeon.*—To proceed to the South Atlantic Quarantine Station for temporary duty, October 28, 1890.

GEDDINGS, H. D., *Assistant Surgeon.*—Granted leave of absence for fourteen days, November 14, 1890.

GROENEVELT, J. F., *Assistant Surgeon.*—To report to the Superintendent of Immigration for temporary duty, October 28, 1890.

THE MEDICAL NEWS.

A WEEKLY JOURNAL OF MEDICAL SCIENCE.

VOL. LVII.   SATURDAY, DECEMBER 6, 1890.   No. 23.

ORIGINAL LECTURES.

ONE YEAR'S WORK IN DISEASES OF THE RECTUM AT THE NEW YORK POST-GRADUATE MEDICAL SCHOOL AND HOSPITAL.

By CHARLES B. KELSEY, M.D.,
PROFESSOR OF DISEASES OF THE RECTUM.

GENTLEMEN: At the close of this, the first year of clinical instruction in diseases of the rectum, it is interesting to glance back over the case-book and see what has been accomplished. If the amount of material has not been as large as it doubtless will be in the future, it is because sufficient time has not yet elapsed to make this new departure in hospital work known to the sufferers who are benefited by it. And yet those of you who have been with me any length of time have had a chance to see almost all diseases of the rectum and the operations for their relief.

We have had 125 patients, showing 131 cases of disease of the rectum. These in the order of their frequency are as follows:

Hæmorrhoids	42	Deep pelvic abscess		3
Fistula	15	Congenital malformations		3
Fissure	10	Polypus		2
Benign stricture	9	Recto-vaginal fistula		2
Ulceration	6	Recto-vesical fistula		2
Pruritus	6	Paralysis of rectum from		
Superficial abscess	5	spinal disease		2
Cancer	5	Urethral fistula and abscess		1
Prolapse	4	Foreign body		1
Papilloma	4			

For these various affections 67 operations have been done before the class, as follows:

Hæmorrhoids	17	Excision of rectum		3
Fistula	12	Polypus		2
Fissure	8	Plastic operation on anus		2
Colotomy	6	Recto-vaginal fistula		1
Abscess (superficial)	4	Deep pelvic abscess		1
Prolapse	3	Proctotomy		1
Ulcers	3	Foreign body		1
Papilloma	3			

You will observe at once that the number of severe and unusual cases (cancer, benign stricture, congenital malformations, etc.) is out of all proportion to the whole number of cases seen, probably because our medical friends are kindly sending us these cases, while the simpler ones take care of themselves. As a natural consequence our death-rate has been high—3 cases in 125—much higher than will be met in practice, as cases generally run. Without the least desire to explain away this rate of mortality or make it appear less than it is, it is instructive to call attention to it more fully. In one case we did an inguinal colotomy on a man at the point

of death, regardless of statistics, but in the desperate hope of prolonging his life. You remember the case of the man whose stricture was divided by a deep posterior incision three months ago. Contrary to my usual practice, the incision was not continued outward through all the soft parts about the anus for drainage, but a drainage-tube was carried backward from the stricture through the skin at the tip of the coccyx. This procedure has served me well in other cases, and saves much time in the healing of the cut, but I advise you against it. The drainage is by no means as perfect as when the anus is divided, and a fistula may remain in the track of the tube. I do not know that the character of the drainage had any effect in this particular case, but on the third day an immense phlegmon appeared on the left side of the anus and in the perineum—a true septic periproctitis. Free incisions were at once made and constant antiseptic irrigation kept up, while for many days large sloughs of cellular tissue worked their way out through the cut. The patient went very near to death's door at that time, but rallied after a fortnight, and seemed on the point of recovering, when a diarrhœa began which never ceased. Six weeks before his death we tried to put the abscess in a condition to heal, and discovered, under ether, the frightful destruction it had caused. The superficial openings were turned into one, the cavity was cleared of its unhealthy granulations, but the finger passed into the ischio-rectal fossa and up into the pelvis parallel with the gut, and no limit to the suppurating cavity could be reached. There was a large opening between the rectum and the abscess just within the anus, and another higher than the finger could reach, which allowed all of the fæces to escape from the rectum into the abscess cavity. The attempt to excite reparative action failed, the abscess steadily extended into the pelvis, and as was shown by frequent hæmorrhages, vessels were opened up, and, finally, a few days before death, a communication was made with the bladder. At first the flow was entirely from the bladder into the abscess, but twenty-four hours before death signs of acute cystitis began to show themselves, and for this, as a last resort, colotomy was done. Those of you who saw the operation remember with what extreme rapidity it was performed (seven minutes from the first incision to the dressing), and how little shock attended it. The patient rallied well and seemed none the worse, but later on sank quietly and died the same evening. You can therefore judge as well as I of the influence of the incision upon the result.

In another of the fatal cases following colotomy the influence of the operation was, I think, absolutely *nil*. The woman had a cancerous stricture of the rectum, with secondary deposits throughout the abdomen in the mesentery and omentum. As it was impossible for her to relieve the bowels, the left inguinal operation was done, and we had great difficulty in finding any coil of gut, small or large, sufficiently free from cancerous adhesions to permit its being drawn to the surface. The sigmoid flexure was, however, finally attached to the wound and the dressing applied without incising the gut. Forty-eight hours after the operation the patient suddenly developed all the signs of severe illness—chill, high temperature, and immediate collapse. Thinking that the acute obstruction at the site of the incision might be the explanation of the condition, I hastened to open the gut, but the intestine was not at all distended, and no gas escaped, as is usually the case. It being manifest that no obstruction existed at the point of operation, the case was supposed to be one of septic peritonitis, and the collapse and general cancerous infection decided us against further surgical interference. At the autopsy it was found that the patient died of acute intestinal obstruction, which was, however, entirely unconnected with the operation and in no way due to it. At the splenic flexure of the colon, many inches above the wound, the gut was tightly bound down and sharply flexed by a cancerous mass in the mesentery, and against this point a lump of solid fæcal matter had impinged and completely obstructed the lumen. In her feeble condition the fatal result followed in a few hours.

The third death was no less interesting and instructive. In this case we excised a cancerous rectum, the disease reaching high up, but not beyond the limit of digital examination. Excepting the presence of chronic intestinal obstruction the patient was in good condition and the case a favorable one for operation. After the disease had been removed a complication occurred which I was unable to explain at the time, but which became very evident at the autopsy on the following day in the dilated sigmoid flexure. A large mass of fæces, in fact an impaction as large as a child's head, was found, which I removed, piece by piece with the fingers before suturing the ends of the gut. No force was used, and yet before all had been removed there was free hæmorrhage, not from the wound, but from the inside of the upper end of the gut. After all of the collection had been scooped out the bleeding still continued, and after suturing the divided ends and putting in the drainage-tubes, it was necessary to apply a tampon of charpie within the bowel in order to check the flow of blood. As the ether passed off the patient began to complain of most violent abdominal pain, and after twelve hours, during which no relief could be given him, he died in collapse. At the autopsy a rent was found in the upper part of the rectum, but not connected with the wound, through which fæcal extravasation had taken place. The rent was in the middle of a part of the gut which had become as thin as blotting-paper from the ulceration, caused by the direct pressure of the fæcal mass.

Of the three deaths, then, it seems but fair to say that though they all followed within a few hours of capital operations, two were in no way due to the operation, and the third was not prevented by it.

In our other four colotomies we have had good results, both immediate and remote, as a result of this procedure. Two of the cases you have seen to-day, namely, the doctor with the non-malignant ulceration and stricture high in the bowel, which was incurable by any other method of treatment, and the little child of seven

months born with an imperforate anus. This case I should not have been surprised to see die after the operation, so weak and marasmic was he, and so great was the distention of the abdomen. You remember how, when the incision was made, nearly the entire intestinal tube came out through the wound, the large gut distended to about the size of two thumbs and the small one shrivelled and contracted. The child was born with no anus at all, and at the time of birth a deep incision was made which reached the blind rectal pouch. As is always the case, the little patient had with difficulty been kept alive for seven months, suffering about equally from obstruction and the efforts made by bougies to overcome it. At the time of the colotomy it had gone several days without any passage, and then had unloaded the gut by five or six fluid stools, due to one of those violent intestinal convulsions by which nature so often overcomes for the time a chronic obstruction. These are not favorable conditions for the operation of colotomy, and yet the child has done well; nor, should it live, need it be so great an object of sympathy, for if adults in the higher walks of life are contented in this condition and grateful for the relief afforded, surely it may be borne by one who has never known a different condition.

We have been especially fortunate in the number of cases of this sort of congenital malformation brought to the clinic in the year. Many men in active practice have never seen a single case, and yet we have had three. Both of the others were simple fibrous partitions between the rectum and anus, which allowed the escape of a small amount of fæces, and might have been relieved, at least for a time, by division and subsequent dilatation, had the parents consented; but this case was of a more serious character, and left us no hope of prolonging life for any great length of time except by more radical measures.

I show you the case again to-day, one week after the operation, and the difference in the child's general appearance is very marked. You would hardly believe that it has reached the age of seven months, so small and marasmic is it; but the vomiting, restlessness, and fretful crying have ceased, and the little patient is dividing its time between eating and sleeping. I have been asked, rather sarcastically, whether it was not possible to relieve the obstruction in this case without cutting the baby open, and for answer I point to the child. One gentleman has introduced his finger into the cicatricial tissue which forms the anus, and at about an inch from the surface feels an obstruction which he rightly believes could be cut through. There is no doubt about this; but, after cutting, the stricture must be kept open by dilatation, and the results of seven months of this treatment are shown in the present condition of the baby. Does a few months more of the same treatment bid fair to restore the child to health? In this matter we have been guided not only by the manifest dying condition of the child, but by the recorded experience of such men as Brodie, Benjamin Bell, Velpeau, and Van Buren, each of whom has recorded his experience that the struggle is always a hopeless one, and after a few years ends fatally for the patient. Had I desired to give only temporary relief to the obstruction I should have cut and dilated the stricture; but wishing to see this child grow to adult age, I have made an entirely new outlet for the fæces; and preferring to do this with the least possible shock and immediate risk, have made that outlet in the left inguinal region.

I want to call your attention to the differences in appearances between this anus and the one in the adult patient just seen. Here you see the wire suture which was passed through the abdominal wall and mesentery, and by which the gut was raised and held almost entirely outside of the abdominal cavity and bent on itself at an acute angle, still in position. We will remove it. You see also that the edges of the opening in the gut have been cut away so that you are looking directly into the interior of the gut. In the other case the gut was not drawn out of the abdomen to such an extent and none of its wall was sacrificed. This has been done with an object. The adult is suffering from benign stricture and ulceration at about five inches from the anus, which has rendered life miserable for nine years, and is incurable by any sort of local or general treatment save colotomy. But after this operation the ulceration is very likely to heal, and, being a physician the patient may at first use bougies, either through the natural or artificial anus, and come back after a year or more to have the artificial opening closed. The opening has been made with the especial object of being able to close it in the future by a plastic operation, and without resection and suture.

In the baby there is no such hope, and the anus has been made so as completely to occlude the gut, leaving only a small opening into the distal portion to introduce the tip of a syringe for the purpose of washing out what fæcal matter may have been in the rectum at the time of operation.

Perhaps the most interesting, and certainly the rarest, case shown you was the girl of thirteen, with well-developed and advanced lupus of the ano-vulvar region and consequent stricture of the rectum, sent to us by Dr. Lee, of Newark. As far as I am acquainted with the scanty literature of this affection it is the only case on record in a child, and in this one it had existed since the age of seven years. Although the history is imperfect and the parents deny syphilis, it would seem that this case must have had a specific origin from the great improvement which has taken place after eight months' treatment by Dr. Lee with anti-syphilitic remedies. The child was shown again a few days ago and the ulceration had certainly been greatly diminished in extent, while the induration so strongly resembling elephantiasis which is characteristic of the disease had in great measure disappeared. The case when first seen seemed only suitable for colotomy, while now it appears in a fair way to recover.

Of benign strictures you have seen almost every variety, and likewise almost every mode of treatment. The congenital forms have been referred to. We have also had syphilitic stricture, stricture in a man associated with the practice of unnatural vice, that due to pressure of pelvic exudation in a woman, and that caused by simple ulceration neither lupoid, dysenteric, or tubercular—ulceration impossible to account for except by some such simple traumatism as may be caused by the lodgement of scybalous masses of fæces, or by childbirth. I have again and again called your attention to the small proportion of cases in which it was possible to discover any venereal origin of the disease, and have tried to impress upon you the danger of jumping to the conclusion that a stricture must of necessity be either cancerous or syphilitic.

In the way of treatment you have seen colotomy for the bad cases, excision where it was applicable, and simple proctotomy. What you have not seen are the results which may follow this last measure, when patiently and intelligently carried out, and supplemented by systematic dilatation in a better class of cases than are seen here. This is the one method which should be relied upon in a large number of cases, and by it many patients may be made comfortable for life; but, unfortunately, it is seldom applicable to the poor in hospital practice. It is a method for the rich, and one covering years of patient work; but by it I have seen the nearest approach to a cure of the disease. Proctotomy is only the beginning of the treatment, and you have seen that done here. But the patient has not returned to us, and we know that by this time she is preparing to go to some other hospital for something else.

In the treatment of hæmorrhoids the clamp and cautery operation has been used in all cases except one, and the question of its advantages has been left entirely to the decision of the class. You know what is claimed for it here—quicker recovery and less pain than by any other method of cure. You have seen the patients again and again able to come down stairs to the out-patient room forty-eight hours after the operation, and heard them say that after the first few hours there was only a sense of soreness and some pain on defæcation. You have seen physicians leave the hospital and start in comfort on long journeys on the fourth day, though you have never heard me advise such a procedure. Usually the patients stay in the house for one week; seldom do they wish to stay longer. Almost invariably they are able to urinate without the use of the catheter. Accidents have not occurred, and it has been impressed upon you that the surest way to avoid them is to cauterize thoroughly the stump held in the clamp after cutting off the body of the hæmorrhoid with the scissors; and to see that there is no bleeding from the cauterized surface. After the operation is finished, a large speculum is introduced, and the rectum well irrigated with bichloride solution. If there is no bleeding then, there is no more likelihood of secondary hæmorrhage than there is after the ligature; and if there is bleeding (not from the cutaneous cuts with the scissors, but from the cavity of the gut), the operation is simply not finished, and the bleeding point must be secured. The cutaneous bleeding is controlled by direct pressure with pad and bandage, as in the ligature operation.

Carbolic acid injections have been used in one case where this method seemed specially indicated. The woman was at the end of the third month of pregnancy and was covered with a syphilitic eruption, and operation was therefore out of the question; but she was suffering greatly and bleeding profusely with each act of defæcation. A few drops of a ten-per-cent. solution of carbolic acid were injected into two of the hæmorrhoids, and a third one, with an eroded strawberry-like surface, was painted with nitric acid, and all of the bad symptoms ceased. But I explained to you that the woman was certainly not cured, as she supposed herself, and that what was done was not free from serious risks of sloughing and abscess, though less likely than a radical operation to produce a miscarriage.

The same thing may be done in many cases with the same happy results. It is a fascinating procedure to both patient and surgeon till the bad case comes along ; but after causing one severe phlegmonous inflammation of the peri-rectal cellular tissue the *surgeon* generally abandons it for methods attended by less risk and by permanent results.

Of fistulæ we have had all varieties from the simpler ones which were cut in the out-patient room without ether, to those extending deep into the pelvis, and the case of combined recto-vaginal and vesico-vaginal openings, due probably to chancroidal ulceration. In the one case of large recto-vaginal fistula associated with an abscess behind the uterus, in which the attempt was made to reach and suture the opening by a Kraske's incision, the operation was a failure, due, perhaps, to the difficulty in getting at an opening so near the body of the uterus, or perhaps to the presence of the abscess discharging into the vagina at the site of the fistula.

Another bad case of fistula-in-ano, extending deep into the pelvis, was the one due to carious bone on the anterior and lateral surfaces of the sacrum. The first operation here also was a failure, because the incisions, though deep, were not deep enough. At the second trial the coccyx and lower sacral vertebræ were removed, the incision was carried along the side of the sacrum to about its middle, and the diseased bone scraped away. Tracks were then found running around the deep urethra on both sides behind the triangular ligament, which were also scraped out with the finger. The patient still reports to us occasionally with the wound entirely healed except a small sinus just admitting a probe, which leads to the stump of the sacrum.

ORIGINAL ARTICLES.

THE TREATMENT OF ENTERIC FEVER, WITH SPECIAL REFERENCE TO THE METHOD OF BRAND.[1]

BY J. C. WILSON, M.D.,
PHYSICIAN TO THE HOSPITAL OF THE JEFFERSON MEDICAL COLLEGE AND TO THE GERMAN HOSPITAL, PHILADELPHIA.

A FRENCH medical writer has said, "When I see a young man die from typhoid fever, I experience the sensation of having witnessed a homicide." Here, as always, something of the truth is sacrificed to the desire to be epigrammatic, but no one who has carefully studied the subject, can fail to enter into the spirit which suggested this forcible statement.

In the first place, enteric fever, in theory at least, is a preventable disease. Our knowledge of its causation is to-day sufficiently extended and accurate to make it a preventable disease in practice. That it is not prevented in communities where it is endemic is largely due to the absence of positive

convictions as to the material nature of the infecting principle and the possibility of destroying it or preventing its spread. It is the highest duty of the doctor to see to it that no new cases of infectious disease arise, by direct or indirect contagion, from any patient under his care. In enteric fever we have to do with a disease in which this is wholly practicable. Not only may the spread of the contagium be prevented, but the infecting principle can be wholly and absolutely destroyed. It is not too much to say that this disease, the great fever of the present historical epoch, is among the scourges of mankind which can, by organized effort, be stamped out ; not in the wide sense that in the history of the past two centuries the plague was driven from Western Europe, that typhus disappeared from ships, jails, and armies, and that leprosy died out in Great Britain, but in a much more narrow and literal sense. There is abundant evidence in medical literature to show that organized prophylaxis, dealing with the water-supply, the milk, the drainage, and the excreta of individual cases, is capable of eradicating enteric fever from restricted localities.

In the second place, enteric fever is a curable disease. I use the word curable in an equally literal and narrow sense. It is my purpose here, having some slight personal knowledge of the matter, to endeavor to demonstrate that this proposition is true. I am not sure that I shall succeed. It is no easy thing to unsettle established convictions and to gainsay the conclusions of experience which seems to be based upon the daily observation of facts. Nor, indeed, have I the warrant of a sufficiently extended personal observation to do so.

Certain recent experiences in this disease have, however, greatly modified my views as to the part played by treatment, and it is because the treatment of which I am about to speak is, as a plan, so different from that generally employed, and because the results, as shown both by the course of the disease in individual cases and by the diminution of the death-rate, are so striking, that I feel impelled to urge this plan upon the attention of my professional associates who have not yet had an opportunity to try it. I know that enteric fever destroys, in the aggregate, more lives that could be saved than does any other acute infectious disease. I believe that, in the words of Baruch,[1] "We are standing to-day on the threshold of a great epoch in the treatment of this disease."

What has been the treatment up to the present time? Among innumerable plans, a host of drugs, and countless modifications of the methods of administering them, we may distinguish four general methods of treatment.

---

[1] Read before the Lycoming County Medical Society, at Williamsport, Pennsylvania, November 4, 1890.

[1] Reprint from the Transactions of the New York State Medical Society, February, 1889.

First, *the expectant plan*. Under this head must be included pure expectancy and those methods in which measures or medicaments are employed which are incapable, either by reason of want of force or by minimum dosage, of producing any physiological or therapeutic effect whatever. The disease is practically left to run its course, the duty of the physician being confined chiefly to regulating the hygiene and the diet.

Second, *the expectant-symptomatic*, or so-called *rational plan*, which is an extension of the expectant plan in that symptoms, as they arise, are treated by measures of more or less energy especially directed against them. Under this plan the physician's duties are manifold and perplexing, and the therapeutic measures, instituted in response to various indications, are complex, difficult, and often at variance among themselves.

Third, *the antiseptic plan*. This method has its origin in the fact that the evolution of the disease is due to the development within the organism of pathogenic germs, a process which continues until the soil is practically exhausted and the germs cease to grow. It recognizes the splitting up of complex chemical compounds entering into the formation of the fluids of the body, with the result of the production, on the one hand, of the pabulum necessary to germ-growth, and, on the other hand, of toxic substances foreign to the organism, to which the fever and the other symptoms are chiefly due. This plan of treatment claims to do all that the expectant and the expectant-symptomatic plans do, and undertakes to anticipate the development of unfavorable symptoms, by at least holding in check the cause of those symptoms. It embraces, first, intestinal antisepsis, and second, in theory, at least, constitutional antisepsis, and under certain forms has appeared to exercise a favorable influence upon the course and mortality of the disease.

Fourth, *the antipyretic plan*. This plan is based upon the theory, long since formulated by Griesinger, that the fever in great part controls the situation. It demands as an essential of treatment the restriction of the temperature-rise within limits, and insists upon the use of therapeutic measures to reduce the temperature whenever it attains a certain degree of elevation varying according to the views of different practitioners. These measures are, first, antipyretic drugs, and second, the external application of cold water. Under this plan the attention of the physician is directed to high temperature as at once the most serious symptom and the chief indication for treatment.

While these plans are in the main essentially different, it cannot be said that the boundary-line between them is absolutely fixed. Thus as intestinal antisepsis unquestionably exerts a favorable

influence upon the intestinal symptoms, it constitutes to a certain extent a symptomatic treatment. And in the same way the symptomatic and antipyretic methods overlap.

Under one or the other of these four plans, or under some combination of them, enteric-fever cases are treated.

There are two tests of the efficiency of treatment in serious acute diseases ; first, the effect upon individual symptoms and upon the clinical course of cases taken together in series; and second, the influence upon the death-rate. Submitted to these tests, none of the four general plans can be said to yield satisfactory results. Making due allowance for the fact that the enteric fever of childhood, from the second until the twelfth year, is a mild disease, with an extremely low mortality, and making further allowance for the large number of mild cases among adults which tend to recover without treatment, we all regard the disease under consideration as a serious one, often protracted, grave in itself, liable to dangerous complications, frequently followed by serious sequelæ, and terminating in a protracted convalescence. Many practitioners, having decided upon some one of the above plans of routine treatment, of which the details are modified to suit individual cases, come to regard it as the proper plan and to consider the results as on the whole satisfactory. Such confidence is occasionally seriously shaken. But the force of habit, the lack of a better method, and of the criteria by which to judge any plan, forces a return to the old method. Indeed, in testing the influences of therapeutics in the acute infectious diseases a wide experience and a critical scientific spirit are essential. If here and there a practitioner of large experience is satisfied with his results in the management of this disease, the same cannot be said of the profession as a whole. The very multitude of plans and remedies which overcrowd the journals shows a continued unrest and dissatisfaction with existing methods of treatment.

When we come to apply the second test, namely, the influence upon the death-rate, dissatisfaction with existing methods finds ample warrant. The rate of mortality in private practice is unquestionably lower than that among persons treated in hospitals. This is chiefly due to the previously better condition of private patients, and to the fact that they come earlier under treatment than do hospital patients, it being a matter of common observation that the mortality of cases neglected in the beginning of the disease is very much higher than that of those who early come under treatment. The statistics of private practice, however, are limited and difficult of access and are commonly based upon an insufficient collection of facts. Hospital statistics are more trustworthy; they are derived from facts observed by many different physicians, and in sufficiently large collections. They are, however, open to the objection that they probably indicate a death-rate somewhat too high.

The following reliable statistics collected from the great mass which is available indicate the hospital death-rate:

	Cases.	Deaths.	Mortality.
London Fever Hospital (21 years) .	8000	1519	18.9
" " " (9 years) .	500	80	15.9
Pauper Hospital at Homerton . .	1509	255	16.8
Stockwell Pauper Hospital . .	1223	301	22.6
St. George's " . .	387	76	19.6
Guy's " . .	295	57	19.3
University College " . .	163	29	17.7
St. Bartholomew " . .	635	104	16.3
St. Thomas " . .	445	70	15.7
Middlesex " . .	461	72	15.6
King's College " . .	318	39	12.2
Total number of cases in the London Hospitals . .	13.936	2602	17.8

Dr. Murchison found that of 27,051 cases collected from various sources, many of which have been included in the foregoing list, 4723 proved fatal, a death-rate of 17.45. Jaccoud, with a collection of 80,140 cases treated in Europe on the expectant plan, observed a mortality of 19.23 per cent. The General Hospital of Vienna, with 17,000 cases, has a mortality of 22.5; the hospital at Basle, with 1718 cases, a mortality of 27.3; and the principal Continental hospitals have, according to Dr. Cayley, a mortality varying between 16 and 25 per cent.

The English army statistics for six years, ending in 1877, are as follows:

	Cases.	Deaths.	Mortality.
On home service . . .	545	131	24
On foreign service . . .	1383	564	40.7
The Royal Navy for a period of six years, ending 1878 . . .	1414	110	26.5
Massachusetts General Hospital .	303	42	13.5

The statistics of the *Medical and Surgical History of the War of the Rebellion*, from 1862 to 1866, inclusive, show:

	Cases.	Deaths.	Mortality.
Among white troops . . .	75,368	27,056	35.9
Colored troops, 1864–1866 inclusive .	4094	2280	55.6

In the New York hospitals,[1] between January, 1877, and October, 1883, there were 1305 cases, with a percentage of mortality estimated by years, varying between a minimum of 20.1 per cent. in 1879 and a maximum of 30 per cent. in 1880.

The foregoing figures, covering a period terminating in 1884, show in general the results of the expectant and symptomatic treatment of enteric fever, although they probably include a small proportion of cases treated upon special antiseptic or antipyretic plans.

A second series of statistics, overlapping to some

[1] Delafield: Medical Record, November 17, 1883.

extent the foregoing in time and reaching down to the present, gives better results. They show the influence of the external application of cold as a therapeutic measure. Thus, Brand collected from various reliable sources 19,017 cases, treated by all kinds of cold baths, with a mortality of 7.8 per cent; Bouveret and Teissier, with a mixed expectant-symptomatic and antipyretic treatment (1873 to 1881), 629 cases, mortality 16.5 per cent.; and 1882 to 1887 inclusive, cold baths in severe cases, 376 cases, mortality 6.9 per cent.

Vogl's statistics, from the Military Hospital in Munich, are as follows: Expectant treatment from 1841 to 1868, 5484 cases, and a mortality of 20.7 per cent.; intermediate, with water, 1868 to 1881, 2841 cases, mortality 12.2 per cent.; and baths and internal antipyretics, 1875 to 1881, 702 cases, with a mortality of 7.6 per cent.

. Ziemssen's statistics from 1877 to 1887 (graduated cold bath and antipyretics), show 2000 cases, with a mortality of 9.6 per cent.

In startling contrast to the above is a third series of statistics, dating back more than a quarter of a century, and including, first, the cases of Brand, and later of those who, under the force of incontrovertible facts, have gradually fallen into the line of treatment devised and so long advocated by him. Thus:

Teissier, 1887, strict cold bathing, 139 cases, mortality 5 per cent.

Vogl, in 1880, strict cold baths, 428 cases, mortality 2.7 per cent.; 1882 to 1887, strict cold baths, 141 cases, mortality 3.5 per cent.; 1882 to 1887 (a second series), increasing baths and the abolition of internal antipyretics, 144 cases, mortality 4.1 per cent.; Naunyn, strict cold baths, 145 cases, mortality 6.9 per cent.; Brand, cases collected from various sources, with strict cold baths, 2198 cases, mortality 1.7 per cent.

The last-named observer shows from an analysis of the same cases, omitting those not treated before the fifth day, 2150 cases, without a death.

The general statistics of the strict cold-water treatment show a reduction of the mortality to 3.9 per cent. These figures are obtained by Brand from twenty-three German and French designated sources with 5573 cases, this number undoubtedly containing many imperfectly-managed cases. (Baruch.)

The number treated strictly according to the method of Brand by himself, Jurgensen, Vogl, and others up to January, 1887, amounted to 1223 cases, of which 12 died, a mortality of 1 per cent., not one of the fatal cases having come under treatment before the fifth day.

That the modifications of the expectant-symptomatic method brought about by the use of antiseptics and antipyretics have not greatly reduced the death-rate is shown by the fact that in Philadelphia during the year 1889 there were reported to the registry office of the board of health 4631 cases, with 736 deaths, a mortality of 15.9 per cent.

The mortality statistics of enteric fever studied in connection with the prevalent methods of treatment justify the conclusions that under pure expectancy recovery will take place in about seventy per cent. of the cases; that about fifteen per cent. will die despite the treatment; and that the result in the remaining fifteen per cent. will depend to some extent upon the management of individual cases.

It is impossible to foresee at the onset of any particular case what its course is going to be, either as regards intensity or complications. The real objection to the expectant-symptomatic treatment is that it is not directed against the cause of the morbid manifestations. Too often the appearance of grave symptoms indicates mischief that is already past remedy. The aim of treatment should be not to control serious symptoms as they arise, but by acting upon the cause of the disease from the beginning to anticipate their development. This I have for some years insisted upon in speaking of the treatment by carbolic acid and iodine, originally suggested by Bartholow. If the claims made by Brand and his followers, that under the strict cold-bath treatment the course of the disease is essentially modified, that the symptoms are milder, that complications and sequelæ do not arise, and that the death-rate, as shown by large series of cases reported by a number of competent observers, undergoes the startling reduction indicated by the figures I have cited—if these claims can be substantiated, there can be no question as to the duty of the profession toward the sufferers from this disease.

We cannot disregard the array of facts marshalled in the literature of the past five years. That a routine treatment so novel should be officially recognized by the Prussian War Department is important testimony to its value. Still more important is the fact that French military surgeons who, as prisoners at the close of the Franco-Prussian war, had the opportunity to observe Brand's treatment at Stettin, adopted, and have since practised, this treatment in the military hospitals of their own country.

What, then, is the method of Brand? It consists in the following systematic procedure:

Whenever the temperature taken in the rectum reaches 102.2° F. (39° C.) the patient is placed in a bath of 65° F. A compress, wet with water about five degrees lower, is placed upon the head, or water at a lower temperature is poured upon the head and shoulders. The patient remains in the bath fifteen minutes, during which time he is systematically rubbed by the attendants and encouraged to rub himself. At the expiration of that time, he is removed from the bath, and wrapped in a coarse linen sheet over which a blanket is folded, the extremities being thoroughly dried and rubbed. A little wine or spirits is then given. This is repeated every three hours, unless the temperature remains below 102.2° F. The alimentation is liquid, nutritious, and carefully regulated. No drugs are administered.

Glénard[1] gives the following outline of the technique of the treatment by cold baths:

"If the diagnosis of typhoid fever is probable, recourse should be had to the baths, whatever may be the symptoms. The full tub should be placed in the ward or chamber, parallel to the bed at a distance of one or two metres, the floors properly protected by oilcloth, and a screen placed between the bed and the bath-tub. A sufficient quantity of water should be used to cover the patient's body to the neck. It should be of a temperature of from 64.4° to 68° F. (18° to 20° C.). The baths should be prepared without disturbance or noise. There should be placed on the floor near the head of the tub two pitchers of cold water of a temperature of from 46.4° to 50° F. (8° to 10° C.), each containing four or five quarts (litres). A glass of water should be at hand. The first bath should be given preferably about four o'clock in the afternoon, unless there is some urgent reason for selecting a different hour, and the physician should be present. The rectal temperature is taken, the urine is voided, and the patient is assisted into the full tub, the screen having been removed. If there is perspiration the patient is dried before entering the bath. Cold water from the pitchers is poured upon the head and the back of the neck, for one or two minutes, the amount being from two to three quarts (litres). Then a swallow of cold water or red wine is given. This being done, the whole surface of the body is briskly rubbed with a sponge or brush and the patient is made to rub his abdomen and chest. These frictions stimulate the peripheral circulation, prevent the accumulation of heat at any one point, moderate the sensation of cold, and help to pass the time; they are not indispensable. Shivering appears, as a general rule, in between eight and twelve minutes; this is a necessary evil to which too much attention is not to be paid. Toward the middle of the bath, or at its termination, cold water is again poured over the head and neck. The time occupied ought to be at least fifteen minutes, longer if the head is still warm and the cheeks red, or if the temperature of the patient was very high before the bath.

"The patient should leave the bath without precipitation. He cannot take cold. thoracic complications are caused by typhoid fever and not by

[1] Le Bulletin Médicale. February 26, 1888.

chilling. The air of the apartment should be pure and not too warm ; the window should be opened in the intervals between the baths, during the bath it ought to be closed. On leaving the bath, the patient should be gently dried with a towel. The bed should be carefully made during each bath. If on returning to the bed shivering takes place, the limbs should be rubbed and a hot bottle placed at the patient's feet. A cold compress, covered with oil-silk or flannel, should be placed over the abdomen, and a little warm nourishment administered.

"Three-quarters of an hour after the bath the rectal temperature should again be taken. If, however, it is found to be below 101° F. (38.5° C.), it is not necessary to take it again for three hours.

"Alimentation should consist of the following articles : Milk diluted with coffee or tea or cocoa (a quarter of a litre at each administration) ; thoroughly cooked gruel, oatmeal, tapioca, or vermicelli ; veal, mutton, or chicken broth, freed from fat when cold and reheated at the moment of administration. As a drink, pure cold water should be given; the indication for wine or spirits is urgent only in cases that are subjected to this treatment late in their course. If the patient does not sleep, or sleeps badly, he is to have a draught of iced water, and the abdominal compress is to be changed every quarter of an hour. The discharges from the bowels are to be preserved for inspection, and the total quantity of urine may be collected in the same vessel. Neither age, sex, menstruation, pregnancy, nor sweating (except that which occurs at the end of defervescence) in any way modifies the treatment. In women who are weaning their children, cold compresses should be applied to the breasts and frequently renewed. If diarrhœa persists, it is to be combated by cold compresses, which may be kept cold by the aid of a bladder of ice. If there is constipation, it is to be treated by cold enemata, and, if these fail, by enemata consisting of one part of cold water and one part of fresh ox-gall.

"When the temperature before the bath is very high, or if the fall forty-five minutes after the bath is less than 1.8° F. (1° C.), the bath must be prolonged to eighteen or twenty minutes. It is very rarely necessary to modify the general formula. After the temperature does not exceed 102.2° F. (39° C.), but yet reaches 101° F. (38.5° C.), it is necessary to treat these slight exacerbations by baths of 68° F. (20° C.), and of five minutes' duration in order to prevent the prolongation of the fever or the occurrence of relapse, and to shorten convalescence. If relapse occurs, it must be treated according to the general formula. When the temperature no longer exceeds 101° F. (38.5° C.), defervescence being established, the baths are discontinued, and the patient should be treated as convalescent, but

is to be kept in bed until the temperature has not exceeded 100.4° F. (38° C.) for four days. He may then rise and in a short time walk in the open air ; he may prolong his promenades according to his strength, and one will be struck by the rapidity with which his strength increases after every outing. Proper precautions are to be taken against cold. As to alimentation, already during defervescence there may be added to his soup, milk, or bouillon, either one or two raw eggs daily, or, a little later, one or two teaspoonfuls of scraped raw meat or a little toasted bread or biscuit ; but the aliment must always be given in liquid form.

"The régime of the convalescence should be gradually established, and may consist of solid food after the temperature has not risen above 100.4° F. (38° C.) for four days. At this period the intervals between the feedings should be at first three hours during the day ; afterward one regular meal daily may be given ; and a little later the patient may have roast beef and fish, morning and evening, and bread in small quantities. The appetite is excellent, and it is necessary to control it. For the first two days of the convalescence the temperature is to be taken as before, after that, for a week, morning and evening. At the end of that time temperature observations may be discontinued.

"During the treatment by baths, one attendant is required for the day and one for the night ; these duties may be fulfilled by members of the family. In a hospital one bath-tub may be made be used for a dozen patients, but it is better to use one for six patients. Two attendants are sufficient for twelve patients. It is not necessary to renew the water of the bath every three hours ; once in twenty-four hours is sufficient. The patient treated from the beginning in this manner, never suffers from fæcal incontinence. As a rule, the patient should pass his water before entering the bath. During epidemics, the water of the bath, if it is not soiled, should serve for several patients, and should only be renewed two or three times a day."

This is the line of treatment to which, rigorously carried out, the extraordinary results which I have indicated are ascribed. That it seems heroic, thus briefly stated, cannot be denied. That it is heroic to those who see it practised for the first time, is more than true. Preconceived notions in regard to the management of typhoid cases are violated. The frequent disturbance for the purpose of taking temperatures and bathing, the fact that the patients are compelled to rise from their bed and with the aid of the attendants to step into the bath, the pallor, shivering, and the blueness of the extremities which shows itself during the course of the bath and continues for a varying time after the patient is put to bed, demand conviction on the part of the physician, and the courage of conviction to continue.

It is only when the favorable effect upon the condition of the patient is seen, and when we reflect that in every hundred cases at least ten lives which would be lost under the expectant-symptomatic treatment are saved by strict cold bathing, that we dare to proceed.

What is the effect upon the course of the disease in cases treated from the beginning, that is, before the fifth day? Brand declares that the classical picture of typhoid fever is no longer seen. It may be objected to this that we do not get our cases before the fifth day; and even if they come under observation so early a positive diagnosis cannot always be made at that time. Only in garrison life and in epidemics will a treatment so radical be justifiable at the onset of a vague febrile disease. But Brand's statement is true of cases in which treatment is instituted at a later period, even so late as the middle of the second week. After six or eight baths the familiar picture is no longer seen. Delirium ceases, stupor gives way to light somnolence from which the patient is easily aroused with a bright expression and a clear mind. The tongue becomes moist and clean and remains so. There is desire for food, and very commonly a complaint of hunger. The abdomen is not tympanitic. Diarrhœa is rarely excessive or troublesome. In short, there remains, in the words of Brand, of the ordinary picture of typhoid nothing more than (*a*) a moderate fever, (*b*) an unimportant bronchial catarrh, (*c*) enlargement of the spleen, (*d*) the rose rash, and (*e*) infiltration of the intestinal glands. Everything else is prevented, and what might have been a severe case runs its course as a mild one if the patients are brought under treatment sufficiently early. Exceptions to this statement occur only when complications develop at the onset. There are rapid wasting and progressive anæmia, as in all prolonged febrile diseases, but severe enteric fever is changed to mild, the mild to a still milder form. This is brought about through the control of the temperature and by preventing disturbances of normal functions. The treatment is directed against the typhoid process as an entirety.

It does, it is true, not only reduce the temperature; the repetition of the bath also *controls* the temperature and keeps it down. But the bath does much more than this. It acts upon the nervous system in such a manner as to enable it to withstand the toxic influences of the infecting principle and the products of its evolution. This it doubtless does by the action of cold water upon the peripheral nerve-endings, a reflex stimulus being transmitted to the nerve-centres presiding over the circulation, respiration, digestion, excretion, and nutri-

tion. This general reinforcement of function is shown by improved action of the heart, the first sound continuing distinct, the pulse being slower and more regular, and the improvement in the arterial tension showing itself by an absence of dicrotism ; by persistence of appetite and digestive power, permitting freer alimentation without gastric disturbances ; by deepening and slowing of the respiration ; and by the absence of nervous symptoms, the increased excretion, the prevention of complications, and the rapid convalescence.

As was pointed out by Jürgensen, every attempt to deviate from the routine treatment as above laid down is followed by less satisfactory results. The treatment thus stands by itself as a definite procedure, to be distinguished from treatment by graduated baths, the cold pack, cold affusions, spraying, and other hydro-therapeutic measures. It is especially to be looked upon as something distinct and different from the antipyretic treatment. Upon this Brand and his followers insist.

In a service at the German Hospital of Philadelphia, extending from February 1st to July 15th of the current year, I had the opportunity to treat fifty cases of enteric fever. Of these, ten, for reasons chiefly connected with my want of experience in cold bathing, were treated either upon the expectant method or by means of carbolized iodine. The remaining forty were treated in accordance with the method of Brand, with two modifications : First, each case admitted prior to the tenth day of the attack received one or two laxative doses of calomel ; second, the temperatures being taken in the axilla or mouth instead of in the rectum, the bath was regularly administered every three hours so long as the temperature reached 101.5° F. Otherwise the routine method above described was carried out in every particular.

Of the ten cases treated according to the old methods, one died, the patient being a man aged thirty-three years, admitted at the end of the second week of the attack, and already suffering from an intestinal hæmorrhage. Death occurred on the third day after his entrance to the ward.

Of the forty cases treated by bathing, all recovered. One case suffered two relapses and was much protracted. A second case suffered a single relapse. Intestinal hæmorrhage occurred in two cases. Upon the supervention of hæmorrhage bathing was discontinued. The average number of baths in each case was forty-two, the smallest number, ten, the largest number, one hundred and thirty-eight. These cases showed the favorable effects of bathing in every instance. As a rule, the patients did not object to the baths. When they did so, the objections ceased after a few baths had been administered. Complications were trifling, there were no sequelæ, and in every case the convalescence was rapid and satisfactory.

As I have already taken up much time, I reserve an analysis of the details of these cases for future publication. Suffice it to say that the statements made by European observers were fully realized in this series of cases. Severe symptoms were mitigated, and mild cases ran a most favorable course.

For the sake of comparison I submit the statistics of some of the hospitals in Philadelphia for the same period of time and for a corresponding period of last year.

Hospital.	Year.	Number of cases.	Average number of days in hospital.	Number of deaths.	Percentage of mortality.	Treatment.
The Pennsylvania Hospital,[1]	1889	31	38	5	16.1	Expectant-symptomatic.
Do.	1890	46	37	6	13.04	
The Episcopal Hospital.	1889	69	44	9	13.04	Mixed, intestinal antiseptic. Internal and external antipyretic; no baths.
Do.	1890	40	50	5	12.5	
St. Agnes Hospital,	1889	19	36	2	10.5	Expectant-symptomatic.
Do.	1890	15	34	4	26 6	
The German Hospital,	1889	41	36.5	4	9.75	Expectant-symptomatic.
Do.	1890	50	36.9	1	2	10 cases carbolized iodine; 40 strict cold baths.

Two hundred and seventy-one cases on expectant-symptomatic treatment with some antiseptics and applications of cold water, and with 36 deaths, a mortality of 13.29 per cent.; 40 cases with strict cold bathing; no deaths.

Since the 15th of July the strict cold-bath treatment has been uniformly followed in the German Hospital by my colleagues, Dr. Trau and Dr. Wolff, twenty-four cases having been treated without a death. The statistics of the German Hospital then as regards enteric fever are, from February 1, 1890, to this date, sixty-four cases treated by the cold baths without a death.

In conclusion, the objections which have been urged against this method of treatment are of the general nature of those usually brought forward against radical departures from established therapeutic customs.

First, the statistics are questioned. This objection can no longer be sustained. A large number of independent observers have fully confirmed the general results obtained by Brand.

' For these statistics I beg to express my thanks to Dr. Meigs, attending physician, and Dr. Scott, resident physicians of the Pennsylvania Hospital; to Dr. Knight and Dr. L. H. Adler, of the Episcopal Hospital; Dr. Grove, of St. Agnes; and Dr. Frese, chief resident physician at the German Hospital.

Second, it is asserted, *a priori*, that the typhoid of this country is not sufficiently severe to demand so radical a treatment. The statistics which I have presented sufficiently disprove this statement. Furthermore, it must be insisted upon that it is impossible to foresee the severity of any particular case at the outset of its course. The treatment by the method of Brand tends to make every case a curable one.

Third, another *a priori* objection is that patients in this country do not bear cold bathing as well as the French and Germans. It is a matter of surprise that this can be seriously urged as an objection to a treatment incontrovertibly shown to be as efficient as the one under discussion. Furthermore, our experience in the German Hospital of Philadelphia does not bear this objection out. It is true that certain cases do not react promptly, and that women react less promptly and less satisfactorily than men. In no case in my series, however, did the delay in reaction after the patient was put to bed cause the slightest apprehension on the part of the attendants.

Fourth, it is inconvenient, and demands an amount of experience and labor on the part of the attendants not easily to be had in private practice and in some public institutions. Objections of this nature cannot stand against the lowered rate of mortality.

Finally, the opposition of the patients themselves and of their friends may be urged as an obstacle to any attempt on the part of medical men to introduce the treatment into private practice. This is no real objection; it is a mere difficulty that will vanish so soon as the profession generally recognizes in the method an efficient means of saving many lives, and lends its weight to the advocacy of the plan among the people. These remarks are intended to contribute to that desirable end.

TREATMENT OF GENERAL SEPTIC PERITONITIS.[1]

BY W. L. ROBINSON, M.D.,
OF DANVILLE, VA.

THE subject of the treatment of general septic peritonitis is full of interest to every surgeon, for prompt decision and action determine the fate of the patient. No wonder, then, that the alarm is repeatedly sounded to warn the general practitioner. It is not alone the cases that are lulled to rest and deceptive security by opiates which confront us, but often the most dangerous condition is that in which the patient is, without opiates, quiet, non-febrile and contented, expressing himself as much better, sub-

1 Read before the Southern Surgical and Gynecological Association, November 12, 1890.

sequent to a chill and fever. In such conditions either suppurative peritonitis or a secondary abscess has probably commenced to form.

I recall two cases of appendicitis, abscess, and suppurative peritonitis which I was called to see during the last few months. One had used salines and opium alternately for a week, and had had fever and a chill on the day that I saw him. On the next day he was perfectly comfortable, he had no fever, the pulse was quiet, the tenderness had diminished, and there seemed to be improvement. An operation was performed, followed by irrigation and drainage, but the patient died two days later from septic peritonitis and secondary abscess.

The other case on the second day of the attack had a chill, which recurred in six hours, and was followed by collapse and delirium. After restoration by the use of hot bottles, hypodermic injections of whiskey and strychnine, I urged an operation, but freedom from pain, diminished tenderness, absence of fever, a fairly good pulse, some appetite, and no nausea, prevented the attending physician from consenting to an operation until the third day, when, although there was no change save an increase in the size of the tumor, he yielded. There was a considerable amount of pus in a sac, which was as thin as paper and formed by adhesions. The cavity was irrigated and drained, but the patient died in two days. At the autopsy a gangrenous condition of the intestines and suppurative peritonitis were found. Why this sudden cessation of pain and fever and the comfortable condition of the patient?

We all have noticed in puerperal peritonitis the absence of pain and the disproportion between the pathological condition and the slight amount of tenderness on pressure. Septic conditions may cause fever, restlessness, prostration, etc., but seldom pain; and when pain is present in puerperal peritonitis, it is only from pressure in a distended sac. Indeed, in this disease pain is so uncertain a symptom that he who relies upon it in diagnosis will, I fear, often be misled.

I believe that in the adult the three principal causes of general septic peritonitis are gunshot wounds, appendicitis, and pelvic inflammations. Of course, many other causes indirectly produce it, such as a blow resulting in abscess, tubercular inflammations, etc.; indeed, any internal or external influence producing an abscess, which ruptures, may cause it.

I fully concur with the views that Dr. Lydston has expressed in a recent article, in which he denies the existence of idiopathic peritonitis in children, and regards blows, falls, etc., as causes of suppurative peritonitis and appendicitis. I believe, as he does, that suppurative peritonitis is more frequent than we imagine, and that we often recognize it too late.

I will refer to gonorrhœa as a cause of septic peritonitis in women, and state that I have had case after case in which I could trace the peritonitis to nothing else. Now, it may be asked. Why does not gonorrhœa always produce septic peritonitis? One reason is, I think, that adhesions form between the ovaries and the tubes, and that these adhesions confine the gonorrhœa to the tubes. Gonorrhœa in the female does not always invade the uterus any more than in the male it invariably attacks the bladder.

Now, as to the treatment. I would first say that preventive operations should not be neglected. If either appendicitis, hepatic abscess, or pus-tubes is diagnosed, or if pus in the abdominal cavity is suspected, operate. Exploratory incisions may be dangerous, but far less so than inattention to either of the above conditions. If there is one fact established in surgery, it is the importance of evacuating pus, no matter in what part of the body it is found. Abdominal section, irrigation, and drainage is the accepted treatment.

You will often find not only extensive adhesions, but pus-sacs. Insert your fingers as gently as possible, separate the intestines carefully, yet effectually, irrigate thoroughly, and if bleeding is excessive pack the cavity with iodoform-gauze; if bleeding is not excessive, use drainage-tubes. The gauze can be removed in small amounts every day. The drainage-tube should be cleaned antiseptically every six or eight hours, and gently rotated. The time to remove it will be indicated in each case. Pus-sacs should be aspirated or, if possible, brought to the surface and emptied. Always be prepared, in case of injury to the bowel, to resect, anastomose, or treat as may be indicated. After operations I usually give a saline daily to prevent adhesions from re-forming.

In some cases you can do only a partial operation. In such cases you tear as many adhesions as is prudent, irrigate, and after improvement in the general condition of the patient you will be able to complete the operation.

Again, in those cases in which there is extensive and distressing tympanites, there is a most troublesome condition to deal with. The muscular coat of the bowel is paralyzed by overdistention, and purgatives have little effect. In such cases I would be disposed to adopt the suggestion of Dr. Davis, namely, open the bowel and flush out with hot water.

Illustrative of the good that can be accomplished by the partial separation of adhesions, I will report a case which I was called to see in consultation three or four weeks ago:

The patient was a young married woman, and had never been pregnant. She had been treated for two weeks for fever, and was seemingly better, but later developed peritonitis, which spread rapidly, and was accompanied with constant pain, much aggravated by defæcation and urination. At the expiration of the fourth week I saw her. The doctor said she was better, yet 150 drops of laudanum had failed to give relief the previous night. Her stomach would retain nothing. Her abdomen was swollen, tympanitic, and fluctuating. I elicited from her husband that he was convalescing from an attack of gonorrhœa. I obtained consent to operate on the next day, and gave a saline, which caused two movements. I should have stated that the temperature was 102°; pulse 130. On the following day the temperature was still high, the pulse more frequent and feeble. The physicians present did not think she would live through the operation. However, I operated. The tissues bled at every cut. The peritoneum was firmly adherent to the abdominal walls; the bowels were generally adherent, and it was with great difficulty that I was able to introduce my finger. I broke up the adhesions as gently as possible, partially irrigated, and put in a drainage-tube. The breaking up of the adhesions caused considerable bleeding, the blood being mixed with pus. She reacted slowly, but on the following morning her pulse was less than 100 and temperature 99°. She continued to improve, a saline being given daily to prevent the adhesions from re-forming. On the seventh day I was confined to my bed and remained there a week. The patient, on my return, was suffering from pain, especially during defæcation and urination, but said that she had had no movement of the bowels, except a small one that morning, for five or six days. I gave her a full dose of sulphate of magnesium, and after six stools all her symptoms disappeared, and she was sitting up when I left her. I know I did an incomplete operation, but to have done more would have killed my patient. Should it become necessary, I can complete it now that she is more able to stand it.

Regarding gunshot wounds of the abdomen, I will only say that he who has once opened an abdomen for such an injury will not hesitate to operate when his second case is presented.

OPERATION FOR ANKYLOSIS OF THE TEMPORO-MAXILLARY ARTICULATION.

BY CHARLES B. PENROSE, M.D., PH.D.,
SURGEON TO THE GERMAN AND GYNECEAN HOSPITALS, AND TO THE OUT-PATIENT DEPARTMENT OF THE PENNSYLVANIA HOSPITAL, PHILADELPHIA.

ANKYLOSIS of the temporo-maxillary articulation may be the result of an injury, such as a severe sprain or concussion; or it may be due to arthritic inflammation, followed by plastic adhesions, which become converted into fibrous, cartilaginous, or osseous tissue.

If the ankylosis is caused by fibrous bands, these can be divided subcutaneously with a tenotome

passed into the articulation, as has been done by Spariton.[1] The condyle has also often been excised, and with favorable results in most cases.

Mears[2] has proposed the operation of dividing the ramus of the jaw by an Adams's saw introduced through the mouth, and excising, in this way, the condyle with the coronoid process and sigmoid notch.

The operation, first proposed by Esmarch, of making an artificial joint in the lower jaw by the removal of a wedge-shaped piece of bone, has been successfully done a number of times. Indeed, most of the operations which have been performed for the relief of ankylosis of the temporo-maxillary articulation have had a fair percentage of successful results, though the methods varied. Even the plan of Rizzoli, of merely cutting through the jaw with powerful forceps introduced in the mouth, without removing any portion of bone, has been attended with success. The operations, however, in which a portion of bone is removed, and thus the formation of a false joint is facilitated, are preferable.

. When there is complete ankylosis with entire loss of motion of the jaw, it is often difficult to determine on which side the lesion exists. And though the stiffness may have been primarily confined to one temporo-maxillary articulation, yet the other joint may become secondarily ankylosed from the changes following long-standing disease. It is probable that this occurred in the case which I am about to report, for the ankylosis must at first have been confined to that side, since the first operation, performed on this side alone, was followed, for a short time, by good motion of the joint.

A man twenty-eight years old was admitted to the Pennsylvania Hospital, April, 1890, with complete ankylosis of the temporo-maxillary articulations. The upper teeth were firmly set upon the lower teeth, and he was unable to pass the blade of a penknife between them. He could take only liquid food. He suffered constantly from dyspepsia and from sore-throat, which could not be relieved by local treatment. His family history and his general personal history were good. Four years previously he had had an attack of acute articular rheumatism of several months' duration. Most of the joints of the body were affected, those of the jaw being the last attacked. The movements of the jaw rapidly became stiff, and by the time convalescence was complete he was unable to open his mouth at all. Four months after the appearance of complete ankylosis he was operated upon in New York, and, as he states, the condyle of the lower jaw on the right side was removed. After this he had fair motion of the jaw, but the stiffness gradually returned, and in two months was as complete as before operation. The scar of this operation was barely perceptible

1 Lancet, April 16, 1881.
2 American Journal of the Medical Sciences, October, 1883.

upon the right cheek. The incisions were evidently similar to those which I subsequently made. There was no pain and no swelling of either temporo-maxillary articulation, and it was impossible to determine whether the ankylosis existed on only one or on both sides. He said that he thought the left joint was normal and that his disability was caused by ankylosis of the right side, as at the time of the first operation. There was no perceptible muscular rigidity or stiffness.

Operation.—A vertical incision was made in front of the right ear, and a horizontal one meeting the upper end of the first incision was carried along the lower border of the zygoma. The flap thus formed, with the parotid gland, was drawn down, and the posterior fibres of the masseter muscle were cleared away with a periosteal elevator. The position of the temporo-maxillary articulation was thus exposed. There was complete bony union between the neck of the lower jaw and the temporal bone, and no condyle was discovered. A small trephine was applied to the centre of the ramus immediately below the sigmoid notch, and a button of bone was removed. The bridges of bone on each side of this opening were then divided by a chisel.

As, notwithstanding this division of the right ramus, it was found impossible to open the mouth, and as the difficulty did not appear to be caused by any muscular contraction, a similar incision was made upon the left cheek. The upper part of the left ramus was exposed, and there was found to be firm bony union between the condyle and the temporal bone. A portion of the neck one-third of an inch in thickness was resected by means of a chain saw. As there then appeared to be some contraction of the temporal muscle which prevented free opening of the mouth, the attachment of this muscle to the coronoid process was divided. After this it was possible to separate easily the upper and lower incisor teeth a distance of more than one inch.

There was free, though easily controlled, bleeding during the operation. The wounds were drained with small rubber-tubes and closed with silkworm-gut sutures. Primary union took place. Seven days after the operation all dressings were removed, and the patient was able to eat the ordinary hospital diet, which included beefsteak of the average toughness.

As during sleep he was unable to keep the jaw in motion, and thus prevent union or adhesion and contraction, the jaws always became stiff during the night, and in the morning he found difficulty in opening the mouth to the same extent as on the previous evening. He was, therefore, given a wedge of rubber varying in thickness from one-half to one inch, to place between the teeth on retiring. Three weeks after the operation he was etherized and the mouth was forcibly opened to the fullest extent, in order to break thoroughly whatever adhesions might have formed. He continued to use the rubber wedge for four months, when the tendency to stiffness at night disappeared and he was able to do without it. When last seen, six months after the operation, he could eat any kind of food ; he constantly chewed tobacco ; and he had three-fourths of an inch space

between the incisor teeth. He was perfectly comfortable, except that after much chewing he had slight pain in the region of the artificial joints. There seemed to be no tendency to any further closure of the mouth, and the scars upon the cheek caused no disfigurement.

A SUCCESSFUL CHOLECYSTECTOMY FOR IMPACTED GALL-STONES AND INTRA-MURAL ABSCESS OF GALL-BLADDER.

BY J. L. DAWSON, JR., M.D.,
PROFESSOR OF THE PRINCIPLES AND PRACTICE OF MEDICINE AND OF CLINICAL MEDICINE IN THE MEDICAL COLLEGE OF THE STATE OF SOUTH CAROLINA, CHARLESTON, S. C.

OPERATIVE procedures for the removal of the gall-bladder are sufficiently rare to render the following case of interest, and successful results are so seldom obtained that I desire to place this one on record :

History.—Mrs. L., white, aged thirty years. Always suffered from hysteria at her menstrual periods. She was under constant observation, needing medical aid at every menstrual flow. She was the mother of two healthy children. Vaginal examination disclosed a prolapsed left ovary, subacutely inflamed. At her menstrual periods she became very nervous, complaining of great pain in the left side of the pelvis, and having frequent convulsions, hysterical in their nature. Being susceptible to mental shock, the most trivial anxiety, such as the illness of her children, or any slight worry, would produce an hysterical attack. She was of costive habit, but to no great degree, and she had no disorder of the digestive tract. She went to the mountains during the summer of 1889, and gained several pounds in weight.

On June 2, 1890, I was summoned to see her and found that she had just returned from Savannah, Georgia, where three days previously she had been caught in a shower, during which her clothes became soaked. Her menstrual flow, which had just begun, was immediately checked. She had also received a severe mental shock by the sudden disclosure of some family secrets. I was not surprised to find her in an hysterical convulsion, and did not examine very carefully into the cause of the abdominal pain of which she complained. This pain was dull and aching in character, not acute or spasmodic. She was put upon the bromides, and things went well for seventy-four hours. when she had a severe rigor, followed by a rise of temperature to 104°, and profuse sweating. These symptoms presented themselves on the next day at about the same hour, and again on the third day, the temperature falling after the sweat.

Presumably a case of malarial quotidian fever, she was given quinine. This drug had no effect and the rigors became more frequent, the temperature remaining above 102°, and nearly stationary. A mercurial purgative was given, which emptied the bowels, and the temperature was controlled with phenacetin. On June 15th I discovered a tumor in the right hypochondriac region extending obliquely to the middle line, and reaching an inch below the umbilicus. Its outlines were clearly definable, it being pear-shaped, with the base downward and forward. Her rigors and the elevation of temperature continuing, with the advice of Dr. Manning Simons, whose opinion as a consultant I sought, we passed a fine aspirating needle into the swelling and removed a few drops of sanious fluid. The abdomen was very tender, the slight manipulation necessary for this operation causing exquisite pain. The stools, which were frequent throughout the illness, were carefully examined. They were fluid, stained with bile, and threw no light on the diagnosis.

On the following morning the aspirating needle was again inserted, this time not in the base of the tumor, but in the side and from the median line. We now readily obtained a clear watery fluid of low specific gravity, and no color. This fluid was examined chemically and microscopically. It consisted of a strong solution of sodium chloride, and was devoid of albumin. The microscopical examination was negative, nothing being found save a few epithelial cells. Subsequently a large Dieulafoy's aspirator was used. The needle was entered at the point of the last puncture and two ounces of a thin muco-sanious fluid were obtained. This fluid contained a slight amount of pus and blood, otherwise the composition was the same as that previously obtained. For thirty-six hours the patient's condition improved. The temperature fell from 104° to 99°, and the rigors ceased. Locally the tenderness over the seat of the tumor increased, due probably to the punctures.

On the evening of June 22d the temperature again rose to 104° after a severe chill, and it was thought advisable to temporize no longer.

Operation, June 23, 1890.—The patient was anæsthetized with chloroform and placed upon the operating-table. An incision three and one-half inches in length was made over the tumor parallel to the median line, and corresponding to the centre of the right rectus muscle. It extended from the margin of the last true rib to one inch below the umbilicus. After the hæmorrhage was thoroughly controlled the peritoneum was divided on a director to the full length of the wound. The tumor lay just beneath the centre of the incision and extended upward along the under surface of the liver toward the posterior border. It was slightly adherent posteriorly, at its neck, and quite adherent superiorly to the under surface of the liver. After being carefully detached from these adhesions by passing the finger around it, the pedicle was transfixed and securely ligated with a stout silk ligature. The pedicle was then cut through and the tumor removed. The hæmorrhage, which was a slight general oozing, was readily controlled by the pressure of sponges soaked in hot bichloride solution. The peritoneum, which had become very much thickened by inflammation, was united with catgut and the edges of the abdominal wound were brought into perfect apposition with deep silver and superficial catgut sutures. The wound was dressed with iodoform-gauze and absorbent cotton supported with a flannel roller. The strictest antiseptic precautions were used throughout.

The tumor was the gall-bladder hypertrophied and thickened by inflammatory products. Its walls were from three-fourths to seven-eighths of an inch thick, and contained an abscess cavity posteriorly about the size of a large filbert. This abscess had opened into the cavity of the gall-bladder and had thinned its walls so that rupture into the general cavity of the peritoneum was imminent. The sac contained three large gall-stones, weighing respectively, seventy-nine, eighty, and eighty-one grains. These stones were polyhedral and showed well-marked facets. They completely filled the cavity and occluded the orifice of the duct. The cavity also contained two drachms of muco-pus unstained with bile, and no trace of biliary coloring matter was discernible. The hypertrophied cyst measured four and three-quarters inches in length by two and one-half inches in its greatest width.

Result.—The patient reacted well from the operation. On the third day a large evacuation of the bowels followed the administration of an enema. The fæces were well formed and of a bright yellow color. She retained nourishment well. On the morning of the fourth day she passed about four ounces of almost pure blood from the bowels. This hæmorrhage occurred again during the subsequent night. She then began to improve rapidly, her whole aspect becoming better. Her temperature, however, did not become normal, rising a degree to a degree and a half every evening.

At the end of a week the wound was dressed. It had healed superficially, but there was a suppurating tract extending upward through which flowed a considerable quantity of creamy pus. In a few days this pus became thin and mixed with bile, a temporary biliary fistula being established.

The flow of bile through the wound ceased in about ten days but the fistula remained patent. The temperature continued to rise in the evening and the case became complicated by a large bedsore which formed over the sacrum. On the forty-eighth day after the operation the silk ligature passed out through the fistulous tract. The temperature then returned to normal and the patient made a good recovery, being now, three and one-half months after the operation, quite well, and having gained twenty pounds in weight. Her bowels act well and the stools contain the usual amount of bile. She has had no return of hysterical symptoms.

REMARKS.—The diagnosis in this case was an extremely difficult one. We had a patient known to have a subacute ovaritis, presenting symptoms of sepsis and concealed abscess, with no sign of derangement of the liver or intestinal tract. The appearance of the tumor and the fluid aspirated therefrom suggested a hydatid growth which had broken down and suppurated. The gall-bladder had not performed its function for years and yet there had been no evidence of the fact.

The abdominal section was, therefore, from the very necessity of the case, more or less of an exploratory operation. That an abscess would be found was almost certain, and when the true nature of the case was revealed the gall bladder and contained gallstones were removed with the most gratifying result.

Monotony of detail must be forgiven in the history of this case, as the minutiæ are of more than ordinary interest.

CAUSES WHICH IMPERIL THE HEALTH OF THE AMERICAN GIRL, AND THE NECESSITY OF FEMALE HYGIENE.[1]

BY GEORGE J. ENGELMANN, A M., M.D.,

PRESIDENT OF THE SOUTHERN SURGICAL AND GYNECOLOGICAL ASSOCIA-
TION AND OF THE ST. LOUIS OBSTETRIQAL AND GYNECOLOGICAL
SOCIETY; PROFESSOR OF DISEASES OF WOMEN IN THE MIS-
SOURI MEDICAL COLLEGE AND POST-GRADUATE SCHOOL;
FELLOW OF THE AMERICAN GYNECOLOGICAL SOCIETY,
OF THE BRITISH GYNECOLOGICAL SOCIETY,
OF THE LONDON OBSTETRICAL
SOCIETY, ETC.

To guide woman in greater safety through the dangers which beset her path in life is one of the highest and most sacred duties of our profession, as we may say that the care of woman is the care of the nation; the good health, mental, moral, and physical, of the woman and mother is the very foundation of our national growth and prosperity; and the conditions which tend to undermine that health cover a field of such extent and importance that the reader will readily realize the necessity of a limitation of my remarks.

I shall speak of the girl, the coming mother; of adolescence, the most important and interesting period of woman's life—the period of greatest functional activity, during which the foundation of future health is laid.

Girlhood is the most dangerous period, during which the organism, the budding mind, the developing system are susceptible to disturbing influences from without and within. It is the time when the clay is soft and the vessel is forming, when it yields most readily, and when trifling impressions are permanently recorded. It is in this period of school-life, the period of beginning social life, the period of learning trades, that the nervous energies of the female are most fully engaged, and her activity is concentrated on the brain-function, to the detriment of other functions, above all the developing sexual function, the central and most important, and at that time the most readily disturbed.

That I speak of the American girl is but natural, and I need hardly say that she is, moreover, subjected to a far greater number of disturbing influences than her sister in other lands, and more recklessly exposed to the very injuries which react most violently upon the female function.

[1] The President's Address to the Southern Surgical and Gynecological Association, November 11, 1890.

True as it generally is that woman is the exponent of a nation, and indicative of its development, of its growth, and of its depreciation, the American woman is more closely linked with the state and fate of her nation than the women of other countries.

Woman shares the febrile activity of our existence; she is a factor in our social and political economy; she participates in the rush and crush of the times to the utmost extent of her nerve-force and brain-power; but especially is this true of the American girl, as compared with the girls of other countries.

When I speak of the American girl I speak not of the extremes, not of the rich or the poor, but of the American girl of the great middle class of our cities—the typical American girl. Compare her to her hearty, strong-boned English sister; to the French girl raised within convent walls, carefully guarded, removed from the world until her marriage; or to the average German girl, reared amid the calmness of her surroundings, taught the solid rudiments of learning, and educated in household duties. Compare her even to her sister of the village or country, if the latter still be free from contaminating influences—from the nervous life of the city or boarding-school. You will recognize her at once. You will recognize the effect of brain-work and nerve-strain, the rush and mental activity of the day, the want of muscular training, the want of harmony in life, in training and education—mental, moral, and physical.

Whilst I will not agree with Ploss in his descriptions of the characteristics of the American girl, when he records the statements of an ungallant Yankee, that the American girl has no bones, no muscle, no vitality—only nerves; and what should we expect, he asked, when in the place of bread they eat chalk, in the place of wine they drink ice-water, when they wear tight corsets and shoes.

Even now one of our greatest authorities, and one of our keenest observers, Dr. S. Weir Mitchell, says that the American woman is unfit for her duties as a woman—not quite up to what nature asks of her as a wife and mother.

I believe that the essential causative factors to which the ill health of the American girl must be referred, are functional neglect or ignoring of her functions, excessive brain-work, and over-exertion of the nerves and emotions, with imperfect development of the muscular system, a want of harmony between development and exertion—physical, mental, and moral.

The peculiar organization of woman is too much ignored. It is claimed that woman is equal to man in her primitive state, and that her functions are physiologically and naturally not in want of any particular attention. Are these functions of such paramount importance, and do they so completely control woman's life? This is a physiological problem upon the solution of which depend the relative capacity of woman for labor, mental and physical, and an understanding of the causes, influences, and remedies of diseases. The answer is readily found, if we observe with an unprejudiced eye the existing conditions.

Throughout both of the great kingdoms of nature the importance of the reproductive function in the female is demonstrated: it is strikingly demonstrated in the vegetable as well as in the animal life; it was recognized by the intuitive keenness of the most primitive people, and distinct expression is given to these fundamental facts in nature by the great lawgivers of ancient times.

Differences in sex are more or less well marked throughout the vegetable kingdom, and the supremacy of the reproductive function in the female, with the necessity of additional vitality for its perfect performance, is distinctly characterized. This is well exemplified in our common hemp, which, when the seed is moderately distributed over fertile soil, develops more than fifty per cent. of male plants, as a superabundance must be provided for the necessary waste which follows the distribution of the male pollen by the winds. If the seeds are thickly sown, so that the nutrition is insufficient or scant, the number of female plants will be diminished, as the supply requisite for their greater vitality is wanting; and, if densely crowded, the female plant may be altogether unable to develop. To the fruit-grower the great demand of vitality for the reproductive function is well known. The apple-tree with vigorous growth and foliage bears no fruit, its vitality being directed toward the one function of vegetable growth. To reduce this the tree is girdled, when, with a diminution of growth and foliage, it bears fruit. This harmonious development of the function is as necessary for the symmetrical growth of the plant as it is to the perfect development of the human being.

The great importance of the peculiar function of women, which it is the tendency of our enlightened nineteenth century to ignore, was fully appreciated by the people of olden times, and the necessity of functional hygiene for the welfare of the community was recognized to such an extent that it was made obligatory by laws of custom or of religion; and the highest penalties—expulsion from the community, everlasting damnation, and even death were imposed for certain transgressions which are thoughtlessly practised to-day by the refined and enlightened beings of our advanced civilization. The essence of such laws and customs of the savages of to-day, in fact of all primitive people from past to present, was rest, functional rest.

Instinct and experience have taught primitive people these truths, which in our day are but imperfectly realized even by medical science, and are denied by some who call the susceptibility of the woman of to-day to her ailments unnatural, and claim them to be altogether the result of civilization.

It is asserted that woman in her natural state is the physical equal of man, and the primitive or savage woman is constantly pointed to as an example of this supposed axiom.

Do those who make these assertions know how well the savage is aware of the weakness of woman and of her susceptibilities at certain periods of her life, and with what care he protects her from harm at these periods so that health may be retained? Religious superstition and the anger of the gods were invoked to secure this simple, but effective female hygiene—much-needed rest. Rest by isolation during the periods of functional activity, for nine days of each month, from thirty to ninety days after childbirth, and for five months at puberty. The budding of the maid into woman among savages is marked by a long period of rest and isolation, and her return to her tribe is celebrated by ceremonies of various kinds.

The importance of surrounding woman with certain precautions during the height of these great functional waves of her existence was appreciated by all people living in an approximately natural state, by all races at all times, and among their comparatively few religious customs, this one, affording rest to women, was among those most persistently adhered to. This idea was so deeply impressed that a mere touch at such periods was regarded as contaminating, and the girl was accordingly obliged to desist from all ordinary duties of life, and was removed from exertion and excitement by forced isolation. Where isolation is not customary, as we find it among people approaching civilization, a certain characteristic mark or signal is worn, for the wearer a passport of safety. In Eastern India young girls show their condition by a small piece of linen steeped in blood, and worn at the neck, as I myself have seen in the Nautch girls brought to this country for the purpose of exhibition. The Woloff negress wears a bright-colored folded cloth upon the cheek.

In the same manner the necessary rest is accorded to woman during the period of susceptibility for from three to four and even five days of each month throughout functional life. We find that either a hut is erected at some distance from the village, as among the Bedas in Cambodia, and on the isle of Yap, one of the West Caroline islands; or that a certain house is assigned as a place of seclusion within the village, as in New Caledonia, upon the coast of Guinea, and among the Kaffirs, the Hottentots, and the American Indians. The Hindoos, the Nayers of Malabar, and others, assign to the woman a separate room in the house. In Japan, likewise, she is confined in a separate room, not permitted to eat with the family, and forbidden to visit even the temple, and given no possible excuse for leaving the house. Work of every kind and bathing are strictly forbidden, the dangers of cold water at this time being thoroughly appreciated by all these people, whilst it is an essential part of their religious teachings that the women should bathe before returning to their families and the village after the wave has passed. The laws of Moses and Zoroaster are almost identical, pointing to these great functional waves of woman's life as a working of the gods.

The laws of Zoroaster necessitated a seclusion of four nights for women, and, what is remarkable, she was then forced to determine her condition by examination, and if the flow had not completely ceased, indicating an abnormality, additional precautions were observed—she must remain five more nights, to which nine days were added, after which time she might cleanse herself and return to life.

The life of woman does not run smoothly like that of a man. It is characterized by marked periodicity, by ebbs and floods, by great life-waves, which are dominant in the sphere of her especial functions; waves of vascular tension and nerve excitement, marked by a heightened activity and susceptibility of her entire being, distinctly indicating that woman's periodical activity is not a local process, as we have been taught, but one involving the entire organization, as it was held to be by the ancients, and exerting a permanent influence upon that organism of whose condition and development it is indicative. The menstrual function involves the entire vascular and nervous systems, and may be said to be the central exchange of that great network of wires, the vasomotor nerves, the great sympathetic linking it most intimately with the brain and spinal cord and with every part of the system.

The most persistent period of nerve and vascular excitement is that of developing womanhood, when for months the system is in a period of unusual activity, and consequently of the highest susceptibility, which does not cease as speedily as its outward tokens disappear. Then follow the cyclical changes of mature activity, varied by the higher waves of active reproduction.

The functional wave slowly rises, accompanied with an increase of nerve activity and vascular tension, and a rise of temperature, as Mary Putman Jacobi tells us, of from 0.01° to 0.8° F., until it reaches the highest point; and it is during the decline of this wave that the depletion takes place,

23*

the distended vessels rupture and nature relieves herself, the temperature steadily falls, but does not reach the normal until after the cessation of all external symptoms.

Are we to believe that a function which so deeply implicates the entire system can be so completely disregarded? That it does not demand special care —greater care than functions less general, less susceptibie, less intimately connected with the organism? Are we to believe that this function can be ignored; and are we to be guided by the dangerous arguments of those who claim that precautions are unnecessary at this period?

In considering the initial causes of disease and their effect upon woman, we must analyze not alone this one function, but we must consider the entire being of woman, in order that we may apply the proper standard, and that we may not measure her capacity for labor, mental or physical, or her powers of endurance, with those of man.

Woman—the woman of our civilization—cannot be properly compared with man; differences of many kinds exist, the most obvious of which are of course external and anatomical. Her form and shape differ; her organism is a different one; individual organs are said to be more vascular and to contain more nerves; she is more emotional, more readily exhausted, and less able to bear continuous and prolonged application; more blood is produced, and the circulation and respiration are more active. The period of puberty is shorter and more marked, and the last stages of development are reached at an earlier period of life.

Consider her lighter frame, her nervous organization, her emotional nature; consider the constant activity of the reproductive functions, the influence of this sphere which dominates her entire being; consider the intimate connection of every organ, above all the spinal cord, with this reproductive centre, and then, need we wonder that injury befalls this sensitive organization when exposed to the intense and continuous nerve- and muscle-strain of our present system of education and labor, which is upon a basis of male vigor?

Whilst the evil is great, I am happy to say that an improvement in the physique of the American girl of the better classes has become evident in late years, due to progress of the science of hygiene, and its better understanding by the educated public, and perhaps by the introduction of sound physiological and hygienic doctrines in some of the more advanced schools, but above all to the new fad, the increased popularity of outdoor sports.

In the higher classes we mark this change, and we may be thankful for the change of fashion which has produced the result. The girl must have a good color, a healthy figure, a brisk walk, to be " in the swim''; riding and walking, lawn tennis and rowing, even fencing, have become fashionable, and are working wonders upon the health of the American girl who can afford these luxuries—the same girl who twenty years ago drank vinegar to acquire a fashionable pallor and an early grave. Compare the swinging gait of the girl of to-day with the mincing walk and the Grecian bend of some years ago.

A beginning has been made, but the greatest difficulties are still to be overcome; the American girl has a just claim to the most perfect and harmonious development, mental, moral, and physical, by virtue of the invigorating influence of an intermingling of race and blood, the favorable hygienic possibilities of her life, and the freedom she is given. But the average girl is not what she might be, and I repeat that this is due to our habits of life and our methods of labor and education.

We must of necessity inquire whether the health of the girl suffers during school-life, or, rather, whether functional life is impaired by our present methods of education, and I must unhesitatingly say that it is, unfortunately, a question which is asked in different ways and distorted by the partisans of higher education for women.

Statistics of functional health during school-life are out of the question, and we must refer to a few general facts, and to our individual observation. How commonly do we see the once healthy girl returning from school—above all from the pernicious boarding-school—neurasthenic, with flushed face, cold feet, impaired digestion, backache, and painful and disordered functions, all of which symptoms gradually fade with the enjoyment and recreation of vacation, and return with the next session of school.

It is the American idea of "putting one through" which lays the foundation of evils which not only follow the individual through life, but pursue her descendants. It is the idea of finishing her education before the pleasures of society can be anticipated. It is the source of beginning functional disturbances. She is straining every nerve for the dangerous struggle of supremacy, and, cost what it may, her ambition must be gratified; she must graduate with honor before making her début in society, and even now her emotional nature is excited by the foretaste of its pleasures. Evenings which should be devoted to rest are given to boy visitors and dancing parties. Healthy recreations, outdoor exercise, and the necessary sleep are neglected; school gymnastics, calisthenics, or official recreation do not afford the healthful exercise needed. An increased quantity of blood is diverted to the brain, whilst the general supply is diminished and the circulation impaired; lassitude, malaise,

and local trouble follow. Is it to be wondered at that she breaks down, and that the mothers best fitted to produce capable children fail to fulfil their destiny?

In boarding-schools enervating routine takes the place of social dissipation, but the results are the same, if not worse, as the girl is removed from her natural guardian and adviser—the mother. One statement from the pen of Dr. Goodell will best indicate the frequency of the injury. He tells us that he has been repeatedly asked by physicians attending such institutions whether it were possible that laundresses could have drugged the scholars unknown to them, in order to avoid the washing of soiled napkins: so common is the complete cessation of that essential function in the most critical period of the girl's life when she is removed from home influence with a view to securing the supposed better advantages. This is the state of affairs in common schools and boarding-schools, at the most critical epoch, from the age of twelve to eighteen years.

Let us see what the results of so-called higher education are. The showing is a better one, as we may see from the report of the Association of College Alumni who have investigated the present health of female college alumni as far as practicable. The health of these girls was very much the same as that of their parents, but was three per cent. better, constitutional weakness being mostly the cause of the disorders that existed. Overwork, accidents, and bad sanitary conditions would explain others. Among the college graduates the deterioration in health is two and one-half per cent. less than in the working girls of Boston at the same time.

Worry over studies alone caused no decline in health, whilst worry over personal affairs caused deterioration of health in ten per cent. of the students, and worry over studies and personal affairs combined, in fifteen per cent., but the health of those who declined while in college has more than recovered in later years. We find but a very slight falling off, and that only from excellent to fair health, in college life, as we might expect if we consider that it is only the healthier and stronger girls who venture upon higher education, and that one-half of these avoided exertion during the menstrual period, and saw but little society. We must bear in mind that college education is an innovation of recent date, in the establishment of which modern hygiene has been consulted, and the study and recreation as well as the health of the pupil, are subject to constant medical supervision; moreover, in some of the more advanced institutions, good health is made a condition of admission, and yet Miss Howe, of the College Alumni Committee, finds that only four hundred and ninety-six out of one thousand graduates married between the ages of fifteen and sixty, and she comes to the conclusion that the tendency of higher education for women is to celibacy. Whether this is from choice or from necessity—for reasons moral or physical—she does not say; it appears to be the natural result of misdirected culture.

The injurious effect of our present system of education upon the essential function of woman must be apparent if we bear in mind that in the period of life from twelve to eighteen, and eighteen to twenty-one years, nutrition should be directed to the essential organs of female life, whilst all other organs are in active growth, and are demanding increased supply. It is then that an increased expenditure of vital energy is demanded, and that the brain concentrates upon itself the nutrient fluid; it is at this time when the system is most susceptible to disturbing influences of all kinds, and in an almost explosive state during one week of each month, that it is subjected to the greatest strain, to excessive brain-work, nervous and emotional excitement, and even physical injuries.

Are the results not natural when we consider that girls in this dangerous period of life spend more time in study than boys, and that boys do have healthy recreation, that the Greeks even withheld male children from study until the tenth year, while laying a solid foundation for a healthy physical system and a harmonious development of the functions.

Injuries are wrought by our systems of education, and very similar are the injurious effects of our systems of labor upon the developing girl and the reproductive functions, but less obscure and more marked than those of education, for the reason that the unfortunate sufferer cannot, like the school-girl, withdraw at will, or when the evidences of injury are distinctly felt. She is obliged to continue until she is prostrated. It is not manual labor only; it is not alone wear and tear on muscle which tells—nervewear is still worse. The effects are seen in girls in the employments now so much affected as a so-called higher class of female labor—in telephone and telegraph offices—clerks, type-setters, and stenographers. Examples of this kind we unfortunately see every day.

A most interesting report is given by the Bureau of Labor Statistics of 1875, on the special effect of certain forms of employment on the health of women. From this I shall quote, as it is, perhaps, the first effort to regard the cardinal re'ation which labor bears to essential attributes of the forming woman, on which hinge all other vital results. The alarm-bell, the first evidence of coming trouble, is menstrual disturbance; and how rapidly nerve-strain reacts upon the functions we may see by the effects of an unexpected rush of business suddenly befalling

a female clerk in good health, during the period of functional activity. Complete cessation of the flow, and general prostration follow, with slow and imperfect recovery.

In the main these functional disturbances are produced by over-work, with innutritious food and nonsanitary association—labor of both body and mind—the effects of disease primarily produced by early employment during animal growth, the regular and long-continued employment of the plastic, undeveloped girl, and the long day's work with unremitting attention. As causative errors in the management of mental or manual labor are mentioned in this most admirable report the following:

1. a. Youth unequal to the work.
   b. Impairment of animal growth.
   c. A constrained position.
2. a. A disregard of ultimate injuries.
   b. Unbroken application without vacation for a long term.
   c. Depression and disease inviting demands on immature vitality.
3. Employment in unsuitable occupation for condition of body and mind.
4. a. Unduly long hours.
   b. Concentration of vital energies, involving extreme nerve-tension.
   c. Unfavorable sanitary surroundings.

Constant injury is wrought by the error of system in schoolroom and workshop, but potent and more directly evident causes of ill health and functional disturbance in the growing girl exist in our daily life, our social customs, and our habits of dress. To them I will not refer; they are too well known.

The constriction and compression of the corset, the dragging weight of the skirt, the circulation-impeding garter, the insufficient covering of low-necked dresses, and of thin stockings and shoes, the total absence of protection where it is most needed, and the absence of drawers.

Among our social customs there are many which bring ruin to woman. I cannot even touch upon them all; there is but one of which I shall speak, and that is the most dangerous of all, more or less underlying all other causes of disease; it is the ignoring of the function of woman by woman—the mother's ignorance of its import. Fearful are the consequences of woman's ignorance, the calamities which follow the course of the misguided mother, swift, certain, and lasting the penalties inflicted upon the unadvised or ill-advised girl, whose one great misfortune is ignorance. She steps into the unknown sphere of womanhood, and in darkness she pursues its irregular path; and fortunate is she who by chance does not stumble.

Many who might be saved by proper management during the transition from adolescence to maturity, now fall victims to their ignorance, and no words of mine could be more convincing than the data given by Tilt as far back as 1853, in his admirable work on the *Elements of Health and the Principle of Female Hygiene*, which shows how many are injured by the unexpected appearance of the unknown function.

Great is the danger in all classes, be it from ignorance or modesty, and most susceptible is the highly-strung nervous system of refined organization. Even though the bark float in safety through that first stormy epoch of life, it is constantly endangered, most of all from the ceaseless crash of the ever-recurring waves of functional activity, and it remains in need of guidance until it has passed through a final storm into calmer waters. The mother is the pilot, and functional hygiene the guiding chart, and the physician the engineer who maps it out.

I cannot exaggerate the danger to the health of the susceptible girl, from each wave of functional activity. The greatest danger is during the height of the wave—that period of greatest activity throughout the entire system, the period of vascular pressure and nerve excitement, which threatens her functions as well as does the era marked by local depletion and depression, the decline of the wave.

So common are the injuries to the health of woman at this epoch, that I need state but a few of the examples which have come under observation during the writing of this paper,—in fact, I may say, almost upon this very day. Fright, nervous and emotional excitement, and exposure to cold have brought injury to many at this time. What is more natural than that the anxious girl should seek to check the bleeding wound, as she supposes? For this purpose the use of cold washes and applications is common, and some even seek to stop the flow by a cold bath, as was done by a now careful mother, who lay long at the point of death from the result of such indiscretion, and slowly by years of care, regained her health. The terrible warning has not been lost, and mindful of her own experience she has taught her children a lesson which but few are fortunate enough to learn.

How many, passing in safety through the first ordeal, are ruined by an indiscretion, or an exposure at a later period. Many a vigorous frame has been broken, health has been ruined, and death even caused, by disturbance of the function during its period of activity, by exposure, by cold, by physical or mental exertion, by nerve or emotional excitement. A cold foot-bath during the period, a dance in a low-neck dress, a walk in rain or snow, a hard day's work of mind or muscle, and excitement of heart or head has made an invalid of many a previously healthy girl, by its influence on this omnipotent function.

CONCLUSION.—I have endeavored to show that the health of the American girl is threatened and impaired by causes more or less avoidable, as they are due to our methods of life, of training, and of education; that the physique of this girl, who is most favorably situated, is imperfect; that her brain is overworked, her nerve power exhausted, her function impaired, and reproduction endangered; all by reason of the susceptibility of her peculiar organization, and the increased impressionability of the sensitive system during the years of development, in which it is subjected to the most severe strain.

Such is the fact: What is the remedy? Condition and cause make the remedy self-evident. Let me briefly review the conditions as we have found them. A perfectly-organized being, in the very beginning of woman's existence, waning with the rise of the great wave of functional life during the period of functional development; showing nerve and physical prostration, with impaired circulation and digestion, imperfect menstruation, and diminished reproductive power; neurasthenia and functional disturbances constantly intermingled as cause and effect. These unfortunate results are brought about, in the main, by more or less similar influences, viz.: 1. Excessive brain-work and nerve-strain, with neglect of the physical system in education. 2. Nerve-strain and partial or incomplete muscular activity in labor; both influences which are inseparably connected with, and complicated by, independently potent causes. 3. Ignoring and neglecting functional hygiene. 4. The physical and emotional strain of society, and the improprieties of dress and over-stimulation of the senses.

The remedy is attention to woman's peculiar organization and to the cyclical waves of her dominant function; or, in other words, harmonious development and occupation of nerve and muscle; diminished brain-work and nerve-stimulation with increased and coördinate physical exercise; increased protection and diminished compression of dress; and self-knowledge and individual care during periods of heightened susceptibility. Changes are necessary in custom and fashion, in methods of labor and education. Whilst each individual, and each calling, is a law unto itself, I may say, in a general way, that we should endeavor to obtain the end of education in its widest senses, the development of all functions and faculties, to render the girl in every way fit for the life she is to enter—"to render youth beautiful, healthful, strong, and honest."

An approximately harmonious co-education of mind and body should be reached with coincident maintenance of proper hygienic conditions. The nerve and emotional strain of class competition must be abolished; the stress of constant work, the train of thought and the routine of regulation must be broken; lungs and heart should be educated, rather than memory; the nerve-strain varied by healthful pleasure and physical exercise in the open air, and relieved more or less, according to individual necessities, during periods of heightened susceptibility.

Whilst the initial causes of ill-health in the school-girl may be readily overcome, the dangers which beset the laboring girl, though equally evident, are more difficult to remove. The same necessity exists for individual care, upon the height of the functional wave and during its period of decline; and the same necessity for a proper coördination of labor, physical and mental. There is the same danger from constant application, from the strain of one part, one function or organ, to the exclusion of others. Nerve-tension is even more continuous and intense, and muscular exertion limited to individual muscles. The years of development should be respected and the continuity of labor broken, and rest and change afforded frequently for short periods. Much good might be done by changes in dress, and last, but not least, by self-knowledge.

I will close with a plea for the self-care of the girl, and for her proper physiological instruction by the mother, which alone will mitigate or remove the initial cause of many of her ailments. I wish to impress upon the mother that the perfect development of the female function, and the maintenance of this function, once developed, in a healthy condition, are essential to the perfect development of the girl and the perfect health of the woman; that self-care and well-regulated hygiene form the foundation of her well-being, and that it is the mother's first duty so to guard herself and so guard her daughter.

MEDICAL PROGRESS.

The Treatment of Boils. — VEIEL (*Monatshefte für praktische Dermatologie*, Oct. 15, 1890) admits that we already have efficient antiseptic means for the treatment of furuncle, such as Biddle's method of injecting with a hypodermic syringe three-per-cent. carbolic acid solution, Lewin's method of cauterizing with nitrate of silver, and the application of Unna's sublimate paste; but he thinks that these methods are too painful for general use, particularly when more than one boil is present. In the place of these the author uses a paste composed of equal parts of zinc oxide and vaseline, and four per cent. of boric acid. The ointment is thoroughly rubbed into the skin around the boil three times daily, and is also thickly spread upon lint and applied. In cases of general furunculosis the whole body is rubbed with the ointment.

Treatment of Cholera Infantum. — DR. LEONARD G. BROUGHTON, of. Reidsville, N. C., recommends the following mixture in severe cases of cholera infantum with profuse and watery stools:

R.—Salicylate of bismuth . . 2 drachms.
   Sulpho-carbolate of zinc . . 4 grains.
   Chalk mixture . . . 1 ounce.
   Paregoric } of each . . ½ " .—M.
   Water }

One drachm of this should be given every two hours until the bowels are controlled, after which the following is prescribed:

R.—Calomel . . . . . 1 grain.
   Sulpho-carbolate of sodium . . 20 grains.
   Saccharated pepsin (P. D. & Co.) . 19 "

Divide in ten powders and give one every three hours. If the stomach is not irritable, sulpho-carbolate of zinc is substituted for the sodium salt in the last prescription. —*Therapeutic Gazette*, November 15, 1890.

Treatment of Hæmorrhoids by Cold Water. — According to *La Semaine Médicale*, DR. ALVIN employs very cold water for the pain, tenesmus, and spasm of the sphincter ani muscle provoked by congested hæmorrhoids. The water is applied to the anal region by means of a sponge. This method is very successful when continued for a number of days, and as a result the growths decrease in size, and there is general relief from all the unpleasant symptoms. These results are practically identical with those obtained by Dr. J. William White, of Philadelphia, whose paper appeared in THE MEDICAL NEWS some months ago.

An Efficient Method of Removing Foreign Bodies from the Nose. — DR. S. JOHNSON TAYLOR (*Lancet*, November 8, 1890) describes the following method of removing foreign bodies from the nose, which was successful in the case of a child of three years with a large bead in the nostril. The procedure is simply Politzer's method of inflation through the unobstructed nostril:

The nozzle of the Politzer bag is introduced into the nostril which does not contain the foreign body, and if the patient is old enough he is requested to swallow a mouthful of water. During the act of swallowing the bag is vigorously compressed, the escape of air from around the nozzle being prevented by grasping the nose with the thumb and forefinger. At the moment of compressing the bag the foreign body will probably be blown out. In the case of a young infant the compression should be made while the child is crying.

The Treatment of Enlargement of the Spleen. — MOSLER (*Wiener medicinische Wochenschrift*) writes that all enlargements of the spleen, irrespective of their nature, size, and duration, are frequently associated with a hæmorrhagic diathesis, which may not have become apparent. For this reason he disapproves of any operative procedure for the removal of the organ, and for some time has used a variety of other measures, chiefly injections, to reduce the swelling. He at first tried parenchymatous injections, by means of a syringe with a long needle, of weak carbolic acid solution. Later he injected pure Fowler's solution with better results—decrease in the size of the organ. Injections of iodine and of quinine he considers dangerous and he has not tried, nor does he approve of the injection of ergot and its preparations. He believes that the cases suitable for injection are those in which the spleen is hard and not associated with extreme anæmia. Fowler's solution, he thinks, is better than the numerous other drugs which have been recommended for the purpose. The dangers of the injection are diminished by applying an ice-bag to the splenic region for an hour or two before and after the operation. — *Centralblatt für Chirurgie*, October 11, 1890.

The Use of Small Doses of Antifebrin.—In the treatment of fevers which are accompanied with cyanosis and collapse, PROFESSOR SAHLI, of Berne, employs minute doses of antifebrin, believing that the effect on the temperature can be thus obtained without the disagreeable symptoms attending the administration of large doses of quinine. Antifebrin acts rapidly and effectively in small quantities ; on the contrary, quinine has no action on the febrile state when administered in minute doses, and may produce untoward effects from its accumulation in the system. Sahli's observations, comprising eleven cases, have been collected by Favrat in a recent work, and show that antifebrin in small doses is very efficient in combating fevers. The drug was given in doses of from 5 to 10 centigrammes in the form of pilules. Cases of pulmonary phthisis and of typhoid fever were decidedly influenced by antifebrin, and while the drug reduced the temperature, it produced at the same time a sensation of comfort. It prevented sudden exacerbations, and only in two cases were untoward effects noticed, such as cyanosis, but vomiting and digestive troubles were never observed. The same good results were obtained in the treatment of typhoid fever. In young children the initial dose should not exceed two centigrammes. The drug, of course, does not influence complications, and in phthisis, for example, neither the progress of the disease nor the cough is prevented. It is the fever.alone that antifebrin attacks, and thus prepares the organism, as it were, to resist more successfully the other symptoms of the disease. The higher the temperature the more decided is the action of antifebrin. It was observed that a temperature of 39° C. could be reduced 1.9° C. by a dose of 10 centigrammes. In the period of decline the drug appeared to exercise the same action, but less markedly.—*La Médecine Moderne*, September 25, 1890.

Injection for Seat-worms.—The *Annales of Gynæcology and Pædiatry* quotes the following prescription to remove seat-worms :

℞.—Tincture of rhubarb . . . 30 drops.
　　Carbonate of magnesium . . 3 grains.
　　Tincture of ginger . . . 1 drop.
　　Water . . . . . 4 ounces.

The mixture should be warmed and used as an injection, repeating three or four times in twenty-four hours.

A Simple Method of Estimating Fat and Casein in Milk.—DR. J. B. NIAS (*Lancet*, November 15, 1890) has devised the following convenient method of estimating the fat and casein in milk in connection with the feeding of infants :

Place some of the milk in a test-tube with a piece of red litmus-paper, add a drop or two of liquor potassæ—enough to render the milk distinctly alkaline as shown by blueing of the litmus paper—and boil. Set aside in a warm place, when the fat will rise to the top, a small but constant percentage remaining behind. The proportions can be determined by a graduated rule placed at the side of the tube. Remove the layer of fat with a small glass pipette, add sufficient acetic acid to redden the litmus-paper, boil, and set aside in a warm place. The whole of the proteids will be precipitated and the relative proportion can again be determined by the graduated rule.

Albuminuria in Children.—DR. SEYOURNET (*L'Union Médicale du Nord-Est*) describes a form of albuminuria in children which he thinks is not infrequent. It differs from scarlatinal albuminuria. He has studied the disease in children between the ages of eleven and sixteen months. Many of the patients were bottle-fed and had been given improper food, which caused distention of the stomach, intestinal catarrh with vomiting and diarrhœa, or in a few instances enlargement of the liver. The author believes that the albuminuria is toxic and due to certain substances generated by abnormal fermentation in the intestines, the absorption of these substances causing congestion or inflammation of the kidneys. The disease was usually accompanied with anuria, and in some cases the daily amount of urine did not exceed one-half ounce. A marked symptom was œdema of the feet, occasionally extending to the eyelids and face. The duration of the disease was two to four weeks. The treatment consisted in the administration of milk to which lime-water was sometimes added ; salicylate of bismuth to disinfect the intestines ; gentle aperients when there was vomiting, and systematic massage of the lumbar region in order to reduce the congestion of the kidneys.—*Lancet*, November 15, 1890.

Injection for Cancer of the Bladder.—

℞.—Iodoform ⎫
　　Glycerin ⎭ of each . . 1 ounce.
　　Distilled water . . . 1 drachm.
　　Gum tragacanth . . 2 grains.—M.

Add a teaspoonful of this mixture to a pint of hot water. The bladder is first to be washed out with water as hot as can be borne, after which the iodoform mixture just named may be injected, and then permitted to escape. These injections should be repeated three times a day ; and it is worthy of remark that after three or four injections very great relief generally ensues.

Prescription for the Prevention of Dental Caries.—

℞.—Tannic acid . . . . 75 grains.
　　Tincture of iodine . . 1 drachm.
　　Tincture of myrrh . . 1 "
　　Iodide of potassium . . 15 grains.
　　Rose-water . . . 6 ounces.—M.

Make into a solution and use a teaspoonful in a wineglassful of hot water as a mouth-wash.

THE MEDICAL NEWS.

A WEEKLY JOURNAL
OF MEDICAL SCIENCE.

COMMUNICATIONS are invited from all parts of the world. Original articles contributed exclusively to THE MEDICAL NEWS will be liberally paid for upon publication. When necessary to elucidate the text, illustrations will be furnished without cost to the author.

Address the Editor: H. A. HARE, M.D.,
1004 WALNUT STREET,
PHILADELPHIA.

Subscription Price, including Postage.

PER ANNUM, IN ADVANCE . . . . $4.00.
SINGLE COPIES . . . . 10 CENTS.

Subscriptions may begin at any date. The safest mode of remittance is by bank check or postal money order, drawn to the order of the undersigned. When neither is accessible, remittances may be made, at the risk of the publishers, by forwarding in *registered* letters.

Address,   LEA BROTHERS & CO.,
NOS. 706 & 708 SANSOM STREET,
PHILADELPHIA.

SATURDAY, DECEMBER 6, 1890.

PYOKTANIN IN DISEASES OF THE EYE.

ALTHOUGH a mass of clinical and experimental evidence in regard to the antiseptic and therapeutic qualities of pyoktanin has been published since its introduction by Stilling, we are by no means in a position to know the exact value of the drug. We are confronted on the one hand by the claims of the discoverer that pyoktanin is devoid of injurious effects upon the animal economy, that it is destructive to microörganisms, and that it is rapidly diffusible in healthy and in diseased animal tissues; and on the other by those who not only have failed to obtain the usual results from its use, but warn against its indiscriminate employment. The many diseases of the external coats of the eye and its appendages, probably largely dependent upon microbic infection, should afford an excellent field for studying the effects of this new claimant for antiseptic and therapeutic favor. Here we are at once met by discordant views. Stilling, as we all know, reported rapid cure of blepharitis, eczema of the lids, conjunctivitis—simple and phlyctenular—corneal ulcer, marginal and parenchymatous keratitis, serous iritis, and even disseminated choroiditis. Bayer, after its use in forty-six cases of scrofulous pannus, various types of corneal ulcer, dacryocystitis, parenchymatous keratitis, iritis, and sympathetic iridocystitis, came to the conclusion that· the excellent qualities attributed by Stilling to this aniline dye did not exist in fact ; and, moreover, in addition to disagreeable discolorations, positively harmful results might follow its application.

Quite recently some very careful clinical observations have appeared on this side of the water. Thus Dr. G. M. Gould (*University Medical Magazine*, December, 1890) reports his results in the eye wards of the Philadelphia Hospital, results which are particularly valuable, because this observer, wherever possible, treated one affected eye with pyoktanin, and the other with either nitrate of silver or bichloride of mercury. In trachoma the drug was without noticeable effect, and in some instances, owing to a species of desiccating effect, injurious. In gonorrhœal ophthalmia nitrate of silver was the preferable drug, and in corneal ulcerations other substances, especially eserine, produced far better results. In dacryocystitis, lachrymal conjunctivitis, unhealthy orbital cavities, and chronic soft leucomata, the sequelæ of interstitial keratitis, pannus, and like affections, pyoktanin did excellent service. Dr. Gould is particularly strong in his praise of the efficacy of the drug in chronically unhealthy conditions of the lachrymal excreting apparatus. Dr. W. Cheatham (*The Cincinnati Lancet-Clinic*, November 15, 1890) observed numbers of cases of the milder conjunctival affections readily yield to solutions of pyoktanin, and instances of trachoma, unaffected by the usual remedies, showed remarkable changes for the better under the daily application of the pyoktanin pencil. Cheatham and Gould are in accord that the remedy is of unusual service in muco-purulent inflammation of the tear-sac.

It will be remembered that Stilling states that pyoktanin dilates the pupil. One of Cheatham's cases affords an interesting confirmation of this fact —an example of interstitial keratitis in which atropine failed to produce its physiological effect upon the pupil, but when it was employed in conjunction with pyoktanin the desired mydriasis was secured.

We have used pyoktanin quite freely, and are in entire accord with those observers who find it of excellent service in diseases of the lachrymal passages, and believe that we have never obtained equal results with any other drug. It is a good application in the various types of inflammation of the conjunctiva associated with the formation of pus, but not better than several other standard remedies. We have failed to observe any curative effect in other diseases of the eye.

Pyoktanin may be prescribed either in the form of the blue or the yellow variety, and used in a solution, as a pencil, or in powder. Solutions are most desirable in acute conjunctivitis, dacryocystitis, etc., but in chronic ophthalmia, trachoma, and old fistulous openings into the lachrymal sac, the direct application of the pencil would seem preferable. The intense discoloration which blue pyoktanin produces is an objection, but the stains may be removed from the skin by scrubbing them with alcohol and water.

KOCH'S DISCOVERY.

THE dispatches which are being constantly received from Berlin tell us nothing of importance in regard to the emyloyment of Koch's remedy for tuberculosis, and time has not elapsed in which to determine the value of the treatment. No one beyond the boundary-line of Germany has as yet received any of the lymph, except Dr. Watson Cheyne, of London, and one or two Viennese physicians. The introduction of a quantity of it into France, sent to Pasteur by Koch, was prohibited on the ground that it was a medicinal agent of unknown composition.

In other columns will be found accounts of various cases treated by von Bergmann, Levy, Fräntzel, and Gerhardt which are of great interest.

We are glad to announce that of the first three American physicians to register in Berlin, our special correspondent, Dr. John Guitéras, the Professor of Pathology in the University of Pennsylvania, is one, that Dr. Dixon, representing the Jefferson Medical College, is the other, while Dr. Herring, of New York, is the third.

Dr. Guitéras goes to Berlin prepared to keep our readers fully informed of Koch's work and its results by letter and cable.

CORRESPONDENCE.

ATLANTA.

To the Editor of THE MEDICAL NEWS,

SIR: The Southern Surgical and Gynecological Association, which recently met here, was a great success, and, in the language of Dr. Hunter McGuire, "the Association came into the world a lusty infant, and its cry was heard all over the South." The papers read and the discussions would have done credit to any medical body. The officers have been uniformly efficient. Dr. Hunter McGuire, who was the first President of the Association, has an international reputation as a surgeon. The Secretary of the Association—in fact, almost the organizer

of it, Dr. W. E. B. Davis, of Birmingham, Alabama, is one of the most tireless and enthusiastic workers in America. He is a man of high literary attainments and great personal magnetism, and he has linked with his magnetism an unsurpassed energy.

Perhaps no man was better fitted to occupy the executive chair than the retiring President, Dr. George J. Engelmann, of St. Louis. Dr. Engelmann was born in St. Louis in 1847. He was graduated from Washington University, and from that college received the degree of Master of Arts. To obtain his medical education he studied for six years in Europe. He is a graduate of the Berlin University, from which he received the degree of Doctor of Medicine. He is also a graduate of the Vienna University, which conferred upon him the degree of Master of Obstetrics. During the greater part of the Franco-Prussian war he served before Metz, in the hospitals of Lyons, and in the reserve hospitals in the University of Berlin. At the close of the war he returned to this country, resuming the practice of medicine in his native city in 1873, and has since been connected in various capacities with the medical colleges there. He is now Professor of Gynecology in the Missouri Medical College, President of the St. Louis Obstetrical and Gynecological Societies, and was Honorary President of the Gynecological Section of the International Medical Congress, which met at Copenhagen. Dr. Engelmann commenced practice as a general practitioner, but gradually drifted into gynecological work. Finding his work in this direction assuming gigantic proportions, he abandoned his general practice, and has since devoted his entire attention to obstetrics and diseases of women.

His successor as President of the Southern Surgical and Gynecological Association, Dr. L. S. McMurtry, is a native of Kentucky and a graduate of Centre College of that State. He was graduated in medicine by the University of Louisiana, and afterward studied at the University of the City of New York. He was Professor of Anatomy in the Kentucky School of Medicine for several years, and is now Surgeon to the Saints Mary and Elizabeth Hospital of Louisville. Two years ago he was President of the Kentucky State Medical Society. Dr. McMurtry has made numerous contributions to medical literature, chiefly relating to abdominal surgery and the diseases of women. He is a Fellow of the Obstetrical Society of Edinburgh, and is about thirty-eight years of age.

The Association is now in the third year of its existence, it having been organized in Birmingham, Alabama, in 1887. It has been successful from its inception, and is steadily increasing in membership, which will be limited to one hundred. It is a Southern organization, but it is not sectional in the *political* meaning of the word. It will take in all good men, whether from the North or South. But the intention of its organizers was that all its meetings should be held in the South. The North has its organizations, from which Southern men have in the past been practically frozen out, and they have been unable to obtain the benefit of an interchange of views and mutual discussions of important medical and surgical questions.

Dr. Engelmann tendered a lunch to the members of the Association, while the Capital City Club held a reception and tendered the Association a banquet, which was one of the most elaborate affairs of its kind ever given in Atlanta.

Many visiting members of the Association were entertained by resident members.

Dr. Hunter P. Cooper has just been appointed surgeon for the Georgia Railroad, and will enter upon the discharge of his duties at once. He is one of Atlanta's most successful and popular physicians, and thoroughly worthy of the position.

CHICAGO.

To the Editor of THE MEDICAL NEWS,

SIR : A small pamphlet of one hundred and thirty-seven pages has just been published by Mr. James C. Strain, Ex-warden of the Cook County Hospital, and is entitled *Medical and Surgical Reports of the Cook County Hospital, Chicago, for the six months ending July 1, 1890.* It includes a history of the hospital and the registrar's report, the surgical and medical abstracts being well illustrated. It is the first medical report of the hospital that has been issued. The Cook County Hospital is just twenty-five years old, having been organized in 1865, though it did not begin its work until January, 1866. Previously to that time the city cared for its sick at the Mercy Hospital. But in January, 1866, it fitted up two wards in the old City Hospital, at the corner of Eighteenth and Arnold Streets, and moved to them twelve patients from the Mercy Hospital. These wards were rapidly filled, and additions to the building were erected. But these, too, soon became overcrowded, and in 1876 the institution was removed to its present location, at the corner of West Harrison and Wood Streets. The new structures, not all of which were erected at the same time, consist of a long administration building of imposing appearance, and a pavilion of four wards with a wing of three wards on each side. There is plenty of space between all these buildings, conducing not only to their appearance, but to the light, ventilation, and comfort of the wards. The grounds contain twelve acres. In the administration building are the main office, the examining room for patients, the drug store, the office of the custodian, the office for coroner's inquests, the offices of the warden, the registrar, the chief clerk, the hospital committee, and the medical board, and the private apartments of the warden, internes, and druggist. In the rear of this building are the instrument-room, the office of the training-school for nurses, and the amphitheatre.

The wards are thirteen in number, and of these, three are men's medical wards, five are men's surgical wards, one is a woman's medical ward, and two are women's surgical wards, one is an obstetrical ward and one a ward for children. The pavilion wards are large, being 120 feet long and 30 feet wide. There are in each of them about forty beds. The wing wards are 40 feet long and 15 feet wide, and contain about thirty beds. They are lighted by windows on three sides, and each ward has in connection with it a bath-room, a nurse-room, a linen-room, a kitchen, and a dining-room. The surgical wards have, in addition, operating-rooms. The beds are iron, with woven-wire springs. The floors of the wards are of Georgia pine, and the floors of the corridors are paved with tiles.

During the six months ending January 4, 1889, there were received and treated 3255 cases, and during the six months ending July 1, 1889, 3903 cases, showing an increase of 648. As there were 435 patients present on January 1, 1889, and 488 on July 1, 1889, the number in the hospital during the two periods, respectively. was 3690 and 4391. So that it is only a matter of time when the vast accommodations of the hospital will have to be increased to keep pace with the growing wants of our city.

The September grand jury of Chicago, after visiting the public institutions, recommended that a crematory be built at the Hospital, and that some of the inmates of the infirmary should be sent to the State institution.

The registrar's report contains analytical tables of the diseases treated, of the patients admitted, of the conditions in which some of them were discharged, and of the number of those that died. This report is followed by a long and interesting dissertation on the "Treatment of Empyæma," by Dr. Bayard Holmes, editor of the *North American Practitioner.*

The surgical abstract includes cases of compound fracture, bullet wounds of the hand, injury of the musculo-spiral nerve, fracture of the larynx from falls, death from œdema of the glottis, fracture of the trachea, resection of the ulnar nerve, nephrorraphy, and many other interesting subjects. The medical abstract contains many interesting cases, including carcinoma of the œsophagus, rupture of the portal vein from a fall, chylous ascites, Hodgkin's disease, thoracic aneurism, Landry's paralysis, etc.

Dr. William N. Hibbard, of this city, died on October 29th. The cause of his death is said to have been ptomaïne-poisoning, and the attendant circumstances were peculiarly distressing.

About a week before his death Dr. Hibbard ate some oysters, which, doubtless, contained the poisonous substance. The paroxysmal efforts of his digestive system to rid itself of the poison brought on intussusception, and his physicians decided that his life could be saved only by an operation. The patient, however, was too weak to rally, and died while under the influence of the anæsthetic.

Dr. Hibbard was born December 16, 1858, at Freeport, Illinois. He was prepared for college in the Hyde Park High School, and entered the University of Vermont at Burlington, of which both his father and grandfather were graduates. He was graduated in the class of 1880. He taught for three years in the High Schools of Chicago and then entered the Chicago Medical College, from which he was graduated in 1886. He was then appointed an interne in the Cook County Hospital, serving for eighteen months, after which he began the practice of medicine in Hyde Park, and was shortly after appointed Demonstrator of Anatomy in the Chicago Medical College. Few young physicians had brighter prospects, or a larger number of friends. After his graduation from the Chicago Medical College he married Miss Mary Barker, of Kenwood, who, with a son two years old, survives him.

At a recent meeting of the Chicago Medico-legal Society, Dr. M. H. Lackersteen read a paper entitled "The Scientific Aspect of Medical Hypnotism." He asserted that of all modern therapeutic measures hypnotism has caused the most debate and excited the most prejudice. He believed that the dreams of hypnotism are no more dangerous or injurious than are those of normal sleep, and denied that hypnotism leads to mental derangement or to paralysis. There are few remedies, he said, that are not dangerous when carelessly used, and this is also true of hypnotism. The fact that ignorant persons can exercise the hypnotic influence is no argument against the usefulness of hypnotism. He regretted that quacks and impostors have taken advantage of the new discovery and brought it into disrepute. There are few people, he said, that are not susceptible to the hypnotic influence, and some can be influenced even by a letter. A case was cited in which a physician frequently wrote to a certain patient telling him to fall asleep at a certain hour. The order was never disobeyed.

During many years of life in India, Dr. Lackersteen had an opportunity to witness the results of hypnotic treatment as practised by Indian doctors. They aecomplished by charms, incantations, and superstitions, cures which would baffle the most skilled, scientific physicians.

DR. GOODELL'S ARTICLE.

To the Editor of THE MEDICAL NEWS,

SIR : In your issue of last week, my article entitled "What I have Learned to Unlearn in Gynecology" contains a serious error, which was overlooked in the proof-reading. In the first column of page 562 the word *not* should be erased, and the sentence should read: " I have learned to unlearn the idea—and this was the hardest task of all—that uterine symptoms are always present in cases of uterine disease ; or that, when present, they necessarily come from the uterine disease."

Yours truly,

WILLIAM GOODELL, M.D.

NEWS ITEMS.

Koch's Method.—The special correspondent of the *British Medical Journal* gives the following account of von Bergmann's, Levy's, Fräntzel's, and Gerhardt's cases :

Dr. v. Bergmann's anxiously-expected address and exhibition of cases treated by Professor Koch's method took place on Sunday evening, November 16th, before a numerous and select audience of invited guests. The Minister of Public Instruction, Herr von Gossler, and amongst other celebrities Professors Virchow, Gerhardt, Liebreich, Waldeyer, and Olshausen were present. In beginning his address Professor v. Bergmann referred in stirring words to the intense emotion which, since Koch's publication, had seized not only suffering but also healing humanity. He then discussed the cases that had come under his own observation, which were cases of (1) lupus, (2) glandular tuberculosis, (3) tuberculosis of the joints and bones, and (4) tuberculosis of the larynx. Five lupus patients were exhibited, to whom a subcutaneous injection of one centigramme of Koch's remedy had been given in the morning between 8.30 and 9.30 ; all these five cases showed the general and local symptoms spoken of by Koch—namely, fever

and inflammation. The lecturer remarked that the unerring certainty with which an attack of fever, aecompanied by rigors, followed the application of the remedy, was of the highest interest from a medical point of view. This general reaction was invariably accompanied by a marked action on all tuberculous parts of the body— visible in cases of lupus. Of the patients exhibited some showed temperatures of 41.0° C., and even higher. The lupus spots were enormously swollen and very red, this reaction being more marked in recent cases. One of the patients had suffered from the disease for twenty years and one for twenty-nine years. On Sunday morning, before the subcutaneous injection was given, Professor Gerhardt had designated the first of these as a slight and superficial one ; nevertheless, an enormous reaction followed the injection, tending to prove that there was more lupus than had yet been found, and that Koch's remedy finds the most secret places and nests of tubercle bacilli.

The next five patients exhibited were treated in presence of the assembly by Stabsarzt Dr. Pfuhl, subcutaneous injections in varying doses being applied to the back. One of the patients was a sickly-looking lad of seventeen, who had been under Professor v. Bergmann's and the late Professor Volkmann's treatment for the last fourteen years. " Now the poor fellow will have relief at last," said Professor v. Bergmann, smiling.

The next set of three patients exhibited had been under treatment for some time, and had gone through a course of subcutaneous injections, the reactions becoming weaker after each injection. Here partial cure was already visible ; but the application will be continued until no reaction at all can be observed.

Professor v. Bergmann resumed his address by remarking that the value of the remedy was enhanced by the control experiments that could be made in the case of healthy subjects, or those affected by other diseases, which were all-important for diagnosis. He illustrated this by exhibiting a patient suffering from an affection of the cheek, which might have been considered tuberculous. The experimental subcutaneous injection produced no feverish reaction. Probably this case was syphilitic.

The second group exhibited contained two cases of glandular tubercle, in the person of two little girls of scrofulous appearance. Here the reaction was marked.

The third group comprised sixteen cases of tubercle of the joints and bones, with suppuration, fistulæ, and similar phenomena. Some of these, to whom a first injection had been applied, showed the usual symptoms ; the joints were much swollen and highly colored, and movement was scarcely possible. Others had been treated by repeated injections. One of these, who suffered from consumption and tuberculous inflammation of the knee-joint, was so severely affected by the injections (intermittent pulse, faintness, etc.), that there seemed cause for anxiety. He had, however, recovered, and was progressing favorably.

The last patients exhibited excited special interest, as they were cases of tubercle of the larynx. Professors Gerhardt and von Ziemssen had in both cases found serious lesions of the larynx. And here the remedy showed its diagnostic value as a means of distinguishing cancer from tuberculosis.

In summing up the cases exhibited, Professor v. Bergmann said that from the local and general phenomena which had already shown themselves the prognosis was decidedly favorable. Nevertheless, in many cases surgical operations would still be unavoidable, as abscesses and dislocations could be cured by mechanical means only. In these cases it would be of the highest importance to guard against relapse by the repetition of Koch's treatment, and thus both methods united gave the brightest prospect of success.

The *Therapeutische Monatshefte* publishes a supplement containing an account of cases treated by Koch's new method in Dr. Levy's clinic. The report, written by Dr. H. Fielchenfeld, Levy's assistant, is here summarized: The treatment was begun on September 22d, that is, not quite two months ago. This comparatively short time has sufficed to show in what cases complete recovery may be hoped for, and where only amelioration of symptoms can be expected. No definite opinion can be formed as to the length of time necessary for perfect recovery. Fielchenfeld cites three cases of lupus, one of which is a sort of test-ease, and has already beenme celebrated in the history of the investigation. In this case all the phenomena of reaction took place in the typical form with which Koch's paper has made the world familiar. A complete cure seemed to have been effected—it was as though the diseased tissue had been cut away with a chisel. Further subcutaneous injections, however, proved that the end of the trouble had not been reached, and that in spite of superficial cicatrization there was considerable tuberculous tissue below awaiting destruction. Even now the patient cannot be considered cured. In a second case of lupus the general condition of the patient became much worse after each subcutaneous injection, and severe pains persisted, especially in the bones of the affected arm.

A third case of lupus is interesting because, of all cases treated in Levy's clinic, it is the one furthest advanced toward recovery. In this case the subcutaneous injections no longer produce a reaction. Here too, however, Dr. Fielchenfeld speaks of "provisional cure" only, as no final verdict can be given after two months in a disease which runs its course so slowly as tuberculosis does.

In cases of tuberculosis of the bones and joints, cures were effected ; that is, no reaction followed the subcutaneous injection of even large doses. The same result was obtained in cases of glandular tuberculosis. Turning to his cases of consumption, Dr. Fielchenfeld states that three patients in the first stage of phthisis were dismissed as cured, their sputum having been found free from bacilli, and the auscultatory signs having considerably decreased. Dr. Fielchenfeld, however, does not consider these two facts a complete proof of definite cure. Bacilli may disappear from the sputum to reappear after a time.

As regards the more advanced forms of phthisis, where cavities have already formed, Dr. Fielchenfeld remarks that no complete recovery has been observed. But the general symptoms of the disease—night-sweats, etc.—disappeared promptly. Even in the worst cases there was a diminution of expectoration. There was no increase of weight, even when the general condition was much improved. On the other hand, no loss of weight was observed, even in the most advanced and desperate cases.

At Monday's meeting of the Verein für innere Medicin, Professor Fräntzel gave an account of the cases treated in his clinic by Koch's method. He divided them into two classes: (1) those in the first stage of phthisis; (2) those in advanced stages of the disease (disintegration of tissue, cavities, etc.). In the latter group no change of condition could be observed. Two patients died during treatment ; their cases were desperate from the beginning. The *post-mortem* examination showed no indication of the commencement of recovery. Fräntzel utters a word of warning against using large doses at the beginning of treatment in advanced cases, and cited one case in which death ensued after twenty-four hours. As regards the first group of patients—early stages of consumption—Professor Fräntzel was able to record decided improvement. Expectoration was easier and more abundant after the injection, while the cough decreased. The general condition visibly improved ; the appetite became keener, the weight increased, and the night-sweats disappeared. The microscopic examination of the sputum demonstrated first a decrease, and secondly a change of the bacilli. They seemed stunted ; nevertheless, their vitality was not destroyed. Fräntzel is of opinion that the treatment, even in the most successful cases, must be continued for a considerable time to guard against relapse.

In a clinical lecture given in the presence of many distinguished physicians on Tuesday, November 18th, Professor Gerhardt gave an account of his experiences with Koch's remedy. He exhibited three cases specially fitted to illustrate the progress made in the diagnosis and treatment of tuberculosis. The first case was one of tuberculosis of the throat, in which various methods had been tried without effect. On Sunday, two milligrammes of Koch's fluid were injected, and a decided reaction was observed on Monday. Considering the success which has attended a similar case in v. Bergmann's clinic, Professor Gerhardt thinks that recovery is possible. The second case was in the initial stage of consumption, whilst the third patient showed an affection of the apex of the lung which aroused suspicions of tuberculosis. Tubercle bacilli had not been found, but this is no absolute proof of the non-existence of tuberculosis. Koch's fluid was injected on Sunday ; no reaction ensued, which is a conclusive proof that the affection is not tuberculous. Professor Gerhardt, in conclusion, spoke some serious words of warning. He said it was absurd to imagine that Koch's treatment was of so simple a character that by subcutaneous injection consumption could be simply driven out of the body ; on the contrary, in order to apply it successfully, the physician would have to use the most careful discrimination.

Professor Koch's Syringe.—We have received from the maker, Herr E. Kraus, 55 Kommandantenstrasse, Berlin, an electrotype of the syringe used by Professor Koch and his colleagues in their antituberculous inoculations. As will be seen, it is a slightly modified form of the ordinary Pravaz's hypodermic syringe.

The instrument consists (1) in an exactly-graduated glass cylinder of the capacity of two grammes, with a conical nozzle for the reception of the hollow needle ;

(2) a stopcock of German silver with an elastic ball; (3) two hollow needles. When the stopcock is closed, the upper part of the glass cylinder filled with injection fluid

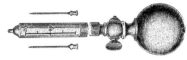

is fixed into the hermetically closed cone of the German-silver stopcock. After the canula is introduced, the stopcock is opened and the remedy injected by pressure on the India-rubber ball.—*British Medical Journal*, November 22, 1890.

DR. HENRY MORRIS desires us to state that he has not been and is not a candidate for the Chair of Therapeutics and Materia Medica at the Jefferson Medical College.

Mutter Lectures of the College of Physicians of Philadelphia.—The course of lectures on surgical pathology provide in accordance with the will of the late Professor Thomas D. Mütter, will be delivered during 1890–91, by Professor Roswell Park, of Buffalo, New York.

The first series of five lectures will be given in the Hall of the College of Physicians, corner of Thirteenth and Locust Streets, on December 4th, 5th, 6th, 8th, and 9th, at 8.15 P. M.

The subjects are as follows:

1. Introductory. Study of the blood and of some phases of the inflammatory process. Thrombosis, Embolism, Hæmoglobin, Oligochromæmia, and Ptomaïnes. Conditions predisposing to infection.

2. A study of pus and of pyogenic organisms, obligate and facultative.

3. Surgical sepsis and the organisms which produce it. *Résumé* of experimental work, Surgical Fever, Intestinal Toxæmia, Sapræmia, Septicæmia, and Pyæmia.

4. Peritonitis—forms and causes. Testing the relative values of antiseptics.

5. Tetany and Tetanus.

The medical profession are cordially invited to be present.

WILLIAM HUNT,
Chairman of the Committee.

D. HAYES AGNEW,
President

Prize of the New York State Medical Association.—Dr. J. G. Orton, ex-President of the New York State Medical Association, has offered a prize of $100 for the best short popular essay on some subject connected with practical sanitation, under the following conditions:

1. Competition to be open to all.

2. Essays to be forwarded to the Secretary of the Association, Dr. E. D. Ferguson, Troy, N. Y., not later than August 1, 1891, accompanied by the name of the author under separate seal.

3. Examination and award to be made by a committee appointed by the Council of the Association.

4. The successful essay to be read at the next annual meeting of the Association, and, if approved by the

Council, to be offered for publication in the secular press, and issued in tract form or otherwise for general circulation.

5. Authors of essays, unsuccessful so far as the prize is concerned, but found worthy of special commendation, to receive intimation as to a proper disposition to be made of them.

The Congress of Hygiene and Demography.—The Congress of Hygiene and Demography will be held in London during the week beginning August 10, 1891.

The governments of all countries and municipalities, and all public health authorities, universities, colleges, and societies occupied in the study of the sciences more or less immediately connected with hygiene are invited to coöperate and appoint delegates to represent them at the Congress. The Prince of Wales will preside.

A committee of organization has been formed, of which Sir Douglas Galton is chairman, and Professor W. H. Corfield and Mr. Shirley F. Murphy are honorary secretaries. An exhibition of articles of hygienic interest will be held in connection with the Congress. The last of these congresses was held in Vienna in 1887, and was attended by more than 2000 persons, and it is expected that the London meeting will be one of great magnitude and importance.

OFFICIAL LIST OF CHANGES IN THE STATIONS AND DUTIES OF THE MEDICAL CORPS OF THE U. S. NAVY FOR THE WEEK ENDING NOVEMBER 29, 1890.

CRAWFORD, M. H., *Passed Assistant Surgeon.*—Ordered to the Receiving-ship " Independence."

MARSTELLER, E. H., *Passed Assistant Surgeon.*—Ordered to the U. S. S. " Petrel."

NASH, FRANCIS S., *Passed Assistant Surgeon.*—Resigned from the U. S. Navy, to take effect November 23, 1891.

CORDEIRO, F. J. B., *Passed Assistant Surgeon.*—Granted extension of leave for four months, with permission to leave the United States.

LANSDALE, PHILIP, *Medical Director* (Retired).—Granted one year's leave, with permission to leave the United States.

ADRIAN, RICHARD ALFRED.—Commissioned an Assistant Surgeon in the U. S. Navy, from November 24, 1890.

OFFICIAL LIST OF CHANGES OF STATIONS AND DUTIES OF MEDICAL OFFICERS OF THE U. S. MARINE-HOSPITAL SERVICE, FROM NOVEMBER 15 TO NOVEMBER 22, 1890.

FESSENDEN, C. S. D., *Surgeon.*—Granted leave of absence for fourteen days, November 22, 1890.

AUSTIN, H W., *Surgeon.*—Detailed as Chairman of a Board of Medical Officers to convene, December 1, 1890, in Washington, D. C., November 19, 1890.

IRWIN, FAIRFAX, *Surgeon.*—Detailed as a member of a Board of Medical Officers to convene, December 1, 1890, in Washington, D. C., November 19, 1890.

KINYOUN, J. J., *Assistant Surgeon.*—Detailed as Recorder of a Board of Medical Officers to convene, December 1, 1890, in Washington, D. C., November 19, 1890.

WOODWARD, R. M., *Assistant Surgeon.*—Granted leave of absence for fourteen days, November 21, 1890.

CONDICT, A. W., *Assistant Surgeon.*—To proceed to Cairo, Ill., for temporary duty, November 19, 1890.

STIMPSON, W. G., *Assistant Surgeon.*—To proceed to Cape Charles Quarantine, for temporary duty, November 20, 1890.

PROMOTION.

KINYOUN, J. J., *Passed Assistant Surgeon.*—Commissioned as Passed Assistant Surgeon by the President, November 21, 1890.

APPOINTMENT.

COFER, L. E., *Assistant Surgeon*—Commissioned as Assistant Surgeon by the President, November 21, 1890.

THE MEDICAL NEWS.

A WEEKLY JOURNAL OF MEDICAL SCIENCE.

| VOL. LVII. | SATURDAY, DECEMBER 13, 1890. | NO. 24. |

ORIGINAL LECTURES.

THE CURE OF PROCIDENTIA UTERI.

*A Clinical Lecture
delivered at the Woman's Hospital of Chicago,
October 20, 1890.*

BY HENRY T. BYFORD, M.D.,

PROFESSOR OF CLINICAL GYNECOLOGY IN THE WOMAN'S HOSPITAL;
PROFESSOR OF GYNECOLOGY IN THE CHICAGO POST-GRADUATE
MEDICAL SCHOOL; GYNECOLOGIST TO ST. LUKE'S HOSPITAL;
SURGEON TO THE WOMAN'S HOSPITAL OF CHICAGO.

LADIES AND GENTLEMEN: While our patient is being anæsthetized I will call your attention to the conditions upon which procidentia uteri depends. The first conditions to be taken into consideration are, of course, the natural position and attachments of the uterus. The normal viscus is small, weighs but four ounces, and is situated well up in the pelvis, with the os pointing backward toward the lower end of the sacrum. Its supports may be divided into three sets: the superior or sustaining, the inferior or retaining, and the external or supplementary.

The pelvic organs are roofed over by the peritoneal membrane, which is reflected about them like gables, and which, with the muscular and fibrous tissue in and under them, constitutes the sustaining supports or ligaments. The bladder, uterus, and rectum project upward through this roof of peritoneum like domes, towers, or chimneys, and, as you know, are held in place by a great abundance of connective tissue. Were it not for the variable abdominal cover them they would be adequately sustained by these attachments. But when the ordinary pressure is augmented by the muscular action of the individual, this elastic connective tissue is stretched, and the organs come down against the pelvic floor. Here they are retained until the cessation of this additional pressure allows them to be drawn back into place. The pelvic floor consists of the levator ani muscle and fascia, the coccyx, and the tissues of the interior pelvic walls.

The bladder, the uterus, and the rectum each constitutes a chamber in the structure, and each has its outlet, viz., the urethra, the vagina, and the anus. These outlets terminate at the pelvic portico or perineum proper, which, as Emmet has told us, acts as their support—but supports the uterus only in a supplementary manner. The perineum consists mainly of the triangular ligament, and the levator vaginæ, constrictor cunni, transversus perinei, and sphincter ani muscles, with their fasciæ. Now if the perineal body be torn, the urethra, vagina, and rectum having lost a part of their support, tend to protrude, and in protruding weaken the contiguous portions of the pelvic floor and connective tissue. Lacerate the pelvic floor also, and the uterus has nothing to prevent it from protruding under increased ab-

dominal pressure except the elastic superior supports, which, in turn, are weakened by the laxity of contiguous tissues under them. Now let the uterus, particularly its cervical portion, become enlarged from chronic disease; or let it remain in a state of subinvolution, along with subinvolution of the other pelvic tissues; or let a chronic diarrhœa, or proctitis, or a general condition of debility, impair the integrity of the pelvic connective tissue, and procidentia will result.

Our patient, as most of you can see, is the one upon whom we performed a high amputation of the cervix two weeks ago. She acquired lacerations of the cervix and perineum in childbirth, followed by subinvolution of the uterus and vagina, and most of the time during the nine or ten years that have followed, she has suffered from diarrhœa. Two weeks ago the fundus lay on the relaxed perineal body, and the enlarged and lacerated cervix protruded about three inches from the vulva, bringing the vagina, bladder, and rectum down also. The uterus measured four inches in length. The pelvis would hold no pessary, and her condition was one of extreme misery.

As it would have been unscientific to attempt to keep a uterus and vagina of that size in this pelvis, I made an oval incision around the cervix and about half an inch away from it, so as to cut off some of the vaginal walls. I then dissected up the connective tissue as high as the uterine arteries, ligated these arteries with strong catgut, and continued the separation of the connective tissue as high as the internal os. Drawing the uterus well out, I put an elastic ligature about it and the protruding vagina, and proceeded to amputate the cervix near its junction with the corpus. I then drew the vaginal walls together over the stump and stitched the edges to each other and to the cervical mucous membrane. As is often the case, the internal os was very small, even though the uterus was enlarged, and the cervix had been lacerated and everted. I then tamponed the uterus in position for twenty-four hours, and have subsequently kept the woman in bed, using one-per-cent. carbolic acid douches after each urination. The uterus is about the normal size, and has been in a normal position ever since. I may say that the two weeks she has been in bed, and the four that she will remain in bed after to-day's operation, constitute quite an important part of the treatment. The vagina, as is apparent to you, has contracted in the upper part as a result of the first operation, and our endeavor to-day will be to contract its lower portions and the perineum. At the same time I will give it a new attachment to the tissues at the sides of the pelvis over the deeper portions of the levator ani muscles, by a procedure somewhat different from those that have been employed by other operators.

Having cleansed and disinfected the field of operation, I remove a strip of mucous membrane nearly one inch wide from the left lateral vaginal wall just above the sulcus and extending from the carunculæ about two inches back toward the cervix. The wound bleeds profusely, as I knew it would, but the bleeding does not matter, as I shall immediately close the wound with uninterrupted catgut sutures. The stitches are passed deeply into the fascia at the upper edge, then out into the wound, then into the bottom and through the lower edge, so as to gather up the looser tissue and lower edge, and bring them to the upper edge and firmer fascia. Having completely closed this wound, I put in two silkworm-gut sutures to relieve the strain upon the catgut. I now quickly excise a similar strip from the right vaginal wall, and close it in the same way. The posterior vaginal and anterior rectal walls are now drawn well up in their proper places and firmly held, while the vagina has become quite narrow, except under the neck of the bladder.

There is one point in connection with this operation on the lateral vaginal wall that deserves your attention, namely, it is not merely a denudation but a removal of the entire thickness of the mucous membrane, and opens into the cellular tissue. The vagina is thus not only narrowed, but the connective-tissue attachments are in part restored. This is an idea that has been overlooked in the various operations for prolapse. But the frequent failure of methods which are designed merely to narrow the vagina and build a perineal body afford convincing proof of its importance.

With this long-handled needle I now pass a silk suture around a circular space of sagging vaginal wall, about the size of a silver half-dollar, just under the neck of the bladder, cut out the mucous membrane within the circle, and draw the edges together with the silk puckering string, as if it were the mouth of a purse. Now all is tight internally, and we have but to reconstruct a perineal body externally.

For our present purpose nothing is better than Tait's flap-operation. Entering the point of the scissors high on the inside of the left labium, and a short distance external to the vaginal sutures, I cut deep into the tissues, and carry the point of the scissors down the labium, across the perineal body, a little above the sphincter ani, and upward on the other labium. With a few additional snips I lay open the tissue quite deeply, catch up the centre of the superior edge of the wound with forceps, and draw it well up so as to make the wound more perpendicular than transverse. You will observe that this wound has no connection with the lateral vaginal wounds previously sutured, being entirely below them. Commencing at the upper end of the labial incision, I pass silkworm-gut sutures into the raw tissues under, but not including, the edge of the skin, and bring them out on the other side, also under the edge. Now that they all are in, I find it more convenient to tie from below upward, and the patient is ready to be cleansed and put to bed. Plain vaginal douches will be given after each urination for forty eight hours, then douches of one-percent. carbolic acid solution. In four weeks she will be permitted to get up and go home.

It is well for me to remind you that this procedure will not do for every case. Had the uterus remained retroverted after the amputation of the cervix, I should have performed Alexander's operation. The reason that the latter operation cannot always be depended upon is because the round ligaments are often stretched to such an extent that they cannot be found or utilized. The popular objection that the ligaments are not strong enough to hold up the uterus is based upon ignorance of their action. They merely hold the fundus forward so that abdominal pressure will be exerted upon the posterior surface of the uterus, the retention of which, after it is placed in this advantageous position, is the work of other supports.

When the inguinal canals are opened during the Alexander operation, it becomes an easy matter to suspend the prolapsed bladder. We may cut through the posterior walls of the canals, separate the loose connective tissue from the pubic bones, pass sutures down through the vaginal walls on either side of the neck of the bladder, draw up the prolapsed vesico-vaginal septum, and stitch it behind the pubes. I prefer to use silkworm-gut sutures, and include a portion of the vaginal walls and pillars of the external inguinal ring in each.

Shortening the sacro-uterine ligaments has been done in various ways, both through the vagina and in the abdominal cavity. Cauterization of the vagina, incomplete closure by uniting the denuded anterior and posterior walls, or the denuded lateral walls; removal of almost the entire anterior or posterior wall, etc., have been tried with varying success. Our time is too valuable to allow us to describe the numerous forms of denudations in use, such as triangles, quadrilaterals, pentagons, circles, ovals, parallelograms, monograms, butterflies, and other figures of professorial fancy.

In order to extricate our minds from this confusion of methods, we should never forget that in each case there are certain defects either of the superior, inferior, or supplementary supports which must be remedied. The perineal body, pelvic floor, connective-tissue attachments, uterine ligaments, or the vagina and uterus themselves, must be thought of, while the Chinese puzzle of denudation, as figured in many of the textbooks, should be duly treasured as an interesting relic of mediæval art.

In some slight cases Thure Brandt's uterine massage, by restoring tone to the muscular fibres, suffices for a cure.

In case of diseased ovaries, we may be justified in opening the abdominal cavity, removing them with as much of the relaxed broad ligaments as possible, and stitching the stumps to the anterior abdominal walls. An operation upon the sacro-uterine folds would also be justifiable at such a time.

Removing the entire uterus *per vaginam* will, of course, cure the procidentia uteri. But if we confine ourselves to that, the relaxed tissues will be apt to permit the vagina and intestines to protrude, and thus fail to cure the patient. I have, in fact, had to perform some of these operations after the uterus had been taken out. If, however, we decide to remove the uterus for procidentia, we should at the same time remove all the redundant vaginal wall in such a manner as to secure lateral connective-tissue attachments.

The Buffalo Medical College.—It is said that the buildings of the Buffalo Medical College will soon be remodelled and enlarged.

ORIGINAL ARTICLES.

THE USELESSNESS OF SPLINTS IN FRACTURE OF THE LOWER END OF THE RADIUS.[1]

By JOHN B. ROBERTS, M.D.,

PROFESSOR OF SURGERY IN THE PHILADELPHIA POLYCLINIC AND IN THE WOMAN'S MEDICAL COLLEGE OF PENNSYLVANIA.

THE treatment of fracture of the lower end of the radius is exceedingly satisfactory, because the character of the injury seldom varies and because the results obtained are usually good both in rapidity of cure and in perfect restoration of function.

This statement is, perhaps, unexpected, since it is not unusual to find the opinion expressed in text-books that this fracture is troublesome to treat, and very liable to be followed by deformity of the wrist and stiffness of the fingers. I am convinced that such unfortunate results usually come from mismanagement of the fracture, and are due to a want of appreciation of the nature of the lesion, and of the necessity for forcible reduction immediately after its receipt. These errors of judgment and treatment are perpetuated by the current belief that the essential treatment of a fracture is the application of a splint.

I propose to show that in the great majority of cases fracture of the lower end of the radius needs no splint; and hence that splints for this injury are usually useless. If the tendency to use a splint impels the practitioner to neglect the all-important reduction of the fracture, my position, it seems to me, is strengthened.

The innumerable forms of splint devised for fracture of the lower end of the radius show how much this very common injury has interested the profession. Some of these splints have done great harm because they have misled the practitioner as to the nature of the lesion. A few of them are very good, in that they have been devised in accordance with the anatomy and pathology of the osseous lesion. As, however, in the vast majority of cases, none of them is really needed they are practically useless. The fact that positive harm is liable to be done by their use is a point in advocacy of the abandonment of all such appliances.

The usual cause of the injury is forced extension of the radio-carpal joint, which produces a transverse disruption through the lower end of the radius from three-eighths to one-half an inch above the articular surface. The characteristic deformity is caused by the fracturing force driving the lower fragment upward and backward upon the shaft, or thrusting the shaft downward and under that fragment; so that it is caught or impacted upon the dorsal edge of the shaft-fragment. Occasionally

[1] Read before the Philadelphia Academy of Surgery, November 3, 1890.

there is a tendency to lateral or antero-posterior obliquity of the line of fracture, but this is rather uncommon. The displacement sometimes occurs much more markedly at the radial than at the ulnar side of the lower fragment, which is then tilted obliquely backward, carrying the styloid process of the radius upward and backward, so that it is on a level with, or even higher than, the styloid process of the ulna. This angular displacement tends to throw the articular surface with the attached carpus upward and backward to the radial side, causing thereby undue prominence of the lower end of the ulna.

Muscular action has nothing to do with the production or continuance of the deformity. In cases in which the fracturing force has not been sufficient to cause displacement, no deformity exists, and in such instances the diagnosis rests upon a localized point of great tenderness about half an inch above the wrist-joint.

Sometimes comminution of the lower fragment takes place so that lines of fracture enter the radio-carpal joint. The ligaments and cartilages are sometimes extensively injured, and sometimes there occurs actual loss of substance by crushing and pulverizing of the bone tissue. These complications, except that of comminution, are quite rare.

Reduction of the fracture, the most important element in the treatment of the injury, is often ineffectually accomplished, or, indeed, not attempted. This is owing to ignorance rather than carelessness on the part of the attendant. When reduction is once thoroughly accomplished, displacement is not apt to recur, because the broad rough surfaces of bone are held together by their serrations, and because there are no muscular masses tending to displace the fragments.

The condition, it will be observed, is quite different from oblique fracture of the shaft of a bone, in which it is often difficult to maintain accurate apposition because of the muscular displacing forces. Hence if reduction, which is the essential in treatment, is properly performed, no splint is needed. On the other hand, if reduction is neglected, no splint will act as a substitute for it. If reduction has been properly accomplished, an improper splint may displace the lower fragment and cause recurrence of the deformity. Hence, abandonment of splints is usually the proper course to pursue, and probably the most judicious method of treatment to advocate and teach.

Comminuted fractures, of course, need more support than do non-comminuted ones; but even here, the simple support of a bandage applied in a circular manner, or of strips of adhesive plaster wound around the wrist like a collar will usually be found sufficient.

In uncomplicated fractures treatment is required for about three weeks.

Perfect function of the wrist and fingers may be expected in nearly all cases; provided that reduction has been properly effected immediately after the injury, and provided that the fingers have not been restricted in motion at any time during the treatment. Slight stiffness of the wrist may be expected for a few weeks in complicated cases; and in such injuries some thickening about the seat of the fracture will persist for two or three months. Slight shortening of the radius, due to loss of tissue by crushing and absorption, occurs in most cases, but the resulting inclination of the hand to the radial side in well-treated cases of average severity can usually be detected only by very close scrutiny.

The statement of some authors that long-continued disability of the wrist and fingers is to be expected is absolutely untrue in the average case of fracture of the lower end of the radius; and is due to observation of cases improperly treated.

The danger of many of the splints advocated for this fracture is due to the non-recognition by their respective inventors of the curved or arched shape of the palmar surface of the lower third of the radius. The dorsum of the bone when covered with the tendons is straight, but the palmar surface is curved. It is readily understood, therefore, that the application of any straight splint (such as that called Bond's splint) to the palmar surface of the broken radius has a tendency to displace the lower fragment upward again, as soon as the bandage which retains the splint in position is applied. A straight splint may, however, be applied with propriety to the back of the wrist. I have used with satisfaction two or three pieces of whalebone held in position by a strip of adhesive plaster. Any rigid article, such as a piece of steel or wood, half an inch wide and five or six inches long, will answer the purpose. The truth is, however, that in a person of ordinary intelligence, who will avoid subjecting the bone to severe strains, there is no need of any splint or rigid support. Exceptions to this rule may perhaps be found in the case of refractory children and of ignorant or stubborn adults. The fact that these persons are liable to use the hand at an early period, and in such a way as to cause a *slight* risk of displacement of the fragments, is evidence of the simplicity and painlessness of the injury and of the satisfactory manner in which union takes place, if reduction has been properly effected.

That the treatment of this fracture is misunderstood by many practitioners is evident to me from the fact that I have repeatedly been obliged to refracture and reduce partially-united fractures of this kind after several weeks' treatment in splints. In a number of instances an exceedingly good splint had

been applied though the fracture had not been reduced. A quite recent experience of this kind in which I refractured the bone eight weeks after the injury has forcibly brought the subject to my mind.

Osteotomy, for the purpose of correcting such deformities, is seldom if ever required. I have known a deformed fracture of the radius to be broken for re-adjustment five and a half months after the injury. To do this requires considerable power, but it can generally be accomplished by forcibly bending the bone across the operator's knee.

A few years ago, while holding a position as out-patient surgeon in one of the hospitals of this city, I had occasion to treat, within less than three months, forty-two cases of fracture of the lower end of the radius. Some of these were treated with the moulded metal splint recommended by Dr. Levis; others were dressed with a straight dorsal splint of wood; while in some the wrist was immobilized by means of a single strip of steel, or two or three strips of whalebone applied to the dorsum of the joint by means of adhesive plaster encircling the limb. A few were treated during a part of the time by applying to the palmar surface a curved steel strip, such as the "husk-bones" of corsets.

The accompanying table gives a brief account of the treatment, the time the splints were worn, and the results in these cases. In a few instances no results were recorded in the case-book, either because the patient discontinued attendance or because no unusual condition was found. It is very probable that in the latter case there was not much deformity or disability, else it would have been mentioned. There are a few other cases in the table in which the record is deficient in detail, because the patients were still under treatment when my term of service was completed.

It will be observed that six cases came to me with the lower fragment still unreduced, although in each instance a splint had been applied. In five of these cases Levis's moulded splint, the best splint manufactured for this fracture, had been applied. This fact proves my assertion that it is the custom of many to apply a splint, and often a very proper one, without reducing the fracture. It is this belief in the therapeutic value of the splint which causes many physicians to have bad results in the treatment of this fracture. If the profession were made to understand that no splint can be constructed which will take the place of reduction, better results would be more frequent.

It is interesting to note that all, or nearly all, of the cases tabulated had been originally dressed by the resident physicians belonging to the wards of the hospital. It is also worthy of comment that these residents belonged to a hospital with which at the time were connected two surgeons who have

TABLE OF FRACTURES OF THE LOWER END OF RADIUS.

Age.	Sex.	Treatment.	Days splint worn.	Result.	Remarks.
70	F.	Metal splint	...		Diagnosed sprain at hospital.
21	M.	Metal splint	8		
50	M.	Metal splint	17		
16	M.	Metal splint	9	Good union; no stiffness of fingers of wrist.	
63	M.	Metal splint.			
12	M.	Metal splint	17	No deformity; good motion; no stiffness.	
12	M.	Dorsal straight splint . . .	17		Palmar surface was vesicated by in-
60	F.	Metal splint	20	Good motion.	flammation; hence, used dorsal
24	M.	Metal splint	10	Good motion; no deformity.	splint.
65	M.	Metal splint	9	No deformity; good motion.	
38	F.	Metal splint; twelve days later steel strip on dorsum.	18		
40	F.	Metal splint	5	No deformity; no stiffness.	Examined five and a half weeks later; slight stiffness of wrist; some shortening on radial side.
19	M.	Dorsal straight splint put on November 3d, when I first saw him; had Bond's splint on previously.	13	No stiffness; some shortening on radial side.	Weak flexion of fingers; had palmar wound, but not down to fracture.
15	M.	Metal splint	14	Good motion; some bowing at lower end.	
16	M.	Metal splint; three days later, steel strip on dorsum.	7	Motion perfect.	Fracture three days old when first treated, and no deformity then existed.
55	F.	Metal splint	20	Some deformity; slight stiffness of forefinger.	Kept at home by illness; not seen regularly.
13	M.	Metal splint; one day later, steel strip on dorsum.			
68	M.	Metal splint	25 ?	Considerable stiffness.	
48	F.	Metal splint	...		When fracture was two days old re-duced again; much comminution: no record to show that it was properly reduced before I saw her.
18	M.	Metal splint; two days later, steel strip on dorsum.	10	Deformity from callus; good mo-tion.	Great deformity before reduction.
44	F.	Metal splint, two days ago, outside; but not reduced. Reduced, applied curved corset steel to palmar surface.	10		The time given is from the time I reduced the fracture.
17	M.	Metal splint; six days later whalebone strips to dorsum.	13	No deformity; perfect motion.	Great deformity before reduction under ether.
35	M.	Metal splint	14	No deformity; perfect motion.	
70	F.	Metal splint; two days later, curved cor-set steel to palmar surface.	15	No deformity; perfect motion.	
14	M.	Curved corset bone to palmar surface on day after injury; metal splint for one day.	8		
25	F.	Metal splint, three days ago, outside, but not reduced. Reduction, metal splint for one day, then curved corset steel to palmar surface.	7		The time given is from the time I reduced the fracture.
15	F.	Metal splint	17	As no note was made, probably good result.	Treated in hospital; on admi-sion great deformity, and had scalp wound; came to out-patient de-partment after union had occurred.
26	M.	Metal splint, three days ago, outside; nar-row curved corset steel to palmar surface	10	No deformity; no stiffness.	
39	F.	Metal splint.			
45	F.	Metal splint; three days later, curved corset steel to palmar surface.	13	Good result.	
35	F.	Metal splint			
54	F.	Metal splint; four days later, steel strip on dorsal surface.	...	No deformity.	
55	M.	Metal splint	...	Good result.	
35	F.	Metal splint; eleven days later, steel strip on dorsal surface.	...		Not seen after first dressing until eleven days had elapsed; Sick in bed at home during that time.
48	F.	Metal splint, two days ago, outside, but not reduced. Reduction.			
29	F.	Metal splint, two days ago, outside, but not reduced. Reduction.			
25	M.	Narrow corset steel on palmar surface, as there was no deformity.			
30	M.	Metal splint.			
52	F.	Metal splint.			
50	F.	Metal splint.			
40	F.	Bond's splint outside, but not reduced. Reduction, metal splint.			
48	M.	Metal splint	15	No deformity; perfect motion.	Much pain during treatment; chloral and morphine g ven; said to have been broken two years before.

written and done most effective work in teaching the pathology and proper treatment of this particular injury.

The table is instructive, I think, as showing that perfect motion without special deformity was obtained in almost every case. It must be remembered, in addition, that these records were made a few weeks after the receipt of the injury, and that the results, so good at that time, probably became more perfect after the lapse of a longer period.

At the present time I should be inclined in nearly all cases to treat the fracture without using any splint at all; or, at most, I should employ only a thin strip of steel or zinc, or a couple of pieces of whalebone, six inches long, applied to the dorsum of the wrist, and held in place by strips of adhesive plaster.

When the tabulated cases were treated the time during which restrictive dressings were continued was probably less than would be advocated by most surgeons. I have seen no reason to alter my practice in this regard, except perhaps to shorten the time still more. I am now convinced that a roller bandage or a strip of adhesive plaster applied to the wrist in a circular manner is all that is necessary, except in unusually complicated fractures. All ordinary forms of splints should, as a rule, be discarded as useless or dangerous.

The proper treatment of fracture of the lower end of the radius is *reduction*. Little else is required in the ordinary cases.

DISCUSSION.

In discussing this paper DR. WILLIAM HUNT said that he fully agreed with Dr. Roberts that the proper treatment of these fractures is prompt reduction, and that it makes very little difference what splint, if any, is used afterward, provided the pathology and the anatomy are kept in mind. He, however, advocated the use of a splint of some kind in nearly all cases, if only to relieve the patient of pain through the sense of support. He also said that the majority of Dr. Roberts's cases were last seen two or three weeks after they were discharged, whereas, it is six months or a year after the accident that the deformity usually becomes most manifest, as a result of the subsidence of the œdema. We may think that the result is perfect, but when the swelling passes away we may find that there is distinct deformity.

Years ago he had an opportunity to study the pathology of this fracture in a case in which it was necessary to amputate the arm on account of an injury of the elbow-joint. There was at the same time a characteristic radial fracture. In his account of the condition found he stated that there was no displacement of the ulnar side in ordinary cases, but that the hand, losing the support of the radius, falls away, leaving the ulna projecting. This is the deformity which in most cases becomes more apparent five or six months after the injury, and in the majority it is unavoidable. It does not, however, interfere with the use of the hand. Although the treatment

of fractures of the lower end of the radius is reduction, we should nearly always put the part at rest with a splint of some kind.

DR. O. H. ALLIS regretted that Dr. Roberts was not present to take part in the discussion. One of the saddest experiences in the duties of a physician is learning that he is not at liberty to do that which in his judgment is best; and this is especially true in the treatment of fractures. There is no department of medical or surgical practice so likely to drag the surgeon into the courts as that of fracture. There are defects other than deformity over which a surgeon has no control, and if a surgeon were to treat a fracture of any kind without splints, and deformity, paralysis, or any permanent disability ensued, the patient would have a strong case in the courts; and very few of the defendant's medical witnesses would be able to sustain him in his course.

THE PRESIDENT, DR. AGNEW, said that probably all would agree with Dr. Roberts that these fractures are badly reduced, and that if properly adjusted it matters little what splint is employed to maintain the fragments in position. To allow the patient, however, to go without any means for protecting the parts, is dangerous, and calculated to expose the surgeon to a suit for damages in the event of an accident, especially with a careless patient, who might take unwarranted liberties with the arm. It must not be overlooked that there are several tendons attached by loops of fascia to the bone, and one tendon implanted upon the latter, though Dr. Roberts states that there are no muscles to cause displacement. It will be difficult to persuade the profession, many of whom have had years of experience in the management of these fractures, to leave the bone without some fixed support.

DR. ALLIS said that with Dr. Roberts he recently attended a clinic of Dr. Pilcher's, in New York. A case was exhibited which had been treated without a splint. This was the first case he had seen treated in this manner, and he thought that it required a good deal of courage on the part of the surgeon. The necessity for a splint is less if the surgeon can see his cases frequently, than as in the country, where the cases cannot be seen so regularly.

DR. L. W. STEINBACH believed that he had seen almost all the cases to which Dr. Roberts referred, and that splints, in the proper sense of that term, were not used, although a strip of adhesive plaster was sometimes applied to remind the patient of the injury. Dr. Roberts sometimes used a corset steel with the curved end applied to the inferior part of the forearm and the hand.

He thought that Dr. Roberts made an important point when he said that the physician's mind should be disabused of the idea of the necessity of a splint. The physician often thinks that when he has applied a splint he has done his entire duty, and rarely dwells upon the importance of reduction. In many of the cases reported in the table a splint had been applied before the fracture was reduced.

DR. DEFOREST WILLARD, while recognizing that the splint does not cure the fracture and that reduction is the important element in the treatment, yet could see no reason why in the majority of cases of careless boys and men, and in fact in nearly all cases, we should not endeavor to maintain the fracture in position after reduction. Both the injury and muscular action aid in displacing the fragments. Splints are of use in maintaining the reduction, and are safer than leaving the individual simply with a piece of adhesive plaster, which, while it is a reminder, yet will not prevent injury from blows.

DR. JOHN B. DEAVER agreed with Dr. Roberts in some particulars, but said that if he did not know Dr. Roberts so well he would question the diagnosis in some of the cases of fracture of the lower end of the radius treated without splints. In the majority of his own cases the line of fracture was oblique and involved more than one-fourth of an inch of the radius—sometimes as much as one inch or one inch and a half. The extensor muscles of the thumb and the extensors of the carpus aid in producing deformity. He believed that in some of these cases the muscular fibres . become entangled between the fragments. Under such circumstances it would be almost, if not entirely, impossible to keep the parts in position without support. One of the cardinal principles in the treatment of fracture is immobilization of the joints on the proximal and distal sides of the fracture. This is just as true in fractures of the lower end of the radius, as it is in fractures of both bones of the forearm. He would not permit a fracture of his own radius to be treated without a splint, and he would not treat a patient in that way. It is contrary to all anatomical and pathological teaching. A simple transverse fracture—which is rare—in an intelligent person, requires only a light splint.

In the correction of deformities due to badly-set fractures he believes that osteotomy is more scientific than re-fracture and causes less injury to the soft tissues.

DR. J. EWING MEARS said that the subject was an interesting one. It reminded him that years ago he in connection with the other resident physicians of a large hospital came to the conclusion that the binder after labor was of no service and that it had simply a moral effect. During their term of service they tied a string around the abdomen after labor and believed that the effects were the same as those of a binder. He does not now believe that anything was gained by this, and thinks that patients would complain if obstetricians failed to apply a binder.

In regard to fractures of the lower end of the radius two points were dwelt upon. First, that there is no fracture in the body which is so often treated badly as this. It seems natural for the physician to suppose from the peculiar character of the splint usually employed that its simple application effects the reduction. Secondly, a properly-reduced fracture may result in deformity by reason of a badly-adapted splint. The treatment of fracture is reduction, and retention of the fragments by means of some appliance. The views expressed by others cover the entire ground. Dr. Hunt referred to an important point, namely, the comfort to the patient derived from a properly-applied support. And the President sounded a note of warning with regard to suits for malpractice in cases in which deformity may result.

DR. HUNT said that every hospital surgeon of large experience studies individual cases, and he could recall no ordinary fracture that he has not in some instances treated without splints. In these cases the fracture is reduced, placed in proper position and closely watched.

DR. ALLIS referred to the case of a man injured by a
24*

fall from a great height, who was brought to the Presbyterian Hospital, and died in about twenty hours. Among the injuries was a fracture of the lower end of the radius, which he dissected. The injury to the soft parts and bone was so great that if the man had lived the resulting inflammation would have unified all the tendons of the wrist so that no finger could move independently of the others. There was a fracture about three-fourths of an inch above the end of the bone, which ran part of the way across, then downward. The bone was broken into small pieces, as though the fragments had been forcibly rubbed together. The fragments were not interdigitating, and if placed in position would not have remained so. On the dorsal aspect, far removed from the seat of fracture, blood was found in the sheaths of the tendons and also in the bellies of the muscles. In cases of fracture we never know how much injury has been done at the time of the fracture. He has treated a woman who had a severe injury to the wrist from falling down stairs. It was compound, but at once made simple by organized blood-clot. The injury occurred three or four years ago, but the woman is still unable to close her hand. In other cases apparently with the same injury, the result is a perfect cure. The explanation of these cases is found in the different extent of the injury at the time of the accident.

THE MEDICAL TREATMENT OF PERITONITIS.[1]

BY JOSEPH EICHBERG, M.D.,
OF CINCINNATI, OHIO.

THE treatment of peritonitis must necessarily be adapted to the cause, and varies greatly as we are dealing with a primary or a secondary form of the affection. Yet, in many cases, the search for the cause is neither easy nor successful; and while uncertainty on this point may exist, our duty to the patient demands prompt action. The whole history of this affection is so recent that it is rather to be marvelled at that the plan of treatment now generally adopted has been matured in so short a time, and that, if properly carried out, it will in many cases prove so successful, independent of the causal condition.

A moment's consideration of the natural function of the peritoneum will help us considerably to understand why certain measures must be used to attain a favorable issue. As a delicate, smooth investment of nearly all the important organs of the abdominal cavity, its presence greatly facilitates those constant changes of size, position, and mutual relation that result from the various phases of the digestive process; its surface, kept constantly moist by the lymph that finds its way into the cavity, is never with an excess of fluid, because of stomata, or little lymph-mouths, that readily afford exit into the lymphatic circulation of any fluid that may

[1] Read before the Southwestern Ohio Medical Association, October 7, 1890.

accumulate in undue proportions—under physiological conditions.

With the appearance of inflammation the smooth, pliant, moist covering of the abdominal viscera becomes turgid and roughened, its surface covered with a viscid rather than a liquid product, its stomata closed, its cavity filled with the accumulated inflammatory exudations, for which there is no escape. It is now that the necessity for treatment arises. The patient, in the great majority of cases, experiences that symptom, common to many affections, of pain, and pain in a most severe and intolerable form. It is here that we have an indication both causal and symptomatic, for pain itself is prostrating, and pain will kill. The organs covered by the peritoneum are richly supplied with nervous connections, and through these they influence by reflex action the heart and circulation. We know the sudden, it may be fatal, collapse that follows a severe blow or injury upon the abdomen, and it is not difficult to believe that an irritation of less intensity and longer duration would bring about similar results. The pain in peritonitis is continuous, exaggerated by every movement, by. every breath; it excludes every other consideration, and prevents sleep and needed rest. It is here that opium comes to our aid—the sheet-anchor, as it has been called, in peritonitis, the splint to the wounded peritoneum. I speak now of cases of acute diffuse peritonitis, the cases that are commonly met with.

It has seemed singular to me, after all that has been written and spoken upon this subject, that it should so frequently be necessary to encourage physicians to a more ready resort to this agent. It would seem that the proper amount of attention has not been given to the teachings of Alonzo Clark, who has summed up his own therapeutic experience of more than fifty years in the article upon this subject in Pepper's *System of Medicine*. Why it is that where such obvious indications for a remedy exist, so many medical men manifest an ill-founded timidity I cannot understand. Assuredly, it can not be the fault of their teaching; and if they only dared to use it properly, their first experience with opium in peritonitis would soon give them the needed confidence to do right by their patients. I feel very strongly upon this point, because it has happened to me to see several cases that made a lasting and very unfavorable impression. In one of these, a case of puerperal peritonitis, seen in consultation not long ago, the patient had been receiving for six days—mark it well—an average of one-fourth of a grain of morphine daily. She had not slept one hour in all that time, and, it is almost needless to say, she died. In another case of acute peritonitis in a boy of fourteen years, I was assured by the attending physician that he gave a hypodermic injection of an eighth of a grain of morphine as often as he thought necessary—as though it were not necessary every half-hour !

The average medical graduate leaves college with the carefully-acquired information that the dose of opium is from one-fourth to one-half a grain, every three or four hours, but that there are marked idiosyncrasies, and that its administration must be anxiously watched. He will, accordingly, treat his case of peritonitis on this plan, constantly feeling uneasy lest in his absence the patient develop narcotism. Finding that no symptoms of poisoning develop he will rest satisfied that he has done the full measure of his duty, and will repeat the small dose every three or four hours in his next case.

It is no imaginary picture that I am drawing; it is what I myself have seen; and it is time that the profession learned to regard this timorous, fainthearted misuse of opium, deceiving alike to the practitioner and the patient, as malpractice; as criminal as the neglect to recognize a fracture, and place it in a suitable dressing. It has been said that there is no dose of opium for pain. This may be extended, and it may be as truthfully said that the smallest suitable dose of opium in peritonitis is that which will promptly carry the patient to the limits of narcotism, and that the frequency for its repetition is to be determined solely by the degree of narcotism. It is not conscientious regard for the patient's life that prevents the physician from following this plan. It is his own lack of courage which sacrifices the patient.

I am fully aware of arguments that have been advanced in answer to Dr. Clark's report of the case, who, at the height of the attack, received for six days the equivalent of from 421 to 467 grains of opium every twenty-four hours. It is said that of all this large amount but the smallest fraction was absorbed; that to get the proper dose it should be given hypodermically, etc. Supposing it was necessary to give 467 grains to obtain absorption for the amount required to cure the patient, then 467 grains was the proper dose in that case. Hypodermic medication, is unnecessary, as morphine can easily be given in concentrated solution by the mouth, and most of it will be absorbed before it enters the stomach, to say nothing of the intestines. The basis of some of the opposition is, that in the inflamed condition of the peritoneum, the mesentery and its contained vessels, and the intestines and their lacteals, are unable to perform their physiological duty. The full measure of their physiological duty, we will admit, but certainly not a large fraction of it, else how could nutrition be maintained ?

A word more as to the opium treatment. To secure its best effect it must be given early. It has for some time been my rule in every case commencing with fever, prostration, and an acute, localized, continuous pain, to begin the treatment at once with opium or morphine, without regard to the possibility of existing constipation. Should the painful symptoms subside in the course of a day or two the bowels may be opened by a mild saline cathartic, or, by what seems preferable to me, repeated minute doses of calomel; but opium first, and all the time, until convinced that peritonitis, in its diffuse form, has not developed. Little attention need be paid to the bowels at the start. Clark says that he has allowed patients to go for fourteen days without a stool.

The use of opium does not always prevent the regular evacuations, and I have seen a patient who had one movement daily during the entire course of the disease, though for two weeks he was receiving half a grain of morphine every hour, and, doubtless, many similar instances could be narrated. These cases should be regarded as exceptional, since the effect of the opium, as usually observed, is to retard greatly, if it does not wholly arrest, intestinal movements. By diminishing the frequency of respiration the opium tends to eliminate another source of pain, as well as to prevent that rapid spread of the disease which the constant attrition of diseased against healthy portions of the peritoneum will almost surely entail. Upon the circulation, too, the action of the opium must be regarded as largely beneficial. The slowing of the heart-beats with the rise in arterial tension following its use, are ample testimony that, if properly controlled, it is a cardiac tonic. We obtain this result at once, but it is necessary to carry the patient beyond this point, and to induce a sedative action on the circulation.

How are we to judge of the proper degree of narcotism, seeing that it is easy to carry the patient beyond the desired point, especially while employing such large doses? Not by the relief of pain, for this result may be attained early; nor by the contracted pupil, which also shows itself after very moderate doses. The index of the proper degree of narcotism is furnished by the respiration, the pulse, the continual drowsiness of the patient, and the partial relaxation of the abdominal wall. The frequency of the respirations, increased by the embarrassment of the abdominal movements, should be brought down to twelve or ten per minute, and maintained at this rate as long as the symptoms persist; should it fall below this limit, the interval between two successive doses can be lengthened. The pulse of peritonitis is hard and wiry; under the influence of these full doses of opium it becomes slow, soft, and compressible. The drowsiness of the patient is a symptom that should be watched by the physician himself, and not trusted to either

nurse or attendant. It should be a drowsiness from which the patient can be readily roused, and should never be allowed to become a stupor. It is well in connection with this, to bear in mind that the maximum effect of any dose of opium or its derivatives is not obtained until three hours after administration—a safe criterion in deciding the frequeney of repetition of our doses. With the patient fairly narcotized, there is slight relaxation of the abdominal muscles, the tympanites become less, with corresponding relief from the feeling of tension.

One effect incidental to the use of opium remains to be mentioned, and that is, its influence upon the secretions. It diminishes the saliva and the urine promptly and decidedly; it slightly increases the amount of the perspiration, and thus may aid in counteracting an excessive elevation of temperature. With regard to its use in peritonitis Brunton says that "Opium, by its action on the vaso-motor centre, and by its action also on the peripheral terminations of vaso-motor nerves, will prevent or diminish the reflex dilatation of the vessels, which the local irritation would otherwise produce; congestion will thus be diminished, and inflammation will be relieved." The action of opium in peritonitis is, therefore, probably twofold: First, it lessens peristaltic movements of the intestines, and thus diminishes local irritation; secondly, it lessens reflex activity of the centres through which local irritation causes dilatation of the vessels, and thus it diminishes peritoneal congestion.

The unpleasant effect of opium and its derivatives upon the secretions has led me to combine with it minute doses of a drug at one time very generally used in the management of this disease, but latterly decried on all sides: I refer to a salt of mercury, the mild chloride being the form commonly employed. The physiological effects of mercury and its salts upon the saliva and the urine are directly antagonistic to that of opium, both of these secretions being increased by its use. By combining with our opiate a small quantity of calomel we are frequently enabled to avoid the furred tongue, the dry lips, the pasty and unpleasant taste in the mouth, that so frequently attend the employment of large doses of opium. Nor need there be much fear of ptyalism when the two drugs are combined, as each in a measure counteracts the effects of the other. It is certain that mercury is tolerated better and for a longer time when combined with opium than when given alone.

Upon the urinary secretion the action of the mercurous salt is no less welcome. With the diminution of the secretion and the blunting of sensibility in the bladder, and with the impairment of muscular strength in the wall of this organ from the existing inflammation of its outer tunic, the expulsion of the urine is often effected with the greatest difficulty; at times, indeed, it becomes impossible. It is in relieving these symptoms that calomel often assists, especially when combined with digitalis in small doses.

It seems to me that calomel has yet another virtue that entitles it to particular consideration here, namely, its action upon the intestine and intestinal contents. It cannot longer be gainsaid that mercury and its salts in physiological doses act as cholagogues. As Brunton says in his admirable work upon pharmacology, "The real action of mercury as a cholagogue consists, not in its stimulating the liver to form more bile, but in removing more readily from the body the bile which is already present in excess." It appears to perform this function by stimulating the upper part of the small intestine, and thus causing the evacuation of the bile before time has been allowed for its reabsorption. The reasons for this supposition are: (1) That mercury is so beneficial in bilious disorders; (2) that it does cause the appearance of bile in the stools, for Buchheim has proved by analysis that the green stools which occur after purgation by calomel owe their color to bile; and (3) that in the stools passed after mercurial purgatives, leucin and tyrosin, the products of pancreatic digestion, have been found.

Now we know that one office of the bile is to promote peristalsis. If we can assist in regularly transmitting to the lower part of the intestine some of this fluid we counteract by just so much the obstinate constipation that, if too long continued, may in itself constitute a menace to the patient suffering from acute peritonitis. Bile also has a tendency to prevent decomposition of the residual alimentary mass, and it is assisted in this by the presence of mercury, which acts as a disinfectant of the intestinal contents. In peritonitis this tendency to decomposition is greatly assisted by the sluggish movement or inaction of the bowel, by the temporarily increased local temperature, and by the presence of a large amount of inflammatory fluid, and any remedy which can counteract this tendency is useful.

It has been my practice to combine one-tenth of a grain of calomel with each half-grain of morphine, and to continue the administration of both drugs until the bowels are easily moved. This result is generally obtained on the fourth or fifth day, when several stools are apt to follow in quick succession. Should the tendency to diarrhœa become annoying, the calomel is discontinued and the patient given a little of Hope's camphor mixture.

The only contraindication for the use of opium may be furnished by the condition of the kidneys. Chronic interstitial nephritis, so insidious in its onset that the patient himself has never received any warning of its presence, is very apt to be revealed by the excessive effect of a single moderate dose of an opiate. The tendency to uræmia seems to be favored, if manifested before, or even to be developed, when not previously indicated, by the use of opium. Even in peritonitis, where there usually exists so remarkable a tolerance for this drug, the ill effects have not been wanting; so that patients suffering from peritonitis, occurring in the course of chronic Bright's disease, have quickly passed into a state of uræmic coma, with no symptoms of narcotism, and have died comatose, without rallying from the first attack.

My preference for morphine has always been strong, and I am in the habit of giving it in the form of a standard solution in cherry-laurel water, one grain to the drachm. Of this solution a sixth, fourth, third, or half can easily be given, and the cherry-laurel water acts in part as a gastric sedative, preventing the tendency to vomit which morphine produces in some patients. Where this tendency nevertheless exists I have given the morphine by suppositories or have substituted codeine, which must be given in doses four times greater than those of morphine, but is easy to administer, and little likely to produce gastric derangement.

With symptoms that from the beginning are chiefly local, it is but natural that local measures should have early occupied a prominent place in treatment. The local application of leeches, the use of blisters and other powerful counter-irritants have had their place and are now, happily, no longer relied upon. Not so with topical applications intended, by their temperature, to influence the course of the inflammation. Cold applications, hot applications, turpentine stupes, flaxseed or other poultices have had their champions, and are still very commonly used. It is sometimes difficult to decide what form of application may be best suited to the individual case, but it is a safe rule, in every instance, to consult the comfort of the patient, and to let that influence the selection of hot or cold applications. All of these applications are open to one serious objection, namely, that they require to be constantly changed—the cold applications, lest they get too hot, the warm, lest they grow too cool; and in these frequent manipulations the tender abdomen is liable to fresh injury.

It was formerly the practice in acute peritonitis, when mercury stood high in favor as the preliminary step in all kinds of treatment, to apply freely mercurial ointment to the abdomen, the ointment being spread upon flannel or some other soft fabric and left in contact with the abdomen. In the reaction following the excessive use of mercury the drug in all its forms was practically banished from the materia medica, save for a few specific purposes, and this use of it in peritonitis was banished with the rest. But the pendulum has swung a little too far in the other direction, and, I think, we must again return to many of the things that were found useful by our fathers in medicine. For the last three years every case that has come under my care, in hospital or private practice, has been treated by the free application of mercurial ointment over the whole abdomen. It has promptly relieved the feeling of rigidity and painful distention; the immediate effect has been cooling and pleasant to the patients and the tympanites has subsided as quickly as after any other local application. It constitutes a dressing that easily adapts itself to the shape of the abdomen; it does not annoy by its weight; there is no wetting of the bedclothes, and the patient is not disturbed for its frequent removal, the ointment being renewed but twice in twenty-four hours. In all of these particulars it possesses decided advantages over other local applications: The mercury is evidently absorbed very slowly, for I have yet to see a case of ptyalism from its use; and in many instances it has remained in contact with the skin for two or three weeks.

Of the individual symptoms but two require especial mention in connection with the treatment, namely, the vomiting and tympanites. The former, which frequently ushers in the whole train of symptoms, is often so severe at the outset as to suggest intestinal obstruction; yet it is promptly controlled, as a rule, by large doses of opium. When occurring later in the disease, cracked ice taken freely into the mouth, small quantities of iced champagne, alone or in combination with aromatic spirit of ammonia, or half-drop doses of creasote in emulsion of sweet almonds, usually succeeds in controlling the trouble. Champagne has the advantage of being a stimulant and at the same time a gastric sedative; it is readily taken by children as well as by adults, and its use can be continued through the entire course of the disease.

Tympanites is always present to a greater or less degree but rarely, except in peritonitis of septic origin, and especially in those forms incident to the puerperal period, does it become excessive. The abdominal distention may, however, attain such proportions that the upward pressure of the diaphragm becomes a dangerous impediment to the circulation and respiration, and calls for immediate relief. A rectal tube carried high into the bowel, and left there, may accomplish all that is necessary; but this result cannot be confidently expected, since the gaseous distention is found mainly in the small intestine. Under these circumstances it has been recommended to puncture the bowel with a hypodermic or aspirator needle through the abdominal wall. I cannot regard such a plan as wholly devoid

of danger, and should resort to it only in extreme cases, selecting a needle of the smallest calibre to be found. It is true that puncturing a healthy bowel is a matter of very little moment, since the muscular layer quickly contracts about the minute orifice, thus preventing the escape of liquid or gaseous intestinal contents; not so when puncture becomes necessary as a curative measure. Is not the tympanites itself evidence of paralysis, or great loss of tone of the bowel; and would not the increased pressure within the intestine tend to favor the escape of some of the intestinal contents as soon as the needle is withdrawn? Such considerations call for the exercise of the greatest care and discrimination with regard to this step.

The diet should be liquid, easily assimilated, and of a kind likely to leave but little residue. Some form of peptones, or peptonoids, now readily obtained, or, if need be, prepared by artificial digestion, constitutes at once a palatable drink and a food. A little alcoholic stimulant, brandy or whiskey, may be added from the first, and will help to sustain the patient. There should be plenty of fresh air, with a limited number of attendants. Above all I would enforce rest and quiet; and the constant stream of visitors that besets so many a sick-room is to be wholly interdicted.

I have made no reference to surgical measures, because I have been here dealing with what is known as acute idiopathic peritonitis, and surgical treatment is never called for in this disease, unless the case ends in abscess or diffuse suppuration. But with prompt resort to the treatment as here outlined such a termination is unlikely; and even in many of the secondary forms, occasioned by typhlitis or perityphlitis this treatment will obviate the necessity for an operation, which, however brilliant its results, is yet a very grave step for the patient, and not to be undertaken rashly. Despite the almost reckless manner in which the peritoneum is now treated by surgeons, we have the opinion of so brilliant and renowned an operator as Schede, advising against surgical intervention in peritonitis, simple or acute, and in perityphlitis during the height of the process, unless it can be pretty clearly shown in the latter case that perforation and a distinct tendency to sacculation exist.

The treatment of chronic peritonitis need occupy us but briefly. It may, indeed, well be questioned if such a disease as chronic peritonitis ever occurs, excepting that due to tubercular or cancerous infiltration. In both of these conditions supporting treatment, fresh air, good hygienic measures, and, in case of tubercular disease, the selection of a suitable climate, indicate the extent of the physician's power.

In cases of tubercular or cancerous peritonitis it frequently becomes necessary to interfere, by surgical means, owing to great distention of the abdominal walls by fluid effusion. The operation of tapping is the classic remedy for this condition, but abdominal section, in the tubercular variety, seems to promise better results, as by means of it some cases have been cured. It is a question for pathologists whether these cases have really been tubercular in character, or whether the miliary nodules may not have been of the character of the tumors described as endothelioma, of which the peritoneum is the most frequent seat. At all events, we have not had records of every case successfully treated by incision, in which an autopsy subsequently revealed the return of the affection, nor can we understand from carefully-acquired knowledge of the life and habits of the tubercle bacillus how the mere exposure to the air for a few moments, and the contact with a warm solution of boric acid or plain boiled water, should permanently alter the conditions upon which its vitality depends. This question trenches, however, on the surgical aspects of the disease.

I am well aware that there can be no claim of novelty in the treatment here outlined, but it is sometimes desirable to burnish our old silver, and let the treasure appear in its true light.

THE EMPLOYMENT OF SPANISH MOSS (TIL-LANDSIA USNEOIDES) AS A SURGICAL DRESSING.

BY LOUIS McLANE TIFFANY, M.D.,
PROFESSOR OF SURGERY IN THE UNIVERSITY OF MARYLAND,
BALTIMORE.

THE holding of raw surfaces in accurate apposition, the abolition of dead spaces, and the exercise of physiological pressure over a wounded area, are essential to rapid healing. To abolish dead space and exert the proper amount of pressure is not always easy and is largely dependent on the material used as a dressing. During the early spring of 1889, when on a plantation in Louisiana, it occurred to me that the moss which hung from the trees would be a soft and elastic wound-dressing, so I brought some home with me. I found later that it could be obtained in a sufficiently clean condition at any upholsterer's, and since the date mentioned I have continued to use it with great satisfaction.

The moss, which hangs in festoons from the branches of trees throughout the Southern States, is of the pineapple family—sub-order, *Tillandsia;* species, *usneoides.* Stems thread-shaped, branching and pendulous; leaves thread-shaped; peduncle short; one-flowered. (Gray.) On the trees it is of a gray color, very curly, and is prepared for commerce by being dried and beaten so as to free it from bark. After this process it appears to consist of black, elastic, tough fibres, resembling curled hair.

I usually have the moss made into cushions or pads of about six inches by four inches, and two inches thick, cheesecloth being the material employed as a covering. The pads have been made of other dimensions; in one or two cases of mammary extirpation with extensive axillary dissection, pads large enough to envelop nearly one-half of the thorax were employed, but I find no advantage in the use of such large cushions, and the size given has proved very generally applicable.

The pads are adjusted outside of a gauze-and-cotton dressing, and the bandage applied snugly, the elasticity of the moss serving to distribute the pressure evenly. About the chest wall, as after a deep axillary operation, I have been especially pleased with the pads. A fact of a good deal of importance is that when exposed to the action of moist heat in a sterilizer, the moss remains elastic, so that the cushions are prepared with the other dressings for each operation.

AN ADDITIONAL NOTE ON THE EMPLOYMENT OF ANTIPYRINE IN PERTUSSIS.[1]

BY J. P. CROZER GRIFFITH, M.D.,
INSTRUCTOR IN CLINICAL MEDICINE IN THE UNIVERSITY OF PENNSYLVANIA.

TWO facts are to be prominently borne in mind in the employment of any drug in the treatment of disease. First, that no method of treatment is infallible, and that every drug will at times fail to produce the desired effect. Second, that success will sometimes depend on the adoption of *prudent courage,* and that a medicine should not be condemned as useless unless we are sure that it is the drug itself, and not the method of its employment which is at fault.

Soon after Sonnenberger's announcement[2] of the value of antipyrine in the treatment of whooping-cough, and stimulated thereto by his experience, I published[3] the reports of a number of cases treated in this way. Many of these proved that the drug is capable of exerting a very powerful influence upon the course of the affection. Since that time I have used the remedy in many cases, and usually with more or less improvement in the condition of the patient. In some instances the disease was favorably influenced in a remarkable manner, the paroxysms being greatly reduced in frequency, or in intensity, or in both. A large number of cases have been under my observation, however, in which this plan of treatment, now so generally in favor, was totally without effect, although as large doses were employed as I have, as a rule, found useful.

It has usually been my custom to begin the treat-

[1] Read before the Philadelphia County Medical Society, November 26, 1890.
[2] Deutsch. med. Wochenschr. 1887, 280.
[3] Therapeutic Gazette, February, 1888.

ment with 2 grains of antipyrine, given every three hours, in patients two years of age, or from 3 to 4 grains at four years of age, and to increase this somewhat if necessary. These doses seem at first sight somewhat large, but it is, I think, certain that children bear drugs of the antipyretic series much better, and in much larger doses, than do adults, whether in febrile or afebrile states. I have never seen bad results follow these doses, and believe that much larger ones could sometimes be employed with advantage in bad cases. It is possible that some of the patients whom I have recorded as unyielding to this form of treatment would have been relieved by a more heroic dosage. At any rate, it is beyond dispute that many of those physicians who have reported adversely regarding the administration of antipyrine in whooping-cough have erred in the manner of administration. In a very severe and fatal endemic outbreak which occurred in an institution in this city within the past few years, infants received an amount which could only be considered useless, and as no fair test of the value of the drug. Of course, in the instance referred to it was without effect. Quite recently, in another local outbreak, children of from two to nine years of age were given only from 1 to 2 grains three times a day, and were, of course, entirely unrelieved by it; the remedy consequently being regarded as useless in the treatment of whooping-cough.

I am led to report the following case because several physicians of my acquaintance, who have had a large experience in the diseases of children, have failed to obtain satisfactory results from antipyrine in the affection under consideration ; and the suspicion has arisen in my mind that the failure was, perhaps, due to an improper method of administration. The case is an instance of the advantage of a bold trial of large doses after small ones had proved useless :

Katie McD., four months old, only fairly well nourished and rather feeble, was brought to the Out-patient Department of the Children's Hospital, May 6, 1890. She was said to have been coughing for four weeks (although the exact time was uncertain), and was growing worse. It seemed that she was certainly approaching the height of the disease. The paroxysms were very frequent and very severe. As the child was evidently severely sick, and demanded vigorous treatment, this was commenced by giving ¾ grain of antipyrine every three hours; although this dose was so much larger than I had been in the habit of giving at this age, that I confess I was somewhat anxious lest the amount should prove injurious.

May 10. The child was no better, and was now having attacks of intense cyanosis and loss of breath after the paroxysms. These were so severe that the mother feared the child might die in one of them. As the antipyrine seemed to have failed to relieve,

and as the mother was prejudiced against it, my assistant in my absence replaced it by extract of belladonna $\frac{1}{18}$ grain, alum ½ grain, whiskey 30 drops every three hours.

19th. The attendant at the clinic rushed excitedly into the room, followed by the mother with the child in her arms. It had just had a severe paroxysm, and was, when seen, deeply cyanosed, entirely unconscious, and with its head hanging forward on its chest. Respiration had entirely ceased. The child was in fact apparently dead, and I feared that it was actually so, for only after some moments could respiration be induced. The mother reported that the child had been much worse, and had been having attacks similar to, though probably not so severe as this, every quarter-hour or half-hour during the preceding night. She was evidently much feebler, and the prognosis was most unfavorable. In truth, I never expected to see the little girl alive again. Feeling that treatment had been absolutely without service, and that nothing but the most energetic and rapidly-effective remedies could save the life of the patient, I returned to antipyrine, increasing the dose to *1 grain every three hours*, believing that if the medicine did not kill the patient the disease certainly would.

21st. The mother returned to the clinic with the little patient lying quietly asleep in her arms. The thought arose that she might be too depressed by the drug, or by the exhaustion from coughing, to stir, but inquiry showed that her strength and liveliness were greatly improved. During the remainder of the day of her last visit, May 19th, the cough did not improve. On May 20th she was still coughing, but evidently with much less severity, for there were no attacks of cyanosis. During the night of May 20th the child *had not coughed at all* until five o'clock in the morning, and from that time until seen in the clinic (after 11 A.M.) *there had been no paroxysms whatever.*

28th. The medicine was administered until May 25th. The child then whooped about four or five times a day, and slept at night.

This case is, of course, a remarkable one, and such sudden and complete recovery from so desperate a condition will probably seldom be observed under any method of treating pertussis. The treatment was heroic, but necessarily so. Antipyrine given in doses of this size cannot be without danger, and such doses are not to be generally recommended. Nevertheless it seems hardly questionable that in cases of life or death it is better to dare than to watch inactively our patients die. That large doses of antipyrine will save the life of every patient with whooping-cough is not to be expected, but that it may be of the greatest benefit to some is proved by this case. The drug may be expected at least to mitigate the intensity or the frequency of the paroxysms in a considerable proportion of cases. I have known it relieve children who were rapidly losing ground on account of inability to retain sufficient food to nourish them, and to relieve them to such an extent that they promptly regained strength. In some instances, as in this, the disease, while in the full vigor of the second stage, was either entirely, or almost entirely, checked. The administration of the remedy should be commenced in full doses and gradually increased, bearing in mind that though depression, and even collapse, may occur, yet the probability of these is exceedingly slight in afebrile cases as compared with the danger of it in febrile conditions.

TIN PLATES IN THE TREATMENT OF INDOLENT ULCERS.

BY E. R. MORAS, M.D.,
OF CEDARBURG, WIS.

ULCERS are perhaps the most tedious and unsatisfactory cases in minor surgery that the physician is called upon to treat. Although this applies more particularly to varicose ulcers of the leg, yet one meets with ulcers in other localities, and of different origin, which are very difficult to heal, such as many of the ulcerated surfaces remaining after freely-incised septic wounds of the hand, arm, foot, or leg, after suppuration following amputations, and, in fact, after any wound, accidentally or intentionally inflicted, in which the granulations from lowered vitality of the tissues fail to cicatrize.

The various methods of treating indolent ulcers, and the remedies used both in and out of the profession, are surely too numerous to mention, but they can be generalized thus:

1. The moist treatment: Ointments, pastes, washes, wet antiseptic dressings, etc.

2. The dry treatment: Iodoform, iodol, boric acid, oxide of zinc, bismuth, and other powders.

3. Compression: Flannel bandages, rubber bandages, adhesive plaster, and silk elastic stockings.

These may be considered the usual methods. In addition rest of the part is sometimes enforced.

4. Skin-grafting: Small grafts repeatedly applied, or large grafts, after the method of Thiersch.

5. Transplantation of a flap.

6. Tin-plate treatment.

The latter mode of dealing with ulcerated surfaces is probably a novel one to many, and in this paper the writer will claim that in ulcerated wounds, which do not heal kindly, the tin-plate treatment is more certain, more satisfactory, and less tedious, and effects quicker results, than the first three methods of the foregoing summary, and that it is much simpler and more generally applicable than the fourth and fifth methods. And this is claiming only what is proven by facts. Of the cases which were thus treated I will report two—one a hospital case, the other a case in private practice:

CASE I.—L., a man aged about fifty years, who I saw a year and a half ago in the Cook County Hos-

pital, Chicago. He was the first patient on whom the experiments were conducted. Each leg was the seat of an extensive, irregularly-shaped, foul ulceration, the results of a burn received two years before. One ulcer covered nearly one-third of the leg between the ankle and the knee. All forms of treatment had been tried for two years. To judge better of the effects of the tin plate I applied it over only a portion of one ulcer, selecting for the purpose the least promising one, situated over the inner aspect of the tibia. The remainder of the ulcer was treated with powdered iodoform. Four days later the dressings were removed, and the difference between the granulations covering the area over which the tin plate was used and those on the remaining surface was surprising. The former were smoother, cleaner, and healthier in appearance.

I now applied the plate over the entire surface of both ulcers. One week later the dressing was renewed, and an addition of one-fourth of an inch of new epidermis around the ulcer was found. Intervals of nine and ten days elapsed between this and the next two dressings, and finally the plate was left on for two weeks twice in succession. The smaller ulcer was then completely healed, and of the other a spot scarcely as large as a silver half-dollar remained. Satisfied that this would heal in a week or two, the patient asked to have the tin plate reapplied, and to be given his discharge.

CASE II.—A. L. received an injury to the left leg some twenty years ago, resulting in a chronic ulcer, which has since been almost constantly "running," and caused frequent disability. His occupation compels him to be on his feet during working hours.

When he submitted himself (which he did with great misgivings) to the tin-plate treatment, the leg was decidedly œdematous, excruciatingly painful at the ankle, and presented two scooped-out, gangrenous ulcers, measuring respectively 1⅜ by 1¼ inches, and 1¼ by 1 inch.

Simple washing with a 1-to-1000 bichloride solution was used, and the tin plate applied—the patient going to his work as usual. Four days later the sloughs had separated, and were removed with ease, the base of the ulcers already showed signs of activity, and their margins revealed a faint attempt at epidermization. In five more days the bases had attained the level of the skin, a decided growth of skin had taken place, there was but little œdema, and the pain had entirely disappeared. The dressings were subsequently renewed every sixth or seventh day, and both ulcers were found completely healed by the fifth week, the patient having lost not a single day of work.

REMARKS.—In the first case, ulcers which for two years manifested no inclination to heal under other forms of treatment disappeared under the use of the tin plates, and the time occupied in healing (about two months) was short enough to meet the most sanguine expectations. I may here remark that in this case Thiersch's method would have been at least partly a failure, owing to the condition of that portion of the ulcer corresponding to the inner aspect of the tibia, for there could be no hope of grafts "taking" upon that area until some means had been devised to cover it with fresh, healthy granulations.

In the second case healing progressed without interruption *while the patient followed his usual avocation.*

From both of these cases we may infer that no operative procedure is required, and the annoyance of frequent dressings may be done away with.

Now, as to the details of the treatment. Bichloride of mercury solution, 1-to-1000, oiled silk or rubber-tissue protective, common sheet tin, surgeon's adhesive plaster, dressing material, and bandages, are required.

away the offensive discharges surrounding the tin plate with plain warm water, or an antiseptic solution.

No preparatory treatment of the ulcer is needed, unless the granulations are unusually elevated above the skin, when they may be levelled by one application of lunar caustic.

The primary dressing should be renewed on the fourth or fifth day after its application. Owing to the effects of the pressure the ulcer may seem larger than before, and, according to the former character of the granulations, it is found covered with a thin layer of creamy exudate or with a layer of slough. Even if the ulcer was formerly very indolent, it will already show signs of physiological activity; new, healthy granulations will be seen here and there, and on close observation a narrow border of very delicate

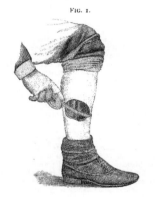

FIG. 1.

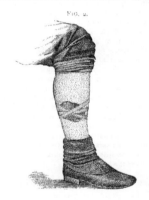

FIG. 2.

With ordinary strong shears cut a piece of tin corresponding to the shape and size of the ulcer, but large enough to overlap one-fourth of an inch of the surrounding skin. Slightly evert the sharp edge of the plate, and cut a piece of oiled silk or rubber-tissue protective, of the same size. These are placed in the bichloride solution. The ulcer and surrounding surface are washed with bichloride solution; the protective is then placed over the ulcer, the tin plate over the protective, and firmly fixed with adhesive strips. Be careful that the plate is adjusted with uniform pressure.

It is best not to encircle the part with the strips of plaster, which would interfere with the circulation, and, as happened in my first case, produce a new wound by the adhesive strips cutting into the integument. As a rule, only a light dressing, such as one of gauze, is necessary, for when the secretions are profuse the patient himself may be allowed to renew the outer dressing every second day, and wash

bluish-red epidermis may be seen creeping over the periphery of the wound, while the skin immediately surrounding it appears whitish and spongy. The same process continues between subsequent dressings, the granulations assuming a healthier appearance and activity, and epidermization advancing more rapidly.

When the ulcer is entirely healed it is advisable to reapply the tin plate for a week longer, that the delicate centre may have protection while it is becoming firmer. In cases which require it an elastic stocking of flannel bandage should be worn during the day as long as necessary.

The same piece of tin is used throughout the treatment, and is trimmed to meet the requirements of the varying size and shape of the ulcer. The first two, or possibly three, changes of the primary dressing are made at intervals of four or five days, after which it will seldom be necessary to change oftener than every eighth, ninth, or tenth day.

The good results will vary with the care and judgment used in fitting and fastening on the plate. Apply it snugly, and in such a way that the movements of the part will not displace it. Be careful that the edge of the tin is properly everted.

The tin and oiled silk, or rubber-tissue, might be perforated. I used them thus in the hospital, but not often enough to notice any special benefit resulting therefrom.

Were I to state the varieties of ulcers in which this plan of treatment gives the most satisfactory results, I would say that in varicose and other ulcers of the leg, in ulcers about the feet, hand, arm, and in amputation-stumps, it has given satisfaction.

The *modus operandi* of the tin plate in promoting the healing of indolent ulcers, which I have outlined for myself, may be an incomplete one. Some of the peculiarities of these ulcerations are : (1) That the granulations are raised above the level of the adjoining skin, which cannot creep over them ; or, (2) the granulations are depressed below the skin, and lack the vitality necessary to fill the hollow ; or, (3) they are constantly bathed in a profusely foul discharge ; or, (4) they are wanting in the proper stimulation that would enable them to accomplish their physiological purpose. It would seem that the tin plate remedies these defects in two ways, namely, as a stimulant and as a compressor. Being a smooth foreign body it acts as a gentle stimulant, and, by compression, it prevents profuse oozing, and keeps the granulating surface to the exact level of the skin, or the skin to the level of the granulations, and thus affords the epidermis an opportunity to spread over the ulcer.

TWO CASES OF PROSTATECTOMY.

BY J. WILLIAM WHITE, M.D.,
PROFESSOR OF CLINICAL SURGERY IN THE UNIVERSITY OF PENNSYLVANIA ; SURGEON TO THE UNIVERSITY AND GERMAN HOSPITALS.

DR. BELFIELD'S original operation, followed by Mr. McGill's admirable work in the removal of portions of the prostate in those cases in which catheterization has become impossible, or has ceased to give relief, and in which cystitis has developed and septicæmia or uræmia is imminent, have attracted the attention of surgeons everywhere, and vastly increased the number of cases submitted to similar operative procedures. It is, therefore, of special importance at this time that all such cases, with their results, favorable or unfavorable, should be published, in order that we may arrive, as soon as possible, at some definite conclusion as to the indications and contra-indications, as well as to the scope and limitations of this operation, so exceedingly important on account of the large number of men who are the subjects of prostatic hypertrophy, and because in aggravated cases the suffering is so great and the disability so complete. For these reasons I desire briefly to place upon record the following cases :

CASE I.—I. S., aged sixty-eight years, white, a hotel-keeper ; family history of tuberculosis ; always a moderate drinker, recently intemperate, Urinary symptoms began sixteen years ago ; catheter has been required at intervals for eight years ; for four years he has been unable to urinate at all without catheterism. Pain in hypogastrium has been progressively increasing until now it is constant and excruciating ; pain is also felt at the end of the penis and in the rectum. He has lost flesh rapidly, having gone down from about 170 pounds to 120 pounds. Is sallow and pinched in appearance ; has chronic bronchial cough ; eats and sleeps poorly. Urine scanty (20 ounces in twenty-four hours) and loaded with pus and vesical débris ; contains hyaline and granular casts. Physical examination *per rectum* reveals a prostate enormously enlarged both laterally and longitudinally, the finger being unable to reach its upper limit. The bladder contains a soft phosphatic stone of medium size. Mitral murmur of heart ; bronchial catarrh, with evidence of beginning consolidation at left apex.

The case seemed very unfavorable, but the patient's suffering was so great, and his condition so steadily deteriorating, that it appeared to be justifiable to run considerable risk in attempting to relieve him. An operation for the removal of the calculus at least was clearly required. Litholapaxy was slightly contra-indicated by the intense cystitis which existed, and by the probability of recurrence, as the calculus was phosphatic, and strongly by the fact that the retention would remain unrelieved. Perineal lithotomy was negatived on account of the size of the prostate, and because of the very insufficient digital exploration of the bladder which it would permit. Suprapubic lithotomy was therefore decided upon. The question of further operative interference, in case it was found practicable, with the object of removing the obstruction, was then submitted to the patient, with a fair statement of the attendant risks, which he promptly decided to accept.

The patient was carefully prepared by rest in bed, milk diet, attempted sterilization of urine by boric acid administered both by the mouth and by vesical irrigation, full doses of quinine, etc. At the time of operation the bladder was rendered accessible and opened in the usual manner. An oval rectal bag was used, and filled with eight to ten ounces of water. Ten to twelve ounces of warm boric-acid solution were injected into the bladder, which was reached by a linear incision three and a half inches long just above the pubes. The walls were transfixed with silk threads held by an assistant. The stone, which lay in the bas fond, crumbled down under the touch of the forceps, and had to be removed by the finger and a scoop. It was then found that both the middle and lateral lobes were greatly enlarged and projected far into the bladder. The mucous membrane was at places was snipped through with scissors, and the major portions of the projection removed by enucleation with the finger.

This required the exercise of only moderate force, and was not attended by any considerable hæmorrhage. The pieces removed, eight in number, varied in size from a hickory-nut to a large walnut, and weighed three ounces. A large drainage-tube was inserted into the bladder and held in place by a stitch through one wall of the wound. A suture was inserted at each angle. The patient was returned to bed, with the wound dressed, fifty-five minutes after the incision was made, some delay having been caused by the difficulty in extracting the fragments of calculus from the deep parts behind the prostate. He was moderately, but not dangerously, shocked, and in ten hours had a normal temperature and a pulse of 100.

For three days the outlook was most favorable. There was not a single alarming symptom. The temperature reached 100° once on the second day, but fell again to normal, and subsequently was normal throughout with the exception of a few hours on the fourth day, when it again rose to 100°. Milk was taken freely, the patient was rational and comfortable. About the middle of the fourth day, however, he suddenly developed a maniacal delirium with excessive restlessness, wakefulness, jactitation, etc. He obstinately refused food, took off dressings when he had an opportunity, and had to be kept in bed by force. His tongue became dry and dark, and his pulse increased in frequency, but there was neither chill, sweating, nor rise of temperature. The urine continued to flow from the wound, which was irrigated daily with boric acid, with listerine, with phenol sodique. Various sedatives and hypnotics were used without effect, attempts at stimulation were equally useless, and the patient finally passed into a condition of stupor and died seven and a half days after the operation.

The following are the notes of the autopsy: Man, five feet seven; emaciated, pallid. Wound, two and one-half inches long in the linea alba, extending upward from symphysis pubis. Walls healthy, granulating. Genito-urinary organs and rectum removed together. Bladder shows granulating surfaces where portions of prostate were removed, but these are much smaller and much less noticeable than might have been expected. Lower portion of prostate and wall of bladder intact. No injury to rectovesical septum or to urethra. No other foci of suppuration or ulceration present. Bladder capacions and moderately hypertrophied. Ureters distended to nearly the size of the wrist. Kidneys almost completely disorganized, containing multiple purulent collections, showing scars of previous abscesses, and rendered almost useless by chronic nephritis, scarcely any secreting structure remaining. Abdomen, organs healthy. Thorax, tubercular changes in both lungs. Cranium not opened.

REMARKS.—As I look back upon the case I may make the following criticisms of my own course:

1. It would have been wiser in the presence of scanty urine, tube-casts, and rapidly-increasing emaciation, and with a history of sixteen years of obstructive disease, to be content with supra-pubic lithotomy and permanent drainage. In only one of Mr. McGill's twenty-four cases had the symptoms extended over sixteen years or more. In that case only a portion of the prostate the size of a pea was removed, the patient was not much relieved at the end of six weeks, and his further history was not traced. The next case in order of duration of symptoms had extended over fourteen years. Three portions the size of a bean were removed. The patient died the following day. His kidneys were healthy. None of the other cases approached these in length of continuance of urinary symptoms. It may certainly be assumed that the possibility of the existence of serious disease of the urinary tract above the bladder increases in every case in a direct ratio with the duration of obstructive disease anterior to that organ. Indeed, we know that even frequency of micturition is of itself a competent cause of ureteral dilatation, hydro-nephrosis, etc., and when to these factors are added such grave vesical changes as occur in these cases, it becomes a matter of astonishment that healthy kidneys are ever found in these patients.

2. I should probably have used chloroform instead of ether in view of the renal disease which I knew to exist, and which might have been fairly supposed to be extensive. It will be noticed that death did not occur from any form of septicæmia or pyæmia. It was undoubtedly uræmic, and it may have been hastened or precipitated by the employment of 10½ ounces of ether, many of the recorded ether-deaths having occurred in patients with chronic nephritis.

3. After the prostatectomy was decided upon and was begun, I might perhaps have been content with a much less thorough and extensive operation. Just here is emphasized the need of a large collection of similar cases reported in considerable detail, such as is now being made by Dr. Belfield.[1] I did not know then how much of the projecting prostate it was necessary to remove to insure subsequent spontaneons evacuation of the bladder. The risk of hæmorrhage, of shock from prolongation of the operation, of septic trouble from a larger absorbent surface, are all directly increased with the amount of the prostatic overgrowth which is removed, and it will be quite important in the future to know how little we may do with a reasonable prospect of resulting benefit.

In none of Mr. McGill's cases, where the weight of the portions removed is given, did it reach three ounces. In one both lateral lobes were removed in seven pieces, weighing two ounces and thirty grains.

---

1 Since writing the above, Dr. Belfield's summary of cases has been published, and cannot fail to help us greatly in the attempt to arrive at definite conclusions as to the indications for and the value of the operation.

The patient died some months later. In another the piece removed weighed two ounces and forty grains. The patient died in thirty hours. We have not even now enough cases to generalize from, but it is significant that of the three deaths in Mr. McGill's table directly due to the operation, one was in a patient who had had symptoms for fourteen years; two underwent the removal of *large* portions of the prostate; and all three had bladders with thickened and hypertrophied walls. It is probable that we will find in these facts a valuable guide to our future work in this direction.

CASE II.—A year ago, discovering a small, hard stone in the bladder of a gentleman sent to me from a neighboring city, I advised median lithotomy. The patient was forty-three years old; had been a free liver; came from a gouty family; had had gonorrhœa twice in his youth, and with one case had an attack of acute prostatitis as a complication. He had a urethral stricture, calibre 23 French (normal calibre about 32), four and one-half inches from the meatus. His urinary symptoms had for years been referred to that, and he had never before been examined for stone. On introducing the vesical sound I had some difficulty in passing it through the prostatic urethra, but as he was hyperæsthetic and very nervous, I was not clear as to the cause. Examination *per rectum* disclosed a prostate which I noted at the time in my case-book as "very moderately enlarged, but distinctly indurated." His urine showed quantities of pus and phosphates and oxalates in great excess, but there were no tube-casts. I advised lithotomy on account of the existence of the stricture, the presence of the cystitis, and the hardness and small size of the stone, which was presumably a mulberry calculus. Measurement by introduction of a very small lithotrite (child's size) showed that the stone was not more than a half to three-quarters of an inch in diameter, and confirmed the impression of its density given by the sound. The passage of the lithotrite was likewise difficult, gave rise to extreme pain, and was followed by profuse bleeding—facts which also influenced me in my selection of lithotomy, the small size of the stone leading me to choose the median variety of that operation.

A few days later, after the usual preparatory treatment, I cut him at his home. As the knife passed from the membranous to the prostatic urethra I remarked upon the almost cartilaginous density of the tissue through which I was cutting, and upon the great increase of the "perineal distance"—the distance from the junction of the membranous and prostatic urethras to the most distant point of the median enlargement within the bladder.[1] This distance, I should think, was not less than three and one-half inches, and it was only by having the hypogastrium strongly depressed that I could reach the bladder with the tip of my middle finger. A small pair of forceps was introduced, and after a

little difficulty the stone was caught and extracted. Further digital exploration showed that the middle lobe of the prostate was enlarged, distinctly pedunculated, and projected directly upward. I seized this projecting portion, which was really intravesical, first on one side of my incision and then on the other, with strong forceps, and by dissection with my finger-nail, and by dragging and twisting strongly with the forceps I succeeded, with some trouble, in removing two small particles, each the size of a hickory-nut, and looking to the naked eye, and on section with the knife, not unlike scirrhous carcinoma. As the patient bled freely, and the separation of the fragments required the use of so much force, and as I had not discussed with him or his family the propriety of any operation except that of lithotomy, I decided to refrain from further interference. I did so, however, without much hope of having given him permanent relief from his urinary symptoms.

The specimens were submitted to Dr. John Guitéras, Professor of Pathology in the University of Pennsylvania, who reported the growth as "a pure fibro-myoma with no admixture of suspicious elements of any sort." The patient convalesced without a bad symptom, and was out of bed with the wound healed in two weeks. He was in my office within a few days on account of a recent urethritis, and reports himself as free from all vesical symptoms.

REMARKS.—In this case, as I saw the patient but once before the operation, I neglected to inquire into the existence of residual urine. The absence of any lateral prostatic overgrowth, as revealed by rectal touch, prevented me from attaching much importance to the prostatic hardening which I did feel. The difficulty in the introduction of instruments seemed sufficiently explained by the great sensitiveness of the patient and by possible urethral and prostatic spasm dependent on the stricture and the calculus. If it had not been for these circumstances I would doubtless have discovered the prostatic growth earlier, as I was, of course, aware that intravesical growth sufficient to cause marked urinary symptoms frequently exists without any appreciable enlargement toward the rectum. I am not at all sure, however, that such a discovery would have been to the advantage of my patient. If a prostatectomy in addition to a lithotomy had entered into my calculations I would probably have selected the suprapubic route for the performance of both operations. Indeed, after having made the median incision and discovered the depth of the perineum I would have been justified, according to excellent authority,[1] in employing hypogastric section and cystotomy then and there. I could by no possibility, however, have had a better result.

Perineal prostatectomy as an accidental or inter-

---

[1] Watson: The Operative Treatment of the Hypertrophied Prostate.

[1] Watson: loc. cit. Belfield: American Journal of the Medical Sciences, November, 1890.

current complication of perineal lithotomy has been known since the days of Fergusson, and has never had a large mortality. Its usefulness, however, is confined to the class of cases like this one, in which the obstructive cause consists of an enlarged and pedunculated middle lobe. The other varieties described by McGill (and by Brodie, Cadge, Thompson, and others before him), viz, the collar enlargement, the hypertrophy of the lateral lobes, or of either of them alone, or the hypertrophy of all three lobes, are unquestionably to be dealt with most satisfactorily by suprapubic cystotomy; but it must be noted that the latter operation has a mortality of 16 per cent. as against 9 per cent. by the perineal method.[1] It seems to me that one explanation of this fact lies in the comparatively moderate interference with the prostate which this method permits of. I feel sure, at any rate, basing my opinion on general surgical principles, that some of the recent teaching on the subject touches too lightly on the increase of danger which must necessarily be associated with more extreme removals of portions of the prostate. Belfield, speaking of the possibility of return, says, for example:[2] "An important deduction from these considerations is the indication for thorough enucleation of all circumscribed masses within as well as above the general prostatic surface. Such tumors can be enucleated with surprising rapidity." "An important advance in the removal of prostatic obstructions is the enucleation of all accessible masses in the substance of the organ instead of a simple levelling off, etc." McGill[3] and Mayo Robson[4] write in the same vein. I believe in the future of the operation, and think that in carefully-selected cases it is likely to have a progressively smaller mortality, but I do not think it one to be undertaken lightly, and I am quite sure that it is not proper to adopt it as a routine method of treatment in all prostatics.

A considerable proportion of patients with obstructive prostatic enlargement can be made perfectly comfortable by the use of a Nélaton or Mercier catheter, provided the instrument is scrupulously sterilized before and after each introduction. It should be employed by the patient himself from one to three times daily, according to the amount of residual urine. Such patients may go on for years in this manner with little or no difficulty, and do so with increasing frequency since the importance of urinary antisepsis has been realized and its details perfected. In spite of every precaution, however, a number of cases break down, the catheter cannot be passed without distress, or without causing troublesome bleeding, or occasionally cannot be

passed at all. The urine becomes ammoniacal and stinking. Vesical tenesmus is constant and severe. These are the symptoms which, above all others, indicate the performance of prostatectomy, viz., difficult and painful catheterization and the occurrence of marked and persistent cystitis.

In the presence of those symptoms, in a person of average strength and vitality, the surgeon should, in my judgment, proceed in one of the two following ways:

First: Introduce Syme's staff into the bladder, and make a small incision through the perineum and the membranous and prostatic urethra. Introduce the finger into the bladder. If a pedunculated middle lobe is found, enucleate it with the finger, or twist it off with forceps, as in the above case. Put in a large drainage-tube, and allow it to remain for a week or two.

Or, second, make a suprapubic cystotomy, remove only such portions of the prostate as are manifestly obstructing the urethral orifice, and then if the urethra is not free complete the operation by doing an external perineal urethrotomy

Statistics are not yet numerous enough to allow us to be dogmatic as to the relative merits of these plans, but I am inclined to think that in the majority of cases the second is the one to be preferred.

In cases markedly feeble, and especially in those with chronic nephritis, it is best to be content with establishing perineal drainage.

HOSPITAL NOTES.

CYSTITIS.

Abstract of a Clinical Lecture delivered at the Chicago Policlinic.

BY WILLIAM T. BELFIELD, M.D.,
PROFESSOR OF SURGERY.

DR. BELFIELD presented six cases which were sent to him with the diagnosis of cystitis, but which illustrated the fact that cystitis is a secondary affection, and that therefore the first step in the treatment must be a search for the cause, that is, the primary morbid process. We should remember, he said, that cystitis is—like jaundice and dropsy—a result, a symptom of disease, and not the primary disease itself; and that the cause of the trouble may be found anywhere in the urinary tract from the meatus to the capsule of the kidney.

CASE I.—A robust man, twenty-one years old, who had had for the past six months gradually-increasing frequency of, and pain during urination. He now evacuated the bladder every hour, day and night, the act being accompanied with pain along the entire urethra. On standing, the turbid urine deposited a slight amount of pus.

Examination excluded morbid conditions of the meatus and prepuce, stricture, and stone. The right epididymis presented, however, a hard, painless swelling, in places distinctly nodular, a condition which the patient

[1] Belfield, loc cit.   [2] Loc. cit.
[3] British Medical Journal, October 19, 1889.
[4] Ibid., March 9, 1889.

first noticed nearly three years ago. This swelling was evidently tubercular, and gave a clue to the cause of the cystitis, the tuberculous process having doubtless found a foothold at some point in the genital outlet near the bladder.

Upon rectal examination a distinct hard thickening near the right seminal vesicle at the apex of the prostate was found. The process probably extended to the vesical surface of the prostate, where it could be recognized by means of the cystoscope.

CASE II.—A man, fifty-five years old, whose symptoms dated back one year. After the patient had urinated Dr. Belfield introduced a soft catheter and withdrew one ounce of residual urine. Rectal examination showed an increased vertical diameter of the prostate. This case was evidently one of chronic retention from prostatic obstruction.

CASE III.—A man of thirty-five years, with a history of cystitis for three years. Examination of the pelvic and external organs was negative, but a hard painless body was discovered just below and adjoining the right kidney. The disease was tuberculosis of the kidney, and illustrated the fact that symptoms of cystitis are frequently produced by morbid conditions of the pelvis of the kidney.

CASE IV.—A boy of nineteen years, who was sent to Dr. Belfield eight weeks previously with the history that for six years he had usually been obliged to urinate at least once every hour, though occasionally enjoying a respite for a few days. His urine contained a small amount of pus. A sound entered the urethra to the prostate without obstruction, but was stopped in the prostatic urethra, as determined by the finger in the rectum. No instrument could be made to enter the bladder except a small flexible bougie. Perineal urethrotomy was performed, and the obstruction found to be a hypertrophied prostatic ring (internal sphincter), an unusual condition in young men. The body of the gland was not enlarged. The constricting ring was thoroughly stretched with forceps and with the operator's fingers.

The patient stated that since the operation he has been able to retain his urine for from three to five hours without discomfort, and has gained fifteen pounds in weight and feels perfectly well.

CASE V.—A man of twenty-seven years, who had had the usual symptoms of cystitis, associated with considerable aching in the perineum, for two years. Dr. Belfield said that the last symptom suggested the condition which, upon examination, was found to exist, namely, chronic inflammation of the posterior urethra. During the last month he had given the patient twelve deep injections of nitrate of silver solution of a strength of seven grains to the ounce. The symptoms have almost disappeared.

CASE VI.—A man of forty-three years, of full habit, who for three years had been treated by different physicians by nearly all the usual remedies for cystitis, both local and general. After a careful examination some three months ago, Dr. Belfield suspected a calculous pyelitis of moderate extent. Treatment with the object of relieving this produced, however, no improvement, but within two weeks an attack of severe renal colic occurred, and was followed by the expulsion of three uric-acid calculi—the largest of which was about

the size of a bean. Complete recovery from the " cystitis " ensued.

MEDICAL PROGRESS.

Treatment of Gastric Ulcer.—DONKIN (*Wiener medizinische Presse*, November 2, 1890) thinks that the best results in the treatment of gastric ulcer are obtained by giving the patient neither food nor medicine by the mouth, and relying upon rectal alimentation. He does not believe that gelatin suppositories and peptonized preparations have any advantages over beef-tea and milk in rectal feeding. The patient should receive at intervals varying in different cases 2½ ounces of beef-tea and from ½ to 1 ounce of brandy either with or without the yolk of an egg. An equal amount of milk may be substituted for the beef-tea, or the enema may consist of equal parts of each. It is necessary to wash out the rectum before each injection and if it becomes very irritable a few drops of laudanum may be given with each enema. By the mouth, the patient may be occasionally given a small piece of ice but absolutely nothing else. Morphine, given subcutaneously to allay the pain, the author considers the most useful drug that we have in the treatment of gastric ulcers.

In Donkin's experience this treatment causes the gastric symptoms to disappear in from ten to nineteen days, when in addition to the enemata small quantities of milk and bouillon may be given by the mouth. The author has also adopted this method in the treatment of many obstinate cases of dyspepsia.

Guaiac as a Laxative.—MURRELL (*Medical Press and Circular*) thinks that guaiac is a valuable laxative. His attention was drawn to the subject, two years ago, by casually prescribing guaiac lozenges made up with blackcurrant paste, for a man suffering from rheumatism. The man continued taking the lozenges long after the pain had ceased, and in explanation said that they did him good by acting on the liver and bowels, and said that one or two of the lozenges taken in the morning before breakfast produced a stool promptly and without inconvenience. The author ordered the lozenges for others of his patients suffering from constipation, and what is conventionally called "biliousness," and the results were equally satisfactory. The lozenges not being available for hospital use, he had a confection prepared containing ten grains of guaiac resin to one drachm of honey. This, for the last two years, he has used extensively not only as a purgative, but in the treatment of chronic rheumatism, sciatica, tonsillitis, dysmenorrhœa, and allied affections. He gives from one to two drachms three times daily. The purgative effect is very pronounced, and in one case the patient had fifty-six evacuations in one week. In another case it produced a well-marked rash, covering the arms and legs with an eruption which forcibly reminded one of a copaiba rash. It was accompanied by intense itching which disappeared on discontinuing the drug. The guaiac not infrequently gives rise to a burning sensation in the throat, and to obviate this he prescribes ten grains of the resin in half an ounce of extract of malt. He believes that a trial of guaiac, either as a laxative or purgative, according to the dose employed, will be found satisfactory. It is possible that if the drug were triturated with cream of tartar, or with some inert substance, such as sugar of milk, its efficacy would be increased, and that it would produce the desired effect in smaller doses.—*London Medical Recorder*, November 20, 1890.

Iodide of Potassium in the Treatment of Urticaria.—STERN has successfully treated five cases of chronic urticaria by the administration of iodide of potassium, four of the cases having been rebellious to all the measures usually employed in this disease. The fifth case was one of acute urticaria of a few days' duration. None of the patients were syphilitic and all were rapidly cured. In one case which had lasted for four months the intolerable itching disappeared on the second day of treatment, and a complete cure was obtained after two and a half drachms of the iodide had been administered. In two other cases, one of two years' and the other of six years' duration, the effect of the iodide was equally good, cure following the administration of six and eight drachms respectively.—*London Medical Recorder*, November 20, 1890.

Somnal.—As a result of several experiments upon animals and fifty-four administrations to man DR. W. GILMAN THOMPSON (*New York Medical Journal*, Nov. 29, 1890) comes to the following conclusions:

1. The effects of somnal are much more striking and certain than those of urethan, and far less depressing than those of chloral.

2. There is no vertigo or depression after taking somnal, such as may follow the use of sulphonal.

3. The action of somnal is usually very prompt, and doses of half a drachm disguised in a little syrup of tolu or whiskey are always well borne, easily taken, and entirely without deleterious effects.

4. The drug in doses of a drachm is not powerful enough to control decidedly delirium tremens, maniacal delirium, or severe pain.

5. In doses of from thirty to forty minims somnal is a safe and reliable hypnotic for ordinary insomnia.

Creolin in Diseases of Children.—SCHWINZ has used creolin in the treatment of a number of infantile diseases. In ten cases of purulent ophthalmia in the newborn irrigations with a one-per-cent. solution were practised. In two of these cases in which the disease was not very intense there was complete cure at the end of six days. In the eight remaining cases irrigations were continued for four or five weeks but the results were not satisfactory, and recourse was had to solutions of boric acid and nitrate of silver. A solution of the strength of one or two per cent. of the latter was used by instillation and caused less pain than the creolin solution.

Eleven cases of thrush and aphtha which had been treated for a long time with potassium chlorate, potassium permanganate, and boric acid without appreciable results were cured by irrigations of the mouth and pharynx with one-per-cent. solution of creolin.

In cases of umbilical periphlebitis the use of an ointment of creolin was followed in four days by complete disappearance of the inflammation. The author also writes that the use of pure [?] creolin by friction will give gratifying results in the treatment of erysipelas.

In five cases of acute gastro-enteritis creolin was given according to the following formula, and caused the symptoms to disappear in from three to six days:

R.—Creolin . . . . 3 drops.
Canella water . . . 2½ ounces.
Syrup of mallows . . . 6 drachms.

Dose for very young children, a small teaspoonful every hour. For older children the creolin may be given in powders thus:

R.—Creolin . . . . . 15 minims.
Sugar . . . . . 75 grains.—M.

Divide in ten powders and give one or two daily.

In the surgical diseases of children creolin, according to the author, may be used in the strength of from one-half to one per cent. to produce asepsis of the surface and cavities of the body without fear of poisoning.—*Archives of Pediatrics*, December, 1890.

Pambotano: a Substitute for Quinine.—According to *Le Progrès Médicale*, a decoction of pambotano, the root of the *Calliandra Houstoni*, is proposed as a substitute for quinine. Very few cases in which it was used have been reported, and it is impossible as yet to form any opinion of its value.

Application for Chronic Pharyngitis.—The *Canada Lancet* quotes the following prescription for the treatment of chronic pharyngitis:

R.—Ergotin . . . . 15 grains.
Tincture of iodine . . 1 drachm.
Glycerin . . . . 1 ounce.—M.

To be applied three times daily, with a soft brush.

Strophanthus in the Treatment of Exophthalmic Goitre.—In a paper read before the New York State Medical Association (*New York Medical Journal*, November 8, 1890), DR. E. D. FERGUSON reported several cases of exophthalmic goitre in which the administration of strophanthus afforded prompt relief, the patients being able to return to their ordinary occupation. As was expected, however, in no instance was either the exophthalmia or the goitre removed, although in each there was decided improvement. The pulse-rate and the rhythm of the cardiac contractions improved even in cases in which there was undoubtedly dilatation of the left ventricle, and in the latter cases all the signs and symptoms of dilatation disappeared. The only preparation of the drug used by Dr. Ferguson was the tincture, which was given by the mouth three times daily during meals, the initial dose being from eight to ten drops, which was increased, if necessary, to reduce the frequency of the pulse, to fifteen, twenty, or even twenty-five drops.

Insoluble Tablets of Antipyrine.—According to DR. ARNOLD, of Zug (*British Medical Journal*, October 4, 1890), many of the tablets of antipyrine, antifebrin, and other new preparations, pass through the alimentary canal undissolved. This fault is easily remedied by having a thin layer of powdered sugar or tragacanth interposed between the layers of the tablet. He advises that physicians from time to time test the solubility of these tablets by placing them in water.

THE MEDICAL NEWS.

A WEEKLY JOURNAL
OF MEDICAL SCIENCE.

COMMUNICATIONS are invited from all parts of the world. Original articles contributed exclusively to THE MEDICAL NEWS will be liberally paid for upon publication. When necessary to elucidate the text, illustrations will be furnished without cost to the author.

Address the Editor: H. A. HARE, M.D.,
1004 WALNUT STREET,
PHILADELPHIA.

Subscription Price, including Postage.

PER ANNUM, IN ADVANCE . . . . $4.00.
SINGLE COPIES . . . . 10 CENTS.

Subscriptions may begin at any date. The safest mode of remittance is by bank check or postal money order, drawn to the order of the undersigned. When neither is accessible, remittances may be made, at the risk of the publishers, by forwarding in *registered* letters.

Address,   LEA BROTHERS & CO.,
Nos. 706 & 708 SANSOM STREET,
PHILADELPHIA.

SATURDAY, DECEMBER 13, 1890.

DR. BILLINGS AND THE SURGEON-GENERALSHIP.

THE President of the United States is again called upon to fill the high office of Surgeon-General. The task is not an easy one, and we feel it our duty to speak briefly but strongly upon the question. From an early day the principle of seniority has been discarded in filling this office. Barnes and Crane were promoted over the heads of a considerable number of seniors, and we hold that it is essential for the good of the country and the service that this policy should be followed. The best man for the place should be chosen irrespective of seniority. The great scientific and sanitary questions which agitate the medical world to-day have important bearings upon the medical service of the Government, and may require a man who is thoroughly abreast of the times, and fully equipped with the latest attainments of science. The office is not wholly, or perhaps chiefly, a scientific one, however ; the Surgeon-General has important executive and administrative duties as well. The general supervision of the great National Museum, and of the famous Library of the Surgeon-General's Office, and of the Government hospital system throughout the country, are among the matters which devolve upon him. He must have strict financial methods, and should be a man of business training and ability. He must be a good judge of men, and able to make his appointments so as to get the right men in the right places, and to get the greatest amount of work out of all of his assistants and associates. Our national medical service now enjoys a high reputation the world over, and it is the duty of the Government to make an appointment at the present juncture that will not only maintain, but enhance this good reputation.

For all the reasons above urged we hold it of the first importance that DR. JOHN SHAW BILLINGS should be named Surgeon-General. Born in Indiana fifty-two years ago, he was graduated from The Medical College of Ohio. He was graduated in medicine in 1860. He entered the army at the opening of the war and saw hard service, including the battles of the Wilderness. As an organizer and executive of hospitals he achieved an early and a high reputation. Under Surgeon-General Barnes he disbursed during eight years many millions of dollars with the greatest satisfaction to his superiors, and in the organization and development of the Library of the Surgeon-General's Office he has shown executive and administrative talents of the highest order.

It is needless to refer to the high position he has attained as an authority upon sanitary science. At the present time he is officially connected with Harvard University, the University of Pennsylvania, Columbia College, and Johns Hopkins University. He has received the highest recognition from abroad. Oxford, Cambridge, Edinburgh, and Munich have conferred honorary degrees upon him, and his career is full of instruction and encouragement to the profession. The special duty to which he has been detailed so long in Washington has not been used as a means of leisure or personal gain. No medical man in the country has worked harder, or to better effect, and the Government would honor itself by rewarding this distinguished man with the highest medical gift that is in its power to bestow. The President and his advisers may rest assured that no appointment they can make will be regarded so favorably by the Medical Corps of the Army and by the medical profession at large.

KOCH'S DISCOVERY.

SINCE our last issue a number of physicians in this country have received a supply of Koch's lymph, and will doubtless soon be ready to present to their professional brethren the results of their experiments. As already announced, Drs. Chittenden and Foster, of New Haven, were the first in the field by some days, and they will be followed by Dr. Jacobi and Dr. A. McLane Hamilton, of New York, as well as by Dr. Bennett and a committee appointed by the University of Pennsylvania in Philadelphia. We are glad to announce that the reports of Professor Chittenden and Dr. Foster, Dr. Hamilton, and Dr. Bennett have already been secured for publication in THE MEDICAL NEWS ; and a number of other gentlemen who have just begun their work with the liquid have promised to contribute reports from week to week. Information derived from widely-separated sources, and obtained primarily by investigators thoroughly qualified to complete such studies, cannot fail to prove of interest to our readers.

In another column will be found a general summary of news concerning the character and effects of the fluid, which, while it conveys no definite information concerning the character of the liquid, shows the direction of thought in Europe in regard to its possible composition.

CORRESPONDENCE.

LONDON.

Koch's Treatment of Tuberculosis—A Case of Sleeping Sickness.

KOCH'S method of treating tuberculosis is still creating great excitement, and almost every day we see in the papers some fresh proof of the widespread desire for advertisement. Meanwhile the first reports of enthusiastic but utterly untrustworthy newspaper reporters have by no means been substantiated, for so far from cases of lupus being cured in a few hours and almost under the eyes of the observer, we have not been shown a single instance in which a cure was effected. That the new treatment exercises a most remarkable influence upon lupus there can be no doubt, for several medical men who have returned from Berlin agree upon that point, and I hoped that last night we who stayed at home would have an opportunity to see. one of the cases, for it was expected that Mr. Malcolm Morris would exbibit at the Clinical Society the patient whom he took to Berlin three weeks ago. But it seems that the cure is not sufficiently advanced, and the patient is still there. As, however, Mr. Watson Cheyne and Dr. Heron have returned with some of the precious fluid, and have commenced inoculating patients, we shall not have to wait long before we can judge of the results.

A good deal of abuse has been vented upon the College of Physicians for not sending delegates to investigate the subject, but it seems to me that the College has taken the right position, for at present no facilities are given for investigation ; and if such an investigation were permitted, I am by no means sure that the College of Physicians is the proper body to undertake it. The matter is of such great importance that, I think, the Government, and not private parties, should

set on foot the inquiry. At present, however, Koch has declined to divulge his method, and although this is contrary to all scientific tradition, no one can compel him to do so. His ostensible reason for secrecy, namely, that incompetent persons would at once prepare a fluid which would not give the expected results, and so bring the treatment into disrepute, is clearly a mere excuse, because it will also apply whenever he does make public his mode of preparing the " brown fluid." The general belief here is that Koch is working at the cure of other infectious diseases on the same lines, and that he is afraid that if he now describes his methods someone will precede him in discovering a cure for the other diseases.

A fortnight ago Dr. Stephen Mackenzie showed a case of the so-called " sleeping sickness " of the Congo, at the Clinical Society. The patient was a negro, aged twenty-two years, who had spent all his life in the neighborhood of the Congo, and had come to England in order that his malady might be thoroughly studied, though not with any expectation of being cured. Nearly all of the members of his family have succumbed to the disease, and in the district where he lived it is well known and much dreaded, for it is believed to prove invariably fatal. As the name implies, a lethargic tendency is the chief characteristic, and is accompanied by progressive weakness. Dr. Mackenzie's patient has been under observation since june, and has had continuous fever. When he arrived he was able to go about and even do light work, but tremulousness gradually came on, and now he is so weak that he can do nothing. His mental powers have grown gradually weaker, so that it is difficult to get him to answer a question. He almost constantly falls asleep, but never sleeps long at a time, either during the night or day. One important feature in the case remains to be mentioned, and that is, the presence of filariæ in the blood. Contrary to the usual rule, these show no periodicity, and are always present—a fact that Dr. Mackenzie is inclined to attribute to the febrile condition. He is doubtful of any connection between the filariæ and the lethargic attacks, as filariæ have not been observed in other cases ; but it must be remembered that very few cases have been carefully observed, and probably none so carefully as this one. The blood is, in other respects, normal, and the patient is not the subject of any form of malaria. The case is obviously progressing to a fatal termination, and the report of the autopsy should be of much interest.

PARIS.

The Production of a Biliary Fistula for Disease of the Liver—Sudden Death in Diseases of the Abdominal Organs—Intestinal Antisepsis —Observations on a Guillotined Man.

AT the last meeting of the Academy of Medicine Professor Terrier reported an interesting case of exploratory abdominal section to ascertain the condition of a diseased liver. The history of the case is as follows :

The patient, a man, was admitted to the hospital with the diagnosis of hepatic cyst, but an exploratory puncture showed that there was no cyst, and the diagnosis remained obscure, there being intense jaundice with clay-colored stools and general symptoms. Professor Terrier determined to open the abdomen. At the operation the liver was found enlarged and congested, but no tumor or calculus was discovered, either in the gall-bladder or ducts. Professor Terrier then determined to make a biliary fistula, and to do this he sutured the mucous portion of the gall-bladder to the abdominal parietes and made an opening sufficiently large to admit a No. 10 catheter. The results of the operation were excellent. Two days later the fæces were of a natural color, while the general symptoms gradually disappeared, and one month later the patient left the hospital with the biliary fistula still open. The liver remained somewhat enlarged.

Dr. Jacquemard has lately made a study of the cause of sudden death in cases of abdominal diseases. The results are of great scientific interest and are important from a medico-legal point of view. The mechanism of sudden death in certain abdominal lesions, such as cancer of the stomach, hepatic cirrhosis, and cancer of the liver and pancreas has heretofore been obscure. Some authors believe that it is the result of cardiac degeneration and consequent syncope ; others believe that death in such cases is due to sudden reflex inhibition of the heart. The two following histories are interesting in connection with the subject:

The first case was that of a man, forty-five years old, suffering from carcinoma of the lower curvature of the stomach. He was not cachectic, and his general appearance was excellent ; he had no marked cardiac symptoms except a murmur of the right heart. He died suddenly, and on post-mortem examination the tricuspid opening was found dilated—admitting three fingers. The cardiac muscle appeared healthy.

The second patient was suffering from interstitial nephritis of the right kidney, and also from tuberculosis of the right suprarenal capsule. He died suddenly during sleep after a few convulsive movements of his extremities. At the autopsy no lesions were found in the brain or lungs. During life the heart presented no abnormal symptoms, yet at the autopsy the parietes of the right heart were found in a state of myocarditis, the left heart being normal.

The cardiac lesions alone in these two cases, according to the author, were not sufficient to produce sudden death, which, he thinks, was caused by some abdominal reflex. The effect on the heart of a reflex starting from a sudden and prolonged irritation of the filaments of the solar plexus is without danger or gravity if the heart is healthy, but a sudden arrest of cardiac action is probable where there are lesions of the organ.

Professor Debove has presented before the Société Médicale des Hôpitaux a new mode of treating tubercular peritonitis. Spencer Wells, in 1862, opened the abdomen of a case of tubercular peritonitis believing he had to deal with an ovarian cyst. The patient, however, improved after the operation, and since then some surgeons have recommended opening and washing out the cavity for this disease. Dr. Debove, thinking that abdominal section could be dispensed with in such cases, simply tapped, in the case of a woman, aged twenty-eight years, who suffered from tubercular peritonitis, the diagnosis being confirmed by injecting the peritoneal fluid in three guinea-pigs which became tuberculous. As soon as the patient was tapped, the peritoneal cavity was washed out with a saturated solution of boric acid. Eight days later her condition had very much improved—she has gained twelve pounds, and is now considered cured.

At the Société de Biologie Dr. Féré recently presented photographs of a patient suffering from epilepsy treated by large doses of bromide of potassium, which greatly diminished the number and severity of the fits, but caused most serious cutaneous lesions. These lesions disappeared under the use of intestinal antiseptics—naphthol, associated with the salicylate of bismuth. In a number of similar cases Dr. Féré has seen digestive troubles disappear under the influence of the same treatment, permitting one to increase progressively the dose of bromide.

Dr. Gley has presented the results of his observations on a guillotined man whom he had the opportunity to study a minute and a half after death. The heart was flaccid, but still beating regularly. The anterior interventricular groove was mechanically excited by means of needles, which produced that state of the ventricles known as tremulation. The auricles after this excitation also presented tremulation ; but, contrary to what took place in the ventricles, their rhythmical movements started again. After a second irritation the right auricle again showed tremulation, while the left auricle continued to beat rhythmically until the fourteenth minute after death. Dr. Gley has observed rhythmical contractions of the diaphragm even three-quarters of an hour after death.

Before closing this letter, let me give you two or three of the most common formulæ used in the Paris hospitals as intestinal antiseptics.

Professor Bouchard recommends the following in cases of gastric and intestinal fermentation as found in cases of gastric dilatation, in poisoning by decayed or diseased meats, in typhlitis, dysentery and typhoid fever, and in diseases in which there is insufficient renal secretion :

R.—Beta-naphthol, finely pulverized ½ ounce.
  Salicylate of bismuth . . 2 drachms.—M.

Divide into thirty wafers, and give from three to ten daily.

Professor Dujardin-Beaumetz recommends the following :

R.—Pure bisulphide of carbon . 35 grains.
  Essence of peppermint . . 30 drops.
  Water . . . . . 15 ounces.

The mixture is placed in a large bottle, shaken, and allowed to settle : 8 to 12 tablespoonfuls are to be given daily in half a tumblerful of water and wine, or in milk.

Dr. Huchard recommends:

R.—Salicylate of bismuth ⎫
  Salicylate of magnesium ⎬ of each 75 grains.
  Benzoate of sodium ⎭ —M.

Divide into twenty wafers, one of which is given before each meal.

ROME.

The Third Italian Congress of Internal Medicine.

THE third annual Italian Congress of Internal Medicine was held this year at Rome between October 20th and 23d. Several interesting papers were read, of which I will give a brief account.

The subject of the etiology and treatment of pleurisy occupied the first day of the meeting. Dr. Patella gave a short review of the present status of the subject. He said that ten years ago only three kinds of pleurisy were described—the rheumatic, the traumatic, and that due to extension of the inflammatory process from the lung. We have now also pleurisies of microbian origin. The sero-fibrinous pleurisy is still considered as rheumatic, but another agent besides cold is necessary for its development. The cold probably prepares the organism for microbian infection by modifying the circulation in the blood and lymphatic vessels. The way in which germs penetrate into the pleura is still obscure, but Fränkel has demonstrated that one of the microbes of purulent pleurisy—the encapsulated lanceolated micrococcus—is found in the tonsils, and from there it may reach the pleura through the lymphatic channels. According to Ziemssen, certain pleurisies are not of microbian origin, such as, for instance, those appearing in acute rheumatism. A bacteriological examination of the products is often difficult, and some positively tuberculous pleurisies present no bacilli on examination. Maragliano states that a tubercular pleurisy can give rise to a serous effusion. On the other hand, Dr. Patella has observed non-tuberculous pleurisy in tuberculous patients, the pleurisy being due to Fränkel's diplococcus. The speaker concluded with the following summary: 1. There are sero-fibrinous pleurisies caused by Fränkel's encapsulated micrococcus. 2. There are pleurisies with extensive effusion, probably of tuberculous origin. 3. In tuberculous subjects, pleurisy of non-tuberculous origin may occur. 4. There also exist pleurisies of *chemical* origin, which are not yet understood. 5. It is safer to rely on clinical symptoms than on bacteriological examination to determine the causes and nature of primitive pleurisies. 6. The etiology of pleurisies secondary to acute pulmonary inflammation, meta-pneumonic pleurisies, is certainly that of the pneumonia. Their prognosis is generally more favorable than that of primitive pleurisies. 7. The spontaneous absorption of pus in cases of purulent pleurisy is possible when the pleurisy originates from Fränkel's diplococcus, and whenever this microbe is found we are justified in expecting a cure.

Dr. Luzzato, of Padua, after discussing the subject in a general way, said that the pathogenic agents in purulent pleurisy are the staphylococcus, the streptococcus, the tubercle bacillus, and, in rare cases, the typhoid-fever bacillus, and that sero-purulent pleurisies are rarely associated with tuberculosis. In the treatment of pleurisy, the author rejects mercury and bloodletting, the former having never given him good results, while the latter increases the amount of the effusion. The salicylates, antipyrine, flying blisters, and poultices give some relief. Aspiration must be resorted to when the liquid reaches the level of the third rib.

Dr. Bozzolo, of Turin, then said that the typhoid-fever bacillus could be found in pleurisies oftener than is ordinarily believed. As to the treatment of purulent pleurisy, he very much prefers the operation of excision of part of a rib to simple aspiration.

Dr. Maragliano spoke of the association of pneumonia with pleurisy. He thinks that all cases of fibrinous pneumonia are accompanied by a pleuritic exudate between the third and fifth day of the disease. To be able to diagnose a small quantity of liquid in the pleural cavity, he places his patient in the genu-pectoral position. In order not to mistake the splenic dulness for that of effusion the patient is directed to lie upon the side opposite to that in which the effusion is thought to exist. In doing this the dulness of the spleen is displaced forward, while the pleuritic effusion moves toward the vertebral column. Among 216 cases of pleurisy he has observed 20 hæmorrhagic ones, only 7 occurring in tuberculous subjects, which shows that tuberculosis is not a *sine qua non* of hæmorrhagic effusion. Most of the hæmorrhagic cases were in alcoholics. In regard to treatment, he believes in an early aspiration, which he usually practises between the second and third week of the disease. Contrary to Dr. Maragliano, he thinks that purulent pleurisies should not always be evacuated by resection of a rib, spontaneous resorption being possible.

Dr. Bacelli, of Rome, said that by auscultation eight ounces of liquid can be demonstrated in the pleural cavity; that costal resections should not always be practised in cases of empyæma, and that a simple aspiration may be all that is needed. In cases of encapsulated purulent effusion, resection is indicated, but one must not forget that such operations are often followed by atrophy of the thoracic muscles.

Dr. de Renzi, of Naples, said that the etiology of pleurisy was variable, sometimes Fränkel's diplococcus being the cause, at other times a streptococcus, and, as an example, he mentioned the last epidemic of influenza, during which all pleurisies showed the presence of the streptococcus. He believes that tubercular pleurisy can be cured. Thoracic aspiration often immediately relieves the fever. The influence of pleurisy upon pulmonary tuberculosis may be either good or bad. It will have an unfavorable influence if the pleurisy appears on the healthy side, but if it develops on the same side as the pulmonary disease it may have a very favorable influence. This the author has observed in two cases in which all symptoms due to pulmonary tuberculosis disappeared after the evacuation of a pleuritic effusion.

Dr. Tomaselli, of Catane, recommended wet cupping at the beginning of acute pleurisy; he also employs blisters and the milk diet, aspiration being used only when the effusion persists too long.

Dr. Archangeli, of Rome, spoke of the success of surgical interference in purulent pleurisy, and said that Dr. Maneso, of Rome, has obtained 49 cures out of 52 operations.

Dr. Marino, of Messina, said that he had treated pleuritic exudates by compressed air, but the results were absolutely negative as regards increasing the rapidity of absorption of the exudate, and he thinks that aërotherapy should be reserved for the thoracic retraction consecutive to empyæma, especially in children and adolescents. Dr. Foazio, of Naples, thought aërotherapy very valuable in the treatment of pleuritic effusions.

Dr. Rovigli, of Modena, speaking on the subject of the displacement of pleuritic effusions by the change of position of the patient, said that among 40 patients which he examined for this purpose, only 14 presented a movable effusion, while in 12 of these the effusion was very slightly movable. He thinks that the instability of a pleuritic exudate depends more upon the quantity than on the nature of the effusion.

Dr. Bianchi, of Florence, gave a short description of the clinical history of colloid cancer of the pylorus. He has found that this cancer is more frequent in men than in women; that it does not ulcerate very readily, and is not painful. Vomiting and dilatation of the stomach are absent, because the pyloric orifice remains open. As differential signs the author enumerated the following as belonging to this affection: When the patient lies on his right side liquid taken into the stomach rapidly passes into the intestine; again, when the patient is standing, if liquid is introduced into his stomach, it rises no higher than the level of the pyloric orifice, if one continues to introduce liquid, on account of the open pylorus. The only rational treatment is extirpation of the growth.

Dr. Filetti recommended a new way of staining fresh blood by means of dried methyl-blue, which colors the nucleus of the white corpuscles. Mr. Gualdi, of Rome, saw no advantage in this process over the one of Dr. Celli-Guarnieri, in which the methyl-blue is dissolved in ascitic fluid or serum.

Dr. Marchiafava, of Rome, spoke on the subject of pernicious intermittent fever, with symptoms of acute paralysis. This form of paralysis, he claims, is quite frequent, but is rarely fatal, as the lesions of the central nervous system are only secondary and dependent on a blood-stasis in the cerebral vessels.

Dr. Mya read a paper on the pathological value of the presence of urobilin in the urine. He has found that in patients suffering from pneumonia, acute rheumatism, typhoid fever, and anæmia, and in intoxication by antipyrine, pyridine, antifebrin, and other antipyretics, the quantity of urobilin is very great, which indicates a destruction of blood-corpuscles. In serious liver diseases we find only traces of urobilin, while in renal lesions urobilin is not found in the urine, but only in the blood.

Dr. Queirolo, of Genoa, spoke of the value of diaphoresis in the treatment of infectious febrile diseases. He said that in experiments undertaken by him 100 grammes of sweat from a healthy man produced no effect when injected in rabbits, while one-third less than that quantity of sweat obtained from patients suffering from typhoid fever, smallpox, etc., produced death. The latter result being obtained with sweat that had been sterilized, the infection cannot be due to a virus, but to a chemical substance, which, however, may be the product of pathogenic microbes. This fact encouraged the author to experiment on the elimination of poisons by the skin, and for this purpose he placed some of his patients in a sweating-room, with favorable results; the patient immediately felt better, and there was a remarkable change observed in the temperature, pulse, respiration, and nerve functions.

Dr. Farina, of Naples, in connection with this remarked that in Africa, where patients suffering from infectious diseases are subjected to sweating on account of the climate, diseases such as scarlet fever, typhoid fever, and measles terminate more rapidly than in Europe.

Dr. Masini, of Genoa, reported six cases of pulmonary tuberculosis treated by intratracheal injections of twenty-per-cent. solution of creasote in oil. Two patients were absolutely cured, although no bacilli had been found in their sputum; two were considerably improved, the fever disappeared, and the sputum and bacilli diminished in quantity, while in the two remaining the improvement was less marked.

Dr. de Lollis said, as a result of his observations on animals, that tannin is not incompatible with opium; and that an enema of opium and tannin will kill an animal as rapidly as an enema of opium alone.

NEW YORK.

To the Editor of THE MEDICAL NEWS,

SIR: It has been said that every new operation usually passes through three distinct stages before it takes its final position among the recognized resources of surgery: First, a period following its announcement, when it is enthusiastically praised; secondly, a stage of reaction, when all sorts of objections and adverse criticisms are heaped upon it, and when it is branded as nearly useless, if not in many cases actually harmful; thirdly, a stage of restitution, when reason again asserts itself, and, reinforced by the results of time and experience, places the operation in its true position before the profession. This description seems appropriate to many discoveries in medical science, and, perhaps, to none more than to Koch's great discovery of the tubercle bacillus. The many special systems of therapeutics which sprang up like mushrooms, almost before the scientific world had recovered from its surprise, have been but a "nine days' wonder," and we now hear fewer fascinating theories and more sober science. Dr. E. F. Brush, in a recent paper entitled "The Mimicry of Animal Tuberculosis in Vegetable Forms," has drawn some interesting lessons from the vegetable kingdom. Nut-galls are really tuberculous processes, affecting the breathing apparatus and nutritive channels of a plant. The gall-fly punctures the leaf and deposits an egg, injecting at the same time a minute drop of what has been called a poison, but which is, in all probability, a digestive ferment. This fluid gives rise to such changes in the nutritive process of the leaf that the irritation which the egg would otherwise cause is entirely overcome. This egg may be likened to the giant-cell of a tubercle in the human subject. An important lesson in therapeutics is to be found in a study of the pest known as the phylloxera, for this is a tuberculous disease due to a bacillus; yet, although its life-history is well understood, and the diseased parts are easy of access, treatment has been futile. It is not enough, therefore, to know that there is a germ constantly present in a mass of morbid material. But, if we have been disappointed in our therapeutic efforts to cure tuberculosis, our pathological studies are teaching us more and more how often Nature puts a stop to a tuberculous process which threatens to invade the whole system.

Dr. H. M. Biggs, not long ago, showed a specimen of tuberculosis of the pericardium. The two layers of the pericardium were adherent, and between them were several cheesy masses. The case was apparently one of primary tuberculosis of the pericardium, in which recovery had taken place, the tubercles having been surrounded by connective tissue, while the peritoneum had subsequently become involved, and presented the usual lesions of tuberculosis. There were extensive adhesions binding down both lungs, but no tuberculous lesions were found here.

Aside from the unusual type of tuberculosis presented in this case, Dr. Biggs thought that it was of especial interest, as experience was gradually teaching him that there was apparently no form of tuberculosis which might not terminate in recovery. So, although gaseous enemata, heated air, and other similar " fads " have almost passed out of notice, Nature is constantly showing us how much she can accomplish in staying the hand of disease, if we will but assist her by maintaining good nutrition and providing the patient with proper hygienic surroundings.

The discussion at the Academy of Medicine the other evening on the subject of hydrophobia was something of a failure, if the object of those who arranged for it was to present a clear and authoritative statement of our present knowledge and beliefs concerning this disease, and of the plan of preventive treatment introduced by Pasteur; but the radical differences of opinion which were brought out, not only as to the efficacy of this special mode of treatment, but even as to the very existence of such a disease as hydrophobia, were ample justification for devoting an evening to the discussion. Incidentally, the newspapers and the Pasteur institutes came in for their share of adverse criticism, the former for the sensational accounts which they are continually publishing concerning the wonderful cures said to have followed the antirabic treatment, and the latter for their loose methods of investigation and of keeping the records from which their much-quoted statistics were compiled. In connection with this subject, it may not be amiss to note that in a very recent communication from Dr. Paul Gibier, Director of the Pasteur Institute of New York, he states that since it was opened on February 18, 1890, 610 persons who had been bitten by dogs or cats applied for treatment. In 130 of these the existence of hydrophobia in the animals was demonstrated, either by a veterinary examination or by inoculation experiments, and in many cases by the death of some persons or animals who had been bitten by dogs suspected of having rabies. All these persons were subjected to the anti-rabic treatment, and all remain in good health.

The annual meeting of the New York State Medical Association was held this Fall in its new home, the Mott Memorial Hall, 64 Madison Avenue. This building also contains the Association's library, which has grown very rapidly from a small beginning made in June, 1885, at the Carnegie laboratory. A little over five months later, the library contained 3448 books, and 4000 pamphlets. In December of last year it was decided to accept the offer of the trustees of the Mott Library to consolidate the two collections, and on May 5th of the present year the library was opened in its present location. There have been a number of large additions by bequests, and at present the library contains 8788 volumes, which with the 4000 volumes of the Mott collection, make a total of 12,788 books, besides about 5000 pamphlets. The library needs contributions of the recent medical, surgical, and obstetrical publications, a larger list of exchanges, and a permanent fund, which when invested will yield a sufficient sum to maintain and increase the number of books. The central location of this hall, and its quiet surroundings, make it a desirable retreat for the searcher into medical lore.

Progress in the direction of simplifying the practice of antiseptic surgery has been very rapid. Five or six years ago it was thought necessary to deluge the operating-field constantly with an antiseptic solution, and so zealously was this done, that some of our surgeons found it expedient to attire themselves in waterproof garments. Gradually the quantity of fluid employed was reduced, until now occasional sopping of the wound, or a final irrigation with bichloride solution, is considered sufficient. Antiseptic dressings are also less complicated, the Lister protective and the mackintosh being seldom used, while the eight layers of carbolized and resinous gauze have given place to soft bichloride "handkerchiefs," or to simple absorbent gauze, which has been previously steamed in a "sterilizer." Notwithstanding all this simplification, the list of bottles, dressings, dishes and other accessories necessary for the performance of any large operation according to modern ideas, is sufficiently formidable to make many a surgeon's assistant yearn for still greater simplicity. I recently saw a very convenient instrument-dish made of rubber, and capable of being inflated with air like an ordinary rubber ring bed-pan, or of being flattened out and packed away for transportation.

NEWS ITEMS.

Koch's Discovery.—Very little of interest has been developed during the past week concerning the discovery of Koch for the cure of tuberculosis. In this country a number of physicians have been fortunate enough to obtain some of the fluid for experimentation, Professor Chittenden and Dr. Foster, of New Haven, being the first to receive the fluid and to study its action by at least a week. They are now carrying out a series of experiments on three patients, one of whom is suffering from lupus, one from pulmonary phthisis, and one from laryngeal phthisis.

THE MEDICAL NEWS during the past week sent a correspondent to New Haven for the purpose of discovering whether anything unusual had been noticed in the cases in that city after the injection of the fluid, but he was assured by the gentlemen who are using it that the symptoms noted were identical with those described in Koch's original paper, which was published in this journal.

Just as we go to press we hear that Dr. Jacobi and Dr. A. McLane Hamilton, of New York, have begun a series of studies with the liquid and that the committee of the University of Pennsylvania, consisting of Dr. Pepper, Dr. White, Dr. Musser, and Dr. Tyson, has done likewise.

Correspondence from Berlin, combined with newspaper dispatches, show that the possibility of a general distribution of the lymph for curative purposes, particularly in this country, will not be possible for several weeks. It is stated in one of the New York papers that the German Government will have the liquid for sale by the 15th of this month, but so far as we can learn, this is merely a newspaper report, based on very little authoritative information.

Several of the physicians who were in Europe at the time that Koch announced his discovery, have returned to this country, after having gone to Berlin to investigate the value of the remedy. They all are in accord in stating that the hypodermic injections of the fluid act most favorably upon lupus, and they all insist that it is without value in pulmonary phthisis excepting in its earliest stages.

The latest reports of the cases of lupus under Levy and von Bergmann show that as time goes by the lesions are continually undergoing favorable changes, but these investigators very properly do not claim any permanent effects as yet, this being impossible in the case of a disease which is so slow in its formation as is lupus.

Dr. Dengel has published a paper in the *Berliner klinische Wochenschrift* which, while it endorses the opinions so far expressed, particularly emphasizes the harmfulness of the lymph in well-advanced cases of tubercular disease of the lung.

Much discussion has also been resorted to by the medical journals in Europe as to the composition of the liquid. Thus, Nencki and Sahli have published a paper in the *Correspondenzblatt für Schweizer Aerzte* upon " Enzymes in Therapeutics " with the idea of throwing some light upon Koch's remedy. They point out that the intravenous injection of these soluble ferments in various other diseases produces changes closely allied to those brought about by the liquid of Koch in tuberculosis. It is stated that the favorable action that follows the inoculation of the *streptococcus erysipelatus* into malignant tumors is probably due to the presence of the soluble ferment produced by the cocci. Again, the *Wiener medizinische Presse* publishes an article upon a similar subject, and argues that bio-chemical processes are involved in the production of the liquid, also pointing out that Sewall and others have proved that preventive inoculations with the poison of the rattlesnake finally render the organism capable of withstanding the poison. On the other hand, the *British Medical Journal* reminds its readers that, while these statements are of course very interesting, the possibility of heating Koch's liquid without destroying its specific action seems to render it unlikely that it has any such origin. The *British Medical Journal* also refers to a case, under the care of von Bergmann, in which the lupus disappeared under the use of the fluid, and was reported cured, but nevertheless recurred with great intensity a fortnight after the injections were stopped.

All the physicians who have returned so far from Berlin insist upon what THE MEDICAL NEWS has already insisted upon in previous issues, namely that it is exceedingly inadvisable for either doctors or patients to go to the German capital at the present time, owing to the number already striving unsuccessfully for opportunity to study or receive the liquid.

A number of the regular profession have been fearful ever since the publication of Koch's results lest charlatans should use some bogus liquid upon patients who are only too eager to be treated for consumption, and it seems that in Germany itself this fraud has been first attempted. It is stated that a janitor, named Meyer, who is employed in the Central Hotel, of Berlin, has been accused of selling to some foreign doctors 5 grammes of what he alleged was Koch's lymph, for 300 marks.

Cholera Rife in India.—Despatches from India to the New York *Herald* say that while the Second battalion

of the Third Ghoorkha regiment was on the march in the Chin Hills several of the men were stricken with cholera. The troops went into camp at Guatheit, where thirty men, out of a total of sixty attacked, succumbed to the disease. The battalion subsequently broke camp and proceeded to Rangoon. During the march many more soldiers were attacked by cholera.

OFFICIAL LIST OF CHANGES IN THE STATIONS AND DUTIES OF OFFICERS SERVING IN THE MEDICAL DEPARTMENT, U. S. ARMY, FROM NOVEMBER 25 TO DECEMBER 8, 1890.

By direction of the Secretary of War, CHARLES B. EWING, *Captain and Assistant Surgeon*, in addition to his present duties, is assigned to duty as Examiner of Recruits at St. Louis, Mo.—Par. 7, S. O. 275, *Headquarters of the Army, A. G. O.*, November 24, 1890.

By direction of the Secretary of War, EUGENE L. SWIFT, *First Lieutenant and Assistant Surgeon*, is relieved from further duty and station at Fort McDowell, Arizona Territory, and assigned to Fort Thomas, Arizona Territory, where he is now on temporary duty.—Par. 16, S. O. 282, A. G. O., *Washington, D. C.*, December 3, 1890.

By direction of the Secretary of War, JAMES E. PILCHER, *Captain and Assistant Surgeon*, now on leave of absence, will report in person to the commanding general Division of the Atlantic, for temporary duty at Fort Columbus, New York Harbor, during the absence on leave of William E. Hopkins, Captain and Assistant Surgeon.—Par. 3, S. O. 278, A. G. O., *Washington, D. C.*, November 28, 1890.

By direction of the Secretary of War, leave of absence for six months, is granted WILLIAM E. HOPKINS, *Captain and Assistant Surgeon*.—Par. 2, S. O. 278, A. G. O., *Washington, D. C.*, November 28, 1890.

OFFICIAL LIST OF CHANGES IN THE STATIONS AND DUTIES OF THE MEDICAL CORPS OF THE U. S. NAVY FOR THE WEEK ENDING DECEMBER 6, 1890.

ATLEE, L. W., *Assistant Surgeon.*—Ordered to examination preliminary to promotion.

MARTIN, H. M., *Surgeon.*—Placed on the Retired List, December 4, 1890.

ALFRED, A. R., *Assistant Surgeon.*—Ordered to the Naval Hospital, Norfolk, Va.

WHITFIELD, J. M., *Assistant Surgeon.*—Detached from the Hospital at Norfolk, and ordered to the U. S. S. " Chicago."

McCORMICK, A. M. D., *Assistant Surgeon.*—Detached from the U. S. S. " Chicago," and wait orders.

KEENEY, J. F., *Assistant Surgeon.*—Ordered to the U. S. S. " Minnesota."

HARRIS, H. N. T., *Assistant Surgeon.*—Detached from the U. S. S. " Minnesota," and wait orders.

OFFICIAL LIST OF CHANGES OF STATIONS AND DUTIES OF MEDICAL OFFICERS OF THE U. S. MARINE-HOSPITAL SERVICE, FROM NOVEMBER 24 TO DECEMBER 6, 1890.

FESSENDEN, C. S. D., *Surgeon.*—Leave of absence extended seven days, December 4, 1890.

BAILHACHE, P. H., *Surgeon.*—Granted leave of absence for twenty days, November 28, 1890.

HUTTON, W. H. H., *Surgeon.*—To proceed to Solomon's Island, Md., on special duty, November 29, 1890.

SAWTELLE, H. W., *Surgeon.*—Granted leave of absence for ten days, December 2, 1890.

PECKHAM, C. T., *Passed Assistant Surgeon.*—Granted leave of absence for ten days, December 1, 1890.

HUSSEY, S. H., *Assistant Surgeon.*—When relieved, to proceed to New Orleans, La., for duty, November 24, 1890.

GROENEVELT, J. F., *Assistant Surgeon.*—When relieved, to rejoin station, November 24, 1890.

COFER, L. E., *Assistant Surgeon*—Ordered to temporary duty at Boston, Mass., November 24, 1890.

EXTRA EDITION.

MEDICAL NEWS.

A WEEKLY MEDICAL JOURNAL.

Vol. LVII. No. 25.
Whole No. 936.   SATURDAY, DECEMBER 20, 1890.   SUPPLEMENT.   Per Annum, $4.00.
Per Copy, 10 Cents.

Sir JOSEPH LISTER
ON
KOCH AND HIS METHODS.

SPECIAL CABLE DISPATCH TO THE MEDICAL NEWS.

KOCH AND HIS METHODS.[1]

AFTER some preliminary remarks about his journey to Berlin, Sir Joseph Lister said that the effects of Koch's treatment upon tubercular disease were simply astounding. As an example, he cited cases of extensive lupus of the cheek, in which two days after the injection the diseased surfaces became covered with crusts of dried serum, with no inflammation elsewhere. In cases of strumous glands in the neck the injections caused swelling of the glands with redness of the skin over them and pain. In gelatinous disease of the knee-joint similar effects are observed, only the tubercular tissue being affected.

The systemic effects which follow the injections are severe for a few hours, and consist in transient fever, pains in the limbs, shivering, nausea, and sometimes vomiting. The usual dose of the lymph is one-thousandth of a gramme diluted with water to one gramme. The method is useful in the diagnosis of suspected latent tuberculosis. The therapeutic effects on lupus are separation of the crusts, leaving a more or less sound scar. In tubercular joints the swelling diminishes. In phthisis the sputa becomes scantier and more mucous, the bacilli diminish in number, the sweats disappear, the patient gains in weight, and the physical signs of pulmonary tuberculosis vanish. The important questions are, How far are the effects permanent, and What are the limits to the curative power? Diseased tissue is expelled by

[1] Abstract of an address published in the London Lancet of December 13, 1890.

sloughing or is absorbed; spontaneous expulsion of deep-seated caseous masses being impossible, fresh infections would demand further and indefinitely prolonged treatment for the production of immunity from tubercular infection.

If it is true that the living but diseased tissues surrounding the tuberculous masses are acted on by the remedy, and are rendered capable of resisting the development of bacilli, then caseous masses would remain harmless as regards further infection, and tubercular disease would be definitely cured, for immunity is wanted to make the treatment perfect. Immunity has been attained in guinea-pigs by very large doses, and perhaps could be attained in man by gradually increasing the size of the doses. Acquired tolerance is best shown by the greatly increased dose borne after several injections. It would seem probable that by steadily pushing the dose a degree of tolerance might be attained equal to immunity.

Sir Joseph Lister then continued as follows:

There is another line of inquiry from which I cannot help hoping for good results. Through Koch's great kindness I had the opportunity of penetrating into the arcana of the Hygienic Institute of Berlin, where I saw most beautiful researches carried on in that institution, of which Koch is the inspiring genius. I saw things which, while they excited my admiration, made me also feel ashamed that we, in England, from one circumstance or another, are so greatly behind our German brethren.

The researches to which I desire especially to refer are still in progress, and fresh facts are accumulating day by day though they have not yet been published. I am not at liberty to mention details, but there can be no harm in my saying this much, that I saw in the case of two of the most virulent infective diseases to which man is liable, the course of the otherwise deadly disease cut short in the animals on which the experiments were performed, by the injection of a small quantity of a material perfectly constant in character, an inorganic chemical substance, as easily obtained as any article in the materia medica. Not only this, but by means of the same substance these animals were rendered incapable of taking the disease, and under the most potent inoculations perfect immunity was conferred upon them.

I suspect that before many weeks have passed the world will be startled by the disclosure of these facts if they can be applied to man, although our experience of the different behavior of Koch's fluid in guinea-pigs and in the human subject makes this a matter of uncertainty until tested by experiment. But if they can be applied to man, the world will be astonished, and the beneficence of these researches will be recognized everywhere.

At the present time Koch is engaged in the earnest endeavor to produce his remedy for tubercle by some process which could be divulged without the risk of the public being supplied either with material useless from its inertness, or, on the other hand, a deadly poison. Koch, I believe, would not have published his method had it not been for the great pressure brought to bear upon him, until he could produce it in a form capable of being revealed in every detail.

It is nothing but the fear that by publishing now the specific mode of preparing this material he might do immense harm instead of good that prevents him from making it known, and I must say that the carping criticism against Koch, on account of what is spoken of as a "secret remedy," can only proceed from absolute ignorance of the beautiful character of the man. If it should happen that, as with the other diseases to which I have referred, so with tubercle, complete immunity should be obtained by means of some inorganic chemical substance which anyone can prepare, then would be achieved the complete triumph of the treatment of tuberculosis; and, for my part, I rejoice that we are permitted to look forward with hope to that glorious consummation.

AMERICAN REPORTS ON KOCH'S METHOD OF TREATING TUBERCULOSIS.

THE following reports have been received from physicians in New York, Baltimore, and Philadel-phia, and are of interest, not only because of the importance of the subject, but also for the reason that they are the first authentic publications of American experience :

REPORT OF CASES TREATED BY KOCH'S LYMPH.

BY DR. FRANCIS P. KINNICUTT, M.D.,
PHYSICIAN TO ST. LUKE'S HOSPITAL, NEW YORK.

UP to the present date fifteen patients suffering from various forms of tubercular disease have been inoculated by me with Koch's lymph, in the wards of St. Luke's Hospital.

The cases were carefully selected with the view to study thoroughly this method of treatment. All of them will remain under my personal observation in the hospital during the entire period of treatment, and a detailed report of their histories, subsequent to inoculation, will be published from time to time.

The cases are as follows: Two cases of lupus of the face; one case of lupus of the hand, accompanied by tuberculous infiltration of a limited portion of one lung; two cases of tuberculous glands (cervical); three cases of hip-joint disease, with intermittently-discharging sinuses; one case of tuberculous disease of the tibia and fibula, with open sinus; one case of prostatic surface tubercular disease; four cases of pulmonary tuberculosis in its early stage and limited in area; one case of doubtful diagnosis is embraced in the above group.

Thus far 0.001 gramme of the lymph has been used for the initial inoculations in all adult cases, and 0.005 in children. Decided reactions have been obtained in all patients but one of the fifteen inoculated. The reactions have been varied in the time of their appearance—from four hours after inoculation to twenty four; also in their intensity and duration. The longest duration of the reaction has been forty-six hours. The highest temperature recorded during the reaction has been 104° F. The increase in the pulse- and respiration-rate has been proportionate to the rise in temperature. The local changes in the cases of lupus have corresponded very exactly with those recorded by the Berlin observers, and have been of the greatest interest. The differential diagnosis in the doubtful case mentioned lay between lupus of the throat and a tertiary specific lesion. No reaction followed the inoculation of 0.001 gramme, and a second of 0.002 gramme, and the case was accordingly regarded as one of specific disease. No symptoms which could occasion any apprehension have been observed in any of the cases. Tables are appended showing the symptoms and signs observed during and following inoculations in three patients presenting different forms of tubercular disease. The local changes observed in the case of lupus are kindly described by Dr. George H. Fox, by whom the patient was sent to me.

The diagnosis of tubercular disease of the prostate in Case II. was made by Dr. Keyes, by whom the patient was referred to me. The reaction obtained would seem to be corroborative of this diagnosis.

At the present moment, in the stress of increased time and labor demanded by the treatment and observation of the large number of new cases admitted to the wards of the hospital, only the above brief notes are possible.

NOTES ON CASE III. *Lupus vulgaris of left ear.*—On December 11th, at 3 P.M. (date of first injection of lymph), the case presented the following appearance :

The left auricle was considerably thickened, of a dull-red hue and partly covered by adherent flakes of dead epidermis. Below the ear was a rounded, circumscribed patch of lupus, about the size of a silver dollar, the smooth surface of which presented well-marked cicatricial lines, the result of previous scarification. This patch extended for a short distance up behind the ear. Between the paler lines the dull-red hue of the lupoid tissue was still apparent. During the patient's two weeks' residence in St. Luke's Hospital there had been no sensation of pain, burning, or itching in the affected part.

On December 12th, at 3 P.M., there was so marked a change in the appearance of the ear that it was noticeable at first glance, even at a distance. The affected part appeared as though it were acutely inflamed or erysipelatous. The auricle had assumed a bright-red hue, and was considerably swollen. The patch beneath and behind the ear was notably elevated, and the redness had increased to such an extent that the cicatricial appearance of the surface was no longer apparent. At the margin of the patch there was a narrow zone of hyperæmia and a number of prominent red points which had not been noted on the preceding day, and which doubtless indicated the most recent infiltration of the healthy tissue. The patient stated that a burning sensation had occurred during the previous night, and the ear had felt quite painful toward morning. It now felt as it looked, swollen and inflamed.

On December 13th the elevation of the patch and swelling of the auricle had subsided, and the color was less inflammatory. The burning sensation had gone. The epidermic flakes, especially upon the helix of the ear, were dry and whitish. At a single point on the patch below the ear a serous exudation was noted. A second injection of lymph was made.

On December 14th there was not much change in the affected part. There was a slight increase of inflammation, but by no means so marked as after

the first injection, although double the dose had been employed.

There was no elevation of the margin of the patch, and the lobe of the ear felt a trifle softer. Below and behind the ear there was a slight moist discharge, with a tendency to honey-like crusting. The patient stated that during the previous night she experienced "a heavy, stupid, sick feeling," and felt a sharp pain in the ear as after the first injection, but the sensation of burning and swelling was much less this time.

On December 15th it was simply noted that the surface of the affected part presented more of an eczematous appearance.

CASE I. *Tubercular infiltration of apex of right lung.*—Female, aged forty years. Sputa contain very numerous tubercle bacilli. No rise of morning or evening temperature during two weeks previous to inoculation. General condition good.

First inoculation, December 10th, 11 A.M., 0.001 gramme. Reaction developed five hours after inoculation ; slight chilliness, headache, general malaise, fever. Duration of reaction twenty-one hours. Highest temperature 101.2°. Amount of sputum for twenty-four hours preceding inoculation, 11 drachms; for twenty-four hours following inoculation, 13 drachms; for second twenty-four hours following inoculation, 18 drachms; for third twenty-four hours following inoculation, 3 ounces. Urinary examination : a trace of albumin present before and after inoculation. Physical signs consisted in crepitation over affected area more marked, with mucous râles in larger tubes of same ; no enlargement of spleen.

Second inoculation, December 13th, 3 P.M., 0.001 gramme. Reaction developed thirteen hours after inoculation. Duration of reaction nineteen hours. Highest temperature 101.2°, seven hours after beginning of reaction. Amount of sputa for twenty-four hours following inoculation, 3 ounces. Urinary examination : trace of albumin, otherwise negative. Physical signs : bronchial element of respiratory murmur distinctly more marked, and physical signs of infiltration obtained over an increased area ; no enlargement of spleen.

Third inoculation, December 16th, 3 P.M., 0.001 gramme.

CASE II. *Prostatic surface tubercular disease.*—First inoculation, December 11th, 3.30 P.M., 0.001 gramme. Temperature normal. Reaction developed seven and a half hours later ; rigors, headache, pains in limbs, general malaise, fever. Duration of reaction thirty-one hours. Highest temperature 104°. Local symptoms, pain and uneasiness over region of bladder, increased irritability of same. Urinary examination : small amount of albumin present before inoculation ; distinctly increased during reaction.

Second inoculation, December 13th, 3.30 P.M., 0.001 gramme. Reaction developed four hours later. Duration of reaction thirty hours. Highest temperature 101⅘°. Local symptoms similar to those following first inoculation. Urinary examination same as preceding, with a few hyaline casts.

Third inoculation, December 16th, 3.30 P.M., 0.001 gramme.

TEMPERATURE (CASE II.).

December 11th,	4	o'clock P.M.	. . .	99$\frac{4}{5}$°
"	"	5	"	"	. . .	99$\frac{3}{5}$
"	"	6	"	"	. . .	99$\frac{3}{5}$
"	"	8	"	"	. . .	99$\frac{1}{5}$
"	"	10	"	"	. . .	99$\frac{1}{4}$
"	"	12	"	"	. . .	101
"	12th,	1	"	A.M.	. . .	102$\frac{1}{4}$
"	"	3	"	"	. . .	102$\frac{2}{5}$
"	"	5	"	"	. . .	102$\frac{1}{2}$
"	"	7	"	"	. . .	102
"	"	9	"	"	. . .	101$\frac{4}{5}$
"	"	11	"	"	. . .	101$\frac{3}{5}$
"	"	12	"	"	. . .	103
"	"	2	"	P.M.	. . .	102$\frac{4}{5}$
"	"	4	"	"	. . .	102$\frac{4}{5}$
"	"	6	"	"	. . .	103$\frac{1}{5}$
"	"	7	"	"	. . .	103$\frac{1}{5}$
"	"	8	"	"	. . .	102$\frac{4}{5}$
"	"	9	"	"	. . .	101$\frac{2}{5}$
"	"	10	"	"	. . .	100$\frac{4}{5}$
"	"	11	"	"	. . .	101$\frac{1}{2}$
"	13th,	1	"	A.M.	. . .	100$\frac{4}{5}$
"	"	3	"	"	. . .	100
"	"	4	"	"	. . .	99$\frac{3}{4}$
"	"	6	"	"	. . .	99$\frac{3}{5}$

CASE III.—Female, aged twenty-two years. *Lupus of ear and contiguous portions of face and neck, of twelve years' duration.* Under treatment for the greater portion of this time.

First inoculation, December 11th, 3 P.M., 0.001 gramme. Temperature normal. Reaction developed nine hours later; slight rise of temperature and burning sensation in affected ear. Duration of reaction twenty-one hours. Highest temperature 99.8°. (Local signs described in appended note.) Urinary examination negative. No enlargement of spleen.

Second inoculation, December 13th, 0.002 gramme. Reaction developed eleven hours later; slight fever, decided burning sensation in affected ear. Duration of reaction twenty-two hours. Highest temperature 100.6°. Local signs described elsewhere. Urinary examination: trace of albumin, otherwise negative. Physical signs negative; no enlargement of spleen.

Third inoculation, December 16th, 0.003 gramme.

PRELIMINARY REPORT ON KOCH'S LYMPH.

BY WILLIAM OSLER, M.D.,

PROFESSOR OF THE PRINCIPLES AND PRACTICE OF MEDICINE IN THE JOHNS HOPKINS HOSPITAL.

AT the meeting of the Johns Hopkins Hospital Medical Society, December 15th, Dr. Osler made a preliminary report on the cases—eleven in number—under treatment by Koch's method. He said: "In the presence of an alleged discovery of such importance we should neither display a blind credulity nor an unreasonable scepticism. The extraordinary enthusiasm which has been aroused in the profession by the announcement is a just tribute to the character of Robert Koch, who is a model worker of unequalled thoroughness, and whose ways and methods have always been those of the patient investigator, well worthy of the unbounded confidence which every expert in pathology places in his statements. The cold test of time can alone determine how far the claims which he has now advanced will be justified, and meanwhile the solution of the question—so far as human medicine is concerned—has been transferred from the laboratory to the hospital wards, in which the careful observations of the next few months should give the necessary data for final judgment.

"In the selection of cases of pulmonary tuberculosis we have begun with patients not far advanced in the disease, and with little or no fever—cases, too, which we have had under observation for some time, and in whose sputa bacilli and elastic tissue have been repeatedly found. We began on Friday, December 12th, the day on which we received the lymph, through the kindness of Dr. Billings, to whom, as stated in a communication from Professor Koch, the first sample of the fluid was sent in America. One-tenth of a cubic centimetre of a one-per-cent. solution was used for the first injection, and as no reaction followed 0.2 c.cm., and then 0.5 c.cm. were used. With the latter strengths the reaction has, in each instance, been fairly characteristic. Hourly observations have been made in each instance, and there has been within six or eight hours a rise in temperature of three or four degrees. In one case there was a slight chill. The constitutional disturbance has not been great, and the chief complaints have been of restlessness, sleeplessness, and slight pains in the back and limbs. In three cases the cough was greatly aggravated. So far, no change of note has been observed in the sputa. The physical signs will be recorded only once in each week, as it is believed that any changes can be better appreciated after these intervals. Two cases of pleurisy—one chronic and one acute—have received injections for purposes of diagnosis. The chronic case was suspected to be tuberculous, but there are no signs of affection of the lung and no expectoration. He is showing reaction after the third injection. The acute case, as yet, has no special symptoms. No advanced cases have been treated, nor is it thought that much can be expected from the method after large cavities have formed and when numerous foci of softened tissue exist in the lungs. No unpleasant effects have, as yet, followed the injections."

Several of the male patients were shown to the Society, and the charts of the hourly observations passed around for the inspection of its members.

[*For conclusion of the reports see page 670.*]

THE MEDICAL NEWS.
A WEEKLY JOURNAL OF MEDICAL SCIENCE.

| VOL. LVII. | SATURDAY, DECEMBER 20, 1890. | No. 25. |

ORIGINAL LECTURES.

ON THE FORM OF CONVULSIVE TIC ASSO-CIATED WITH COPROLALIA. ETC.

*Clinical remarks made to the Post-graduate Class in Medicine,
Johns Hopkins Hospital, Baltimore, October 11, 1890.*

BY WILLIAM OSLER, M.D.,

PROFESSOR OF THE PRINCIPLES AND PRACTICE OF MEDICINE,
JOHNS HOPKINS UNIVERSITY.

GENTLEMEN: There is a curious disease—or perhaps, more correctly, symptom-group—met with chiefly in children, to which attention has been called of late by French writers, which is characterized by irregular, spasmodic movements, the utterance of involuntary explosive sounds or words, and mental defects of various sorts. It is not a very common affection in this country, and I take this opportunity to bring to your notice a case which we have been studying for the past few weeks.

The cases have usually been described as chorea, or "habit-spasm," both of which conditions are simulated very closely by the irregular movements; certain instances also have been reported as hysteria.

Unfortunately Charcot and his pupils, Guinon and Gilles de la Tourette, have given to this affection the name *maladie des tics convulsifs*. I say unfortunately, for here and in England we use the term *convulsive tic* to characterize a totally · different affection, involving usually the facial muscles and of either central or peripheral origin, but not necessarily coming on in childhood and not characterized by the other features presented by the disease of which we are at present speaking; and thus it happens that if we turn to the recent editions of French books we find under *tic convulsif* a disease very different from that described by the same name in English and American works.

The history of our patient is briefly as follows :

Mary ——, aged thirteen years, applied at the out-patient department, July 10th, and was under observation there until September 16th, when she was admitted to ward G. Her mother brought her to the hospital on account of irregular involuntary movements and curious barking-sounds.

Her family history is good. Her mother is a bright, intelligent woman, a German by birth, and has had ten children, none of whom have been affected as is this girl—the third child. There is no tendency to mental disease in the family. The birth of the child was normal and there is no history of convulsions in infancy. She has had scarlet fever, but has not had rheumatism.

Since her fifth year she has been subject to involuntary jerking movements of the arms and head, which vary very much in intensity, sometimes better, sometimes worse, and they have usually been called by the doctors chorea. They have not interfered with her development or her education. She has not yet menstruated. For the past year she has been making curious sounds; beginning by saying "hah" very frequently. Sometimes she would bark like a dog. She would also call out the names of people, and if she heard a new name she would be apt to repeat it.

Her condition on admission was as follows : A bright, intelligent child ; well educated, writes nicely, takes an interest in her books and has evidently been ambitious at school. She is nervous, the right arm occasionally twitches and the head jerks. There are no grimaces, but on several occasions she seemed to mimic movements of the face. Every now and then she calls out "hah," "Bridget," or "stools," or says in sharp, clear tones "bow, wow." There are no disturbances of sensation, and the special senses are unimpaired. Examination of the heart and lungs was negative; the thyroid gland is slightly enlarged.

Throughout the latter part of July and in August attempts were made to treat the case by hypnotic suggestions, at first with success, but subsequently without any improvement.

On September 8th her mother wrote the following letter, which illustrated a new phase of the child's malady :

"Mary makes use of words lately that make me ashamed to bring her to you or take her out of the house ; it is dreadful, such words as ——, ——, ——, etc. She was always a modest child, and it almost kills me for to hear her use such words."

Her mother was asked to bring her again and was told that this was really a part of the affection, and, like the movements, involuntary in character. The child seemed more depressed, had lost flesh and, her mother said, had changed mentally. She was very obstinate, and almost invariably did what she was told not to do, and had threatened to take poison. She will say the bad words aloud or mutter them to herself.

On admission to the hospital she was placed in a room by herself, kept in bed, and encouraged in every way to cease making the sounds and to stop the use of the bad words. During the first two weeks she improved very much. The movements were reduced in frequency and sometimes during my visit they would not be noticed at all. They most commonly affected the right arm, which, with the hand, was drawn up in a sudden electric-like jerk. The head and neck would jerk simultaneously or alone. Sometimes there was combined movement of the neck and chest-muscles. The involuntary expressions of which she made use were those mentioned above; a sharp bark was the most frequent sound, which, from its ringing quality, could be heard at a considerable distance.

She was so much better that she was allowed to get up and another patient was placed in the room with her. This seemed to excite and worry her, and shortly afterward the barking sounds became much more frequent, occurring every one or two minutes, and she complained of great soreness of the muscles of the chest and abdomen. The movements, however, did not increase. She was again placed in seclusion and in bed, and again improvement followed, but she still barks and she has not given up entirely the use of bad words.

She is a docile, intelligent child, and seems anxious to get well. She has kept a diary, which displays no special peculiarity. She writes verses, which are not worse than those usually composed by girls of her age.

The patient, as you see, is a bright, intelligent child, and there are still to be seen occasional lateral jerkings of the head, and now and then the right arm is elevated with great quickness. You have also heard the peculiar sharp sound which she makes from time to time, which sometimes resembles a hiccough. More commonly it has a barking quality, which is not nearly so marked as it was some weeks ago, when usually two of the sounds succeeded each other with rapidity. In addition, this child has presented several of the symptoms which Charcot and his pupils regard as characteristic of the affection.

I have just spoken of the emission of involuntary sounds and words. The use of bad words, for which the ingenious expression *coprolalia* (fæcal speech) has been invented, is present in very many of the cases, forming a feature very distressing to the relatives.

You can judge from the letter of this child's mother how grievously troubled she was over our patient's "slips of the tongue." She cried bitterly when she told us of it, and said that she wished her daughter would die. In some of the reported cases, even children of five or six years have persistently used words of the most obscene character.

A second peculiarity of a similar nature is the repetition of any sound or word heard, for which the name *echolalia* is employed by Charcot. It is a veritable echo, and the word is repeated by the patient so soon as heard. In our case this did not often occur, but, on hearing a new name, she would be apt in a short time to repeat it very often ; thus, on first coming into the hospital, she used for some time the word "nurse," which she was constantly hearing.

The facial mimicry was noticed on several occasions, but has not been a special feature. This curious imitation of muscular movement has been described, not only in the face muscles, but in those of the extremities, and simulates closely those of the remarkable Malay disease known as *latah*. The term *echokinesia* has been applied to this mimicry of movements.

So far, our patient has not presented any symptom of mental disorder, unless indeed her extreme obstinacy and her addiction to poetry could be so considered. Upon this aspect of the affection Charcot lays great stress, and thinks that sooner or later the cases invariably show psychical changes. By far the most common mental change is the existence of fixed ideas, and Guinon, whose article in the *Dictionnaire Encyclopédique* is the most extensive on the subject, describes these as very often a fear of impending trouble, or a fear of places (*agoraphobia*). In other instances there is "*folie pourquoi*," in which the patient incessantly demands the reason for the performance of even the simplest actions of life.

"*Folie du doute*" and the curious, irresistible impulse to touch certain objects, may also be present. Another form of this obsession which has been noted in some instances, is what has been termed *arithmomania*, in which the patient is possessed with an irresistible desire to do some special mathematical problem, or to count up to a certain number before doing a certain action.

In brief, the main peculiarities of the disease are : the involuntary uttering of words or cries, coprolalia, mimicry of words or movements, and, in very many instances, mental symptoms, chiefly some form of obsession. The majority of the cases present only the first two or three of these features, and it is not until the more advanced stages that the mental symptoms become marked.

The prognosis, according to Charcot and his pupils, is extremely grave, and very few cases recover, but years may elapse before the onset of mental symptoms. The diagnosis is easily made in cases such as the one before you ; but there are several conditions which in certain features simulate the disease very closely. Thus coprolalia and the irresistible tendency, on all occasions, even the most solemn, to use obscene words have been described apart from any motor phenomena. There is the oft-quoted case of the Marquis of Dampierre, who, from early youth to his ninetieth year, involuntarily uttered, even under circumstances the most solemn, the words "*merde !*" and "*foutu cochon !*"

Still more common is the existence, particularly in children and youth, of a fixed idea. One of the commonest is the "*dilirie de toucher*," which impels the individual to touch certain objects, and of which the great Dr. Johnson, as is well known, was a subject. One of the most graphic accounts, probably autobiographical, of this imperative impulse to touch objects is given by George Borrow in his *Lavengro, the Scholar, the Gypsy, and Priest*, in which the practice was followed in order to prevent evil happening to the lad's mother.

In many points the affection has a close resemblance to the common habit-chorea or habit-spasm, with which indeed the involuntary movement of convulsive tic is identical. I do not remember, however, to have seen at the Philadelphia Infirmary for Nervous Diseases, among the numerous cases of habit-spasm which came to our clinics, particularly to the clinic of Dr. S. Weir Mitchell, a single instance in which other symptoms developed.

I had one case with facial spasm, in which the lad put his middle finger into his mouth and bit it severely, and at the same time with the index-finger compressed the tip of his nose. This habit had continued for a long time, and had resulted in the production of a thick callosity on both surfaces of the second phalanx of his finger. A somewhat similar trick is reported to have been practised by Hartley Coleridge when a boy, only, if I recollect aright, he was in the habit of biting his arm. And quite recently there was at the clinic a girl nine years old, who, during convalescence from chorea, developed the curious trick of first smelling and then blowing upon anything she took into her hand.

With hysteria the relations of the disease are not thought to be very close by Charcot and his pupils. The affection usually sets in at a period of life earlier than that at which hysterical symptoms begin, and very many of the cases show no manifestations of hysteria

The utterance of loud involuntary cries and anomalous sounds is, however, a special feature of certain cases of hysteria which may thus present a resemblance to this form of convulsive tic. They, however, are not necessarily associated with involuntary movements, and are usually of a more bizarre character. I remember a remarkable case of the kind which was brought into Professor Waguer's clinic at Leipsic. A child, aged about fourteen years, had for several weeks uttered the most remarkable inspiratory cry, followed by a deep-toned expiration, both of which were audible at a great distance. They persisted during the day with each respiration, but ceased during sleep. The child was worn to a skeleton.

Dr. Gapen, of Omaha, brought to the hospital last year a phonographic cylinder, on which was recorded a most remarkable hysterical cry which the patient, a young girl, had been in the habit of uttering for many months, and which was loud enough to be heard at a distance of several blocks. These cases, however, usually present other features which make the diagnosis clear.

As was the case in this patient, the affection begins at an early period, in a majority of the cases, according to Guinon, from the sixth to the twelfth year. They are commonly regarded as chorea.

An hereditary neuropathic taint has been present in many instances.

We have treated this child in the hospital by seclusion and rest in bed, and have made moral rather than physical efforts to improve her condition. She is certainly better, particularly in the matter of the use of bad words.

ORIGINAL ARTICLES.

THE TREATMENT OF PNEUMONIA.[1]

By J. C. WILSON, M.D.,
PHYSICIAN TO THE HOSPITAL OF THE JEFFERSON MEDICAL COLLEGE, AND TO THE GERMAN HOSPITAL, PHILADELPHIA.

THE subject of the treatment of pneumonia is trite and well worn, I admit; but its earnest consideration enters into the everyday life of all of us. Those among us whose views as to the proper treatment of this familiar disease are definitely settled are few, and friendly interchange of opinion upon the subject is likely to be useful. What I shall have to say relates solely to croupous pneumonia, and has no special bearing upon so-called catarrhal pneumonia, broncho-pneumonia, or any form of secondary pneumonia whatever.

Croupous pneumonia occurs with great frequency in connection with other diseases. It is not uncommon during convalescence from acute infectious processes. Those who suffer from chronic Bright's disease and from valvular and degenerative diseases of the heart and from organic diseases of the nervous system are especially prone to it. It

not unfrequently occurs as the terminal condition in these affections and in other constitutional diseases, such as diabetes mellitus and pulmonary phthisis. Under these circumstances, it preserves, however, its own clinical and anatomical characters, and must be regarded, not as a mere complication of preëxisting pathological processes, to which it has no essential causal relation, but as an entirely independent intercurrent disease.

When we consider the modifications of pneumonia under these circumstances and in the different periods of life from childhood to old age, and in alcoholic subjects, we are impressed with the uselessness of attempts to show by statistics the value of different plans of treating the disease. No general percentages of mortality can be relied upon as indicating the efficacy of a treatment, unless they are on a large scale and in connection with a critical analysis of the condition of the patients. It is a question of the seed, which is probably always the same, and the soil, which is infinitely modified. The only reliable test of the value of treatment is its effect upon the general course of the disease, a test which is much influenced by the personal equation of the observer. For this reason plans of treatment once in vogue, credited with surprising results in reducing the mortality of the disease, have failed to stand the test of time and have passed into disuse. And while the profession unites in striving after some specific treatment for other infectious diseases, the present drift of opinion in regard to croupous pneumonia seems by common consent to be in the direction of a vigilant expectancy with active treatment of symptoms as they arise.

Whether we regard acute lobar pneumonia as a specific inflammation, or, in the language of the day, as an acute infectious febrile disease, of which the pulmonary lesions are merely a localization, we recognize in its causation three factors—a pathogenic bacterium, a predisposition, and an exciting cause—in other words, the seed, the soil, and the implantation. Nothing in the process is more obvious than its specific nature. Against this neither the existing uncertainty as to the actual bacterium which causes it, nor the fact that the local lesions sometimes terminate in gangrene or in abscess, militates in the slightest degree.

Pneumonia cannot be regarded as a simple inflammation. This being the case, the antiphlogistic treatment of former times scarcely deserves discussion. Indiscriminate bloodletting as a routine treatment for a specific pathological process, the natural history of which shows it to be self-limited and of comparatively short duration, is not in accordance with modern therapeutic principles. Still less are repeated venesections and bleeding *ad deliquium*. Patients recovering after such treatment

[1] Read before the Alumni Association of Jefferson Medical College, November 25, 1890.

do so, not as a result of it, but despite it. In connection with this, one turns with interest to the words of Trousseau: "The necessity, the utility, even, of bleeding does not appear to me to have been made out so clearly as is believed by the majority of physicians, to whom the denial of the efficacy of extracting blood in pneumonia would seem the denial of a demonstration." The investigations of Magendie, Dietl, Niemeyer, and others into the natural history of croupous pneumonia had already called attention to the uselessness and dangers of indiscriminate bleedimg. In recent years attempts have been made to show that the disuse of bloodletting in pneumonia has resulted in a notable increase of the death-rate as made manifest by a comparison of recent with older statistics. The unreliability of mortality statistics in pneumonia has already been alluded to. The special error in the statistics of this disease arises from the fact that prior to the middle of the present century the diagnosis of croupous pneumonia was by no means an exact one, and many other pathological processes affecting the chest were very commonly set down as pneumonia. Furthermore, Townsend and Coolidge have shown from a critical analysis of a thousand cases, treated in the Massachusetts General Hospital, from 1822 to 1889, that the increase in the death-rate is misleading for other reasons. The average mortality was twenty-five per cent. This gradually increased from ten per cent. in the first decade to twenty-eight per cent. at the present time. But the average age of the patients has been increasing from the first to the last decade. The relative number of delicate and complicated cases has also been increased, as has the relative number of foreigners. These authors do not regard the treatment, which was heroic before 1850, transitional between 1850 and 1860, and expectant and sustaining since the last date, as having influenced the mortality-rate, the duration of the disease, or its convalescence.

We all recognize the occasional necessity for venesection in the early stages of croupous pneumonia. It often gives relief from urgent dyspnœa and pain, and sometimes even appears to save life. It cannot, however, be considered as a specific treatment. It must be regarded as symptomatic, like wet cups and leeches, which likewise give relief under similar circumstances in a way that is not understood. In the same manner we condemn the treatment by tartar emetic in large doses, and with it is to be relegated to the limbo of discarded medicaments in pneumonia Trousseau's lauded *kermès*. The treatment by large doses of veratrum viride in the early stages, which still survives and finds in many quarters earnest advocates, is based upon the same antiphlogistic idea and has little to commend it. To add the depressing effect of a

powerful drug to the pathological influences already depressing the heart is now recognized as increasing the danger of cardiac failure. In fact, if, as our knowledge of croupous pneumonia indicates, many of the symptoms are due to a toxæmia, it were better to bleed the patient, if he is to be bled at all, into a basin than into his own vessels. To depress the heart by veratrum viride or aconite in the first stage, and to harass it by digitalis at a later period are among the vagaries of a therapeutics which takes pleasure in vaunting itself as rational. To give cardiac depressants in croupous pneumonia is always of doubtful expediency, and digitalis as a cardiac stimulant should be administered only in response to special indications. Of the latter drug Brunton says, "It is of little use in pneumonia."

Efforts to discover a specific, *i. e.*, an antiseptic or germicide treatment for croupous pneumonia have not been followed by success. The most recent attempt in this direction is the suggestion of Bartholow in regard to the use of ethyl iodide by inhalation. The anæsthetic and antispasmodic properties of this drug may render it, when cautiously used, a valuable addition to our resources in the management of pneumonia, but its antiseptic and germicide properties are feeble, and there is no experimental evidence to show that it has, in the high dilution in which it reaches the residual air, any effect upon any of the forms of bacteria present in the pneumonic exudate. Furthermore, there is reason to believe that the pathogenic bacterium has already done its work so far as the lung is concerned when the exudation as manifested by dulness and bronchial respiration is established.

It remains to speak of the treatment of pneumonia by systematic repeated cold or tepid bathing, as practised by Jürgensen at Kiel and Tübingen. Notwithstanding the fact that this treatment, as shown by certain series of statistics, has resulted in an apparent reduction of the mortality amounting to fifty per cent., it has never come into general use, either in Germany or elsewhere. A partial explanation for this undoubtedly lies in the fact that a large proportion of the cases recover under ordinary methods of treatment, and, further, the application of every bath is a disturbance to the patient, which is at least troublesome. Finally, in the absence of conclusive evidence of the efficacy of bathing as a plan, it is impossible to overcome the traditional objections to it on the part of the people.

As yet, we know no remedy of which it can be positively said that it is capable of controlling or aborting the pneumonic process. In affirming this I do not overlook the fact that large doses of quinine given early in the disease are thought by many to exert a favorable influence upon the subsequent course of the attack.

The milder cases run a favorable course and get well without the use of perturbating remedies. The treatment must, therefore, in the present state of knowledge, be expectant. But this expectancy is not idle; it it alert and vigilant, and abundant in resources. It is expectant-symptomatic.

I will speak briefly of the hygiene of the sick-room. The room itself should be large and well lighted, but so arranged that the lighting can be controlled to suit the sensations of the patient. It should be well ventilated, care being taken that the patient is not exposed to draughts. The ideal room for the treatment of pneumonia, or, in fact, almost any of the acute infectious diseases, is like that described in the newspapers as occupied by the Iron Chancellor—large, airy, and well lighted, without furniture, except a military bedstead, a small table, and a chair for the attendant. The patient is not liable to take cold, and requires, above, all an abundance of fresh air. The bed-clothing should be light, but occasionally varied in accordance with the sensations of the patient. The food should be of the simplest and most digestible kind, and during the earlier stages administered sparingly.

A laxative dose of calomel, from three to five grains, at the beginning is useful. It may require repetition later.

The prominent symptoms after the initial chill are the fever, with or without delirium, the pain in the side, the difficulty and distress in breathing, and the cough. The chief danger lies on the side of the circulation, the cause of death in the majority of fatal cases being heart-failure.

The most striking peculiarities of the fever of pneumonia are the suddenness of the rise and its extent; but the importance of the high temperature of pneumonia has been overrated. Welch, in his *Cartwright Lectures*, 1888, carefully analyzes the experimental and clinical data bearing upon this subject. He shows that animals may be kept at a high temperature for at least three weeks without manifesting serious symptoms. The functional disturbances to be attributed directly to the influence of elevated temperature are increased frequency of the respiration and quickened pulse. No definite relation can be established between the variations of arterial tension which occur in fever and the height of the temperature. Though prolonged high temperature is an element in the causation of fatty degeneration of the heart, there are other factors, such as infection, concerned in the production of the lesion. The lessened perspiration, the renal disorders, and the digestive disturbances, with the possible exception of constipation, are always referable chiefly to other causes than the increased temperature. Both experimental and clinical observations strongly support the view now widely accepted that the disturbances of the sensorium, which constitute so prominent a part in the group of so-called typhoid symptoms, are dependent in a far greater degree upon infection or intoxication than upon the heightened temperature. In support of the conclusions derived from the experimental study of the effect of heat upon men and animals, Dr. Welch called attention to the absence of all serious symptoms in many cases of relapsing fever, and in the so-called aseptic fever, in spite of prolonged high temperature. In conclusion he emphasized the fact that those fevers, such as typhoid fever and pneumonia, in which the height of the temperature is undoubtedly a most important index of the severity of the disease, there exists no such parallelism between the temperature and the nature and severity of the other symptoms as we should expect if these symptoms were caused by the increased heat of the body.

It is a matter of common observation that in the so-called typhoid pneumonias, which constitute one of the groups in which the mortality is excessive, and which are of gradual onset, the temperature usually attains a very moderate elevation, 101° to 103° F.

A large dose of quinine given in the beginning and the early administration of calomel exert a favorable influence upon the temperature.

Sometimes it may become necessary to administer internal antipyretics. Among these antipyrine, not less on account of its sedative action upon the nervous system than on account of its antithermic influence, is preferable. Very large doses are to be avoided, lest they depress the action of the heart.

On the continent of Europe cool bathing is resorted to in the treatment of pneumonia with excessively high temperature. The bathing exerts a remarkable effect upon the nervous system; it is at once stimulant and calmative. The baths should be administered at a temperature of from 85° to 90° F., or even higher; or, in the case of strong people with high fever or severe nervous symptoms, as low as 77° F. Strümpell advises that not more than two or three baths should be administered daily, and that they should not be given at night, except in the event of threatening symptoms. Refreshing sleep is said to follow the application of the bath, with quieter and deeper breathing, and a remarkable sense of relief and refreshment. I have had no personal experience with the use of baths in pneumonia, except in the pneumonias of infancy; but I have repeatedly seen very marked benefit follow cold affusions to the head and chest in severe pneumonia of young adults with high temperature and a tendency to stupor.

A fall in temperature must not always be attributed to the action of an antipyretic drug which may have been given, since the natural history of croupous pneumonia shows a decided pre-critical fall as well as the abrupt defervescence at the crisis.

It is important to relieve pain. This may be accomplished by small doses of Dover's powder, from three to five grains, or the tincture of ipecacuanha and opium in corresponding doses, repeated at intervals of three or four hours, or by hypodermic injections of morphine repeated at intervals of six or eight hours. The doses should be so ordered as to produce a slight amount of continuous somnolence. Mental agitation and anxiety are thus also avoided. Under the influence of these remedies the patient's breathing is often notably improved.

Early in the case, leeches over the consolidated lung often seem to exert a favorable influence. Turpentine stupes may be applied at intervals of four hours, or warm wet compresses covered with oiled silk may be used. Sometimes the application of an ice-bag gives relief. I believe poultices are less used at present than formerly. Certainly unless well made and carefully applied they have very decided disadvantages. The cotton jacket is a good substitute for them, or, still better, a shirt lined with light carded wool, which packs less readily than cotton. Blisters should not be used in the early stages. Dry or wet cupping is sometimes used in place of leeching.

After a time pain ceases to be a troublesome symptom, and the opiates may be diminished either in dose or in the frequency of administration. Carbonate of ammonium may now be given with advantage, partly on account of its stimulant effect upon the respiratory centre, and partly because it appears to exercise a favorable influence as a cardiac stimulant. After the defervescence, it may be replaced by the chloride of ammonium.

In ordinary cases a small amount of alcohol in the form of milk-punch or wine should be systematically administered from the beginning, and in others immediately after the subsidence of the intensity which characterizes the onset of the febrile movement. If the heart flag, alcohol is to be given liberally, the character of the pulse and the first sound of the heart being made the gauge of dosage. Strong black coffee or hypodermic injections of ether or of camphor dissolved in olive oil are to be given upon the supervention of evidences of failure in the circulation. Strychnine is useful as a respiratory stimulant and may be administered hypodermically at intervals of eight or twelve hours.

If there be sleeplessness notwithstanding the administration of small doses of opiates, chloral, in doses of from seven and one-half to fifteen grains, proves a most serviceable hypnotic.

In severe cases of pneumonia I am in the habit of administering throughout the attack the mixture of one part of oxygen with two parts of nitrogen monoxide, sold in the shops under the name of Walton's oxygen. These inhalations, systematically repeated at intervals of one or two hours, and sufficiently prolonged, have appeared to exercise an admirable influence upon the respiration and circulation and are often, in cases of great restlessness or agitated delirium, followed by a period of quiet sleep.

Upon the supervention of defervescence there is occasionally observed a tendency to collapse which demands the application of external heat and the free use of diffusible stimulants both by the mouth and hypodermically. If resolution be delayed or if pleural pains continue to be troublesome, flying blisters over the affected side are indicated. Convalescence is, in the absence of complications, usually short and satisfactory.

Insidious pneumonias beginning centrally, the lesion progressing little by little, are often difficult alike to diagnose and to treat. These are the so-called typhoid pneumonias. They often run a protracted course and are of unfavorable prognosis. Death usually occurs from asthenia; sometimes from the mere mechanical circumscription of the respiratory tract, as, for example, when upon the third or fourth day after the appearance of consolidation throughout one lung, the same process is set up in the other lung. When the lesion in the second lung is extensive, the case is not usually amenable to treatment and speedily terminates in death.

MECHANICAL OBSTRUCTION IN DISEASES OF THE UTERUS.[1]

BY GEORGE F. HULBERT, M.D.,
OF ST. LOUIS, MO.

MY observations of and experience with the diseases of the uterus in which mechanical obstruction, or its congener, stenosis of the canal, is considered to be the malady is so at variance with the consensus of medical opinion and practice, that I wish to make it a matter of record and open the door to criticism and correction, if such are deserved.

It may be somewhat startling to many of those men whose reports of cases and operations relating to the subject under consideration so frequently appear in our medical journals, when we say that in more than ten thousand women coming under our care in hospital and private practice, a large proportion of whom suffered from uterine disease, we have not seen a single case which satisfied us that mechanical obstruction existed or was the disease, although the phenomena supposedly attendant upon that condition were frequently observed; and

[1] Read at the sixteenth annual meeting of the Mississippi Valley Medical Association, Louisville, Kentucky, October 8, 9. and 10, 1890.

that in over three hundred autopsies in which the pelvic contents and conditions were carefully examined, we have not found a single case which positively demonstrated that during life mechanical obstruction existed —that condition which has occupied so much of the time and attention of gynecologists, and has been the *fons et origo* of so much operative procedure and instrumental paraphernalia.

Such being our declaration, it becomes incumbent upon us, in explanation, to present the reasons for "the faith that is in us." In doing so, we shall consider the subject under the following heads :

1. The normal or natural order of things, as related to structure and function.

2. The abnormal, pathological, or unnatural order of things, as related to structure, and the possibility or impossibility of, or interference with, the performance of function.

3. The phenomena usually considered as due to "mechanical obstruction" and their accepted explanation.

4. Our criticism and reconciliation of inconsistencies, based upon the facts and phenomena observed by us during life and in the dead-house.

5. Conclusions.

First. We may question if menstruation, as observed to-day, is a perfectly normal or natural phenomenon as far as it relates to the quantity of fluid discharged. Reasoning by analogy and from the purely physical standpoint, it certainly seems a strange straining of that universal uniformity of law and order in nature, that in the highest mammalian this particular element in the functional phenomena should be so greatly and unnecessarily overdone. But it seems from the testimony at hand that such is the fact ; that at the menstrual period in women we do have a more or less free *discharge of fluid*, instead of what seemingly should be a simple elimination or excretion. The conclusion, therefore, which we must reach, is that the organ which we are considering must be competent to discharge fluids. The reason that the uterus is composed of involuntary muscle is at once plain to any one who considers its other peculiar function, gestation ; but the reason for its peculiar form, the arrangement of its cavities, the complicated interlacement of muscular fibres, the dual nervous supply, and the delicately-poised position in the body is not so evident. In our search for a reason for these things, it occurred to us that the uniformity of law and order in nature might be a possible explanation, and that in the physical laws and conditions governing the discharge of fluids would be found the answer to the query. Investigation in this direction led to the conviction that the application of the conic frusta to containers presented the most perfect conditions in order that the greatest

velocity and quantity of discharge of fluids be attained. The laws and principles involved in this particular domain of physics presented a striking adaptation to the uterus, and seemed to offer a clear explanation.

By reference to Fig. 1 this application may be seen. We have four apertures of exit, at D, E, C, and A. At the aperture of the Fallopian tubes ; at the internal os or sphincter, extending down to the line B ; and at the external os extending into the vagina, we see the principle of the conic frusta applied with peculiar perfection. As to form, we see this at the internal os, C. It is also to be observed that that part of the entire canal which approaches each

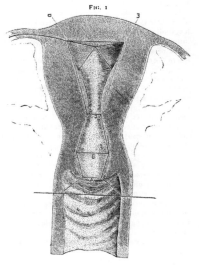

Fig. 1

aperture is more or less perfectly tubular in form, thereby assuring a *column* of liquid above and pressure in the axis of exit. We also find that each aperture is provided with a well-developed muscular sphincter, covered with a thin, closely-adherent mucous membrane, which insures the even closure of the lips of the apertures, save at the external os, where other principles come into play. namely, that of aspiration by the contact of the os with the vaginal mucous membrane. and the elastic play insured by the uterine ligaments. the movements of respiration. and the general movements of the body.

In estimating the capacity of the normal uterus by means of the above principles of hydrodynamics, it was found that the uterus was capable, with one-fourth of an inch aperture at the point of exit and one inch depth of cavity, with the resultant pressure of the column of liquid contained therein, of discharging 0.64541 cubic inch per second, or 38,624.4 ounces during the twenty-four hours. Reducing the diameter of the aperture to one-thirty-second of an inch, we find a capacity equal to 603.493 ounces for twenty-four hours. In menstruation the average flow for twenty-four hours is from three to five ounces of fluid with a temperature of 100° Fahr. and a specific gravity of 1.055. This gives the uterus a capacity to discharge about 600 ounces more than it is required to discharge, with an aperture of one-thirty-second of an inch.

It is also necessary to recall the peculiar arrangement of the muscular elements of the uterus, namely, longitudinal, oblique, and transverse muscular fibres intimately interlaced, establishing conditions which, in the presence of proper innervation and nutrition, insure the certainty of play of force. With peculiar strength is the fact of the dual nerve-supply, namely, a direct spinal supply to the cervix and a ganglionic supply to the body of the uterus, brought to mind in our application of these principles. The cervix, responsive to immediate reflex influences at the internal sphincter, especially concerned in permitting exit and entrance under proper conditions; the body, under ganglionic innervation, concerned in the wonderful phenomena of creative energy, in the to-and-fro play of its forces annuls sufficient of the necessary antagonism to establish equilibrium in the performance of function, and menstruation becomes an unconscious experience in the life of women, save to the sense of sight.

In the circulatory arrangement we see a still further application of our principles, in that the quantity of fluid is governed by a power inherent in the organs, so that in the presence of equilibrium of all else the supply and discharge are under perfect control.

As a last point under this head, we will recall the *rhythmical intermittent discharge* of the fluid during menstruation, dependent upon the physiological action of the uterine circulation. It may be well termed the evidence of a *uterine respiration*, so to speak, by which the life of function is maintained.

Second. From a pathological point of view, the conditions accepted as being the cause of mechanical obstruction are those that produce narrowing or closure of the uterine canal. These so far as described are flexions, conical cervix, pinhole os, and congenital or acquired partial or complete stenosis, the latter being synonymous with atresia. Some consider displacements without distortion of the canal as mechanical obstruction, but the presence of the open canal makes such claims inconsistent.

However, those who have taken the latter position have made progress, and, in reality, their inconsistency has brought them nearer the truth.

The condition of flexion of the uterus has generally been considered the typical one for mechanical obstruction; and we are presented with the flexed rubber tube as illustrating the condition. But this fails to illustrate the conditions as they actually exist.

The manner in which a flexion is brought about is, we believe, in perfect accord with mechanical laws. Given that vicious constitutional condition, of which the local expression is debility of the uterine tissue and its supporting ligaments, called *softness* by Graily Hewitt, without which the development of a flexion is impossible, the first step is an excessive amount of blood in the parenchyma of the organ and its adnexa. This means lack of muscular tone and increased weight, causing the uterus, as a whole, to rest on the posterior and lower part of the pelvic floor; or, if the conditions are so fortunate, on the lower uterine ligaments. The descent persisting and increasing, owing to the angle at which the cervix meets resistance, or to pressure on the fundus, the cervix or body must move either forward or backward, and the result is a flexion. This is a matter of time; there is not sudden violent bending of the uterus, as occurs in the rubber tube, and the degree of bending is determined by the conditions of the uterine tissue. This bent position having been produced, a process of atrophy at the

FIG. 2.

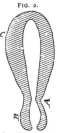

At *A* is seen the indentation where the normal tissue has atrophied. *B* and *C* show the hypertrophy in the posterior wall.

concavity of the angle, and of elongation and hypertrophy at the convexity, at once begins, and *pari passu* with the bending the atrophy and hypertrophy proceed, so that in the process, when completed, that factor which is the essential cause in producing closure in the rubber tube, namely, the V-shaped wedge of tissue at the convexity of the angle, is not present. This is shown by the accompanying cut (Fig. 2).

The hypertrophy of the posterior wall is due, no doubt, to the constant efforts exerted to accomplish the function of menstruation under the changed conditions, and also by the constant irritation produced at the point of impact on the floor of the pelvis.

The atrophy of the anterior wall at the angle is in accordance with the well-known effects of pressure and interference with nutrition. The disappearance of this wedge of tissue in the anterior wall at the site of the angle, in the final rearrangement and adaptation for function, results in the longitudinal and oblique fibres, anteriorly, having instead of two points of departure in contracting, as at the fundus and extremity of cervix, three points, namely, from fundus to angle, and from the angle to the extremity of the cervix, the ultimate result being the same in either case—pulling forward of the anterior segment of the tissue at the site of the angle. The posterior segment would follow, as it does in the rubber tube, on the simultaneous contraction of the longitudinal and oblique fibres, *but for the interposition of the lateral segments, which does not occur in the rubber tube.* Thus it is seen that with a fairly coördinate action of all the fibres in any particular transverse plane of the uterine body closure of the canal is simply impossible. Any angle in the direction of the canal must be more or less straightened, this result being dependent upon the area of uterine tissue brought into action. A perfect *en masse* contraction of the organ must produce more or less straightening and patency of the canal dependent upon the amount of force exerted.

This is illustrated by Fig. 3:

FIG. 3.

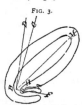

Extreme degree of flexion—45°: *O*, showing the atrophy in the anterior wall at the site of flexion; *M, O, A*, points of departure on the contraction of longitudinal and oblique fibres in the anterior wall. The interposition of the lateral wall between the anterior segment at *O* and the posterior at *B* makes it impossible for the inner surfaces at *A* and *B* to come in apposition, save by a dominant contraction of the sphincter fibres.

To this antagonism of forces we can attribute the fact that in the most acute flexions the canal is not bent at an angle, but maintains the direction of the segment of a circle.

In our examinations to determine the degree of flexion we frequently deceive ourselves, and speak

25*

of acute angles. As a matter of fact, it is rare that we meet with a flexion more acute than a right angle, and in an acute-angled flexion during life we not only would be sure to find the fundus in the position of an anteversion, but the os would be toward the meatus urinarius.

Fig. 4 illustrates what would be present in a right-angle flexion:

FIG. 4.

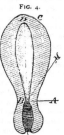

If the central line, *D B* (Fig. 4), of the fundus was brought forward, and placed on the line *C B*, Fig. 3, we would have the fundus about in the normal position in the body. Now, moving the central line of the cervix forward so that it rests on *B, F*, we would find that the prolongation of this line would make its exit at the anterior edge of the anus. This would represent a flexion with a right angle. Now place *D B* on *M B* (Fig. 5, *a*), and the central line of the cervix on *B F*, and we have an angle of 45°. In this case a prolongation of the central line of the cervix would pass out through the posterior commissure of the vulva.

FIG. 5.

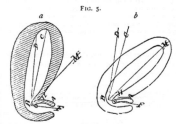

The last illustration shows an extreme degree of flexion, which is found only in the minority of cases. The proof of the disappearance of the tissue at the concavity of the angle of flexion is found in autopsies, and is demonstrated by straightening the bend and comparing the anterior and posterior walls. We have seen some specimens in which the healthy tissue at the concavity was only one line in thickness.

In order that the rubber tube should accord with the existing conditions, it is necessary to select one corresponding in the thickness of its walls and in its calibre with the normal uterus at the internal sphincter, one which is elastic, one in which there is some means of producing the effects of the longitudinal and oblique fibres, and, lastly, one in which a sufficient amount of the wall at the concavity of the angle shall be removed corresponding to the absorbed and atrophied tissue at the site of the angle in the deformed uterus. This done, the bent rubber tube will in a fair degree illustrate what takes place at menstruation in a flexed uterus.

The action of the longitudinal fibres, as far as the anterior wall is concerned, can be produced by passing a few threads through the calibre of the tube, fixing it in the angle desired, which is usually not more acute than a right angle, and making traction on the threads in the line of each arm of the bent tube. It will be found that the obstruction even with this imperfect arrangement will be overcome, and that water will flow through the tube.

This is illustrated by Fig. 6:

FIG. 6.

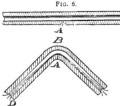

The upper illustration shows the prepared tube; at *A*, V-shaped wedge of the anterior wall removed. The lower illustration represents the same tube, bent at a right angle, and the effect produced by traction on the threads in the line of each arm of the bent tube. The arms are firmly fixed in position in any sustaining apparatus, as a glass tube is slipped over and held by an assistant.

Fig. 7 illustrates the usual faulty method, save that the tube is of the proper dimensions to use in the above experiment.

FIG. 7.

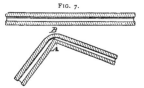

The closure on bending at *B* is readily understood, and the effect of removing the wedge-shaped piece of the anterior wall at *A*, as well as the influence of the longitudinal threads, is possibly better appreciated by the comparison.

From the foregoing we conclude that in the abnormal deviations of direction which are found in flexions, nature in her conservatism still utilizes the principles and agencies present in the normal state, and thereby perpetuates the operation of natural laws and insures the performance of function.

Only by this conception are we able to account for the phenomena of normal menstruation so frequently found, certainly in fifty per cent. of women who have well-marked flexions. We have frequently seen women in whom it was possible to pass into the uterus only a small wire probe, who had at no time suffered from inconvenience during the menstrual flow.

Upon the other conditions productive of mechanical obstruction there is this observation to make, namely, that *at times there exists the capacity to discharge fluid blood*, save in only one condition—atresia. All that the uterine canal can justly be called upon to permit to pass through it is *fluid blood*. If the passage of clots, mucous plugs, shreds of membranes, etc., are the evidences needed to establish the conditions for mechanical obstruction, then we are, indeed, undone. We respectfully submit that such a demand is unreasonable, illogical, and unscientific. We conclude, therefore, that the passage of fluid blood is positive proof that there exists a capacity in all the above conditions, save that of atresia, for the performance of function.

Third and fourth. Such being our conclusion, how do we account for the symptoms usually ascribed to mechanical obstructions, namely, pain, intermittent and scanty flow, relief from pain when the flow is present, and inability to pass the uterine sound? The most radical of those who claim that flexions produce mechanical obstruction, freely admit that where menstruation is normal and painless obstruction is not present. Stenosis being the condition considered necessary, by the "obstruction philosophy," in the absence of the diagnostic symptoms mentioned above, there is, consequently, no stenosis; hence these diagnostic symptoms must be explained.

We have seen from what has been presented the importance of that harmonious, perfect, involuntary, and unconscious rhythm of circulatory, muscular, and nutritive action found in health. As the dominant energizing factor we must look to the inherent quality of nutritive and nervous capability, and to this alone; and in grasping the full meaning of this we must go back to the quality of protoplasm before our position becomes rational. This is a universal principle so frequently lost sight of by us as gynecologists, that it is no surprise to see so much error and disappointment in our therapeutics, be they surgical or otherwise.

We must go to the nervous system, especially the sympathetic, for the all-governing factor : to nutrition, as a whole, we must go for stability of function. The nerve-tone coupled with the resultant nutritive activity and power, both impressed, under favorable environment, with the capacity for a higher standard, determines what shall be the future of every organism or part thereof.

A woman born with and maintaining a standard degree of health will never be cursed with any of the conditions we are considering. But in those who are born without the standard, or who, by the vicissitudes and accidents of life, depart from perfect health, in proportion to the deviation we will find the liability to and acquisition of these conditions. In these deviations from the standard degree of health we find lowered nerve and nutritive tone, manifested by irregular and erratic innervation, resulting in irregular, incoördinate action, increased irritability, irregular circulation and muscular action, pain, spasm, and relaxation, alterations of secretion, rapid exhaustion, slow recuperation, imperfect repair, insuring debility, fatigue, pain, and disorder in the accomplishment of function. These are the real factors in the dysmenorrhœa of so-called mechanical obstruction. These, and not stenosis, are the disease.

In the functional antagonism between the cervix and the body of the uterus we find the immediate cause of all the symptoms attendant upon mechanical dysmenorrhœa. Irritation or dilatation of the cervix produces contraction of the cervix. This physiologically and anatomically demonstrable fact, which, if sought for, is always found antedating and associated with mechanical dysmenorrhœa, when followed to its reasonable and logical conclusion, proves that mechanical obstruction, as at present generally accepted, does not exist save in that condition termed atresia.

The constitutional condition means increased local irritability and lowered nutrition. This begets irregular and spasmodic muscular and circulatory action, with altered excessive or scanty secretion and excretion. The excessive flow, the blood-clots, the membranes, and the mucous plugs are due to the influences mentioned, and their expulsion produces severe suffering. Such cases are used by some as an argument in support of the idea of mechanical dysmenorrhœa, especially when a flexion is present. It is unnecessary to answer such arguments. It would be perfectly consistent for these men to assume mechanical obstruction as a disease, in the delivery of a fœtus. But given menstruation with fluid blood as the substance to be expelled in a woman who presents the symptoms of mechanical dysmenorrhœa, what facts will aid us in the present discussion? Excluding atresia, it matters not what the local condition is, we find the general devia-

tion from the standard degree of health. A fat and apparently well-nourished woman may present symptoms at her menstrual period similar to those presented by another woman in the opposite condition of general health. In the first instance, innervation, motor power, is at fault ; in the second, the fault is in both innervation and nutrition. In both the local conditions are alike. Now, take either of these women and place her under methods of treatment that will allay irritation, produce coördinate action, and improve the general health, and we find that *without any local treatment* all the symptoms indicative of mechanical dysmenorrhœa disappear, and still the flexion, pinhole os, elongated cervix or stenosis, remains. Let the woman return to the original diseased condition, and the symptoms of mechanical dysmenorrhœa again appear. Furthermore, in the worst cases, in which the flow is usually very scanty, we find that in spite of the *persistent stenosis*, as they approach the standard degree of health the flow increases and the suffering decreases and eventually disappears. Manifestly, we must look elsewhere for the cause of the symptoms, and we find it in lowered nutrition and increased irritability, expressed by hyperæsthesia and erratic muscular and circulatory action. It is nerve-ache, muscle-ache, nerve-tire, muscle-tire. It is the cry for quietude, harmony, and rest from the ceaseless and persistent wants of the physiological rhythm of forces. That the local condition in its development has no influence on the systemic we do not affirm. In the progress of every case the time arrives when the local condition, by reflex influences, becomes a very important element in the process : first, from general to local ; second, from local to general, until the poor sufferer cries out in agony, afraid to move, afraid to laugh, afraid to lie down ; tenderness and pain in all parts of her body, and in constant fear of the monthly onslaught of what should be to her an unconscious relief. This is not enough, it seems, but she must be further accused of carrying around with her a disease called "mechanical obstruction," and be subjected to sponge-tents, and incision and divulsion of the cervix, followed by the use of a stem-pessary.

Especially bearing upon the interpretation of the pain in conditions of supposed mechanical obstruction, we desire to direct attention to a condition in which the pain is of the same character and in which mechanical obstruction cannot be present, namely, the "after-pains" of parturition. We are of the opinion that as far as the location, character, and manner of onset of the pain are concerned, there are no differential features between the pain of mechanical dysmenorrhœa and the "after-pains" of labor, yet in the presence of only *fluid blood* severe "after-pains" frequently occur. There being no stenosis after a parturition, the severity of "after-pains" in the absence of blood-clots is considered dependent upon nervous, nutritive, circulatory, or muscular influences, even by the most radical supporters of mechanical obstruction in menstruation.

In considering the question of spasm of the internal sphincter as a factor in producing the phenomena of mechanical obstruction, we are impressed with the desperation of many in striving to retain the mechanical idea of dysmenorrhœa. Correctly understood, this frequent and ever-ready action of the internal sphincter serves but to establish our position in antagonizing the mechanical idea. The presence of the spasmodic element is proof positive of unnatural and incoördinate muscular action, as well as increased local irritability. This, coupled with the antagonism existing between the cervix and body of the uterus, readily explains why during menstruation, the spasmodic action should occur, and also why there is no flow until the spasm is relieved. In spasmodic or neuralgic dysmenorrhœa the menstrual flow is almost *nil.* This is not due to a damming back by the spasmodic closure at the sphincter, but is due to the fact that there is no menstrual fluid in the cavity of the uterus, and it is only when coördinate action is accomplished that blood exudes from the endometrium. This is readily proven by the introduction of a tube into the uterine canal during the menstrual period, insuring beyond a doubt patency of the canal.

The diminution or disappearance of pain when the flow is established is now readily understood, when we say that it is due to the rhythm of forces finally accomplished, to nervous, muscular, and circulatory factors, within the tissues, and not to the forcible expulsion of retained fluid. The failure to pass the probe or sound is a mere matter of diagnosis and dependent upon the hand that manipulates it.

Finally, we appeal to post-mortem investigations. Any one who has labored in the dead-house, investigating the pathology of those conditions which are considered active factors in the production of mechanical obstruction will meet with one stubborn fact, namely, that the conditions found after death are far different from those that would be expected from the severity of the symptoms during life. Consider, for instance, endometritis, and in the dead-house specimen, macroscopically, is hardly distinguishable from one obtained from a subject who had never during life suffered from such a disorder. Microscopically we find the difference, and in the vast majority of cases are forced to conclude that this difference is more a functional than organic one. Take also any specimen and study the subject of stenosis of the canal, and how often, unless there is stenosis from scar-tissue in the mucous tissue lining the canal or

congenital atresia, will you find a contraction that fluid blood would not find its way through; certain it is that fluid blood will travel through the capillary system, and the uterine canal, save in atresia, has a diameter equal to at least several capillary vessels. We also find in post-mortem examinations that the uterine canal, even in the presence of great deviations in surrounding structures, or extreme distortion and displacement of the organ, is free from acute angles, and that the cavity is tubular, especially at the site of the internal sphincter. These facts are readily proved by sections in any direction, and are readily accounted for if we accept the influence of the muscular elements and correctly interpret the mechanical laws at work in the form and structure of the uterus in their relation to the performance of function.

In the attempted demonstrations of the existence of mechanical obstruction by its supporters, the fact that they were dealing with a *dead* organ seems to have been lost sight of; for in no other way can we explain the usual methods of attempting to prove mechanical obstruction *during life* by forcing a *lifeless flexed uterus* into a greater degree of flexion, for even dead as it is it will not remain in the forced position. It would seem unnecessary to remark that pickled specimens are not suitable for demonstration, either affirmative or negative, yet they are frequently presented as showing the state during life.

The therapeutic measures which are successful in relieving and curing mechanical dysmenorrhœa demonstrate beyond all doubt the correctness of our position. And in using the expression therapeutic measures, we wish it distinctly understood that we exclude all local, surgical, or mechanical treatment to relieve the supposed stenosis of the canal. The use of reconstructives, such as good, palatable food, the elegant gluten and malt preparations, and the hypophosphites and bitter tonics, for the purpose of restoring the standard nutrition; the employment of narcotics, anodynes, anti-spasmodics, such as opium, compound spirit of ether, antipyrine, viburnum opulus and viburnum prunifolium, alætris farinosa, helonias dioica, cimicifuga, scutellaria, laterifolia, and gelsemium; the valuable anti-congestive drug, hydrastis; the coördinating muscular tonics, ustilago maydis and quinine; and last but not least, electricity, are attended with results eminently successful. The intelligent and persistent use of these means will, in the absence of atresia, cause all the phenomena of mechanical obstruction to disappear, while the local deviation, as far as form and displacement are concerned, may remain. The local state, as far as secretion and function are concerned, will be restored to a normal condition.

Furthermore, it is a matter of daily observation,

that all surgical and mechanical methods of treating dysmenorrhœa which are not assisted by pronounced improvement in the systemic, nervous, and nutritive forces of the patient are ineffectual.

We respectfully submit the following conclusions:

1. That in the natural order of things we find the uterus in form and structure endowed with a capacity for the performance of the function, menstruation, so far in excess of any legitimate demand, that with a diameter of the canal of one-fourth of an inch at the sphincters the excess is 7724.8 times the demand, and with a diameter of one-thirty-second of an inch the excess equals 120.7 times the requirement.

2. That in the pathological conditions considered essential for mechanical obstruction we find that the conservation of force so regulates the conditions that this capacity is not abolished, but persists in an eminent degree, so that in the presence of the normal physiological energy the function is accomplished, unless there is atresia.

3. That the phenomena considered as dependent upon mechanical obstruction are not due to the forcible expulsion of retained fluids through the uterine canal, but are produced within the tissues, and are dependent upon *disturbed* rhythm of physiological forces evolved by abnormal innervation, muscular action, and circulation.

4. That the demand upon the uterus for the passage of blood-clots, membranes, mucous plugs, uterine sounds, sponge-tents, uterine dilators, etc., in order that the diagnosis of mechanical obstruction may be made, is not only vicious in the extreme, but irrational, illogical, and unscientific.

5. That the correct and rational interpretation of the testimony offered by symptomatology, pathology, and therapeutics, removes mechanical obstruction from the domain of gynecology as a demonstrable fact, save in atresia uteri.

3026 PINE STREET.

THE MEDICAL EXPERT.[1]

BY J. T. ESKRIDGE, M.D.,
OF DENVER, COLORADO.

AT a recent meeting of the Medico-Legal Society of Denver, the President appointed several committees to report before the approaching session of the Legislature of Colorado, on certain necessary changes in our laws in relation to the establishment of a State Lunacy Commission and a State Board of Charities. Committees were also appointed to consider and report on the medical expert, the care and protection of our insane, prison reform, and the necessary statutory changes to make official autopsies more scientific and thorough.

[1] Read before the Medico-Legal Society of Denver.

These several committees are expected to report on the various subjects committed to them, so that the Society's Committee on Legislation, after hearing the discussion by members of the Society, may be prepared to enter upon their duties, and endeavor to secure legislative enactments in accordance with the Society's wishes.

No one who has compared the laws of many of the Eastern States of this country on the above subjects with the meagre legislation, or the absenec of legislation, on the same in Colorado, can doubt the propriety and timeliness of the Medico-Legal Society's action upon these neglected but important subjects.

As a preliminary to the report of the Committee on the Medical Expert, I wish to consider the status and necessary qualifications of the medical expert most in demand by the majority of the legal fraternity, together with some suggestions looking to a partial prevention of the confusion resulting from the present method of employing medical expert testimony.

According to decisions of various courts of law, anyone who possesses special knowledge of medicine and subjects relating thereto, whether he be a graduate in medicine or not, and regardless of the school of medicine to which he belongs, may be called to testify in court as a medical expert. It seems, then, impracticable for any State to enact a law to prevent either side of a case from calling any medical witness desired, and the jury must be left to judge of the fitness of the expert and the value of his testimony.

There are several causes which aid in producing the unsatisfactory results obtained by the present method of using medical expert testimony. In the majority of instances the attorney for the plaintiff secures experts that best serve his purpose in the case, and the lawyer for the defence likewise endeavors to fortify his side of the case by the testimony of witnesses with different opinions. We cannot blame the lawyer, whose whole training has been to win the cause of the client rather than to guide the case and to see simple justice done. If he can secure the services of respectable witnesses who will testify in favor of his client, it seems to him proper and right. He leaves the witness to justify his own testimony. I am loath to believe that all lawyers, or even the majority of them, are anxious to gain their cases regardless of right, but I am convinced that many bright and honest legal advocates are deceived by the misrepresentation of their clients. A lawyer once impressed with the justness of his side of a case (I do not say absolutely convinced), is in sympathy with his client, and apparently without examining into the merits of each side of the case, he seems to think and act as if every means tending to support his side is justifiable and should be employed.

The position of the medical witness should be directly opposite to that usually assumed by legal advocates. In impartiality he should rival the most upright judge and the ideal juror. In the medical aspects of a case he should take pains to inform himself without reference to the side on which he is to testify. He is but human and should not be subjected to the slightest mercenary temptation that might in anyway bias his judgment. If the medical witness should be as impartial as the judge and jury, and I think no one will deny this postulate, he should not be subjected to temptations from which they are free. How ridiculous it would seem to allow plaintiff and defendant each to choose and pay his jurors and judge I Yet, the medical expert is required to testify to, and in a certain sense, sit in judgment upon facts which neither the learned judge nor the jury "just and true " claim to be able to understand.

The habit of separate and independent examinations by medical witnesses often leads to erroneous conclusions, because, in these days of the rapid accumulation of medical literature observation and scientific investigation, no one person can become thoroughly conversant with every department of medicine. To comprehend all the facts pertaining to a difficult and obscure case, the specialist and the general practitioner, both of medicine and of surgery, are often necessary. What one fails to observe, the other will very probably see. No two minds follow exactly the same train of thought. If the examination of a person is made by a physician subpœnaed to testify for one side, he, in the majority of instances, is alert to discover symptoms more favorable to the side that has employed him than to the opposing one. Imperfect or partial examinations are more likely to result, and the personal equation of the examiner is in greater danger of being magnified, when the examination is made separately than when the physicians examine and consult together as a board. One physician may be thorough in certain departments of medicine and not in others, or he may hold certain theories which carried to their ultimate conclusions become mere vagaries. Such defects may be partially obviated by joint examinations. The editor of the *British Medical Journal* [1] writes:

"In Leeds, the custom has, we believe, long obtained among the leaders of the profession to refuse to give expert evidence on any case until after a meeting of the experts on both sides; and this practice has worked so well that the Leeds Assizes are notable for the absence of the conflicts of scientific testimony which elsewhere have done so much to discredit such testimony in courts of law."

---

[1] March 1, 1890.

To meet the objections against the present system of employing medical expert testimony, Dr. Morton Prince, of Boston, in an able article entitled "The Present Method of Giving Expert Testimony in Medico-Legal Cases,' [1]" makes the following suggestions:

" 1. The examination of all claimants should be made by experts on both sides, but in conjunction with each other and acting as a Board. The examination should be conducted as frequently as the Board should determine. This would not prevent preliminary and individual examinations by either side.

" 2. The Board of Experts after thus acting should make a sworn written report to the court in accordance with a specified form; that is, the report should contain a distinct and separate statement of the medical history, objective facts, and finally the opinion of the experts.

" 3. If the Board is unable to agree on the purely objective facts (for example, whether there was or was not paralysis, loss of sight, fracture of bone, etc.), the court should, at its discretion, direct one or more official State experts to examine the claimant in conjunction with other experts, and report likewise in writing their opinions.

" 4. A number of experts in each department of medicine should be appointed by the Governor, and from them the court should select experts at its discretion.

" 5. At the request of either side of a case, the court should direct one or more State officials to make an examination.

" 6. All experts should be examined in court as now."

It is easier to criticise the suggestions made by Dr. Prince than to suggest better ones. There are, however, many objections to State medical experts, and to their appointment by the Governor. If the appointing power rested with the Governor, it would become a part of the political machinery of the State, and candidates for positions on the Board would receive their appointment more on account of their political influence than because of scientific qualifications for the work.

Further, there would be a temptation for ambitious, but unscrupulous, physicians to seek such appointments on account of the prestige it would give them to be recognized as State medical experts. Any ignoramus in Colorado, be he a graduate in medicine or not, might be sure of such an appointment if he, or his friends, could control a few hundred votes. Men should be sought for such positions and should not seek the positions. Again, the influence that such a Board would have with a jury would be as great if composed of unqualified persons as it would be if none but the most competent men in the State were on the Board. If such a body of official experts should have no further qualifications for their positions than would be necessary to secure their appointment through political influence, it might lead to exorbitant awards or unjust punishments. It seems to me that in Colorado, at least, an official Board of experts, appointed

---

[1] Boston Medical and Surgical Journal, January 23, 1890.

annually or less frequently, would probably be productive of more harm than good.

Might not the benefits expected from a State Board of medical examiners be obtained by other, and less elaborate means, without incurring the objections against such a State organ? Much of the confusion resulting from conflicting expert testimony might be avoided if the court were required to name experts to testify in a given case, regardless of the wishes of the lawyers for either plaintiff or defendant, and guided solely by the qualifications of the experts for the particular case. This would not prevent the attorneys from calling physicians of their own selection, provided that no expense beyond the ordinary witness fee were incurred by the county for these witnesses The experts named by the court should have a definite fee for their services, regardless of their opinion in the case. Testimony from experts so appointed and paid would be entirely unprejudiced by mercenary considerations, and would deservedly have more weight with a jury than the testimony of physicians selected and paid by either the plaintiff or the defendant.

If we had a law making it obligatory upon the court in every case requiring medical expert testimony to appoint one or more experts, the number depending upon the importance of the case and the wishes of the counsel for each side, then the experts appointed by the court, and those chosen by the attorneys, if any were so selected, should be required to examine jointly all such persons whose claims might be under investigation, and consult together as a board. The number of examinations should be determined by the majority of the board. Individual and preliminary examinations should not be denied if consented to by the attorneys and by the person whose claims might be under investigation.

It is remarkable how infrequently physicians disagree in consultation, either in hospital or private practice, and equally remarkable how frequently physicians employed by opposing counsels disagree in their testimony on the witness-stand. Much of this difference of testimony occurs from the one-sidedness of the physician's information of a case. Were examinations made jointly and consultations held afterward, this source of error would be excluded.

The following is the report of the Committee on Medical Experts appointed by the President of the Medico-Legal Society of Denver:

1. "That it is the sense of this Society that its Committee on Legislation should endeavor to have a law enacted at the approaching session of the State Legislature empowering and requiring the judge, before whom a case necessitating medical expert testimony is to be tried, to select one or more medical experts, the number depending upon the importance of the case, the wishes of the attorneys for both sides, and upon the approval of the presiding judge.

2. "That the Board of Physicians so selected by the court be required to examine the claimant or defendant jointly as a Board, and that other physicians selected by the attorneys for either side be permitted to be present and participate in the examinations and discussions of the Board.

3. "That the physicians selected by the court be required to testify in court concerning their examination and submit to cross-examination as is now the custom.

4. "That a definite expert fee be allowed by the court and paid by the county for each of the physicians selected by the judge.

"All of which is respectfully submitted.

J. T. ESKRIDGE,
H. A. LEMEN,
A. H. WYCOFF,
Committee.

THE DIAGNOSIS OF EARLY ECTOPIC GESTATION.

BY J. M. BALDY, M.D.,
OF PHILADELPHIA.

IN following me into a discussion of this subject I wish it to be distinctly borne in mind that what I have to say is applied to ectopic gestation only in its earliest stages, namely, in that period when the rupture is liable to take place from the tube into the broad ligament, or into the abdominal cavity, as well as the period immediately following the rupture.

It would seem from this that I accept the views of Mr. Tait as to the pathology of extra-uterine pregnancy, and, with a few reservations, this is the fact. My whole line of argument will be based on the premises that conception has taken place in one or other of the Fallopian tubes, or has subsequently found its way there, and has there developed. I do not wish to be understood as denying that there is such a condition as ovarian or abdominal pregnancy, but for our present purpose we may safely ignore that phase of the question altogether, because in the early stages of the disease with which we are dealing the three conditions could hardly be differentiated. It is certain that an overwhelming majority of the cases are tubal in their incipiency, and if an occasional case is either of the other two varieties, it cannot make the slightest difference from a diagnostic and therapeutical point of view.

In this discussion I propose to ignore, to a great extent, the ancient literature of the subject. However valuable this has proven in times past in establishing the pathology of extra-uterine pregnancy, it is to-day of far less value from the point of view of this paper than the experience and literature of the last few years. I infinitely prefer the testimony of men who have made their observations with a pretty clear idea of the pathology and frequency of this and allied diseases, to that of men who were groping in the dark with little or no idea of this or any of the many diseases with which it may be and has been confounded. With the recent data, then, to supplement my own personal experience of more than twenty cases of early ectopic gestation, I shall be satisfied to draw my conclusions.

The symptoms of this disease have been variously classified, and it is claimed that if a certain number of them be grouped together in the same patient, the presence of the abnormal gestation is assured. In considering these symptoms we. will take them as nearly as possible in the order of their importance.

Menstruation.—This may be absent for one or two periods, and then a spurious flow appear which is at first lighter and finally darker in color than normal. It is irregular, prolonged, and contains, after awhile, clots and shreds. There may be no missed period at all—simply a prolongation of the normal flow, with the above characteristics. I have had patients in whom this spurious menstruation did not appear at all; in whom there was neither a scant nor prolonged flux. To a great extent this depends on the period in which the patient is seen ; the earlier, the less likelihood of irregularities. Often the patient gives a history of similar irregularities, and one is very apt to be misled by this fact.

Pain.—This pain is of a somewhat different character from other pains to which women are liable. Early in the growth of the gestation-sac the pain is slight, and occurs at long intervals, and as a rule not much notice is taken of it. Often it disappears altogether for a few weeks, and would be forgotten but for its reappearance in redoubled force. It is intermittent in character, cramp-like, becoming more and more severe, and more and more frequent. At times it becomes so severe as to cause syncope. Its situation is almost invariably pelvic, and low down in the abdomen. It can be safely said that this symptom is invariably present. As a rule, it is the one thing which forces the patient to seek the advice of her physician. Of all the individual symptoms this one has proven of most value to me in recognizing the true condition. This almost characteristic behavior of the pains in connection with the behavior of the menstrual discharges when they are abnormal should always put one on his guard, and force him at least to weigh carefully all the *pros* and *cons* before dismissing the possibility of ectopic gestation.

Expulsion of decidua.—The decidua may be thrown off in the shape of shreds, and mixed with clots of blood, or, which is more usual, after a few days the shreds may come away in one good-sized mass. This symptom is theoretically of the greatest importance, and when it is demonstrated is conclusive (of pregnancy). Practically, its value is in the majority of cases lost. As a rule, we must depend on the statements of the patient in regard to the matter, and these statements are too often worthless. I find that patients do not observe closely enough, or are so ignorant as not to be able to distinguish between blood-clots and other things. Again, the decidua is often lost in the water-closet or in a vessel-full of clots. I have known women to declare they were discharging shreds, when a careful examination failed to reveal a sign of one. Taking it all in all, I do not attach much value to this sign—realizing, however, its great importance when it can be properly demonstrated. Its absence is usually in the early weeks of the disease.

General signs of pregnancy.—As a rule, these are the reflex, gastric, and breast symptoms of normal pregnancy, as well as the bladder and rectal disturbances of the same condition. The same symptoms may be present in women who are not pregnant, and may arise from almost any cause of irritation in the genital canal, and are only too frequently present in such diseases as ovarian cyst, pyosalpinx, etc. Standing alone they are worthless for determining pregnancy, especially the extra-uterine variety.

Period of sterility.—As a rule, the patient gives the history of having had a child or miscarriage some years previously, and of being sterile since then. This is not always the history, however, as some women conceive with the foetus extra-uterine soon after the first pregnancy.

Vaginal discoloration.—The vagina almost invariably has the usual discoloration of pregnancy.

Cervix.—The cervix is usually enlarged and soft, and the os is patulous ; but I have noticed an absence of these symptoms in several cases, and they cannot be considered as at all constant.

Body of uterus.—The fundus is enlarged and softened, and usually crowded either far forward against the pubic bone or pushed to either side. It is more or less immovable. Like the cervical signs, however, these conditions are not constant. I have studied patients for several weeks at a time, in whom the uterus was normal in every particular, trying to arrive at a diagnosis, and yet ectopic gestation was finally proven to be present.

Uterine appendages.—At times an examination of the appendages of one side is absolutely negative, while on the opposite side a tense, adherent, tender cyst is present. In several cases I have found this cyst almost in the median line, posterior and apparently so continuous with the cervix as to make it impossible to find any dividing-line between them. In one case the fundus was so high and so far back as to seem to be a part of the cyst. On the other hand, cystic masses (apparently characteristic) will be found on both sides, one proving to be an ovarian cyst, an ovarian abscess, a pyosalpinx, or a dermoid cyst, the other being demonstrated to be a tubal pregnancy. All these conditions I have seen, and have studied with the specimens in my hands. The local condition is so varied and deceptive that only corroborative evidence can be obtained from it. The ectopic gestation-cyst, if kept under observation, increases very perceptibly in size from time to time, but it is exceedingly dangerous to wait and watch for this symptom.

Pulsation of the cyst.—I have studied the disease with reference to pulsation, and in spite of what others have said as to its importance, I have been unable to find the slightest thing characteristic about it. The pulsation is present in so many pelvic conditions, especially in distended Fallopian tubes, that I have found it worthless as a diagnostic sign in this disease. In proven cases of ectopic gestation, in my experience, it was present in some and absent in others.

Ballottement.—I have never been able to observe this sign in any case, nor have I seen a specimen earlier than the third month in which I think it could have been demonstrated. The number of cases in which it is claimed that it has been observed is small, and to me it is of very doubtful value as a diagnostic aid.

The patient considers herself pregnant.—In the majority of cases that I have seen the women did not think they were pregnant, or at least were very uncertain when questioned on this point. Only two or three of my patients stated positively that they thought themselves pregnant, and we all know how often women think themselves so when they are not. I cannot believe that this point is of much value in diagnosis.

Temperature and pulse.—A number of times I have noticed a persistent and considerable rise of temperature and increased pulse-rate, and the patients have occasionally complained of feeling chilly. The elevation of temperature is due, no doubt, to the local pelvic inflammation which so often accompanies this condition, and which causes the adhesions almost always met with.

When we come to the period of rupture, symptoms of great pain, followed by collapse, and all the signs of concealed hæmorrhage, make the presumptive diagnosis easy, especially when taken in connection with the past history.

It would be natural to suppose that if a number of these symptoms presented themselves in the same patient a diagnosis of extra-uterine pregnancy could readily be arrived at. Such is the belief of some of the profession. Reeve[1] states that "in a patient presumably pregnant, having had more than one such attack as this (he refers to the paroxysmal pains), and having a tumor to be felt *per vaginam*, there could scarcely be a doubt of the existence of extra-uterine pregnancy." My own experience has taught me the fallacy of this, and I am coming more and more to regard my position taken in a previous paper[2] as the true one. In that paper I made the three following propositions:

1. In a certain proportion of cases of extra-uterine pregnancy, in the early stages, the diagnosis is easy and unmistakable.

2. In a certain (quite large) proportion of cases sufficient symptoms are present more than to warrant a diagnosis of extra-uterine pregnancy, such a pregnancy not being present.

3. In a certain other proportion of cases the symptoms, until rupture has occurred, are entirely wanting, or are of such dubious character as in nowise to warrant such a diagnosis.

The following history is that of a patient who passed under my observation:

CASE I.—Mrs. X., aged twenty-six years; married for seven years. Had one child six years ago. Puerperal trouble followed confinement, and she has not been pregnant since. Two and a half months ago she missed her menstrual period, and soon began to develop symptoms which made her think she was pregnant. In the course of about six or seven weeks she began to have a bloody vaginal discharge, which finally contained shreds and clots. About this time pains, which had been present in slight degree, became severe and paroxysmal. On account of the bleeding and pain she applied to me for advice. On close questioning she acknowledged having passed a mass, but was doubtful whether it was blood-clot. A vaginal examination revealed a softened cervix, a slightly-enlarged uterus, with a tense, adherent, tender cyst on the right side, the uterus being crowded to the left. A diagnosis of tubal pregnancy was made, and the gestation-sac removed two days afterward.

This case presents a line of symptoms which apparently could lead to but one conclusion, and so the event proved. But contrast this case with the two following, which occurred in my practice.[3]

CASE II.—The patient presented general and reflex symptoms of pregnancy, such as swollen and painful breasts, containing milk; morning nausea; enlarged abdomen; frequent micturition; constipation, etc.; and had missed one or two periods. The patient thought herself pregnant, though she had not been pregnant for some years. There was

---

[1] American Journal of the Medical Sciences, July, 1889.
[2] Medical Record, September 21, 1889.
[3] Ibid.

irregular bleeding for a week or two, with colicky pains in the abdomen, and the passage of blood and shreds *per vaginam.* Examination showed a cystic tumor to one side of the uterus, painful to the touch. The patient was seen by Dr. J. Price, and several other men, all of whom concurred with me in the diagnosis of undoubted extra-uterine pregnancy. Several days afterward an operation disclosed an ovarian cyst as large as an orange.

CASE III. presented general and reflex signs of pregnancy almost the same as in Case II. She had not been pregnant for years, when she missed a period ; had profuse bleeding with clots and shreds, and severe pelvic pains of a colicky character. Examination disclosed a pelvic mass at the side of the uterus, evidently a distended tube. A diagnosis of extra-uterine pregnancy was made by Dr. Kynett, several other men, and myself. Operation in a few days by Dr. Penrose disclosed pyosalpinx.

The following cases simply emphasize what my own cases prove :

CASE IV.—Mrs. D. ;[1] a patient of Dr. Weeks, of Trenton, N. J. ; married for four years ; never pregnant ; menses always regular, and not painful. One week after her January period she noticed dull pain in the lower part of the abdomen, followed in another week by sick stomach and all the symptoms of pregnancy. Her menses were absent for six weeks, when she was suddenly seized with severe pain and a flow. The woman finally took to her bed. The discharges seen by both doctor and nurse were lochial in character, and contained shreds. A tender cystic mass was found to the left and posterior to the uterus ; the fundus was crowded forward and to one side. A diagnosis of extra-uterine pregnancy was arrived at, and I was asked to see the patient. I found everything as narrated, and verified the diagnosis. Two days later abdominal section disclosed a large pelvic (intra-peritoneal) abscess. The Fallopian tubes and ovaries showed no signs of having been impregnated.

CASE V.—Mrs. K.,[2] a patient of Dr. B. C. Hirst, aged twenty-five years. Her last child was born two years ago ; menses were absent for two periods, but had returned some time before being seen by Dr. Hirst. History of discharge of clots and membrane, with great pain in pelvis and abdomen. Examination showed the uterus enlarged, and displaced to the right side ; os patulous ; and a tumor in left broad ligament the size of an egg. Extra-uterine pregnancy was diagnosed. At the operation which followed a broad-ligament cyst was removed. The woman afterward passed remnants of an abortion.

Dr. Joseph Price,[3] in a patient sent to him by Dr. Garrett, of Germantown, found a mass on the left side of the pelvis as large as a three months' uterus. The woman had been married for ten months ; the menses ceased three months after marriage, and she had all the symptoms of pregnancy. There was absence of two periods, followed by hæmorrhage and pain. Extra-uterine pregnancy was diagnosed. Abdominal section revealed a small suppurating cyst of the right ovary, with an adherent hydrosalpinx.

Dr. H. C. Coel reports the case of a woman whom he saw in consultation. She had missed two menstrual periods, and presented the subjective symptoms of pregnancy. One day she had an attack of violent pain in the abdomen, with evidences of collapse. A mass was found on the right side of the uterus, which gradually increased in size week by week. She had a bloody discharge from the vagina. A sound was passed into the enlarged uterus a number of times, and both the galvanic and faradic currents were applied. The uterus was enlarged, the cervix soft, and the os patulous. The tumor was fixed and fluctuating. Finally, she had another attack of pain, with apparent collapse. Extra-uterine pregnancy was diagnosed. Abdominal section revealed a normally-pregnant uterus, with a large adherent ovary on the right side.

Dr. G. W. Johnston reports[2] the case of a patient, aged twenty-two years, who, shortly after the cessation of a monthly period, began to suffer from nausea, frequent micturition, and colicky abdominal and pelvic pains. Her breasts were tender, the uterus enlarged and anteposed ; on the right side of the uterus and posterior was a round, exquisitely tender, semi-fluctuating tumor, the size of a lemon. The attacks of pain were paroxysmal, and on several occasions were almost followed by collapse. She had a vaginal discharge which contained shreds. Extra-uterine pregnancy was diagnosed. Abdominal section revealed a tubo-ovarian cyst the size of a lemon.

W. Gill Wylie[3] says that he has operated on three cases in which the diagnosis of extra-uterine pregnancy had been made, in two of which a supposed cure by electricity had been recorded, and at the operation no sign could be found of ectopic gestation having existed. The cases were simply those of Fallopian tubes dilated with fluid, one tube containing over two pints of fluid.

An article by Vander Veer[4] discloses two cases (Mundé and Janvrin) of pregnancy in one horn of a bicornate uterus, which were mistaken for ectopic gestation. He also reports two cases (Warren and Vander Veer) of normal pregnancy, mistaken for ectopic gestation.

It certainly is unnecessary to produce more evidence than this in order to convince the most sceptical that the symptoms of extra-uterine pregnancy are very often present when the disease is

---

[1] Annals of Gynecology, May, 1890.
[2] Personal communication.
[3] Annals of Gynecology, March, 1890.

[1] American Journal of Obstetrics, January, 1890.
[2] Ibid., August, 1889.
[3] Ibid., January, 1890, p. 71.
[4] Ibid., November, 1889.

anything but an ectopic gestation. I am ready to grant that all the symptoms which we have considered as being produced by this disease were not present in each of the cases presented; but in what disease in the whole range of medicine are all the symptoms present in one case?

The most prominent and valuable points are noted in each case, viz.: the subjective signs of pregnancy, the pains, the missed menstrual period, and the bloody vaginal discharge containing shreds or masses, together with the cystic tumor in the region of the broad ligament. A study of these cases will show most decidedly that no other conclusion could have been arrived at in any single case, and in addition, the names of the attending physicians are a sufficient guarantee that the symptoms and history were carefully weighed. There are many more such cases on record, and very many which are not but should be.

It is interesting in connection with this to note the large number of diseases which have been mistaken for ectopic gestation in its early stages. Dr. T. Gaillard Thomas says: "There are few pelvic conditions which develop in the female, from phantom tumor to fæcal impaction, which I have not seen confounded with ectopic gestation." Amongst the few cases I have reproduced in this paper the mistake was made in cases of ovarian cyst, pyosalpinx, pelvic abscess, broad-ligament cyst, ovarian abscess, normal pregnancy, pregnancy in one horn of a bicornate uterus, and tubo-ovarian cyst. These are not all of the diseases which may be so mistaken. If the mistake is to be made in one class of cases oftener than another, I believe it will be in patients in whom an abortion has taken place, followed by a pelvic tumor (abscess or pyosalpinx)—or a pelvic mass may have existed formerly and unknown—the facts of the abortion being unknown or concealed. The case of Dr. Weeks, as quoted above, was such a one.

Now, with all these chances of mistake in diagnosis, have we considered all the possible errors? By no means. We still have to consider those cases in which extra-uterine pregnancy exists, but is not suspected, and cases in which it was taken into consideration, but was dismissed for lack of sufficient evidence. The following two cases which occurred in my own practice illustrate these points very well:

CASE VI.—Mrs. R.[1] came to me complaining of abdominal and pelvic pain. After giving a negative history she was put on the table, a diagnosis of pyosalpinx was made, and an operation advised. One week later she sent for me, and I found her upon her bed. She said she had had abdominal pains during the entire week. She arose from her bed in order to obtain a letter. While on her feet

she was seized with colicky pain. As I watched her the idea suddenly seized me that possibly this might be extra-uterine pregnancy. I carefully examined her with this possibility in view.

She had been bleeding, at times, for more than two weeks; the flow was pure blood, with no shreds or clot. She had not the slightest general or reflex signs of pregnancy; her husband had been away for only three weeks; she had not missed a period, nor had she had a scant one; and she had had children for the past six or eight years at regular intervals.

The examination showed the uterus in good position, and the cervix perfectly normal for a multipara. There was a mass posterior to and apparently continuous with the cervix, so that I had not been able clearly to feel the fundus anteriorly. I should have considered the mass the fundus. The only symptoms I had then for diagnosis were the bleeding and the pain. These symptoms are such constant and almost invariable companions of all serious pelvic troubles, that without something more to sustain the diagnosis it had manifestly to be given up. Dr. R. H. Hamill made a most careful examination for me, and could find nothing more on which to base a diagnosis; in fact, he did not think that it was a case of ectopic gestation. Our reasons for the diagnosis of pyosalpinx were the absence of symptoms of extra-uterine pregnancy, and the facts that the woman had been complaining of pelvic pain for the past three or four years, had pain at her menses, and painful coition and defæcation. She had had more or less leucorrhœa, which had suddenly become profuse, with itching about the vulva and painful micturition. She was in that condition of life in which one would expect her husband to infect her almost certainly with gonorrhœa. She had a high temperature and pulse, and chilly creeps. Taking it all in all, the indications were clearly for pelvic inflammatory trouble, and against extra-uterine pregnancy. It proved to be pregnancy of the fimbriated end of the tube.

CASE VII.—Mrs. T. C.,[1] aged twenty-four years, married for nine years. Has had two children, and no miscarriages. The last pregnancy was six or seven years ago. After this labor she was in bed for eight weeks with a "sore and swollen belly," and since then she has never been free from pelvic and abdominal pain. Her menstruation has been regular but profuse, lasting eight or nine days. In the interim between her first illness (following the birth of her child) and the present, she had an attack of abdominal pain, which confined her to bed for a week or more. On November 15, 1889, she came to me stating that her regular menstrual period had come on five weeks previously, and that she had been bleeding more or less ever since. The constant pain she had been having had become worse. She had the appearance of a very sick woman, her temperature was elevated, her pulse quick, and she was having chills and creeps. An examination of the pelvis showed the uterus in fair position and of normal size. There were irregular cystic masses on each side, the larger being on the right. A diagnosis of chronic double pyosalpinx, with an acute attack of pelvic peritonitis, was made, and an operation advised. I removed from the right side a tubal pregnancy (verified by microscopical examination) which had advanced to about the sixth or seventh week ; from the left side an ovarian cyst the size of a hen's egg.

The results of the operation were a complete surprise to me. My diagnosis of pyosalpinx, which was concurred in by Dr. T. Hewson Bradford, was made with the utmost confidence, and we had not the slightest doubt that it would prove to be correct. Ectopic gestation never entered into consideration. As soon as the patient was well enough I questioned her closely to see wherein we were at fault in our deductions. The questioning disclosed the following facts : At no time during the past year had she missed a menstrual period, nor had there been a scant or delayed one. At no time had she any signs of pregnancy, such as she suffered from when she was previously impregnated. In fact, she does not even now believe that she was pregnant, basing this scepticism on the absence of a missed period and the early signs of pregnancy. Her breasts were of normal size, the areolæ were not enlarged or changed in color ; there was no tingling or itching about the breasts, though they contained a small quantity of milk—however, she states that such had been their condition since the birth of her last child. There was no decidual discharge ; the only thing she passed besides blood was "a piece of whitish matter," such as she was in the habit of passing at the end of each menstrual period. This point has been most carefully inquired into, and she answers very intelligently. In addition to her statements we have those of a carefully-trained nurse. The patient was in the hospital two or three days before the operation, bleeding constantly. The nurse declares that the napkins were soiled with a discharge entirely free from clots or shreds. Stomach symptoms were entirely wanting. The pains were, according to her statement, not different from those she had with her previous attack of probable pelvic peritonitis.

In addition to these cases of my own, I will emphasize my position by reference to a few others occurring in competent and skilled hands.

G. M. Tuttle[1] reports the case of a woman who was under observation for several months. A diagnosis of double pyosalpinx was made. The operation revealed a pyosalpinx on the left side, with a tubal pregnancy on the right side.

H. T. Hanks[2] records a case on which he operated. The physician who sent him the patient said that she had suffered very little, and advised that no treatment be instituted. After reaching New York, however, she began to suffer, and a diagnosis of pyosalpinx was made. At the operation which followed a tubal pregnancy was removed.

J. P. Tuttle[1] records a very interesting case. After carefully studying all the symptoms, he discussed the case at length with an experienced physician in New York, and after weighing the evidence *pro* and *con* they decided against ectopic gestation. The fœtus was afterward delivered through the rectum.

E. W. Cushing[2] mentions a case which had been operated on for an ill-defined tumor. The cyst was opened after the operation and a fœtus was found. There had not been a suspicion of pregnancy.

Smith[3] reports a case in which the patient died, and a post-mortem examination showed the right Fallopian tube distended into a sac, and containing a three months' embryo and placenta ; the sac had ruptured, causing the death. He says, " In this case extra-uterine pregnancy was not suspected until I received the history of the symptoms immediately preceding death, nor can I see anything after reviewing the case which would have justified the diagnosis of tubal gestation. There was no attempt at abortion, no hæmorrhage, no pain referable to the uterus or tubes."

William T. Lusk[4] recently operated on two patients, and found extra-uterine pregnancy. In either case, under ordinary circumstances, it would have been impossible to make a diagnosis. He has in the last few years changed his views very considerably on this subject, and he now believes " that the number of cases in which we can diagnose extra-uterine pregnancy in advance is really very small."

Dr. Joseph Price in a recent discussion before the Philadelphia Obstetrical Society stated that he had failed to make a diagnosis in four out of the last five cases of ectopic gestation he had operated on.

I could quote many other similar cases, but I have already produced sufficient for my purpose.

It is here interesting to note the mixed character of the trouble in a number of the cases. My second case was complicated by an ovarian cyst on the opposite side. The case of Dr. G. M. Tuttle had pyosalpinx on the side opposite to the pregnancy. Cases have been reported where there was an ovarian cyst on the same side. Medical literature is full of such mixed conditions.

The class of cases we have been considering form no small proportion of the total number of cases of ectopic gestation on record, and in all human probability the vast majority of such cases are unrecorded. To give some idea of the immense proportion of mistakes which have been made in diagnosis during even the past few years, let us

1 American Journal of Obstetrics, January, 1890.
2 Ibid., January, 1890.

1 Annals of Gynecology, February, 1889.
2 Ibid., November, 1889, p. 87.
3 American Journal of Obstetrics, March, 1889, p. 259.
4 Journal of the American Medical Association, April 12, 1890.

compare some approximate figures. It is fair to assume that the total number of cases of extra-uterine pregnancy in its early stages which have been put on record in the United States during this period does not much exceed two hundred, if it reaches this point. At the end of the year 1888, Hanks[1] tells us that there were in the previous three years ninety-seven cases of extra-uterine pregnancies of all stages reported in all the journals published in the English language. It is also fair to assume that there were very few cases in this period of time which were diagnosed and not recorded. Add fifty cases to cover this possible discrepancy and we have an approximate total of two hundred and fifty cases diagnosed during this period of time. Now compare these figures with those of the other side of the story. With merely a superficial glance over only a part of the literature, I have found some twenty cases recorded (a few of which I have quoted above). It must be remembered that this does not by any means represent all the mistakes which have occurred, as men will conceal their blunders in spite of anything which can be said. In addition to these, which in themselves form a formidable percentage of the total number diagnosed (20 as against 250, or 12½ per cent.), I have the word of the coroner's physician of Philadelphia, Dr. H. F. Formad, that he has in his possession the specimens from more than thirty women who died from rupture of an ectopic gestation-sac (and I myself have seen and studied many of the specimens). These cases had been under the care of one or more physicians, and yet none had been diagnosed, and a post-mortem examination by the coroner's physician was necessary in order to ascertain the cause of death, it being supposed in many of the cases that they had been the victims of foul play. No reasonable man will contend that such cases occur only in Philadelphia, and if we make a calculation on a population of fifty millions or more we have an approximate total in the United States during the past few years of about 1500 deaths from undiagnosed extra-uterine pregnancy. Of course these figures are only approximate, and it would take a great deal of time to verify them. However, they are sufficiently accurate to give a thinking man plenty to reflect upon, and must carry conviction to the minds of most. Now, in addition, take into consideration all those cases in which the disease has existed, but was overlooked, and those, again, in which the diagnosis was made, and the disease did not exist, and our chances for a correct diagnosis fade to a minimum. I do not wish to be understood as thinking that it is always impossible to make a correct diagnosis in the early

stages of extra-uterine pregnancy, because it has been accurately made, and I myself have made it, and verified the correctness of my diagnosis; the impression I wish to create is that in the great majority of cases the diagnosis can only be an approximate one, and when it is once made we are oftener likely to find ourselves mistaken than not. I think the evidence here produced more than sufficient to uphold that opinion.

THE USE OF ESSENTIAL OILS IN SURGERY.[1]

BY CARL E. BLACK. M.D.,
OF JACKSONVILLE, ILL.

SINCE the germ-theory of the cause of sepsis and infection became generally accepted, the minds of surgeons, experimenters, and money-makers have been actively engaged in seeking new and more efficient antiseptics and disinfectants. An antiseptic to meet the needs of many cases must fill several requirements.

1. It must fully inhibit the growth of or destroy microörganisms.

2. It must not be very irritating, and must not destroy the tissues.

3. It must be convenient to prepare and carry.

4. It must have a diversity of application.

The wider the "range of value" the more desirable is the antiseptic, and a non-poisoning antiseptic is more desirable than a poisonous one.

Further, antiseptics may be either stimulating or sedative to the tissues to which they are applied. This makes it necessary for us to have at least two antiseptics for everyday use. As a sedative antiseptic there is probably none better than carbolic acid, although there are several objections to it; namely, it is a poison, will destroy tissue, has a disagreeable odor, and considerable caution must be exercised in its employment. For general use, antiseptics which are stimulating without being irritating are more desirable; and for this purpose it seems probable that our best agents will be found among the essential oils.

For comparison we will refer to two or three antiseptics which are in common use. The following are the results of some experiments made by Dr. G. V. Black, with cultures of microörganisms submitted to the action of drugs in solutions of known strength for definite periods of time. Carbolic acid was found effective in the proportion of 1 : 300, or in the proportion of from 1 : 8 to 1 : 15 of a five-per-cent. solution. That is, one part of pure carbolic acid to three hundred of the culture-medium in which the microbes were growing, inhibited their growth; or one part of a five-per-cent. solution of

[1] Transactions of the American Gynecological Society, 1888, p. 360.

[1] Read before the District Medical Society of Central Illinois, October 28, 1890.

carbolic acid to from eight to fifteen parts of the culture medium was equally effective.

A saturated solution of boric acid was found effective in the proportion of from 1 : 4 to 1 : 6.

Mercuric chloride was found effective in the proportion of from 1 : 25,000 to 1 : 50,000, or from 1 : 50 to 1 : 100 of a 1-to-500 solution.

Let us compare these figures with those obtained from similar experiments with the essential oils. Oil of cassia was found effective in the proportion of from 1 : 3000 to 1 : 5000, or from 1 : 2 to 1 : 8 of a saturated solution.

Oil of cinnamon was found effective in the proportion of 1 : 2000 or from 1 : 1 to 1 : 3 of a saturated solution.

Oil of cloves was found effective in the proportion of from 1 : 1100 to 1 : 1200, or in from 1 : 1 to 1 : 2 of a saturated solution.

Oil of mustard was found effective in the proportion of from 1 : 1000 to 1 : 1500, or from 1 : 1 to 1 : 2 of a saturated solution.

Oil of turpentine was found effective in the proportion of from 1 : 500 to 1 : 600, or in 1 : 1 of a saturated solution.

These experiments show mercuric chloride to be the most effective antiseptic, but its corrosive and poisonous qualities make it undesirable for general use. Both carbolic acid and boric acid are less effective than any of the essential oils named. Next in power to mercuric chloride is oil of cassia, made from the Chinese cassia bark. It is commonly sold as oil of cinnamon in our shops. One part of this oil to 4000 of the culture-medium was shown to be uniformly effective in inhibiting the growth of microbes. The Ceylon oil of cinnamon, made from the buds, is only about one-half as effective as that made from the Chinese bark. The other oils named are effective when used in larger proportions. One difficulty in the use of mercuric chloride is that it is not effective in the presence of albumin. All the albumin must be precipitated before the mercuric salt becomes active. Therefore in weak solutions its effects are uncertain, and in strong solutions its poisonous properties become dangerous.

The experiments with the essential oils were made about two years ago, and have recently been fully confirmed by the experiments of Dr. W. D. Miller, of Berlin, a member of the Imperial Board of Health of Germany.

It would consume too much time to give in detail the experiments, and the practical application of the results is more interesting. My experience has been almost exclusively confined to the oil of cassia, which was chosen because it was shown to be more effective and to have a wider "range of value" than any other of the oils, and in fact than any of the antiseptics in common use, excepting mercuric

chloride. A review of a few of the cases in which I have used it will be of interest.

For more than a year I have relied on a solution of oil of cassia, the aqua cinnamomi of the Pharmacopœia, for cleansing the hands, instruments, patient, etc., in all obstetrical procedures, and always with good results. The same solution was used in all cases in which a wound was made, and primary union invariably followed. In cases of suppuration or necrosis the solution seems especially useful. In the case of a large cancer of the breast, involving the axilla, in which sloughing had extended to such an extent that the closed hand could be placed in the abscess cavity, the cassia solution soon diminished the suppuration and sloughing, and reduced the septic fever. In this case it was also efficient in relieving the disagreeable odor which accompanies the breaking down of carcinomatous tissue.

Another case was that of a man suffering from locomotor ataxia, who severely injured his foot. A few weeks later the bones of the second phalangeal articulation of the little toe were found necrosed. All the dead bone was scraped away and the wound cleansed with the solution of the oil of cassia. Healing promptly occurred, which, considering the general condition of the patient, was surprising. In a boy ten years old, who had had an abscess of the tibia for eight weeks, several sinuses were incised and the whole cavity thoroughly curetted, and dressed with the oil of cassia solution. The wound healed rapidly.

A rectal abscess was treated in the same way and with equally good results.

In a patient with necrosis of one and three-fourths inches of the outer plate of the body of the inferior maxilla, three sinuses were opened, the necrosed bone was scraped away, and the cavity washed with an emulsion of oil of cassia. In this case the entire wound healed at once and without further formation of pus.

In several cases of herpes circinatus the disease promptly disappeared after being thoroughly rubbed two or three times with the pure oil of cassia.

As an antiseptic wash in many forms of chronic nasal and pharyngeal inflammation the cassia solution gave excellent results, and at the same time was agreeable to the patient.

For a number of years dentists have used what is known as the " 1, 2, 3 " mixture, as an antiseptic for cleansing cavities and pulp-chambers, and for the treatment of alveolar abscesses. This mixture contains one part of carbolic acid crystals, two parts of oil of cassia, and three parts of oil of wintergreen. It seems in the light of recent experiments and experience, that the oil of cassia is the most active ingredient of the mixture, and that the same results, so far as antisepsis is concerned, would be obtained if it was used alone.

A number of physicians and surgeons have used oil of cassia with results similar to those I have reported, so that the proof of its effectiveness is complete. The late Dr. David Prince chiefly relied upon the oil of cassia as an antiseptic, and used it in all his later abdominal operations.

The oil will inhibit the growth of or will destroy microörganisms. In solutions of effective strength it is not irritating, and will not destroy tissue. It has a "wide range of value," being exceeded only by mercuric chloride in the absence of albumin. It is not poisonous unless considerable quantities of the pure oil are used. The solution is convenient to prepare and carry, and has an agreeable odor. It has a considerable diversity of application.

An emulsion of oil of cassia causes some smarting at the juncture of the mucous membrane and skin, and irritates the tissues of the eye. The pure oil rubbed on the skin twice a day causes marked redness and a few blisters will appear about the third day.

The most common form in which oil of cassia or any of the essential oils is used is a watery solution, prepared by placing enough of the oil in distilled water to form a saturated solution, or by making the aqua cinnamomi of the Pharmacopœia.

The emulsion may be made by beating up the desired quantity of the oil in water. For local application it may be used in any strength for one or two applications, but is liable to cause irritation if applied frequently.

The oil may be mixed with powdered boric acid and applied as a dry dressing, or it may be made into an ointment with vaseline. In nasal diseases a favorite application is the oil of cassia dissolved in fluid cosmoline and applied by means of an atomizer.

It seems to me that no other antiseptic offers us so wide a range of adaptability with so few objections as the oil of cassia. In special cases some other antiseptic may be more desirable, but for general use this has many points in its favor.

MEDICAL PROGRESS.

Treatment of Keloid.—M. VIDAL (*Annales de Dermatologie et de Syphilographie*) has observed that the cicatrices of scarifications made in keloids not only disappear rapidly, but that the keloid-tissue disappears with them. In recent growths one scarification may suffice, but the treatment of large growths must be continued for several months, and many patients are not willing to submit to the treatment for a sufficiently long time. If the treatment ceases when only a small nodule remains the growth will rapidly re-form; the scarifications must therefore be continued until the scar is everywhere soft and thin. The incisions should be made about one-fourth of an inch apart and "cross-hatched" either at

right angles or obliquely, and should penetrate through the keloid, but must not extend for more than one-fourth of an inch beyond its borders. Previously to operating Vidal produces local anæsthesia by means of liquefied chloride of methyl, painting the surface with this until congelation causes the skin to whiten. As soon as the color begins to return the chloride of methyl is again applied, experience having shown that successive applications cause the anæsthesia to penetrate more deeply. The scarifications may usually be made to the depth of three-eighths of an inch without pain.

The loss of blood is not great and is immediately stopped by the application of absorbent wool saturated with boric acid solution. On the following day the surface is dressed with diluted mercurial ointment.—*Practitioner,* November, 1890.

Treatment of Ringworm of the Scalp.—According to the *St. Louis Medical and Surgical Journal,* QUINQUAND has devised the following method of treating ringworm of the scalp:

The hair is cut very short and the circular areas covered with scales and spores are scraped. The scraping induces a slight superficial dermatitis, and should be repeated at intervals of from five to eight days. During the intervals between the scraping the following solution is continuously applied:

R.—Biniodide of mercury . . 0.2 part.
　　Bichloride of mercury . . 1 "
　　Alcohol . . . . 4 parts.
　　Water . . . . 25 " —M.

On the fifth day after scraping, the following ointment is applied to the entire scalp in order to reach all new foci of the disease:

R.—Chrysarobin ⎫
　　Salicylic acid ⎬ of each . . 2 parts.
　　Boric acid ⎭
　　Vaseline . . . . 100 " —M.

After applying this ointment, the scalp is covered by a linen or rubber cap, held in place by means of Unna's zinc-glue. This is removed after forty-eight hours and the entire process is then repeated. In about a month epilation is practised and repeated, and the cure should be complete.

Errors in the Diagnosis of Infectious Diseases.—According to Russell, the following table derived from hospital statistics of Glasgow, shows the number of errors which have been made in regard to the diagnosis of contagious diseases:

Scarlet fever .	. 508 cases	15 errors.
Measles . .	. 368 "	3 "
Whooping-cough .	. 248 "	42 "
Typhoid fever .	. 36 "	16 "
Typhus " .	. 38 "	9 "
Diphtheria . .	. 64 "	2 "
Erysipelas .	. 3 "	3 "
Puerperal fever .	. 3 "	3 "

In other words, there were 7.6 errors for each 100 cases, and prompt diagnosis, important in order that isolation might be practised for the prevention of the spread of disease, was in this number of cases wanting.

THE MEDICAL NEWS.

A WEEKLY JOURNAL
OF MEDICAL SCIENCE.

COMMUNICATIONS are invited from all parts of the world. Original articles contributed exclusively to THE MEDICAL NEWS will be liberally paid for upon publication. When necessary to elucidate the text, illustrations will be furnished without cost to the author.

Address the Editor: H. A. HARE, M.D.,
1004 WALNUT STREET,
PHILADELPHIA.

Subscription Price, including Postage.

PER ANNUM, IN ADVANCE . . . . $4.00.
SINGLE COPIES . . . . 10 CENTS.

Subscriptions may begin at any date. The safest mode of remittance is by bank check or postal money order, drawn to the order of the undersigned. When neither is accessible, remittances may be made, at the risk of the publishers, by forwarding in *registered* letters.

Address, LEA BROTHERS & CO.,
Nos. 706 & 708 SANSOM STREET,
PHILADELPHIA.

SATURDAY, DECEMBER 20, 1890.

LATEST INFORMATION CONCERNING KOCH'S DISCOVERY.

ASIDE from the abstract of the paper of Sir Joseph Lister, which we print as a special cable dispatch, in the EXTRA attached to this number of THE NEWS, we are glad to be able to give our readers other information from American investigations and foreign journals concerning the progress of this remarkable discovery. (See extra and page 670.)

It is very evident, as time goes on, that Dr. Koch has acted wisely in refusing to divulge the character of the anti-tubercular liquid, and it now appears that the criticisms which have been made concerning the secrecy of its preparation were exceedingly unjust to the great bacteriologist.

On November 7th, in other words a week before Koch's paper appeared, the distinguished investigator had a long discussion with the Prussian Minister, Herr von Gossler, in the presence of two witnesses, in which he stated that it was his desire to publish everything in connection with his research, including the method of preparation of the fluid. From the explanation which Koch gave to the Minister, it became evident to this official that a description of the preparation of the drug could only be followed by disastrous effects, if those who were not skilled in its manufacture should attempt to follow the directions given, for the method is so difficult in its details that it must either be seen or else be independently discovered by experiments, which, according to Koch's calculations, would take an experienced experimenter six months. For these reasons Herr von Gossler advised that this part of the discovery be kept a secret, and volunteered to take the responsibility of the information being withheld.

In his speech before the Prussian Diet von Gossler stated that in the present stage of organic chemistry the remedy cannot be analyzed with any degree of certainty, and that the method by which the remedy is obtained will probably render it applicable to other infectious diseases. He also stated that Koch himself lays special stress upon the chemical aspect of the subject.

The difficulties which exist in the manufacture of the remedy on a large scale are so great that the Prussian Government has been urged to put its authoritative stamp upon all of the liquid which was given out for experimentation in order to prevent fraud and to avoid the production of serious results by the use of impure material.

INFECTION FROM THE INTESTINAL CANAL.

IT is very generally believed that failure to procure healing *per primam* of tissues not previously infected can invariably be attributed to carelessness on the part of the surgeon or his assistants. This is doubtless a satisfactory rule of thumb, since it is in the great majority of cases strictly true, and since its tendency is to make more careful those in whose practice secondary local complications occur after operation. It should be recognized, however, that this rule has its exceptions, since dogmatic assertions to the contrary might not only cast undeserved reproach upon the most careful surgeons, but might even subject them to action at law to recover damages for a sequel to operation entirely beyond their control.

It is well known, for instance, that pathogenic microbes may gain access to the circulation by means other than those offered by the instruments of the operator, and may cause characteristic local effects in spite of rigid and successful antisepsis. Indeed, this has been so frequently observed in trauma not accompanied by surface-loss of continuity that the possibility of its occurrence in the operating-room must be admitted.

In addition to infection by the well-recognized

pyogenic microbes, it now seems probable that the bacterium coli commune may, exceptionally, play an important part in interfering with the healing of wounds. The possibility of wound-infection by microörganisms gaining access to the circulation by means of the intestines has long been maintained, especially by those interested in abdominal surgery. It is very generally admitted that in ulcerative conditions of the mucous membrane of the alimentary canal systemic infection may occur. But when the intestines are healthy, or subject to no greater alteration than that accompanying moderate catarrhal inflammation, proof has been wanting as to the possibility of harmful germs penetrating into the lymphor blood-channels.

In this relation the communication of TAVEL (*Correspondenzblatt für Schweizer Aerzt.*) is most important. He calls attention to a former paper in which he demonstrated the intestinal origin of two cases of acute goitrous inflammation. In both were discovered pure cultures of a gas-forming bacterium very similar to one found in the large intestines. The chain of evidence was incomplete, however, since he was not able to obtain the identical microörganism from the alvine evacuations.

Kocher many years ago expressed the opinion that inflammation in goitres was frequently secondary to an enteritis, but this has remained without positive proof till the present communication by Tavel. The chain of evidence in his last reported case seems complete. In January, 1890, Kocher operated upon a goitre containing two cysts. One was enucleated—this was accompanied by much bleeding, checked only by sponge-packing; the other was enucleo-resected. The wound was drained, closed, and dressed with sublimate gauze. The following day the drainage-tube was removed. Gelatin into which portions of the tube were dropped remained sterile for several weeks; then a small colony of cocci, commonly found on tubes which have remained in contact with the skin, developed. These cocci were obtained from nearly all wounds which united by first intention. Healing took place rapidly. Eight days after operation, the wound having in the meantime completely closed, redness about the cicatrix and fluctuation were observed. Hæmatoma was suspected; an incision was made, and a brownish, bloody fluid, containing no clots, escaped. Microscopical examination was not made, but cultures showed an abundant growth of a short bacillus which proved to be the bacterium coli commune.

The cavity from which this liquid escaped was found to have grayish necrotic walls. No pus was discharged at any time. As healing was exceedingly slow, the curette was freely used. During this manipulation another cavity was opened and was found to contain a fragment of sponge. This cavity corresponded to the enucleated cyst. Small fragments of the portion of sponge showed that the latter was absolutely sterile. The proof that the bacillus observed in the completely-cicatrized wound was of intestinal origin would seem to rest upon the fact that the drainage-tube, when removed, was found to be practically sterile, that the piece of sponge removed from another portion of the field of operation was still sterile although it had remained in the tissues for a month; hence that infection had taken place after complete closure of the wound, consequently from within and not from without. A further indication of the origin of this infection rests upon the circumstance that nutritive enemata were required for a few days after the operation and that they had to be discontinued on account of a fœtid diarrhœa which seemed to be caused by them. On account of the very large loss of blood during the operation intravenous saline injections were practised in this case, and it might possibly be claimed that in this way the bacillus entered the circulation. The drainage-tube was not removed, however, for twelve hours after these injections had been made, hence had they been the direct cause of infection the presence of the bacterium would probably have been shown in the cultures from the drain.

Still another case of local infection of intestinal origin, though not following operation, is reported by Nicaise. In this case the patient suffered from a subacute cervical adenitis, which upon incision discharged a peculiar form of muco-pus. The author considers that the intestinal origin of this local trouble is exceedingly probable, from the fact that no cause could be found about the throat, head, or upper extremity, and that the patient was at the time suffering from a severe enteritis. It must be admitted that proof in this case is entirely wanting. It would also seem to be especially unlikely that, even were the general system affected, the local manifestation would appear in the neck.

Troisier, however, has shown that there exists some definite relation between the viscera and the cervical lymphatic glands, since enlargement of the latter is so common in cases of intra-abdominal malignant disease that it is at times of diagnostic importance.

Whether or not the cases of local infection recently reported have really depended upon pathological conditions of the intestines, the fact remains that microbes can readily traverse intestinal walls which are in an abnormal condition. This would point to the very great importance of carefully attending to the condition of the alimentary canal, not only in abdominal surgery, but in all severe operations on any part of the body ; and it would seem unwise to practise surgical intervention, save in cases of urgent necessity, upon those suffering from obvious intestinal disorders.

SPECIAL ARTICLE.

REPORT OF THREE CASES TREATED BY KOCH'S LYMPH.

BY WILLIAM H. BENNETT, M.D ,
OF PHILADELPHIA.

THE following records of cases treated with Koch lymph are, with one exception, incomplete, because the patients are still under treatment ; and though they are of no value in indicating its curative effect, they are published at this time because of the great interest felt in every experiment made with the lymph.

The records will be completed in future numbers of THE MEDICAL NEWS, if the amount of lymph at my disposal proves sufficient. The specimen of it employed was obtained in such a way that it could not possibly have been diluted before reaching me, and it still retains its perfect transparency. It will, however, be seen that somewhat larger doses were required to produce the effects than those stated by Koch, and it is likely that the lymph slightly deteriorates either from age, or on its voyage across the Atlantic.

The first case well illustrates its value in diagnosis :

Mrs. C., a lady of seventy-nine years, weakened by age, a chronic intestinal catarrh, and a malignant disease of the face, was the first in Philadelphia to receive an injection.

The disease of the face had been pronounced lupus by a distinguished microscopist to whom had been submitted a portion of tissue removed last May. Although there was some doubt as to the correctness of this diagnosis, it was decided to test the question by an injection of the lymph.

The disease has existed for more than twelve years, but it has made very little progress until within the past eight months. During the latter period six operations have been performed by Professors Agnew and Ashhurst, with a view to check its inroads. It

consists of an ulcer of irregular quadrilateral form, extending from a little to the right of the median line of the nose one and a half inches to the left, and from the lower edge of the nose nearly to the eyebrow. There is a hard, hemispherical nodule, half an inch in diameter, involving the inner half of the lower eyelid, and a similar smaller one on the inner edge of the upper lid. The flat surface of the hemisphere in each case forms part of the quadrilateral ulcer. The principal activity of the disease is in these nodules. The floor of the ulcer is covered with granulations showing no tendency to cicatrize. The right-hand border has on it a few warty papillæ, and from it extend, here and there, into the sound tissue, grayish lines, indicative of the invasion of the disease into other regions.

At 5.30 P.M., December 10, 1890, in the presence of Professors Agnew and Ashhurst, I injected between the shoulder-blades 0.002 c.cm. of lymph which had just been diluted with boiled distilled water. There was only the ordinary pain of a hypodermic injection The following is a record of the pulse and temperature :

Time.	Pulse.	Temperature
P. M.		
5.45	80	98.4°
6.15	76	98.4
6 45	76	98.4
7.15	75	97.
7.45	72	97.6
8.15	74	97.6
8.45	78	97.6
9.15	—	97.6
9.45	—	97.6
10.45	—	97.8
11.45	78	97.8
A. M.		
2.15	—	97.8
8.45	91	98.4

There has not been at any time a change in the appearance of the ulcer, except that, in consequence of the removal of all dressing and exposure to air, it becomes dryer and darker. The site of the injection could not be discovered at 6.45 P.M. It had become slightly red and tender by 8.45 A. M., December 11th. The patient at that time seemed in better condition than before the injection.

At 9 30 A.M., December 11th, a second injection was given, consisting of 0.005 of lymph. The following is the record of pulse and temperature :

Time	Pulse	Temperature
A. M		
10.00	80	98.4°
10.30	87	99
11.00	87	99.1
11.30	87	98.4
12 00	84	98.8
P M.		
1.00	76	98
2.00	94	99
3.00	100	98.8
5.30	90	99
9 00	94	99 4
10.00	93	100
12.00	79	99.6
A. M.		
9.00	91	99.6

By 2 P.M., December 11th, the site of the first injection had become quite red over an area of one and a half inches in diameter, and two lymphatic glands near the shoulder were enlarged and tender. The second injection produced some disturbance of the system, shown by a rise of temperature to 100° and a general feeling of malaise. The ulcer was in no way affected, and there were no other symptoms worthy of note.

A third injection of 0.01 c.cm. of the lymph, freshly diluted, was given at 12.30 P.M., December 13th, the temperature at that time being normal. The following record was made:

Time. P. M.	Pulse.	Temperature.
Dec. 12th. 1.30	88	99 °
2.30	89	99 2
3.30	91	99.2
4.45	82	99.4
6.00	83	99.2
8.15	93	99.4
10.00	91	98.3
A. M.		
Dec. 13th. 9.00	90	99.4

The effect of this injection upon the system was hardly appreciable, and again the sore showed no change.

The following note was made of the condition of the sites of the injections, December 13th:

No. 1. The redness is fading, and the enlarged glands are growing smaller and less painful.

Nos. 2 and 3 are each slightly red and tender, but no more glands have become enlarged.

December 15th, at noon, a fourth injection was given of 0.02 c.cm. of lymph—a large amount for so feeble a person. The following record was made of the result:

Time. P. M.	Pulse	Temperature	Notes
1.00	72	94.8°	
2.00	77	98 4	
3.00	77	98.4	
4.00	90	98.8	
5.00	91	99	
6.00	100	100	Slight chill.
6.30	112	100.8	
7.10	123	101	
7.40	110	102	
8.15	106	102	
8.45	110	102	
9.15	110	102 2	
9.45	105	102.2	
10.30	110	102.2	
11.00	110	101.4	
12.00	113	102	
A. M.			
Dec. 16th. 1.00	107	102	
2.00	100	100	
10.00	97	98.8	

It will be seen by the above record that there was at this time a decided reaction. The patient complained at 1 P.M., one hour after the injection, of a sudden momentary buzzing in the ears and a feeling as if about to faint. With the slight chill there was a sensation of pulsation in the back of the head

and shoulders. At 7.30 P.M. the respiration became somewhat irregular, and there was a constant effort to clear the throat by coughing. There was at no time actual nausea, but she was "afraid to eat lest it should come on." Between nine and ten she became for a time very restless, and complained of pains in the limbs. She passed an uncomfortable night. having but little sleep. December 16th, she felt better, but weak. The wound did not change at all in appearance, and since the first injection the disease has apparently spread with at least as great rapidity as ever before. It is evidently not lupus.

The second patient treated was a woman of twenty years, suffering from tuberculosis of the lungs. The case is one of a year's duration, with a typical history of heredity, cough, hæmoptysis, hectic, and loss of flesh. A moderate-sized cavity exists in the apex of the left lung, and the sputa are loaded with tubercle bacilli.

December 12th, at 3.10 P.M., I injected between the shoulder-blades 0.005 c.cm. of Koch's lymph. The following is the record made of the pulse, respiration, and temperature:

Time. P.M.	Pulse.	Temperature.	Respiration.
3.10	134	99.8°	25
3.30	126	101.4	24
4.00	126	101.2	29
4.30	122	101.1	30
5.00	120	101.1	28
5.30	114	101.1	28
6.00	120	101.1	26
6 30	120	101.2	26
7.00	124	101.3	26
8.00	120	101.2	25
9.00	120	101.0	24
10.00	118	100.8	24

No record could be taken after 10 P.M, but the patient continued feverish until 3 A.M. In this case there was no decided chill. With the fever there was for a short time slight delirium. The cough was increased, and became very troublesome during the night. There was some nausea. There were pains throughout the body, but especially in the arms and legs, which continued with gradually-decreasing intensity for twenty-four hours. There was no perceptible effect upon the bowels, skin, or kidneys. The morning after the injection the appetite was as good as usual, and with the exception of increased weakness and the lingering pains, the patient was in no way the worse for the injection. The reaction in this instance was characteristic but slight, most of the rise of temperature being due to the daily hectic.

December 14th, at 2.20 P.M., I gave the patient a second injection, consisting of 0.01 c.cm. of lymph, with the following result:

Time. P. M	Pulse.	Temperature.	Respiration.
3 00	120	100.8°	24
3.30	116	100.8	30
4.00	118	100.4	26
4.30	120	100.6	28
5.00	120	100.2	24

Time.	Pulse.	Temperature.	Respiration.
P.M.			
5.30	115	100.2°	28
6.00	114	100	28
6.30	118	100	30
7.00	120	100	30
7.30	120	100 8	30
8.00	112	101.4	26
8.30	120	102.5	28
9.00	130	104	28
9.30	135	105.2	26
10.00	135	104.8	30
10.30	112	105	28
11.00	108	105.1	28

There was nothing of importance to note until seven o'clock, when the patient vomited a little mucus slightly tinged with blood. At 8 P.M. the cough was increased, but was accompanied with very little expectoration. At 8.30 P.M. she complained of slight chilliness of the body, and the hands, which were previously warm, became cool. At 9 they were cold, and the patient still complained of chilliness of the body. At 9.30 this latter sensation had passed away, but the hands were still cool. During a hard coughing spell a little mucus was raised, which contained no blood. A slight pain, lasting a minute or two, was felt in the left chest on rising. At 10 P.M. there was slight pain in the lower part of the back and in the back of the thighs. The patient became somewhat delirious. The cough decreased. At 10.30 there was slight supra-orbital and occipital pain. After 11 P.M. no record could be taken, but the fever gradually abated toward morning, and the next day, December 15th, the patient complained only of weakness. At 2.30 P.M. her pulse was 120, and temperature 99.8°. The following note was made on December 16th: "Since the last injection the patient feels better, and her cough and expectoration are decidedly diminished."

Arrangements will be made for more injections during the ensuing week.

The third case which I have to report is that of a boy five years of age, who was admitted to St. Christopher's Hospital for Children nine months ago with incipient disease of the left hip-joint. His mother died of tuberculosis of the lungs and his sister of Pott's disease.

A periarthritic abscess formed during the past fall, which was opened November 8th by Dr. Simes, the attending surgeon. After discharging freely for three weeks it remained closed for one week, and then about a week ago commenced to discharge again.

At 4 P.M., December 13th, in the presence of Dr. D. D. Stewart and myself, Dr. Simes injected, in the usual place, 0.005 of Koch's lymph. The following record was made of his temperature and pulse.

Time.	Pulse	Temperature.
P.M.		
4.00	88	98.8°
4.30	112	99.2
5.00	104	99.3
5.30	100	98.8
6.00	92	98.4
6.30	92	98.4

Time.	Pulse.	Temperature.
P.M.		
7.00	100	98.2°
7.30	104	98.
8.00	99	98.4
8.30	92	98.4
9.00	100	98.4
9.30	108	98.6
10.00	114	98.8
11.00	116	100.
A.M.		
6.00	130	102.
7.00	130	102.
8.00	144	102.4
9.00	140	102.
10.00	130	102.
11.00	144	102.
12.00	132	101.8
P.M.		
12.30	140	101.6
1.30	136	
3.30	144	101.6
4.30	132	101.9
5.30	132	101.8
6.30	124	
8.00	112	101.6
10.00	116	101.6
A.M.		
6.30	112	99.

The injection was followed very quickly by a slight flushing of the face and an irregularity of the pulse. This irregularity of the pulse was a marked symptom during the whole period of high temperature, and it was also quite marked when, at 6 P.M., the temperature was normal. It disappeared as the child recovered from the injection. The child is free from heart trouble.

There were no other symptoms to note until 9.30 P.M. The child then complained of stiffness and a "sore feeling" in the diseased joint, but not of any pain in the right leg. At ten the joint was slightly swollen and inflamed. At eleven there was a well-marked red ring half an inch broad around the opening of the abscess. Later, the redness extended over the joint, and it became so sensitive that the child feared to have any one touch it. The discharge was slightly tinged with blood. The temperature was not taken during the night, but the child was very restless and feverish, constantly asking for water. At 6.30 the following day he vomited. During that forenoon his face was slightly flushed, his eyes injected, and he complained of headache. He slept much of the time, keeping his eyes partly open. His appetite had failed, his tongue had a brownish coat in the centre and was a strawberry-red along the edges. The urine contained no albumin; it was very turbid on the day following the injection, but quite clear the next day. December 15th, the child was still pale, but he had regained much of his usual animation. The red ring around the opening had become very narrow, and the heat about the joint and its unusual sensitiveness had disappeared.

This case is one of special interest, and further injections will be made and reported as soon as arrangements can be made for continuous and more careful observations.

It will be seen that the symptoms in the foregoing cases corresponded with those described by Koch as developing under similar circumstances, but how far the treatment in the last two will prove curative can only be determined by further injections.

I am indebted to Drs. McCamy and Lawrence, and to medical students Bennett, Woodward, and Van Dyke, for assistance in making the foregoing records.

INOCULATION OF KOCH'S LYMPH AT THE HOSPITAL FOR THE RUPTURED AND CRIPPLED, NEW YORK.[1]

Preliminary Report.

BY ALLAN McLANE HAMILTON, M.D.,
NEUROLOGIST,

AND

VIRGIL P. GIBNEY, M.D.,
SURGEON-IN-CHIEF.

REMARKS BY DR. GIBNEY.—On Tuesday morning, December 9th, Dr. Hamilton notified me that he had a small vial of Koch's lymph and would like to employ it in a case of tubercular meningitis. I replied at once that we unfortunately had no such case at present in hospital, but had any number of cases of bone tuberculosis, and would be glad to have him call in the afternoon to make such experiments as he desired.

CASE I.—At 5.30 P. M., in the presence of two members of the consulting staff, Drs. J. H. Ripley and L. E. Holt, Dr. W. R. Townsend, Assistant Surgeon, Dr. George DeF. Smith, and the members of the house staff, the first inoculation in a public institution in this city was made upon a boy, ten years of age, who had been under treatment in the hospital for several years for tubercular osteitis of the right hip. This case was selected because his general health was good, because the sinuses had closed, and because it was believed that a cure was complete. Dr. Ripley examined his lungs with negative results. His pulse was 76, respiration 20, and temperature 98¼°. The syringe had been previously sterilized and 2 minims of the solution, of the strength of 1 mgm. to 5 minims, were injected in the interscapular space by Dr. Hamilton. At 6.45 P.M. his pulse was 80, respiration 20, temperature 98⅖°. At 7.45 P.M. pulse 76, respiration 20, temperature 98¼°. At 8.45 and 9.45 the vital signs were practically the same. At 10.45 his pulse was 72, respiration 19, and temperature 99°. There was no rise of temperature beyond this. He slept well during the night and kept his bed during the following day, Wednesday. He complained of a little soreness about the puncture and there was a slight area

[1] This report was received from Dr. Hamilton on Friday, December 12th, too late for insertion in the issue of THE MEDICAL NEWS for December 13th.

of redness, but beyond this there was nothing that could be construed as reaction. At 6 P.M., December 10th, 5 minims of the same solution were injected, and up to the present writing there has been no reaction.

CASE II.—A member of the house staff was selected as a healthy subject, lungs examined by Dr. Ripley with negative result, and 5 minims were injected in the interscapular space. Careful records were kept during the evening without any positive result. In the morning the doctor reported that he experienced no change whatever, save a little accentuation of pain around some scratches on his hands, produced by plaster work.

CASE III.—December 10th, boy, aged twelve years, typically tuberculous in appearance, in hospital since May, 1889. Excision of the knee for tubercular disease had been performed last spring. A large portion of bone had been removed, but sinuses remained and these had been treated with the peroxide of hydrogen. In addition to the sinuses, an ulcer, supposed to be tuberculous, existed on the posterior aspect of the thigh. This case also was selected in the hope that the process had been arrested. Dr. John S. Thatcher examined his lungs with negative results. Injection of 5 minims at 6.20. A careful record was made every hour preceding and subsequent to the inoculation, from 5 P.M. to 12 midnight. There was no elevation of temperature whatever. This morning, December 11th, the boy reports himself as feeling quite well; complained during the night of pain in his back, which pain prevented him from sleeping; beyond this, no reaction.

CASE IV.—December 10th, girl, seven years of age; under treatment since May 23, 1890, for dorsal Pott's disease with an abscess about the right hip. This had been opened and treated after Billroth's method. For the past week she has been out of health, had a decidedly "strumous" appearance, and, for the past day or two, has suffered from a phlyctenular conjunctivitis. Her lips were large and flabby and eyes heavy. Dr. Thatcher examined the lungs, pronouncing them healthy. At 6.25 P.M. 3 minims of the same solution were injected, the usual records having been made. At 11 o'clock in the evening, the night nurse reported that the child was suffering from "snuffles," was breathing heavily, and was not resting well. The vital signs, however, showed no change. This morning, December 11th, she is resting comfortably, her vital signs are normal, and she does not complain of any pain about the site of puncture.

Report of Dr. Allan McLane Hamilton.

To the Editor of THE MEDICAL NEWS.

SIR: On Monday, December 8, 1890, I received from Dr. H. Holbrook Curtis, of this city, about four grammes of diluted Koch's lymph, every five minims of which contained one milligramme of the lymph. The attenuation was made on the previous day with sterilized water, by Dr. Curtis himself. Through an unfortunate accident one-half of this solution was lost upon the afternoon of Tuesday the

9th, when I made my first two injections, at the Hospital for Ruptured and Crippled, in the presence of Drs. Gibney, Townsend, J. H. Ripley, L. Emme't Holt, George DeForest Smith, and the house staff. Two more patients were injected on Wednesday, in the presence of several of these gentlemen, as well as Dr. Thatcher. These cases are fully reported elsewhere,[1] and I will not refer to them except to say that the reactions were either absent or trifling, and that one of the cases was nontuberculous and another convalescing. From the fact that other medical men have had decided results with Koch's lymph injected by them, and that Dr. Curtis himself has materially influenced the course of the disease by injections of the same lymph used by me, I am compelled to believe that the barren results from its use in my hands were due either to the smallness of the dose used (2 mgm. to 5 mgm.) or possibly to the fact that the diluted lymph had undergone decomposition. I, however, hope to make other injections toward the end of the week, employing the same patients; when I will forward you my further experiences.

Very truly yours,
ALLAN McLANE HAMILTON, M.D.

NEW YORK, December 15, 1890

CORRESPONDENCE.

CHICAGO.

To the Editor of THE MEDICAL NEWS,

SIR: A new specialty in medicine has apparently been created in Chicago. A certain so-called doctor advertises himself as "the successful obesity specialist: patients treated by mail; no starving, no inconvenience; harmless, and no bad effects." We are informed that this man has a lucrative practice, and that as might be supposed a large proportion of his patients are Germans.

At a recent clinic at the College of Physicians and Surgeons Professor A. Reeves Jackson showed a case of laceration of the cervix, and in commenting upon these injuries said that their pathological importance frequently, though not always, depends upon the degree of eversion which accompanies them. In this case there was no eversion unless the parts were pulled upon and thus separated. The "out-rolling" of the cervical lining is most marked in cases in which the laceration is bilateral, and extends beyond what might be called the crown of the cervix. In such cases it is not unusual to find the internal os at the very lowest portion of the everted tissues. These extreme cases can be cured by plastic operations only. Dr. Jackson regards all cervical lacerations as inviting the development of malignant disease, and when a woman has a cervical tear and is approaching the menopause she should be taught to watch carefully for such symptoms as hæmorrhage, leucorrhœa, or

pelvic pain, for any of these may signify incipient cancer and indicate the necessity for prompt treatment.

Professor Jackson then put the question, "What should be done in the way of treatment in this case?" and added that when Emmet taught us the frequency of this lesion, and the admirable method by which the injury might be repaired, and its effects consequently removed, almost the entire profession agreed with him. Every physician who could do so operated upon every torn cervix when permission could be obtained. But a change has come. The pendulum swung too far in one direction and it is now likely to swing too far in the other. Dr. Jackson believes that the operation is needed particularly in cases in which there is great eversion. We can in some cases effect a cure by local treatment, but even in these if by a procedure of from fifteen to thirty minutes we can in one or two weeks accomplish what would otherwise require many months, the operation should be done. In the case before the class he did not think that an operation would be necessary, and he therefore applied Churchill's tincture of iodine to the interior of the cervix and to the eroded surfaces. This, or carbolic acid, or the two combined, should be applied to the unhealed surface once a week. Between the applications the cervix should be sustained by a vaginal tampon of absorbent wool or cotton, saturated with boric acid and glycerin, and changed every two days. If, however, at the end of a month's treatment, and after involution is complete, the condition is not improved, an operation should be performed.

Dr. G. Frank Lydston recently had an interesting case of non-gonorrhœal double epididymitis. Double epididymitis, as is well known, is rare, and double epididymitis of non-gonorrhœal origin is especially rare.

The patient gave a history of a slight stricture following an attack of gonorrhœa six years ago. This was treated successfully, but since then he has been subject to prostatic irritation, and occasionally suffered from urinary obstruction apparently due to spasmodic stricture. He stated that he had been examined by several surgeons who informed him that his stricture was very slight, but that the prostate was exquisitely tender, a fact which he himself keenly realized when a bougie was introduced. Since the original gonorrhœa there has been no discharge whatever. The patient had been subject to slight muscular rheumatism, and four days before coming under Dr. Lydston's observation he was attacked by what was apparently severe lumbago. On the second day of this attack the right testicle became painful and swollen. On the third day the inflammation of the right testicle subsided somewhat and the left became enormously swollen and acutely painful. Under appropriate treatment the swelling of the left testicle subsided within forty-eight hours, and on the following morning the patient was very comfortable. In the evening, however, the right testicle again became swollen, and it was necessary to give opiates quite freely in order to relieve the pain. The peculiar feature of the case is the fact that a decided decrease followed by a rapid increase in the size of the inflamed organs occasionally occurs within a very few hours. The body of each testicle has become secondarily inflamed.

Dr. Lydston believes the case to be one of rheumatic orchitis and epididymitis, but that there is in all probability some predisposing cause in the deep urethra. He thinks that rheumatic inflammation of the testicle is much more frequent than is generally believed.

Dr. T. Melville Hardie recently contributed a paper to the Chicago Medical Society on the "Local Treatment of Laryngeal Tuberculosis." The paper was largely a review of the work done in laryngeal tuberculosis by Heryng, of Warsaw, and Krause, of Berlin. The frequeney of laryngeal involvement in pulmonary consumption, the existence of primary laryngeal tuberculosis, and the occurrence of frequent cicatrization under treatment were adduced as reasons for departing from the customary therapeutic nihilism. Case-histories were read which showed that at least a partial cure is possible, and that the troublesome subjective symptoms, dysphagia, difficulty in breathing, and hoarseness, can be removed or greatly alleviated. The points requiring attention in the lactic-acid treatment were mentioned and a discussion of the rationale and of the surgical methods employed in the treatment of laryngeal tuberculosis followed. It was insisted upon that the introduction of *curettement* marked an epoch in the treatment of the disease, as it is based upon the conclusions arrived at by modern general surgery with regard to the treatment of tubercular joints. The technical difficulties in the way of the effective accomplishment are not to be urged to its discredit. It is not work for a beginner. Besides *curettement* and treatment by endolaryngeal incision, tracheotomy and electrolysis were briefly discussed. The writer had had no experience with electrolysis.

LONDON.

The Medical Schools—The London Post-graduate Course—Dr. Sharkey on Graefe's Lid-sign—Fatal Obstruction of a Bronchus in an Infant.

THE number of new men in the London medical schools is almost exactly the same as that of last year, but less than that of the preceding two or three years; but those of us who think the profession is already overcrowded will not find any cause for regret in this fact. Of course, St. Bartholomew's Hospital takes the lead, as it has for many years past, and Guy's has resumed its old place as next to the largest school, a position which has been stoutly contested by St. Thomas's in recent years. The new dental school at Guy's is becoming known, and this year quite a number of " dentals " have entered there, but without affecting the number that enter elsewhere ; so I suppose the dental profession also will become overcrowded.

I hear, on good authority, that the London post-graduate course is in a flourishing state, and that the number of names enrolled for the third and concluding series of lectures and demonstrations is equal to that of the two previous series together. This would seem to show that the medical public is awakening to the great advantages which the course offers. I am told that the Government departments are looking upon it with favor, and granting leave of absence to officers in the army and navy who wish to "brush up" by attending the course. Several naval officers have entered, and there

are rumors of a considerable accession of numbers from the same quarter in the course of a few weeks. For some reason, I suppose because it is not yet sufficiently widely known, but very few foreign practitioners have joined, three Canadians and one American representing the total of those who do not hail from the British Isles. An editorial in your journal, August 30th, on the subject of the advantages presented by London as a medical centre was read here with much interest and approval, and probably its effects will soon be shown by the number of men who will stop here instead of hurrying on to Vienna or Berlin.

Dr. Sharkey recently read an interesting paper on Graefe's "lid-sign" before the Ophthalmological Society. This sign consists, as is well known, in the non-descent, or, rather, the imperfect descent, of the upper eyelid when a patient suffering from Graves's disease looks downward. That it is not a constant symptom every physician will admit, but Dr. Sharkey has gone further than this, and shows that it is present in a not inconsiderable number of persons who are not the subjects of Graves's disease at all, and that, therefore, it has not the pathognomonic significance which has hitherto been accorded to it. His reasoning on the cause of the phenomenon was so good that I need make no apology for quoting it : " It is clear," he said, " that there is overaction of the muscles which raise the lid, namely, the levator palpebræ, supplied by the third nerve, and the unstriped muscle of the lid, supplied by the sympathetic. Remak showed that irritation of the sympathetic produced elevation and retraction of the upper lid ; and the fact that one can voluntarily produce this, shows that it can likewise be effected through the third nerve. Constant active spasm rarely results from irritation, though intermittent spasm may. Prolonged spasm most frequently owes its origin to paralysis or weakening of opposing muscles. Is there evidence in Graves's disease of a weakening of the muscles which close the eyes? Stellwag has shown that a very constant symptom of the disease is diminished frequency and incompleteness of the involuntary closure of the eyes, which goes on so continuously in health. The orbicularis palpebrarum which effects this movement and is the opponent of the muscles which raise the lid, being weakened in Graves's disease and losing tone by inaction, the healthy equilibrium of the muscles of the eye is lost, the opening overpowering the closing muscles and producing retraction of the upper lid and Graefe's sign. Thus the infrequency of winking, which Stellwag refers to disease of the nerve-centres, is the primary result of disease, and retraction of the lids and Graefe's sign follow as a consequence."

At the first meeting of the Clinical Society, Mr. R. W. Parker reported a very interesting case and a somewhat unusual form of disease. His patient was an infant, one year old, who was suddenly seized with very urgent dyspnœa, and as the obstruction to respiration was evidently below the larynx, she was naturally assumed to have aspirated a foreign body into the air-passages. Tracheotomy was performed and efforts were made to promote the expulsion of the foreign body, but without success, and the infant died soon afterward. On post-mortem examination it was found that the entrance to one bronchus was completely occluded by a caseous gland, which had ulcerated through the trachea and sloughed into the trachea. Of course, it is common for caseous glands to become adherent to the trachea, and they not infrequently lead to ulceration ; but when perforation has been accomplished the contents of the gland are generally poured into the trachea in a fluid state, and set up a gangrenous pneumonia. The sloughing of the whole gland, such as took place in this case, must be very rare, and the extremely early age at which it occurred is also another point of interest.

Dr. Andrew, the Harveian Orator of the College of Physicians this year, in the course of this address, spoke of the enormous amount of so-called medical literature as the chief of the ills which beset the physician of the present day, and said that this evil would be less prominent if writers paid more attention to the teachings of Harvey, from whom he quoted the following passage in support of his belief : " I had no purpose to swell this treatise into a large volume by quoting the names and writings of anatomists, or to make a parade of the strength of my memory, of the extent of my reading, and of the amount of my pains ; because I profess both to learn and teach anatomy, not from books, but from dissections ; not from the positions of philosophers, but from the fabric of Nature. I avow myself the partisan of truth alone ; and I can, indeed, say that I have used all my endeavors and bestowed all my pains on an attempt to produce something that should be agreeable to the good, profitable to the learned, and useful to letters." It would, indeed, be well if all writers since his day had laid Harvey's precepts to heart and endeavored to act upon them.

NEWS ITEMS.

Opinions of Foreign Journals.—The following excellent summary of the opinions expressed by French and German journals as to Koch's treatment of tuberculosis is taken from the London *Lancet,* December 6, 1890 :

In France the reception of Professor Koch's discovery by the medical press has been fairly cordial. Some journals, as the *Gazette Médicale de Paris* and the *Progrès Médical,* are content with giving abstracts of the recently-published reports from Berlin, the last-named expressing surprise at the moderate and somewhat vague terms in which the action of the remedy is now being spoken of, compared with the more enthusiastic language first used. *L' Union Médicale* (November 27th, 29th, and December 2d) has followed carefully the progress of events. It points out that more caution is being used in the employment of the remedy, especially in view of its liability to induce acute pulmonary œdema in lung tuberculosis, or œdema of the brain in meningeal cases, or of the glottis in laryngeal disease. Surgical cases are more amenable to treatment because of the readiness with which the diseased parts can be completely extirpated after the remedy has exerted its necrotizing effect. It refers to von Ziemssen's opinion that lung cases will require prolonged treatment. M. Villoret, writing from Berlin to the *Semaine Médicale,* insists on there being a certain idiosyncrasy in the manner in which the injections are borne, and cites three cases treated by the same dose, in one of which a typical reaction took place after fifteen hours, in the second an " atypical " one after three hours, and in the third a weak but typical reaction after ten

hours. *L' Union Médicale* thinks that we are still much in the dark, and points to the fact that relapses have already occurred in lupus-cases and that it is an error to believe that we are at all near proofs of its real therapeutic efficacy. At the Laennec Hospital on November 30th, MM. Cornil and Chantemesse inoculated six patients—two being cases of lupus, two of early pulmonary tuberculosis, and two of surgical tubercular affections. In one of the lupus-cases, a man of eighteen years, 0.002 c.cm. was injected, and reaction began five hours after, the temperature reaching its maximum in twelve hours (39.2° C. from 37.2°). The appearances were precisely similar to those described by all who have tried the remedy in lupus.

There was equally marked reaction (maximum temperature 39.4° C.) in a case of early phthisis,with headache and nausea, and slight auscultatory changes attributed to congestion. M. Pean on the 29th inoculated several cases at the St. Louis Hospital. He expressed the opinion that Koch was justified in withholding the nature of the remedy at present, and insisted on the danger of incautious administration. Dr. Moreau, of Algiers, asserts that in some well-marked tubercular cases no reaction has followed injection, and that in some non-tubercular subjects reaction has been observed. In one case of Leyden's the fever set up by the injections continued after these were discontinued. *La Province Médicale* (Nov. 29th) thinks that enthusiasm is giving way to uncertainty, and avers that in pulmonary cases its action is very limited, and that, although it may cause diminution in expectoration of bacilli and in night-sweats, its use is not followed by any gain in weight or strength. Much is required to be known concerning the length of time that such cases have to be treated. The *Gazette des Hôpitaux de Toulouse* defends Koch for his reticence, since he was forced to publish his results prematurely. It says that in showing that the " lymph " has an elective affinity for tubercular tissue, his researches are to be greatly praised. It raises the question as to the desirability of " curing " the phthisical. The *Allg. Wiener med. Zeitung* (Nov. 25th) devotes much space to contributions on the subject, including one by Dr. Buchner, of Munich, who points out that inflammatory action may play the chief part in the destructive process. The *St. Petersburger med. Wochenschr.,* November 17th, states that on November 11th Professor Anrep gave an address on the subject, and inoculated three lupus-cases with some of the " lymph " given him by Professor Koch. Other delegates have also gone to Berlin, and many physicians from all parts of Russia. The remedy has also been used in Professor Baccelli's clinic at Rome.

THE MEDICAL NEWS.

A WEEKLY JOURNAL OF MEDICAL SCIENCE.

VOL. LVII. SATURDAY, DECEMBER 27, 1890. No. 26.

ORIGINAL ARTICLES.

AN INVESTIGATION INTO THE ETIOLOGY AND TREATMENT OF PHTHISIS.

BY HENEAGE GIBBES, M.D.,
PROFESSOR OF PATHOLOGY IN THE UNIVERSITY OF MICHIGAN,

AND

E. L. SHURLY, M.D.,
PROFESSOR OF LARYNGOLOGY AND CLINICAL MEDICINE IN THE DETROIT
COLLEGE OF MEDICINE.

IN a series of papers published by us in the *American Journal of the Medical Sciences* we endeavored to show from the experiments and investigations of many observers, together with our own, that tuberculosis and phthisis pulmonalis are different disease-processes—resting we believe upon distinct pathological and clinical bases. Our therapeutic experiments looking to the discovery of some one agent to act as a specific against these conditions have only confirmed us in the belief. While we have demonstrated to our satisfaction that attenuated cultures will prevent the development of general tuberculosis in guinea-pigs, we have found that such cultures will not in any way prove curative when the disease has started. We have therefore been aiming to discover some agent or agents which will prevent further development in the diseased organ, or organs, and also neutralize in the economy the ptomaïnes circulating at large.

Owing to the various changes which chemicals are apt to undergo in the stomach and intestines before final diffusion, it is obvious that hypodermic medication offers, perhaps, the only rational and accurate method of arriving at desirable results; while the introduction with the inspired air of an agent which will modify and arrest the local process, when situated in the lungs, will most likely assist in cutting off the supply of septic material generated and diffused, as well as prevent further development of disease in the locality.

We have been experimenting continuously for more than two years with a great variety of agents, often with most discouraging results. Of all the agents for inhalation which we have used, we find that chlorine gas is the most effectual in destroying the infective activity of sputum from phthisical patients. Our first experiments with it failed because we exposed the sputum too short a time and used too weak chlorine-water. We found, how-

ever, that if the material were thoroughly exposed to chlorine gas (mixed with it), or thoroughly shaken or mixed with strong, fresh chlorine-water, it soon became innocuous, and animals inoculated with it would not become tuberculous.

In October, at a meeting of the Detroit Medical and Library Association, we showed a healthy guinea-pig which had been inoculated, on February 6, 1889, with chlorinated sputum, while a monkey and another guinea-pig, inoculated at the same time with sputum from the same case, but unmedicated, died in the ordinary way. The fact, however, of chlorine gas being so irrespirable and harmful even when diluted with a large amount of air, rendered its use for inhalation quite out of the question for a time. We have found, however, that when diffused in an atmosphere previously laden with spray of chloride of sodium solution, that patients could inhale large quantities of it without bad effects. Of the many substances used by hypodermic injections, we have found that iodine and iodide of potassium in solution with glycerin and distilled water (all chemically pure) are well borne by the tissues, and exert a marked effect on the course of some forms of phthisis pulmonalis. Our experiments with this combination of substances in 1889, produced terrible abscesses, which we discovered were due to impurity of the drugs, and using too much at first (there should be no residue when the crystals are submitted to sublimation).

Guinea-pigs or monkeys thus well iodinized will not take tuberculosis from inoculation! We have a monkey and several guinea-pigs that were iodinized before inoculation, still living—the control-animals being long since dead. This is also true of the use of the gold and sodium salt. Next to iodine for general use, and superior for some cases, is chloride of gold and sodium, which should be also chemically pure. The injection of this solution causes but little pain. It is most efficient when used alternately with iodine, or mixed with it in the proportion of one-twelfth of a grain of iodine and one-fiftieth to one-twentieth of a grain of gold and sodium. The best place to introduce the hypodermic needle is in the buttocks. The injection in this situation causes less pain, and there is less liability of the formation of abscess.

The injection of iodine causes a little more pain than the solution of gold and sodium. The mixture of the two solutions should be made slowly and carefully; too much of the iodine should not be added, or the insoluble iodide of gold will be formed, which will cause abscesses. We have treated a large number of animals during the past year with very good results so far. We have thoroughly treated since the early part of September of this year up to December, about 25 cases of phthisis pulmonalis in the human being of different types, and 2 cases of general tuberculosis. The latter were advanced cases, and died—although in one there was decided mitigation in the course of the disease. Of the cases of phthisis pulmonalis, 4 were far advanced and died—one being a case of laryngeal phthisis. Four cases (of the subacute variety) not far advanced but showing caseation, etc., have been so positively benefited as to be called "cured." They have remained quite well and resumed their respective avocations. The remaining cases are still under treatment; two of them, however (one laryngeal phthisis and the other subacute pulmonary phthisis, sometimes called pneumonic phthisis), are so much improved that they will leave Harper Hospital in about a week. Of the remaining cases two were well advanced before entering the hospital, but are decidedly better. We have now 21 cases under these plans of treatment exclusively, about one-half of which have been under treatment but a few weeks, and most of them are doing well. We have treated quite a number of cases for only a week or two and then lost track of them; from some we have since heard that they were better. Necessarily many months must elapse and many more cases must be subjected to these plans of treatment before a conclusive clinical test can be attained. We have not as yet had experience enough to formulate any positive rules for the selection of one over another of these agents in the treatment of the different classes of cases. But we submit the following observations for guidance, which up to this time seem appropriate.

In all cases it is better to use the solution of iodine once daily, beginning with $\frac{1}{12}$ grain, and gradually increasing to $\frac{1}{4}$ or $\frac{1}{3}$ grain for about a week, unless symptoms of iodism, or a too rapid diminishing of urine, or expectoration supervene, in which event the gold and sodium should be used instead, beginning with one injection daily of $\frac{1}{30}$ grain, gradually increasing to $\frac{1}{15}$ grain. Cases which have a great deal of cough and little expectoration should be treated *chiefly* with the gold and sodium solution, if not *exclusively*. After a few days' treatment with iodine, cases showing active caseation (gurgling râles, large mucous râles, etc.) with great expectoration should have the chlorine inhalation as well. It may be administered every three or four hours from a face-shield inhaler, or, what is better, the patient should be kept in a room in which there is constantly diffused more or less chlorine with a spray of chloride of sodium. Then, after a week or so of iodine, such cases should receive injections every day, or on alternate days, of the two solutions mixed.

After the third week the injections may be diminished to every second or every third day. Patients with laryngeal phthisis should receive inhalations of chlorine from an inhaler, three times a day, until they complain of a general rawness of the throat, when it should be stopped for some days and inhalations of petrolina or olive oil given instead. Phthisical patients with pulmonary cavities, etc., should receive the inhalation of chlorine, if possible, directly after expectoration so that the gas may reach the diseased surface. The temperature usually keeps elevated for the first two weeks—indeed may go higher than with other plans of treatment. When persistently high it is better to substitute the gold and sodium solution for the iodine for a few days, when both may be used together. With sensitive patients it may be necessary, at first, to precede the hypodermic injection with one of morphine or cocaine. They must not, however, be added to either of these mixtures as a precipitate would follow. We give little or no medicine by the mouth; sometimes some calisaya mixture or compound tincture of cinchona to improve the appetite. Considerable perspiration is a pretty constant attendant on this treatment. The nourishment, it is unnecessary to say, must be looked after carefully.

A CASE OF LEPRA MACULOSA ET TUBEROSA.

By LOUIS A. DUHRING, M.D.,
PROFESSOR OF SKIN DISEASES IN THE UNIVERSITY OF PENNSYLVANIA.

RECENTLY a case of leprosy, illustrating the macular variety, came to my notice in this city. The man presented himself for treatment, and at the time was entirely unaware of the nature of the disease. He had been under the care of a number of physicians, and had been treated for supposed syphilis and other affections, but no one had even intimated to him that the disease was or might prove to be leprosy. When told of the disease from which he was suffering he expressed great surprise, and even doubt as to the correctness of the diagnosis, for the reason that he had not for many years been in a leprosy country or district, and even then only as a traveller; and, moreover, because none of the other physicians who had treated him from time to time had so regarded the disease.

The notes of the case are briefly as follows:

J. A., aged forty-one years, and born in Sweden. There is no family history of interest. He was in Peru and Chili in 1868, and was in the merchant-marine service as a sailor from 1871 to 1888. In 1878, he was in Calcutta and Bombay for a period of three or four months. He frequently went ashore while at Calcutta, but only once while at Bombay. He has never visited other leprosy countries, and during the past eighteen months has lived in a city near Philadelphia, working in shipyards and printworks. He has no idea concerning the origin of the disease, which made its appearance, he states, two and a half years ago, upon the left brow and on the posterior surface of the right thigh, in the same form as it now exists. At first the spots were so faintly discolored and thickened as to be barely noticeable, and they have gradually become more and more pronounced, and have greatly multiplied. At present the disease involves the entire face, the trunk, and extremities, and exists in the form of numerous rounded and ovoidal, coin-sized, dull-yellowish, and dusky-orange, smoky, coppery, and brownish-yellow macules, and tuberose and flat patches of infiltration. The latter are flat or elevated, and in some places even lumpy or nodular, as on the face. The disease is most marked on the face and back. (See cuts.) The face shows the peculiar heavy-looking, severe, leonine expression

spread-out tuberose or flat lesions, such as occur in late syphilitic infiltrations and gummata. The macules and patches are distinctly anæsthetic—some more so, some less—the sticking of a needle into the skin causing no pain. The disease gives rise to no subjective symptoms, nor inconvenience beyond its presence and the consequent disfigurement, and his general health and strength remain good.

The disease portrays mainly the macular manifestation in an advanced stage. The lesions are numerous and extensive, and the entire force of the infective process seems to have expended itself on the skin. Some of the lesions on the trunk well illustrate the so-called morphœa of leprosy, as described by Erasmus Wilson and others of the older authors, and the resemblance to the ordinary morphœa simplex is so marked as to suggest that both diseases have a common starting-point in nerve complication, although, of course, of an entirely different nature. This I feel convinced of, and I have long held this view. Both kinds of cutaneous lesions are due to impaired or altered nerve-supply, the one—lepra—to a known and definite cause, the

FIG. 1.

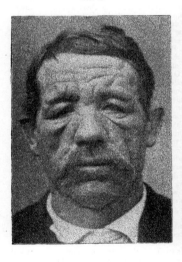

FIG. 2.

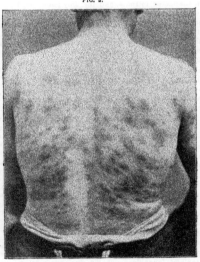

pression so characteristic of this disease, due to the tuberose infiltration and swelling of the cutaneous tissues, and the consequent sinking-in of the normal lines and creases of the skin. The eyelids are much thickened, and droop, as shown in Fig. 1.

There are no circumscribed tubercles present, either on the face or on other regions, the infiltrations, as stated, being in the form of diffuse or

other—morphœa simplex—to obscure and non-specific causes. Both are neuritic.

A piece of infiltrated skin was excised and prepared for the microscope. The examination was made by Dr. M. B. Hartzell, to whom I am indebted, with the following results: The lesion from which sections were made for microscopical examination was situated upon the posterior surface of the upper part of the right thigh, and was one of the earliest signs noticed by the patient, and was therefore one of the oldest. No pathological changes of any kind were found in the epidermis. In the corium an abundant diffuse infiltration of small round cells existed, with here and there slender tracts of unaltered connective tissue. This cellular infiltration was seen to be uniformly distributed throughout all parts of the corium, except that immediately beneath the papillary portion, where it was completely absent. In this part of the corium, beyond a few dilated lymph spaces, no change was noticed. No so-called lepra cells were anywhere found. Numerous sections, stained according to the methods of Weigert and Ziehl, were carefully examined for bacilli, but none were seen.

The man was seen only once, having subsequently failed to return for advice and suggestions as to treatment. The case is interesting from several points of view. First, as to the date and origin of the disease, and as to the mode of infection, upon which questions nothing positive can be stated. The natural supposition would be that the disease was contracted in India, and the only point which renders this doubtful is the long period—ten years— between the time of exposure and the first manifestations. But, it is entirely possible, and even probable, that the disease manifested itself insidiously, perhaps for several years before the attention of the patient was called to it. I think this highly probable, more especially as the man is by no means intelligent or observing. There is no history of contact with other lepers. The patient was amazed when informed of the true nature of the disease, which he had never suspected, and appeared to be anxious to place himself under treatment.

The second point of interest relates to the diagnosis. As stated, he had been seen by many physicians, none of whom informed him as to the nature of the disease, nor instituted or suggested any systematic course of treatment. The disease is undoubtedly lepra, but could be, I can well see, confounded with several affections, notably with granuloma fungoides (mycosis fungoides) in its early stage, to which it bears resemblance, also the infiltrated form of tubercular syphilis; but the wide distribution and the numerous areas of disease, and the bronzed tint of the skin, ought to be sufficient to exclude the latter disease. On the other hand, the dusky-yellowish color is not unlike that seen in granuloma fungoides; but the variegated colors as well as the inflammatory symptoms common to that disease are wanting.

Surgical Dressing for Soldiers.—The *Medical Press and Circular* states that in India the government has authorized a packet of first field-dressing in lieu of a bandage, to be given to soldiers whenever the army is ordered out for active service. Officers also receive the dressings.

REPORT OF A CASE OF GUNSHOT WOUND OF THE ABDOMEN, WITH THREE MESENTERIC AND SIXTEEN INTESTINAL WOUNDS; ABDOMINAL SECTION; RECOVERY.[1]

BY A. B. MILES, M.D.,
SURGEON TO THE CHARITY HOSPITAL, NEW ORLEANS, LA.

ON the morning of September 11, 1890, F. H., while carelessly handling a thirty-two calibre pistol, shot himself in the abdomen, the missile entering in the median line at a point midway between the umbilicus and the pubes. An ambulance was at once summoned, and within half an hour the patient was placed in the operating-room of the Charity Hospital.

His physical condition was, in every respect, excellent. He was a young white man, aged twenty-four years, of slender frame, but strong, and weighed about one hundred and thirty pounds. Fortunately, he had eaten sparingly for several days, owing to some slight indisposition. There were evidences of shock, but not in a marked degree. His pulse was 108. He complained of abdominal pain only.

Having determined that the ball had entered the abdominal cavity, and being convinced that the missile delivered at such a short and direct range, had inevitably injured the viscera or vessels, we at once decided upon active surgical treatment.

The operation was performed in the presence of our resident medical staff, and with the aid of Dr. J. D. Bloom, the assistant house-surgeon, who also with the assistance of Mr. E. D. Martin, conducted most of the after-treatment during my absence from New Orleans.

Median abdominal section was performed, the incision being four or five inches long. There was considerable blood in the peritoneal cavity, and the perforations were soon revealed in the protruding intestines. We at once instituted a systematic search for the bowel wounds, passing the small intestine in review from the beginning of the jejunum to the end of the ileum. The bullet, after entering the cavity, ranged a little to the left, wounded the mesentery in three places, perforated the small intestine sixteen times, and lodged somewhere in the deep muscles of the back. The man having eaten but little for several days, the intestines were practically empty, and this fact alone explains the number of intestinal wounds. A bullet, passing in any direction, could scarcely inflict so many wounds in a bowel even moderately distended. The condition which explains the large number of mesenteric and intestinal perforations also contributed very materially to the successful termination of the case, for aside from a small amount of mucus and blood, nothing escaped from the bowel wounds, and all operators know that in such cases no accident more seriously complicates an operation than faecal extravasation.

The operation was necessarily very tedious, lasting a little more than two hours. The mesenteric vessels were bleeding and their ligation consumed

[1] Read, by title, before the Southern Surgical and Gynecological Association, November 12, 1890.

a considerable part of the time. The intestinal wounds were closed with Lembert sutures of fine silk passed in the direction of the bowel. This plan seems least calculated to contract the calibre of the gut. Hæmorrhage having been arrested and the visceral wounds closed, the peritoneal cavity was douched with sterilized hot water, the abdominal incision sutured with silk and the usual antiseptic dressings of the hospital were applied.

The dressing was removed on the eighth day and the deep abdominal sutures taken out ; the superficial sutures were removed on the twelfth day.

On the evening of September 11th, the day of the operation, the temperature registered $94\frac{4}{5}°$ F., and the pulse was 115. A hypodermic injection of sulphate of morphine ¼ grain and sulphate of atropine $\frac{1}{150}$ grain was administered.

On the evening of the following day the temperature rose to 102° F.; the pulse to 150 per minute. These changes were attributable to our generosity in feeding. The above temperature, representing the highest points of the record, was promptly reduced by 10 grains of antipyrine administered hypodermically. On several subsequent occasions the temperature exceeded 101° F., but during confinement in bed it was usually about 99° F. The pulse was usually in accord with the temperature. After the first week, however, the pulse often beat about 60 and occasionally less (54) per minute.

From the second until the seventh day after the operation the patient was nourished exclusively by rectal alimentation. Only water, in quantities of half an ounce at a time, was given by the mouth. Food by the mouth was allowed on the seventh day, but was given very sparingly—teaspoonful potions of chicken tea, boiled milk, or Dacrois's elixir. The quantity of nutriment by the mouth was gradually increased until the thirteenth day, when the patient was given a breakfast of a soft-boiled egg, crackers, and a cup of coffee. In the meantime the little food given in the natural way was supplemented by rectal feeding.

On September 30th, dietary restrictions as to quality were removed, and the patient was only guarded against an excessive quantity.

On the fifth day after the operation the intestinal gases escaped naturally, and on the twentieth day there was a voluntary fæcal evacuation.

The patient remained in the hospital until October 18th, and from that date until the present writing, November 10th, has remained perfectly well. He affirms that his alimentary functions are in every respect perfectly normal.

This report is intended simply to add one more case to the growing list of successful enterorrhaphies for gunshot wounds, the only remarkable feature in the case being the unusual number of peritoneal and intestinal perforations—nineteen in all.

As we go to press, we learn that the President has appointed Dr. Charles Sutherland Surgeon-General of the United States Army.

LOCALIZED CENTRES IN THE OPTIC THALAMI.

BY HUGO ENGEL, A.M., M.D.,
CONSULTANT ON NERVOUS DISEASES AT ST. JOSEPH'S HOSPITAL,
OF PHILADELPHIA.

J. L., aged forty-three years, came to my clinic at St. Joseph's Hospital, May 5, 1890. Family history showed no hereditary taint. Patient had passed through the diseases incident to childhood without any lasting injury, and remained in good health until twenty-three years of age, when he had typhoid fever. The attack was severe and left him in a weakened condition for a year. Some paretic symptoms, the exact character of which could not be gleaned from the description, affected his lower extremities for several months during the earlier part of convalescence. At last, however, the patient completely recovered and remained well until his thirty-seventh year, when he contracted a primary, single, and indurated venereal sore. This was some months in healing, and was early accompanied by swelling of one of the left inguinal glands. The bubo proved stubborn and, notwithstanding various irritating injections into the enlarged gland, suppuration did not ensue. Within six months after the healing of the initial sore febrile symptoms ushered in an exanthem of roseola syphilitica, and, two weeks later, psoriasis palmaris, mucous patches over the tongue and the lining membranes of the cheeks and lips and angina luëtica formed the phenomena of a typical attack of secondary infection. Whether in consequence of a want of proper specific treatment in the hands of an irregular practitioner, or whether due to the virulent character of the poison, could not be determined, but the constitutional symptoms continued unabated for nearly a year. By the end of that period the eruptions upon the skin and mucous membranes had disappeared under the treatment of a physician in New York, but the throat affection did not heal until deep ulceration had destroyed parts of the palate, leaving an ugly scar.

The therapeutic measures directed by the physician in New York for the cure of the systemic infection evidently were very successful, as the patient remained free from all manifestations of the specific virus for about four years, gained decidedly in weight, and enjoyed the best of health. But he then began to suffer from headache, which always made its appearance about five o'clock in the afternoon, and gradually increased in severity as night approached. During the next few months the headaches came on progressively earlier in the afternoon, still becoming more intense toward evening, and becoming so severe at bedtime that it prevented him from falling asleep until between one and two o'clock in the morning, when the pain ceased, enabling him to obtain about five hours' rest. He never had the headaches in the morning.

He underwent treatment for supposed malaria, then for neuralgia, and finally for chronic meningitis, but without securing the least relief. After he had had the headaches for about three months he experienced a peculiar nervousness, accompanied by such a feeling of lassitude as completely to incapacitate him him for work (that of a foreman in a large machine-shop). The nervousness seized him every afternoon very soon after the beginning of the headache, but these phenomena, as well as some giddiness, which frequently made its appearance about the same time, were ascribed by him and his physieians to the deleterious influence of the torturing headache and the loss of sleep entailed thereby.

The new symptoms also gradually became more intense, until, drifting from one doctor to another in his endeavors to rid himself of his complaint, he finally lauded in my clinic. The group of symptoms enumerated had then been present for nearly a year. Judging from the suffering which the man had undergone, one would have expected to find the consequences of it stamped upon his face, and that his whole system would show the inroad of the disease, but the contrary was noted. When I first saw him he weighed one hundred and seventy pounds, his height being five feet nine inches, and his florid complexion and well-nourished physique gave no evidence of a serious malady. But the skin over the lower part of the forehead between the brows and that over the temples, had that peculiar dirty hue—a yellowish-brown tint in his case, but in other cases varying with the complexion of the individual —which experience has taught me is almost pathognomonic of the luëtic virus when this attacks the nerve-centres, though it is probably met with in most instances of systemic infection by the syphilitic poison.

As I could discover no organic lesion aside from the luëtic affection of the brain which did not appear to me so urgent as to make the postponement of the specific treatment for a few days a weighty matter, and as his digestion was somewhat faulty, and as he did not lead the most regular life, I concluded to place him first under the most favorable hygienic conditions, and to regulate his diet and improve his digestion. It is here that I made a mistake by not recognizing the great danger that he was in.

I asked the patient to return in three days, but I did not see him again until a fortnight later, when his wife called on me and begged me to visit him. Fearfully had the picture of the disease changed within that short period of time! When he came to the clinic there was nothing in his features to denote illness, while two weeks later death had stamped its ineffaceable mark upon the countenance of the man. After a long and patient inquiry I elicited the following:

Three days after he had left the clinic, on awakening in the morning, he felt confused and noticed, on rising, that he staggered, which he ascribed to the fact that he had no feeling whatever in the sole of his right foot. He then also observed the absence of feeling in his right arm, and a further investigation proved to him the total disappearance of all tactile sense on the entire right side of his body. While eating his breakfast he made the discovery that the senses of smell and taste on the right side had suddenly left him. He was sure that these symptoms were not present when he cleaned his teeth before eating and when he washed and dressed himself. He always had been in the habit of using a mouth-wash flavored with teaberry, and he was certain that he would have noticed the absence of taste and smell, and that he would then have examined further, as he did later to see whether hearing and sight were affected, for he was by nature a close observer. Ignorantly ascribing the symptoms to some transient effect of the medicine which I had given him, and even feeling encouraged, as his headache and giddiness, as well as a great deal of the nervousness and lassitude, remained away for the first time in a year, he failed to send for me.

This state of affairs lasted for eight days. On the afternoon of the ninth day, within fifteen minutes, he lost feeling, smell, and taste on the left side also, and very soon after became deaf in both ears. His wife now went to the hospital for me, but was informed—it being Tuesday—that the clinic for nervous diseases would not open again till Friday, though I might be seen at my house. Upon reaching home again she was persuaded by him to wait until Friday, he remarking that he felt generally so well that he did not care to trouble me. But Thursday evening the most alarming phenomenon occurred: he suddenly became blind in both eyes. It was then that they hastened to call me.

There is no doubt in my mind that the symptoms occurred exactly as named. The man first had a primary sore, then a bubo, and within half a year secondary luës, ushered in, as probably all the more virulent cases are, by roseola, preceded by fever. For a year these secondary manifestations did not yield to treatment, but the patient after that enjoyed good health and freedom from symptoms of syphilis for four years. Then headache set in with nocturnal exacerbations, giddiness, nervousness, and general lassitude, the forerunners of nearly all varieties of cerebral luës. When these symptoms had existed for about a year the tactile sense suddenly became extinguished on the right side, followed within an hour by loss of smell and taste on the same side. The senses of touch, smell, and taste, within a few days, were also lost on the other side, and deafness developed in both ears, followed in a few days by complete blindness of both eyes. The headache, vertigo, and nervousness had almost totally disappeared when the special senses became affected.

During Thursday night the patient was taken with convulsions, or, rather, he fell into l'état de mal, during which he died. Immediately preceding the fatal issue he gained consciousness and said, "What has been the m——?" probably intending to continue, "matter with me?"

At that moment the right pupil became widely dilated, the upper lid of the same eye dropped and remained in the state of ptosis, and finally a few lightning-like twitches of the facial muscles announced another convulsion, during which death occurred. The convulsions themselves were absolutely bilateral, and if they presented any especially characteristic point, it was the short duration of the tonic rigidity.

The patient's family assented to an autopsy after a great deal of persuasion, and with the proviso that under no circumstances was I to remove or permit to be taken away any part of the body. Various motives, which it would be out of place to discuss, but which were more or less rooted in superstition, determined the wife to insist upon that condition. Besides two brothers of the deceased, a priest carefully watched Dr. Louis Gruel, the chief of my clinic, and myself, thus making it impossible for us to remove clandestinely any tissue, even had we been so inclined.

Autopsy.—Only the head was opened. The blood-vessels were rigid and in the state first described by Heubner, of arterio-sclerosis syphilitica. Characteristic newgrowths had commenced to form within the lumen of the basilar, middle meningeal, and

smell and taste, and the course of the fibres and their evident prolongation into the respective temporo-sphenoidal convolutions seem to demonstrate the correctness of this view. Fournier has shown that the fornix also connects the thalami with the cortical centres of tactile sensibility. Motor symptoms are always absent when the thalami alone are involved, and in the cases reported as an evidence of motor disturbance, due to disease of a thalamus, the lesions were so near the internal capsule (Ranney) —*i. e.*, its thalamo-lenticular portion (Spitzka)—that the cause of the motor phenomena in these instances is easily explained.

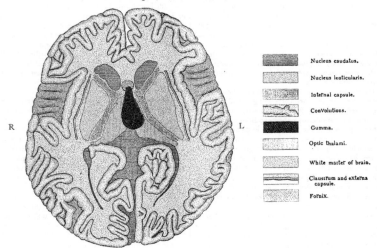

	Nucleus caudatus.
	Nucleus lenticularis.
	Internal capsule.
	ConVolutions.
	Gumma.
	Optic thalami.
	White matter of brain.
	Claustrum and externa capsule.
	Fornix.

R   L

other large arteries at the base of the skull. At the points where the neoplasms were located the vessels were greatly narrowed—the opposite of what occurs in senile sclerosis, in which the stiff walls prevent the vessels from collapsing and the lumen is widened. Although every part of the encephalon was carefully examined microscopically, nothing else abnormal was found until the lateral ventricles were opened. Here was a neoplasm which had formed in the fornix and from thence spread over the optic thalami; the growth being older and more advanced on the left than on the right side. (See cut.) It had the usual characteristics of gummata. As I am not an experienced draughtsman I have taken the normal parts of the drawing from Ranney's and Erb's illustrations. The cut explains itself and clearly shows the extent of the gumma.

REMARKS.—Observers agree that the pillars of the fornix unite the thalami with the cortical centres of

The newgrowth in the case reported here evidently began in the portion of the fornix where, at the posterior end of and between the two caudate nuclei of the corpora striata, it is connected with the most anterior part of the optic thalami. The patient's first symptom was loss of tactile sense, followed by loss of smell and taste on the right side. These symptoms agree with the result of the autopsy, which showed that the disease was more extended and considerably older on the left side of the fornix and in the left thalamus.

Luys has made the most thorough investigation of the functions of the thalami. He discovered in them four isolated ganglia, and Arnold, who at first affirmed the existence of only three, has since been convinced of the presence of a fourth ganglion. These ganglia are arranged in an antero-posterior plane and form successive tuberosities upon the thalamus, giving that body the appearance of a conglomerate gland (Ranney).

Proceeding from before backward these ganglia are:

1. Corpus album subrotundum. This is the most prominent of all and is especially developed in dogs, in which the sense of smell is very acute. By means of the tænia semicircularis it is also connected with the roots of the olfactory nerve. All peripheral olfactory impressions are first condensed in this ganglion, before they radiate toward the cortex.

2. The second centre is said by Luys to be connected with the organs of vision. But the majority of observers now agree, that the posterior part, the pulvinar, together with the external geniculate bodies, is related to the visual tracts, which pass on to the cortical centres of vision in the occipital lobe (cuneus, etc.), while the second ganglion, the fibres of which connect with the side of the internal geniculate body, is brought in direct communication with those temporo-sphenoidal gyri which form the cortical centre of hearing.

Unless a microscopical examination should have shown pressure on other parts or a gradually-extending degeneration of fibres composing portions of the internal capsule, or unless capillaries situated in other regions were the seat of the endo-arteritis first observed by Finger—assumptions which would not agree with the group of symptoms presented *intra-vitam*—the case reported would prove the general correctness of Luys's views, excepting as far as they relate to the second ganglion; concerning the latter the case would confirm the statements of the later authors (Serres, Fleichsig, Wernicke, Monakow, etc.) referring to the pulvinar.

After abolition of the tactile sense and that of smell and of taste, hearing was lost, and later the power of vision; the gumma evidently grew with astonishing rapidity in an antero-posterior direction. If the second ganglion of Luys were connected with the visual apparatus, blindness should have preceded the deafness.

3. The third ganglion, exactly situated in the mathematical centre of the thalamus (Ranney) governs in some way general sensation. It probably is the automatic centre for general sensation or for some special part of sensation, such as touch, so that some impressions belonging to the category of general sensation under certain conditions do not reach the cortex, but are interpreted here, and such impressions proceed further only if the cortical centres (in the parietal convolutions) either exert an inhibiting influence on those situated lower down, or so stimulate them as to cause a further transmission of the sensory impressions.

The lower gray masses seem to have the same relation to the various afferent and efferent tracts

that the strengthening batteries possess to a long telegraphic relay consisting of a number of stations. The current from the cells at the first station is strong enough to carry the current to the next; if the current shall proceed further, it must first pass through wires which bring to it increased electromotive force obtained from another battery, thus enabling the impulse to go on its way undiminished in power. The cells in the cortex must influence in some such way all the various cells situated in the same tract but beneath the cortex. It is then by inhibition or stimulation that an impression is either stopped at some point where the local function of the cells transform the impression into motor acts, or it proceeds to the end and becomes a conscious impression, to be registered in a cortical cell, associated with others and simply recorded as memory —as the wax cylinder of the phonograph retains the indentations made upon it by the recording needle of the diaphragm, which in its turn is set in motion by the waves of sound—or is transformed and interpreted as conscious volition with its efferent result: a motor impulse.

Thus, in an English setter dog, when arriving on the field where partridges are concealed, the cortical centre in the temporo-sphenoidal gyri—probably the most anterior portion of the middle temporal convolution and perhaps the same part of the inferior—sends an impulse to the ganglion of smell in the thalamus and this sets in motion the complicated apparatus which enables the dog to discover the hidden birds, and he then automatically performs his duties.

I omitted in the case of J. L. to examine especially into all the various disturbances of general sensation that may have existed, but he was not conscious long enough to allow me to make such an examination successfully. If the middle ganglion is related to general sensibility, almost all sensation should have been destroyed, unless such afferent impressions pass along a tract which, forming a part of the internal capsule—the third bundle antero-posteriorly from the knee in the thalamo-lenticular portion, between, therefore, the pyramidal and the speech tracts (Wernicke)—proceeds cephalad without connecting with the thalami, ending in the parietal convolutions.

If specific treatment energetically and systematically carried on, had been commenced at once, when J. L. first came to my clinic, the growth of the neoplasm might have been prevented or brought to a standstill—in the latter case absorption would probably have ultimately occurred. His failure to return in three days made the employment of antiluëtic treatment impossible, and thus may be said to have been directly responsible for the sudden fatal issue.

507 FRANKLIN STREET.

ON SOME RELATIONS BETWEEN THE HEART-BEAT AND THE VISCERAL CIRCULATION.

BY HENRY SEWALL, M.D., PH.D.,
OF DENVER, COLORADO.

To the popular mind the heart is, *par excellence*, the central organ of animal life, the engine which keeps the vital forces in continuous play, and the sensitive mechanism of which is readily thrown out of gear. Exact physiological study has in no way diminished the importance in the economy of the cardiac motor, but it has developed the fact that nearly every "functional" disturbance or physiological modification in the activity of the heart is brought about by causes operating not directly on the heart-tissue, but in an indirect way through the nervous system, and especially the vasomotor mechanism.

Every working physiologist has at times been astonished at what may be called the "toughness" of the heart, its tolerance of injury when considered apart from the rest of the body. Among a class of students, wonder is always excited by the spectacle of a living frog's heart isolated from the body, and supplied with a nutrient current of defibrinated blood or diluted blood-serum, beating regularly for hours, and performing an amount of work which would give it a high grade of efficiency among artificial machines.

It is not the design of this paper to enter into a full discussion of the physiological mechanism of the heart, but there are certain general facts concerning it, whether old or new, which have been only imperfectly transmitted from the laboratory to the clinic, and which must be considered if the interdependence of the cardiac and other physiological functions is to be regarded. It may, therefore, not be thought out of place to sum up once more some of the well-known facts of cardiac physiology as a basis for the hypothesis which it is the object of this article to develop.

One of the most surprising facts connected with the study of the heart is the small amount of nutriment on which the organ will continue to perform its work. If a frog's heart be removed from the body, and allowed to remain empty, it will usually cease beating within half an hour; but if a very weak solution of mineral salts, having the qualitative and quantitative relations of the salts in the normal blood plasma, be passed through the heart cavities, strong pulsation may be kept up for five or six hours. If to the salt solution there be added an exceedingly small proportion of appropriate albuminous matter, the heart may continue to beat for a day or two. On one occasion I observed a frog's heart, suspended in a Roy-Gaskell tonometer and supplied by a current of diluted defibrinated blood, keep up its pulsation for more than three days.

26*

It has been found that the addition of drugs, such as acids or alkalies, even in so small a proportion as 1 part to 20,000 parts of the fluid circulating through the isolated heart, profoundly modifies its pulsation, and we should, *à fortiori*, expect that deleterious substances, though present in the normal blood in inappreciable quantities, would have a distinct effect on the action of the heart.

What particularly concerns us here, however, in relation to the direct action of the blood on the heart, is not so much the nutritive value of the fluid as its influence in mechanically distending the cardiac walls; or, in other words, in determining intra-cardiac blood-pressure.

About twelve years ago it was announced by H. P. Bowditch, that if the ventricle of a frog's heart be crushed in a line across the middle, by a pair of small-bladed forceps, the apex of the organ, being thus removed from its physiological connection with the rest of the heart, will remain empty and quiescent, the basal portion alone carrying on the work of circulation. But Foster, in repeating this experiment, found that if the intra-cardiac pressure were raised by clamping the aorta, the previously empty apex would fill with blood and commence rhythmical pulsations.

Many other facts discovered in the laboratory testify in favor of the proposition that increase of intra-cardiac pressure, within limits, acts as a stimulus to the motor mechanism of the heart.

Not only does the intra-cardiac blood-pressure, which is determined, other things being equal, by the ratio of the inflow to the outflow of blood through the heart, have a most important influence on the energy developed by the active isolated organ, but it profoundly modifies the susceptibility of the heart to the reflex impressions which are probably continually pouring into it along the extra-cardiac nerves.

Nearly ten years ago, in association with F. Donaldson, Jr., of Baltimore, the writer published,[1] from the laboratory of the Johns Hopkins University, an account of some experiments undertaken with a view to ascertain the exact relations between the variation of intra-cardiac blood-pressure and the intensity of inhibitory action which the cardiac branches of the pneumogastric nerves exercise over the heart-beat. Most of our experiments were performed on the "slider" terrapin, the heart of which consists of four chambers, namely: a venous sinus, which collects the blood from the tissues and conducts it into one of the two auricles; a second auricle, which receives the aërated blood from the lungs; and a single ventricle, which receives the blood from both auricles. In our experiments the heart was supplied

---

[1] Journal of Physiology, vol. iii., Nos. 5 and 6.

through either auricle by a current of artificial diluted, defibrinated blood, the pressure of which in the heart could be maintained at any desired degree by changing the level of the Mariotte's flask which served as a reservoir for the blood. The vagi nerves being isolated and placed on the electrodes of an induction apparatus, it was ascertained what strength of current was able just to produce an inhibitory slowing of the heart-beat. The intra-cardiac pressure was then changed, and the effect of stimulation was again tried. The invariable results may be stated thus: With increase of intra-cardiac pressure there is a diminution of the inhibitory action of the vagus nerve on the heart-beat; if the intra-cardiac pressure be sufficiently increased, the inhibitory power of the vagus is, for a time, wholly lost. On the other hand, the vagus inhibitory action is intensified by lowering the intra-cardiac blood-pressure. We found this reaction to be extremely delicate, for the susceptibility of the heart toward inhibitory impulses travelling along the vagus was altered by very slight variations in intra-cardiac pressure, as well represented in a column of blood one centimetre or less in height. We endeavored to carry out similar experiments on the dog's heart, isolated according to the "Baltimore method," and though, owing to the vastly increased complexity of the physiological conditions, the results were unsatisfactory, they plainly pointed to conclusions similar to those arrived at in the case of the terrapin.

Subsequently the writer accidentally obtained an interesting confirmation of the foregoing views of the pressure-inhibitory relations in the mammalian heart. A calf was on the operating-table of the laboratory; the excitement of the animal could not be controlled by any reasonable amount of anæsthetic; its circulation was abnormally active and blood-pressure high. It was found that the vagi, stimulated either singly or together by powerful induction currents, were absolutely without control over the rate of the heart-beat. When, however, the blood-pressure was lowered by moderate bleeding, the inhibitory influence of the stimulated vagus was readily manifested.

It is well known among physiologists that it is impossible to produce fatal syncope in animals by artificial stimulation of the peripheral ends of the cut vagi; yet cases are not wanting which indicate that the "shock" which causes death in many casualties is but the expression of powerful reflex inhibition of the heart-beat through the pneumogastric nerves. Thus, Goltz cites the case of a workman who, while asleep after his dinner, was struck on the abdomen by a board in the hands of a playful comrade. The sleeper died instantly, but post-mortem examination failed to show any anatomical lesion. Goltz uses this case as an illustration in the human animal of

the *klopfversuch*—*i. e.*, reflex inhibition of the heart-beat by sharply tapping the intestines—which he had, for the first time, just demonstrated on the frog. It seems exceedingly probable that the reason direct stimulation of the vagi in an animal on the operating-table does not cause death, while reflex inhibition through irritation of the sympathetic system under physiological conditions may do so, lies in the fact that in the former case the cardiac motor system alone is directly affected, the respiratory and vasomotor mechanisms still keeping up their work with even exaggerated activity, so that the heart soon becomes loaded with blood which is squeezed out of the systemic vessels by the spasm of their muscular coats. Thus, in a short time the intra-cardiac tension is so elevated that the inhibitory impulses descending the vagi fall into a motor system so excited as to be insensitive to their influence.

On the other hand, in the case of reflex inhibition, the blow which momentarily stops the heart, at the same time paralyzes the vasomotor mechanism so that the blood collects and stagnates in the widely-dilated vessels of the abdomen; the under-filled heart then lacks the pressure-stimulus of inflowing blood, and, finally, the failure of nutriment in the vital centres is followed by a fatal decrease in their irritability.

Previously to the work referred to above, performed by Donaldson and myself, Ludwig and Luchsinger[1] had carried on somewhat similar experiments.

These authors made the interesting observation that when the temperature of the isolated frog's heart was artificially elevated the effect was to annul the inhibitory influence of the vagi. This suggests, of course, that in fevers the regulating influence of the vagi may be lost in a similar way.

As regards the stimulating effect of intra-cardiac blood-pressure, an interesting fact presented itself in the course of the experiments which have already been cited. The artificial supply of blood was led to the heart by a canula which was tied either in a pulmonary vein or in the sinus venosus, and thus only one auricle directly received the pressure of the inflowing blood, the other auricle being but imperfectly distended by leakage through the cardiac valves. A frequent, if not constant, result of this circumstance was a want of synchronism in the contraction of the two auricles; the systole of the more distended auricle perceptibly preceding that of the less distended auricle. That is to say, increase of the diastolic intra-cardiac blood-pressure in any chamber of the heart hastens the rhythm of pulsation in that part. Building on this fact, we can hardly doubt that in the complex relations under which the heart acts in the normal body, the

---

[1] Pflüger's Archiv, Bd. xxv.

balance of intra-cardiac diastolic blood-pressure in the two auricles is subject to frequent fluctuations, which must be attended by a more or less marked alteration of rhythm in the action of the various cardiac chambers. Such an event would offer an interesting explanation of the origin of those temporary heart-murmurs which ausculation one day reveals and the next finds wanting. Thus it is believed with reason that in the normal cardiac cycle, so soon as the ventricles have emptied themselves, and when the common diastole begins, the blood stored in the auricles immediately begins to flow onward with the effect of floating up the auriculoventricular valves until they nearly meet ; then, at the end of the common diastole comes the short, sharp stroke of auricular contraction, which seems to shoot a current of blood down through the middle of each ventricle, which causes a reverse current to pass along the ventricular wall, lifts the valves and brings them into firm contact ; at this instant the systole of the ventricle begins and regurgitation is prevented by the tightly-closed valves.

Suppose, however, that the rhythm of movement of the auricle and ventricle is altered by the fractional part of a second ; in this case the auriculoventricular valves will have rebounded from their first closure when the ventricle begins to contract, and as a necessary result there will be a regurgitant current of blood and an audible murmur. Any sudden alteration in the volume of blood flowing through the lungs in the normal body would be followed by a corresponding change in the pressure within the left auricle, and give rise to the conditions sufficient to disturb the rhythm of movement in the different parts of the heart.

Such are some of the influences which may cause an alteration in the rhythm of the heart-beat by direct action on the organ. In addition, it may suffice to recall briefly the fact that the nerve-filaments which connect the heart with the central nervous system by way of the vagi and sympathetic nerves, contain physiological fibres of varied function, and which in the normal body are in nearly continual activity.

It has long been a familiar fact, and one already mentioned, that certain nerve-filaments arising in the roots of the spinal accessory, and proceeding to the heart by way of the pneumogastric trunks, carry impulses which exert a cardio-inhibitory influence ; that is, stimulation of them causes a slowing of the heart's rhythm, or even a cessation of the beat. It is, perhaps, less generally known that fibres having an opposite or accelerator function, reach the heart by way of the sympathetic system. Excitation of these causes a quickening of the heart-beat.

In addition there has been established within the last few years the existence of two other sets of cardiac nerve-fibres ; one of these, when excited, causes a progressive weakening or loss of power in the heart-beat, without alteration in the rhythm ; while stimulation of the other set produces the converse effect, or augmentation in the energy of the heart's contraction. All these nerve-fibres belong to the efferent group of nerves; that is, they transmit impulses only from the central nerve-system to the heart.

Of afferent nerves, which carry impulses from the heart to the brain, we as yet know with certainty only one variety, the so-called *depressor* nerve, which, when the heart is over-distended with blood, causes a reflex enlargement of the splanchnic vascular area by inhibition of the vaso-constrictor nerve-centre, thus lowering the resistance against which the heart must empty itself.

But there is little doubt that there exists a full set of afferent fibres corresponding in function with the efferent nerves that have been mentioned.

Such is a brief *résumé* of some of the present certainties of cardiac physiology.

The therapeutics as well as the pathology of the circulation can have a sure foundation only in a physiological scheme which embraces every functional relation of organ to organ and cell to cell. It is this belief, at all events, which is offered as an excuse for the presentation of laboratory data as a basis for clinical inference.

In no organs of the body should we, *a priori*, expect to find more frequent causes of disturbance in the circulation than in the abdominal viscera. Into their vascular area might easily be drained all the blood in the body ; their calls on the output of vital energy are often irregular and excessive ; they are more or less continuously subjected to the influence of poisons physiological and non-physiological; the pressure of a loaded colon and rectum may at any time offer a serious obstacle to the normal current of blood.

The rate and completeness of the circulation, and consequently the character of the heart-beat, must obviously be influenced by each of these conditions; and it is not surprising that long ago there should have been recognized an intimate relation between the state of the bowels and certain symptoms derived chiefly from the circulation, such as vertigo, mental depression, disturbance of vision, flushings, palpitations, and coated tongue ; a group of symptoms which presents itself so frequently as to lead the medical attendants of a certain dispensary to abbreviate the prescription indicated into

R.—Shotgun No. 2.

which being interpreted reads:

R.—Hydrag. chlor. mite   .   .   . 5 grains.
S.—Take at bedtime.

and

R.—Magnes. sulph.   .   .   .   .   ℥ss.
S.—Take in half a glassful of water before breakfast.

In other words, it has been found that simple unloading of the bowels, together with an "alterative" effect of the cathartic, suffices to restore the physiological tone.

It is, however, quite another group of symptoms, the consideration of which has given occasion for this paper. In this group the phenomenon of "heart failure" is most prominent, and I venture to believe the cause would by no means generally be ascribed to the state of the visceral circulation.

The symptoms referred to vary in intensity from a simple feeling of faintness or "goneness" with infrequent, weak, and perhaps irregular pulse, and rather labored, slow respiration, to an attack which in its appearance now resembles syncope, and again somewhat simulates coma.

These phenomena are not necessarily preceded by special symptoms nor by a state of unusual constipation. Patients so suffering have presented an account of more or less frequent recurrence of the attacks, with a history of some previous decided liver derangement, such as that associated with congestion or a malarial attack. Nearly all the cases which have been noted were those of patients in different stages of phthisis; this was, probably, in part due to the large proportion of phthisical patients in the neighborhood where these observations were chiefly made; in part, also, to the modified metabolism and circulatory resistance of the liver in this disease. In no case could any sign of heart lesion be discovered.

The attacks lasted, roughly speaking, from a few minutes to five or six hours, and then gradually subsided.

Unfortunately, in only one case did I witness the disturbance while at its height. In this instance the respiration was deep and labored, and only ten or twelve per minute; the eyes were fixed and staring; the face pale or ashy, and rather drawn and pinched; consciousness was incompletely preserved, and the pulse was weak and slightly rapid. In general, the pulse is characterized rather by weakness than infrequency, and the phenomena, as a whole, seem to indicate morbid feebleness in the circulation and deficient aëration of the blood. The exhibition of cardiac stimulants afforded rather incomplete and temporary relief, and after such treatment the attack might be repeated within a few hours or days; such has been the result even when digitalis was regularly taken in the interim.

On thinking over the clinical history presented by one of these cases, I remembered the picture offered by the dog's heart beating in the opened chest, and the powerless, flapping, spasmodic movement brought about in the organ when the blood-supply was diminished by clamping the venæ cavæ. Following out the analogy it seemed not improbable that the circulatory disturbance in the human subject was likewise the result of diminished blood-flow to the heart. Supposing this to be true, the suggestion was obvious that such a condition depended on a morbid state of the visceral circulation, and the line of treatment indicated was evidently to use the means at command to modify the blood-current through the abdominal organs.

Unloading the bowels by one means or another not only removes a possible mechanical hindrance to the circulation and empties the gland-ducts of their secretions, but the peristalsis excited is, undoubtedly, a most powerful motor factor in the passage of the blood through the portal system.

At all events, in each of the half-dozen cases of what, for want of a better name, I have thought best to call "functional heart-failure," it has been found that judicious catharsis, or rather laxative treatment, has succeeded in giving the surest and most nearly permanent relief from the appalling symptoms which have been discussed.

The cases illustrating my thesis were under observation for periods varying from three weeks to nine months.

1854 RACE STREET, November 1, 1890.

CLINICAL MEMORANDUM.

OPHTHALMOLOGICAL.

Two Cases of Foreign Body in the Eyeball.—These two cases, of recent occurrence, seem worthy of note, on account of the large size of the foreign bodies and the almost entire absence of pain:

P. J. M., machinist, aged thirty years, was struck in the left eye by a piece of cold chisel. The course of the offending body was marked by a nick in the edge of the lower lid, a cut in the lower outer quadrant of the cornea, and a ragged opening in the iris. There was considerable hæmorrhage into the anterior chamber and vitreous, but *absolutely no pain then or subsequently.* Immediate enucleation was advised and consented to by the patient, but his family objected. After two months of varied experiences he returned, and I removed the eyeball, which was softened and had shrunken to one-third its normal size. The bevelled edge of the chisel, about one-eighth of an inch wide and half an inch long, was found on the floor of the eye, imbedded in the degenerated vitreous.

George R., negro, aged ten years, came to me with an injury of the left eye. He said that a boy had fired a buckshot at him from a spring-gun used for killing sparrows. The edge of the lower lid was perforated, and there was a round hole in the lower and inner part of the eyeball, just below the sclero-corneal junction. There was considerable hæmorrhage, but *little or no pain then or afterward.* On the supposition that the buckshot was in the eye, immediate enucleation was advised; but when the boy with the gun insisted that the end of the steel spring had done the injury, it was thought best to wait a few days. At the end of a week the eyeball had softened, and when removed was found to contain the metal end of a large shoestring that had been used for the bowstring of the gun. It was three-fourths of an inch long, and the sharp end was projecting slightly from the eyeball, a short distance below and outside of the entrance of the optic nerve. The sharp, arrow-like tip had transfixed the eye obliquely through the lower half.

JOHN L. DICKEY, M.D.

WHEELING, W. VA.

HOSPITAL NOTES.

KENSINGTON HOSPITAL FOR WOMEN.

SERVICE OF CHARLES P. NOBLE, M.D.

[Reported by A. H. DEEKENS, M.D.]

A CASE OF INTRA-LIGAMENTARY CYST OF THE LEFT OVARY—ENUCLEATION; RECOVERY.

MRS. M., aged fifty-eight years, married, gave a history of abdominal enlargement dating from an attack of dysentery about a year previously. For six months she has had considerable discomfort in her abdomen, while for the last two months her abdomen has been enlarging quite rapidly, and with the increase in size the discomfort became more marked, though at no time has she complained of pain. She had passed the menopause five years before the abdominal enlargement appeared, and for four years enjoyed fairly good health.

Becoming alarmed at the rapid growth of the tumor, which had been complicated by a mild attack of peritonitis with considerable pain, she sent for her physician about a week previously. Dr. Noble saw her in consultation a few days later.

At this time she was stout and apparently fairly healthy, but had a very sallow complexion. She had not been confined to bed, as she said that she felt better when up than when lying down. Upon examination Dr. Noble found a large, hard, multinodular tumor, which nearly filled the abdomen, but was situated more to the right side than to the left. There was doubtful fluctuation. An operation was advised, and the patient entered the Kensington Hospital for Women on the following day, September 9th.

On September 13th, Dr. Noble, assisted by Dr. George M. Boyd, operated in the presence of a number of physicians. The operation proved to be quite a formidable one owing to the numerous adhesions and intimate connections of the tumor with the abdominal organs. A median incision, three inches in length, exposed a multilocular cyst. This was tapped and about eight quarts of the ordinary gelatinous fluid was discharged. The sac was now withdrawn and was found to be an intra-ligamentary cyst of the left ovary. Enucleation was begun by breaking through the peritoneum along the descending colon—the tumor had raised the peritoneum in this locality and was attached to the muscular wall of the colon. The adhesions were stripped or tied off, until the entire tumor was enucleated, and only a slight

attachment to the peritoneum of the broad ligament, near the uterus, remained; this was transfixed, tied *en masse*, and separated from the cyst. A large cup-shaped cavity remained, which represented the original site of the tumor. All bleeding-points were searched for and secured, the pelvic cavity was thoroughly washed out with boiled water and sponged until dry, and a drainage-tube was then inserted and the incision closed. The operation from the beginning of the incision to the tying of the last abdominal suture occupied an hour and twenty-three minutes. The cyst was aspirated in seven minutes and enucleated in fifty minutes. Chloroform was the anæsthetic used. The patient was put to bed with a pulse of 65. This slow pulse-rate was, perhaps, due to the tincture of digitalis which was given hypodermically during the operation.

The woman made an uninterrupted recovery. The drainage-tube was removed on the third day. On the sixth day she was able to sit up in bed, supported by a bed-rest, and the stitches were removed. On September 26th she was able to get out of bed, and on September 30th she walked down stairs on her way to the convalescent wards of the hospital.

Her temperature at no time rose above 100⅘° and was at that point for a brief period only. This elevation was due to constipation, which was relieved by glycerin enemata. Her pulse remained between 80 and 85, once running up to 94 for a short time.

This case is of interest, among other reasons because the patient had not suspected any growth until two months before the operation—she thought that she was merely "becoming fatter"—because there was very slight impairment of the general health, and because the character of the fluctuation was doubtful.

MEDICAL PROGRESS.

Pyoktanin in the Treatment of Gonorrhœa.—LINDSTOERM (*Vratch*, November, 1890) has tried pyoktanin in seventeen cases of gonorrhœa. When injected into the urethra in the strength of from 1 to 4 : 1000 it failed to alleviate the pain, but in all of the cases there was a diminution in the purulent secretion. In a number of cases of chancre he applied pyoktanin with powdered chalk in the proportion of from 1 to 2 : 1000, but found that the effects were no better than those generally obtained from the use of powdered calomel. As a consequence Lindstoerm is not very favorably impressed with the new antiseptic.

Sulphonal in Diabetes.—CASERELLI reports from the Clinic of Professor Grocco that the employment of 30 grains of sulphonal daily in diabetes produces marked diminution in the quantity of both the sugar and urine. He remarks, however, that too large doses of the sulphonal will produce disagreeable symptoms, such as vertigo and excessive somnolence.

Injections for Gonorrhœa in the Male.—LANG, of Vienna, employs injections two or three times daily in both the acute and chronic form of this affection. For acute gonorrhœa he recommends the use of a solution of sulpho carbolate of zinc of ¼, ½, or 1 per cent., the quantity of liquid injected each time being 1½ drachms. For gleet the volume of the injection may be as much as from 2 to 3 drachms. Along with these injections he recommends careful diet, excluding all red meats, and as much rest as possible.

Treatment of Disseminated Acne.—According to HERTZMANN, the following treatment is to be employed in cases of acne indurata et pustulosa. The pustule is to be evacuated and cauterized by introducing the tip of a piece of wood dipped in a solution of perchloride of iron, and frictions of the face are to be made with carbolic acid of the strength of 3 to 5 per cent., in water, and afterward

R.—Salicylic acid . . . . 45 grains.
Alcohol (95 per cent.) . . 5 ounces.
is to be applied to the skin.

For acne papulosa, where the papules are small and numerous, frictions with tincture of green soap are very useful, the prescription being made up as follows :

R.—Green soap . . . . 1 ounce.
Alcohol (95 per cent.) . . 2 ounces.
Spirit of lavender . . . ½ ounce.
Water . . . . . 3 ounces.

After this is applied vaseline or cold cream should be smeared over the skin. Where the disease is very severe the following prescription is advisable :

R.—Naphthol . . . . . 2½ drachms.
Precipitated sulphur . . . 1½ ounces.
Lanolin and green soap, of each 2 "

For seborrhœic acne daily frictions with the following solution are useful:

R.—Flowers of sulphur . . . 2 ounces.
Lime . . . . . 4 "
Water . . . . . 1 pint.

Boil, decant, and keep in a closed vessel. Should application of this medicament produce much irritation of the skin cold cream should be applied.

Tapping and Draining the Ventricles of the Brain.—MR. A. W. MAYO ROBSON (*British Medical Journal*, December 6, 1890) reports a case of localized meningitis, with accumulation of fluid in the lateral ventricles, in a child aged ten years, which was successfully treated by tapping and draining the left lateral ventricle. The fissure of Rolando having been mapped out, the patient was anæsthetized with the A. C. E. mixture, a large semilunar flap was turned down, and the skull was trephined with a one-half inch trephine over the situation of the motor centre of the arm, there being right hemiplegia, aphasia, twitching of the arm, and tonic spasm of the thumb. On raising the dura, which appeared healthy, the surface of the brain was found to be compressed and not pulsating. The needle of an exploring syringe was then thrust deeply in various directions in the hope of finding pus. Failing to find any, the needle was thrust into the posterior extremity of the second frontal convolution and pushed transversely inward and slightly downward into the lateral ventricle. Six drachms of clear fluid escaped, after which the natural pulsations returned to the exposed portion of the brain. The dura was then sutured with

fine catgut, several bone-grafts were placed over it, and the scalp was united, no drainage-tube being employed.

On the following day slight power of movement returned in the right arm and leg, and on the third day the patient could answer simple questions. Within a month all paretic symptoms disappeared. Six months later she was perfectly well, with the exception of occasional slight convulsive seizures, limited to the right arm and unaccompanied by loss of consciousness, which Mr. Robson thinks were possibly due to adhesions at the site of operation. Bromides were prescribed, and when the patient was last seen the attacks were only occasionally returning.

At the close of his remarks the author made a number of suggestions as to the *technique* of the operation, of which the following are the most important :

1. If there is time, a purgative should be given on the day before the operation.

2. The chief convolutions, the fissure of Rolando, and the base-line should be mapped out on the shaven scalp with nitrate of silver, a carbolic acid dressing should then be applied and allowed to remain until the time of the operation.

3. If an anæsthetic is required the A. C. E. mixture should be used.

4. In order not to lose the landmarks after the flap has been turned back, the scalp should be perforated by a small drill which will make a distinct mark on the skull.

5. In simple tapping of the ventricle the trephineopening should be smaller than if a drainage-tube is to be used, and a linear incision, three-fourths of an inch long, in the scalp is sufficient.

6. If drainage is to be adopted the periosteum should be reflected from a circle slightly larger than the circumference of the trephine.

7. The needle or director should be removed and reintroduced for every new puncture, and the large vessels and important parts of the brain should be avoided.

8. The punctures should be made in the course of the fibres and vertical to the surface.

9. If a drainage-tube is to be left in, a fine director should be used, along which a pair of Lister sinus forceps can be pushed and the puncture dilated to receive the tube.

Ichthyol in the Treatment of Gonorrhœa. — KÖSTER (*Wiener medizinische Presse*, November 23, 1890) writes enthusiastically of the use of a one-per-cent. solution of ammonium sulph-ichthyolate in gonorrhœa. He has used it in three cases of gonorrhœa in men and in one case of gonorrhœal cystitis in a woman. In the cases of gonorrhœa he employed injections of the solution three times daily. On the second day of treatment the painful micturition and the painful nocturnal erections disappeared. The discharge ceased permanently in from four to twenty days.

In the case of cystitis, in which the symptoms were severe, four and one-half ounces of the solution were injected twice daily for eight days by means of an irrigator, the solution being retained in the bladder for five minutes, and then permitted to escape through the urethra. After the second day of treatment the pus disappeared from the urine and there was no longer severe pain.

THE MEDICAL NEWS.

A WEEKLY JOURNAL
OF MEDICAL SCIENCE.

COMMUNICATIONS are invited from all parts of the world. Original articles contributed exclusively to THE MEDICAL NEWS will be liberally paid for upon publication. When necessary to elucidate the text, illustrations will be furnished without cost to the author.

Address the Editor: H. A. HARE, M.D.,
1004 WALNUT STREET,
PHILADELPHIA.

Subscription Price, including Postage.

PER ANNUM, IN ADVANCE . . . . $4.00.
SINGLE COPIES . . . . 10 CENTS.

Subscriptions may begin at any date. The safest mode of remittance is by bank check or postal money order, drawn to the order of the undersigned. When neither is accessible, remittances may be made, at the risk of the publishers, by forwarding in *registered* letters.

Address,   LEA BROTHERS & CO.,
NOS. 706 & 708 SANSOM STREET,
PHILADELPHIA.

SATURDAY, DECEMBER 27, 1890.

GOUTY AND RHEUMATIC EYES.

IT is a matter of common knowledge that not infrequently the existence of certain grave constitutional disorders is first discovered by an examination of the eye. The two most noteworthy examples of this fact are albuminuric retinitis in an individual believed to be in good health up to the time of its detection by an ophthalmoscopic examination made because of a complaint of dim vision; and optic neuritis in a person who, before the date of the ocular examination, was not known to be the subject of any of the complaints which may cause the appearance of papillitis. In these instances disease of the intra-ocular end of the optic nerve, or of the retina, leads to the discovery of either a general disease or a gross local lesion in the central nervous system.

In another group of cases some inflammatory disease of the eye precedes the development of the constitutional disorder; that is to say, this inflammation is a symptom that occurs sometimes days or even months in advance of the general outbreak. More than any other two diseases, gout and rheumatism have furnished examples in which the eye has thus become the index of what was to follow.

In a third class of cases the subject of an ocular complaint is attacked not because he himself is at the time afflicted with a constitutional disease in an active state, nor because the eye-symptom which has appeared is a sign that he will become affected with a general malady, but because he is by inheritance the subject of a disorder which makes its first manifestation in him as an inflammation of one or more of the coats of the eye. Leaving out of the question the syphilitic diseases of the eye acquired by inheritance, this class is typified by the remarkable series of cases of iritis almost invariably associated with disease of the vitreous occurring in children and young people, insidious in character and destructive in tendency, described by Mr. Hutchinson. These children of gouty parents, according to this observer, have a peculiar squareness of build, heavy features, florid complexions, and feebleness of the circulation in the extremities.

In the second group of cases the gouty and rheumatic diatheses may present ocular inflammations as their first manifestations, or, in other words, the disease of the eye may reveal these diatheses, previously latent and unsuspected. To this class TROUSSEAU (*L'Union Médicale*, No. 113, 1890) calls attention by the report of some striking examples. The type of these cases is an individual who, up to the age of twenty-five or thirty years, has been in good health; then is attacked with a subtle form of iritis or scleritis, and in spite of repeated questions on the part of the medical adviser the true nature of the malady is undetected until at some later date a manifestation of gout or rheumatism in some distant organ is perfectly evident. As an example Trousseau quotes the case of a patient who had a stubborn episcleritis, which relapsed time and again in spite of the use of salicylates of sodium and lithium, iodide of potassium, and tincture of guaiac. Frequent interrogation failed to extract any history of gout or rheumatism in the ancestors, and a minute examination discovered no trace of arthritic tendency in the patient himself. A continuous course of colchicum was without effect. The actual cautery was employed to arrest the disease, and later the patient was sent to Vichy, where, after some days' residence, he was violently attacked with an acute, frank gout, thus absolutely establishing the diagnosis which had so long remained obscure. As an illustration of the same principle, but more particularly of the fact that the first symptom of gout may appear in the eye, is seen in another case, a woman of twenty-five years, with an iritis associated with hæmorrhage into the anterior chamber, whose father had been gouty, but who herself in her previous life never had suffered from any manifestation of this disease. Rapid improvement followed the administration of salicylate of sodium, but she was unwilling to believe in the gouty origin of her ocular trouble until six months after the cure of the iritis, when a characteristic inflammation of the great toe occurred, with a new attack of iritis. Again, a third case, a man aged forty-one years, without personal or ancestral gouty taint, developed an intense irido-choroiditis, for the explanation of which no satisfactory cause could be found until three months later, when a gouty inflammation of the articulations of the fingers of both hands appeared. Other cases are quoted illustrating how rheumatism may first appear in the eye, in some instances with no sign in either the system generally or in the family history to lead to a suspicion that this was the cause of the local inflammation, and be followed some months later by an attack of rheumatism elsewhere in the body.

Independently of the violent disorders with a tendency destructive to vision, like iritis, irido-choroiditis, vitreous opacities, and even neuro-retinitis, the result of gout, a very much milder inflammation, or rather irritation, may appear in the eye and prove a satisfactory index, if properly interpreted, of concealed gout. This disorder has been more aptly described by Mr. Hutchinson than by any other observer, and to him we are indebted for a name which exactly characterizes the most prominent symptom of the complaint, " hot eye "—which with scarcely an appreciable flush, with a burning sensation unrelieved by local measures, and often entirely unsuspected as far as its etiology is concerned, will worry the patient day in and day out until by accident or otherwise the gouty nature of the complaint is detected. A change in diet, a course of mineral waters, and, usually, some salt of lithium will effect a remarkable change.

The writer of the present note remembers well one woman who several times a year was attacked in the manner just described, who had sought relief in all manner of ways, whose eyes had been douched with various collyria and burdened with all kinds of spectacles, and who barely escaped a graduated tenotomy, when two of her relatives on the paternal side were sent for, one of whom had much deformed fingers, the result of gouty deposits in the joints, and the other a gouty inflammation of the tympanic membrane. The riddle was solved and appropriate constitutional treatment relieved this and all subsequent attacks.

We have called attention to these facts which have so frequently been dwelt upon by Mr. Hutchinson and others, and which are again referred to by Trousseau, because they seem in spite of repetition not always to have made enough impression to result in accurate diagnosis. More than this, they are good examples of the fact that a clinical history alone, however carefully taken, should not be sufficient to eliminate from the mind of the examiner the suspicion of diatheses the presence of which his questioning has failed to reveal, and that in a doubtful case it is well to examine the relatives of the patient under treatment.

SPECIAL ARTICLE.

A SECOND CONTRIBUTION ON THE TREATMENT OF TUBERCULAR DISEASE, BY KOCH'S METHOD, IN ST. LUKE'S HOSPITAL, NEW YORK.

BY FRANCIS P. KINNICUTT, M.D ,
PHYSICIAN TO ST. LUKE'S HOSPITAL, NEW YORK.

AT the end of the second week of investigation of the treatment of tubercular disease by inoculation with Koch's lymph, in the wards of St. Luke's Hospital, the first profound impressions made upon the observer of its potency and elective affinities have only been strengthened.

As a thorough clinical study of a larger number of cases would be impossible, only seven new patients have been inoculated, making the total number of cases at present under treatment twenty-two. The new cases are as follows:

One case of aggravated eczema of the hands, orbiculat in form, inoculated as a control-experiment ; one case of lupus of the uvula and contiguous portions of the throat ; one case of tubercular glands (cervical and submaxillary), with doubtful signs of infiltration at the apex of one lung ; one case of epithelioma of the hand, inoculated with the view of studying the possible effect of treatment ; one case of tubercular disease of the ankle-joint ; one of hip-joint disease ; and one of pulmonary tuberculosis in its incipient stage. The rule has been maintained of making use of 0.001 gramme for the initial inoculation in adults, of 0.0005 gramme in children. The rule is also adopted of continuing the same dosage until reaction ceases to be developed, and of increasing its strength by 0.001 gramme successively as reaction ceases to appear. In cases of lupus, Koch's suggestion that inoculations be given at intervals of a week or longer—that is, only after local reaction has subsided—is now followed.

The observation has been made that the systemic

disturbances in this disease are less severe than those exhibited in other forms of tubercular disease, the inoculations being of similar strength; inasmuch as the reaction in several instances has been delayed as late as twenty-four hours, and has then been characteristic, daily inoculations are not given in any instance. Local irritation at the site of the inoculations has not occurred in any of the cases.

The possibility of obtaining equally good results with a smaller amount of lymph than that used by German investigators has apparently been demonstrated (0.004 gramme is the largest dose used in any case). By this we see that the distressing, if not grave, symptoms of very acute reactions may be avoided. The marked systemic disturbance, aside from the rise in temperature, in a number of patients treated with *small* doses, has been impressive, and has suggested caution in treatment. The appearance and condition of the patient during the period of reaction in many instances have been suggestive of the presence of an acute infectious disease. A low arterial tension has obtained as a rule. The records subsequent to the third inoculation of the three patients whose histories were given in THE MEDICAL NEWS of December 20th, are appended. The histories of two patients, suffering respectively from incipient hip-joint disease and tubercular osteitis of the ankle-joint, have also been selected for the present report, as presenting points of great interest.

CASE I. (*Continued from page 643.*) *Tubercular infiltration of apex of right lung.*—Third inoculation, December 16th, 0.001 gramme. Reaction developed six hours later. Duration of reaction, thirty hours. Highest temperature 103.8° F., eighteen hours after inoculation. Amount of sputa, two ounces. Physical signs: Numerous moist râles in large tubes of affected area, abundant moist crepitation; no appreciable enlargement of spleen. Re-inoculations were made on the 20th and 23d; the reactions being very similar to those previously described. The physical signs observed at the present date are markedly different from those present prior to the first inoculation. They consist in a distinct increase in the moist crepitation, which is heard over a decidedly larger area, associated with large mucous râles and an extension of the limits of broncho-vesicular respiration. The inference is that tubercular infiltration was more extensive than was appreciable by physical signs.

CASE II. (*Continued from page 644.*) *Prostatic surface tubercular disease.*—Third inoculation, December 16th, 0.001 gramme. Reaction developed five hours later. Duration of reaction, twenty-nine hours. Highest temperature 103.8° F. Local signs: Severe pain felt at base of penis. Great irritability of bladder, the urine being ejected every fifteen or twenty minutes through supra-pubic opening (made previous to admission).

Re-inoculations were made on December 19th

and 23d, 0.001 gramme, with the development of reactions very similar to those previously obtained. The only appreciable difference in the patient's symptoms before the first inoculation and at present, consists in the greater freedom from pain in the urethra in passing water.

CASE III. (*Continued from page 644.*) *Lupus of the ear and contiguous portions of the face and neck of twelve years' duration.*—Third inoculation, December 16th, 0.003 gramme. Reaction developed six hours later. Duration of reaction, thirty hours. Highest temperature 103.8° F. Local signs: Very considerable sero-purulent exudation, which crusts rapidly; crusts cover nearly the entire affected area. A hyperæmic areola more than an inch in width surrounds the entire patch. Posterior margin of patch presents a raw fissure, as if the morbid tissue were separating from the healthy skin. It was deemed advisable to permit all local reaction to subside before further inoculations, and none has been made since. The present appearance of the diseased tissue is described by Dr. George H. Fox as follows:

December 22. The crusts having been removed by the application of cotton soaked in oil, the affected part appeared red and smooth, and the cicatricial lines from previous scarification are again apparent. There is a purulent secretion behind and below the ear. The whole ear feels softer; this is especially true of the lobe, which, aside from being hyperæmic, has a normal appearance and feel.

CASE IV. *Incipient hip-joint disease.*—Female, aged six years, in the service of Dr. Newton M. Shaffer, at the New York Orthopedic Dispensary from November 9, 1890, until admission to St. Luke's Hospital. Previous history: Patient had been noticed to limp for three weeks, and had had "night-cries" for about the same period.

Examination showed the characteristic limp, attitude, and reflex muscular protection of the joint.

Although these signs were not of the most prominent type, a diagnosis of incipient hip-joint disease was made by Drs. Samuel Ketch and Newton M. Shaffer, after a very careful examination. A long traction-splint was applied. Admitted to St. Luke's Hospital December 17th. Dr. Shaffer, at my request, has very kindly made daily examinations of the patient, and all further reports of the joint-signs are given in his own words.

Examination by Dr. Shaffer immediately before first inoculation: Patient has no pain, walks with a perceptible limp, the thigh being slightly flexed in locomotion. Examination of joint shows no perceptible swelling. The inguinal fossa on right side not quite so pronounced as on the left. Concussion of the hip-joint gives no pain. There is no deformity present, the flexion above noted disappearing when patient is recumbent. The tests, as applied to the movements of the affected hip, resulted as follows:

Flexion markedly resisted about 10° short of full flexion. When this point is reached the patient "flinches" very decidedly, as is also the case in *abduction* and *adduction* of the thigh, both these movements being limited by reflex muscular spasm a few degrees short of normal. With the thigh flexed to about 135° *rotation in* is very markedly resisted. *Rotation out* in same position resisted only in the extreme. With patient prone, extension of thigh (pelvis being held firmly) is quite noticeably resisted. In this position both *rotation in* and *rotation out* are very much restricted. In all these tests the patient "flinched" very plainly when it was attempted to pass beyond the point indicated by the instinctive muscular protection.

December 17, 1890, 3.30 P. M. First inoculation, 0.0005 gramme. Temperature normal. Reaction developed eight hours later. Duration of reaction, thirty-seven hours. Highest temperature 103° F.

18th. Twenty-four hours later. Hip-joint in position characteristic of hip-joint disease in the *second stage*—that is, the thigh is abducted, apparently elongated, flexed and rotated outward. The joint is very sensitive, the slightest attempt at motion giving pain. By using great care 10° of lateral movement (in abduction and adduction) can be demonstrated. There is a movement of flexion of only 15°. No rotation can be demonstrated. The inguinal fossa is obliterated and there is œdema of posterior swelling. The deformity present was as follows: Thigh flexed at 15°; abduction 20°; rotation out about 30°.

The following peculiar condition was noted, unlike that found in morbus coxæ, in the acute stage. The patient noticed no difference between crowding the joint surfaces together and on making traction on the joint. Each test produced pain and there was no relief from traction.

19th. Joint movements much changed for the better; all movements of the joint can now be made, but they are still greatly restricted. *Deformity:* Flexion 160°; abduction *nil.* Rotation in and out still restricted. Rotation in gives pain. Patient still notices no difference between pressure and traction upon the joint. Swelling still present.

20th. Joint movements very much like those of yesterday. The same may be said of the deformity. Joint can be handled with much freedom. Inguinal fossa still obliterated.

Second inoculation, Dec. 20th, 0.0005 gramme. Temperature normal. Only very slight reaction developed eleven hours later. Duration of reaction, eighteen hours. Highest temperature 100° F.

21st. Twenty-four hours later, motion in joint is more free than yesterday, except in adduction, which can be made of 5°, rotation still being limited. Inguinal glands can be made out. *Deformity:* Flexion 135°. Rotation out unchanged. Muscular resistance at joint well marked. Tenderness of joint diminished.

22d. Examination at 5 o'clock, P.M., Dr. Thomas L. Stedman being present. The following movements of the joint are normal, viz., flexion, abduction, and rotation out. Rotation in, extension, and adduction are approximately normal. Rotation *in* during flexion is slightly resisted.

Another important condition was noted at the examination. The character of the muscular resistance is unlike that observed at the examination of December 17th. The peculiar instinctively muscular check which accompanies hip-joint disease, and which was noticed on December 17th, has disappeared. The muscular resistance to-day can be overcome by gradual and gentle pressure, without pain or flinching, and that which appeared to be a fixed resistance to joint movement disappears. The joint can be handled with freedom without inflicting any pain at all. Still some swelling in inguinal fossa.

REMARKS.—There are four points that seem very instructive. 1st. The diagnostic value of the lymph; 2d. The immediate and wonderful changes produced in all the signs and symptoms; 3d. The fact that though the joint was acutely painful traction gave no relief; 4th. The great change in the character of the muscular protection of the joint. It was deemed best to use the long traction-splint during the treatment, and the immobilization produced by it was of great comfort to the patient. The future history of the patient will be watched with great interest.

CASE V. *Tubercular osteitis of ankle-joint.*—Male, aged six years. Patient under care of Dr. Newton Schaffer in out-patient department of Orthopedic Hospital since 1889. During this period improvement. On admission to St. Luke's Hospital, examination by Dr. Shaffer before first inoculation as follows: Slight thickening about joint; ankle extended to 100°; motion about 3° or 4°; reflex spasm marked; no pain on ordinary manipulation.

December 17. First inoculation, 0.0005 gramme. Temperature normal. Reaction developed ten hours later. Duration of reaction, forty-one hours. Highest temperature 102° F.

18th. Examination by Dr. Shaffer. Joint slightly swollen. Sensitiveness increased. Reflex spasm more marked and more alert.

19th. Joint condition improved; sensitiveness less, though marked when attempt made to flex the joint. Swelling less. Improvement in the equinus deformity.

20th. Second inoculation, 0.0005 gramme. Reaction very similar to that subsequent to first inoculation. Highest temperature 102.3° F.

22d. Examination by Dr. Shaffer. Motion of joint distinctly improved. No pain unless some force is used in flexion. Surface temperature about normal.

FURTHER REPORT ON KOCH'S LYMPH.

BY WILLIAM OSLER, M.D.,
PROFESSOR OF THE PRINCIPLES AND PRACTICE OF MEDICINE IN THE JOHNS HOPKINS HOSPITAL.

THE cases under treatment by Koch's method are progressing favorably. In my wards there are eight selected cases of pulmonary tuberculosis and two of tuberculous pleurisy. The dose in the phthisis cases has been gradually increased, and some of the patients received to-day (December 22d) 1 c.c. of the one-per-cent. solution. Although the febrile reaction in each instance was prompt and definite after the first or second injection, the subsequent inoculations have not been followed by any special febrile reaction, even with the larger quantities injected. There has usually been an increase in the cough, and in several cases a marked increase in the expectoration. A special feature in three of the cases has been the enormous increase in the bacilli in the sputa. The ordinary cover-glass preparation looked, in some instances, as if taken from a pure culture. The change in the appearance of the bacilli, which has been noted by many observers, is quite marked. No definite alterations have, as yet, been detected in the physical signs. In the tuberculous pleurisy, the reaction has been much more intense than in the pulmonary cases.

A very wholesome dread of the treatment has been aroused in the community by the newspaper reports of death. It is remarkable that there have been not more than two or three voluntary applications at the hospital, and several very suitable early cases, which were sent for, refused to subject themment until the method had been more fully tried.

On the surgical side, Dr. Halstead has five cases of bone and joint tuberculosis under treatment, and one of lupus, which has displayed all the characteristic phenomena so often described. In surgical tuberculosis the reaction has been in each instance much more intense than in the phthisis cases.

In Dr. Kelly's ward a case of tuberculous peritonitis is under treatment. The patient some months ago had the tubes removed and at the operation the peritoneum was found covered with tubercles. A condition of tuberculous salpingitis existed. She made a good recovery and left the hospital with a small sinus at the lower end of the abdominal incision. After the injection of one-tenth c. c. of one-per-cent. solution she had intense febrile reaction, reaching to 104°, and the abdomen became tender and slightly swollen. There was no increase in the discharge from the sinus and no swelling of its walls. The fever kept up for three days.

In the pathological laboratory, Professor Welch and Dr. Nutall are making careful studies of the changes in the bacilli and have instituted a series of experiments on guinea-pigs with the sputa of the patients under treatment.

SUMMARY OF TWENTY-ONE CASES TREATED BY KOCH'S LYMPH AT THE MONTEFIORE HOME FOR CHRONIC INVALIDS.

BY SIMON BARUCH, M.D.,
OF NEW YORK.

My data refer to seventy-one injections in twelve male and nine female patients.

The reaction was undoubted in every case, although somewhat less than is announced from abroad.

Several of the cases, male and female, whose temperature had been normal, presented a rise of one to two degrees just before the injection.

Every case of phthisis presented a rise of temperature within twenty-four hours.

In one case of caries of the vertebra, with pneumothorax, the temperature also went up two degrees.

One case of ulceration (of doubtful type) in the left cervical region, with fistulous canal, resisted gradually-advancing injections until 5 mg. were reached, when the temperature rose from 97.8° to 102.4°. To-day it is again 97.4°. There is an increase in the discharge now; no change in patient's general condition.

A jaundiced hue of the skin was noticed in one case of phthisis; also nosebleed, headache, and nausea. Cough and expectoration increased in four cases, was diminished in ten cases, remained the same in six, and appeared anew in one regarded as cured.

Decided nausea and headache occurred in eleven cases.

Every case reached a normal temperature once or oftener in the course of twenty-four hours.

Pulse: The lowest pulse-rate was 44, the highest 134.

Respiration: The lowest recorded was 17, the highest 45.

Temperature: The lowest recorded was 97.4°, the highest 103.2°.

Weight: Of eight patients weighed, one lost one-half pound, one lost one pound, one gained three-quarters of a pound, one gained one-half pound. The others are unchanged.

The most remarkable point in my experience is that in two cases—which were almost ready to be discharged on account of abeyance of symptoms and physical signs, and a gain of weight of twenty-one pounds in one and of thirteen and one-half pounds in the other, under hydrotherapy—one lost one pound and the other three-quarters of a pound since the injection.

These cases would have been regarded as practically cured, had not the injection of 1 mg. of lymph caused decided reaction. One of these cases is, perhaps, more completely prostrated by the lymph than any other. I regard this experience as a complete vindication of Koch's view of the diagnostic value of the injection in suspected tuberculosis.

47 E. SIXTIETH ST., Dec. 23, 1890.

CORRESPONDENCE.

PSOROSPERMOSIS.

To the Editor of THE MEDICAL NEWS,

SIR: In your esteemed journal of November 8th there appeared a clinical lecture by Dr. L. D. Bulkley on *Psorospermosis follicularis cutis*, delivered on October 8th.

The case presented and described is the same one upon which I based my communication to the International Congress in Berlin, August 12, 1890 (*Annales de Dermatologie et Syphilographie*, 1890, p. 707), and which I, together with Dr. L. Weiss, also presented by invitation at the September meeting of the New York Dermatological Society, and was allowed to submit my microscopical preparations for the inspection of the members.

Dr. Bulkley admits the identity, and says in his article : "I am told that Dr. Lustgarten, of New York, gave this patient's disease its present (and probably correct) name and exhibited microscopical sections of the same at the recent Congress in Berlin." It is hardly in accordance with this admission that Dr. Bulkley publishes the case, and it is decidedly unwarranted that in the enumeration of the few hitherto recorded cases he speaks of this case as "my own" and "Case 6 (Bulkley)." As professional custom gives the claim of a case to the man who was the first to diagnose and to describe it, as everyone is well aware, it is evident that the right in this case of literary ownership belongs to me. I can only presume that this gross violation of professional etiquette is based upon an oversight on the part of Dr. Bulkley, which I expect he will rectify by renouncing in your journal the claim which he has put forth.

Respectfully,   S. LUSTGARTEN, M.D.

PARIS.

French Opinions on Koch's Treatment.

AT the meeting of the Société Médicale de Paris, December 8th, which is exclusively composed of hospital physicians, communications were read by Drs. Ferrand, Cuffer, and Chibierge, members of the Society who had been to Berlin for the purpose of observing Koch's investigations. So as to be able to watch the experiments closely, these three gentlemen divided their task into three classes: Dr. Ferrand studied more especially the general action of Koch's remedy, Dr. Cuffer devoted himself to the influence of the remedy in cases of phthisis, while Dr. Chibierge took up the treatment of lupus. All these gentlemen, before making their communications, expressed their thanks for the highly courteous manner in which they were received.

Dr. Ferrand then began on the general action of the remedy. His conclusions are that Koch's agent is capable of producing an elevation of temperature, and that, locally, it excites congestion, which is most marked in tubercular tissues. If one considers the physiological perturbation brought on by Koch's lymph, it is seen that the effects are comparable to those of a muscle-poison ; for symptoms occur which show that the muscular fibres which control the vessels have been paralyzed, and the heart itself, the muscular organ *par excellence*, is involved.

As to the contra-indications of Koch's method in pulmonary phthisis, they are, according to Dr. Ferrand, first, extensive invasion by the tubercular lesions; second, great weakness of the patient, or an adynamic condition ; third, previous pulmonary hæmorrhages; and, fourth, high temperature.

Dr. Senator, of Berlin, says that Dr. Ferrand is the first one to notice these contra-indications, which very much restrict the field of action of Koch's lymph in pulmonary tuberculosis. Dr. Ferrand closed by saying that no fact as yet observed allows one to attribute to this mysterious remedy a curative action on phthisis.

. Dr. Cuffer, who spoke next, recommends all to be on their guard while using the remedy. He has observed several phthisical patients who did not show a trace of reaction after the injection. These cases are, it is true, very few, but sufficient to establish the fact that Koch went a little too far in his first celebrated communication, in which he maintained that whenever he had to deal with a tubercular patient, the injection of his lymph would produce a well-marked reaction. But, besides this, there is a more important fact, namely, that the local reaction produced by the lymph is not always temporary. In Professor Senator's wards Dr. Cuffer has seen several cases of pulmonary phthisis that progressed very rapidly after the treatment, notwithstanding the fact that the injections were made with the greatest possible care. A case of acute phthisis, accompanied by very high fever, sank rapidly as a result of the injections. In other cases there was great aggravation, and the auscultatory symptoms of pulmonary softening increased, as well as the number of bacilli in the sputum. The same bad results have followed the use of the remedy in pleurisy. In one case the patient presented only a slight pleuritic area at the base of the left lung. The first inoculation was followed by extreme prostration and pain so severe in character that for some time Professor Senator thought that he had to deal with pleural and pulmonary gangrene. The author also said that the accidents of the reaction following the injections signify a very intense congestion, and probably, in some cases, acceleration of the pulmonary disease; moreover, complications have been observed in the liver and kidneys, and also albuminuria. Many years ago, the late Professor Lasègue, of Paris, showed how greatly tuberculosis may be accelerated by albuminuria. Dr. Cuffer closed by saying that great improvement following the injection has been announced by some physicians, but that he, during his stay in Berlin, did not see one case in which he could really say there had been improvement, while, on the other hand, cases of aggravation are undeniable.

He thinks that to obtain the best results from Koch's lymph in cases of consumption, provided this remedy is of any use, the proper doses must be carefully studied, and must vary according to the degree of the tubercular lesion, and also according to the resisting power of the patient, his temperament, and whether or not he is subject to congestions. Dr. Cuffer also thinks that to moderate the congestions which occur after injections an anti-congestive and astringent medication should be resorted to.

The effects of the treatment on external tuberculosis as represented by lupus, were next reviewed by Dr. Chibierge, who has had a large experience with tuberculosis of the skin. He said that Koch's lymph produces very intense and peculiar reactive phenomena at the seat of the lupus. It is not certain that these phenomena are curative. During his stay in Berlin he did not see a single case of lupus that was cured, even in patients who had been treated for two months. In a case which was presented as an example of cure, Dr. Chibierge very easily discovered small nodules which were unmistakably lupus-tubercles. The author said that it was very strange that patients suffering from lupus, instead of being placed under the care of specialists in skin-diseases, were placed in medical or surgical wards, or even private clinics. The head of one of these clinics even acknowledged that before becoming an associate of Koch he had never seen a case of lupus. Dr. Chibierge does not say that Koch's method is useless in the treatment of lupus, for he, like others, has noticed the marvellously rapid action of the remedy, and its cicatrizing influence on extensive and rebellious tuberculosis; but he insisted that no one in Berlin was able to show him a single case of cure, or even an apparent cure, and that, on the contrary, he has seen a recurrence and increase of the disease in cases which had been considered as cured. He also advised that the remedy should be used with the utmost care, and never without having obtained the patient's consent.

NEWS ITEMS.

The Characteristic Organism of Cancer.—In an address before the Pathological Society of London on December 2d, and the Medico-Chirurgical Society of Edinburgh on December 3, 1890, Dr. William Russell stated he had been occupied for some years in tracing the mode of growth of cancer in different organs. By this study he hoped to map out the steps of the process, and by learning the manner of its growth to obtain perhaps an insight into the factors determining the departure of the tissues from their normal behavior and arrangements. He had found appearances which he could not fit into modes of cell-growth and nuclear proliferation, and these had so puzzled him in one case that he asked his pathological assistant, Mr. W. F. Robertson, to experiment on it with every possible combination of stains with a view to the possible differentiation of some of these structures. His attempts were soon successful by the following method: 1. Saturated solution of fuchsine in a two per cent. carbolic acid in water. 2. One-per-cent. solution of iodine-green (Grüber's) in a two per cent. carbolic acid in water. Place section in water. Then stain in fuchsine for ten minutes or longer; wash for a few minutes in water. Then wash for half a minute in absolute alcohol. From this put the section into the solution of iodine-green, and allow it to remain well spread out for five minutes. From this rapidly dehydrate in absolute alcohol, pass through oil of cloves, and mount in balsam. By this method it was found that certain structures stained a brilliant purplish-red, while the tissues stained green. Similar bodies were found in a number of cancers then examined, and these, for laboratory purposes, were called "fuchsine bodies."

With this discovery all kinds of possible errors suggested themselves. That they were not accidental impurities in material, bottles, or stains was shown by the fact that tissues from the same bottles and cut at the same time gave no indication of this. That they were not the nuclei of tissue-cells in exaggerated reproductive activity was tested by the cells in organized inflammation of serous membranes not giving the reaction, nor

the cells in tubercle, in typhoid lesion, in inflammatory affections, or in the organs of an embryo. That they were not globes of some degenerative substance was proved by the examination of a great variety of tissues showing different varieties of degeneration. Further, they were not present in the sarcomata, nor in simple tumors, such as fibromata, papillomata, myomata, etc., nor in venereal warts and condylomata, nor in primary syphilitic sores. Sections of a tumor labelled adenoma of the mamma, and rich in adenomatous structures, and a gumma of the dura mater showed the bodies, but of the history of these cases he was ignorant. Another syphilitic case which had defied treatment, and in which there was extensive destructive lesion of the fauces and larynx and the bones of the vertebra behind the fauces, showed a few fuchsine bodies in sections of the larynx. Altogether tissues had been examined from fifty to sixty different cases selected with the purpose of subjecting the positive observations to the severest possible tests. The result was that fuchsine bodies were found in one case of chronic ulcer of the leg, one of tubercular disease of a joint with old sinuses, one of phenomenally severe, destructive, and intractable syphilitic lesion; and in two other cases, of which he had no record—one a case of mammary adenoma, and one a gummatous tumor of the meninges. He indicated possible explanations of these, and that they could not be regarded as sufficient to overthrow the other evidence.

Turning to the positive side of the question, forty-five cases of cancer had been examined, which included malignant epithelial growths of various structure, as epitheliomas of the lips and face, rodent ulcer, scirrhus of the mamma, both primary and recurrent; malignant adenoma of cervical glands, cancers of the stomach, liver, spleen, abdominal glands, supra-renal capsules, uterus, and ovaries. The pathological position of one of these was still uncertain; another was represented by sections dated 1885: in these two no fuchsine bodies were found, but in the remaining forty-three they were present. In individual sections they varied greatly in number, and it was noted that they occurred in special abundance in foci. They might be present in the small-celled infiltration at the margin of the cancer, among or in the epithelial cells, in the stroma, or in the lymphatics. As a rule, they occurred in clusters or groups of two, ten, twenty, or more, and they almost always showed a clear space round them. In shape they were perfectly round. The commonest size was $4\,\mu$, but they might be much smaller or larger. Examined by daylight they appeared homogeneous and structureless.

As there seemed to be no escape from regarding these structures as special organisms, which—so far, at least, as his pathological material was concerned—were practically confined to cancer, the question was, Were they animal or vegetable, and what was their mode of growth and reproduction? To answer this question it was necessary to consider the work which had been done, especially on the Continent, in the study of cancer. He then referred briefly and in detail to the various papers which had appeared in French and German literature, in which it was contended that an animal parasite had been found in some cases of cancer. Summing this up and excluding molluscum contagiosum, it was found that Albarran, Darier, Thoma, Wickham, and Sjöbring had found in cancer an organism which they described as belonging to the protozoa, while Thoma did not commit himself and only Wickham and Sjöbring give figures to aid in forming a judgment on their contentions. He next pointed out the characters of the protozoa, more especially the psorospermiæ or coccidiæ, and indicated that according to the authorities these were unicellular organisms forming in their interior psorospermiæ, which, in turn, developed spores which were usually sickle-shaped bodies, and became free parasites. To meet the necessity of this stage in their life, Sjöbring had figured the spore-formation in the cancers he examined. In short, looking at the work on this subject in the concrete, he regarded some of the figures as having nothing whatever to do with foreign organisms, that others were certainly misinterpreted, while some probably represented the organism with which he was dealing.

Returning to the consideration of the fuchsine bodies, they might be studied by the special method of staining given, or by logwood and eosine, or by Gram's methed with methyl-violet. Each group and most of the isolated individuals were surrounded by a clear area, often having the appearance of being bounded by a definite capsule. In so far as the isolated individuals were concerned one entered an epithelial cell, the protoplasm and the nucleus of which stained with logwood; while the foreign organism lay in a clear area or vacuole in the cell-protoplasm, to which there was no true capsule. Both in the epithelial masses and the vacuoles referred to there might in addition be small fuchsine bodies surrounded by a clear space, and bounded by a capsule or limiting structure. Further, it was to be noted that in the vacuoles there might be several fuchsine bodies; while in others the fuchsine body was granular and had lost its characteristic staining reaction, and showed undoubted spores in its interior. In the epithelium it may also be noted that some fuchsine bodies are surrounded by a vacuole, while others are not.

From the foregoing it might be contended that the organism in question was a protozoon, were it not that in sections stained by Gram's method the mode of reproduction is shown quite diagrammatically. The large fuchsine body is seen to give out a small globular body which increases its distance from the parent body, but remains attached to it by a filament; this bud grows and gives off another and a short chain, or other forms may be produced. The small spores could also be seen in the interior of the lymphoid cells, or leucocytes in the infiltrated area, the effect of this being to clear up the protoplasm of the cell and to produce a clear space or vacuole with a limiting ring.

This, he thought, was the mode of formation of what might be called the free encapsuled organism present among epithelial cells or lying in vacuoles. As to the appearances in the interior of epithelial cells, the foreign body at first had no vacuole round it, but ultimately developed one, and this was to be accounted for by its influence upon the surrounding protoplasm leading to its classification. He said that there could be absolutely no doubt that the organism was a fungus which belonged to the sprouting fungi—*Sprosspilze*—of Nägelè; but the proof of this was not to be readily found in every section, for the usual arrangement was in clusters, especially as demonstrable by the fuchsine and iodine-green method,

which, he thought, acted best when the organism was at a certain stage of its growth.

In conclusion, he said that if the presence of this parasitic fungus in cancer was confirmed by other observers, we had found in it an organism whose nutrition, reproduction, and death in the tissue could hardly be conceived as occurring without producing changes fully equal to the anatomical changes present in cancer.—*Lancet*, December 13, 1890.

Rush Medical College.—A matter that has resulted in the retirement of Dr. Nicholas Senn, of Milwaukee, from the faculty of the Rush Medical College, of Chicago, has caused a number of students at that institution to make pilgrimages to Milwaukee during the past few days. It may be said at the outset that the students are all with Dr. Senn, and that they unanimously desire him to remain at the college. Dr. Senn has for three years been professor of the practice of surgery and surgical pathology at this school. Dr. Charles T. Parkes, who has been a member of the college faculty for about twenty years, is professor of the principles and practice of surgery, and he and Dr. Senn have really filled one professorship, but Dr. Parkes has had charge of the clinical work, while Dr. Senn's instruction has been given almost entirely in the form of lectures. Dr. Senn gave notice that unless he was permitted to take a hand in the clinical work, and give practical demonstrations as well as lectures, he would retire. To this Dr. Parkes strenuously objected, declaring that no one but himself "shall ever handle the knife in the clinic-room of this college." Dr. Parkes holds a large amount of stock in the college corporation and his influence with the faculty is considerable, while Dr. Senn owns no stock whatever.

OFFICIAL LIST OF CHANGES IN THE STATIONS AND DUTIES OF THE MEDICAL CORPS OF THE U. S. NAVY FOR THE WEEK ENDING DECEMBER 20, 1890.

EVANS, SHELDON G., *Assistant Surgeon.*—Ordered to the Naval Academy, Annapolis, Md.
DECKER, CORBIN J., *Passed Assistant Surgeon.*—Detached from the Naval Academy, and ordered to the Naval Hospital, Philadelphia, Pa.

OFFICIAL LIST OF CHANGES OF STATIONS AND DUTIES OF MEDICAL OFFICERS OF THE U. S. MARINE-HOSPITAL SERVICE, FROM DECEMBER 8 TO DECEMBER 20, 1890.

WYMAN, WALTER, *Surgeon.*—Granted leave of absence for twenty days, December 11, 1890. To attend meeting of American Public Health Association, December 12, 1890.
LONG, W. H., *Surgeon.*—Granted leave of absence for seven days, December 20, 1890.
MURRAY, R. D., *Surgeon.*—Granted leave of absence for thirty days, December 20, 1890.
IRWIN, FAIRFAX, *Surgeon.*—Detailed for special temporary duty at Marine-Hospital Bureau, December 10, 1890.
CARTER, H. R., *Passed Assistant Surgeon.*—To attend meeting of American Public Health Association, December 11, 1890.
WASDIN, EUGENE, *Passed Assistant Surgeon.*—To attend meeting of American Public Health Association, December 11, 1890.
KINYOUN, J. J., *Passed Assistant Surgeon.*—Granted leave of absence for thirty days, with permission to go abroad, December 11, 1890.
GEDDINGS, H. D., *Assistant Surgeon.*—Upon expiration of leave, to proceed to New York City for temporary duty, December 13, 1890.

INDEX.

Lightning Source UK Ltd.
Milton Keynes UK
UKHW020625120219
337137UK00005B/529/P